Atlas of
ORTHOPAEDIC SURGERY

Atlas of
ORTHOPAEDIC SURGERY

LOUIS A. GOLDSTEIN, M.D.

Professor of Orthopaedics, Past Chairman, Department of Orthopaedics,
Head, Section of Spine Surgery, University of Rochester School of Medicine
and Dentistry, Past Orthopaedic Surgeon-in-Chief, Strong Memorial Hospital,
Rochester, New York

ROBERT C. DICKERSON, M.D.

Chief Emeritus, Department of Orthopaedics, The Genesee Hospital;
Clinical Associate Professor of Orthopaedics, University of Rochester
School of Medicine and Dentistry,
Rochester, New York

SECOND EDITION
with **1637** illustrations

The C. V. Mosby Company

ST. LOUIS • TORONTO • LONDON   1981

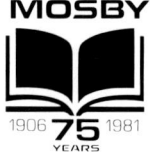

A TRADITION OF PUBLISHING EXCELLENCE

SECOND EDITION

Copyright © 1981 by The C. V. Mosby Company

All rights reserved. No part of this book may be reproduced in any manner without written permission of the publisher.

Previous edition copyrighted 1974

Printed in the United States of America

The C. V. Mosby Company
11830 Westline Industrial Drive, St. Louis, Missouri 63141

Library of Congress Cataloging in Publication Data

Goldstein, Louis A
 Atlas of orthopaedic surgery.

 Bibliography: p.
 Includes index.
 1. Orthopedic surgery—Atlases. I. Dickerson, Robert C., 1929- joint author. II. Title.
[DNLM: 1. Orthopedics—Atlases. WE 17 G624a]
RD733.2.G64 1981 617'.3'00222 80-25987
ISBN 0-8016-1884-3

GW/CB/B 9 8 7 6 5 4 3 2 1 01/C/053

CONTRIBUTORS

RICHARD I. BURTON, M.D.

Professor of Orthopaedics, Head, Section of Hand Surgery of Department of Orthopaedics, University of Rochester School of Medicine and Dentistry, Rochester, New York; Orthopaedist, Strong Memorial Hospital, Rochester, New York

DONALD P. K. CHAN, M.B., B.S.

Associate Professor of Orthopaedics, Co-Director of Spinal Cord Injury Service, University of Rochester School of Medicine and Dentistry; Senior Associate Orthopaedist, Strong Memorial Hospital, Rochester, New York

KENNETH E. DeHAVEN, M.D.

Associate Professor of Orthopaedics, Head, Section of Athletic Medicine, University of Rochester School of Medicine and Dentistry, Rochester, New York; Senior Associate Orthopaedist, Strong Memorial Hospital, Rochester, New York

C. McCOLLISTER EVARTS, M.D.

Dorris H. Carlson Professor of Orthopaedics, Chairman, Department of Orthopaedics, University of Rochester School of Medicine and Dentistry; Orthopaedic Surgeon-in-Chief, Strong Memorial Hospital, Rochester, New York

To
orthopaedic surgery residents,
present and future, who will be the source of future progress
in surgery of the musculoskeletal system

PREFACE to second edition

In this edition, many older operations have been deleted, but an even larger number of newer procedures has been added. This edition has been extensively revised with the help of contributing authors, especially in those chapters relating to surgery of the knee, hip, hand, and spine. As with the first edition, many new illustrations have been redrawn so that all illustrations involving the upper or lower extremity appear consistently throughout the atlas as the right arm or right leg.

The illustrations in this edition are principally the work of Robert Wabnitz, Anita Matthews, and Laura Hayward of the Department of Medical Illustration of the University of Rochester School of Medicine. Other illustrators who have assisted them with this edition include Elizabeth Vanderlinde, Arlette Gagnier, Kirk Moldoff, Susan Brennan, Andrea Crohn, Cynthia Shulman, and Richard Howe.

We want to acknowledge with gratitude the efforts of Dr. P. W. Haake, Marge Cerasoli, Lisa Pauly, and Andrea Arthur, as well as Kathy Falk, Judy Cassidy, and Jeanne Bush of The C. V. Mosby Company, for their added assistance in the preparation of material for this edition.

Louis A. Goldstein
Robert C. Dickerson

PREFACE to first edition

This book has been prepared to provide a comprehensive atlas of orthopaedic operative procedures for practicing surgeons, orthopaedic residents, interns, and students of the musculoskeletal system. The preparation of this atlas has been made possible through the cooperation of the Orthopaedic Attending Surgeons in Rochester, New York.

With few exceptions, the illustrations throughout this atlas have been prepared by the medical illustrator from direct visualization of specific orthopaedic operations as they were actually performed in the operating room. To improve the continuity of presentation of this illustrated material, many of the illustrations have been redrawn so that all illustrations involving the upper or lower extremity appear consistently throughout the atlas as the right arm or right leg.

By permission of the McGraw-Hill Book Company, illustrations previously prepared by the authors and Mr. Wabnitz for *Atlas of Pediatric Surgery*, edited by Dr. Robert White (1965), have been reproduced in this atlas on the following pages: 63, 65, 97, 133, 135, 225, 227, 337, 451, 453, 455, 457, 459, 461, 465, 563, 581, 583, 605, 607, 657, 659, 661, 663, 665, 707, 709, 711, 719, 721, 723, 725, 727, 769, 771, 823, 839, 841, 855, 857, 897, 899, 901, 903, 919, 921, 941, 943, 949, 951, 955, and 957.

The illustrations on pages 253 and 255 are redrawn from *Campbell's Operative Orthopaedics*, edited by A. H. Crenshaw, St. Louis, 1971, The C. V. Mosby Company.

We wish to acknowledge with gratitude the efforts of Diane Bellinger, Richard Howe, and Martha Strain, of the Medical Illustration Department, for their assistance to Mr. Wabnitz in the preparation of illustrated material; and the assistance of Harriet Smith, Laurie DeCamilla, Nancy Selner, and Andrea Arthur, in the preparation of text and bibliographical material.

Louis A. Goldstein
Robert C. Dickerson

CONTENTS

1 SHOULDER, 1

Repair of recurrent anterior dislocation, 2
Repair of recurrent anterior dislocation (Bristow procedure), 9
Repair of recurrent posterior dislocation, 12
Repair of acromioclavicular separation, 15
Resection of lateral end of clavicle, 17
Excision of calcific deposit, 18
Neer anterior acromioplasty, 20
Repair of rotator cuff tear, 23
Open reduction for displaced proximal humeral fractures, 26
Open reduction and internal fixation of clavicle, 28
Transfer of trapezius for paralysis of deltoid muscle, 30
Release of internal rotation and adduction contracture (Sever procedure), 32
Transfer of latissimus dorsi and teres major for Erb's palsy (L'Episcopo-Zachary), 34
Repair of congenital elevation of scapula, 36
Disarticulation of shoulder, 38
Interscapulothoracic resection, 40
Shoulder arthrodesis, 43

2 UPPER ARM, 49

Open reduction and plate fixation for fracture of shaft of humerus, 50
Intramedullary fixation for fracture of shaft of humerus, 52
Curettage and bone graft for benign bone cyst (humerus), 54
Tenodesis of tendon of long head of biceps, 57
Above-elbow amputation, 59
Supracondylar osteotomy of humerus, 62

3 ELBOW, 65

Excision of radial head, 66
Open reduction and internal fixation for fracture of olecranon, 68
Excision of proximal ulna (following olecranon fracture) with reattachment of triceps, 70
Open reduction for displaced fracture of lateral condyle of humerus, 72
Open reduction for displaced fracture of medial epicondyle, 74
Open reduction for supracondylar or T condylar fractures of humerus, 76
Medullary fixation for fracture of shaft of ulna (including Monteggia fracture-dislocation), 78
Repair of rupture of distal tendon of biceps brachii muscle, 80
Steindler flexorplasty, 82

Transfer of triceps tendon, 84
Synovectomy of elbow, 86
Anterior transplantation of ulnar nerve, 88

4 FOREARM, 93

Release of flexor-pronator origin (for cerebral palsy), 94
Open reduction for fracture of proximal radius (anterior exposure), 96
Open reduction for midshaft fracture of radius and ulna, 99
Below-elbow amputation, 102
Tendon transfers for radial nerve palsy, 104
Transfer of flexor carpi ulnaris to extensor carpi radialis brevis, 108
Forearm decompression for impending Volkmann's ischemic contracture, 110

5 WRIST, 113

Tenolysis for de Quervain's tenosynovitis, 114
Release of transverse carpal ligament for carpal tunnel syndrome, 116
Excision of distal ulna (Darrach procedure), 118
Osteotomy of distal radius (for correction of malunion), 120
Open reduction and bone graft for fracture of scaphoid: anterior approach, 121
Open reduction for fracture of the scaphoid, 123
Radial styloidectomy, 124
Surgical correction of radial clubhand, 126
Synovectomy of tendons at wrist, 128
Arthrodesis of the wrist, 129

6 HAND, 137

Incisions, 138
Basic principles of hand dressings, 139
Tourniquet use in upper extremity surgery, 139
Opponens transfer for median palsy, 140
Tendon transfers for clawing of fingers (secondary to ulnar nerve palsy), 142
Tendon transfers for weak or absent first dorsal interosseous, 144
Hinged hand (flexor or extensor tenodesis), 145
Tenolysis for snapping finger (or thumb), 147
Tendon repair of the hand, 149
Removal of donor tendon for tendon grafting, 152
Fasciectomy for Dupuytren's contracture, 154
Repair of swan neck deformity, 156
Repair of boutonniere deformity of finger, 158
Repair of ruptured extensor tendons by tendon transfer, 159
Replacement arthroplasty of the metacarpophalangeal joint, 161
Release of thumb adduction contracture, 164
Repair of collateral ligament of metacarpophalangeal joint of thumb, 165
Volar plate advancement for dorsal fracture-dislocations of the proximal interphalangeal joint, 167
Open reduction and internal fixation for fracture of base of thumb metacarpal (Bennett's fracture), 168
Open reduction and internal fixation for fracture of metacarpal shaft, 170
Open reduction and internal fixation for phalangeal shaft fracture, 172
Osteotomy of phalanx (for rotational deformity), 174
Arthrodesis of carpometacarpal joint of thumb, 175
Arthrodesis of small joints, 177

Repair of syndactyly, 180
Drainage of paronychia, 182
Drainage of felon, 183

7 NECK AND CERVICAL SPINE, 191

Release of sternocleidomastoid for torticollis, 192
Release of scalenus anterior muscle, 193
Resection of first rib (axillary approach), 195
Posterior cervical spine fusion, 198
Occipitocervical fusion, 199
Atlantoaxial spine fusion, 201
Posterior cervical fusion (C3 and below), 203
Anterior cervical spine fusion, 205
Application of cranial halo, 207
Application of pelvic hoop, 210

8 THORACOLUMBAR SPINE, 215

Scoliosis—general considerations, 216
Classification of spine deformity, 216
Idiopathic scoliosis—indications for operation, 216
Selection of the fusion area, 217
  Thoracic curve patterns, 217
    Single major thoracic curve pattern, 217
    Major thoracic curve with compensatory structural upper thoracic and compensatory nonstructural or mild structural lumbar curve, 220
    Major thoracic curve with compensatory significantly structural lumbar curve, 222
    Double major thoracic curve pattern, 224
  Thoracolumbar and lumbar curves, 227
  Double major curve pattern, 229
  Scoliosis with lumbosacral spondylolisthesis, 229
    Reduction of severe spondylolisthesis associated with scoliosis, 229
Methods of correction of scoliosis, 234
  Localizer cast technique, 234
  Posterior spine fusion and Harrington instrumentation, 237
Juvenile kyphosis (Scheuermann's disease), 248
Neuromuscular scoliosis, 251
Congenital spine deformity, 251
Guidelines for the surgical management of certain congenital spine deformities, 253
Posterior lumbosacral spine fusion, 254
Posterolateral spine fusion by bilateral, lateral approach, 258
Anterior spine fusion by retroperitoneal approach to the lumbar spine, 261
Anterior spine fusion by thoracoabdominal approach, 264
Anterior interbody fusion with Dwyer instrumentation, 268
    Ventral derotation system (Zielke), 271
Transthoracic approach to the thoracic spine, 272
Laminectomy (lumbar intervertebral disc lesion), 274

9 PELVIS, 281

Removal of donor bone from iliac wing for bone graft, 282
Acetabuloplasty, 284
Innominate osteotomy, 288
Open reduction and internal fixation for displaced acetabular fracture, 292
Hemipelvectomy, 294
Coccygectomy, 297

10 HIP, 299

Hip pinning for subcapital fracture of femur (multiple pin fixation), 300
Hip pinning for subcapital fracture of femur (telescoping appliance), 304
Hip pinning for peritrochanteric fracture of femur (compression screw fixation), 306
Hip pinning for peritrochanteric fracture of femur (extrastrong nail and bolt fixation), 309
Insertion of femoral head prosthesis, 312
Insertion of femoral head prosthesis (anterolateral approach), 316
Intertrochanteric displacement osteotomy of femur (compression plate fixation), 317
Total hip reconstruction—Charnley-Müller, 319
Total hip reconstruction—resurfacing, 326
Cup arthroplasty, 330
Adductor tenotomy, 336
Release of hip flexion contracture, 337
Obturator neurectomy, 338
Release of iliopsoas, 340
Open reduction for congenital dislocation of hip, 343
Medial approach to the hip joint, 345
Subtrochanteric derotation osteotomy, 346
Transfer of iliopsoas tendon for paralysis of hip abductors (Mustard), 348
Posterior transfer of iliopsoas tendon for paralysis of hip abductors (Sharrard), 352
Transfer of external oblique muscle for paralysis of hip abductors, 356
Transfer of origin of adductor longus and brevis to ischial tuberosity, 358
Drainage of hip joint, 359
Resection of hip (Girdlestone), 362
Disarticulation of hip, 364
Arthrodesis of hip, 366

11 THIGH, 379

Open reduction and internal fixation for femoral shaft fracture, 380
Supracondylar derotation osteotomy (McCarroll), 384
Quadricepsplasty, 386
Quadriceps lengthening, 388
Repair of rupture of quadriceps tendon, 390
Transplantation of hamstrings to femoral condyles (Eggers), 392
Forward transfer of hamstrings to reinforce knee extension, 394
Above-knee amputation, 398

12 KNEE, 405

Arthroscopy, 406
Knee exposures, 408
Medial meniscectomy, 410

Peripheral reattachment of medial meniscus, 414
Lateral meniscectomy, 415
Peripheral reattachment of lateral meniscus, 417
Posterior capsulotomy of knee, 418
Repair for recurrent dislocation of patella (Hauser technique), 420
Elmslie-Trillat patellar realignment, 422
Repair for recurrent dislocation of patella (semitendinosus tenodesis), 424
Repair for recurrent dislocation of patella (Insall technique), 426
Patellar advancement, 428
Repair of fracture of patella, 429
Patellectomy, 431
Epiphyseal arrest of distal femur (epiphysiodesis), 433
Epiphyseal arrest of distal femur (by stapling), 436
Epiphysiodesis of proximal tibia and fibula, 439
Repair of torn medial collateral ligament, 443
Medial collateral ligament reconstruction, 445
Anterior cruciate ligament repair, 449
Anterior cruciate ligament reconstruction, 452
Repair of torn posterior cruciate ligament, 455
Repair of torn lateral ligaments, 457
Modified MacIntosh reconstruction for chronic anterolateral rotatory instability, 459
Lateral ligament reconstruction for lateral and posterolateral rotatory instability, 462
Open reduction and internal fixation for tibial plateau fracture, 465
Drainage of knee joint, 467
Synovectomy of knee, 468
Excision of popliteal cyst, 470
High tibial osteotomy for osteoarthritis of knee, 472
Proximal tibial osteotomy for genu recurvatum, 474
Animetric total knee replacement (nonconstrained), 477
Spherocentric total knee replacement (semiconstrained), 481
Compression arthrodesis of knee, 484

13 LOWER LEG, 493

Open reduction for tibial shaft fracture (anterolateral approach), 494
Open reduction for tibial shaft fracture (posterolateral approach), 497
Intramedullary nailing for tibial shaft fracture, 500
Fasciotomy of anterior tibial compartment, 502
Recession of gastrocnemius (Strayer), 504
Below-knee amputation, 506

14 ANKLE, 511

Tendo Achillis lengthening, 512
Tenodesis of tendo Achillis, 514
Repair of ruptured tendo Achillis, 516
Repair of rupture of anterior tibial tendon, 519
Tarsal tunnel release, 521
Transfer of posterior tibial and peroneus brevis tendons to calcaneus, 524
Open reduction and internal fixation for fracture of medial malleolus, 527
Open reduction and internal fixation for fracture of posterior lip of tibia, 529
Internal fixation for tibiofibular diastasis, 531
Reconstruction of lateral ligaments of ankle, 532

Drainage of ankle joint, 534
Modified Syme amputation, 535
Arthrodesis of ankle (lateral approach), 537
Compression arthrodesis of ankle (anterior approach), 540

15 FOOT, 547

Triple arthrodesis, 548
Subtalar arthrodesis (Grice procedure), 550
Osteotomy of calcaneus (Dwyer procedure), 553
Excision of calcaneal spur, 555
Plantar fasciotomy, 556
Medial soft tissue release (for resistant equinovarus clubfoot), 557
Tarsometatarsal mobilization (for resistant forefoot adduction), 561
Medial transfer of peroneus longus tendon, 562
Lateral transfer of anterior tibial tendon, 564
Excision of accessory tarsal navicular, 566
Excision of tarsal coalition, 568
Transmetatarsal amputation, 570
Intramedullary fixation for displaced metatarsal fracture, 571
Keller procedure, 572
McBride procedure, 574
Reconstructive osteotomy of first metatarsal (for adolescent hallux valgus), 576
Jones procedure for clawing of toe, 578
Excision of tibial sesamoid, 580
Arthrodesis of proximal interphalangeal joint, 581
Proximal phalangectomy, 583
Resection of metatarsal head, 585
Repair for chronic ingrown toenail, 587
Excision of interdigital neuroma, 589
Exostectomy for bunionette, 590
Repair of overlapping fifth toe, 591

16 MISCELLANEOUS OPERATIVE PROCEDURES, 597

Repair of severed artery, 598
Release of superficial tissue contracture (Z-plasty technique), 600
Soft tissue coverage of injured extremity, 601
Closed tube irrigation and drainage of localized musculoskeletal areas, 607
Localization of metallic foreign body, 608
Application of skeletal compression plate fixation, 609
Bone biopsy, 610
Muscle biopsy, 612
Microsurgery and replantation, 613

1

SHOULDER

REPAIR OF RECURRENT ANTERIOR DISLOCATION (Plate 1-1)

GENERAL DISCUSSION. Surgical repair is limited to patients with recurrent anterior dislocation of the shoulder and is indicated most commonly in those younger patients who appear likely to have recurrent difficulty. Surgical repair is seldom necessary in patients over 50 years of age. If the surgeon has not personally treated the patient for the acute episodes of shoulder dislocation, it is imperative to ascertain that the previous dislocations of the shoulder, in fact, have been anterior dislocations of the humeral head before any surgery is undertaken.

Of the multiple operations that have been described for surgical repair of recurrent anterior dislocation of the shoulder, the Putti-Platt type of repair involving shortening of the subscapularis tendon at its point of insertion into the rotator cuff has been satisfactory. The operation may be carried out through either the conventional anterior approach or through an anterior axillary approach to the shoulder joint. Adequate exposure for the critical surgical repair may be obtained through either surgical approach. However, because the conventional anterior approach leaves an unsightly scar, the anterior axillary approach offers a considerable cosmetic advantage with a residual scar that is hardly visible in later years.

DETAILS OF PROCEDURE. For the conventional anterior approach, the patient is positioned supine with a sandbag posterior to the right scapula, and the arm is draped free. A curvilinear incision is made beginning anterior to the lateral end of the clavicle. The incision is continued medially along the anterior margin of the clavicle toward the coracoid process, where the incision is redirected distally onto the anterior aspect of the upper arm as illustrated **(A)**. The dissection is carried down to the deltopectoral groove. The cephalic vein is identified **(B)** and retracted medially with the pectoralis major muscle. The deltoid muscle is retracted laterally, and exposure is facilitated by detaching a portion of the deltoid origin from the anterior aspect of the clavicle. The short head of the biceps and the coracobrachialis muscle are retracted medially, or the origin of these muscles may be carefully separated from the coracoid process **(C)** and tagged with a retention suture, if necessary, for adequate exposure of the anterior aspect of the shoulder joint.

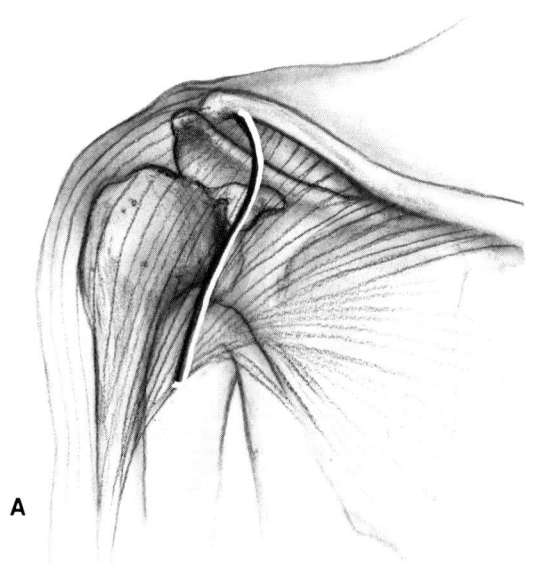

A

(Plate 1-1) REPAIR OF RECURRENT ANTERIOR DISLOCATION

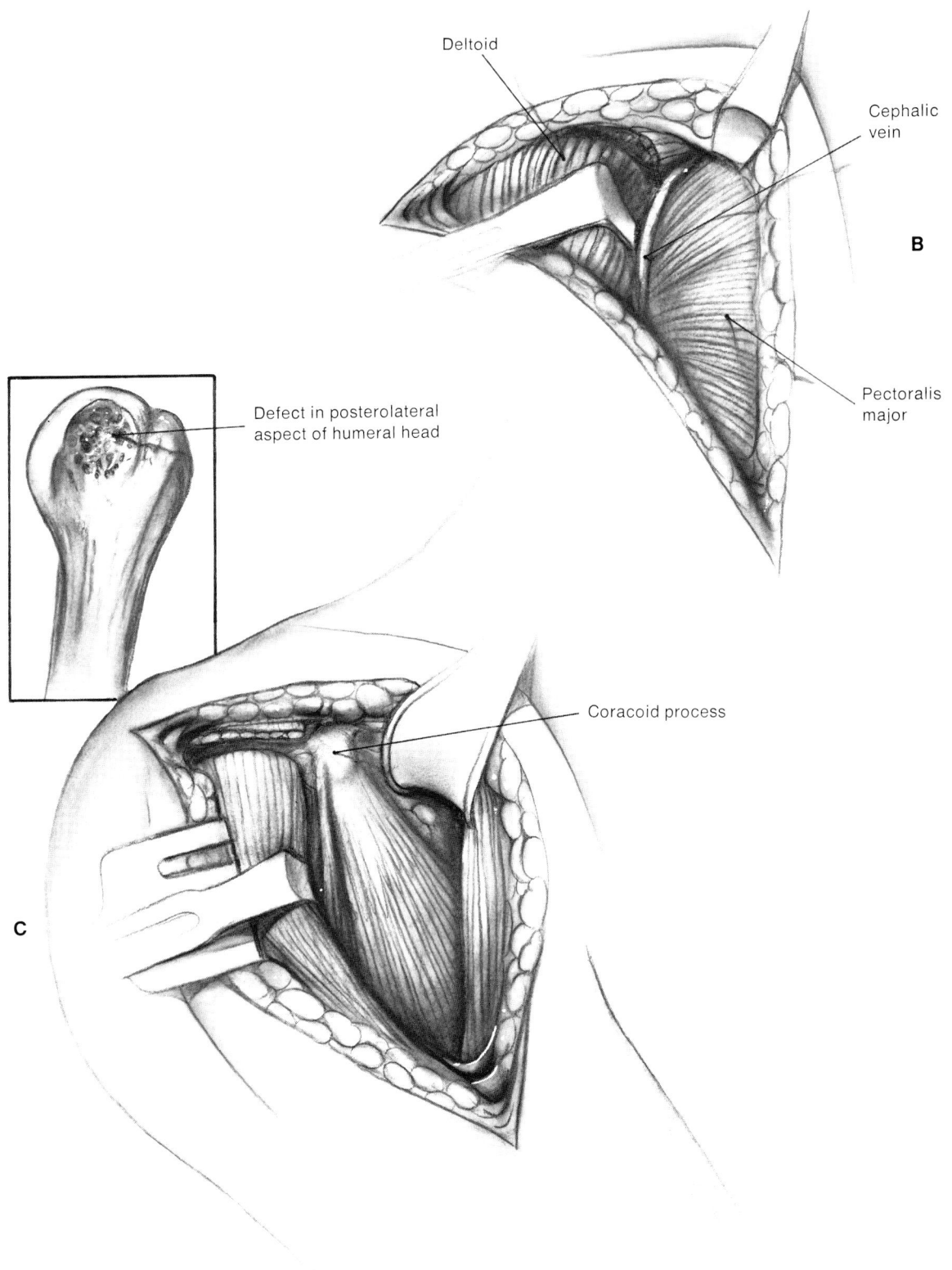

REPAIR OF RECURRENT ANTERIOR DISLOCATION (Plate 1-1)

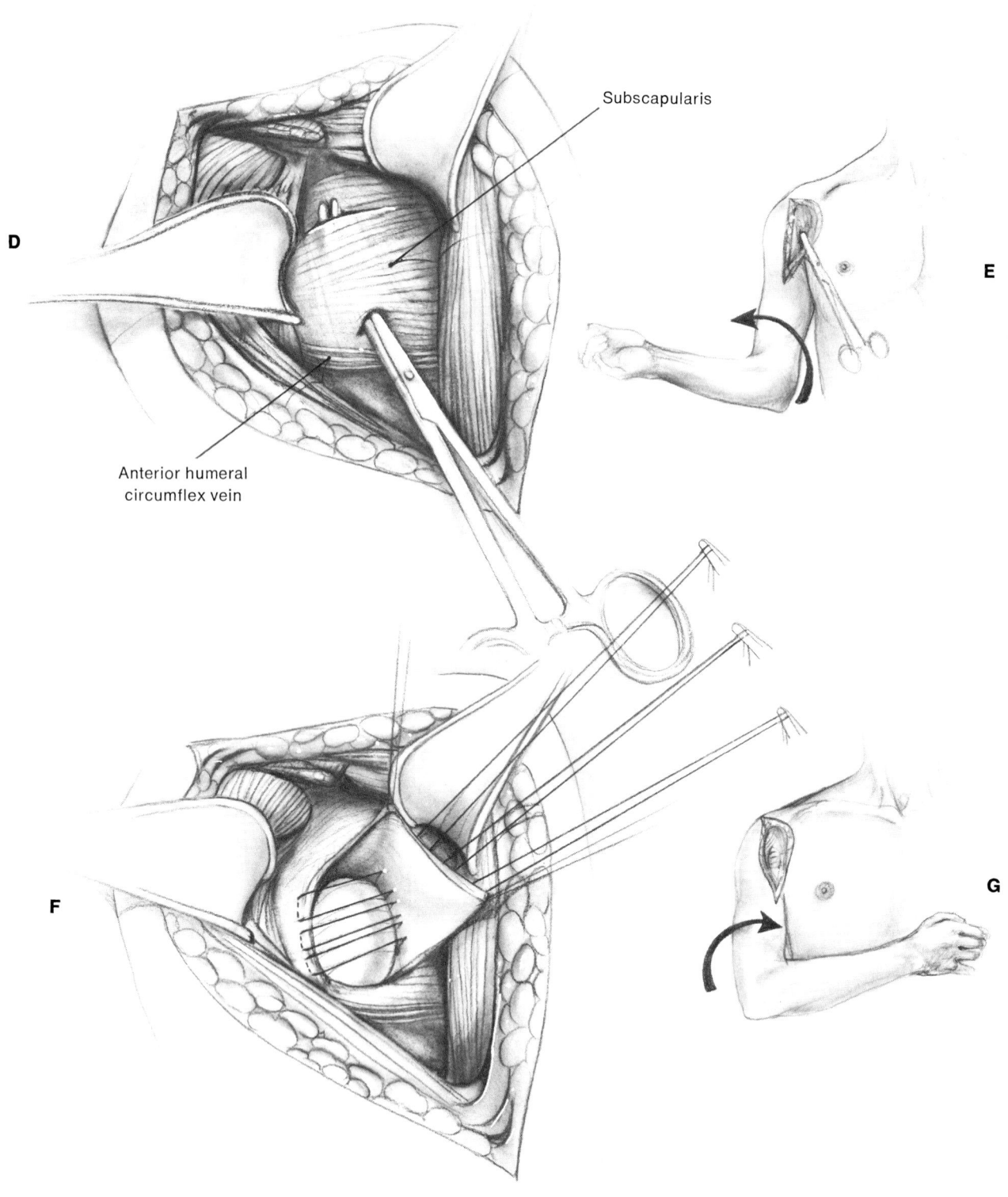

(Plate 1-1) REPAIR OF RECURRENT ANTERIOR DISLOCATION

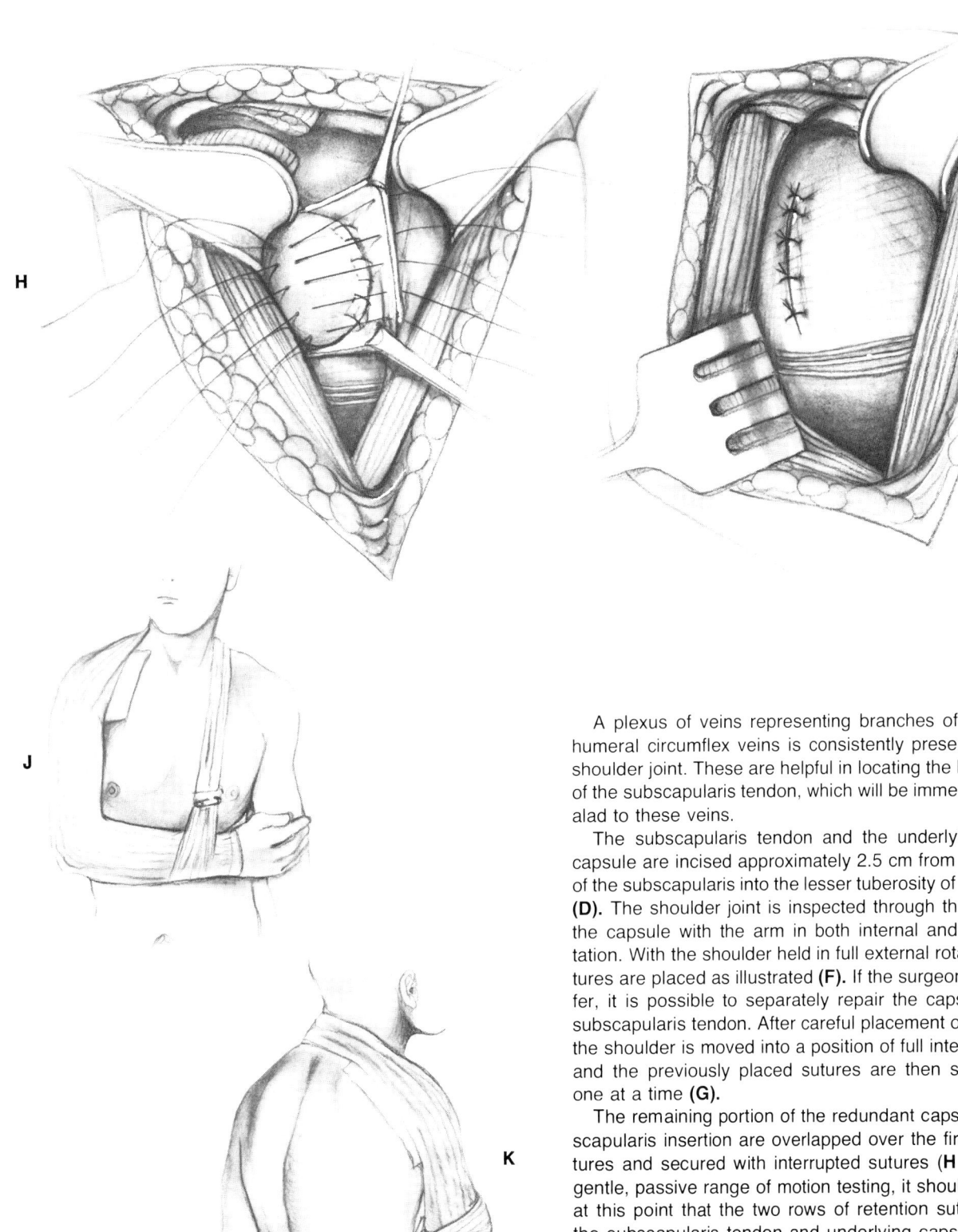

A plexus of veins representing branches of the anterior humeral circumflex veins is consistently present below the shoulder joint. These are helpful in locating the lower margin of the subscapularis tendon, which will be immediately cephalad to these veins.

The subscapularis tendon and the underlying shoulder capsule are incised approximately 2.5 cm from the insertion of the subscapularis into the lesser tuberosity of the humerus (**D**). The shoulder joint is inspected through the opening in the capsule with the arm in both internal and external rotation. With the shoulder held in full external rotation (**E**), sutures are placed as illustrated (**F**). If the surgeon should prefer, it is possible to separately repair the capsule and the subscapularis tendon. After careful placement of the sutures the shoulder is moved into a position of full internal rotation, and the previously placed sutures are then securely tied, one at a time (**G**).

The remaining portion of the redundant capsule and subscapularis insertion are overlapped over the first row of sutures and secured with interrupted sutures (**H** and **I**). With gentle, passive range of motion testing, it should be evident at this point that the two rows of retention sutures holding the subscapularis tendon and underlying capsule now limit external rotation of the glenohumeral joint at a position somewhere between neutral and 10° to 15° of external rotation. The wound is closed in layers and the patient is placed in a sling and swath (**J** and **K**) to retain the shoulder in a position of internal rotation before anesthesia is discontinued.

REPAIR OF RECURRENT ANTERIOR DISLOCATION (Plate 1-1)

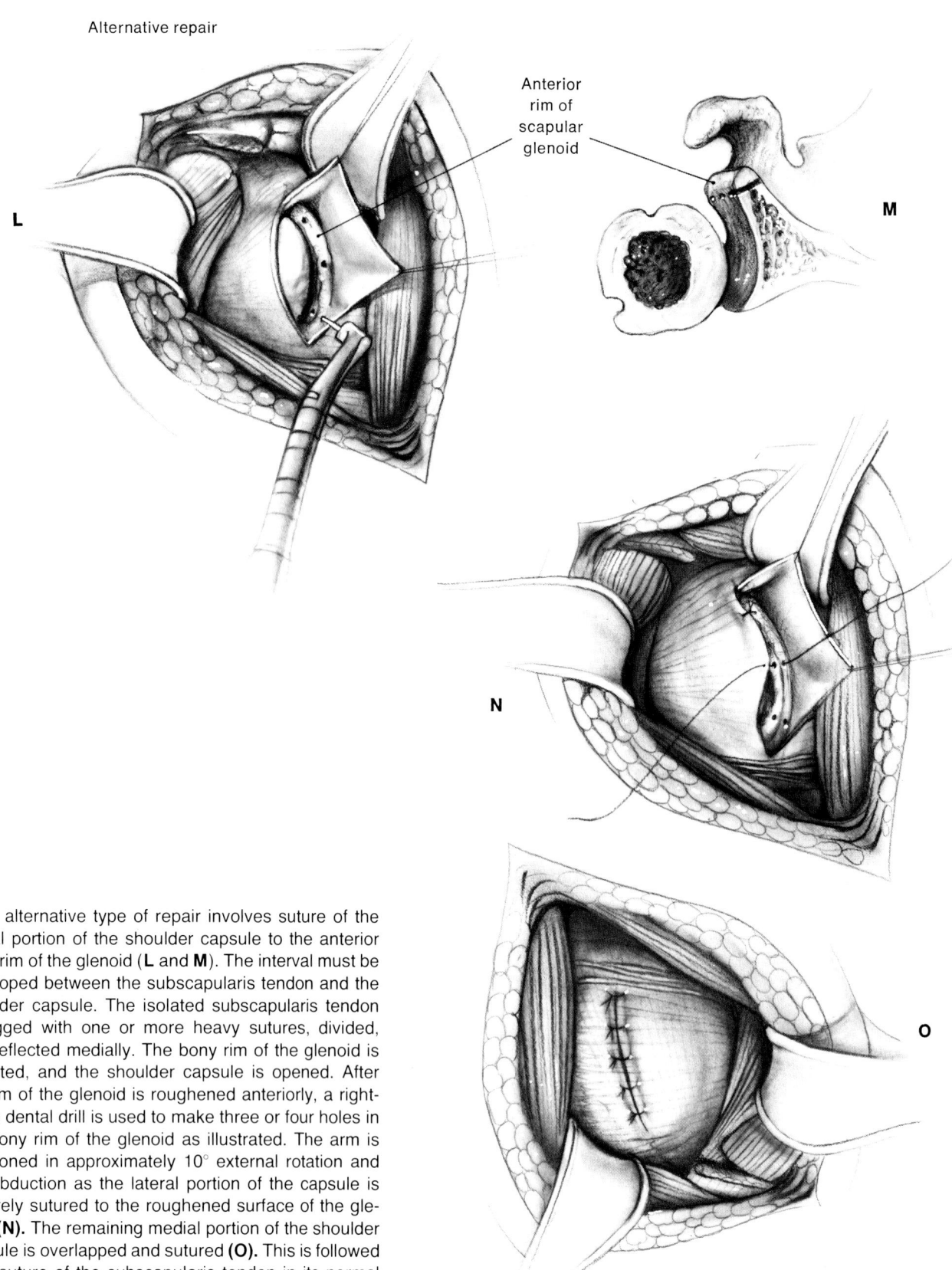

An alternative type of repair involves suture of the lateral portion of the shoulder capsule to the anterior bony rim of the glenoid (**L** and **M**). The interval must be developed between the subscapularis tendon and the shoulder capsule. The isolated subscapularis tendon is tagged with one or more heavy sutures, divided, and reflected medially. The bony rim of the glenoid is palpated, and the shoulder capsule is opened. After the rim of the glenoid is roughened anteriorly, a right-angle dental drill is used to make three or four holes in the bony rim of the glenoid as illustrated. The arm is positioned in approximately 10° external rotation and 45° abduction as the lateral portion of the capsule is securely sutured to the roughened surface of the glenoid (**N**). The remaining medial portion of the shoulder capsule is overlapped and sutured (**O**). This is followed by resuture of the subscapularis tendon in its normal position and wound closure.

(Plate 1-1) REPAIR OF RECURRENT ANTERIOR DISLOCATION

Alternative anterior axillary approach

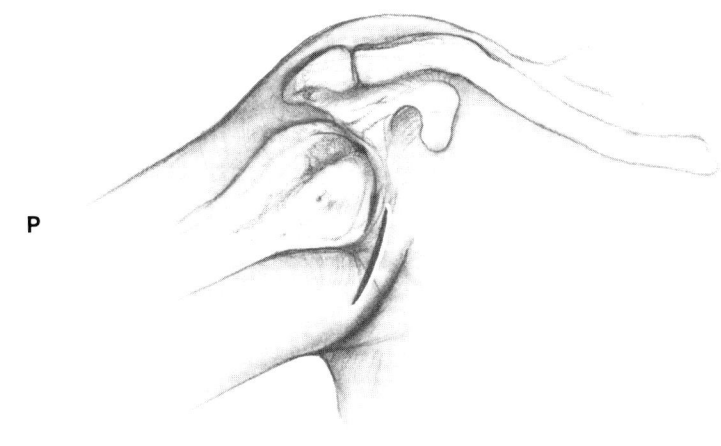

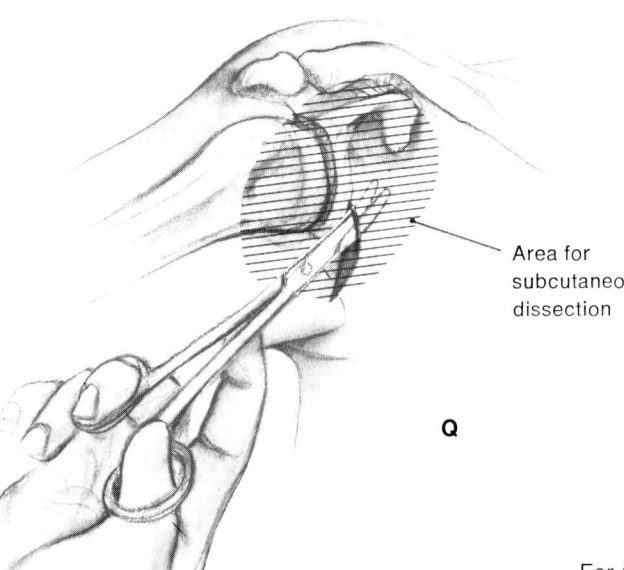

Area for subcutaneous dissection

For the anterior axillary approach the arm is initially positioned in 90° abduction and in external rotation, and the skin incision begins at the midpoint of the anterior axillary fold and then extends 6 cm posteriorly along the axilla **(P)**. Medial, lateral, and superior subfascial dissection is carried out to permit adequate mobility of the wound edges **(Q)**. The cephalic vein is identified in the deltopectoral groove, and the vein is retracted laterally along with the deltoid muscle. The superior border of the pectoralis major muscle is outlined to its insertion along the lateral edge of the bicipital groove. The superior portion of the tendinous insertion (and electively the entire insertion) is divided close to the humerus, and the pectoralis major muscle is retracted medially and inferiorly. The division of the pectoralis major insertion should be close to the humerus and should always be done under direct vision to avoid possible damage to the nearby brachial plexus and brachial artery. Exposure may then be improved by detaching the short head of the biceps brachii and the coracobrachialis from the coracoid process. The subscapularis muscle and tendon will be found just superior to the anterior humeral circumflex veins, which are consistently present along the inferior margin of the subscapularis tendon. The repair with overlapping and shortening of the subscapularis and the underlying shoulder capsule is carried out in the same

REPAIR OF RECURRENT ANTERIOR DISLOCATION (Plate 1-1)

manner as described, with exposure through the conventional anterior approach **(R)**.

Following repair of the subscapularis and shoulder capsule, the divided attachments of the short head of the biceps brachii, coracobrachialis, and pectoralis major are reapproximated, and after wound closure the arm is placed in a stockinette sling and swath. Subcuticular suture for skin closure **(S)** will permit the removal of the skin sutures in the second postoperative week without taking down the stockinette sling and swath or altering the position of the shoulder.

POSTOPERATIVE MANAGEMENT. The patient's shoulder is retained in the position of full internal rotation in a sling and swath for 3 weeks (or a longer period up to 6 weeks if the patient is under 25 years of age). When the sling and swath are discontinued, a program of gradual shoulder exercises is instituted with purposeful avoidance of any passive external force or extreme positions of elevation or external rotation for 3 months postoperatively. Full active shoulder motion except for the limitation of maximum external rotation is usually regained between the second and third month following operative repair for recurrent anterior dislocation of the shoulder.

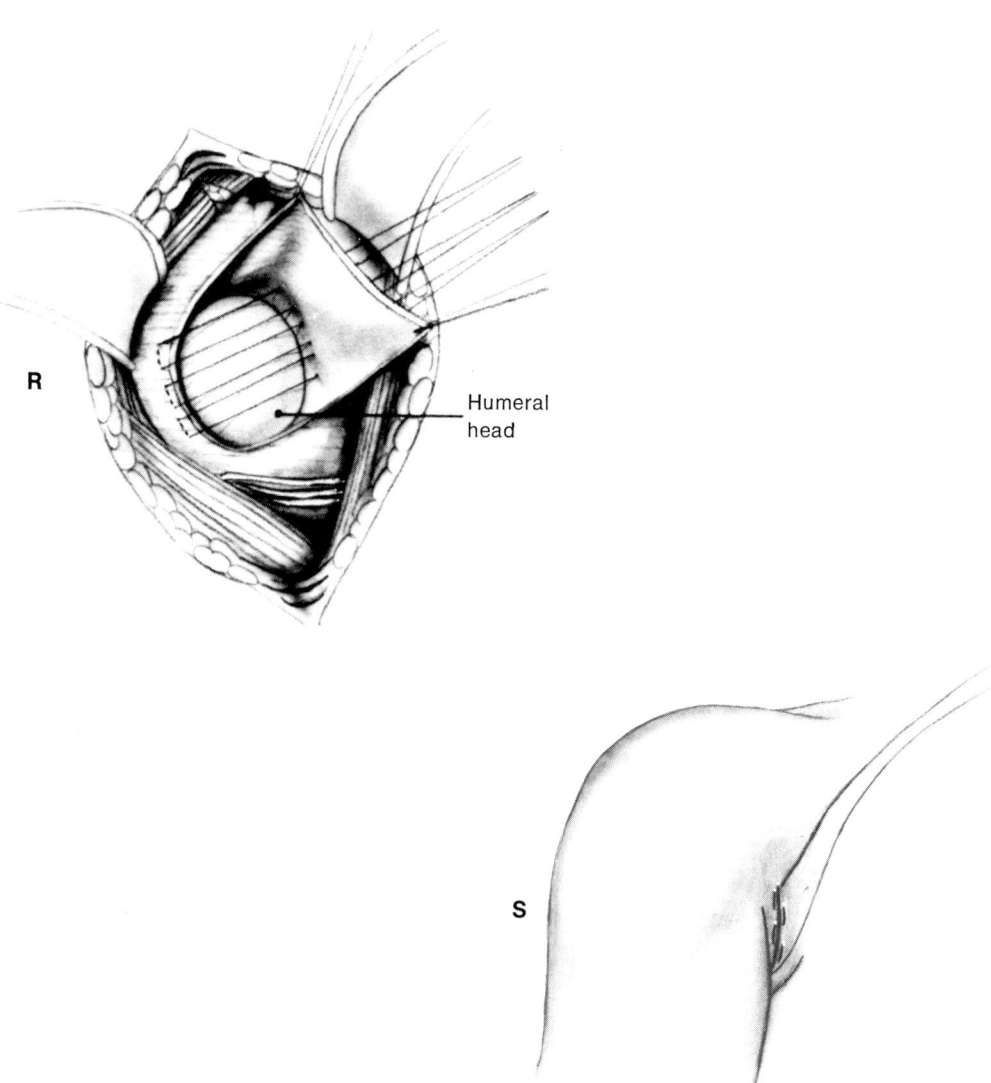

(Plate 1-2) REPAIR OF RECURRENT ANTERIOR DISLOCATION (BRISTOW PROCEDURE)

GENERAL DISCUSSION. An alternative approach to anterior instability is the procedure attributed to Bristow and described by Helfet. The procedure provides for an anterior bone block to obliterate the pathologic anterior glenoid space, and a strong muscular sling consisting of the short head of the biceps, coracobrachialis, and inferior half of the subscapularis to provide dynamic support for the anteromedial capsule. The procedure to be described is based on the technique as developed by Allman, which is slightly modified from Helfit's original description. The results have been gratifying for recurrent anterior subluxation as well as recurrent anterior dislocation, particularly in athletes.

DETAILS OF PROCEDURE. The patient is positioned in the semisitting position with a small bolster under the scapula and the right arm and shoulder draped free. A straight incision is made running from the coracoid process to the anterior axillary fold **(A)**. A muscle-splitting incision is made through the deltoid just lateral to the deltopectoral groove and cephalic vein in an attempt to avoid injury to the cephalic vein **(B)**. The underlying coracoid process is exposed, with the conjoined tendon of the short head of the biceps and the coracobrachialis being delineated from the insertion of the pectoralis minor **(C)**. The tip of the coracoid process is predrilled to facilitate subsequent internal fixation **(D)**.

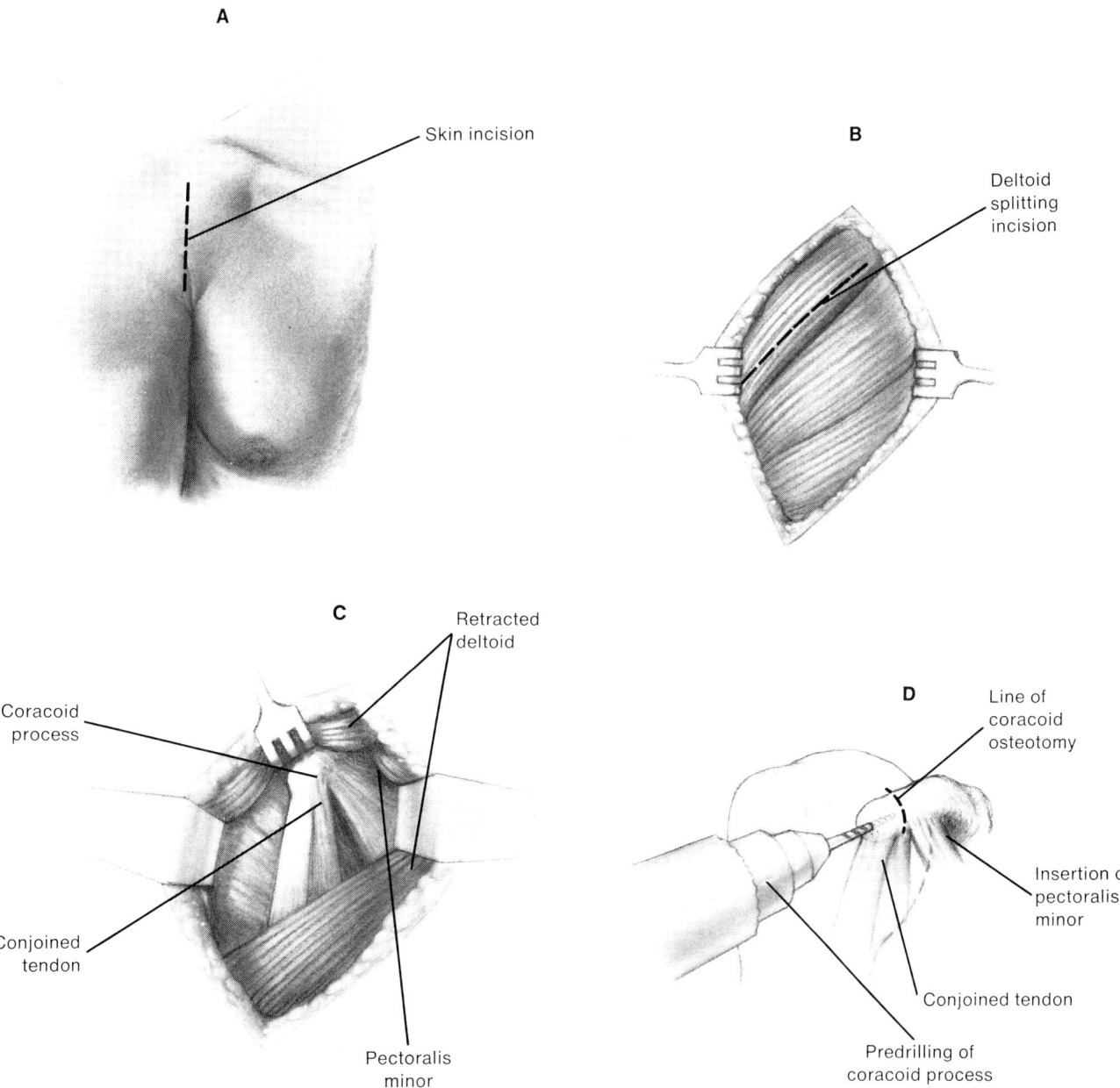

REPAIR OF RECURRENT ANTERIOR DISLOCATION (BRISTOW PROCEDURE) (Plate 1-2)

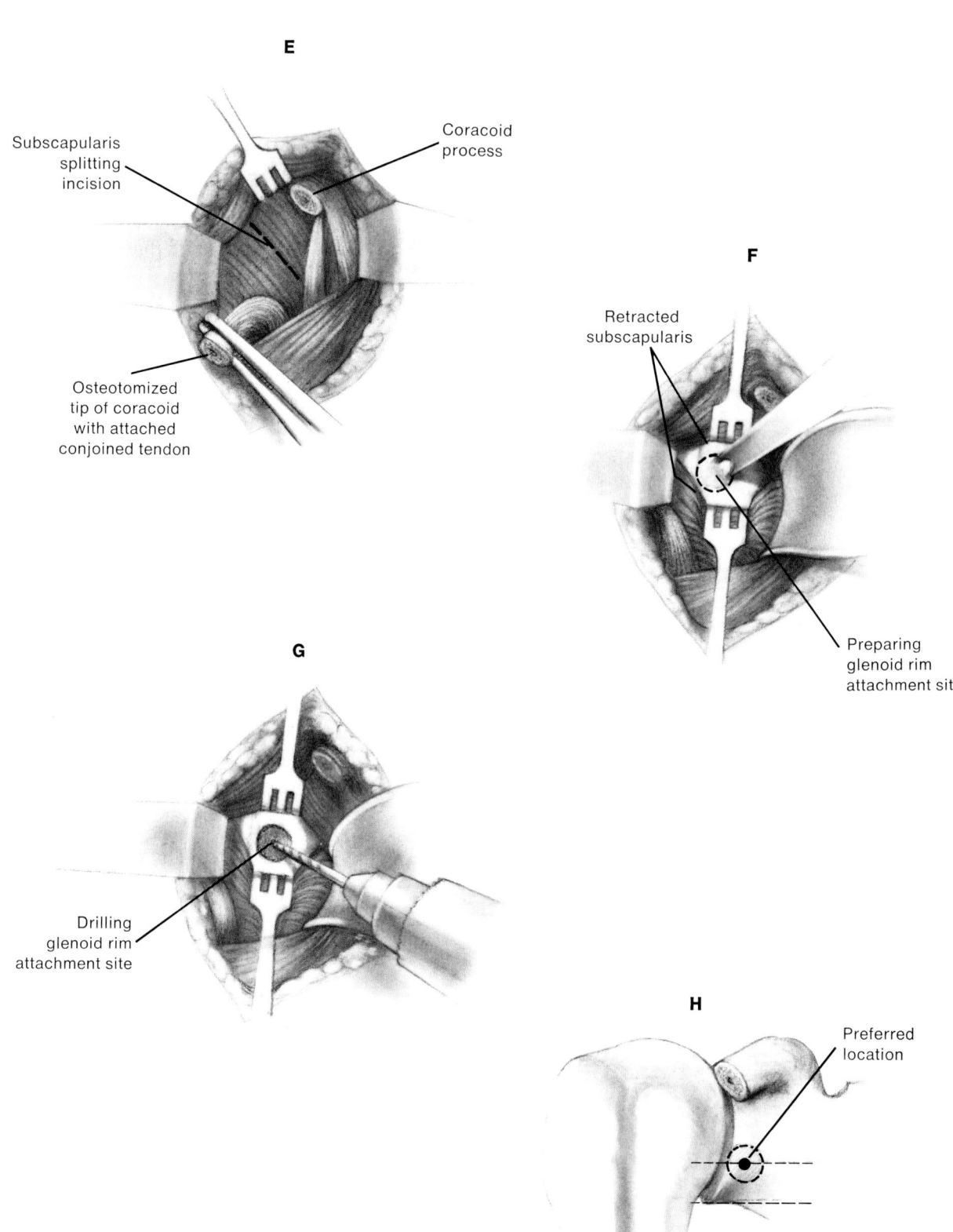

(Plate 1-2) REPAIR OF RECURRENT ANTERIOR DISLOCATION (BRISTOW PROCEDURE)

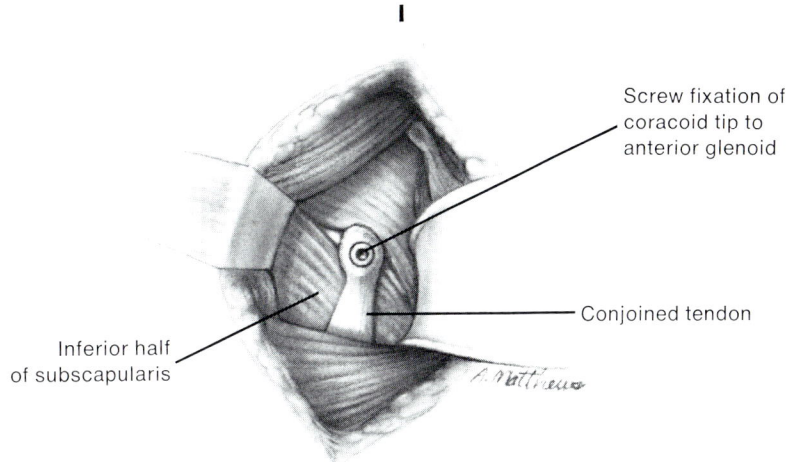

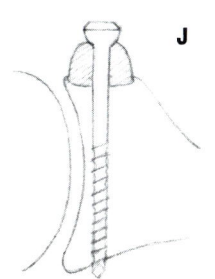

The coracoid process is then osteotomized with the oscillatory saw, and as large a piece of bone as possible is taken, with care to preserve the insertion of the pectoralis minor on the coracoid process. The osteotomized tip of the coracoid with the attached conjoined tendon is then carefully mobilized, with care to protect the musculocutaneous nerve **(E)**.

The arm is then externally rotated to bring into view the muscle belly of the subscapularis, which is split at its midpoint in line with its fibers and retracted both proximally and distally to expose the underlying anterior glenoid and shoulder joint capsule. The capsule is incised in line with the subscapularis incision to allow inspection of the anterior shoulder joint to search for loose bodies and evaluate the status of the glenoid labrum and articular surfaces. The anterior rim of the glenoid is stripped of all soft tissues, and freshened to accept the osteotomized tip of the coracoid process **(F)**. The appropriate site for attachment is selected, ideally just below the midpoint of the glenoid **(H)**. The prepared bed on the anterior glenoid rim is predrilled so that the coracoid tip will not overhang the joint line, and the orientation of the drill bit is kept in the plane of the glenoid **(G)**. Intraoperative roentgenograms in the axillary projection with the drill bit in place in the glenoid will confirm satisfactory positioning and orientation. The osteotomized tip of the coracoid process with attached conjoined tendon is fixed to the prepared bed on the anterior glenoid rim with a compression lag screw **(I)**. The relationship of the bone block and screw to the glenoid is illustrated in the axillary projection **(J)**. Any capsular defect lateral to the bone block is repaired, and after thorough irrigation the wound is closed in layers over suction drainage. Standard sterile dressing and sling and swath are applied.

POSTOPERATIVE MANAGEMENT. The patient is maintained in the sling and swath until the sutures are removed 2 weeks postoperatively. Then the arm is placed in a simple sling, and intermittent passive exercises are initiated, which consist of forward elevation and external rotation with the arm held at the side. If the procedure has been performed on the dominant arm of an active athlete, the intermittent passive motion exercises are initiated 48 hours postoperatively. More vigorous, active rehabilitative exercises are initiated 6 weeks following surgery after roentgenograms confirm that the screw and bone block have been maintained in the proper position.

REPAIR OF RECURRENT POSTERIOR DISLOCATION (Plate 1-3)

GENERAL DISCUSSION. Recurrent posterior dislocation of the shoulder is uncommon. If there has been a posterior dislocation of the shoulder, recurrent posterior dislocations may occur with forward elevation of the shoulder and internal rotation with or without adduction. The shoulder may dislocate each time that it is brought into the unstable position and, therefore, may be a source of significant disability, since the position of forward elevation, internal rotation, and adduction is assumed in many daily activities.

If there is any question about the diagnosis of a posterior dislocation of the shoulder (**A** and **B**), specific additional roentgenographic views of the shoulder may be helpful, that is, an axillary view or an angle-up view. Either one of these views can provide clear evidence of posterior dislocation. For the angle-up view, the cassette should be held parallel to the long axis of the thorax and posterior to the shoulder, and the x-ray tube should be angled cephalad about 35°. Various types of surgical repair for posterior dislocation of the shoulder have been reported by Rowe and Yee, Hindenach, and McLaughlin. The surgical repair that is recommended is similar to that reported by Scott, incorporating an osteotomy of the posterior part of the scapular neck as part of the repair to produce stability in the shoulder without undue disturbance of the congruity of the joint or interference with normal glenohumeral motion.

DETAILS OF PROCEDURE. With the patient in a semi-prone position and with the arm draped free, a skin incision is made extending from the medial border of the scapular spine to the tip of the acromion and then curved distally for approximately 5 cm (**C**). The posterior third of the deltoid is detached from the scapular spine and the acromion process posteriorly (**D**).

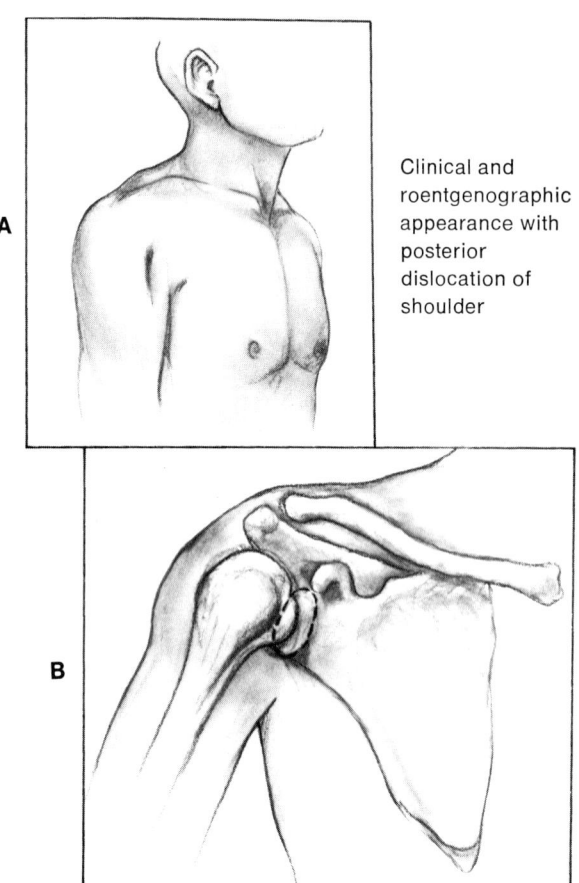

Clinical and roentgenographic appearance with posterior dislocation of shoulder

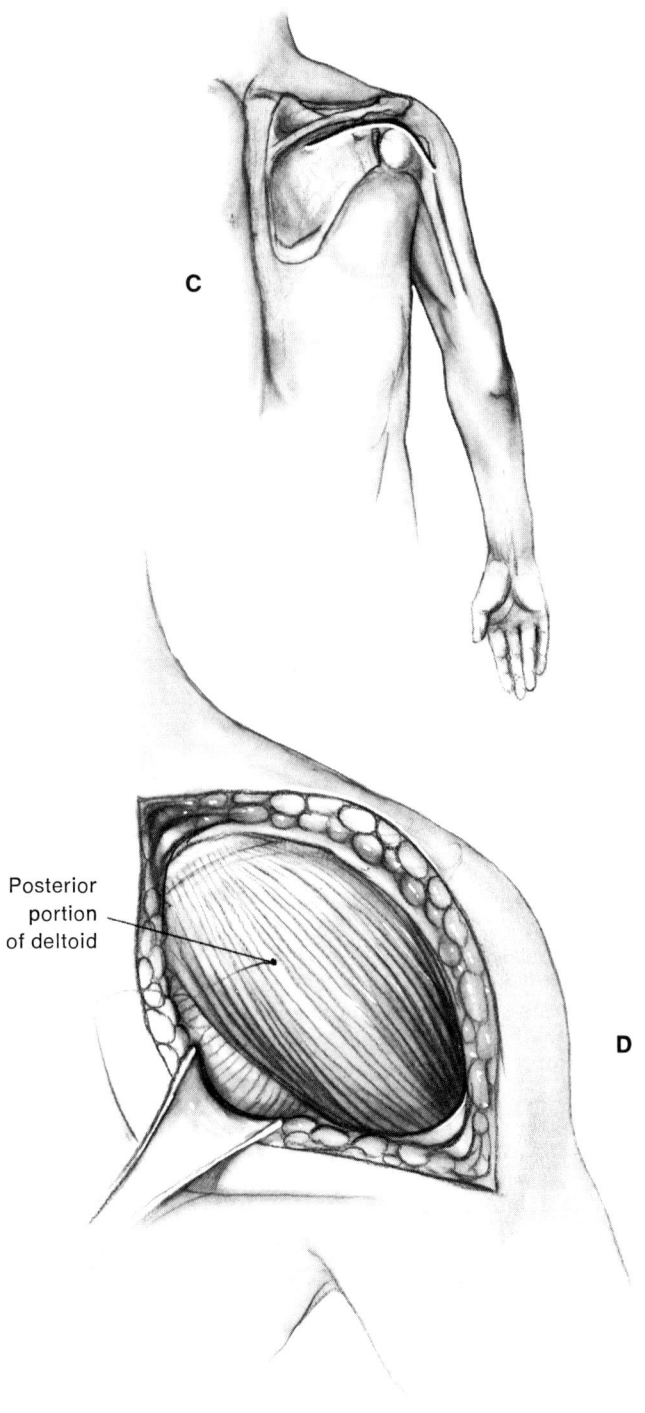

Posterior portion of deltoid

(Plate 1-3) REPAIR OF RECURRENT POSTERIOR DISLOCATION

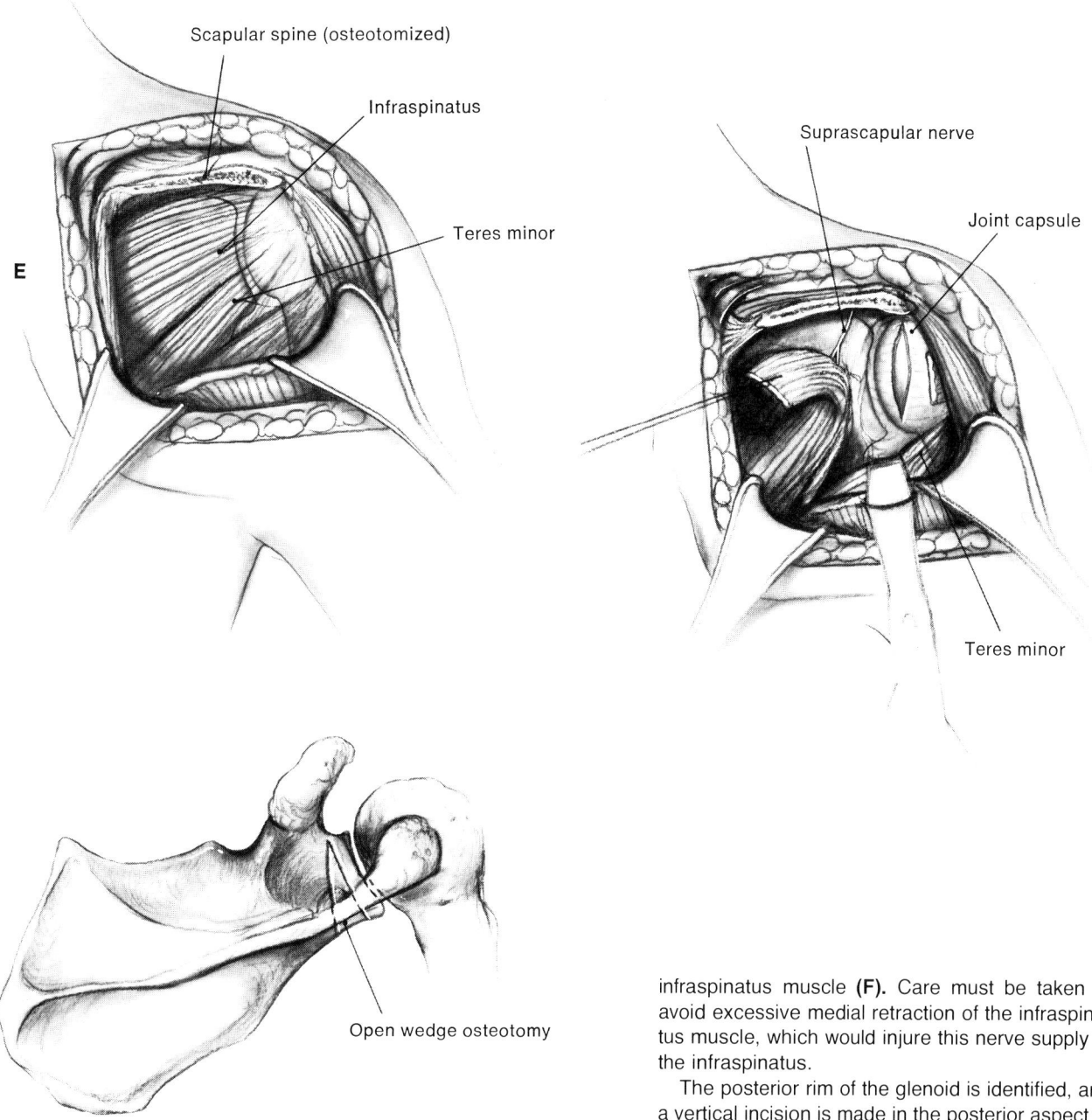

The overhanging portion of the posterior aspect of the acromion is then osteotomized **(E)** and saved for use as bone graft later in the procedure. The interval between the infraspinatus muscle and teres minor muscle is identified. The deltoid muscle is retracted laterally to permit division of the insertion of the infraspinatus as close as possible to its insertion into the posterior aspect of the rotator cuff and greater tuberosity. During retraction of the deltoid, to avoid injury to the axillary nerve, care should be taken to avoid placement of any retractors below the level of the lower border of the teres minor or any forceful retraction of the deltoid. After the insertion of the infraspinatus tendon has been divided, its lateral end is reflected medially and the suprascapular nerve may be visualized as it passes around the base of the scapular spine to enter the inferior surface of the infraspinatus muscle **(F)**. Care must be taken to avoid excessive medial retraction of the infraspinatus muscle, which would injure this nerve supply to the infraspinatus.

The posterior rim of the glenoid is identified, and a vertical incision is made in the posterior aspect of the shoulder capsule, 0.6 cm lateral to the posterior rim of the glenoid **(G)**. Medial extensions from the upper and lower ends of this capsular incision facilitate visualization of the articular surface and concavity of the glenoid. With a broad osteotome, the neck of the scapula is osteotomized and wedged open gradually from the area of the supraglenoid tubercle to the infraglenoid tubercle. This is done carefully while the concavity of the glenoid is periodically visualized through the posterior opening in the shoulder capsule so that the open-wedge osteotomy site may be placed in close proximity to the glenoid concavity, but it must be entirely extra-articular.

13

REPAIR OF RECURRENT POSTERIOR DISLOCATION (Plate 1-3)

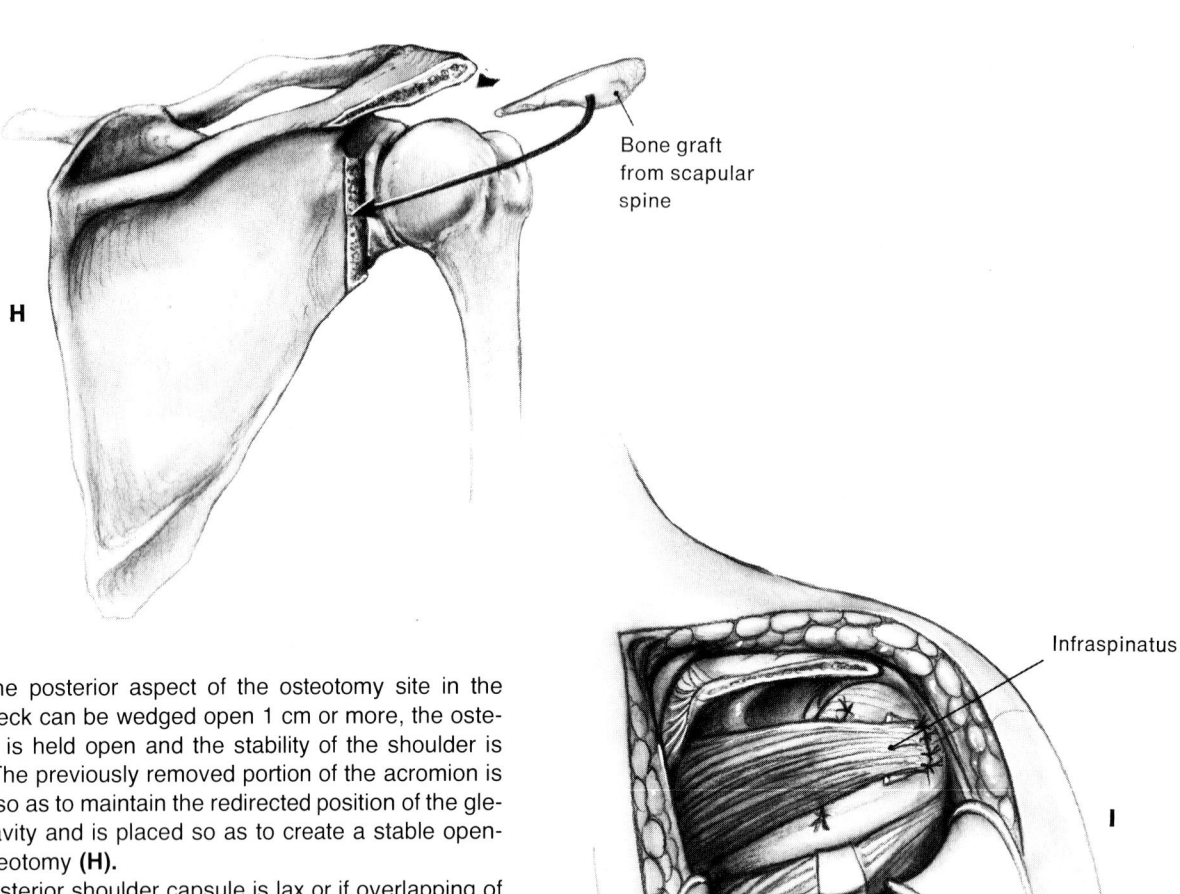

When the posterior aspect of the osteotomy site in the scapular neck can be wedged open 1 cm or more, the osteotomy site is held open and the stability of the shoulder is checked. The previously removed portion of the acromion is fashioned so as to maintain the redirected position of the glenoid concavity and is placed so as to create a stable open-wedge osteotomy **(H)**.

If the posterior shoulder capsule is lax or if overlapping of the capsule opening is possible, closure is made by resuturing the posterior capsule in two layers. The insertion of the infraspinatus tendon is replaced and sutured securely to the rotator cuff, preferably in a more lateral location than its original insertion **(I)**. The deltoid is resutured to the scapular spine and acromion.

POSTOPERATIVE MANAGEMENT. The arm is maintained at the patient's side in a neutral or slightly externally rotated position for 3 weeks to allow the soft tissues to heal. The patient is directed to avoid using the arm in a forceful manner, especially any forceful forward pushing activities, for an additional 3 months.

(Plate 1-4) REPAIR OF ACROMIOCLAVICULAR SEPARATION

GENERAL DISCUSSION. The large majority of acromioclavicular separations require no surgical intervention. When circumstances are such that some type of repair is necessary, this may be accomplished in a manner described by Neviaser of transferring the coracoacromial ligament to make a new superior acromioclavicular ligament. One of the advantages of this procedure is that the clavicle is not held down permanently by a screw or wires, thereby limiting the rotational motion of the clavicle, which in turn would restrict full abduction of the shoulder.

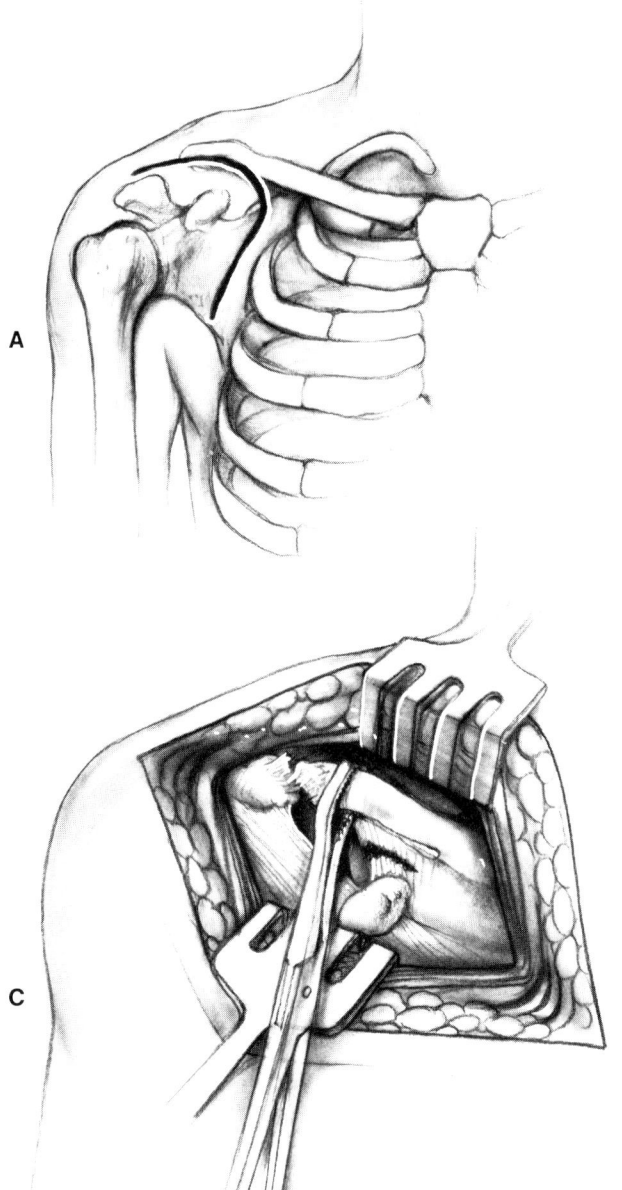

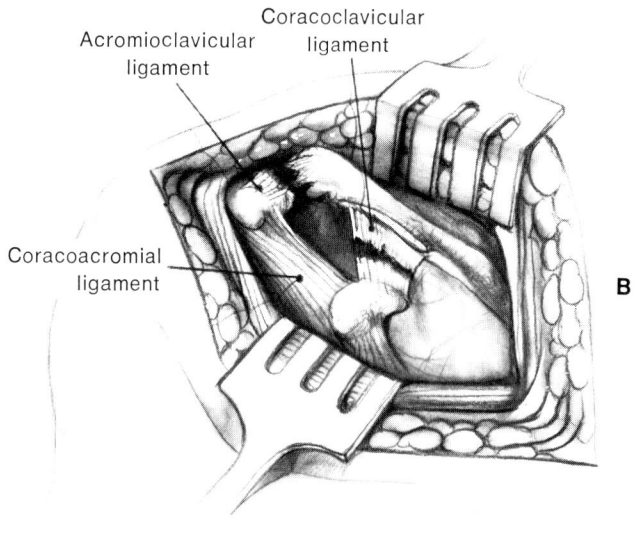

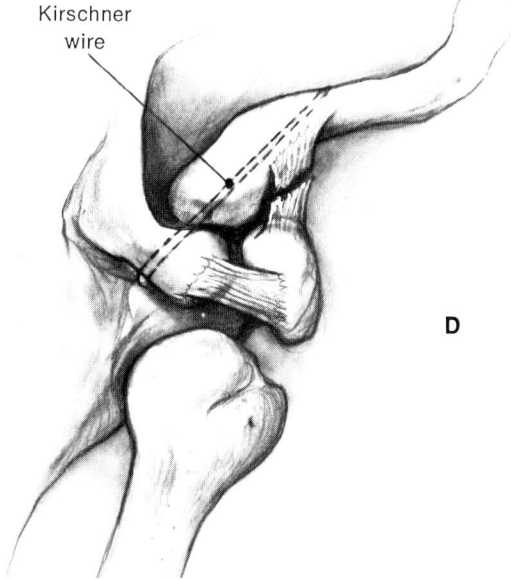

DETAILS OF PROCEDURE. The anterior aspect of the shoulder in the area of the coracoacromial ligament and the acromioclavicular joint are exposed through a slightly curved incision over the anterior aspect of the lateral half of the clavicle extending laterally to the tip of the acromion process **(A)**. The deltoid muscle is reflected from its attachment on the anterior aspect of the lateral third of the clavicle. The disrupted acromioclavicular joint is visualized **(B)** and reduced without disturbing the articular disc that lies between the clavicle and acromion. While the clavicle is held reduced, one or two Kirschner wires are drilled successively through the skin and acromion process and into the clavicle to adequately maintain the reduction of the acromioclavicular joint (**C** and **D**). The lateral end of the wire is bent slightly outside the posterior aspect of the acromion process to prevent its inward migration and is left in this position beneath the skin.

REPAIR OF ACROMIOCLAVICULAR SEPARATION (Plate 1-4)

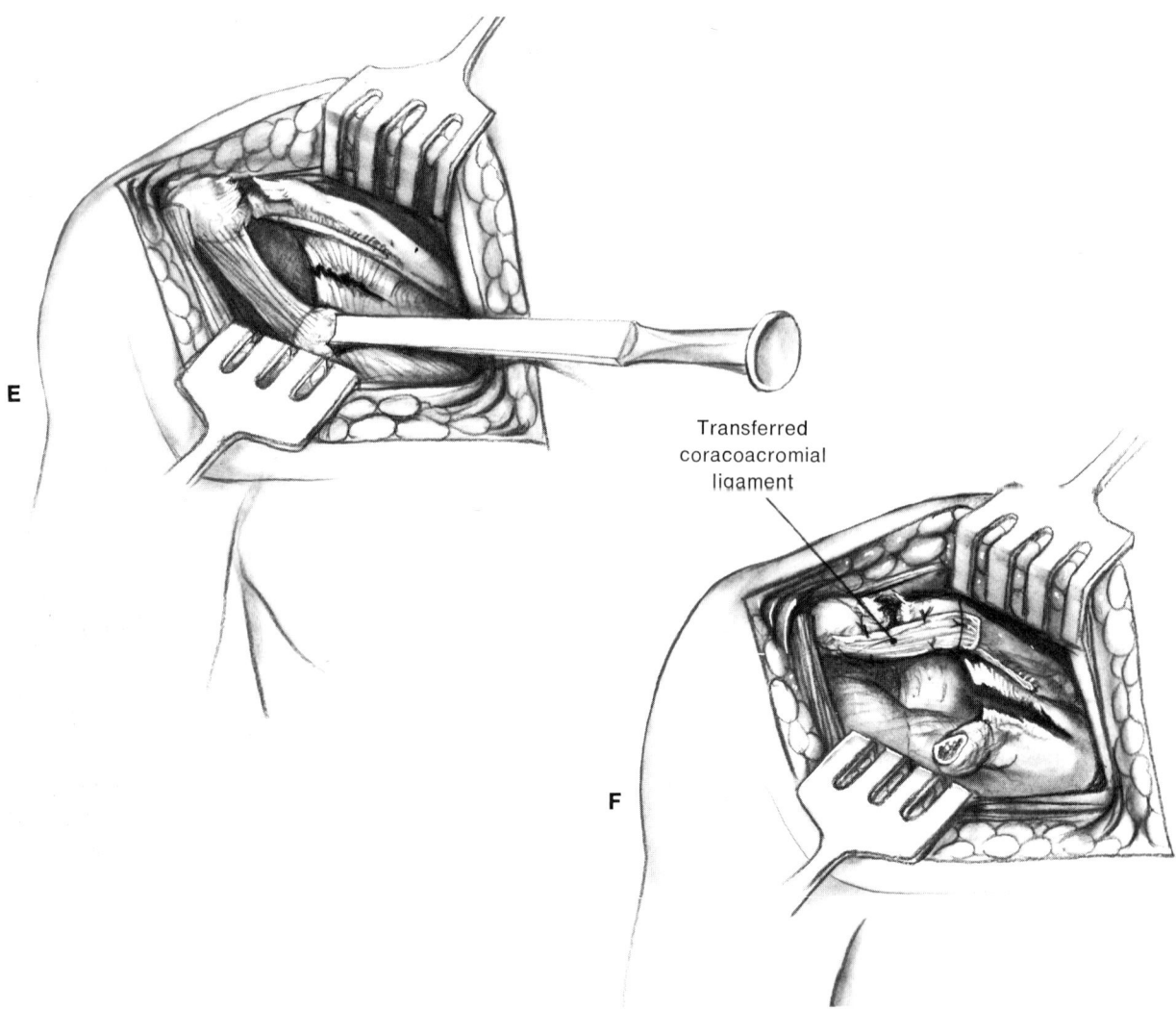

Transferred coracoacromial ligament

When the acromioclavicular joint has been reduced and stabilized with one or two Kirschner wires, the medial end of the coracoacromial ligament is removed by osteotomizing a small piece of the attachment of this ligament to the lateral border of the coracoid process **(E)**. This strong ligament is then reflected laterally to its attachment on the acromion process and then turned over the acromion and placed superiorly over the acromioclavicular joint onto the superior surface of the clavicle. At the area where the shell of bone attached to the medial end of the transferred ligament is to be in contact with the clavicle, the clavicle is roughened with a rasp and the transferred ligament is secured in this position with heavy catgut sutures holding the lateral portion to the fascial tissue over the acromion process and the medial portion to the clavicle **(F)**. Sutures are passed through two drill holes in the clavicle, and a circumferential suture is placed just lateral to the fragment of bone at the medial end of the transferred coracoacromial ligament in its new location on the flat superior surface of the lateral end of the clavicle. The deltoid muscle is resutured to the clavicle, and the patient's arm is placed in a stockinette sling and swath.

POSTOPERATIVE MANAGEMENT. At weekly intervals the patient's arm is removed from the stockinette sling and swath and passed gently through a partial range of motion to minimize subsequent restriction of shoulder motion from the period of necessary postoperative immobilization. At 5 weeks the Kirschner wire or wires used for maintenance of the acromioclavicular reduction at the time of operation are removed. The patient is placed on a progressive active exercise regime for the involved shoulder and is advised to avoid vigorous contact sports or heavy lifting with the involved arm for at least an additional 3 weeks.

(Plate 1-5) RESECTION OF LATERAL END OF CLAVICLE

GENERAL DISCUSSION. For the chronically symptomatic acromioclavicular joint, resection of the lateral end of the clavicle is a relatively simple and reliable procedure for relief of symptoms secondary to an old acromioclavicular separation or for symptoms produced by localized degenerative changes at the acromioclavicular joint.

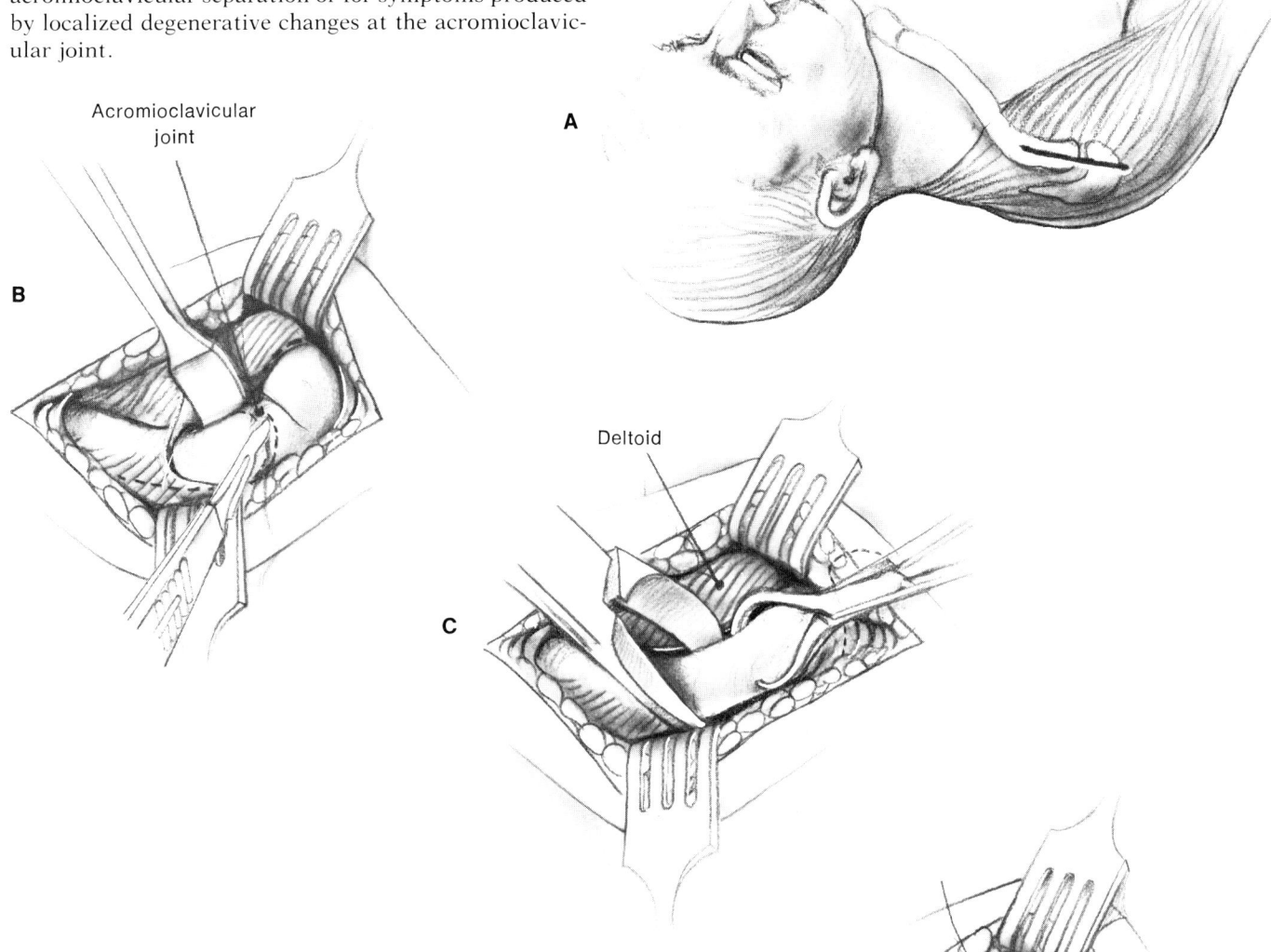

DETAILS OF PROCEDURE. The lateral end of the clavicle is exposed through a short incision **(A)**. The periosteum over the lateral end of the clavicle is incised in line with the clavicle, initially over the superior surface of the lateral end of the clavicle **(B)**. The periosteum is then reflected to expose the outer end of the clavicle, and approximately 2 cm of the lateral end of the clavicle are removed subperiosteally with bone-cutting forceps **(C)** or with an osteotome after multiple drill holes have been made at the desired osteotomy site. The remaining edge of the divided clavicle is smoothed with a rasp with particular attention to the superior surface that will remain in a subcutaneous position. The acromion is not disturbed. The periosteum is resutured to provide soft tissue cover over the raw end of the divided clavicle **(D)**. Following wound closure, the patient's arm is placed in a sling.

POSTOPERATIVE MANAGEMENT. The shoulder is supported in a sling until the patient has become comfortable, usually 7 to 10 days. Active use of the shoulder and arm is then encouraged as tolerated with gradual return to all normal activities.

EXCISION OF CALCIFIC DEPOSIT (Plate 1-6)

GENERAL DISCUSSION. The presence of a calcific deposit may be associated with pain in the shoulder. For the relatively uncommon situations in which nonoperative treatment is ineffective, surgical excision of a calcific deposit may be helpful. This condition is initiated by degeneration of tendon fibers, predominantly those of the supraspinatus, with secondary calcium deposit into this site. Characteristically, there is pain and tenderness, usually lateral to the outer end of the acromion process with painful limitation of shoulder motion and complaint of nighttime increase in the shoulder discomfort. Calcific bursitis is the natural result of tendonitis when calcific debris ruptures into the subacromial bursa.

For any calcific deposit in the shoulder area that is to be excised, it is important to have accurate preoperative roentgenographic localization. A calcific deposit in the supraspinatus tendon will be seen near the tendon's point of insertion on the promontory of the greater tuberosity, and the deposit should move medially with internal rotation of the shoulder. A less common site for calcific deposits in the shoulder area is the infraspinatus tendon, in which case the calcific deposit should be noted by roentgenogram to be localized to the middle third of the greater tuberosity. If the deposit is in the infraspinatus tendon, internal rotation of the shoulder will move the deposit laterally on the anteroposterior roentgenogram. Calcific deposits are still less commonly present in the teres minor tendon. A calcific deposit adjacent to the upper edge of the glenoid fossa that does not move significantly in anteroposterior roentgenograms on rotation of the shoulder may be in the tendon of the long head of the biceps. The calcific deposit inferior to the rim of the glenoid will probably lie in the tendon of the long head of the triceps, and a 30° cephalocaudal view should be able to confirm calcification at this site.

DETAILS OF PROCEDURE. A short incision, which may be longitudinal **(A)** or transverse (the latter exposure leaving a more satisfactory postoperative scar), is made just lateral to the acromion process. The fascia over the deltoid muscle is split longitudinally from the tip of the acromion process distally for approximately 4 to 5 cm. The deltoid muscle is then separated in line with its fibers close to the acromion process **(B)**. Care is taken to avoid injury to the axillary nerve, which passes transversely from posterior to anterior on the deep surface of the deltoid at a level approximately 5 cm distal to the origin of the muscle from the spine of the scapula, acromion, and clavicle.

While the opening in the proximal fibers of the deltoid muscle is gently retracted, the underlying subacromial bursa **(C)** is opened. The calcific deposit in the tendon cuff may be found to be raised above the surface of the supraspinatus tendon **(D)**, and greater visualization may be attained if the shoulder is moved slowly by an assistant to bring adjacent areas of the rotator cuff into view through the opened subacromial bursa. If necessary, serial vertical incisions may be made in the tendon cuff until the calcific deposit is located. In the acutely affected shoulder, the soft tissues will be observed to be markedly inflamed and the calcific material will be soft and white and easily evacuated. If there is any unusual difficulty in locating the deposit, roentgenograms in the operating room can be helpful and should be obtained.

When the calcific deposit is identified, it may be thick, chalky, or somewhat like toothpaste and, if chronic, may be surrounded by a covering of fibrous tissue. The inner elliptic portion of the tendinous fibers immediately adjacent to the calcific deposit should be excised in line with the fibers of the rotator cuff. Any residual calcific material should be removed by curettage if necessary, and the area should be thoroughly irrigated with saline solution. If the coracoacromial ligament has not yet been divided transversely, it should be done at this time. The rotator cuff defect is closed with one or two interrupted chromic catgut sutures, and the fibers of the deltoid muscle are allowed to come back together, interrupted sutures being placed in the overlying fascia of the deltoid muscle **(E)**. Following wound closure, the shoulder may be manipulated if preoperatively there has been chronic limitation of shoulder motion or a "frozen shoulder" syndrome. A light compression dressing is applied to the wound, and the arm is placed in a sling.

POSTOPERATIVE MANAGEMENT. Early active and passive assistive exercises are encouraged, and the sling is discontinued as soon as possible. Return to normal activity should be anticipated within a few weeks except in patients with preoperative chronic "frozen shoulder" difficulty. These patients should regain functional shoulder activity postoperatively at a rate that is progressive but slower than among patients with less chronic shoulder difficulty preoperatively.

(Plate 1-6) EXCISION OF CALCIFIC DEPOSIT

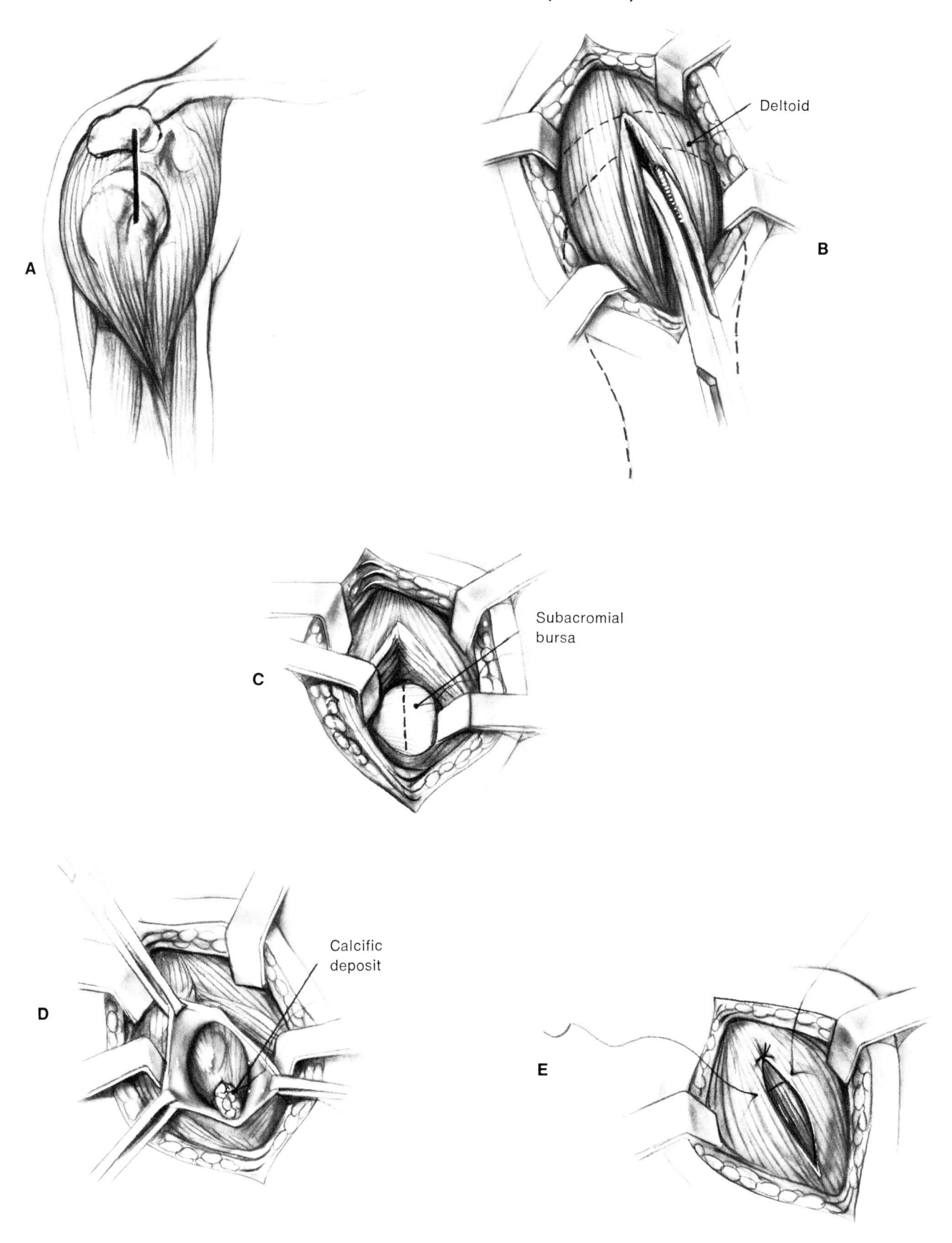

19

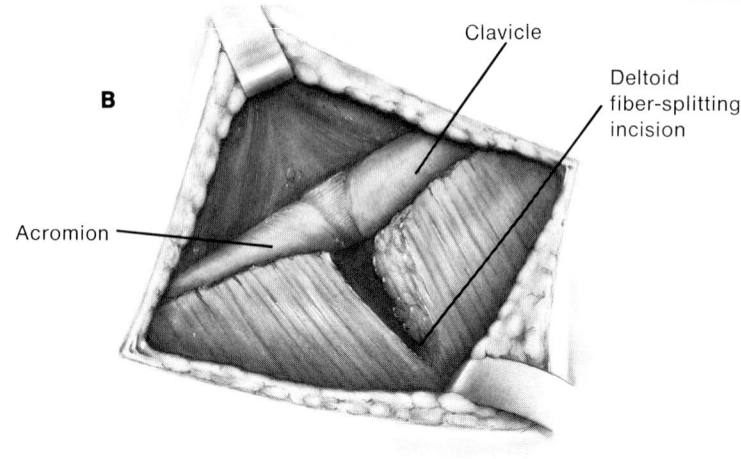

NEER ANTERIOR ACROMIOPLASTY (Plate 1-7)

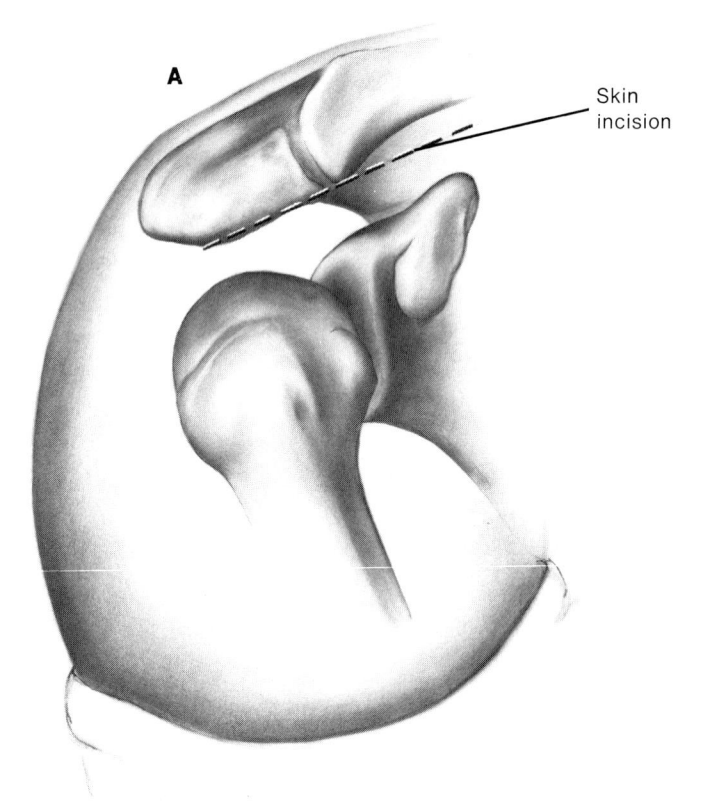

GENERAL DISCUSSION. Chronic inflammation involving the rotator cuff (particularly the supraspinatus), anterior lateral shoulder capsule, and the long head of the biceps tendon leads to chronic thickening of these structures. With shoulder elevation and abduction, the thickened structures must pass beneath the coracoacromial arch consisting of the coracoacromial ligament medially and the inferior surface of the anterior acromion superiorly and laterally. With the thickening of chronic inflammation (including the subacromial bursa), there is insufficient clearance, and the self-perpetuating anterior impingement syndrome becomes established. In long-standing cases there may be associated attritional tears of the rotator cuff. Established cases of chronic anterior impingement syndrome that are recalcitrant to adequate conservative treatment can be effectively treated by the anterior acromioplasty described by Neer, which enlarges the coracoacromial arch to create more room for the thickened capsular and rotator cuff structures. This relieves the physical impingement and allows the chronic inflammation to subside but does not weaken the mechanical advantage of the deltoid muscle because only the inferior portion of the acromion is resected. This procedure is in contrast to acromionectomy, in which the lateral portion of the acromion is resected with resultant decreased arm leverage for deltoid function.

DETAILS OF PROCEDURE. The patient is placed in the supine semisitting position on the operating room table. A horizontal skin incision is made along the anteroinferior border of the acromion and distal clavicle (**A**). The acromioclavicular joint is identified, and a deltoid muscle–splitting incision is made at the level of the acromioclavicular joint (**B**). Then the deltoid muscle is carefully detached from the distal clavicle and anterior acromion and retracted to provide exposure of the coracoacromial arch (**C**). An incision is made through the periosteum and acromioclavicular joint capsule in line with the axis of the distal clavicle and acromion, and carefully reflected superiorly to expose the acromioclavicular joint. If significant degenerative changes are present, the distal 1.5 cm of the clavicle is resected (**C** and **D**).

(Plate 1-7) NEER ANTERIOR ACROMIOPLASTY

C

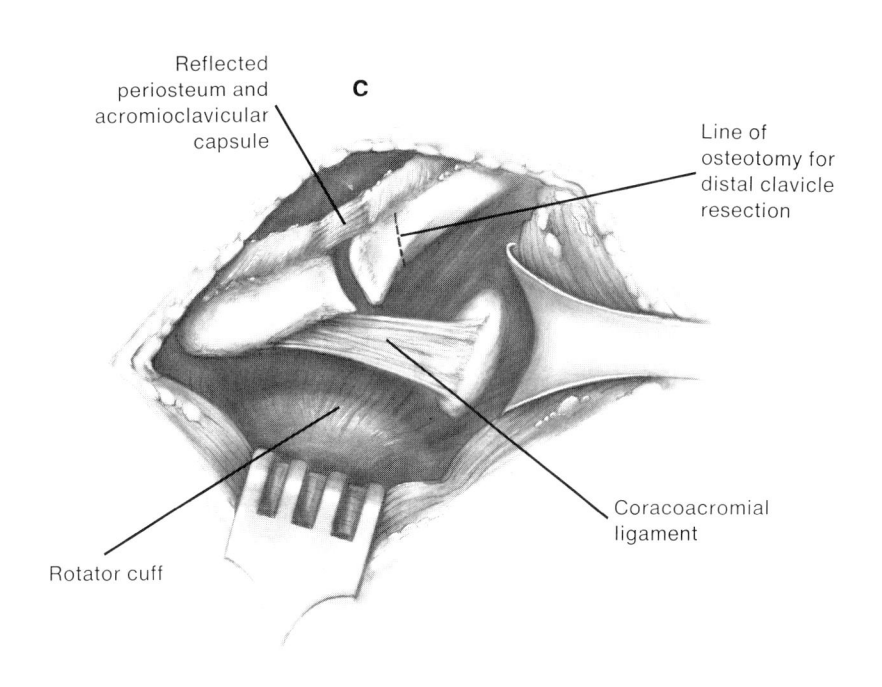

Reflected periosteum and acromioclavicular capsule

Line of osteotomy for distal clavicle resection

Coracoacromial ligament

Rotator cuff

D

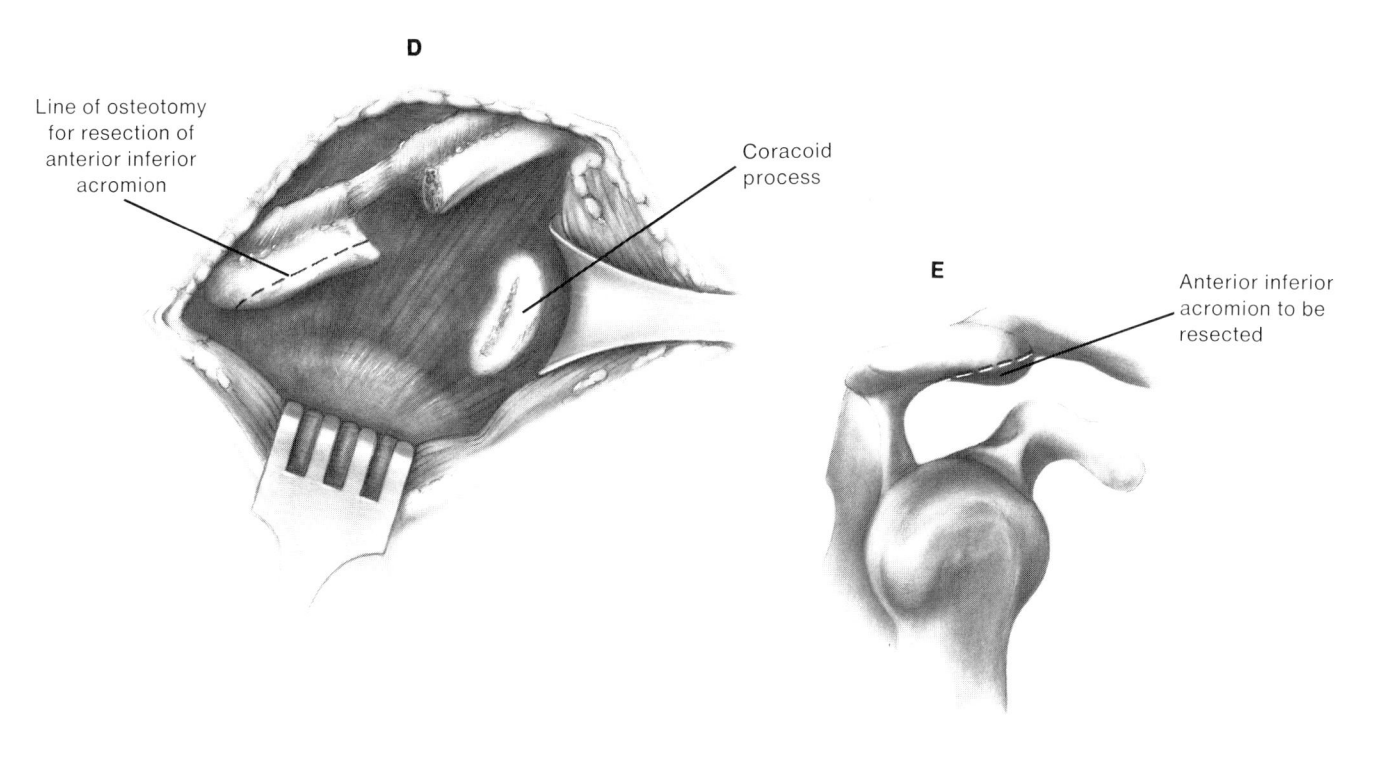

Line of osteotomy for resection of anterior inferior acromion

Coracoid process

E

Anterior inferior acromion to be resected

21

NEER ANTERIOR ACROMIOPLASTY (Plate 1-7)

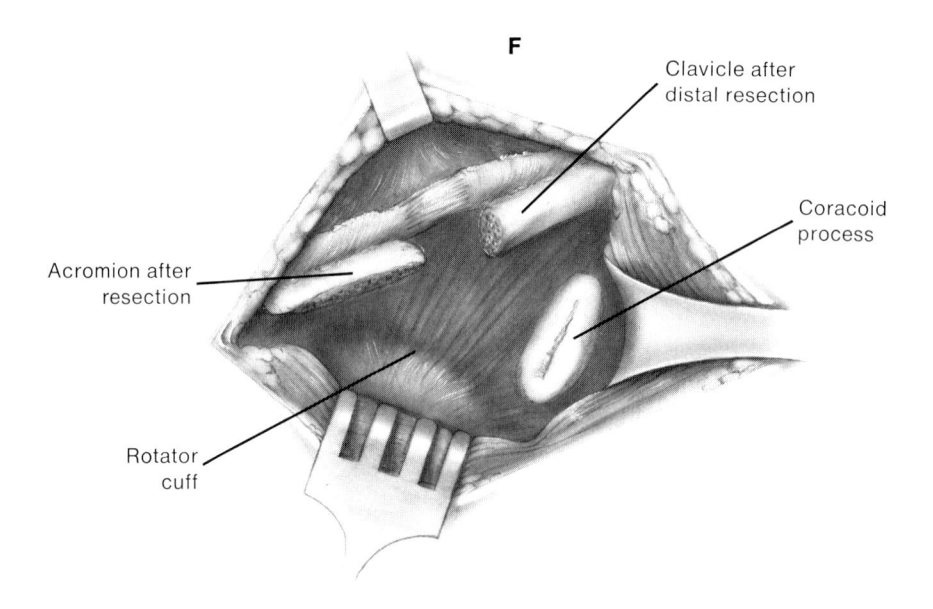

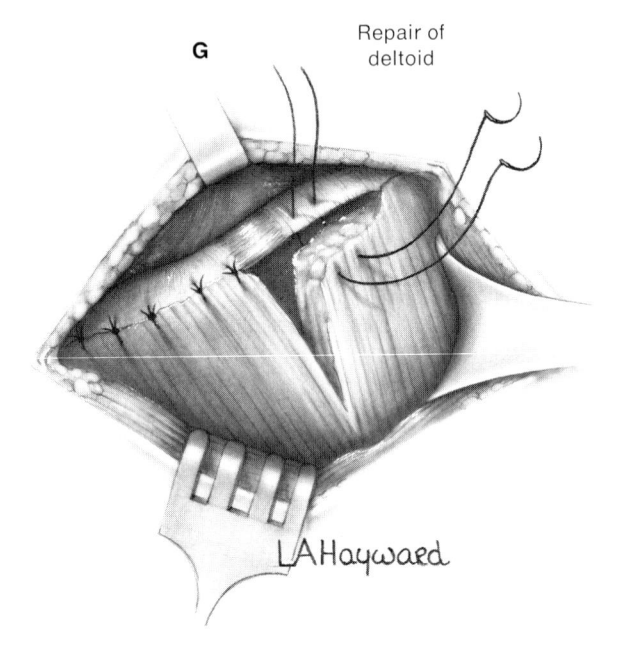

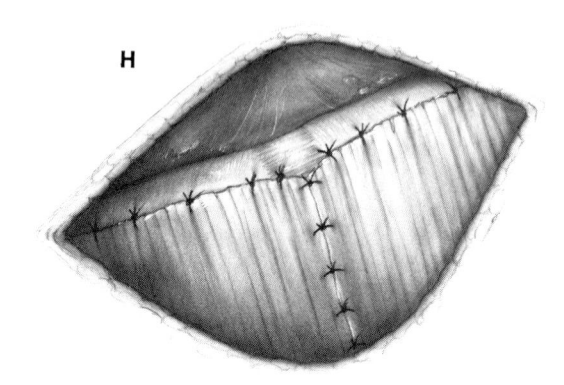

F — Clavicle after distal resection; Coracoid process; Acromion after resection; Rotator cuff

G — Repair of deltoid

LAHayward

H

The coracoacromial ligament is widely resected. The anteroinferior portion of the acromion is then resected with a broad, flat osteotome, the extent and orientation of the resection being indicated by the dashed line (**D** and **E**). The fresh bone surfaces are thoroughly smoothed with a rasp, and forward elevation and abduction of the arm should now demonstrate that the coracoacromial impingement has been eliminated (**F**). The rotator cuff is then carefully examined, and if any tear is present, it is repaired in the usual fashion. The deltoid muscle is securely reattached to the distal clavicle and acromion, with use of the previously preserved periosteal and capsular flap (**G** and **H**). The wound is closed in a routine fashion over suction drainage, and standard sterile dressing and sling and swath are applied.

POSTOPERATIVE MANAGEMENT. Intermittent passive shoulder exercises as described by Neer are initiated 48 hours postoperatively and consist of external rotation of the shoulder with the arm kept at the side and forward elevation. Gentle active exercises are begun 3 weeks after surgery, and vigorous exercises, including progressive resistant exercises are initiated 6 weeks postoperatively.

(Plate 1-8) REPAIR OF ROTATOR CUFF TEAR

GENERAL DISCUSSION. The rotator cuff as a tendon structure is unique in its anatomic location between two bones. The rotator cuff is susceptible to irritation between the acromion and the humerus with active motion of the shoulder, and for this reason the rotator cuff is predisposed to the development of degenerative attritional changes. Small or large tears of the rotator cuff may occur in men or women, the young and the old, and among sedentary as well as laboring-type individuals, but rupture of the rotator cuff is most likely to be encountered in a male laborer past middle age. In young individuals, the rotator cuff is strong and can be disrupted only by great force, but after middle age, a variable degree of degenerative change in the rotator cuff may exist so that it may rupture with relative ease and occasionally with minimal precipitating shoulder exertion or trauma.

In the early, painful period following direct or indirect shoulder injury, diagnosis is often difficult. Even when rupture of the rotator cuff is suspected, early operative repair is not advisable for several reasons (unless, for example, there should be a significant displacement of a tuberosity fracture with an associated rotator cuff tear). Many patients with some degree of rotator cuff tear recover spontaneously if supported with conservative measures, regaining comfortable and full shoulder function—if given the chance. Furthermore, the ultimate end results of early and delayed repair for ruptures of the rotator cuff do not differ to any significant degree.

When rupture of the rotator cuff has occurred, most patients give a history of an injury, although this injury may have been relatively trivial. All patients will have shoulder discomfort and difficulty actively elevating the arm (unless the rotator cuff rupture is very small, that is, 1 cm or less). McLaughlin and others (Inman, Neviaser, and Rowe) have emphasized two findings that are so consistently present that they should be considered necessary for a specific diagnosis of rotator cuff rupture: absence of shoulder contracture and selective muscle atrophy involving the supraspinatus and infraspinatus muscles (atrophy of these posterior scapular muscles will be evident on clinical examination within 2 weeks after any significant rupture of the rotator cuff). Atrophy of the posterior scapular muscles is as necessary for the diagnosis of shoulder rotator cuff rupture as is quadriceps atrophy for the diagnosis of internal derangement of the knee. Many shoulders with a torn rotator cuff may seem stiff, and yet when such a patient is asked to stoop and touch the toes, it will generally be noted that the position of full quadruped extension can be assumed and that no fixed shoulder contracture is present. Furthermore, the coexistence of rotator cuff rupture and presence of a calcific deposit must be rare (MaLaughlin reports that among several hundred shoulders in which ruptures of the rotator cuff were repaired and among a similar number of shoulders from which calcific deposits were removed, these two lesions coexisted only twice).

When there is displacement of one of the humeral tuberosities, the anatomic investment of the tendon fibers of the shoulder rotator cuff muscles is such that some degree of associated tear into the rotator cuff tendon fibers must necessarily also be present (for with an intact rotator cuff, a fracture of either the greater or lesser tuberosity of the humerus cannot be displaced). If there is displacement of a fractured humeral tuberosity in excess of 1 cm, early repair is warranted (late operative repair of a displaced tuberosity fracture is difficult, and the results are likely to be disappointing). If doubt remains regarding the diagnosis of a rotator cuff rupture, arthrography of the shoulder may be useful. If there is an existing tear of the rotator cuff that involves the full thickness of the rotator cuff, radiopaque fluid injected into the shoulder joint may secondarily enter the subacromial bursa as pathognomonic evidence of an existing rotator cuff rupture.

Although many patients with some degree of rotator cuff rupture regain comfortable and satisfactory active shoulder motion when treated nonoperatively (by immobilization of the arm in the early period after injury until pain is under control, followed by gravity-free circumduction exercises and a progressive shoulder exercise program), improvement may be very slow among other patients. These patients may have some persistent symptoms and disability that fail to improve beyond a certain point. When no further improvement is resulting from conservative management and when the situation is sufficiently distressing to the patient to undergo operative repair of the rotator cuff rupture, this procedure may be indicated, but the surgeon must realize that poor degenerative tendinous tissue may be encountered that may be technically difficult to effectively suture and reconstitute. In essence, operative repair for rupture of the shoulder rotator cuff should be undertaken only when the patient has been advised of the cautiously guarded prognosis and when significantly distressing shoulder symptoms and disability persist in spite of all conservative treatment measures.

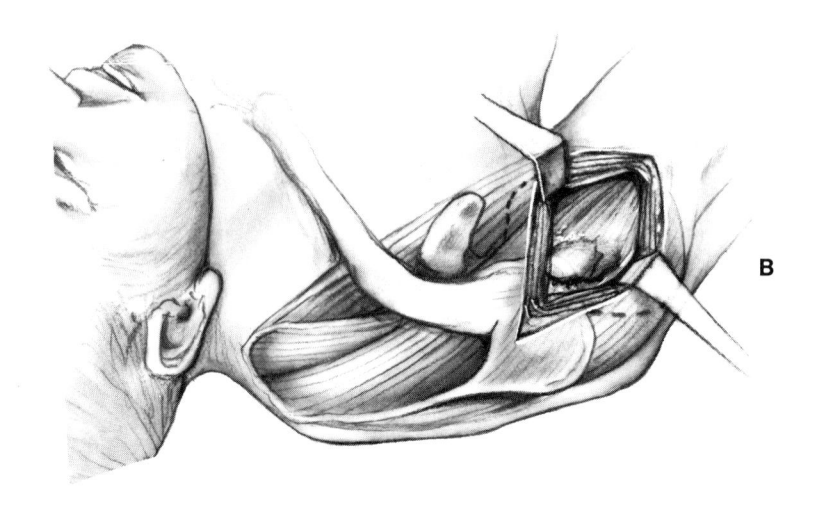

REPAIR OF ROTATOR CUFF TEAR (Plate 1-8)

DETAILS OF PROCEDURE. An incision is made as illustrated **(A)**, ending at a level approximately 5 cm inferior to the level of the acromion process. A large lateral flap of skin and subcutaneous tissue is developed to expose the underlying deltoid muscle. The placement of this incision causes little jeopardy to superficial sensory nerves—sensation medial to the wound is provided by the supraclavicular nerves, and sensory innervation on the lateral side of the wound is accounted for by the upper lateral cutaneous nerve of the arm (or superficial cutaneous branch of the axillary nerve). The muscle fibers of the deltoid may be separated for a very short distance **(B)** no more than 5 cm distal to the acromion process, since any deltoid muscle–splitting approach has the potential disadvantage of endangering the motor nerve supply provided by the axillary nerve that passes transversely along the deep surface of this muscle from posterior to anterior. If a wider exposure is needed, the deltoid muscle should be reflected from its origin along the lateral third of the clavicle and the acromion process.

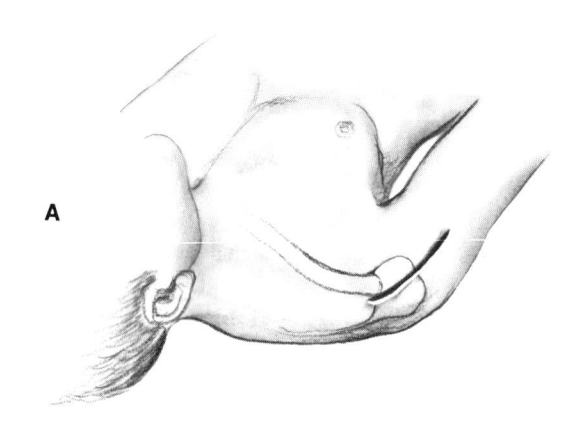

Several important aspects of the operative repair of the actual tear in the rotator cuff should be kept in mind as requisites for successful repair. The edges of the torn rotator cuff will be noted to be fibrotic and avascular and should be incised back to reasonably healthy rotator cuff tissue. The edges of the defect in the rotator cuff are retracted medially by the supraspinatus muscle attachment, forward or anteriorly by the subscapularis, and backward by the infraspinatus muscle inserting into the posterior portion of the rotator cuff. It is important that the final repair be free from tension when the arm is positioned at the patient's side. Medial retraction of the cuff tear will be difficult to overcome without tension, but the forward and backward retraction of the edges of the tear in the rotator cuff should be relatively easy. Therefore it is best to excise whatever abnormal and avascular edges of the cuff tear are necessary to develop an elliptic type of opening with the apex medially **(C)** and to subsequently permit placement of sutures to reapproximate the anterior and posterior edges of the elliptic opening. Strategic placement of skin hooks will help in mobilizing the anterior and posterior edges of the elliptic opening in the rotator cuff to permit placement of reapproximating figure-of-eight sutures to obliterate the defect in the rotator cuff. If the size of the tendon defect or the nature of the remaining tissues is such that it is not possible to obliterate the entire defect without tension, preference should be given to reapproximation and side-to-side suture of the most medial portion of the defect **(D)**. The remaining edge of any persisting defect in the rotator cuff should be inserted into a prepared groove in the humerus to restore continuity between the intrinsic rotator cuff muscles and the humerus **(E)**.

(Plate 1-8) REPAIR OF ROTATOR CUFF TEAR

The superior surface of the repaired rotator cuff should be smooth for subsequent articulation with the undersurface of the acromion process; if this cannot be technically accomplished, it may be desirable to excise the acromion process. If the biceps tendon is unusually enlarged or inflamed immediately deep to or in close proximity to the anterior edge of the defect in the rotator cuff and if it appears that the abnormal biceps tendon will be a continuing source of functional irritation, the intra-articular portion of the long head of the biceps may be excised. If this is done, the distal stump of the biceps tendon is sutured into the bicipital groove or to the adjacent periosteum wherever it is possible to anchor this tendon securely in a location that will remain clear of the overlying acromion process with full anterior or lateral elevation of the arm. An effort should be made to reconstitute the rotator cuff in such a manner that no residual opening remains at the completion of the operative repair. Joint motion will force joint fluid through any opening in the rotator cuff that is not obliterated. The persistence of such an opening between the glenohumeral joint and the subacromial bursa could be the starting point for a new rotator cuff tear.

The deltoid muscle fibers are securely resutured to the clavicle and acromion process. Following wound closure, a stockinette sling and swath is applied for immobilization of the patient's arm and shoulder.

POSTOPERATIVE MANAGEMENT. Complete healing of the repaired rotator cuff will require a period of at least 6 weeks or more, and during this time it is important to begin mobilizing the shoulder carefully as soon as the wound discomfort has sufficiently subsided, usually within 1 or 2 weeks postoperatively. It is important to obtain and maintain full mobility of the glenohumeral joint through gravity-free circumduction exercises and other activities that will not jeopardize healing of the repaired rotator cuff. The operating surgeon should instruct the patient with regard to postoperative shoulder motion and activity. The rapidity with which any passive or active postoperative shoulder motion is progressed should be predicated on the security of the operative repair, the quality of the repaired tissues, the presence or absence of any degree of tension in the final repair, and the understanding and reliability of the patient. For these reasons, there can be no hard and fast postoperative program following repair of a rotator cuff rupture. A guided and specified program of passive and active shoulder exercises and daily living activities will be necessary for several months postoperatively. Maximum recovery is seldom obtained earlier than 6 months after operation.

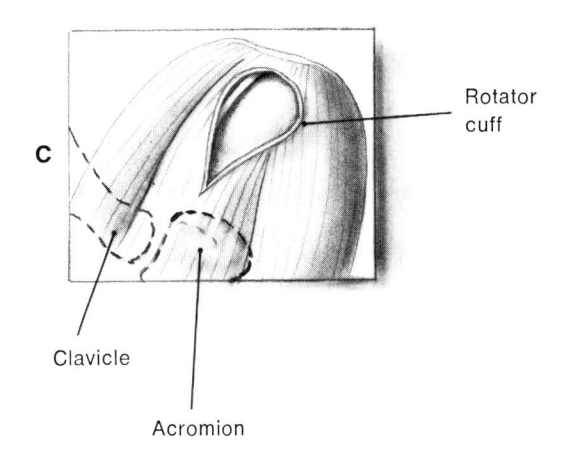

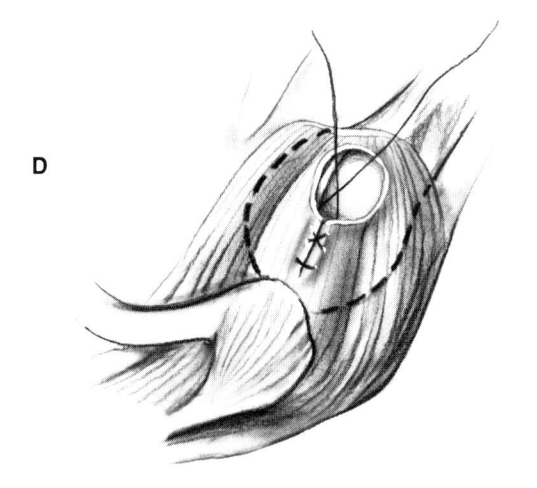

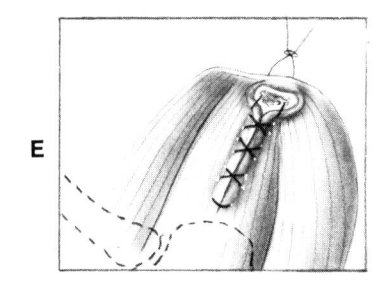

OPEN REDUCTION FOR DISPLACED PROXIMAL HUMERAL FRACTURES (Plate 1-9)

GENERAL DISCUSSION. For active healthy patients, closed management for displaced proximal humeral fractures may be inadequate. With consideration of the classification for displaced proximal humeral fractures recommended by Neer–based on the presence or absence of displacement of each of the four major segments: articular surface of the humeral head, greater tuberosity, lesser tuberosity, and humeral shaft—open reduction may be the preferable method of treatment for three-part fractures, and prosthetic replacement may be considered for four-part fractures. Without open repair of displaced proximal humeral fractures, there is likely to be an element of uncontrollable rotary displacement in three-part fractures and avascular necrosis of the detached humeral head in four-part fractures. When it is apparent that the end result will be unsatisfactory by any closed treatment methods, operative repair for displaced humeral fractures should be undertaken to provide the patient with a more satisfactory end result. With certain severe fractures of the proximal humerus, open repair can result in a satisfactory (although probably imperfect) shoulder and this is more desirable than accepting an inevitable poor result. If operative repair of any such proximal humeral fracture is undertaken, the patient should understand preoperatively that a protracted course of rehabilitation is anticipated, with many months required for maximum recovery. Furthermore, if open repair or reconstruction for displaced proximal humeral fracture is to be carried out, it should be done within several days after the injury. Reconstruction will be difficult at best, and delay in operative repair beyond 2 weeks will render the repair considerably more difficult because of fixed retraction of the tuberosities, early fibrous tissue formation, and softening of the involved bony fragments.

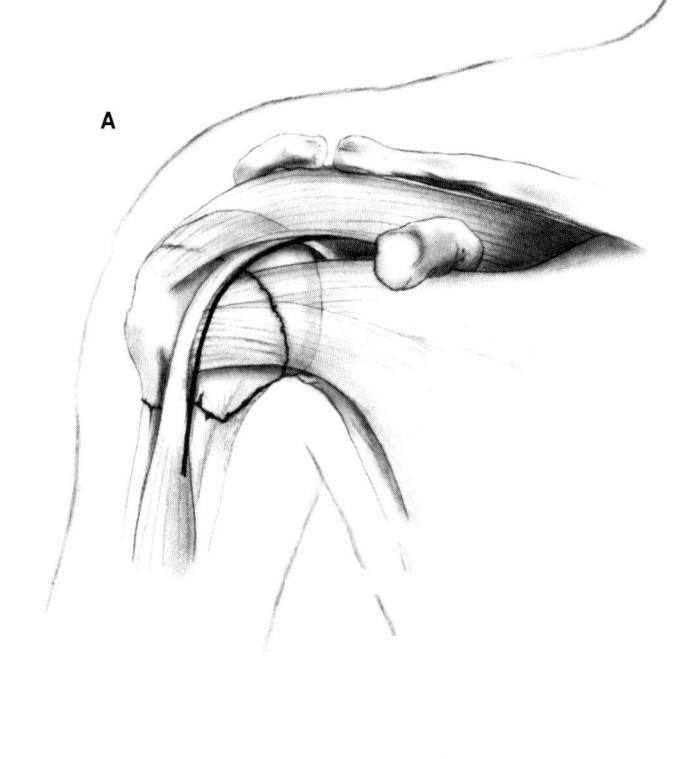

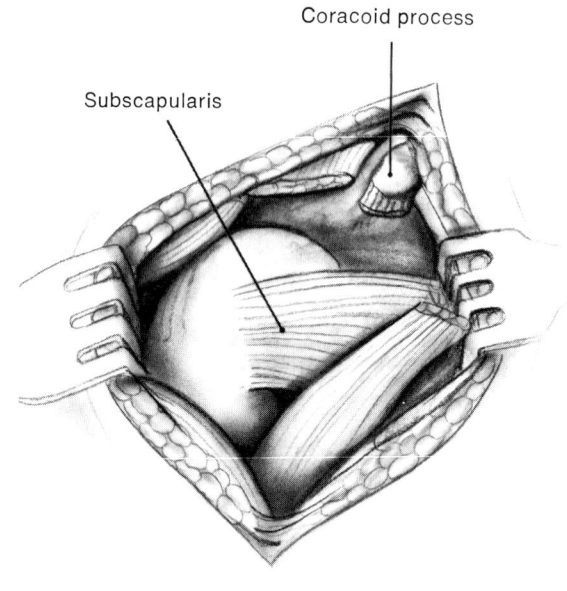

Accurate anteroposterior and lateral roentgenograms of the proximal end of the humerus are imperative preoperatively in planning the reconstructive procedure and must be available in the operating room at the time of the operative procedure.

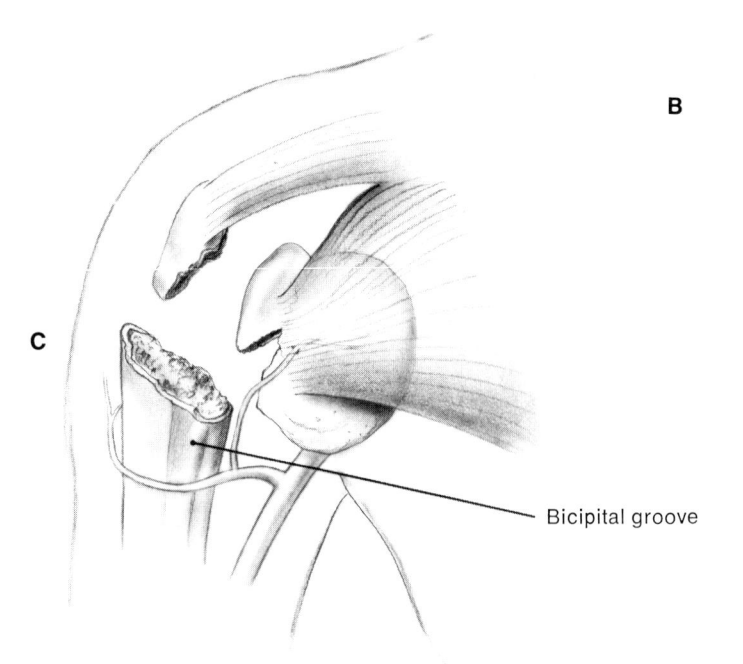

(Plate 1-9) OPEN REDUCTION FOR DISPLACED PROXIMAL HUMERAL FRACTURES

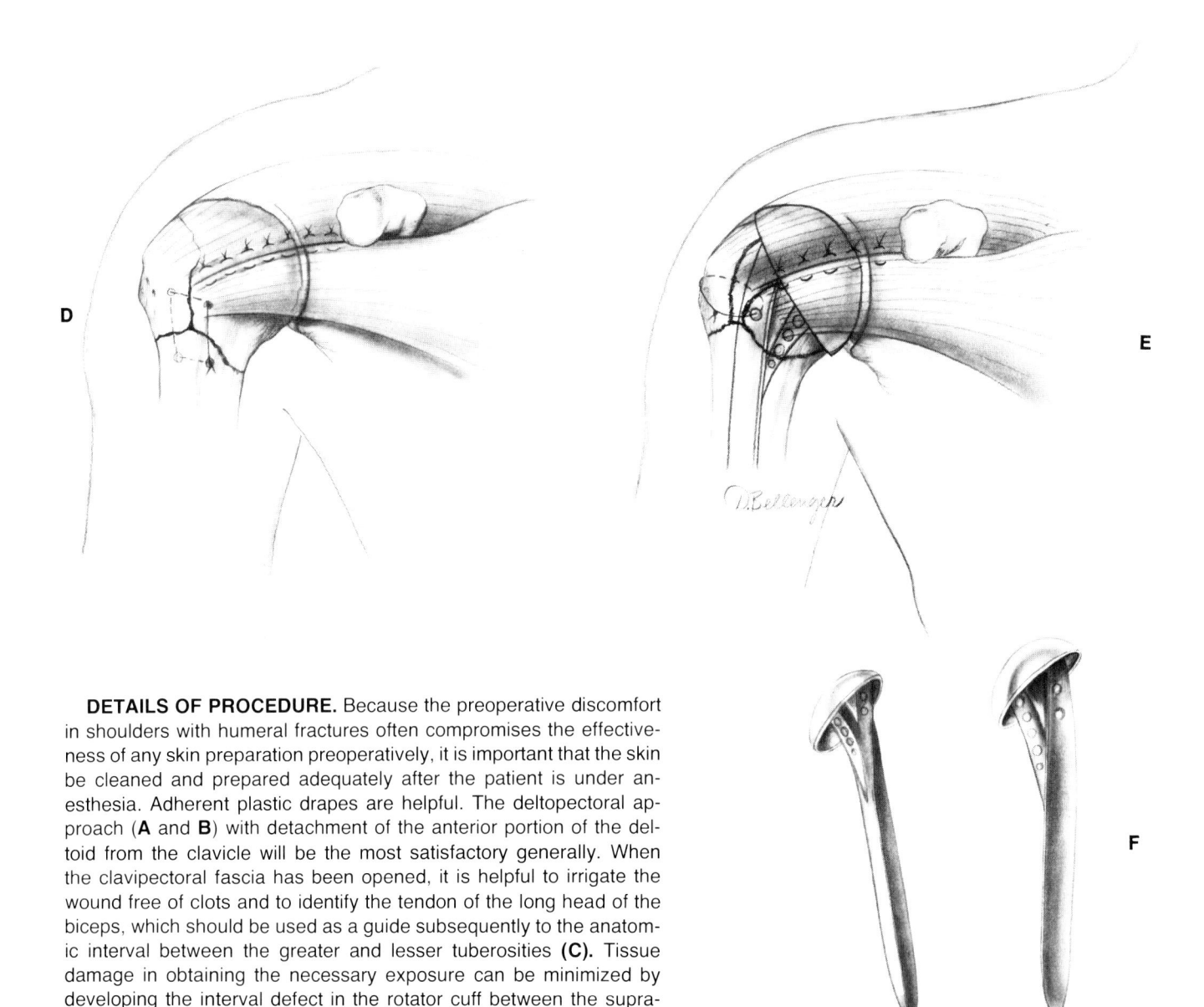

DETAILS OF PROCEDURE. Because the preoperative discomfort in shoulders with humeral fractures often compromises the effectiveness of any skin preparation preoperatively, it is important that the skin be cleaned and prepared adequately after the patient is under anesthesia. Adherent plastic drapes are helpful. The deltopectoral approach (**A** and **B**) with detachment of the anterior portion of the deltoid from the clavicle will be the most satisfactory generally. When the clavipectoral fascia has been opened, it is helpful to irrigate the wound free of clots and to identify the tendon of the long head of the biceps, which should be used as a guide subsequently to the anatomic interval between the greater and lesser tuberosities (**C**). Tissue damage in obtaining the necessary exposure can be minimized by developing the interval defect in the rotator cuff between the supraspinatus and subscapularis muscles.

For open reduction and replacement of bone fragments, fixation by heavy gauge buried wire loops (**D**) will be more satisfactory generally than attempted fixation by nails, screws, or Kirschner wires. After the bone fragments have been secured in position, the associated rent in the adjacent rotator cuff is repaired.

When a proximal humeral prosthesis (**F**) is to be inserted after discarding of the humeral head in four-part proximal fractures, Neer recommends that the articular surface be positioned so as to face in 30° of retroversion to provide stability against dislocation. A secure fit of the stem of the prosthesis within the medullary space of the proximal humeral shaft is essential, and the four available different stem sizes should be on hand to allow the proper stem size selection at the operating table. After placement of the selected proximal humeral prosthesis into the humeral shaft, the fragments of the tuberosities must be approximated beneath the prosthetic head with wire loops, followed by repair of the rotator cuff (**E**).

POSTOPERATIVE MANAGEMENT. Following open repair for displaced proximal humeral fractures, to minimize adhesions, a program of regular exercises should begin at about 4 days postoperatively and progress as rapidly as the type of repair and the condition of the patient will permit. Initially the emphasis is on range of motion and not on regaining strength. In the early postoperative period, assisted external rotation exercises and gradually progressive gravity circumduction exercises are helpful. With a supervised postoperative program of rehabilitative active and passive assistive exercises, a slow but steady improvement should be expected over a period of several months.

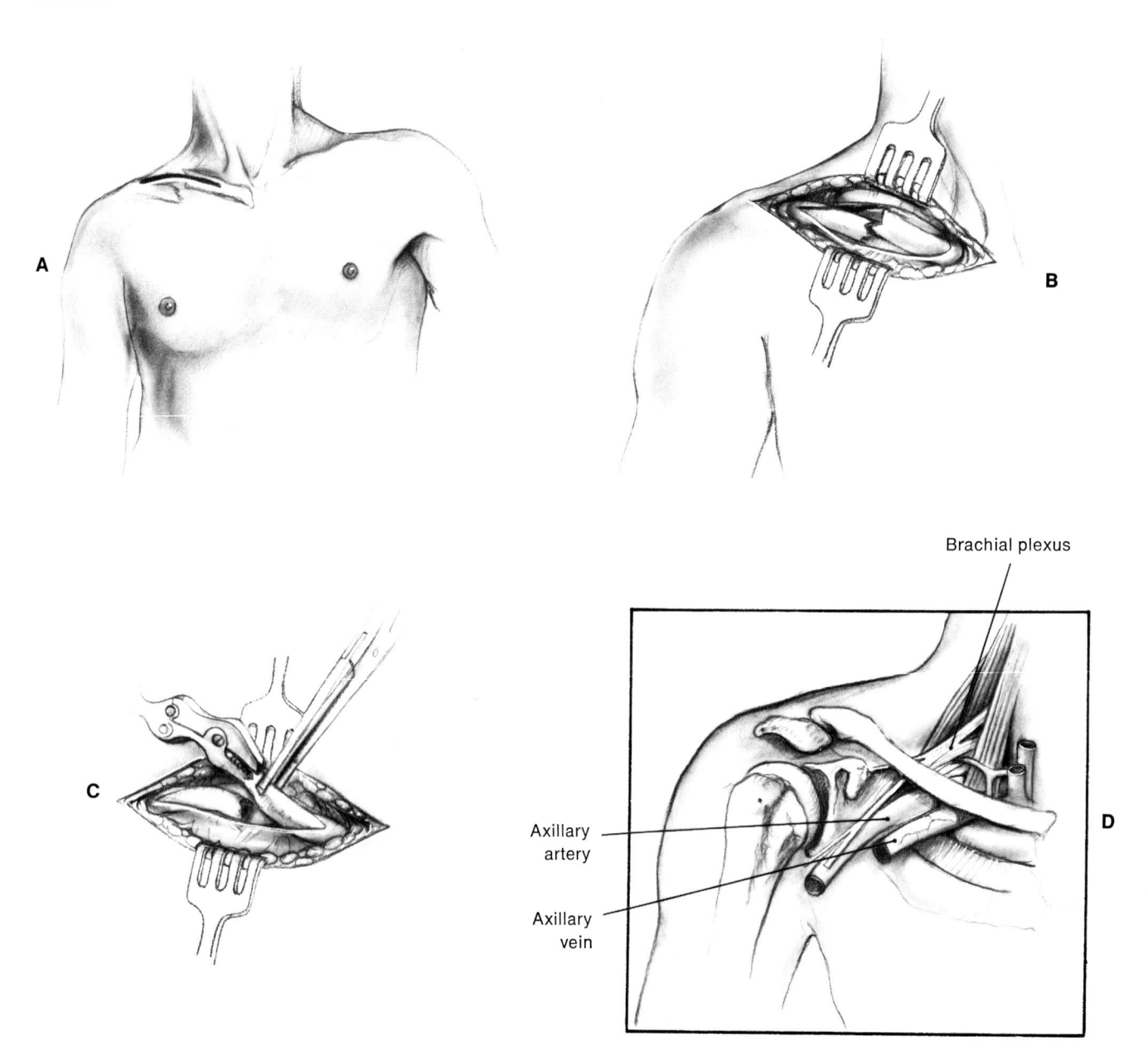

OPEN REDUCTION AND INTERNAL FIXATION OF CLAVICLE (Plate 1-10)

GENERAL DISCUSSION. Almost all fractures of the clavicle are adequately treated by nonoperative management. However, open reduction and internal fixation for a fracture of the clavicle may occasionally be indicated when there is marked displacement or angulation of the bone ends that cannot be reduced by closed means, or if it appears that the bone fragments might perforate the skin or damage the subclavian structures, or for established symptomatic nonunion. Open reduction and internal fixation of the clavicle should not be undertaken lightly, since the unyielding density and instability of the clavicle can make the procedure technically difficult, and the brachial plexus and subclavian vessels are in a vulnerable position in close proximity below the clavicle.

DETAILS OF PROCEDURE. The patient is positioned supine with a folded blanket or sandbag beneath the involved shoulder and plastic skin coverage protecting the area for the surgical exposure. The entire upper extremity must also be draped separately for free movement of the arm during the course of the procedure. An incision at least 8 cm long will probably be needed over the fracture site (**A**). The displaced fragments of the clavicle (**B** and **C**) must be exposed cautiously because of the proximity of the brachial plexus and subclavian vessels (**D**).

(Plate 1-10) OPEN REDUCTION AND INTERNAL FIXATION OF CLAVICLE

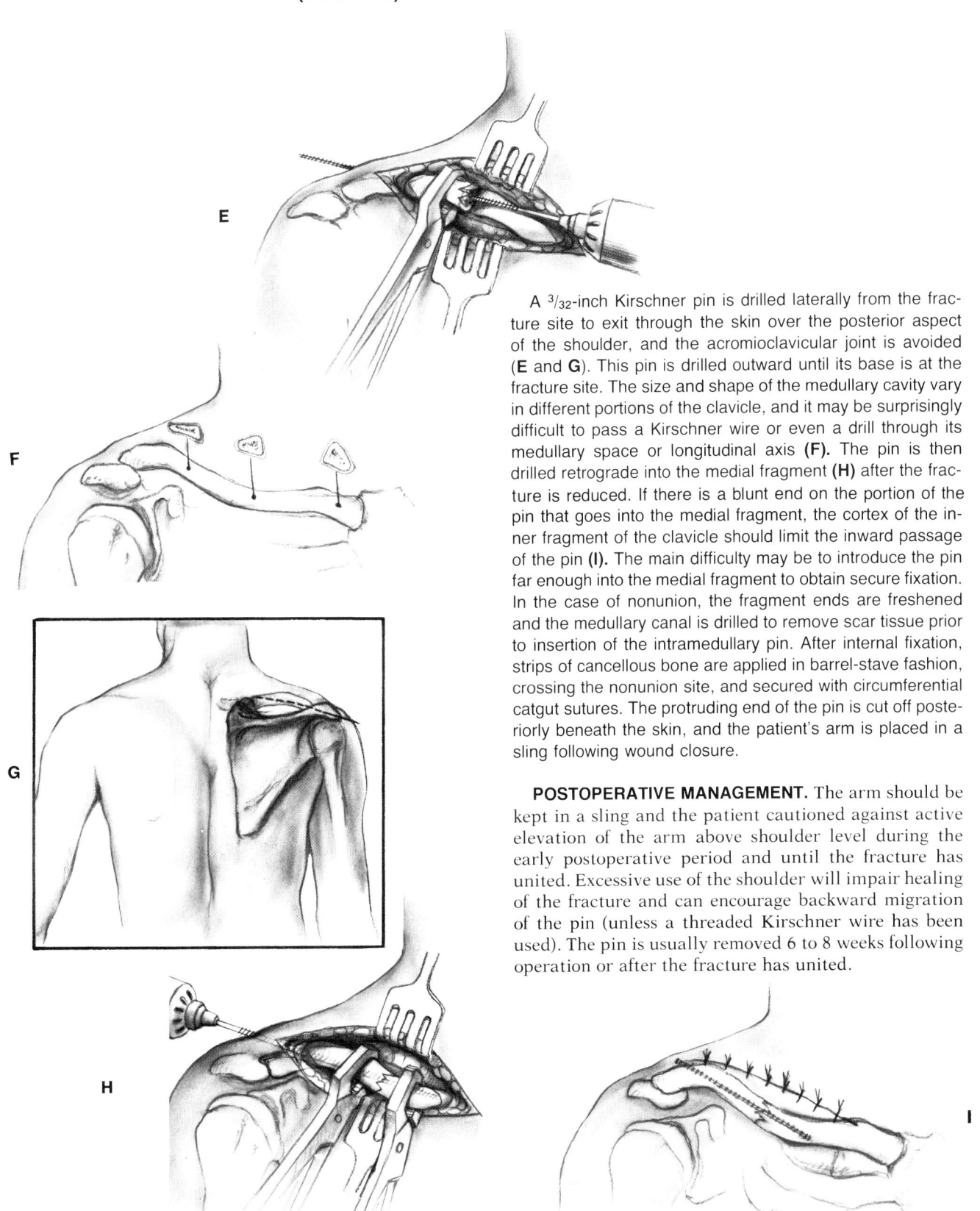

A $^3/_{32}$-inch Kirschner pin is drilled laterally from the fracture site to exit through the skin over the posterior aspect of the shoulder, and the acromioclavicular joint is avoided (**E** and **G**). This pin is drilled outward until its base is at the fracture site. The size and shape of the medullary cavity vary in different portions of the clavicle, and it may be surprisingly difficult to pass a Kirschner wire or even a drill through its medullary space or longitudinal axis (**F**). The pin is then drilled retrograde into the medial fragment (**H**) after the fracture is reduced. If there is a blunt end on the portion of the pin that goes into the medial fragment, the cortex of the inner fragment of the clavicle should limit the inward passage of the pin (**I**). The main difficulty may be to introduce the pin far enough into the medial fragment to obtain secure fixation. In the case of nonunion, the fragment ends are freshened and the medullary canal is drilled to remove scar tissue prior to insertion of the intramedullary pin. After internal fixation, strips of cancellous bone are applied in barrel-stave fashion, crossing the nonunion site, and secured with circumferential catgut sutures. The protruding end of the pin is cut off posteriorly beneath the skin, and the patient's arm is placed in a sling following wound closure.

POSTOPERATIVE MANAGEMENT. The arm should be kept in a sling and the patient cautioned against active elevation of the arm above shoulder level during the early postoperative period and until the fracture has united. Excessive use of the shoulder will impair healing of the fracture and can encourage backward migration of the pin (unless a threaded Kirschner wire has been used). The pin is usually removed 6 to 8 weeks following operation or after the fracture has united.

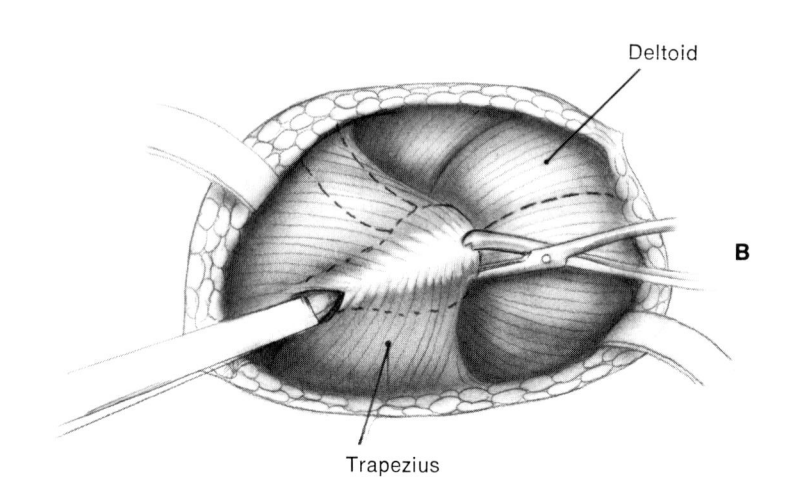

TRANSFER OF TRAPEZIUS FOR PARALYSIS OF DELTOID MUSCLE (Plate 1-11)

GENERAL DISCUSSION. Paralysis or weakness of the muscles controlling elevation of the shoulder may be the cause of significant disability. Depending on the pattern and severity of the muscle paralysis about the shoulder, function of the shoulder may be improved by tendon and muscle transfers if the elbow, forearm, and hand of the same upper extremity are functional.

Transfer of the insertion of the trapezius may be the most satisfactory procedure to improve shoulder function when there is complete paralysis of the deltoid muscle. Before any muscle transfer is carried out, there should be a careful assessment of the postoperative strength of individual shoulder muscles. If the shoulder rotator cuff muscles are also paralyzed, the effectiveness of a single muscle transfer (for example, trapezius) to restore function only of the deltoid will be significantly diminished.

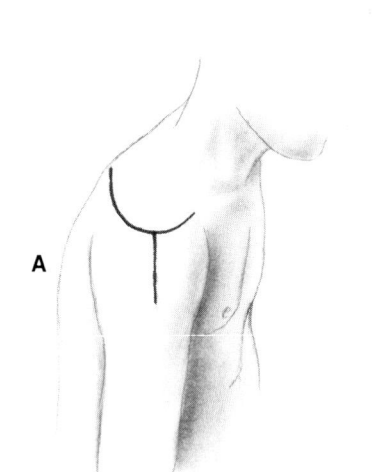

DETAILS OF PROCEDURE. The shoulder is exposed through a T-shaped incision as illustrated **(A)**, with the patient in the prone position. The transverse portion of the incision extends along the scapular spine, over the acromion process, and then over the lateral portion of the clavicle to a point even with the location of the coracoclavicular ligaments. The longitudinal portion of the incision is extended for about 7 cm distally over the upper portion of the deltoid from the acromion process. The flaps of this incision are mobilized, and the atrophic deltoid muscle fibers are separated to expose the rotator cuff and the area of the greater tuberosity of the humerus.

The soft tissues are separated from the undersurface of the acromion and protected in the area of the scapular notch while the posterior and lateral portion of the scapular spine (including the acromion) are osteotomized **(B)** in an obliquely distal and lateral plane to free a broad cuff of trapezius attached to this portion of the scapular spine and acromion. Next, the lateral 2 cm of the clavicle are resected, and the coracoclavicular ligament is left intact. The deep surface of the fragment of acromion and scapular spine is then brought down over the lateral aspect of the proximal humerus below the greater tuberosity with the arm elevated laterally to 90°. The undersurface of the fragment of acromion still attached to the trapezius and the selected area for its attachment to the humerus are separately prepared **(C)**. The fragment of acromion with the attached insertion of trapezius is then anchored as far distally as possible on the lateral aspect of the proximal humerus with two or three screws or with heavy gauge wire while the arm is held in 90° abduction (**D** and **E**). After wound closure, the arm is immobilized in a shoulder spica with the shoulder abducted to 90°.

(Plate 1-11) TRANSFER OF TRAPEZIUS FOR PARALYSIS OF DELTOID MUSCLE

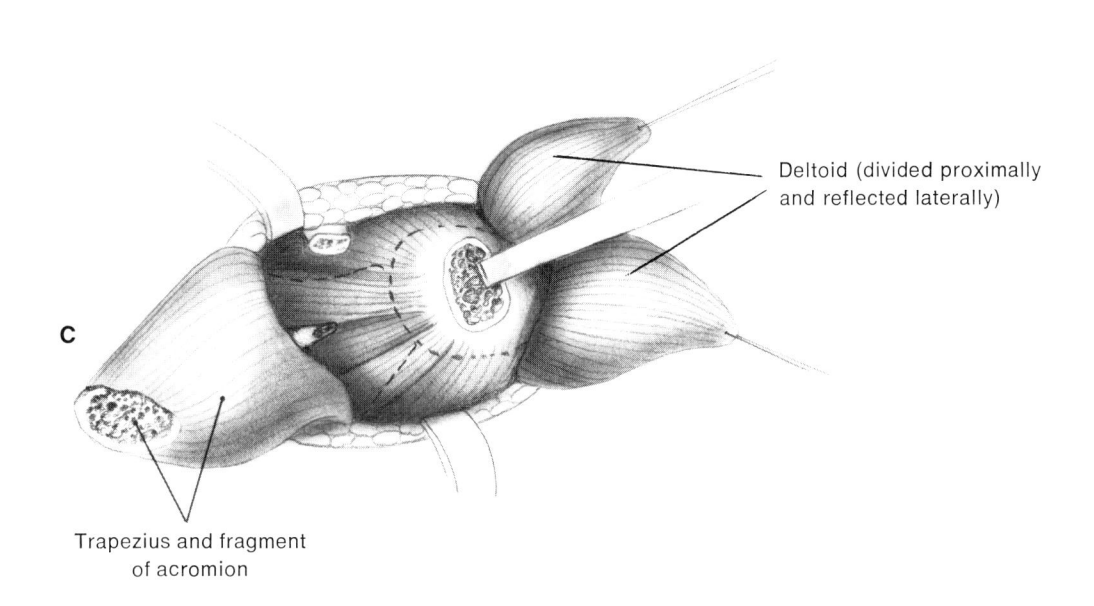

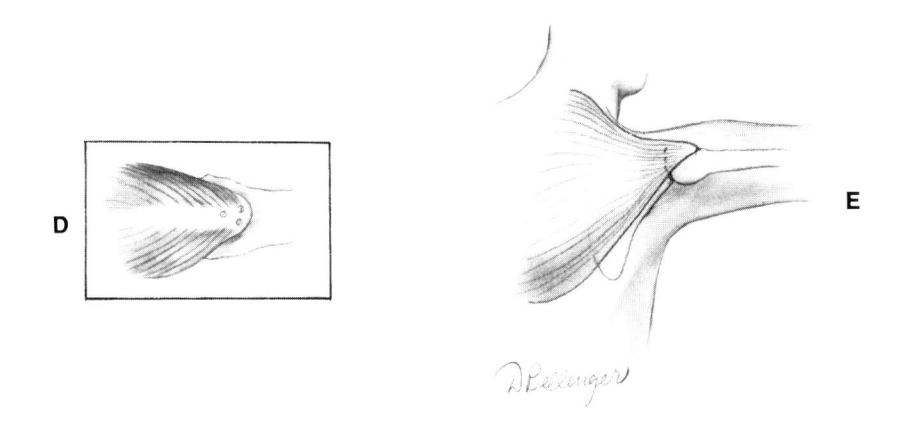

Deltoid (divided proximally and reflected laterally)

C

Trapezius and fragment of acromion

D

E

POSTOPERATIVE MANAGEMENT. Immobilization of the arm in the laterally elevated position is continued for 8 weeks, but the shoulder and arm portion of the spica may be bivalved at 4 to 6 weeks to allow some protected movement of the shoulder on a daily basis until there is evidence that the transplanted acromion has united satisfactorily with the humerus, at which time the entire shoulder spica is removed and the arm is placed on an abduction splint to be gradually lowered to the patient's side. Muscle reeducation exercises are carried out during the weeks that follow.

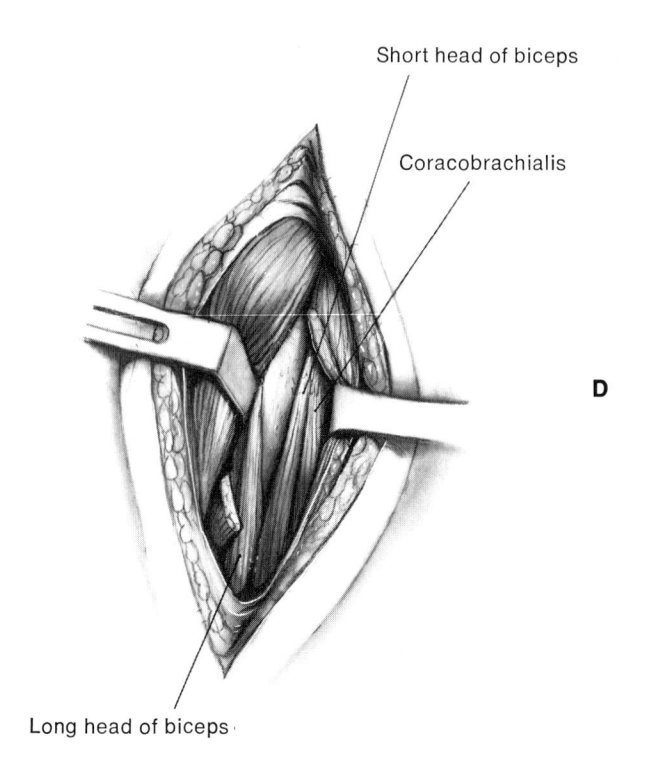

RELEASE OF INTERNAL ROTATION AND ADDUCTION CONTRACTURE (SEVER PROCEDURE) (Plate 1-12)

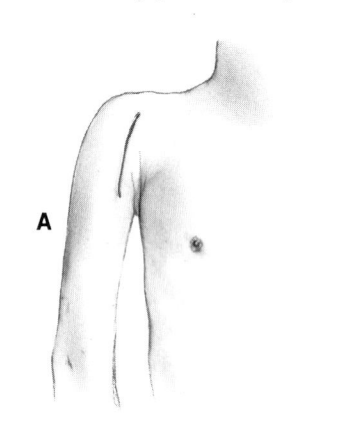

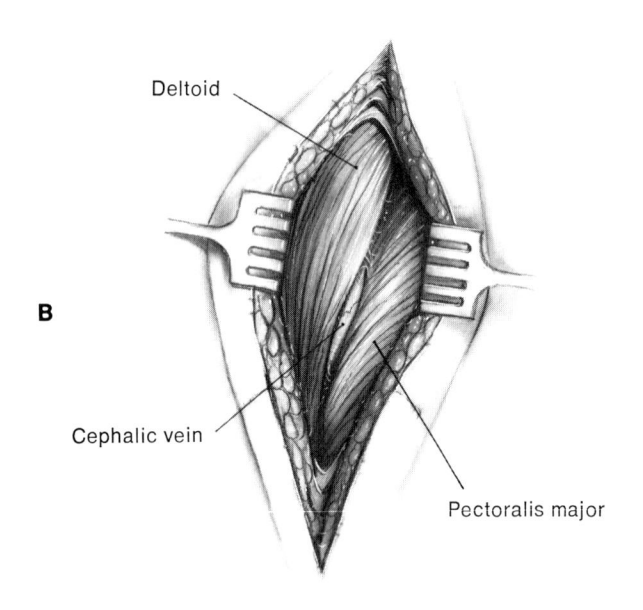

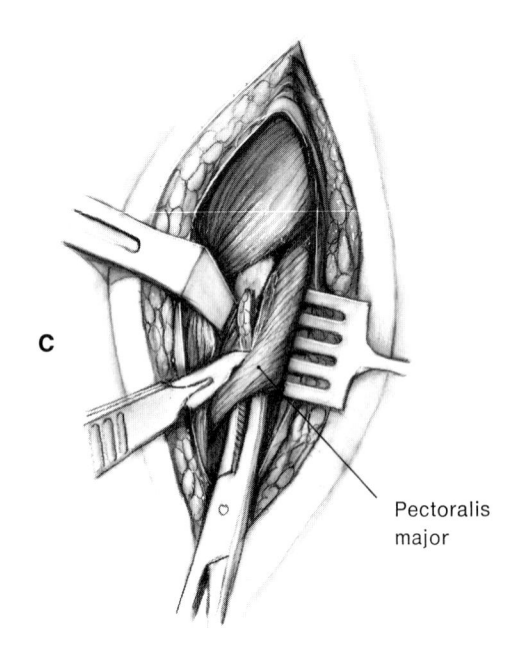

GENERAL DISCUSSION. Release of internal rotation and adduction contracture is most commonly indicated following obstetric palsy with injury to the upper portion of the brachial plexus (C5 root or upper trunk), in which case there may develop the characteristic adduction–internal rotation contracture of the shoulder. Depending on the age of the child and the severity of the contracture, there is frequently an associated deforming prolongation of the coracoid or acromion process, or both, and there may be a posterior subluxation of the shoulder and flattening of the glenoid. If the contracture is established and resists conservative measures, this procedure can be helpful in the child 4 years of age or older.

DETAILS OF PROCEDURE. A longitudinal incision is made from the coracoid process to the lower margin of the pectoralis major insertion (**A**). The deltopectoral groove is identified, and the insertion of the pectoralis major muscle is isolated and completely transected at the humerus (**B** to **D**). The tip of the coracoid process, including all three of its muscle attachments, is osteotomized and allowed to retract.

Next, the subscapularis muscle is identified above the anterior humeral circumflex veins, which are a reliable guide to the lower margin of this muscle. The subscapularis insertion is separated from the underlying shoulder capsule and then completely divided to allow external rotation of the shoulder (**E** and **F**). If the acromion is found to be a hindrance to satisfactory location of the humeral head in the glenoid, osteotomy of the acromion is carried out to allow elevation of the blocking portion of the acromion and to permit proper seating of the humeral head.

(Plate 1-12) RELEASE OF INTERNAL ROTATION AND ADDUCTION CONTRACTURE (SEVER PROCEDURE)

POSTOPERATIVE MANAGEMENT. The arm is held in the corrected position of abduction and extrenal rotation for 2 weeks postoperatively; this is followed by bracing and physical therapy.

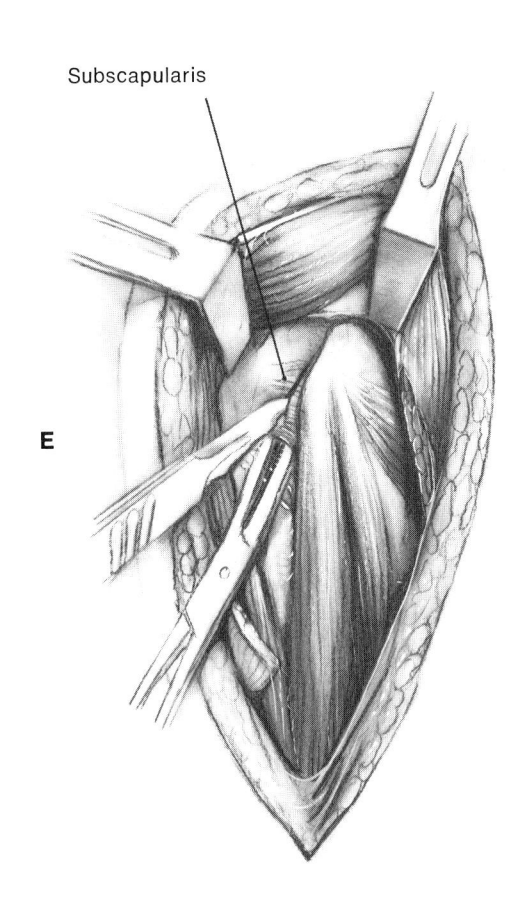

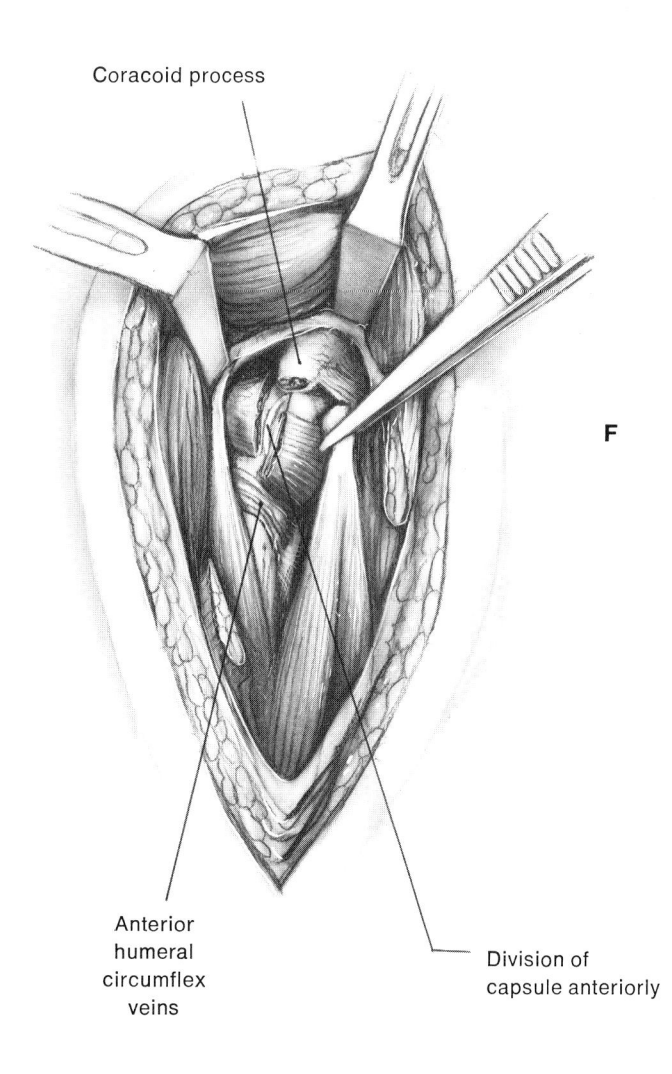

Subscapularis

E

Coracoid process

F

Anterior humeral circumflex veins

Division of capsule anteriorly

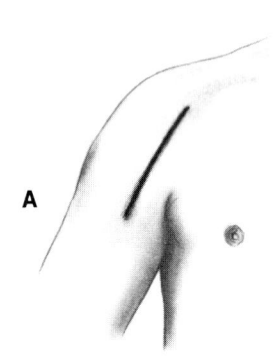

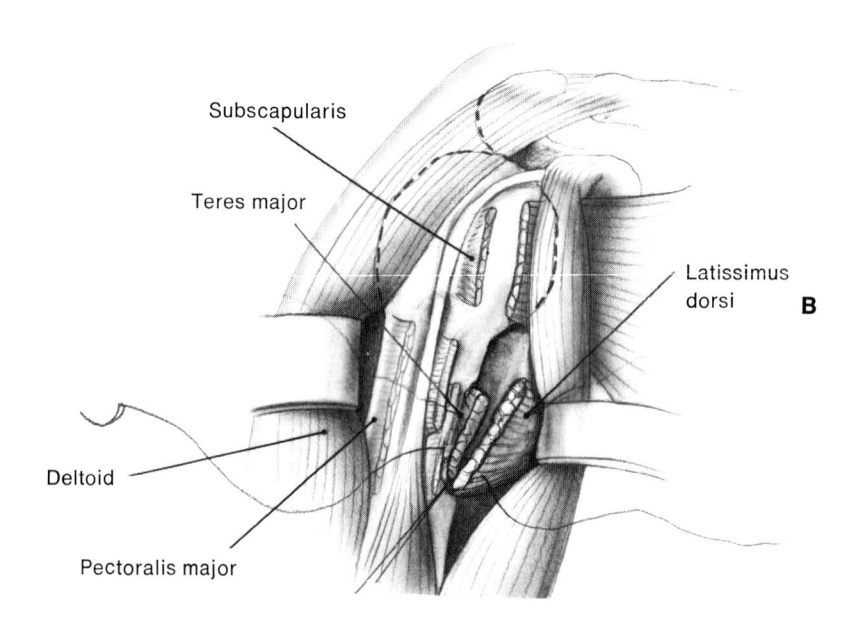

TRANSFER OF LATISSIMUS DORSI AND TERES MAJOR FOR ERB'S PALSY (L'EPISCOPO-ZACHARY) (Plate 1-13)

GENERAL DISCUSSION. Internal rotation contracture and weak abduction in the shoulder following birth injuries of the brachial plexus may produce significant difficulty to the patient in bringing the hand to the mouth or to other portions of the head. Under these circumstances, reconstructive procedures may be considered with the objective of increasing the range of external rotation and abduction of the shoulder. When the glenohumeral joint is free of bony deformities, improvement may be obtained by tenotomies or capsulotomy of the shoulder to relieve the contracted internal rotator muscles and capsule. These procedures may be performed alone or may be combined with transplantation of the teres major and latissimus dorsi to increase the patient's ability and power for active external rotation of the shoulder.

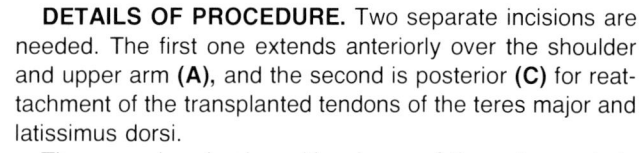

DETAILS OF PROCEDURE. Two separate incisions are needed. The first one extends anteriorly over the shoulder and upper arm **(A)**, and the second is posterior **(C)** for reattachment of the transplanted tendons of the teres major and latissimus dorsi.

The procedure begins with release of the subscapularis and opening of the capsule of the shoulder joint anteriorly. Then the exposure is continued distally along the deltopectoral groove to isolate the tendon of insertion of the pectoralis major, where it attaches to the lateral ridge of the bicipital groove. The insertion of pectoralis major is divided near its attachment to the humerus and is reflected medially to expose the underlying tendons of insertion of the latissimus dorsi and teres major, which are adjacent to each other as they insert near the floor of the bicipital groove and along the medial ridge of the bicipital groove, respectively. The lateral portions of the latissimus dorsi and teres major tendons, which will be transferred jointly to the posterolateral aspect of the humerus, should be sutured to each other through the anterior incision after these tendons have been divided at their insertion into the humerus **(B)** and prior to the transfer of the two tendons to the posterior aspect of the arm.

(Plate 1-13) TRANSFER OF LATISSIMUS DORSI AND TERES MAJOR FOR ERB'S PALSY (L'EPISCOPO-ZACHARY)

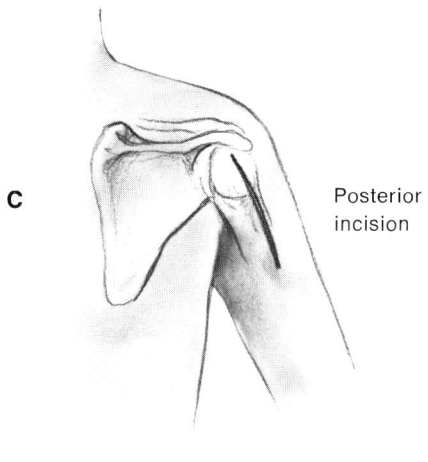

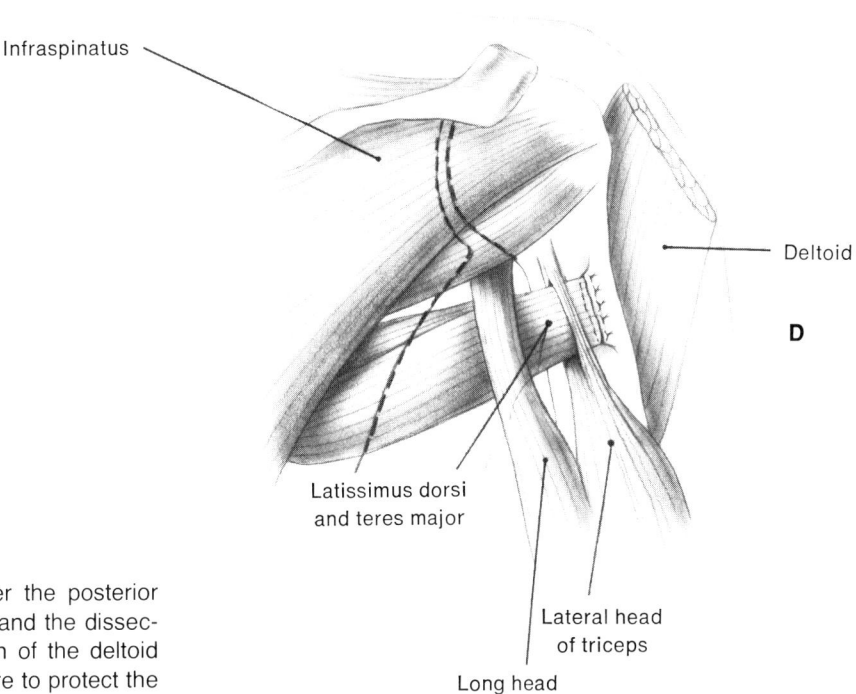

A longitudinal incision is then made over the posterior aspect of the proximal third of the arm **(C)**, and the dissection is continued along the posterior margin of the deltoid muscle, which is retracted anteriorly with care to protect the axillary nerve. The underlying proximal portion of the triceps muscle is identified, and the interval is located between the long and lateral heads of the triceps. The radial nerve is identified and carefully retracted. The two tendons of the previously detached latissimus dorsi and teres major are now passed jointly through a slit in the proximal portion of the lateral head of the triceps **(D)**. The tendons are anchored securely to the posterolateral aspect of the humerus with interrupted sutures to the periosteum or beneath a thin osteoperiosteal flap. After wound closure, a shoulder spica is applied **(E)** to maintain a position of full external rotation and slight abduction.

POSTOPERATIVE MANAGEMENT. The shoulder spica is removed 3 to 4 weeks postoperatively. This is followed by a program of early protected passive assistive exercises initially and, then, gradually increasing range of motion and muscle reeducation exercises.

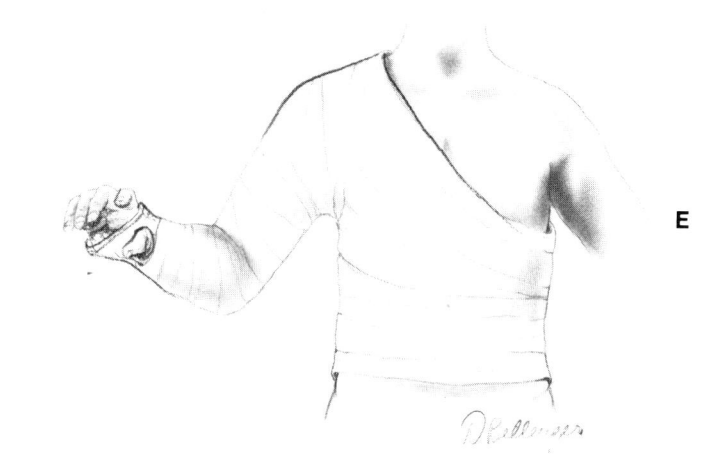

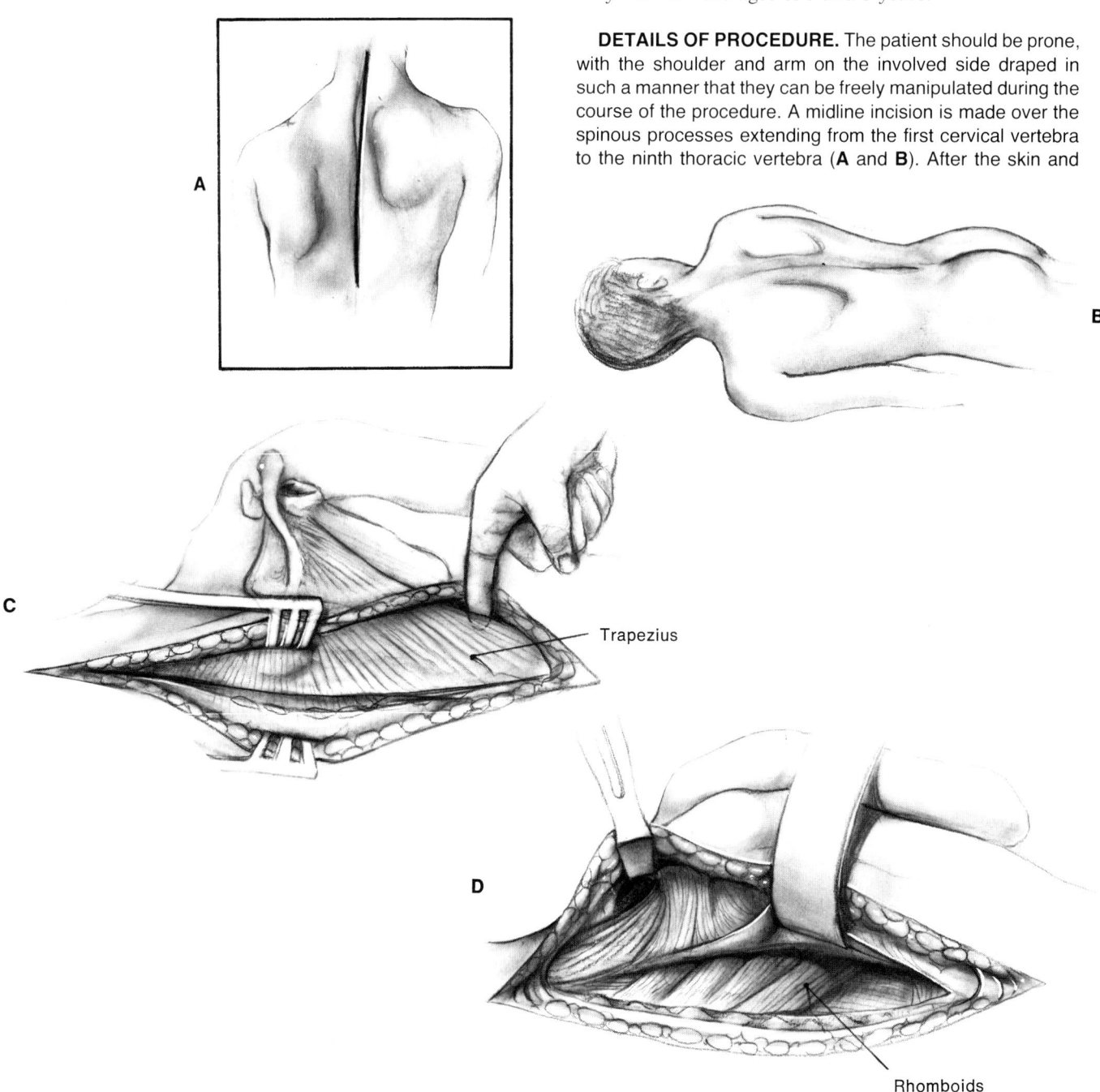

REPAIR OF CONGENITAL ELEVATION OF SCAPULA (Plate 1-14)

GENERAL DISCUSSION. For congenital elevation of the scapula, improvement in the position of the scapula can be obtained and maintained by release and transplantation of the origins of the scapular muscles. In addition to being elevated, the scapula in this deformity is usually hypoplastic and somewhat adducted. There are frequently associated anomalies of the cervical and thoracic spine and ribs. An omovertebral bone, present in approximately one third of these patients, may be found extending upward and medially from the upper margin of the scapula to attach to the spinous process, lamina, or transverse process of one of the lower cervical vertebrae by cartilaginous or fibrous tissue. The levator scapulae muscle may be fibrous and contracted. Limited scapulothoracic motion with a decrease in the range of shoulder abduction will usually be evident by comparison with the patient's normal shoulder. Rotational movement of the neck may also be limited if an omovertebral bone is attached high in the cervical spine or if associated anomalies of the cervical spine are present. Even when there is no significant functional impairment, among older children the appearance may be objectionable and may be associated with psychologic problems. The best time to perform operative correction is probably between the ages of 3 and 5 years.

DETAILS OF PROCEDURE. The patient should be prone, with the shoulder and arm on the involved side draped in such a manner that they can be freely manipulated during the course of the procedure. A midline incision is made over the spinous processes extending from the first cervical vertebra to the ninth thoracic vertebra (**A** and **B**). After the skin and

(Plate 1-14) REPAIR OF CONGENITAL ELEVATION OF SCAPULA

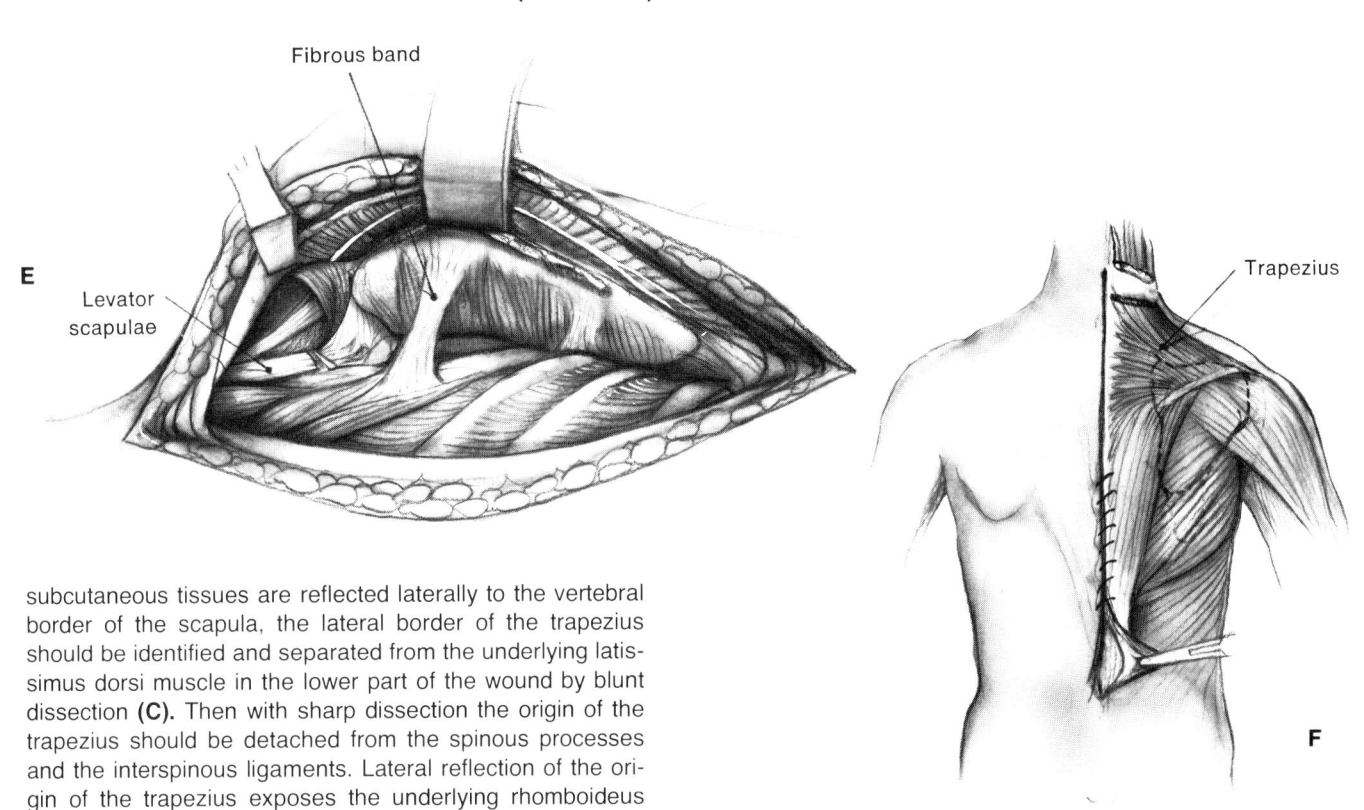

subcutaneous tissues are reflected laterally to the vertebral border of the scapula, the lateral border of the trapezius should be identified and separated from the underlying latissimus dorsi muscle in the lower part of the wound by blunt dissection **(C)**. Then with sharp dissection the origin of the trapezius should be detached from the spinous processes and the interspinous ligaments. Lateral reflection of the origin of the trapezius exposes the underlying rhomboideus major and minor muscles **(D)**, which in turn are also freed from the spinous processes at the origin of these muscles.

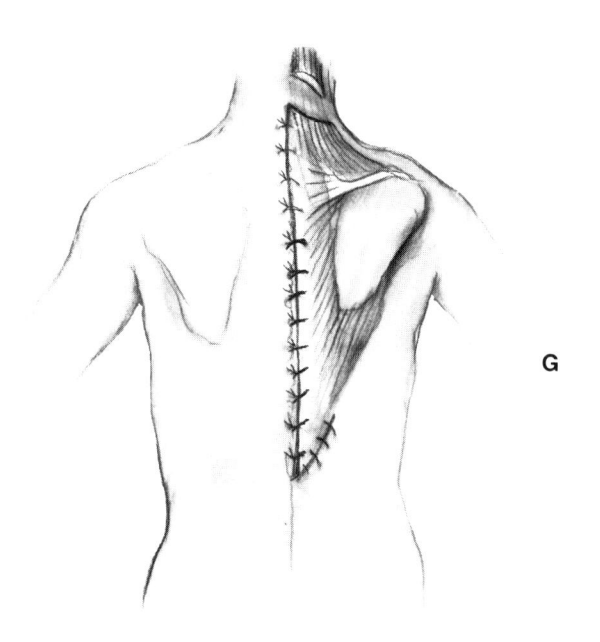

As these muscles (trapezius, rhomboideus major and minor) are reflected laterally, exposing the posterior rib cage, fibrous bands attached to the undersurface of the scapula **(E)**, and possibly an omovertebral bone attached to the superior angle of the scapula, may become apparent. Each of these fibrous bands is excised. An omovertebral bone, if present, is excised by extraperiosteal dissection. If the levator scapulae muscle is found to be contracted, this should be divided. Care must be taken to avoid injury to the spinal accessory nerve and to the nerves to the rhomboids. If the supraspinatus portion of the scapula is deformed, the deformed portion is excised along with its periosteum (this will release the levator scapulae, if it has not already been released). The narrow upper portion of the trapezius muscle is divided transversely at the level of the fourth cervical vertebra. It should now be possible to displace the scapula distally with its attached sheet of muscles until the scapular spine lies at the same level as the scapular spine of the opposite shoulder. It is important to remember that the involved scapula is hypoplastic and one should not attempt to bring the inferior angle of the scapula in line with the opposite side. This would overcorrect the deformity and endanger the brachial plexus. While the scapula is held in the corrected position, the aponeurosis of trapezius and the rhomboids is resutured to the spinous processes and the interspinous ligaments at a more distal level so as to maintain the scapula in the corrected position **(F)**. As this is done, a redundant fold in the origin of the trapezius will develop at the most inferior portion of the wound; this should be incised so the edges of this redundant fold can be overlapped and sutured in place **(G)**. Following wound closure, a stockinette sling and swath are applied.

POSTOPERATIVE MANAGEMENT. The sling and swath are continued for approximately 2 weeks, followed by a directed program of progressively increasing active shoulder exercises.

37

DISARTICULATION OF SHOULDER (Plate 1-15)

INDICATIONS. Disarticulation of the shoulder may occasionally be indicated for a diseased or severely injured limb.

DETAILS OF PROCEDURE. The patient should be in a semisupine position with a sandbag posterior to the affected shoulder and with the affected arm and shoulder draped free. The skin incision should be made as illustrated **(A)**, extending from the area of the coracoid process distally along the anterior border of the deltoid muscle to the area of the deltoid tuberosity and then superiorly along the posterior border of the deltoid to the posterior axillary fold. The two ends of this incision are joined by extending the incision through the axilla. The cephalic vein is identified and ligated in the deltopectoral groove. The deltoid muscle is retracted laterally in the anterior portion of the wound. The pectoralis major muscle is divided near its insertion **(B)**. At this time the neurovascular bundle with the axillary vessels

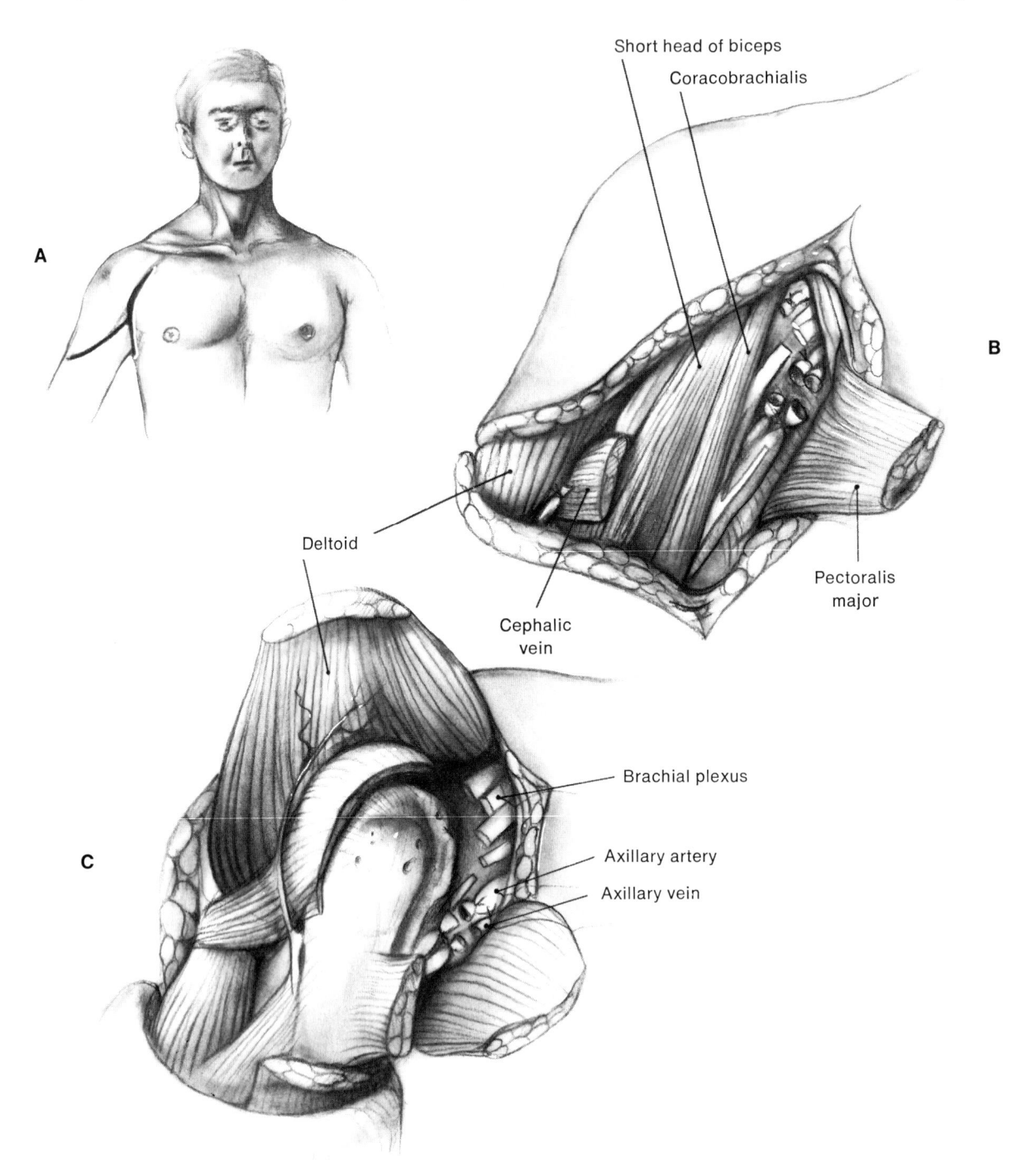

38

(Plate 1-15) DISARTICULATION OF SHOULDER

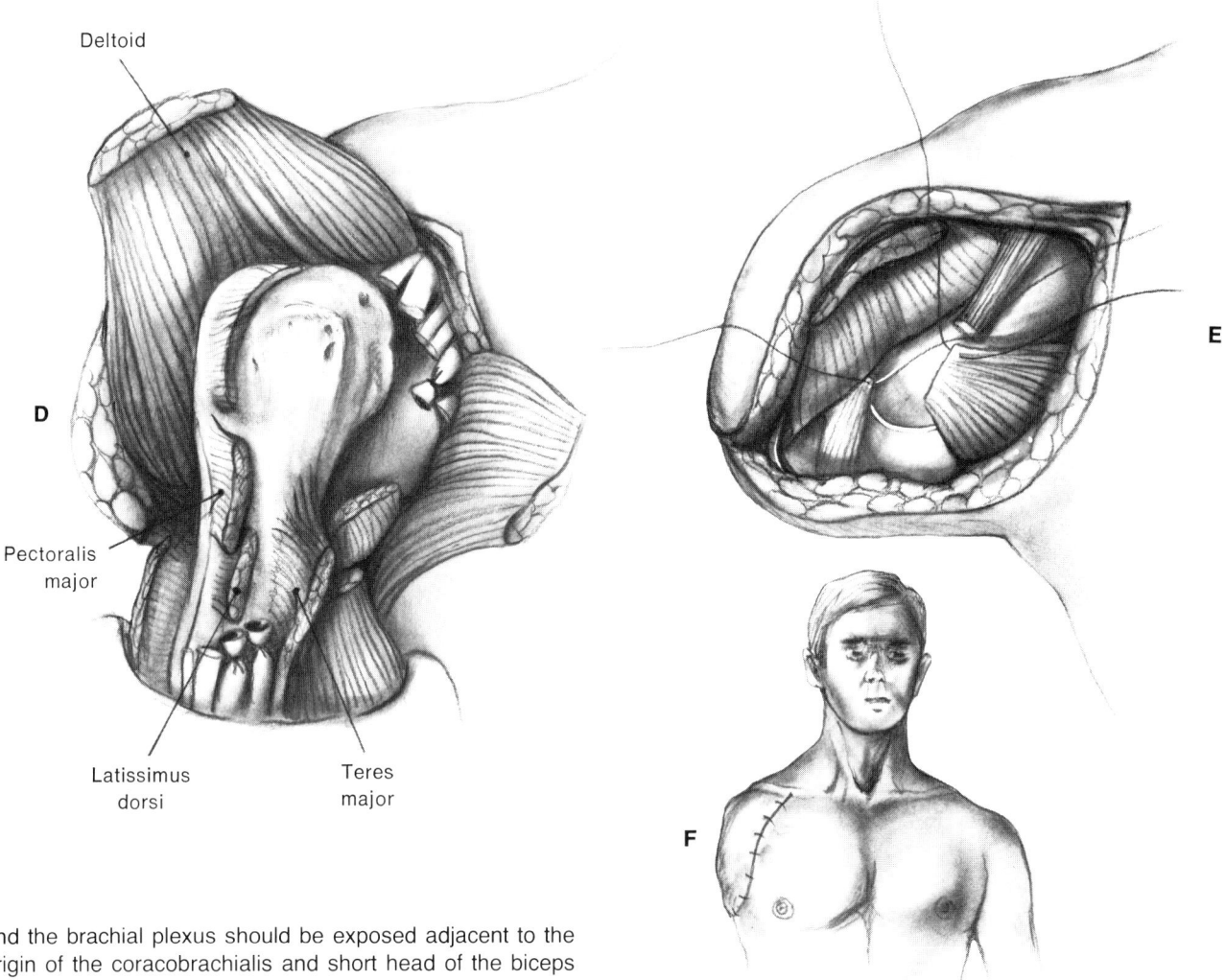

and the brachial plexus should be exposed adjacent to the origin of the coracobrachialis and short head of the biceps from the coracoid process. The axillary artery and vein should be doubly ligated and divided **(C)**, allowing the proximal portion of these vessels to retract superiorly beneath the pectoralis minor muscle.

The individual branches of the brachial plexus are gently drawn inferiorly into the wound and then divided so the proximal ends of these nerves will also retract beneath the pectoralis minor muscle. If the origins of the coracobrachialis and short head of the biceps have not already been detached near their insertions on the coracoid process, this is done at this time. The deltoid muscle is now freed at its insertion on the humerus and reflected superiorly with care to protect the axillary nerve on its inferior surface as the capsule of the shoulder joint is exposed. The teres major and latissimus dorsi muscles are divided near their insertions **(D)**.

With the arm in full internal rotation at the shoulder, the infraspinatus and teres minor muscles are divided near their insertion. The arm is then turned into full external rotation at the shoulder, and the subscapularis and supraspinatus muscles are divided near their insertions. The capsule of the shoulder joint is opened posteriorly, superiorly, and anteriorly. The origin of the triceps muscle from the infraglenoid tubercle is divided and the remaining inferior portion of the shoulder joint capsule is incised to completely sever the limb from the trunk. The cut ends of the muscles of the rotator cuff should be reflected into the glenoid cavity and sutured to each other **(E)** to help fill the cavity left after removal of the arm. The deltoid muscle flap is reflected downward over the sutured ends of the rotator cuff muscles, and the inferior portion of the deltoid is sutured below the glenoid. Any unduly prominent portion of the acromion process should be excised to give the shoulder a more smoothly rounded contour. Drains or tubes for suction drainage are left in place beneath the deltoid muscle, and the skin edges are trimmed and sutured to complete the closure **(F)**.

POSTOPERATIVE MANAGEMENT. The postoperative management, including timing of any prosthetic fitting, will vary depending on individual circumstances.

INTERSCAPULOTHORACIC RESECTION (Plate 1-16)

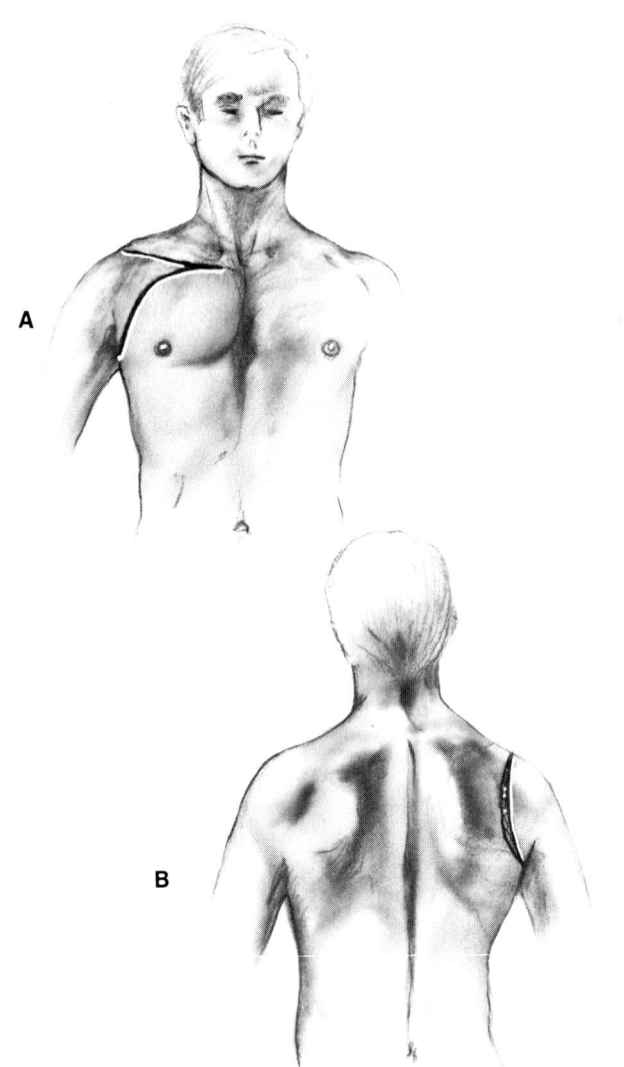

INDICATIONS. Interscapulothoracic resection occasionally may be indicated for a diseased or severely injured limb.

DETAILS OF PROCEDURE. The patient should be in a lateral position on the uninvolved side with the involved arm draped free. The incision is made as illustrated **(A)**, extending along the anterior aspect of the clavicle, across the acromioclavicular joint, along the lateral aspect of the scapular spine, and then distally toward the posterior axillary fold. A second incision is made connecting the two ends of the initial incision, passing through the axilla and extending from the posterior axillary fold to the anterior portion of the initial incision near the middle third of the clavicle **(B)**. The anterior portion of the wound is extended down to the clavicle in its medial portion, and the clavicular origin of the pectoralis major muscle is released from the clavicle. The deep fascia over the superior border of the clavicle is divided close to bone, and, by careful blunt dissection, the soft tissues posterior to the clavicle are separated from the clavicle. The external jugular vein is retracted or ligated and divided. The capsule of the sternoclavicular joint is divided, and the medial end of the clavicle is lifted superiorly and removed after careful separation of the adjacent soft tissues and division of the acromioclavicular joint. The insertions of pectoralis major onto the humerus and pectoralis minor onto the coracoid process are divided. The subclavian artery and vein are isolated, and each vessel is doubly ligated and divided **(C)**.

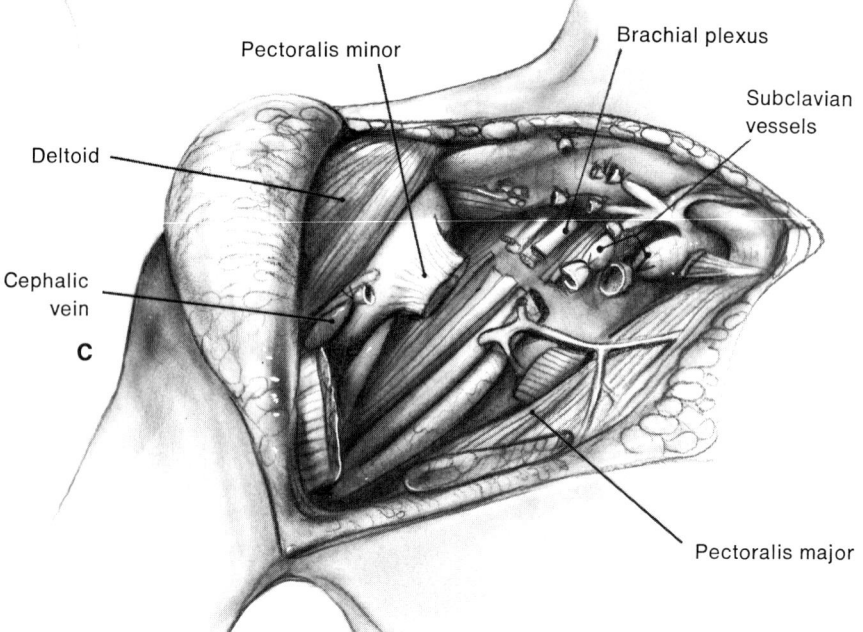

(Plate 1-16) INTERSCAPULOTHORACIC RESECTION

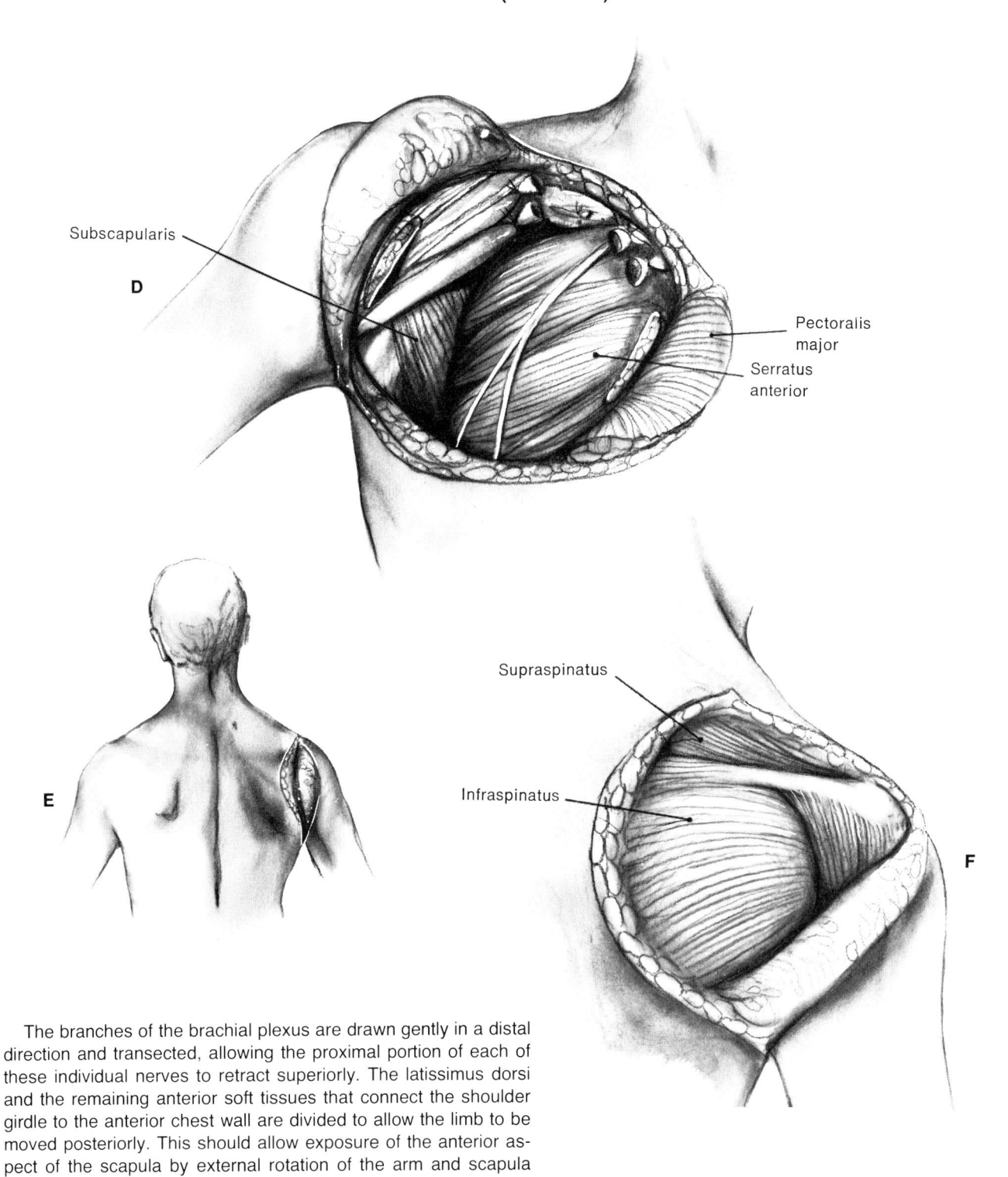

The branches of the brachial plexus are drawn gently in a distal direction and transected, allowing the proximal portion of each of these individual nerves to retract superiorly. The latissimus dorsi and the remaining anterior soft tissues that connect the shoulder girdle to the anterior chest wall are divided to allow the limb to be moved posteriorly. This should allow exposure of the anterior aspect of the scapula by external rotation of the arm and scapula (**D**) before the posterior incision. Now, while the arm is held forward, the posterior incision is deepened, and the muscles that attach the scapula to the spine and rib cage are exposed. These muscles are divided beginning with the trapezius and continuing through the omohyoid, levator scapulae, rhomboideus major and minor, and finally the serratus anterior as these muscles are divided near their insertion onto the scapula (**E** and **F**).

INTERSCAPULOTHORACIC RESECTION (Plate 1-16)

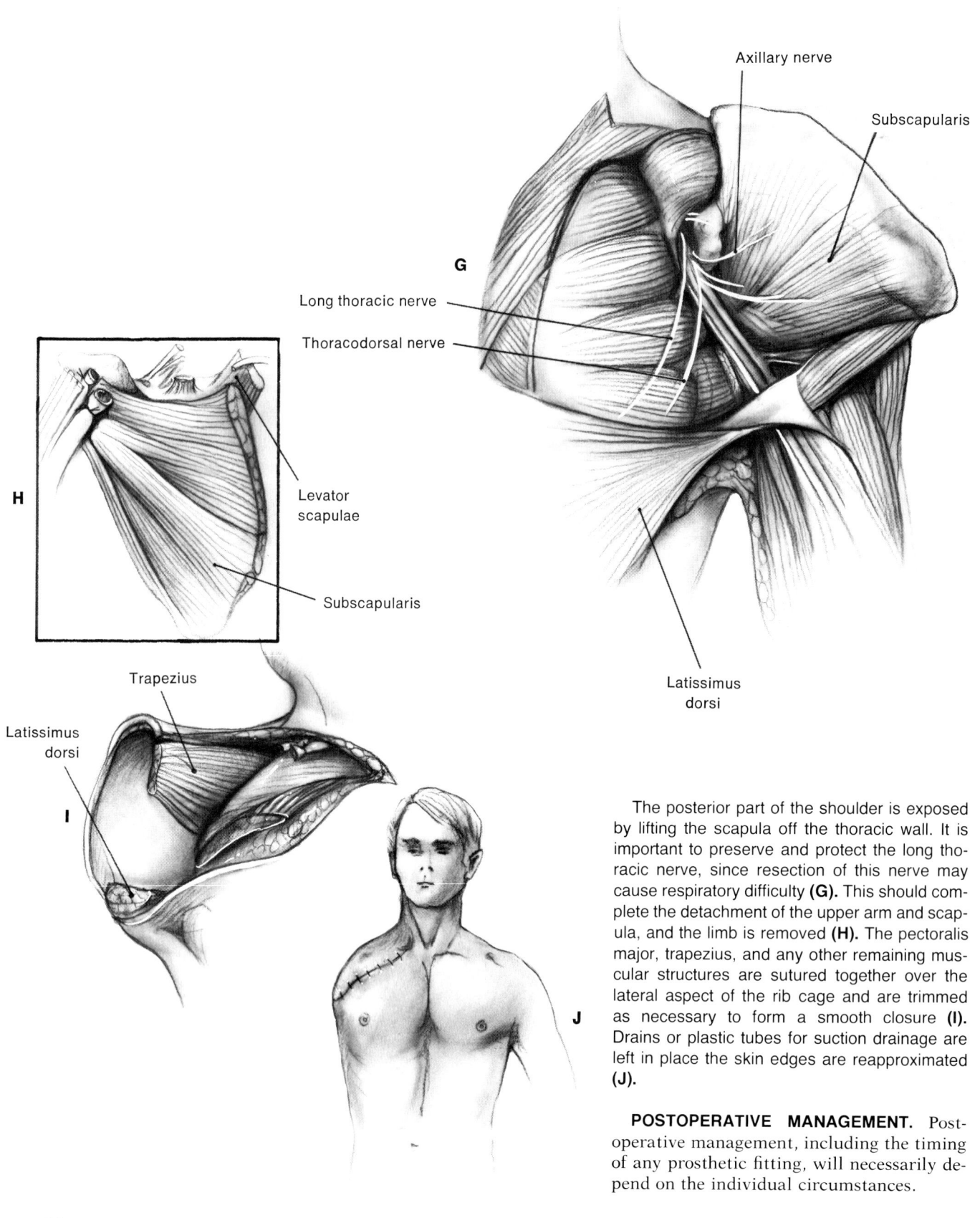

The posterior part of the shoulder is exposed by lifting the scapula off the thoracic wall. It is important to preserve and protect the long thoracic nerve, since resection of this nerve may cause respiratory difficulty **(G)**. This should complete the detachment of the upper arm and scapula, and the limb is removed **(H)**. The pectoralis major, trapezius, and any other remaining muscular structures are sutured together over the lateral aspect of the rib cage and are trimmed as necessary to form a smooth closure **(I)**. Drains or plastic tubes for suction drainage are left in place the skin edges are reapproximated **(J)**.

POSTOPERATIVE MANAGEMENT. Postoperative management, including the timing of any prosthetic fitting, will necessarily depend on the individual circumstances.

(Plate 1-17) SHOULDER ARTHRODESIS

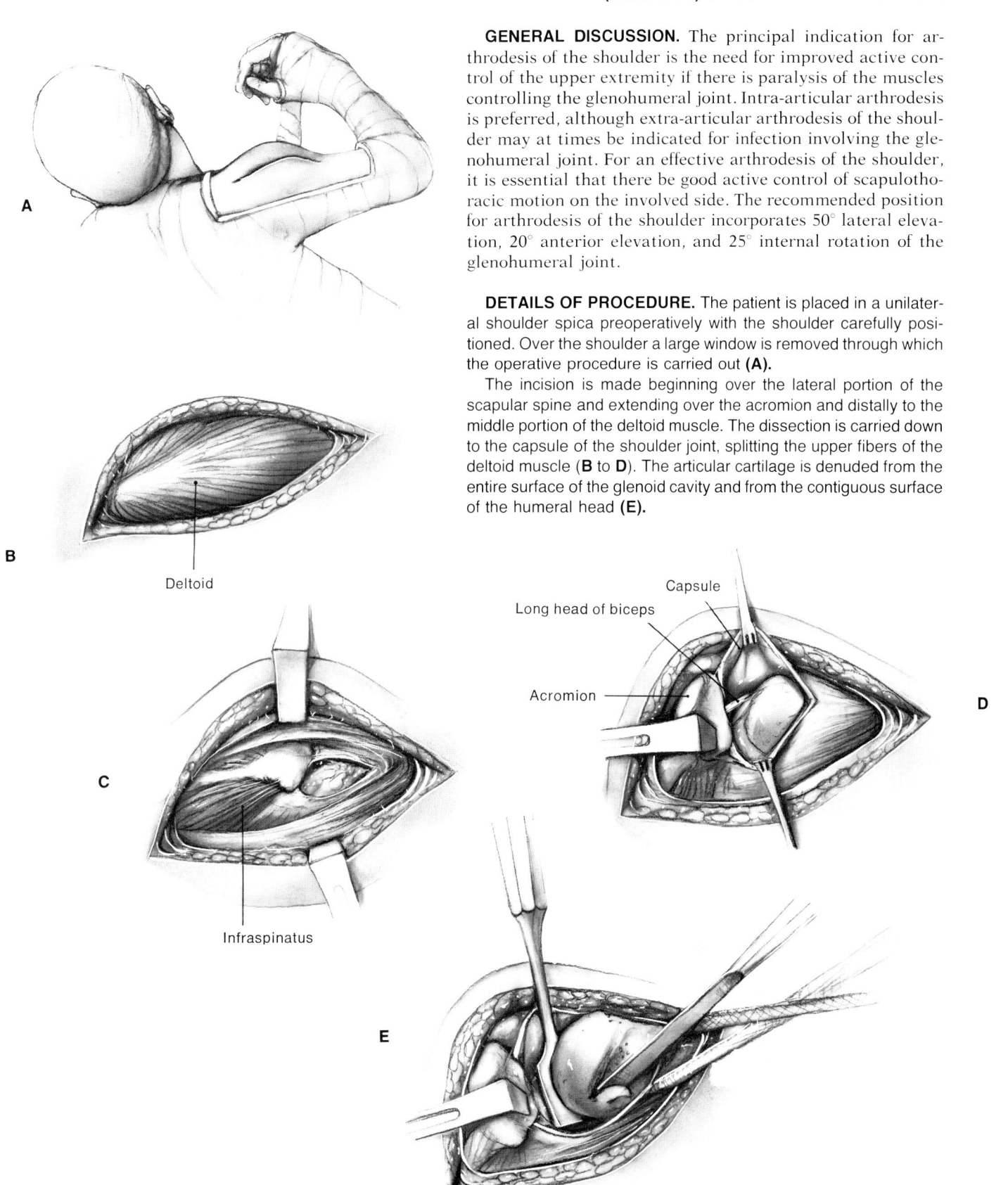

GENERAL DISCUSSION. The principal indication for arthrodesis of the shoulder is the need for improved active control of the upper extremity if there is paralysis of the muscles controlling the glenohumeral joint. Intra-articular arthrodesis is preferred, although extra-articular arthrodesis of the shoulder may at times be indicated for infection involving the glenohumeral joint. For an effective arthrodesis of the shoulder, it is essential that there be good active control of scapulothoracic motion on the involved side. The recommended position for arthrodesis of the shoulder incorporates 50° lateral elevation, 20° anterior elevation, and 25° internal rotation of the glenohumeral joint.

DETAILS OF PROCEDURE. The patient is placed in a unilateral shoulder spica preoperatively with the shoulder carefully positioned. Over the shoulder a large window is removed through which the operative procedure is carried out **(A)**.

The incision is made beginning over the lateral portion of the scapular spine and extending over the acromion and distally to the middle portion of the deltoid muscle. The dissection is carried down to the capsule of the shoulder joint, splitting the upper fibers of the deltoid muscle **(B to D)**. The articular cartilage is denuded from the entire surface of the glenoid cavity and from the contiguous surface of the humeral head **(E)**.

43

SHOULDER ARTHRODESIS (Plate 1-17)

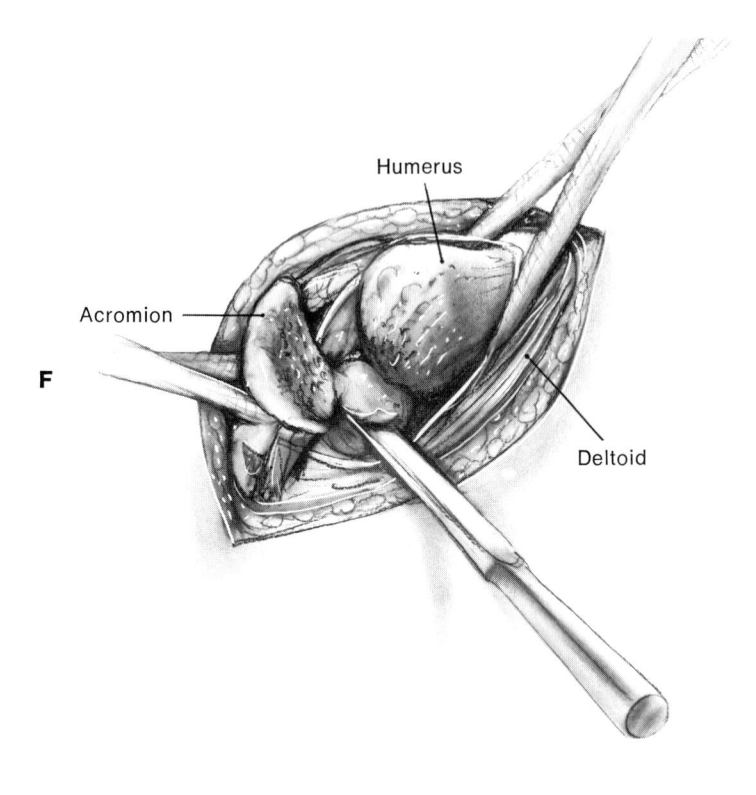

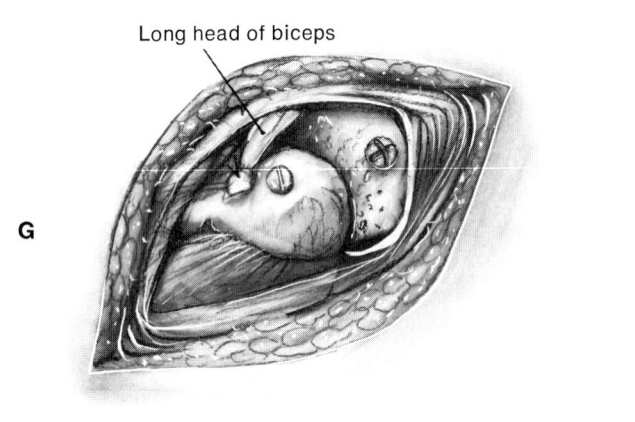

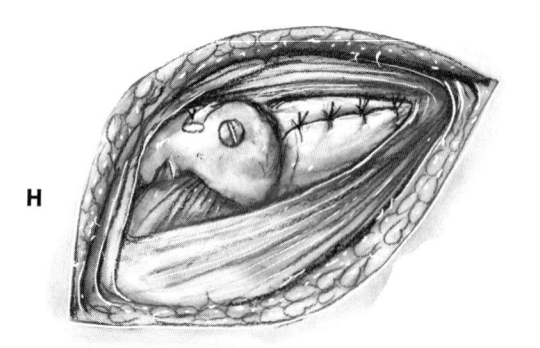

The undersurface of the acromion and the superior surface of the humeral head are similarly prepared, and a partial osteotomy of the acromion is carried out, so as to permit its lateral portion to be reflected downward into contact with a prepared area on the superior surface of the humeral head **(F)**. In the nonparalytic shoulder, resection of the distal 2 cm of the clavicle is performed to improve ultimate shoulder function. A lag screw is inserted through the greater tuberosity and humeral head and into the glenoid and body of the scapula. At a right angle to the transfixing lag screw across the glenohumeral joint, a bone screw is inserted downward through the reflected acromion into the humeral head, **(G to I)**. At this point the denuded surface of the humeral head shoud be firmly in contact with the raw surface of the acromion and glenoid, and there should be no motion between humerus and scapula. The wound is closed in layers, and the lid over the window in the shoulder spica is replaced.

POSTOPERATIVE MANAGEMENT. Immobilization in the shoulder spica is continued until there is evidence of solid union between humerus and scapula; as a rule, this will be at least 10 to 12 weeks after operation.

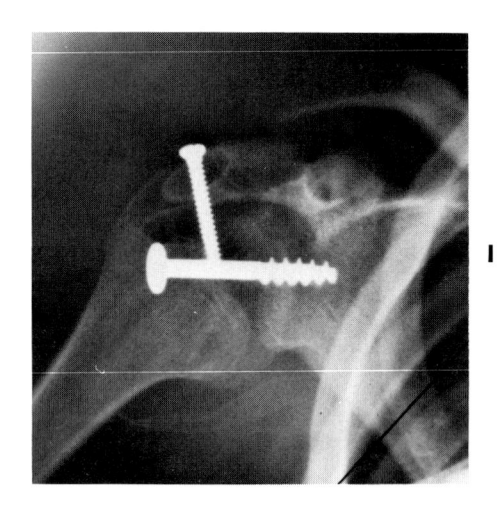

REFERENCES

Abbott, L. C., and Lucas, D. B.: The tripartite deltoid and its surgical significance in exposure of the scapulohumeral joint, Ann. Surg. **136**:392, 1952.

Abbott, L. C., and Lucas, D. B.: The function of the clavicle, Ann. Surg. **140**:583, 1954.

Abbott, L. C., Saunders, J. B. deC. M., Hagey, H., and Jones, E. W., Jr.,: Surgical approaches to the shoulder joint, J. Bone Joint Surg. **31-A**:235, 1949.

Adler, J. B., and Potterson, R. K., Jr.: Erb's palsy, long-term results of treatment in eighty-eight cases, J. Bone Joint Surg. **49-A**:1052, 1967.

Adson, A. W., and Coffey, J. R.: A method of anterior approach for relief of symptoms by division of the scalenus anticus, Ann Surg. **85**:839, 1927.

Alldred, A. J.: Congenital pseudarthrosis of the clavicle, J. Bone Joint Surg. **45-B**:312, 1963.

Allman, F. L., Jr.: Fractures and ligamentous injuries of the clavicle and its articulation, J. Bone Joint Surg. **49-A**:774, 1967.

Allman, F. L.: The Bristow procedure in athletes. A report of 300 consecutive cases, presented at the Annual Meeting of the Association of Bone and Joint Surgeons, Honolulu, 1977.

Armstrong, J. R.: Excision of the acromion in treatment of the supraspinatus syndrome: report of ninety-five excisions, J. Bone Joint Surg. **31-B**:436, 1949.

Babbitt, D. P., and Cassidy, R. H.: Obstetrical paralysis and dislocation of the shoulder in infancy, J. Bone Joint Surg. **50-A**:1447, 1968.

Babcock, J. L., and Wray, J. B.: Analysis of abduction in a shoulder with deltoid paralysis due to axillary nerve injury, Clin. Orthop. **68**:116, 1970.

Badgley, C. E.: Sports injuries of the shoulder girdle, J.A.M.A. **172**:444, 1960.

Bailey, R. W.: Acute and recurrent dislocation of the shoulder, J. Bone Joint Surg. **49-A**:767, 1967.

Bakalim, G., and Pasila, M.: Surgical treatment of rupture of rotator cuff tendon, Acta Orthop. Scand. **46**:751, 1975.

Bankart, A. S.: Recurrent or habitual dislocation of the shoulder joint, Br. Med. J. **2**:1132, 1923.

Bankart, A. S.: An operation for recurrent dislocation (subluxation) of the sternoclavicular joint, Br. J. Surg. **26**:320, 1938.

Bankart, A. S.: The pathology and treatment of recurrent dislocation of the shoulder joint, Br. J. Surg. **26**:23, 1938.

Bankart, A. S.: Discussion on recurrent dislocation of the shoulder, J. Bone Joint Surg. **30-B**:46, 1948.

Bateman, J. E.: The shoulder and environs, St. Louis, 1955, The C. V. Mosby Co.

Bennett, J. E.: Shoulder and elbow lesions of the professional baseball pitcher, J.A.M.A. **117**:510, 1941.

Bost, F. C., and Inmann, V. T.: The pathological changes in recurrent dislocation of the shoulder, a report of Bankart's operative procedure, J. Bone Joint Surg. **24**:595, 1942.

Bosworth, D. M.: An analysis of twenty-eight consecutive cases of incapacitating shoulder lesions, radically explored and repaired, J. Bone Joint Surg. **22**:369, 1940.

Bosworth, D. M.: Acromioclavicular separation; new method of repair, Surg. Gynecol. Obstet. **73**:866, 1941.

Bosworth, D. M.: The supraspinatus syndrome: symptomatology, pathology, and repair, J.A.M.A. **117**:422, 1941.

Boyd, H. B., and Hunt, H. L.: Recurrent dislocation of the shoulder; the staple capsulorrhaphy, J. Bone Joint Surg. **47-A**:1514, 1965.

Boyd, H. B., and Sisk, T. D.: Recurrent posterior dislocation of the shoulder, J. Bone Joint Surg. **54-A**:779, 1972.

Brav, E. A.: An evaluation of the Putti-Platt reconstruction procedure for recurrent dislocation of the shoulder, J. Bone Joint Surg. **37-A**:731, 1955.

Brav, E. A.: Recurrent dislocation of the shoulder. Ten years' experience with the Putti-Platt reconstruction procedure, Am. J. Surg. **100**:423, 1960.

Brown, F. W., and Navigato, W. J.: Rupture of the axillary artery and brachial plexus palsy associated with anterior dislocation of the shoulder. Report of a case with successful vascular repair, Clin. Orthop. **60**:195, 1968.

Carpenter, E. B., and Garrett, R. G.: Congenital pseudarthrosis of the clavicle, J. Bone Joint Surg. **42-A**:337, 1960.

Charnley, J., and Houston, J. K.: Compression arthrodesis of the shoulder, J. Bone Joint Surg. **46-B**:614, 1964.

Codman, E. A.: Complete rupture of the supraspinatus tendon: operative treatment with report of two successful cases, Boston Med. Surg. J. **164**:708, 1911.

Cofield, R. H.: Status of total shoulder arthroplasty, Arch. Surg. **112**:1088, 1977.

Cofield, R. H., and Briggs, B. T.: Glenohumeral arthrodesis. Operative and long-term functional results, J. Bone Joint Surg. **61-A**:668, 1979.

Conwell, H. E., and Reynolds, F. C.: Key and Conwell's management of fractures, dislocations, and sprains, ed. 7, St. Louis, 1961, The C. V. Mosby Co.

Cotton, R. E., and Rideout, D. F.: Tears of the humeral rotation cuff, J. Bone Joint Surg. **46-B**:314, 1964.

Coughlin, M. J., Morris, J. M., and West, W. F.: The semiconstrained total shoulder arthroplasty, J. Bone Joint Surg. **61-A**:574, 1979.

Cranley, J. J., and Karuse, R. J.: Injury to the axillary artery following anterior dislocation of the shoulder, Am. J. Surg. **95**:524, 1958.

Crawford, H. R.: Posterior dislocation of the shoulder, Surg. Clin. North Am. **41**:1655, 1961.

Davis, J. B., and Cottrell, G. W.: A technique for shoulder arthrodesis, J Bone Joint Surg. **44-A**:657, 1962.

Day, A. J., MacDonell, J. A., and Pedersen, H. E.: Recurrent dislocation of the shoulder. A comparison of the Bankart and Magnuson procedures after 16 years, Clin. Orthop. **45**:123, 1966.

Déjerine-Klumpke, A.: Des polynéurites en général et des paralysies et atrophies saturnines en particulier. Étude clinique et anatomopathologique, Paris, 1889, Ancienne Librairie Germer Ballière et Cie.

DePalma, A. F.: Surgery of the shoulder, Philadelphia, 1950, J. B. Lippincott Co.

DePalma, A. F.: Arthrodesis of the shoulder joint, Surg. Clin. North Am. **43**:1599, 1963.

DePalma, A. F., Cooke, A. J., and Probhakar, M.: The role of the subscapularis in recurrent anterior dislocations of the shoulder, Clin. Orthop. **54**:35, 1967.

DePalma, A. F., and Kruper, J. S.: Long-term study of shoulder joints afflicted with and treated for calcific tendinitis, Clin. Orthop. **20**:61, 1961.

Dewar, F. P., and Barrington, T. W.: The treatment of chronic acromioclavicular dislocation, J. Bone Joint Surg. **47-B**:32, 1965.

Dickson, J. W., and Devas, M. B.: Bankart's operation for recurrent dislocation of the shoulder, J. Bone Joint Surg. **39-B**:114, 1957.

Dimon, J. H., III: Posterior dislocation and posterior fracture dislocation of the shoulder: a report of twenty-five cases, South. Med. J. **60**:661, 1967.

Duchenne, G. B.: Physiology of motion (translated by Kaplan, E. B.), Philadelphia, 1949, J. B. Lippincott Co.

Du Toit, G. T., and Levy, S. J.: Transposition of latissimus dorsi for paralysis of triceps brachii. Report of a case, J. Bone Joint Surg. **49-B**:135, 1967.

Eden, R.: Zur Operation der habituellen Schulterluxation unter Mitteilung, eines neuen Verfahrens bei Abriss am inneren Pfannenrande, Dtsch. Z. Chir. **144**:269, 1918.

Ellis, V. H.: The diagnosis of shoulder lesions due to injuries of the rotator cuff, J. Bone Joint Surg. **35-B**:72, 1953.

Elmslie, R. C.: Calcareous deposits in the supraspinatus tendon, Br. J. Surg. **20**:190, 1932.

Fairbank, H. A. T.: Birth palsy. Subluxation of the shoulder joint in infants and young children, Lancet **1**:1217, 1913.

Gallie, W. E., and LeMesurier, A. B.: Recurring dislocation of the shoulder, J. Bone Joint Surg. **30-B**:9, 1918.

Gibson, D. A., and Carroll, N.: Congenital pseudoarthrosis of the clavicle, J. Bone Joint Surg. **52-B**:629, 1970.

Gill, A. B: A new operation for arthrodesis of the shoulder, J. Bone Joint Surg. **13**:287, 1931.

Godsil, R. D., and Linscheid, R. L.: Intratendinous defects of the rotator cuff, Clin. Orthop. **69**:181, 1970.

Goldstein, L. A., and Dickerson, R. C.: Orthopedic surgery. In White, R. R., editor: Atlas of pediatric surgery, New York, 1965, McGraw-Hill Book Co.

Green, W. T.: The surgical correction of congenital elevation of the scapula (Sprengel's deformity), J. Bone Joint Surg. **39-A**:1439, 1957.

Grimes, O. F., and Bell, H. G.: Shoulder girdle amputation, Surg. Gynecol. Obstet. **91**:201, 1950.

Gurd, F. B.: The treatment of complete dislocation of the outer end of the clavicle, Ann. Surg. **113**:1094, 1941.

Hammond, G.: Complete acromionectomy in the treatment of chronic tendinitis of the shoulder, J. Bone Joint Surg. **44-A**:494, 1962.

Hammond, G.: Complete acromionectomy in the treatment of chronic tendinitis of the shoulder. A follow-up on ninety operations on eighty-seven patients, J. Bone Joint Surg. **53-A**:173, 1971.

Haraldsson, S.: Reconstruction of proximal humerus by muscle-sling prosthesis, Acta Orthop. Scand. **40**:225, 1969.

Hardin, C. A.: Interscapulothoracic amputations for sarcomas of the upper extremity, Surgery **49**:355, 1961.

Harmon, P. H.: A posterior approach for arthrodesis and other operations of the shoulder, Surg. Gynecol. Obstet. **81**:266, 1945.

Helfet, A. J.: Coracoid transplantation for recurring dislocation of the shoulder, J. Bone Joint Surg. **40-B**:198, 1958.

Henson, G. F.: Vascular complications of shoulder injuries, J. Bone Joint Surg. **38-B**:528, 1956.

Hill, H. A., and Sachs, M. D.: The grooved defect of the humeral head. A frequently unrecognized complication of dislocations of the shoulder joint, Radiology **35**:690, 1940.

Horelius, L., Thorling, J., and Fredin, H.: Recurrent anterior dislocation of the shoulder. Results after the Bankart and Putti-Platt operations, J. Bone Joint Surg. **61-A**:566, 1979.

Howard, F. M., and Shafer, S. J.: Injuries to the clavicle with neurovascular complications. A study of fourteen cases, J. Bone Joint Surg. **47-A**:1335, 1965.

Howorth, M. B.: Calcification of tendon cuff of shoulder, Surg. Gynecol. Obstet. **80**:337, 1945.

Hybbinette, S.: De la transplantation d'un fragment osseux pour remédier aux luxations récidivantes de l'épaule; constatations et résultats opératoires, Acta Chir. Scand. **71**:411, 1932.

Inman, V. T., Saunders, J. B. deC. M., and Abbott, L. C.: Observations on the function of the shoulder joint, J. Bone Joint Surg. **26**:1, 1944.

Jacobs, B., and Wade, P. A.: Acromioclavicular-joint injury. An end-result study, J. Bone Joint Surg. **48-A**:475, 1966.

Jinkins, W. J., Jr.: Congenital pseudarthrosis of the clavicle. Clin. Orthop. **62**:183, 1969.

Joyce, J. J., III, and Harty, M.: Surgical exposure of the shoulder, J. Bone Joint Surg. **49-A**:547, 1967.

Kennedy, J. C., and Cameron, H.: Complete dislocation of the acromioclavicular joint, J. Bone Joint Surg. **36-B**:202, 1954.

Key, J. A.: Arthrodesis of the shoulder, American Academy of Orthopaedic Surgeons Instructional Course Lectures, vol. 2, Ann Arbor, 1944, J. W. Edwards, p. 276.

Key, J. A.: Calcium deposits in the vicinity of the shoulder and of other joints, Ann. Surg. **129**:737, 1949.

Knight, R. A., and Mayne, J. A.: Communuted fractures and fracture dislocations involving the articular surface of the humeral head, J. Bone Joint Surg. **39-A**:1343, 1957.

Lapidus, P. W., and Guidotti, F. P.: Common shoulder lesions. Report of 493 cases. Calcific tendinitis, tendinitis of long head of biceps, frozen shoulder, fractures, and dislocations, Bull. Hosp. Joint Dis. **29**:293, 1968.

Leffert, R. D., and Seddon, H.: Infraclavicular brachial plexus injuries, J. Bone Joint Surg. **47-B**:9, 1965.

L'Episcopo. J. B.: Restoration of muscle balance in the treatment of obstetrical paralysis, N.Y. J. Med. **39**:357, 1939.

Leslie, J. T., Jr., and Ryan, T. J.: The anterior axillary incision to approach the shoulder joint, J. Bone Joint Surg. **44-A**:1193, 1962.

Litchman, H. M., Silver, C. M., Simon, S. D., and Eshrage, A.: The surgical management of calcific tendinitis of the shoulder, Int. Surg. **50**:474, 1968.

Lombardo, S. J., et al.: The modified Bristow procedure for recurrent dislocation of the shoulder, J. Bone Joint Surg. **58-A**:256, 1976.

Lowman, C. L.: Operative correction of old sternoclavicular dislocation, J. Bone Joint Surg. **10**:740, 1928.

Lusskin, R., Weiss, C. A., and Winer, J.: Role of the subclavius muscle in the subclavian vein syndrome (costoclavicular syndrome) following fracture of clavicle. A case report with a review of the pathophysiology of the costoclavicular space, Clin. Orthop. **54**:75, 1967.

Macnab, I., and Hastings, D.: Rotator cuff tendinitis, Can. Med. Assoc. J. **99**:91, 1968.

Magnuson, P. B.: Treatment of recurrent dislocation of the shoulder, Surg. Clin. North Am. **25**:14, 1945.

Magnuson, P. B., and Stack, J. K.: Recurrent dislocation of the shoulder, J.A.M.A. **123**:889, 1943.

May, V. R., Jr.: Shoulder fusion, a review of 14 cases, J. Bone Joint Surg. **44-A**:65, 1962.

May, V. R., Jr.: A modified Bristow operation for anterior recurrent dislocation of the shoulder, J. Bone Joint Surg. **52-A**:1010, 1970.

Mayer, L.: Transplantation of the trapezius for paralysis of the abductors of the arm, J. Bone Joint Surg. **9**:412, 1927.

McLaughlin, H. L.: Lesions of the musculotendinous cuff of the shoulder: I. The exposure and treatment of tears with retraction, J. Bone Joint Surg. **26**:31, 1944.

McLaughlin, H. L.: Lesions of the musculotendinous cuff of the

shoulder: III. Observations on the pathology, course and treatment of calcific deposits, Ann. Surg. **124**:354, 1946.
McLaughlin, H. L.: Posterior dislocation of the shoulder, J. Bone Joint Surg. **34-A**:584, 1952.
McLaughlin, H. L.: Posterior dislocation of the shoulder, J. Bone Joint Surg. **44-A**:1477, 1962.
McLaughlin, H. L.: Rupture of the rotator cuff, J. Bone Joint Surg. **44-A**:979, 1962.
McLaughlin, H. L., and Asherman, E. G.: Lesions of the musculotendinous cuff of the shoulder: IV. Some observations based upon the results of surgical repair, J. Bone Joint Surg. **33-A**:76, 1951.
McLaughlin, H. L., and Cavallaro, W. U.: Primary anterior dislocation of the shoulder, Am. J. Surg. **80**:615, 1950.
McLaughlin, H. L., and MacLellan, D. I.: Recurrent anterior dislocation of the shoulder: II. A comparative study, J. Trauma **7**:191, 1967.
Meyer, A. W.: Chronic functional lesions of shoulder, Arch. Surg. **35**:646, 1937.
Milch, H.: Partial scapulectomy for snapping of the scapula, J. Bone Joint Surg. **32-A**:561, 1950.
Millbourn, E.: On injuries to the acromioclavicular joint. Treatment and results, Acta Orthop. Scand. **19**:349, 1950.
Miller, D. S.: Brachial plexus lesions in trauma of shoulder, Int. Surg. **48**:270, 1967.
Miller, D. S., and Boswick, J. A.: Lesions of the brachial plexus associated with fractures of the clavicle, Clin. Orthop. **64**:144, 1969.
Morrey, B. F., and Janes, J. M.: Recurrent anterior dislocation of the shoulder. Long-term follow-up of the Putti-Platt and Bankart procedures, J. Bone Joint Surg. **58-A**:252, 1976.
Moseley, H. F.: Ruptures of rotator cuff. Br. J. Surg. **38**:340, 1951.
Moseley, H. F.: Ruptures of the rotator cuff. Springfield, Ill., 1952, Charles C Thomas, Publisher.
Moseley, H. F.: The inferior relations of the glenohumeral joint, Am. J. Surg. **83**:321, 1952.
Moseley, H. F.: Shoulder lesions, ed. 2, New York, 1953, Paul B. Hoeber, Inc.
Moseley, H. F.: Athletic injuries to the shoulder region, Am. J. Surg. **98**:401, 1959.
Moseley, H. F.: The clavicle: its anatomy and function, Clin. Orthop. **58**:17, 1968.
Moseley, H. F., and Övergaard, B.: The anterior capsular mechanism in recurrent anterior dislocation of the shoulder; morphological and clinical studies with special reference to the glenoid labrum and the glenohumeral ligaments, J. Bone Joint Surg. **44-B**:913, 1962.
Mumford, E. B.: Acromioclavicular dislocation, a new operative treatment, J. Bone Joint Surg. **23**:799, 1941.
Neer, C. S., II: Articular replacement for the humeral head, J. Bone Joint Surg. **37-A**:215, 1955.
Neer, C. S., II: Nonunion of the clavicle, J.A.M.A. **172**:1006, 1960.
Neer, C. S., II: Prosthetic replacement of the humeral head. Indications and operative technique, Surg. Clin. North Am. **43**:1581, 1963.
Neer, C. S., II: Fractures of the distal third of the clavicle, Clin. Orthop. **58**:43, 1968.
Neer, C. S., II: Displaced proximal humeral fractures. I. Classification and evaluation, J. Bone Joint Surg. **52-A**:1077, 1970.
Neer, C. S., II: Displaced proximal humeral fractures. II. Treatment of three-part and four-part displacement, J. Bone Joint Surg. **52-A**:1090, 1970.
Neer, C. S., II: Anterior acromioplasty for the chronic impingement syndrome in the shoulder. A preliminary report, J. Bone Joint Surg. **54-A**:41, 1972.
Neer, C. S., II: Replacement arthroplasty for glenohumeral osteoarthritis, J. Bone Joint Surg. **56-A**:1, 1974.
Neviaser, J. S.: Acromioclavicular dislocation treated by transference of the coracoacromial ligament, Bull. Hosp. Joint Dis. **12**:46, 1951.
Neviaser, J. S.: Acromioclavicular dislocation treated by transference of the coracoacromial ligament. A long-term follow-up in a series of 112 cases, Clin. Orthop. **58**:57, 1968.
Nickel, V. L., and Waring, W.: Future developments in externally powered orthotic and prosthetic devices, J. Bone Joint Surg. **47-B**:469, 1965.
Nicola, T.: Recurrent anterior dislocation of the shoulder, J. Bone Joint Surg. **11**:128, 1929.
Nicola, T.: Recurrent dislocation of the shoulder, Am. J. Surg. **86**:85, 1954.
O'Donoghue, D. H.: Introduction, Symposium on treatment of injuries to the shoulder girdle presented by Sports Medicine Committee of the American Academy of Orthopaedic Surgeons 1966, J. Bone Joint Surg. **49-A**:753, 1967.
Osmond-Clarke, H.: Habitual dislocation of the shoulder. The Putti-Platt operation, J. Bone Joint Surg. **30-B**:19, 1948.
Owen, R.: Congenital pseudarthrosis of the clavicle, J. Bone Joint Surg. **52**;-**B**:644, 1970.
Oyston, J. K.: Unreduced posterior dislocation of the shoulder treated by open reduction and transposition of the subcapularis tendon, J. Bone Joint Surg. **46-B**:256, 1964.
Pack, G. T.: Major exarticulations for malignant neoplasms of the extremities: interscapulothoracic amputation, hip-joint disarticulation, and interilio-abdominal amputation. A report of end results in 228 cases, J. Bone Joint Surg. **38-A**:249, 1956.
Pack, G. T., and Crampton, R. S.: The Tilchor-Linberg resection of the shoulder girdle. Indications for its substitution for interscapulothoracic amputation; recent data on end-results of the forequarter amputation, Clin. Orthop. **79**:148, 1961.
Patte, D., Debeyre, J., and Elmelik, E.: Repair of ruptures of the rotator cuff of the shoulder, J. Bone Joint Surg. **47-B**:36, 1965.
Patterson, W. R.: Inferior dislocation of the distal end of the clavicle. A case report, J. Bone Joint Surg. **49-A**:1184, 1967.
Quigley, T. B.: Injuries to the acromioclavicular and sternoclavicular joint sustained in athletics, Surg. Clin. North Am. **43**:1551, 1963.
Rowe, C. R.: Prognosis in dislocations of the shoulder, J. Bone Joint Surg. **38-A**:957, 1956.
Rowe, C. R.: Acute and recurrent dislocations of the shoulder, J. Bone Joint Surg. **44-A**:998, 1962.
Rowe, C. R.: The results of operative treatment of recurrent dislocations of the shoulder, Surg. Clin. North Am. **43**:1667, 1963.
Rowe, C. R.: An atlas of anatomy and treatment of midclavicular fractures, Clin. Orthop. **58**:29, 1968.
Rowe, C. R.: Complicated dislocations of the shoulder. Guidelines in treatment, Am. J. Surg. **117**:549, 1969.
Rowe, C. R.: Re-evaluation of the position of the arm in arthrodesis of the shoulder in the adult, J. Bone Joint Surg. **56-A**:913, 1974.

Rowe, C. R., Patel, D., and Southmayd, W. W.: The Bankart procedure. A long-term end-result study, J. Bone Joint Surg. **60-A**:1, 1978.

Rowe, C. R., Pierce, D. S., and Clark, J. G.: Voluntary dislocation of the shoulder. A preliminary report on a clinical, electromyographic, and psychiatric study of twenty-six patients, J. Bone Joint Surg. **55-A**:445, 1973.

Rowe, C. R., and Sakellarides, H. T.: Fractures related to recurrences of anterior dislocations of the shoulder, Clin. Orthop. **20**:40, 1961.

Rowe, C. R., and Yee, L. B. K.: A posterior approach to the shoulder joint, J. Bone Joint Surg. **26**:580, 1944.

Rybka, V., Raunio, P., and Vainio, K.: Arthrodesis of the shoulder in rheumatoid arthritis, J. Bone Joint Surg. **61-B**:155, 1979.

Sakellarides, H.: Pseudarthrosis of the clavicle, J. Bone Joint Surg. **43-A**:130, 1961.

Samilson, R. L., and Miller, E.: Posterior dislocations of the shoulder, Clin. Orthop. **32**:69, 1964.

Schrock, R. D.: Congenital elevation of the scapula, J. Bone Joint Surg. **8**:207, 1926.

Schwartz, D. I.: Bankart shoulder repair made easier, Clin. Orthop. **56**:59, 1968.

Scott, D. J., Jr.: Treatment of recurrent posterior dislocations of the shoulder by glenoplasty. Report of three cases, J. Bone Joint Surg. **49-A**:471, 1967.

Sever, J. W.: Obstetric paralysis, Am. J. Dis. Child. **12**:541, 1916.

Sever, J. W.: The results of a new operation for obstetrical paralysis, Am. J. Orthop. Surg. **16**:248, 1918.

Simpson, D. C., and Lamb, D. W.: A system of powered prostheses for severe bilateral upper limb deficiency, J. Bone Joint Surg. **47-B**:442, 1965.

Speed, K.: Recurrent anterior dislocation of the shoulder. Operative cure by a bone graft, Surg. Gynecol. Obstet. **44**:468, 1927.

Steindler, A.: Orthopaedic operations, Springfield, Ill., 1940, Charles C Thomas, Publisher.

Steindler, A.: Arthrodesis of the shoulder, American Academy of Orthopaedic Surgeons Instructional Course Lectures, vol. 2, Ann Arbor, 1944, J. W. Edwards, p. 293.

Stener, B.: Dislocation of the shoulder complicated by complete rupture of the axillary artery, J. Bone Joint Surg. **39-B**:714, 1957.

Thorndike, A.: Athletic injuries, ed. 5, Philadelphia, 1962, Lea & Febiger.

Thorndike, A., Jr., and Quigley, T. B.: Injuries to acromioclavicular joint, Am. J. Surg. **55**:250, 1942.

Truchly, G., and Thompson, W. A. L.: Simplified Putti-Platt procedure, J.A.M.A. **179**:859, 1962.

Urist, M. R.: Complete dislocations of the acromioclavicular joint; the nature of the traumatic lesion and effective method of treatment with an analysis of forty-one cases, J. Bone Joint Surg. **28**:813, 1946.

ViGario, G. D., and Keats, T. E.: Localization of calcific deposits in the shoulder, Am. J. Roentgenol. Radium Ther. Nucl. Med. **108**:806, 1970.

Watson-Jones, R.: Extra-articular arthrodesis of the shoulder, J. Bone Joint Surg. **15**:862, 1933.

Weaver, J. K., and Dunn, H. K.: Treatment of acromioclavicular injuries, especially complete acromioclavicular separation, J. Bone Joint Surg. **54-A**:1187, 1972.

Weiner, D. S., and Macnab, I.: Ruptures of the rotator cuff: follow-up evaluation of operative repairs, Can. J. Surg. **13**:219, 1970.

Whitman, A.: Congenital elevation of scapula and paralysis of serratus magnus muscle, J.A.M.A. **99**:1332, 1932.

Wickstrom, J., Haslam, T., and Hutchison, R. H.: The surgical management of residual deformities of the shoulder following birth injuries of the brachial plexus, J. Bone Joint Surg. **37-A**:27, 1955.

Wilson, A. B. K.: Hendon pneumatic power units and controls for prostheses and splints, J. Bone Joint Surg. **47-B**:435, 1965.

Wilson, J. C., and McKeever, F. M.: Traumatic posterior (retroglenoid) dislocation of the humerus, J. Bone Joint Surg. **31-A**:160, 1949.

Woodward, J. W.: Congenital elevation of the scapula. Correction by release and transplantation of muscle origins. A preliminary report, J. Bone Joint Surg. **43-A**:219, 1961.

Zachary, R. B.: Transplantation of teres major and latissimus dorsi for loss of external rotation at shoulder, Lancet **2**:757, 1947.

2

UPPER ARM

OPEN REDUCTION AND PLATE FIXATION FOR FRACTURE OF SHAFT OF HUMERUS (Plate 2-1)

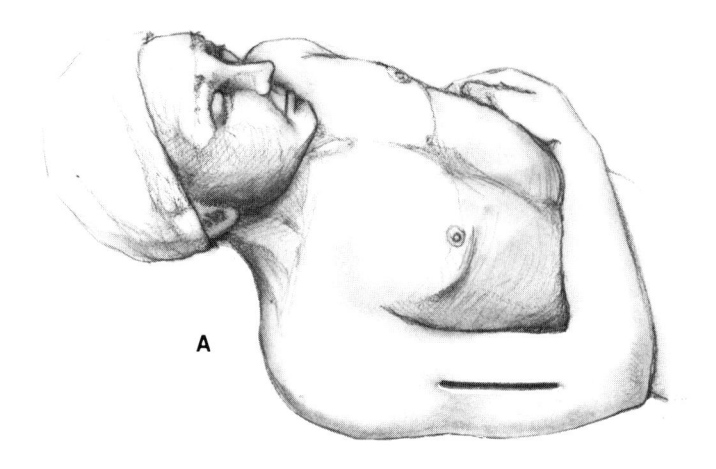

GENERAL DISCUSSION. Most fractures involving the shaft of the humerus are best treated nonoperatively. Under certain circumstances, open reduction and internal fixation for fracture of the shaft of the humerus may be the treatment of choice. Indications for open reduction and internal fixation may include the following: when satisfactory position and alignment cannot be obtained with closed treatment (particularly in segmental fractures); when there are associated injuries that require realy mobilization of the elbow; when the fracture is associated with a vascular injury; when radial nerve palsy develops after manipulation or during closed treatment of the fracture; or when the fracture is pathologic through a malignant lesion in the humerus.

Except for pathologic fractures through a malignant lesion, and occasionally for segmental fractures, internal fixation by plate is preferred when open reduction is necessary.

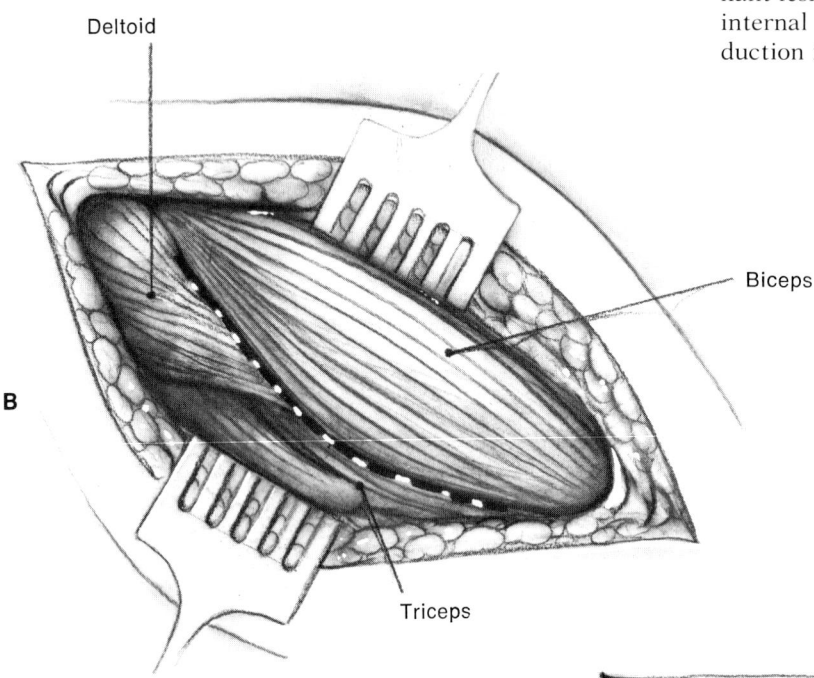

DETAILS OF PROCEDURE. The involved arm should be draped free. The incision for an anterolateral approach to the shaft of the humerus is centered at the level of the fracture (**A**). In the upper portion of the arm the skin incision should be in line with the anterior border of the deltoid muscle and continue distally with the lateral border of the biceps muscle. The cephalic vein may be ligated in the deltopectoral groove. The deltoid muscle is retracted laterally in the proximal portion of the wound. Distal to the insertion of the deltoid, the biceps muscle (**B**) is separated from the underlying brachialis muscle and retracted medially. The muscle fibers of the brachialis muscle are split longitudinally to bone in such a manner that the lateral third of the brachialis muscle can then be reflected laterally by subperiosteal dissection (**C**).

(Plate 2-1) OPEN REDUCTION AND PLATE FIXATION FOR FRACTURE OF SHAFT OF HUMERUS

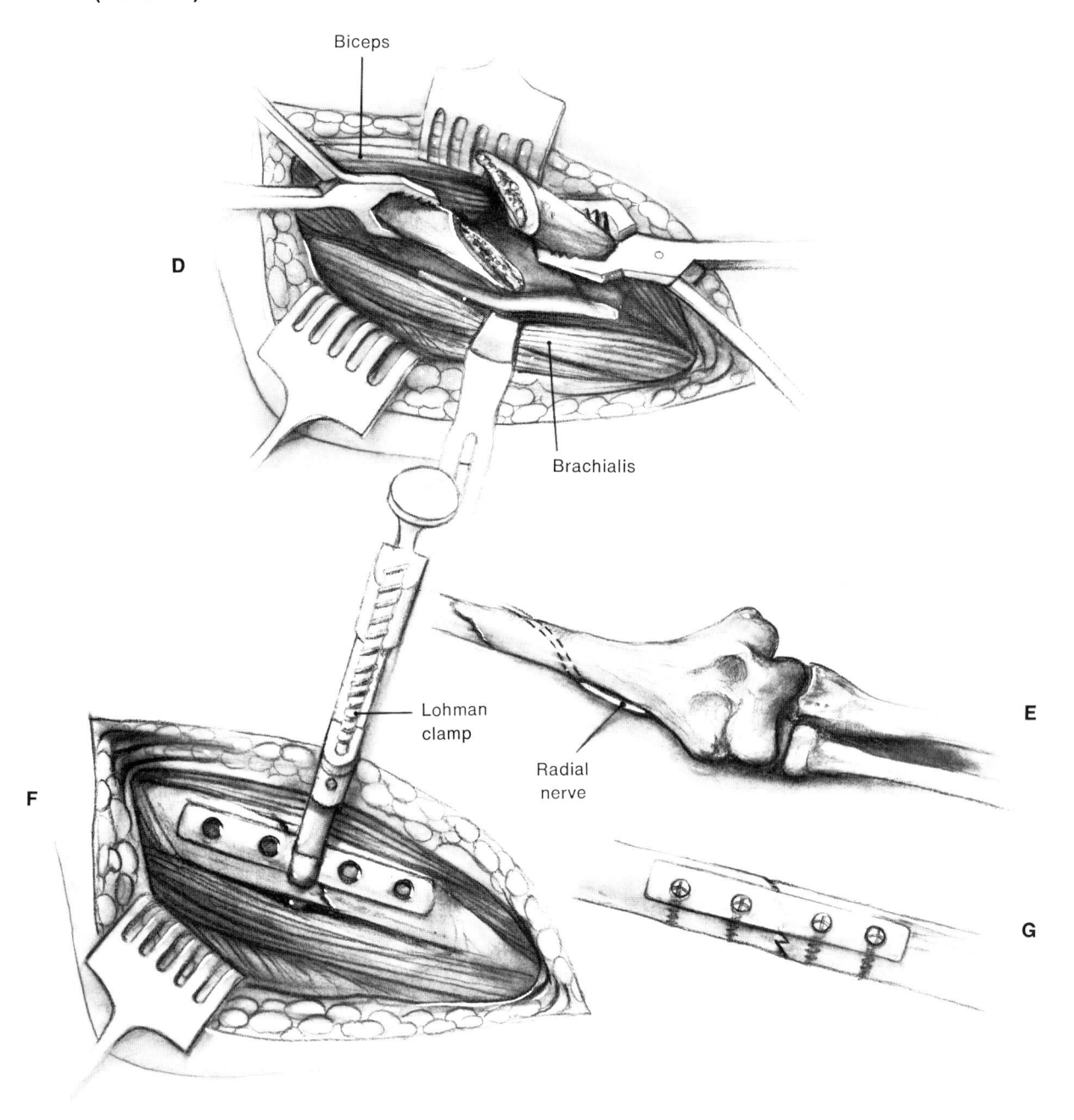

This retraction of the lateral portion of the brachialis muscle is made easier by flexing the elbow to 90°, and the radial nerve (**D** and **E**) is protected in the musculospiral groove of the humerus as the lateral portion of the brachialis muscle is reflected subperiosteally in a lateral direction.

The lateral portion of the brachialis muscle is usually innervated by both the musculocutaneous and radial nerves, which allows this muscle to be split longitudinally without producing any significant motor paralysis of the brachialis muscle. In this manner the shaft of the humerus can be exposed for reduction of the fracture and application of a suitable bone plate for internal fixation (**F** and **G**). The length of the bone plate used for internal fixation should be at least five times the diameter of the bone, and a minimum of two transfixion screws should engage both cortices of the main bone fragments porximal and distal to the fracture. The patient's arm is placed in a sling following wound closure (**F** and **G**).

POSTOPERATIVE MANAGEMENT. The arm is protected, generally in a sling and swath, until there is clinical and roentgenographic evidence of union at the fracture site.

51

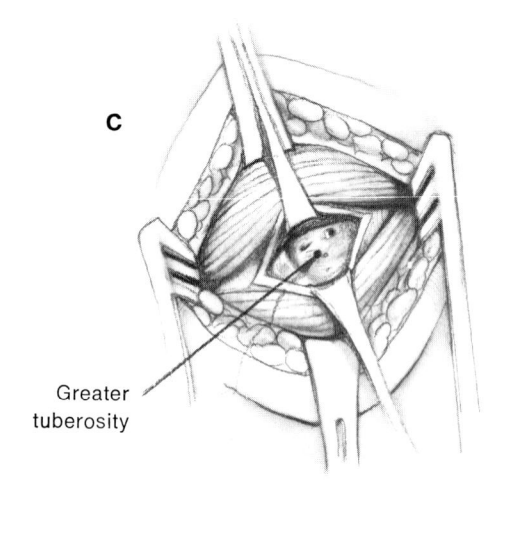

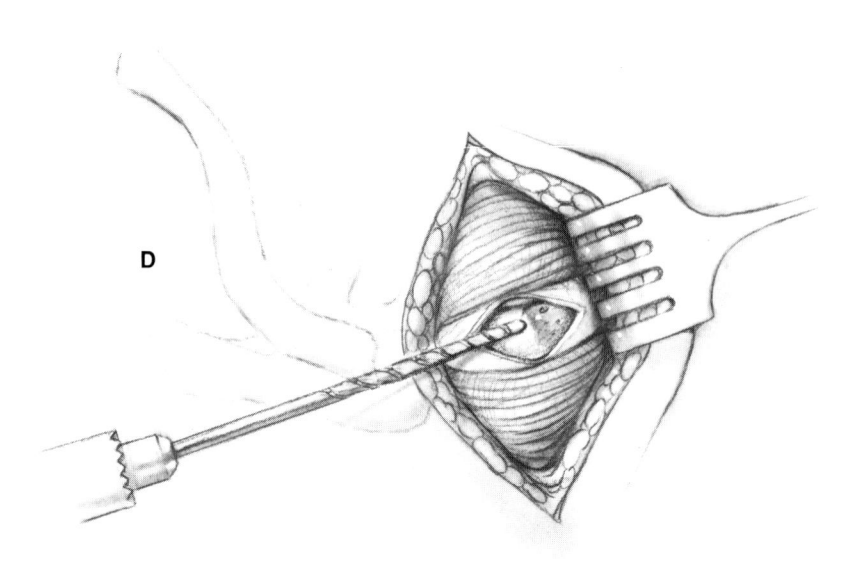

INTRAMEDULLARY FIXATION FOR FRACTURE OF SHAFT OF HUMERUS (Plate 2-2)

GENERAL DISCUSSION. The indications for open reduction and internal fixation for fracture of the shaft of the humerus are the same as with the preceding procedure. Intramedullary fixation for fracture of the shaft of the humerus may be preferred to plate fixation when the fracture is pathologic through a malignant lesion in the humerus or occasionally for internal fixation of a segmental fracture in which satisfactory position cannot be obtained with closed treatment methods.

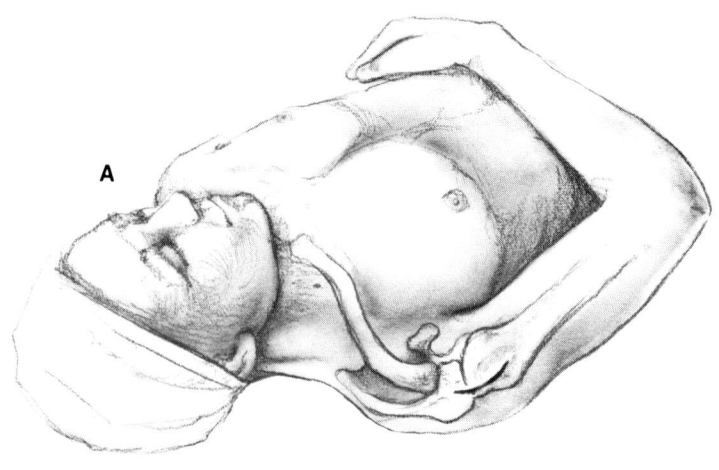

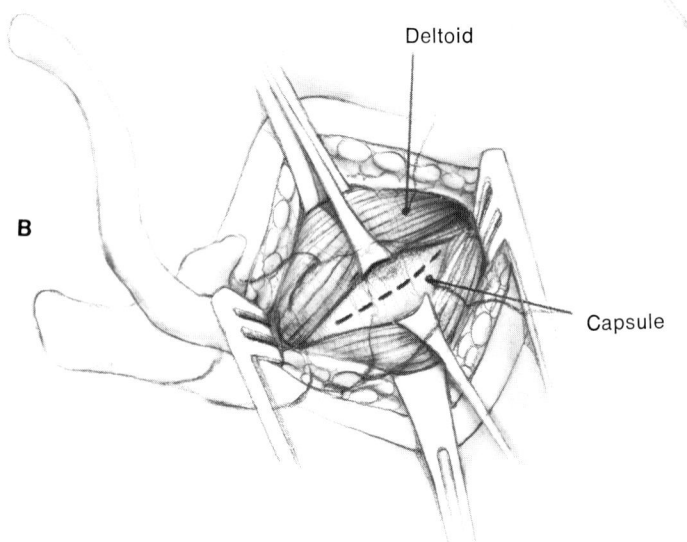

DETAILS OF PROCEDURE. The arm is draped free with the patient in the supine position. With a sandbag located posterior to the involved shoulder, a short longitudinal incision is made beginning over the acromion process, extending distally over the greater tuberosity for a distance no greater than 5 cm with the arm held in internal rotation (**A**). The lateral edge of the acromion is palpated, and the fibers of the deltoid muscle are separated beginning at the acromion and extending distally no more than 3 cm to avoid injury to the axillary nerve supplying the deltoid muscle (**B**). The patient's arm may be moved passively to palpate the bicipital groove and to accurately locate the greater tuberosity. With the arm in internal rotation the capsule is opened with a longitudinal incision over the greater tuberosity of the humerus, and a preparatory drill hole is made in the greater tuberosity at a location that will allow subsequent insertion of the intramedullary nail in line with the shaft of the humerus (**C** and **D**).

(Plate 2-2) INTRAMEDULLARY FIXATION FOR FRACTURE OF SHAFT OF HUMERUS

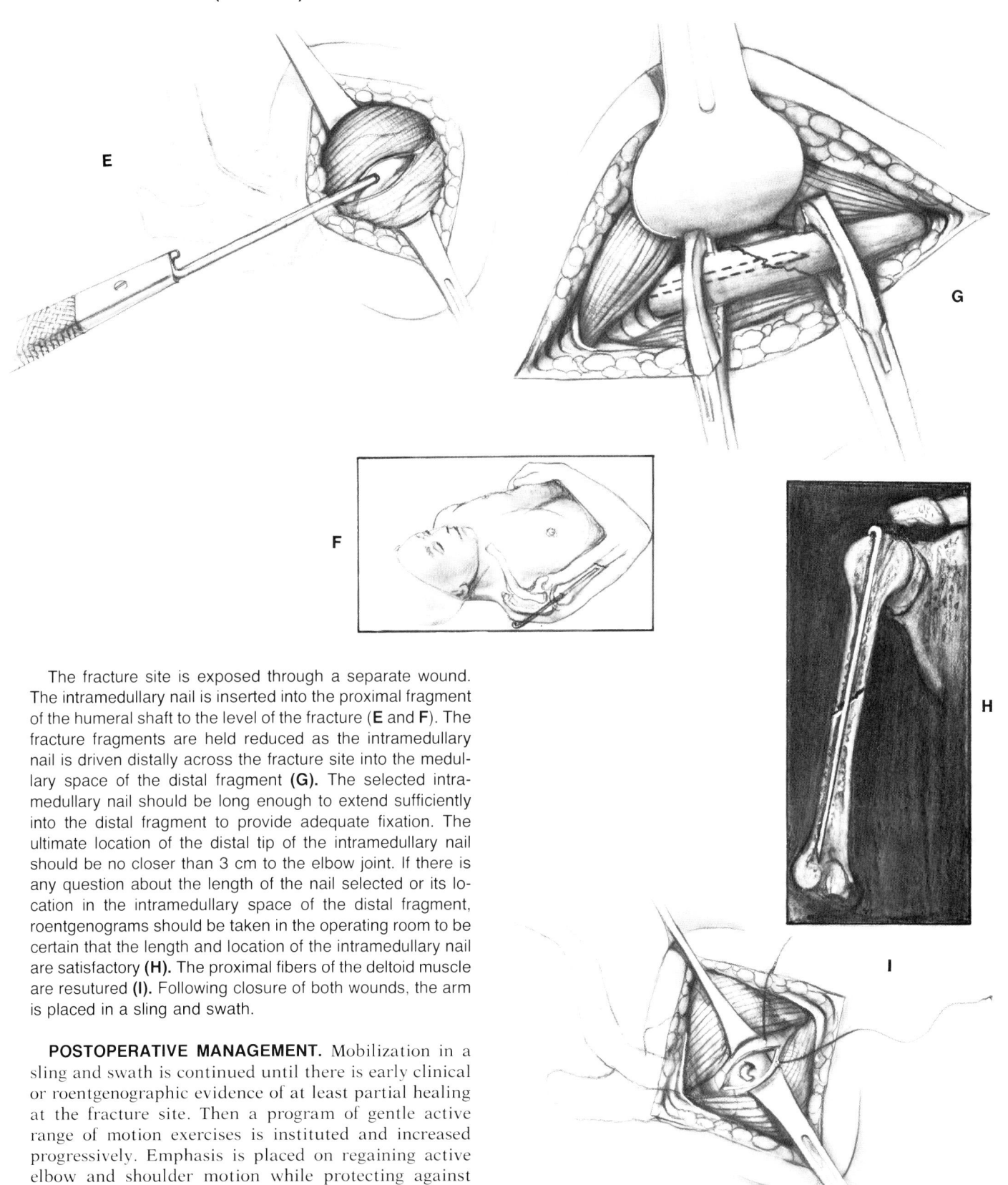

The fracture site is exposed through a separate wound. The intramedullary nail is inserted into the proximal fragment of the humeral shaft to the level of the fracture (**E** and **F**). The fracture fragments are held reduced as the intramedullary nail is driven distally across the fracture site into the medullary space of the distal fragment (**G**). The selected intramedullary nail should be long enough to extend sufficiently into the distal fragment to provide adequate fixation. The ultimate location of the distal tip of the intramedullary nail should be no closer than 3 cm to the elbow joint. If there is any question about the length of the nail selected or its location in the intramedullary space of the distal fragment, roentgenograms should be taken in the operating room to be certain that the length and location of the intramedullary nail are satisfactory (**H**). The proximal fibers of the deltoid muscle are resutured (**I**). Following closure of both wounds, the arm is placed in a sling and swath.

POSTOPERATIVE MANAGEMENT. Mobilization in a sling and swath is continued until there is early clinical or roentgenographic evidence of at least partial healing at the fracture site. Then a program of gentle active range of motion exercises is instituted and increased progressively. Emphasis is placed on regaining active elbow and shoulder motion while protecting against rotational stress at the fracture site until fracture union is solid.

CURETTAGE AND BONE GRAFT FOR BENIGN BONE CYST (HUMERUS) (Plate 2-3)

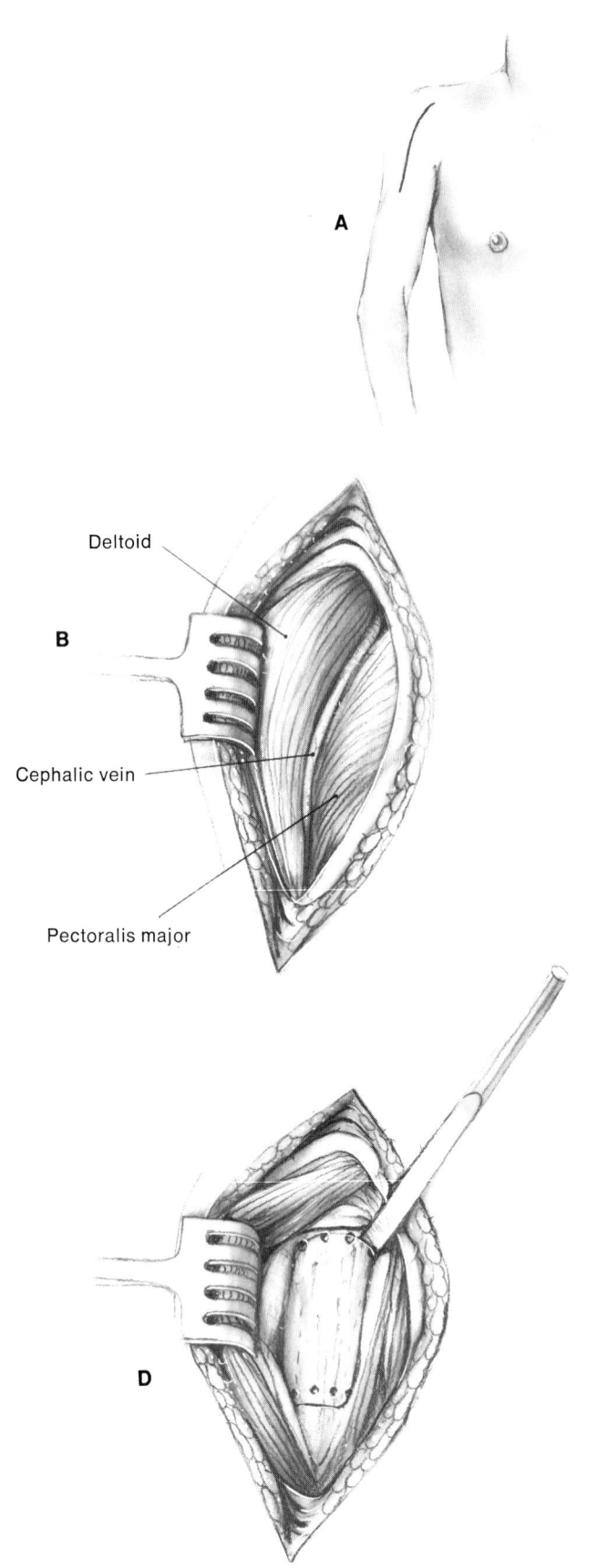

GENERAL DISCUSSION. The solitary bone cyst is characteristically found in the metaphyseal region of the tubular bones. The most common location of this benign bone lesion is in the proximal humerus. The solitary or unicameral bone cyst is often characterized by some thinning and expansion of the cortex, but there will be no periosteal reaction about the cyst unless a recent pathologic fracture has occurred through the cyst wall.

The recommended treatment for a solitary bone cyst is thorough curettage of the bone cyst and packing of the cavity with autogenous iliac bone. The cyst is often first noted after a pathologic fracture, and, if such is the case, it is best to allow the fracture to heal for at least 6 weeks before any definitive treatment of the bone cyst. If the bone cyst is noted in the metaphyseal region of a bone immediately adjacent to the epiphyseal plate, it is advisable, if possible, to delay and definitive treatment until the epiphysis has migrated away from the cyst so as to permit thorough curettage of the cyst without exposure to injury of the epiphyseal plate at the time of surgery.

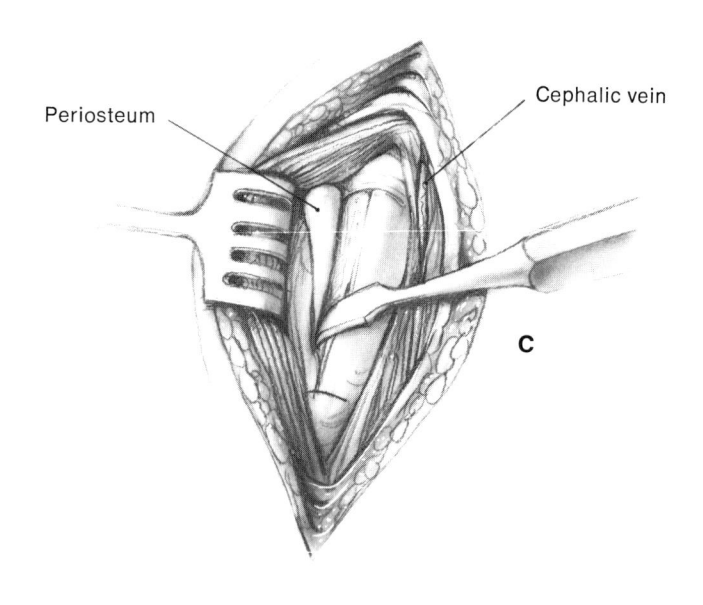

DETAILS OF PROCEDURE. The region of the bone cyst is exposed through an appropriate approach to that portion of the long bone. If the cyst is located in the proximal metaphysis of the humerus, an anterior approach is used **(A)**. The dissection is carried down through the deltopectoral groove, the cephalic vein being retracted medially to expose an adequate area of the anterior cortex **(B)**. The periosteum is reflected, and a large window is outlined with drill holes and then removed to expose the underlying bone cyst (**C** and **D**).

(Plate 2-3) CURETTAGE AND BONE GRAFT FOR BENIGN BONE CYST (HUMERUS)

Sections are taken for pathologic study, and then the entire contents of the cavity are removed, including all portions of any soft tissue lining. Likewise, any sclerotic wall that surrounds the cyst is removed to expose normal medullary bone (**E** and **F**).

Autogenous bone is then taken from the ilium. If the cyst is small, it is packed entirely with fresh cancellous bone (**G**). A cyst that is too large to be packed entirely with fresh autogenous cancellous bone is packed with cancellous bone and cut pieces of cortical bone obtained from one table of the ilium. After all portions of the thoroughly curetted cyst have been effectively packed with fresh autogenous bone, the periosteum and overlying soft tissues are closed in layers (**H**), but the removed window of cortical bone is not replaced. In the case of the proximal humerus, the arm is placed in a sling and swath until healed.

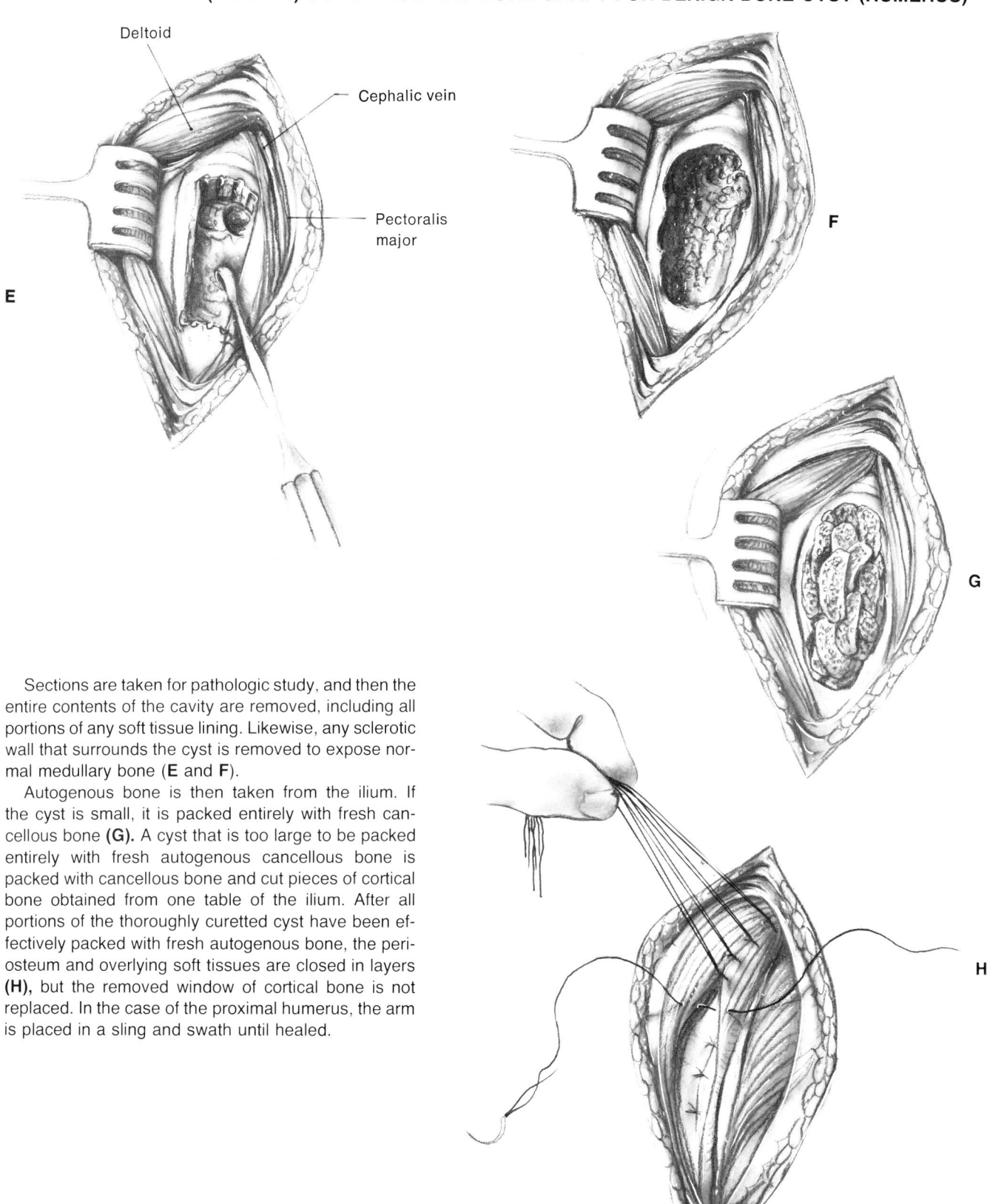

CURETTAGE AND BONE GRAFT FOR BENIGN BONE CYST (HUMERUS) (Plate 2-3)

Fracture through a bone cyst in the proximal humerus is shown in **I**. Early healing of the fracture is shown in **J**. The same area is shown after curettage and packing of the cyst with cancellous bone (**K** and **L**).

POSTOPERATIVE MANAGEMENT. The involved bone is protected in a sling and swath in the early postoperative period and subsequently in a sling alone until there is clinical and roentgenographic evidence of stability that will safely allow resumption of normal functional activity. This may take from 6 to 12 weeks as a rule, depending on the age of the child.

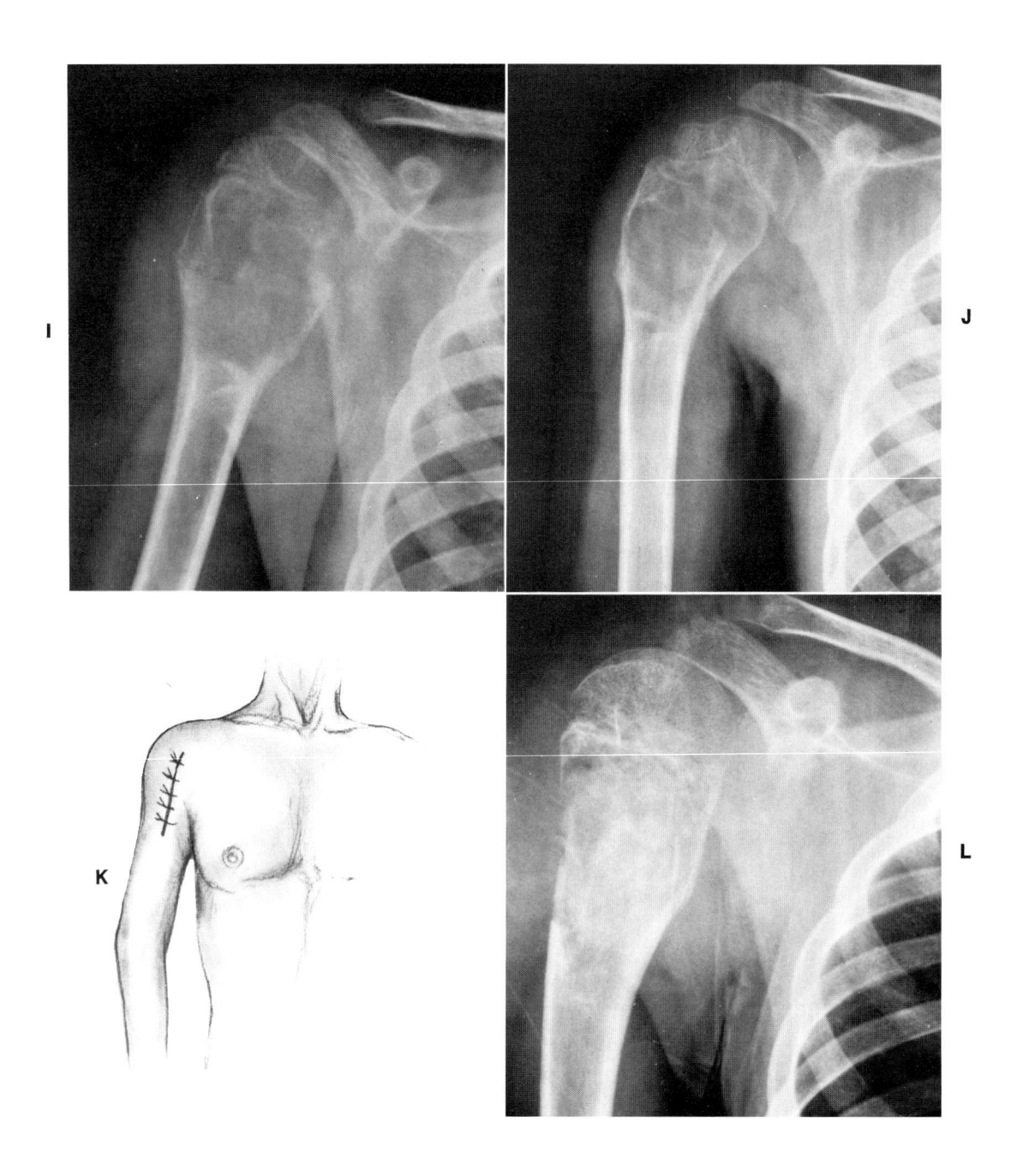

(Plate 2-4) TENODESIS OF TENDON OF LONG HEAD OF BICEPS

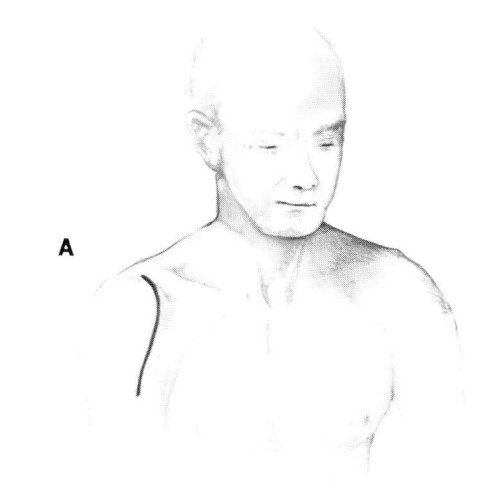

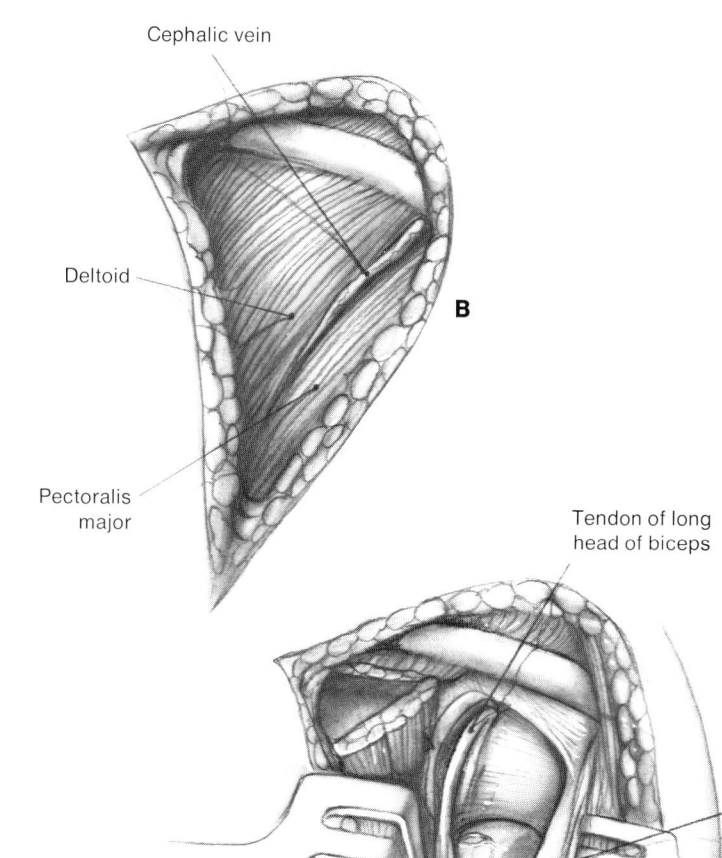

GENERAL DISCUSSION. Bicipital tenosynovitis is only one of many possible shoulder lesions that may produce pain and limitation of movement in the shoulder. When tenosynovitis of the tendon of the long head of the biceps is present (as a primary or secondary cause of shoulder pain) and does not respond to conservative treatment, tenodesis of the long head of the biceps in the bicipital groove can provide relief. Bicipital tenosynovitis is most common in people of middle age or older. Characteristically, the patient will have tenderness to palpation directly over the bicipital groove. Anterior elevation of the shoulder against resistance with the elbow extended will produce pain in the bicipital groove, and, in the early stages, shoulder motion may be normal. Limitation of shoulder motion will be present if there has been symptomatic repetitive irritation of the tendon of the long head of the biceps within the bicipital groove for more than a few weeks.

DETAILS OF PROCEDURE. A curvilinear incision is made to expose the anterior aspect of the humerus from an anterior approach **(A)**. The deltopectoral groove is identified **(B)**. The cephalic vein and pectoralis major muscle are retracted medially. Then 2 to 3 cm of the anterior portion of the deltoid are divided from its attachment to the clavicle to facilitate lateral retraction of the deltoid, if necessary, to expose the underlying long head of the biceps **(C)**. Among patients who have been symptomatic with bicipital tenosynovitis, the position of the tendon of the long head of the biceps may be found medial to its normal location in the bicipital groove (particularly if the arm and shoulder are positioned in full external rotation), and the slope of the medial wall of the bicipital groove formed by the edge of the lesser tuberosity may be shallow.

TENODESIS OF TENDON OF LONG HEAD OF BICEPS (Plate 2-4)

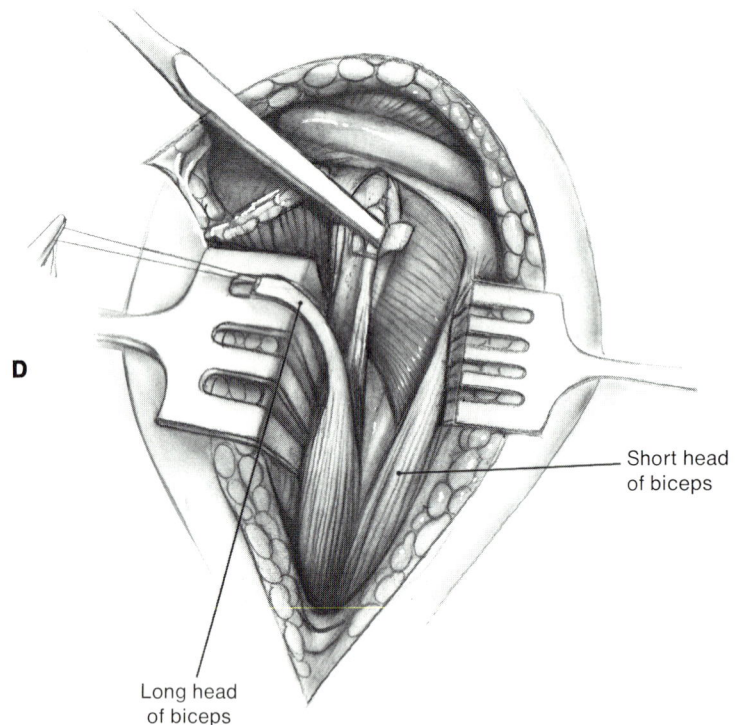

The transverse humeral ligament is incised and the shoulder capsule is opened to allow division of the long head of the biceps as close as possible to the supraglenoid tubercle of the scapula. To accomplish this, it may be necessary to divide the coracoacromial ligament. With a broad, curved osteotome, a bony bed for insertion of the long head of the biceps is created in the proximal humerus about 1 cm lateral to the bicipital groove and parallel to it **(D)**. The location of the area selected for tenodesis of the long head of the biceps into the proximal humerus must be sufficiently distal to the shoulder joint so as to avoid any possible interference with full excursion of the glenohumeral joint. The previously divided long head of the biceps is anchored securely in this trough, and the redundant portion of tendon is excised at the proximal end of the trough **(E)**. The coracoacromial ligament is identified and divided if this has not already been done earlier in the procedure. The wound is closed in layers.

POSTOPERATIVE MANAGEMENT. The arm is placed in a sling with a posterior plaster splint holding the forearm is supination. At 2 weeks the posterior plaster splint is removed and a program of gentle, but progressive circumduction exercises is instituted. The arm is protected in a sling between exercises for an additional 2 weeks. Any forceful active elbow flexion against resistance is specifically avoided for at least 8 weeks postoperatively.

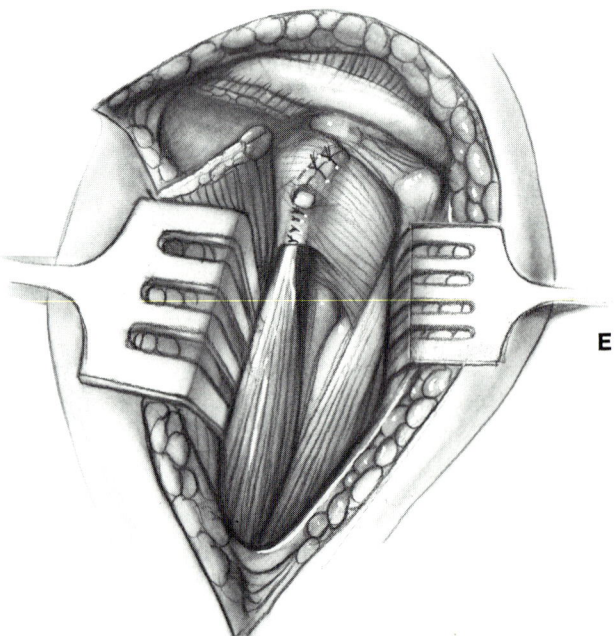

(Plate 2-5) ABOVE-ELBOW AMPUTATION

GENERAL DISCUSSION. Amputation in the upper arm is occasionally necessary for an irreparably damaged or diseased arm.

DETAILS OF PROCEDURE. The arm is extended to the side in a position of shoulder abduction and draped so that the shoulder may be turned freely into internal or external rotation. Anterior and posterior skin flaps are mapped out with the proximal end of incision medially and laterally at a level equal to the level of intended bone division (which should be at least 4 cm proximal to the elbow joint if carried out in the supracondylar area) (**A** and **B**). The neurovascular bundle is identified on the medial aspect of the arm. The brachial artery is doubly ligated and divided. Individual nerves are divided so that the proximal end of each nerve will retract to a level proximal to the end of the stump (**C**). The muscles in the anterior compartment are divided 1 to 2 cm distal to the level of intended bone division, so the retracted level of these muscles will permit a good stump closure.

A

B

C

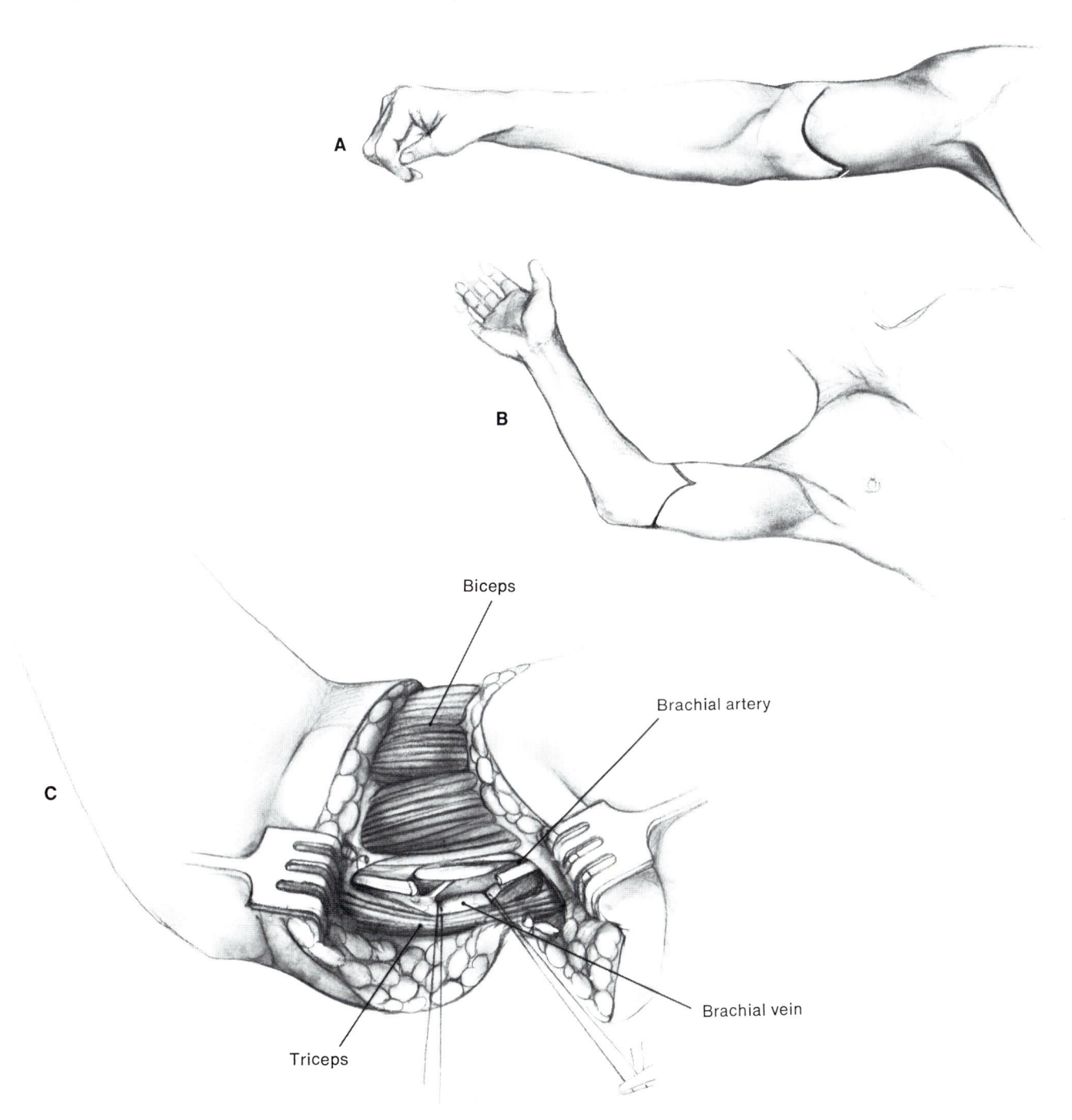

Biceps

Brachial artery

Brachial vein

Triceps

59

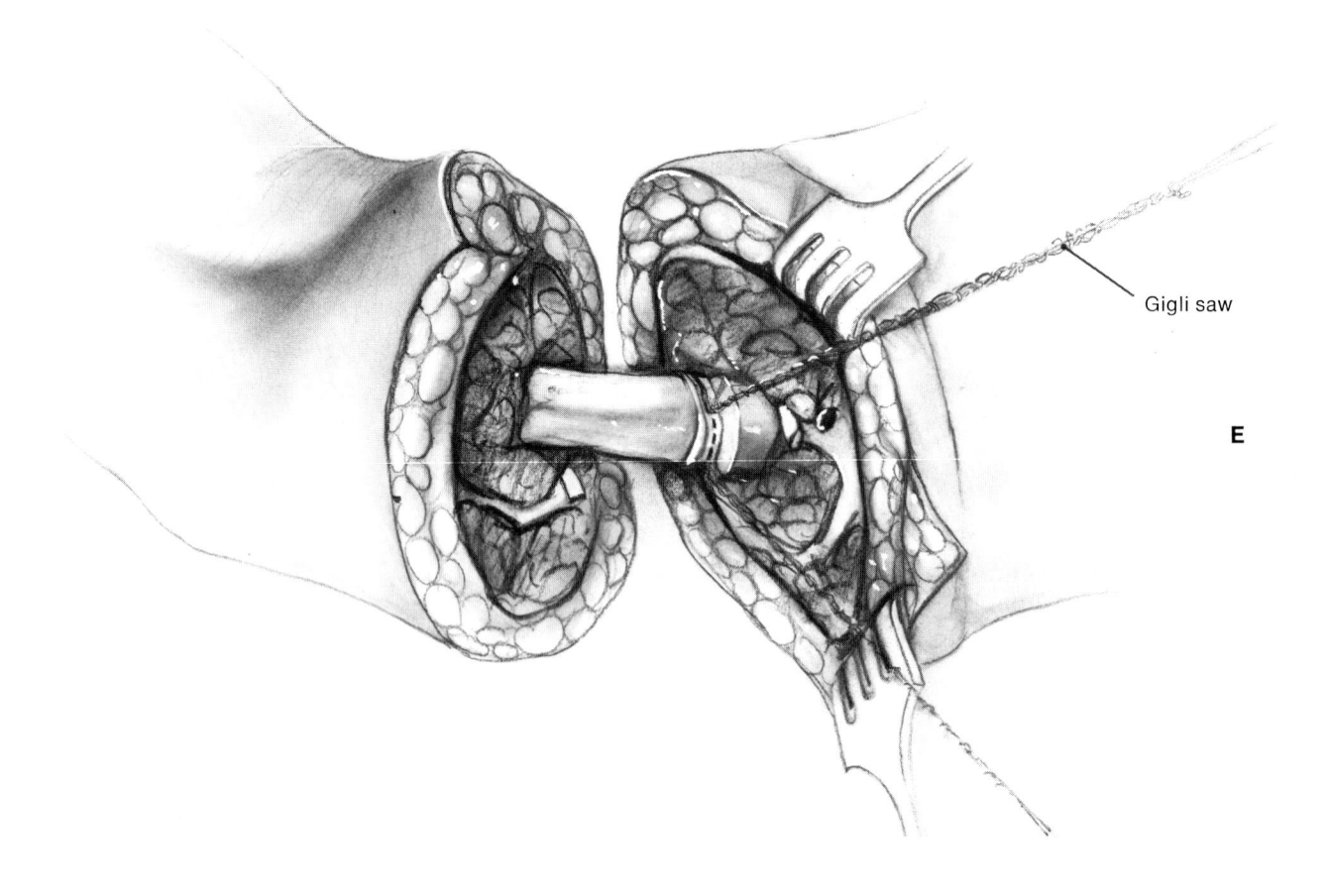

ABOVE-ELBOW AMPUTATION (Plate 2-5)

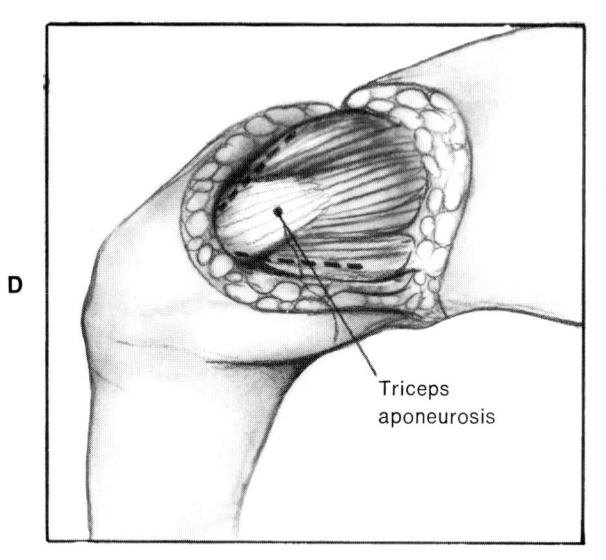

D — Triceps aponeurosis

Shoulder in internal rotation

On the posterior aspect of the arm the skin and subcutaneous tissue are incised in line with the outlined posterior flap. The distal portion of the wound is retracted to allow the triceps tendon to be divided at a more distal level toward its insertion into the olecranon process **(D)**. The humerus is divided transversely at the intended level after all muscles have been divided and the periosteum has been incised circumferentially **(E)**.

E — Gigli saw

(Plate 2-5) ABOVE-ELBOW AMPUTATION

The triceps aponeurosis is sutured to the fascia overlying the muscles anteriorly, and, if needed, a Penrose drain may be left deep to the fascia. The fascia, subcutaneous tissue, and skin are closed in layers with interrupted sutures (**F** and **G**). A light compression dressing is applied.

POSTOPERATIVE MANAGEMENT. The Penrose drain is removed on the first postoperative day, but a light compression dressing is continued. Sutures are removed approximately 2 weeks postoperatively. Early fitting and use of a temporary prosthesis is encouraged while the patient's permanent elbow prosthesis is being fabricated. The permanent prosthesis should include a turntable mechanism to help with rotational positions and an elbow-lock mechanism to permit stabilization of the prosthetic elbow in variable positions between full extension and full flexion.

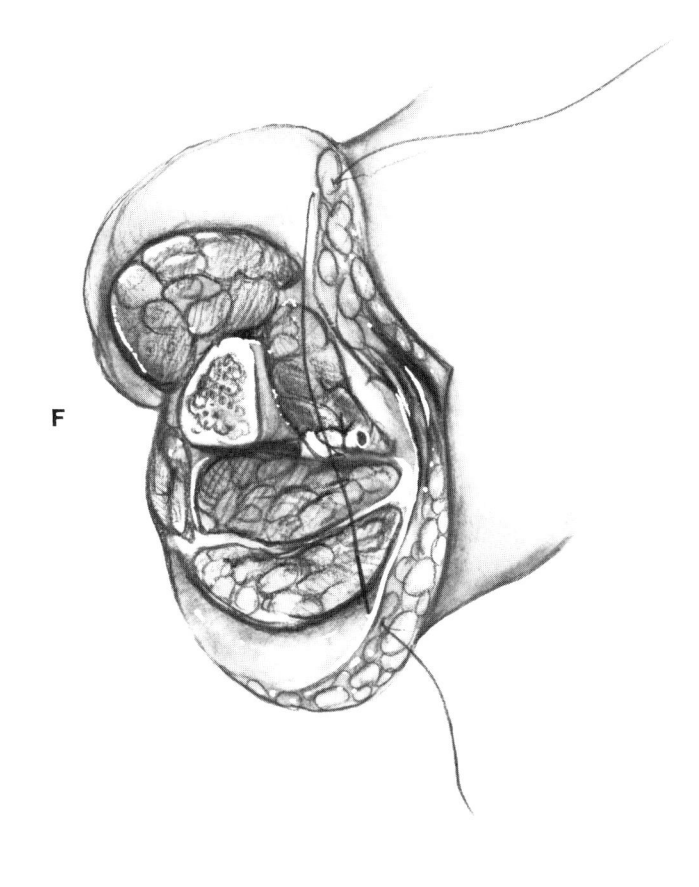

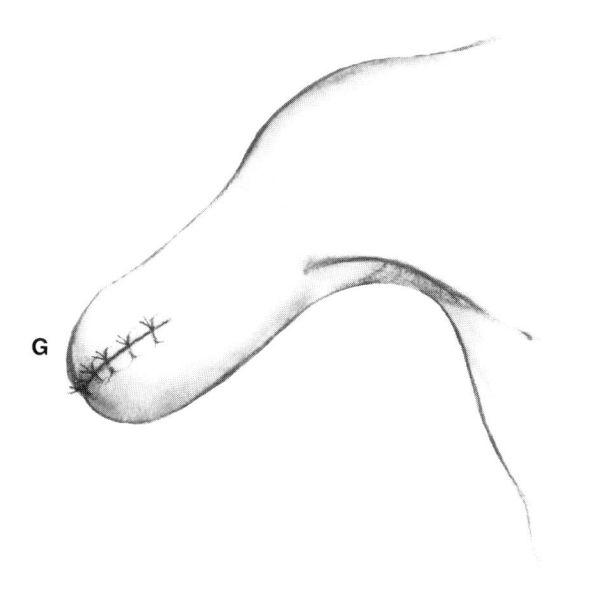

SUPRACONDYLAR OSTEOTOMY OF HUMERUS (Plate 2-6)

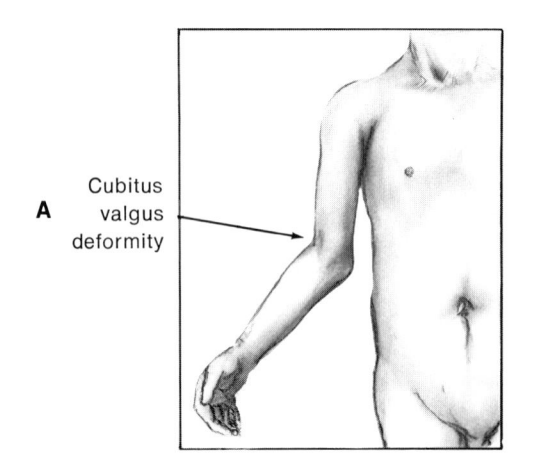

GENERAL DISCUSSION. Angular and rotational deformities may occur after certain fractures about the elbow in children. There may be a pure cubitus varus or cubitus valgus deformity **(A)**, or there may be a combination of angular and rotational deformity. If the deformity is pronounced, it may be unsightly and may represent a handicap functionally. A delayed ulnar nerve palsy may also develop with a cubitus valgus deformity. If ulnar nerve symptoms are present, the ulnar nerve should be transferred anteriorly at the time of the corrective osteotomy. The corrective osteotomy should be planned preoperatively on the basis of a careful clinical and roentgenographic examination of the deformed elbow to correct simultaneously whatever rotational or angular deformity exists, with consideration of the age of the patient and anticipated future growth from the secondary ossification centers about the elbow.

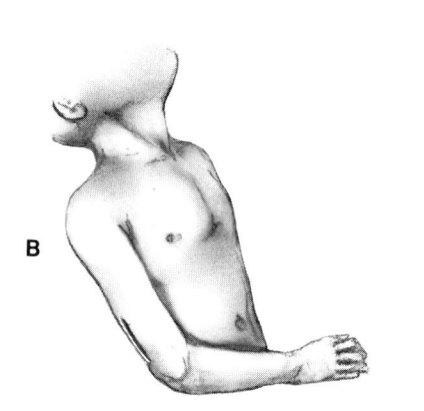

DETAILS OF PROCEDURE. A longitudinal incision is made on the posterior aspect of the distal third of the upper arm **(B)**. The triceps tendon and muscle are split longitudinally in the direction of their fibers, and the distal humerus is exposed subperiosteally **(C)**. The predetermined wedge of bone is outlined with drill holes **(D)** and removed with a sharp osteotome, the surgeon working subperiosteally to avoid damage to the adjacent neurovascular structures. An alternate technique is a dome-shaped osteotomy.

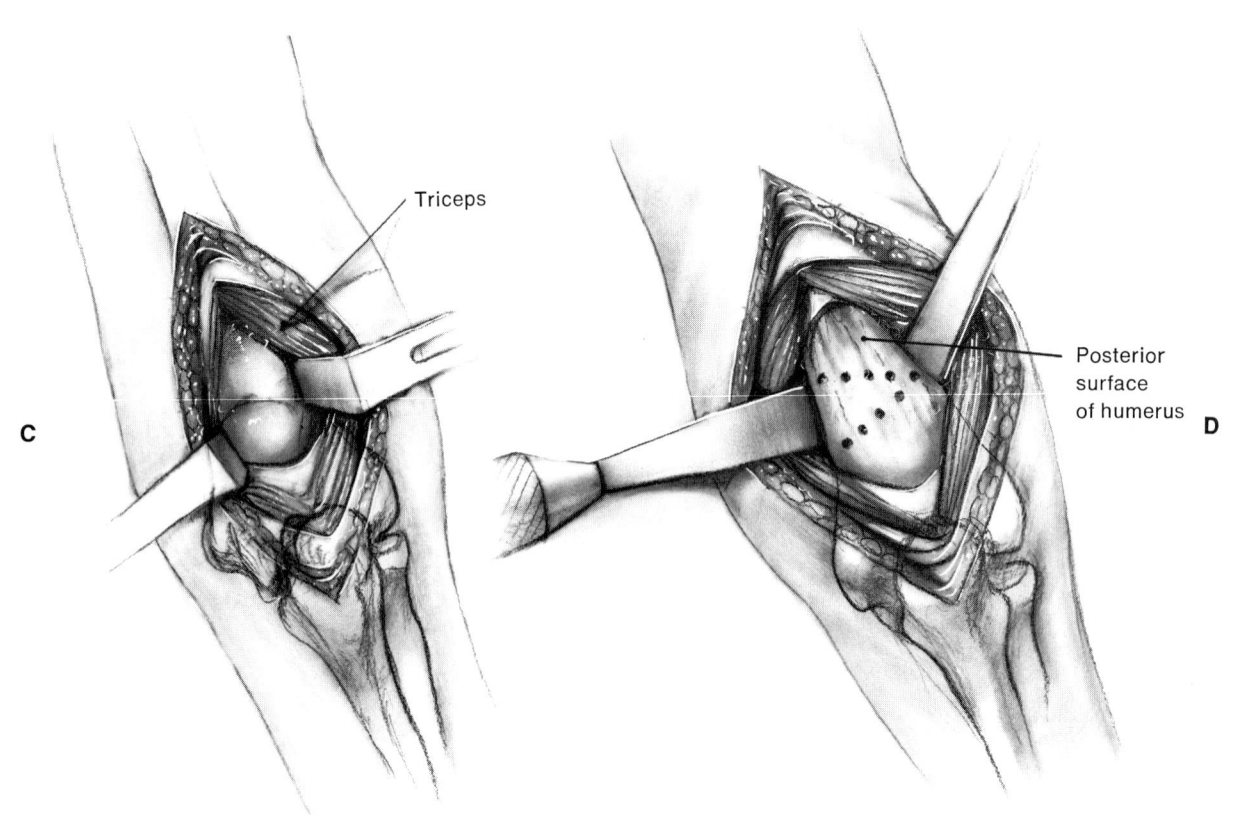

(Plate 2-6) SUPRACONDYLAR OSTEOTOMY OF HUMERUS

E

F

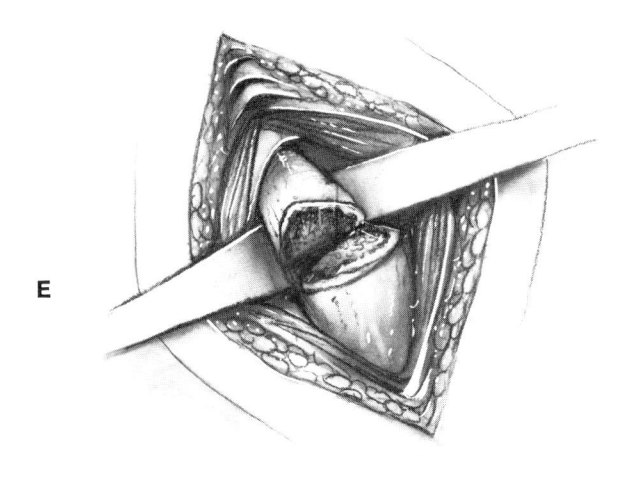

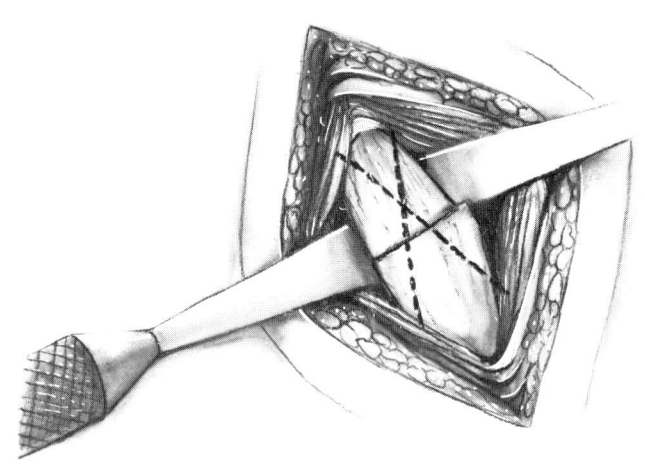

G Postoperative arm position with forearm in supination

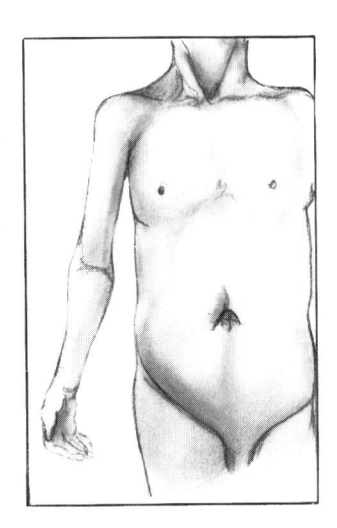

H Kirschner wires

With the wedge of bone removed **(E)**, the existing deformity is corrected manually **(G)**, the two humeral fragments being brought into contact after removal of the bone wedge. Kirschner wires may be used for internal fixation **(F and H)**, or possibly internal fixation may be omitted, allowing postoperative adjustment of the position of the bone fragments by cast change or wedging. The wound is closed in layers, and the arm is immobilized in a long arm cast.

POSTOPERATIVE MANAGEMENT. The upper extremity is protected in plaster and a sling and swath until the osteotomy site is solidly united.

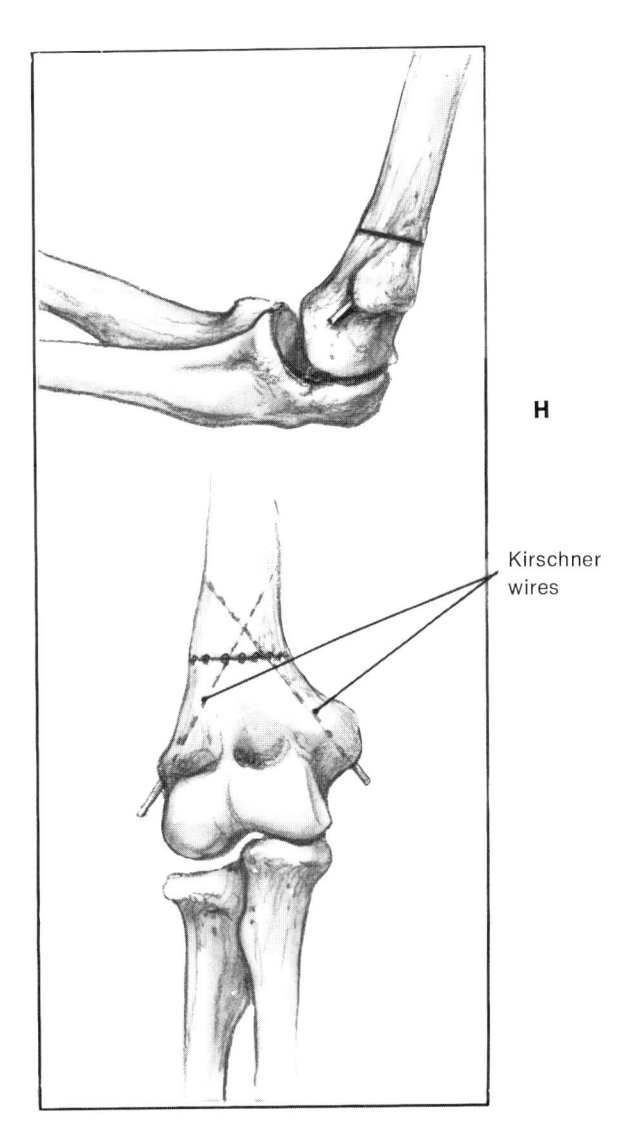

63

REFERENCES

Abbott, L. C., and Saunders, J. B. deC. M.: Acute traumatic dislocation of the tendon of the long head of the biceps brachii; report of 6 cases with operative findings, Surgery **6**:817, 1939.

Alldredge, R. H.: General principles of amputations and artificial limbs in the upper extremity, American Academy of Orthopaedic Surgeons Instructional Course Lectures, vol. 8, Ann Arbor, 1951, J. W. Edwards, p. 232.

Aufranc, O. E.: Nonunion of humerus, J.A.M.A. **175**:1092, 1961.

Boseker, E. H., Bickel, W. H., and Dahlin, D. C.: A clinicopathologic study of simple unicameral bone cysts, Surg. Gynecol. Obstet. **127**:550, 1968.

Burkhalter, W. E., Mayfield, G., and Carmona, L. S.: The upper-extremity amputee. Early and immediate post-surgical prosthetic fitting, J. Bone Joint Surg. **58-A**:46, 1976.

Clark, J. M. P.: Reconstruction of biceps brachii by pectoral muscle transplantation, Br. J. Surg. **34**:180, 1946.

Cohen, J.: Simple bone cysts. Studies of cyst fluid in six cases with a theory of pathogenesis, J. Bone Joint Surg. **42-A**:609, 1960.

Cohen, J.: Etiology of simple bone cyst, J. Bone Joint Surg. **52-A**:1493, 1970.

Coventry, M. B., and Laurnen, E. L.: Ununited fractures of the middle and upper humerus. Special problems in treatment, Clin. Orthop. **69**:192, 1970.

Crenshaw, A. H., and Kilgore, W. E.: Surgical treatment of bicipital tenosynovitis, J. Bone Joint Surg. **48-A**:1496, 1966.

DePalma, A. F., and Callery, G. E.: Bicipital tenosynovitis, Clin. Orthop. **3**:69, 1954,

DePalma, A. F., Callery, G., and Bennett, G. A.: Variation anatomy and degenerative lesions of the shoulder joint, American Academy of Orthopaedic Surgeons Instructional Course Lectures, vol. 6, Ann Arbor, 1949, J. W. Edwards, p. 255.

French, P. R.: Varus deformity of the elbow following supracondylar fractures of the humerus in children, Lancet **1**:439, 1959.

Garceau, G. J., and Gregory, C. F.: Solitary unicameral bone cyst, J. Bone Joint Surg. **36-A**:267, 1954.

Garcia, A., Jr., and Maeck, B. H.: Radial nerve injuries in fractures of the shaft of the humerus, Am. J. Surg. **99**:625, 1960.

Goodfellow, J. W., and Agerholm, J. C.: Simple cysts of the humerus treated by radical excision. J. Bone Joint Surg. **47-B**:714, 1965.

Hall, C. B., and Bechtol, C. O.: Modern amputation technique in the upper extremity, J. Bone Joint Surg. **45-A**:1717, 1963.

Hitchcock, H. H., and Bechtol, C. O.: Painful shoulder. Observations on the role of the tendon of the long head of the biceps brachii in its causation, J. Bone Joint Surg. **30-A**:263, 1948.

Holster, A., and Lewis, G. B.: Fractures of the humerus with radial-nerve paralysis, J. Bone Joint Surg. **45-A**:1382, 1963.

Jacobs, R. J., and Brady, W. M.: Early postsurgical fitting in upper extremity amputations, J. Trauma **15**:966, 1975.

Jaffe, H. F.: Tumors and tumorous conditions of the bones and joints, Philadelphia, 1958, Lea & Febiger.

Johansson, O.: Complications and failures of surgery in various fractures of the humerus, Acta Chir. Scand. **120**:469, 1961.

Johnson, L. C., and Kindred, R. G.: Anatomy of bone cysts (in Proceedings of the Joint Meeting of the Orthopaedic Associations of the English-speaking World), J. Bone Joint Surg. **40-A**:1440, 1958.

King, D., and Secor, C.: Bow elbow (cubitus varus), J. Bone Joint Surg. **33-A**:572, 1951.

Lambert, C. N.: Upper extremity prostheses in juvenile amputees, J. Bone Joint Surg. **38-A**:421, 1956.

Neer, C. S., II., Francis, K. C., Marcove, R. C., Terz, J., and Carbonara, P. N.: Treatment of unicameral bone cyst. A follow-up study of one hundred seventy-five cases, J. Bone Joint Surg. **48-A**:731, 1966.

Shaw, J. L., and Sakellarides, H.: Radial-nerve paralysis associated with fractures of the humerus. A review of 45 cases, J. Bone Joint Surg. **49-A**:899, 1967.

Slocum, D. B.: The present status of amputation surgery of the upper extremity, American Academy of Orthopaedic Surgeons Instructional Course Lectures, vol. 12, Ann Arbor, 1955, J. W. Edwards, p. 207.

Smith, L.: Deformity following supracondylar fractures of the humerus, J. Bone Joint Surg. **42-A**:235, 1960.

Soto-Hall, R., and Stroot, J. H.: Treatment of ruptures of the long head of biceps brachii, Am. J. Orthop. **2**:192, 1960.

Spence, K. F., Sell, K. W., and Brown, R. H.: Solitary bone cyst: treatment with freeze-dried cancellous bone allograft. A study of one hundred seventy-seven cases, J. Bone Joint Surg. **51-A**:87, 1969.

Stewart, M. J., and Hundley, J. M.: Fractures of the humerus, J. Bone Joint Surg. **38-A**:681, 1955.

Wilbur, M. C., and Hyatt, J. W.: Bone cysts: results of surgical treatment in two hundred cases. (in Proceedings of the American Academy of Orthopaedic Surgeons), J. Bone Joint Surg. **42-A**:879, 1960.

3

ELBOW

EXCISION OF RADIAL HEAD (Plate 3-1)

GENERAL DISCUSSION. Early excision of the radial head can improve the functional end result following certain injuries of the radiohumeral joint: (1) displaced fractures involving the articular surface of the radial head with disruption of more than one third of the articular surface of the radial head, (2) severe comminuted fractures of the radial head, and (3) angulated fractures of the radial neck when stable reduction and satisfactory realignment of the radiohumeral and radioulnar joints cannot be achieved by other means. It occasionally may be necessary to excise the radial head when loose bony fragments are lodged within the radiohumeral joint. It is preferable to excise any small bone fragments while leaving the radial head in place if this is feasible with any individual fracture involving the radial head or capitulum of the humerus.

The radial head should never be excised in a growing child. Moreover, excision of the radial head should be carried out with caution if there is any associated proximal ulnar fracture creating relative instability of the proximal ulna. If the radial head is to be excised, it is best to do this within 48 hours of injury. The end result following late excision of malunited fractures of the radial head is likely to be disappointing.

DETAILS OF PROCEDURE. With the patient supine and the elbow supported in 90° flexion, an incision is made beginning just proximal to the lateral epicondyle of the humerus and then along the forearm to end 3½ fingerbreadths distal to the olecranon tip and posterior to the radial tuberosity (**A**). The interval between the anconeus muscle and the extensor carpi ulnaris muscle is most easily identified in the distal portion of the wound (**B**). Development of the plane between these muscles (with care to protect the posterior interosseous nerve) will permit exposure of the capsule of the radiohumeral joint. The capsule of the radiohumeral joint is incised longitudinally (**D**), and the radial head and neck are exposed down to the level of the bicipital tuberosity. When the joint is inspected, the radial head is frequently found to be more severely injured than suspected on the basis of preoperative roentgenograms (**C**).

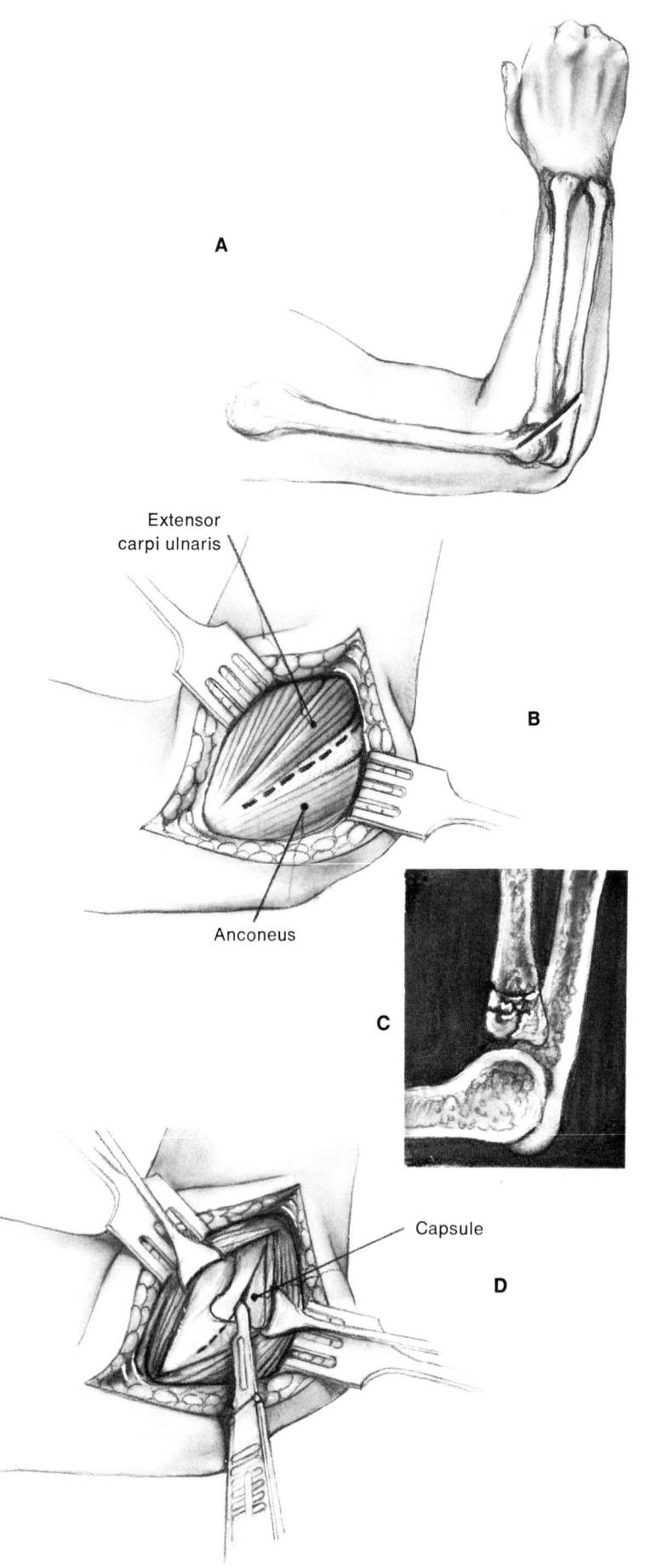

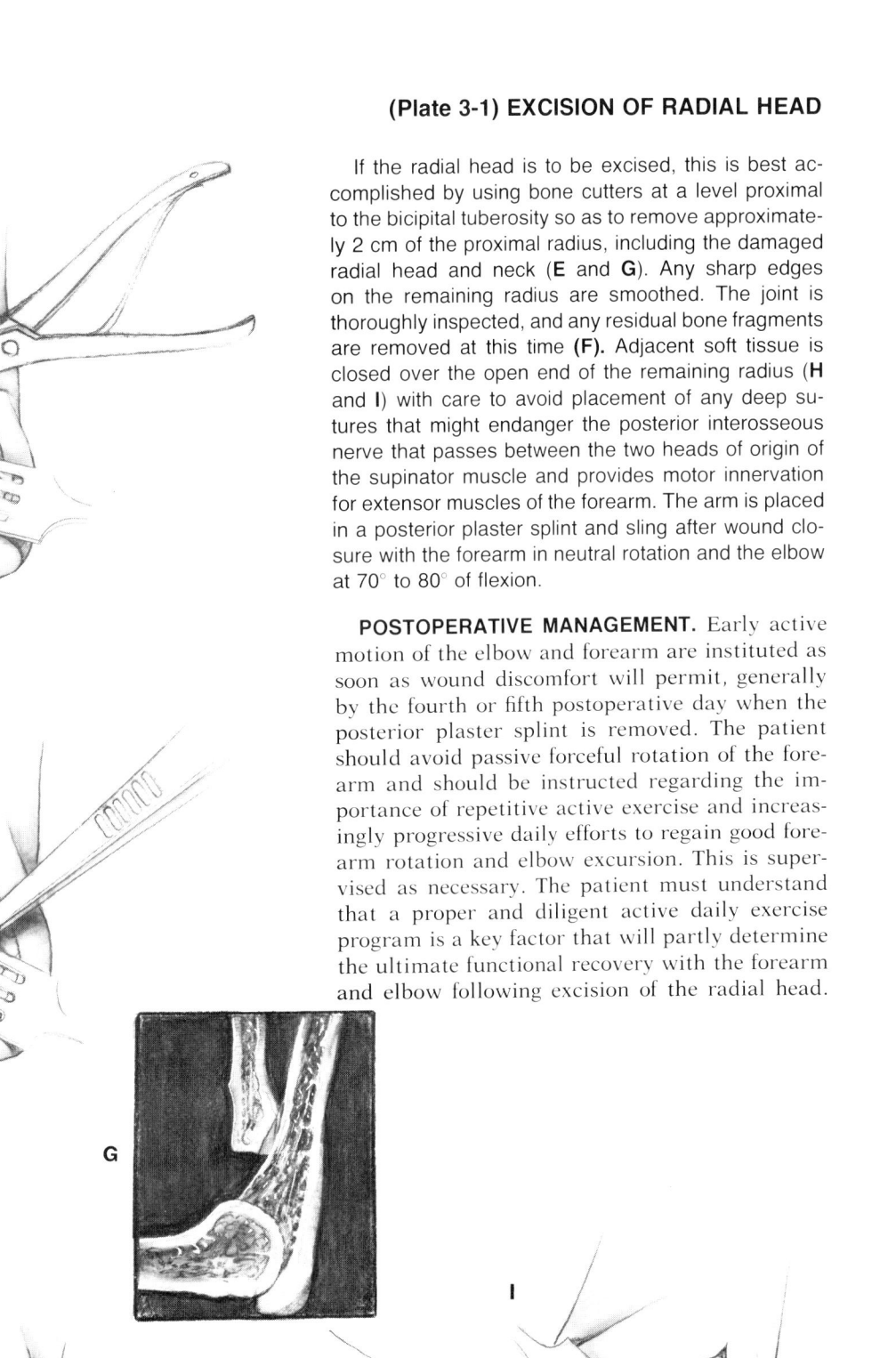

(Plate 3-1) EXCISION OF RADIAL HEAD

If the radial head is to be excised, this is best accomplished by using bone cutters at a level proximal to the bicipital tuberosity so as to remove approximately 2 cm of the proximal radius, including the damaged radial head and neck (**E** and **G**). Any sharp edges on the remaining radius are smoothed. The joint is thoroughly inspected, and any residual bone fragments are removed at this time (**F**). Adjacent soft tissue is closed over the open end of the remaining radius (**H** and **I**) with care to avoid placement of any deep sutures that might endanger the posterior interosseous nerve that passes between the two heads of origin of the supinator muscle and provides motor innervation for extensor muscles of the forearm. The arm is placed in a posterior plaster splint and sling after wound closure with the forearm in neutral rotation and the elbow at 70° to 80° of flexion.

POSTOPERATIVE MANAGEMENT. Early active motion of the elbow and forearm are instituted as soon as wound discomfort will permit, generally by the fourth or fifth postoperative day when the posterior plaster splint is removed. The patient should avoid passive forceful rotation of the forearm and should be instructed regarding the importance of repetitive active exercise and increasingly progressive daily efforts to regain good forearm rotation and elbow excursion. This is supervised as necessary. The patient must understand that a proper and diligent active daily exercise program is a key factor that will partly determine the ultimate functional recovery with the forearm and elbow following excision of the radial head.

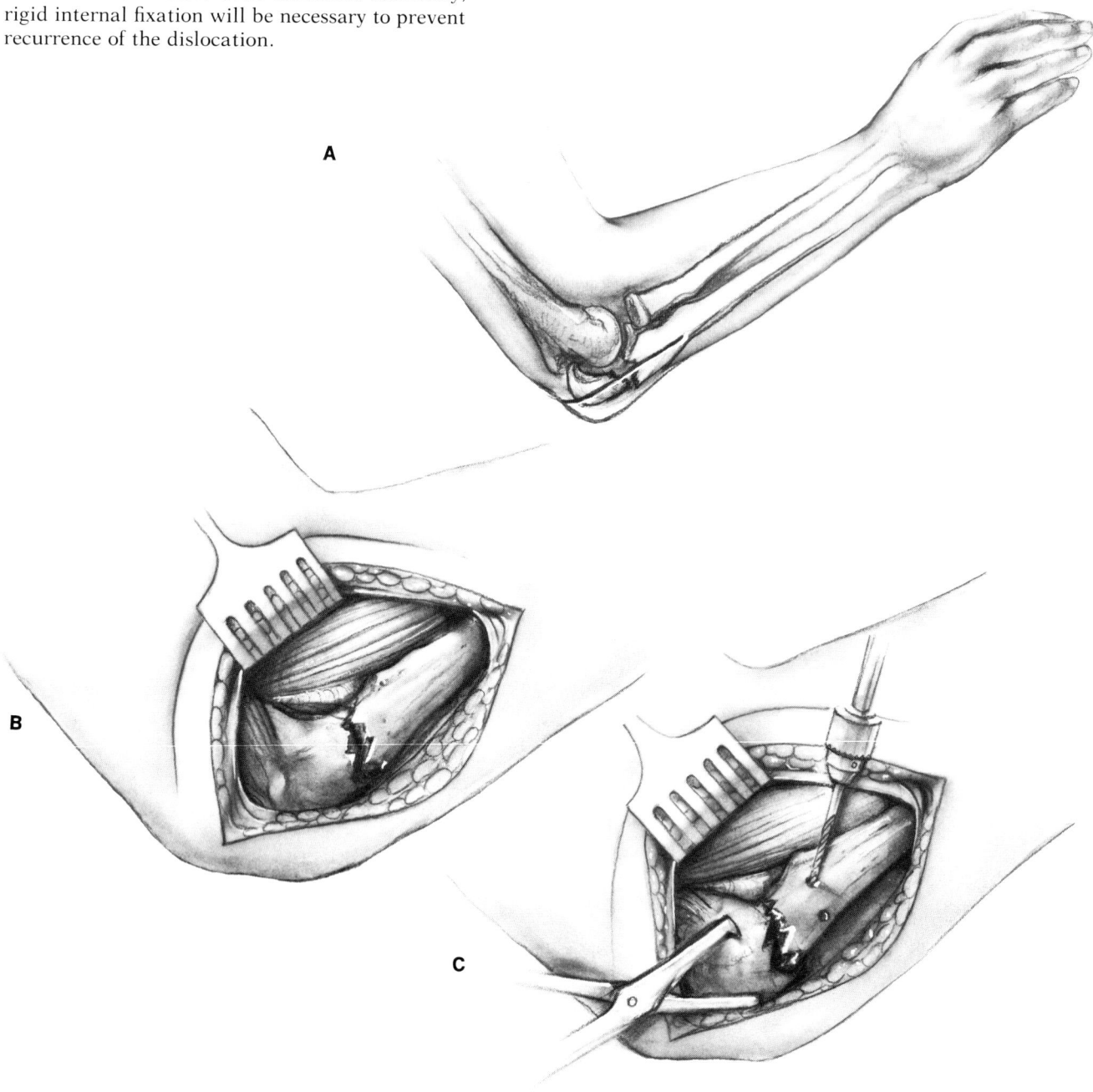

OPEN REDUCTION AND INTERNAL FIXATION FOR FRACTURE OF OLECRANON (Plate 3-2)

GENERAL DISCUSSION. For fractures of the olecranon with separation of the fragments, open reduction and anatomic restoration of the concave surface that articulates with the capitulum of the humerus in addition to restoration of stability of the proximal ulna is important. Intramedullary fixation is preferred, although alternative repair with a figure-of-eight wire loop may be considered for fractures of the olecranon that are not comminuted and when the proximal fragment involves less than half of the concave articular surface of the olecranon. If the head of the radius and proximal shaft of the ulna have been dislocated anteriorly, rigid internal fixation will be necessary to prevent recurrence of the dislocation.

DETAILS OF PROCEDURE. The patient is in the supine position with the elbow flexed at 90° and the forearm across the patient's abdomen. An incision is made across the posterior aspect of the olecranon process and approximately 6 cm distally along the lateral aspect of the olecranon **(A)**. The skin and its thin layer of subcutaneous tissue are retracted together to expose the fracture site. The fracture site is inspected, and any irregular fragments that might prevent anatomic reduction of the fracture are reoriented **(B)**. Any loose fragments of bone within the elbow joint are removed. It is helpful to create two small drill holes adjacent to the fracture in the distal fragment to permit firm seating for the bone-holding clamps (or a Bishop clamp) **(C)**.

(Plate 3-2) OPEN REDUCTION AND INTERNAL FIXATION FOR FRACTURE OF OLECRANON

The olecranon fracture is reduced and held with a Bishop clamp or two separate clamps so placed that they will not interfere with insertion of the intramedullary fixation device. An AOI olecranon screw usually will provide satisfactory fixation for this fracture. If this type of intramedullary fixation device is selected, the entry hole in the proximal fragment of the olecranon must be overdrilled corresponding to the diameter of the selected olecranon screw to allow a subsequent lag effect when the cancellous olecranon screw is tightened in its final position to hold the olecranon fragments. A portion of the cancellous bone within the medullary space is also prepared with a tap prior to insertion of the AOI olecranon screw **(D)**. All threads of the olecranon screw should ultimately be in the medullary space of the distal fragment **(E)**. After final insertion of the olecranon screw, the bone-holding clamps are carefully removed. Security of the internal fixation device may be checked at this time by passively moving the elbow. The wound is closed, and a well-padded long-arm cast is applied with the elbow in 80° to 90° of flexion.

POSTOPERATIVE MANAGEMENT. If the intramedullary fixation was secure when checked prior to wound closure, the cast may be removed at 3 weeks to begin gentle active range of motion exercises. If the nature of the fracture or the degree of stability appears to warrant a longer period of external immobilization, the long-arm cast may be continued as long as 6 weeks. Forceful elbow extension against resistance is avoided until there is clinical and roentgenographic evidence of bony union at the fracture site.

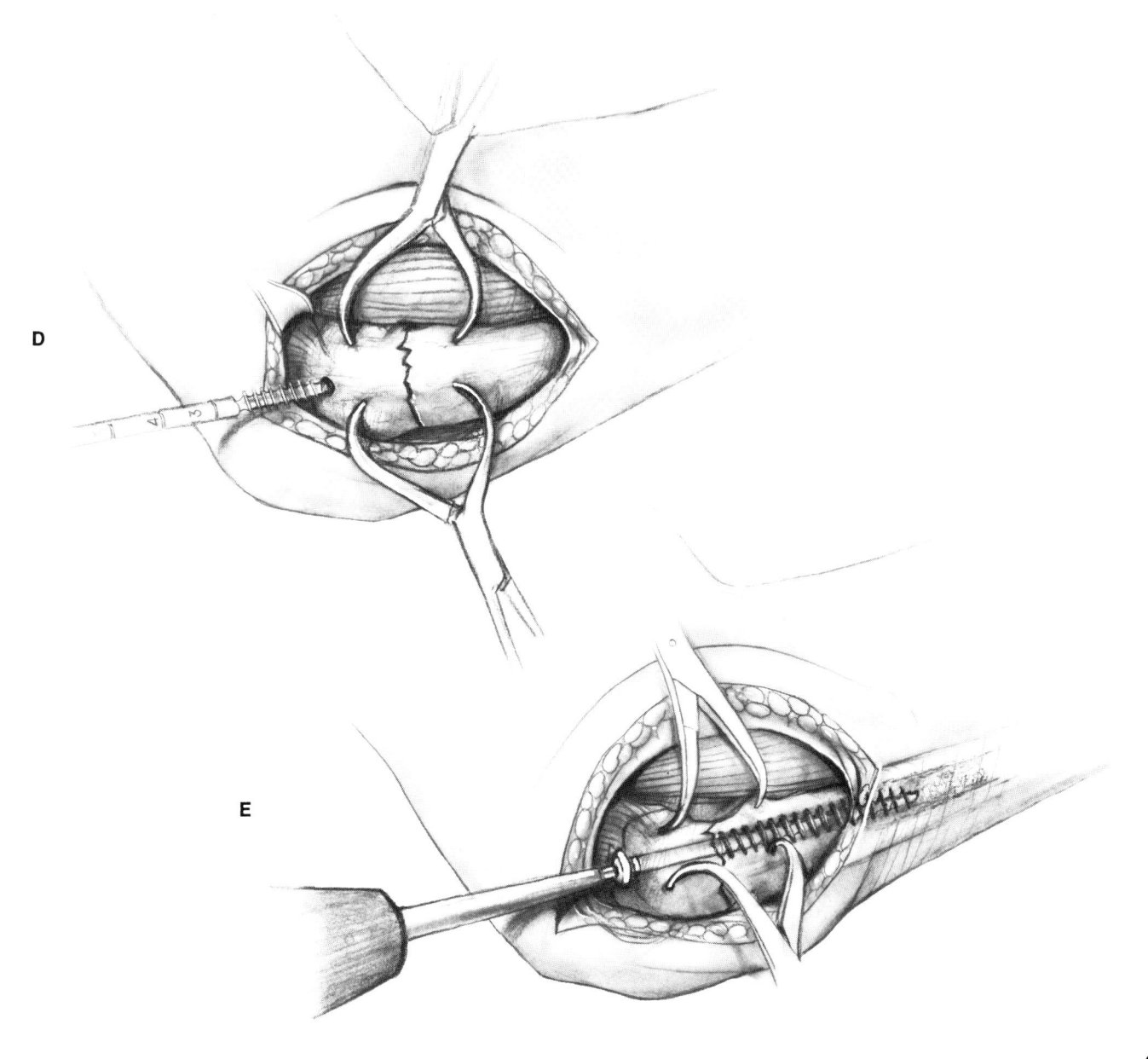

EXCISION OF PROXIMAL ULNA (FOLLOWING OLECRANON FRACTURE) WITH REATTACHMENT OF TRICEPS (Plate 3-3)

GENERAL DISCUSSION. For comminuted fractures of the proximal portion of the olecranon, particularly among patients over 50 years of age who are not required to do heavy work with the involved elbow, excision of the proximal ulnar fragments with reattachment of the triceps is a satisfactory procedure that permits relatively rapid convalescence and can result in good functional recovery and a comfortable elbow. To ensure a satisfactory result, the triceps expansion must be securely reattached to the remaining portion of the proximal ulna.

DETAILS OF PROCEDURE. The patient is in the supine position. The arm is supported with the elbow flexed at approximately 80°. The incision begins over the posterior aspect of the arm approximately 10 cm above the olecranon process and extends distally around the posterior aspect of the elbow joint immediately adjacent to the olecranon process and then distally along the subcutaneous surface of the ulna to a level 3 cm distal to the fracture site **(A)**. Skin and subcutaneous tissue are reflected, and the ulnar nerve is protected on the medial aspect of the elbow **(B)**. The aponeurosis of the triceps is cleared posteriorly, and the broad tongue of this triceps aponeurosis (with its base proximally) is developed down to its insertion into the posterior aspect of the proximal ulna and is reflected proximally.

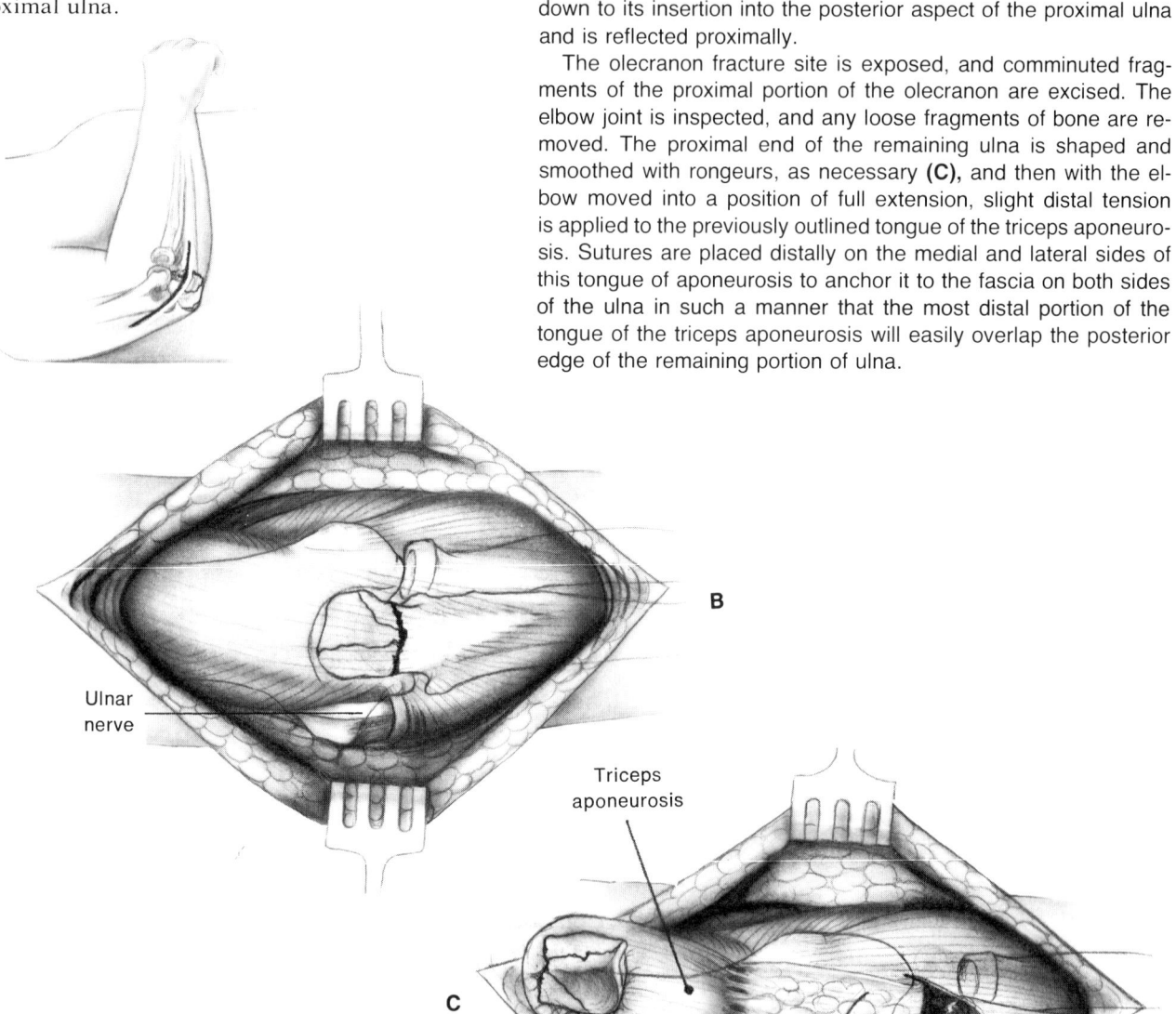

The olecranon fracture site is exposed, and comminuted fragments of the proximal portion of the olecranon are excised. The elbow joint is inspected, and any loose fragments of bone are removed. The proximal end of the remaining ulna is shaped and smoothed with rongeurs, as necessary **(C)**, and then with the elbow moved into a position of full extension, slight distal tension is applied to the previously outlined tongue of the triceps aponeurosis. Sutures are placed distally on the medial and lateral sides of this tongue of aponeurosis to anchor it to the fascia on both sides of the ulna in such a manner that the most distal portion of the tongue of the triceps aponeurosis will easily overlap the posterior edge of the remaining portion of ulna.

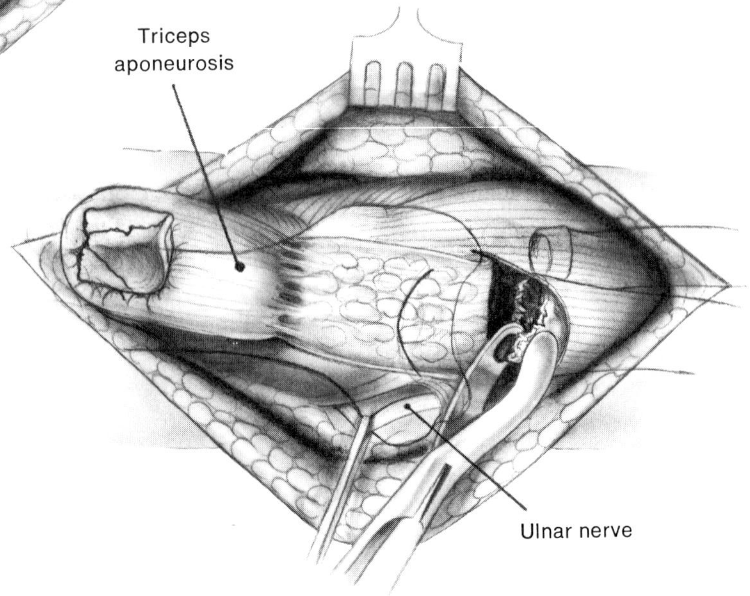

(Plate 3-3) EXCISION OF PROXIMAL ULNA (FOLLOWING OLECRANON FRACTURE) WITH REATTACHMENT OF TRICEPS

The distal end of the aponeurosis is then sutured to the periosteum overlying the ulna, and the remaining proximal edges of the tongue of the aponeurosis are sutured to the adjacent soft tissues (**D**). At this point, gentle passive flexion of the elbow will check the stability of the new attachment of the triceps aponeurosis. Flexion should be possible to at least 110° without undue tension of the triceps reattachment.

The wound is closed, and the arm is placed in a sling with a posterior plaster splint holding the elbow at 70° flexion (**E** and **F**).

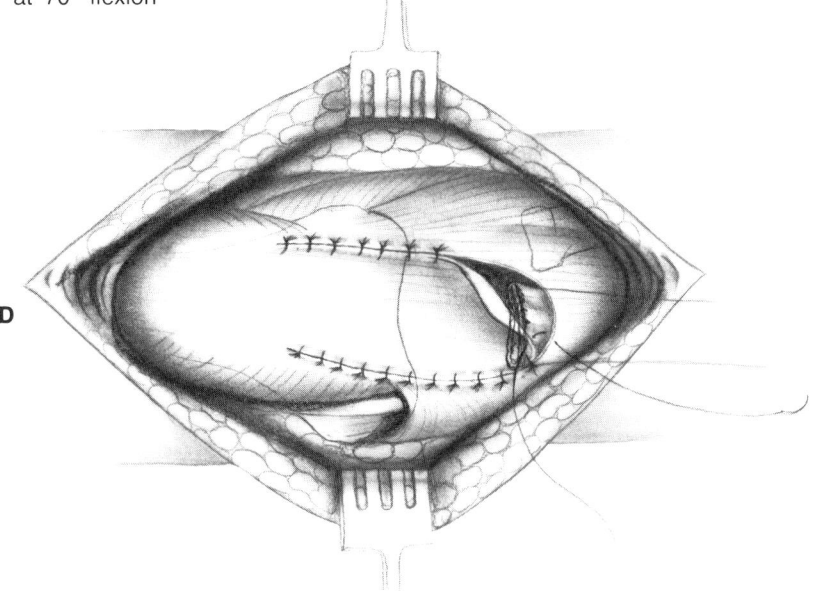

POSTOPERATIVE MANAGEMENT. The posterior plaster splint is removed at 3 weeks, and gentle active elbow range of motion exercises are begun. Passive flexion or forceful active elbow extension is avoided for at least an additional 3 weeks, during which time the patient's arm may be supported intermittently, but not continuously, in a sling.

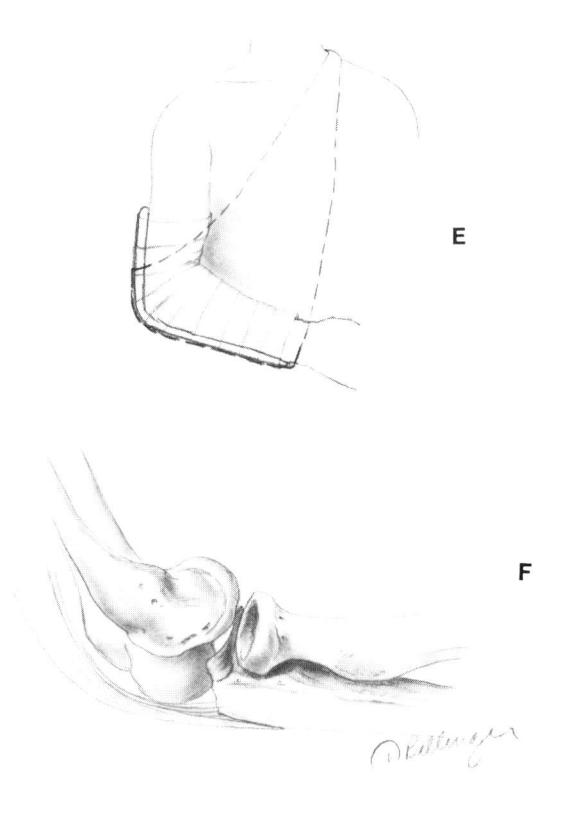

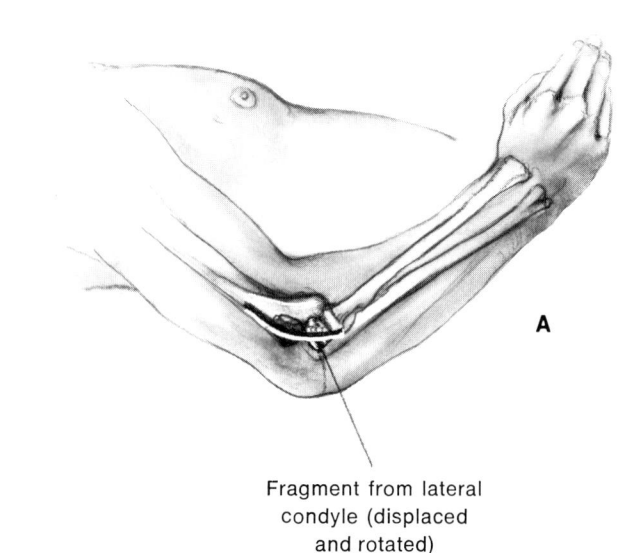

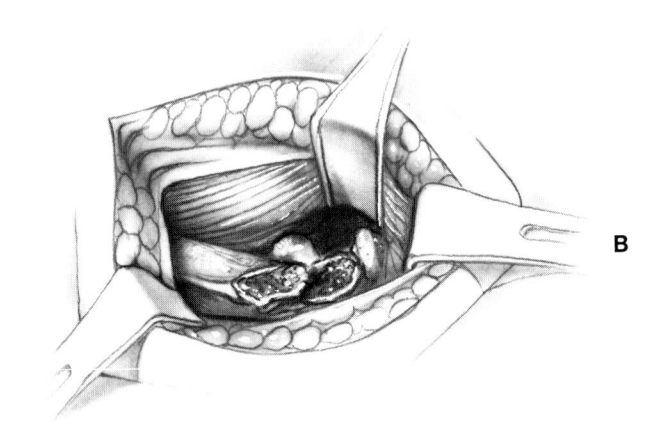

OPEN REDUCTION FOR DISPLACED FRACTURE OF LATERAL CONDYLE OF HUMERUS (Plate 3-4)

GENERAL DISCUSSION. For displaced fractures of the lateral condyle of the humerus, it is important to restore the fragment into anatomic position and to hold it there by means of sutures in the periosteum or by means of Kirschner wires. In very young children, the trochlear process may not have ossified completely, and the only injury seen roentgenographically may be a small crack in the lateral portion of the diaphysis or a change in the position of the small ossification center for the capitulum. The actual fragment will be much greater in size than may be appreciated on the basis of the roentgenogram. The fragment may be pulled distally by the common extensor origin and rotated completely out of its normal position. When displacement and rotation of the fragment have occurred, it will not be possible to restore the fragment to its anatomic position and to maintain it in that position by any closed treatment method. Operative repair will be indicated to restore the fracture fragment into its normal position so the fracture may heal without subsequent functional or developmental disturbance of the elbow.

DETAILS OF PROCEDURE. With the patient supine and the elbow supported in a flexed position, a curvilinear incision is made approximately 7 cm in length and centered over the normal anatomic location of the lateral humeral condyle **(A)**. The fracture fragment (which has been distally displaced and usually rotated) will be located easily just distal to the lateral aspect of the distal humerus in a superficial position and will be larger than it appeared roentgenographically **(B)**. Unnecessary periosteal stripping from the humerus should be avoided, and the dissection should include only that minimal exposure necessary to visualize and control the distal fragment in order to replace it in its anatomic position over the lateral aspect of the distal humerus. A small suction tip is often helpful in evacuating the hematoma and clearly visualizing the fracture surface, its margins, and the orientation of the displaced fragment containing the capitulum while the distal fragment is gently handled with forceps or an appropriate bone-holding clamp.

Fragment from lateral condyle (displaced and rotated)

(Plate 3-4) OPEN REDUCTION FOR DISPLACED FRACTURE OF LATERAL CONDYLE OF HUMERUS

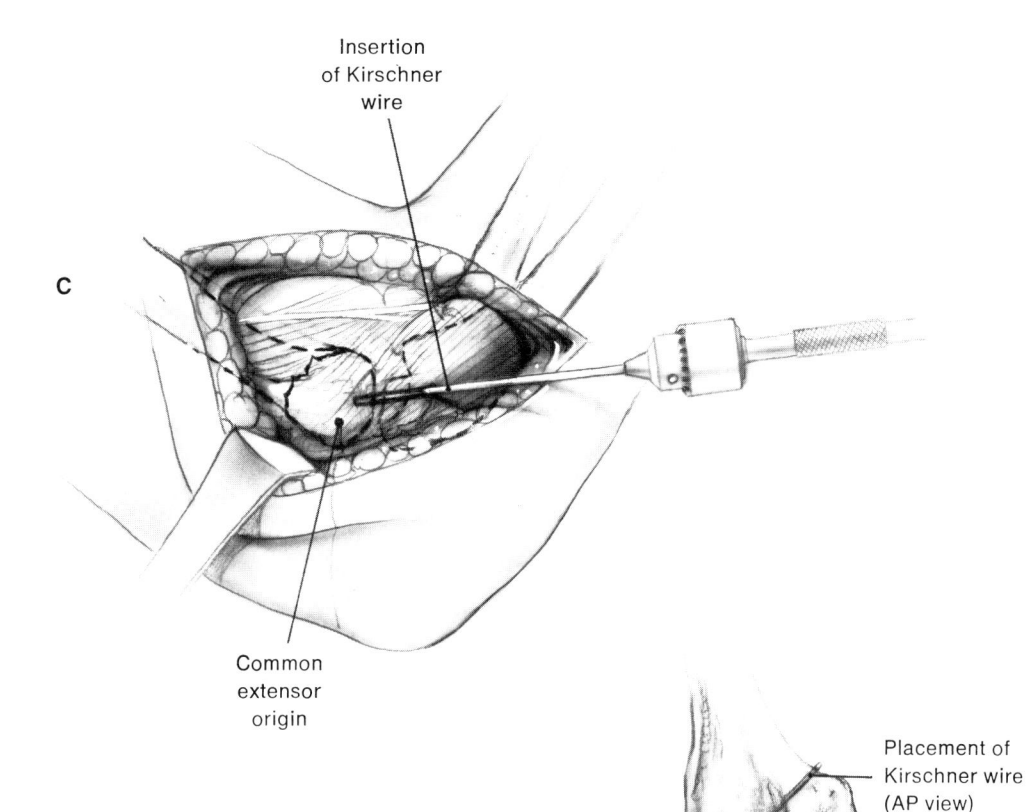

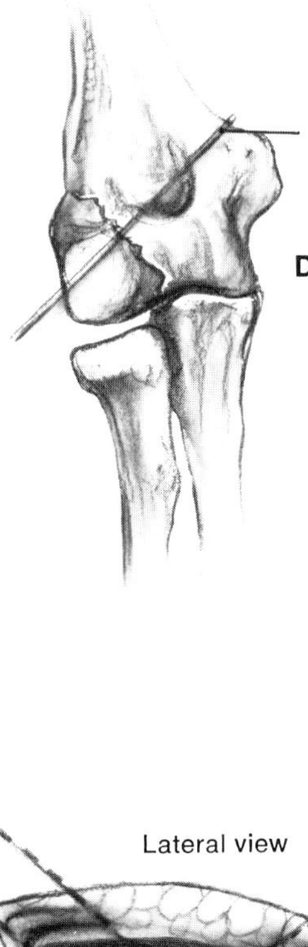

The distal fragment is rotated and replaced proximally in its anatomic position, where it may be possible to place some periosteal sutures to secure the fragment and to maintain it in this position. Otherwise, a Kirschner wire is inserted across the previously displaced fragment as it is held in anatomic position until the Kirschner wire engages the posteromedial cortex of the proximal portion of the humerus (**C** to **E**). The Kirschner wire is then divided to leave approximately 0.5 cm protruding through the attachment of the common extensor muscle origin to the lateral condyle. The stability of the reduction is checked with gentle movement of the elbow and forearm. The reduced position of the fracture is checked with anteroposterior (AP) and lateral roentgenograms prior to wound closure. Following wound closure, the patient's arm is placed in a posterior plaster splint with the elbow flexed at 90°.

POSTOPERATIVE MANAGEMENT. In children the Kirschner wire may be removed at 3 weeks and active elbow and forearm motion instituted thereafter. With anatomic replacement of the fractured lateral humeral condyle, full elbow and forearm function is usually achieved within 3 weeks after removal of the Kirschner wire. In adults any Kirschner wire used for internal fixation should be left in place until there is roentgenographic evidence of bony healing, although some protected elbow motion may be allowed with the Kirschner wire in place if the pin fixation is continued beyond 4 weeks postoperatively.

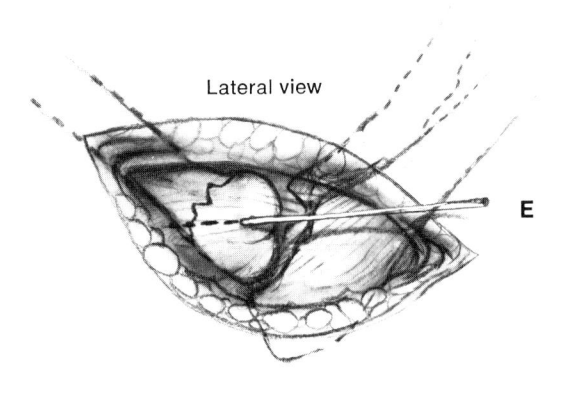

OPEN REDUCTION FOR DISPLACED FRACTURE OF MEDIAL EPICONDYLE (Plate 3-5)

GENERAL DISCUSSION. Displaced fracture of the medical epicondyle is ordinarily an epiphyseal separation. With the common flexor origin of the five superficial muscles of the flexor compartment of the forearm attached to the anterior surface of the medial epicondyle at the humerus, displacement is always in a distal direction. Because there is no effective way by closed manipulation to reduce and maintain reduction of a displaced fracture of the medial epicondyle of the humerus, a fracture of the medial epicondyle with more than 0.5 cm of distal displacement is best treated by open reduction. At the time of open reduction the displaced fragment also is usually rotated, and the fragment may contain a portion of the capsule of the elbow joint. Distal displacement greater than approximately 3 cm ordinarily is prevented by the intact anterior band of the medial ligament of the elbow joint connecting the medial epicondyle and the sublime tubercle on the medial border of the coronoid process. In children the displaced fragment will be larger than the ossified fragment visualized on the preoperative roentgenogram. Prompt open reduction with anatomic replacement and secure fixation should lead to an essentially normal functional end result for the involved elbow.

DETAILS OF PROCEDURE. The procedure is best carried out with the patient prone, the shoulder in full internal rotation, and the wrist of the involved arm resting on the patient's back **(A)**.

A curvilinear incision is made as illustrated **(B)**, crossing the medial aspect of the distal humerus. The fracture surface on the medial aspect of the distal humerus is easily identified. The ulnar nerve should be visualized at the onset of the procedure and be carefully protected throughout the remainder of the procedure **(C)**. The displaced fragment of the medial epicondyle is located and held gently as it is replaced into its anatomic position on the medical aspect of the distal humerus **(D)**. The attached origin of the common flexor muscles may help in orienting the fragment into its normal rotation when the fragment is replaced. The fragment of the medial epicondyle is then sutured to the adjacent periosteum of the distal humerus to hold the fragment securely in place **(E)**, or if soft tissues are such that this is not possible, the medial epicondyle is fixed with a Kirschner wire, which is then cut off to remain in a subcutaneous position following wound closure. A posterior plaster splint is applied that holds the elbow at 90° flexion and the forearm in full pronation.

POSTOPERATIVE MANAGEMENT. If a Kirschner wire was used for internal fixation, in a child it is removed 3 weeks following the open reduction (later in adults). With children the posterior plaster splint is removed 3 weeks postoperatively, and gentle active elbow and forearm exercises are instituted.

(Plate 3-5) OPEN REDUCTION FOR DISPLACED FRACTURE OF MEDIAL EPICONDYLE

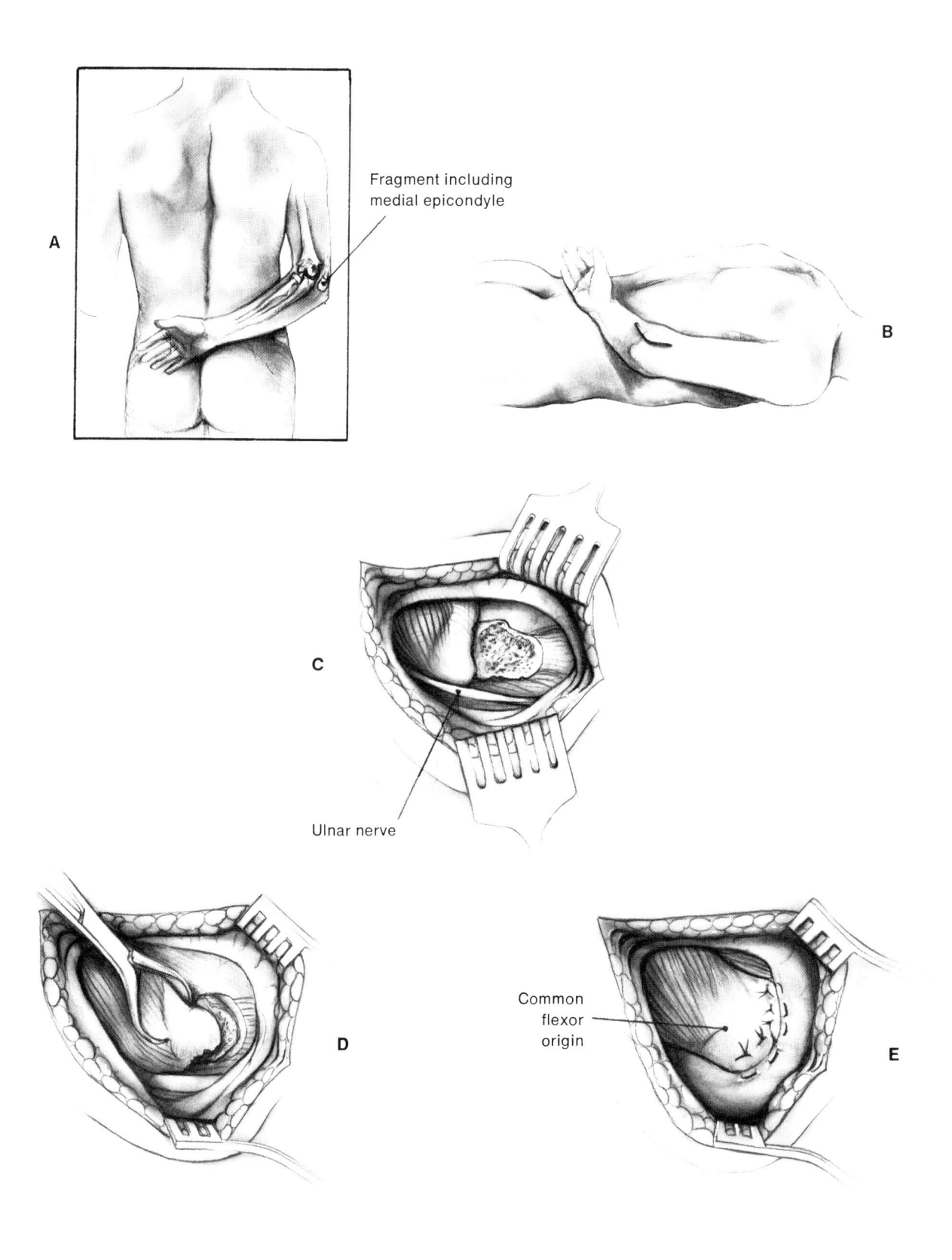

A

Fragment including medial epicondyle

B

C

Ulnar nerve

D

Common flexor origin

E

75

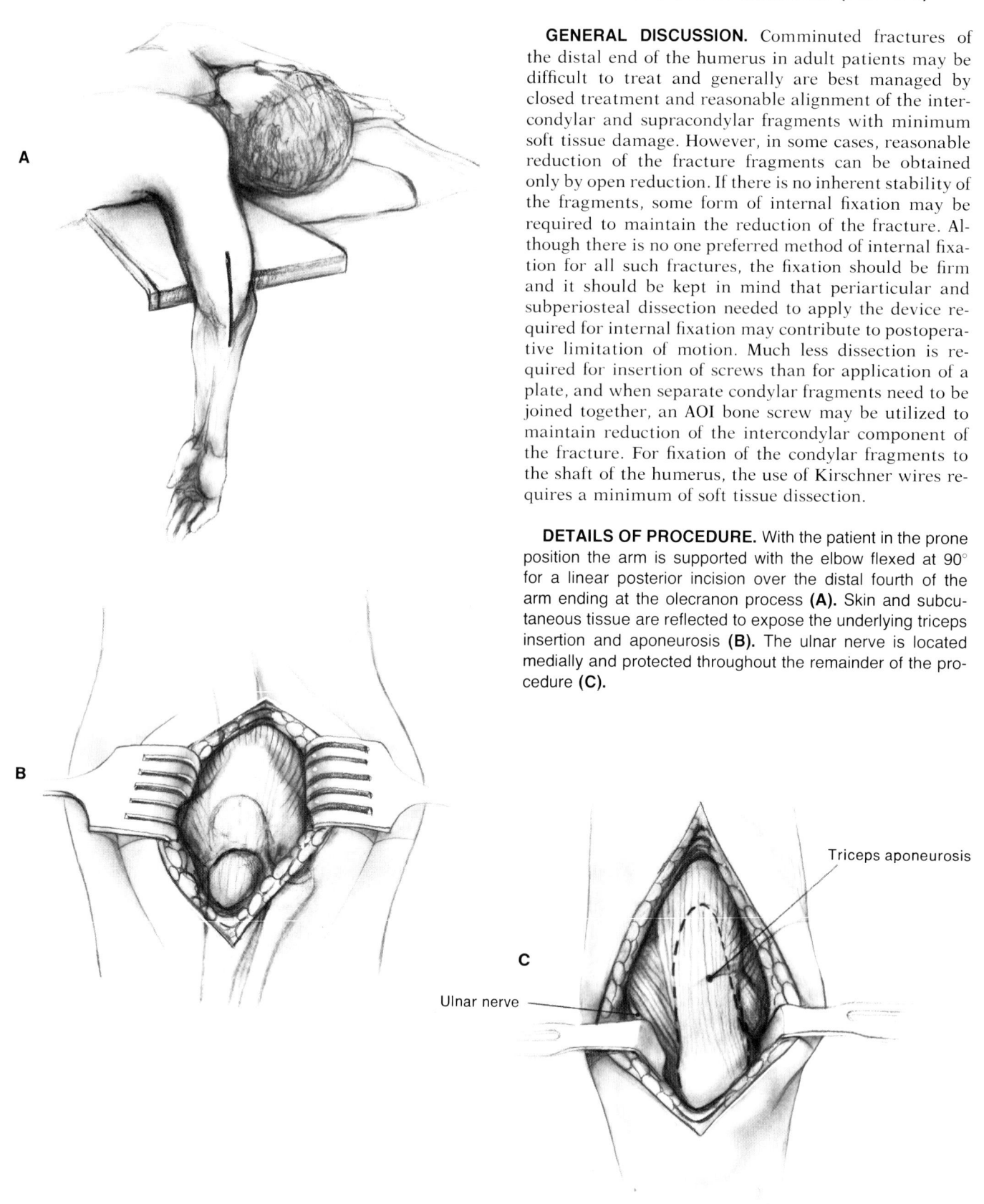

OPEN REDUCTION FOR SUPRACONDYLAR OR T CONDYLAR FRACTURES OF HUMERUS (Plate 3-6)

GENERAL DISCUSSION. Comminuted fractures of the distal end of the humerus in adult patients may be difficult to treat and generally are best managed by closed treatment and reasonable alignment of the intercondylar and supracondylar fragments with minimum soft tissue damage. However, in some cases, reasonable reduction of the fracture fragments can be obtained only by open reduction. If there is no inherent stability of the fragments, some form of internal fixation may be required to maintain the reduction of the fracture. Although there is no one preferred method of internal fixation for all such fractures, the fixation should be firm and it should be kept in mind that periarticular and subperiosteal dissection needed to apply the device required for internal fixation may contribute to postoperative limitation of motion. Much less dissection is required for insertion of screws than for application of a plate, and when separate condylar fragments need to be joined together, an AOI bone screw may be utilized to maintain reduction of the intercondylar component of the fracture. For fixation of the condylar fragments to the shaft of the humerus, the use of Kirschner wires requires a minimum of soft tissue dissection.

DETAILS OF PROCEDURE. With the patient in the prone position the arm is supported with the elbow flexed at 90° for a linear posterior incision over the distal fourth of the arm ending at the olecranon process **(A)**. Skin and subcutaneous tissue are reflected to expose the underlying triceps insertion and aponeurosis **(B)**. The ulnar nerve is located medially and protected throughout the remainder of the procedure **(C)**.

(Plate 3-6) OPEN REDUCTION FOR SUPRACONDYLAR OR T CONDYLAR FRACTURES OF HUMERUS

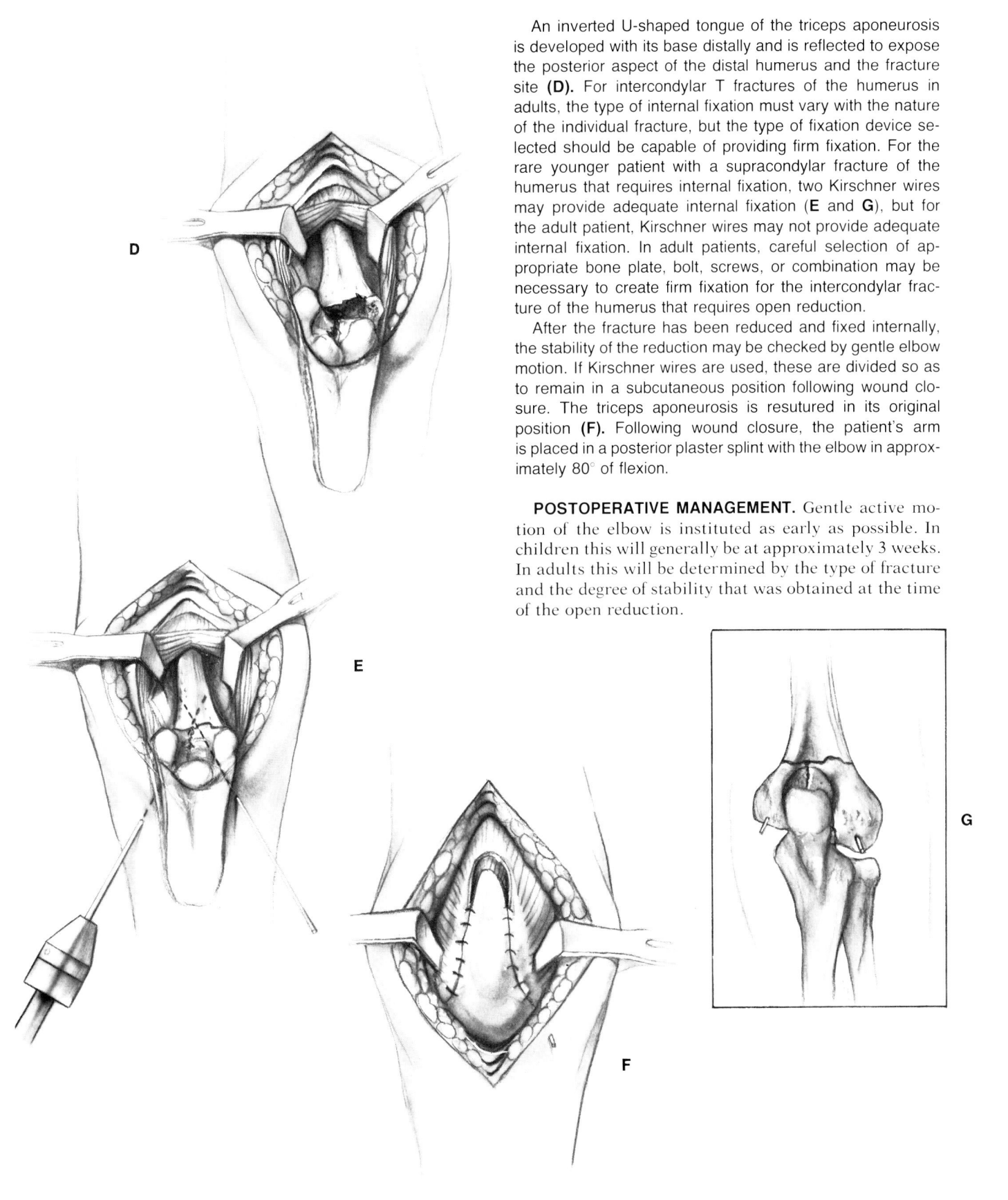

An inverted U-shaped tongue of the triceps aponeurosis is developed with its base distally and is reflected to expose the posterior aspect of the distal humerus and the fracture site **(D)**. For intercondylar T fractures of the humerus in adults, the type of internal fixation must vary with the nature of the individual fracture, but the type of fixation device selected should be capable of providing firm fixation. For the rare younger patient with a supracondylar fracture of the humerus that requires internal fixation, two Kirschner wires may provide adequate internal fixation (**E** and **G**), but for the adult patient, Kirschner wires may not provide adequate internal fixation. In adult patients, careful selection of appropriate bone plate, bolt, screws, or combination may be necessary to create firm fixation for the intercondylar fracture of the humerus that requires open reduction.

After the fracture has been reduced and fixed internally, the stability of the reduction may be checked by gentle elbow motion. If Kirschner wires are used, these are divided so as to remain in a subcutaneous position following wound closure. The triceps aponeurosis is resutured in its original position **(F)**. Following wound closure, the patient's arm is placed in a posterior plaster splint with the elbow in approximately 80° of flexion.

POSTOPERATIVE MANAGEMENT. Gentle active motion of the elbow is instituted as early as possible. In children this will generally be at approximately 3 weeks. In adults this will be determined by the type of fracture and the degree of stability that was obtained at the time of the open reduction.

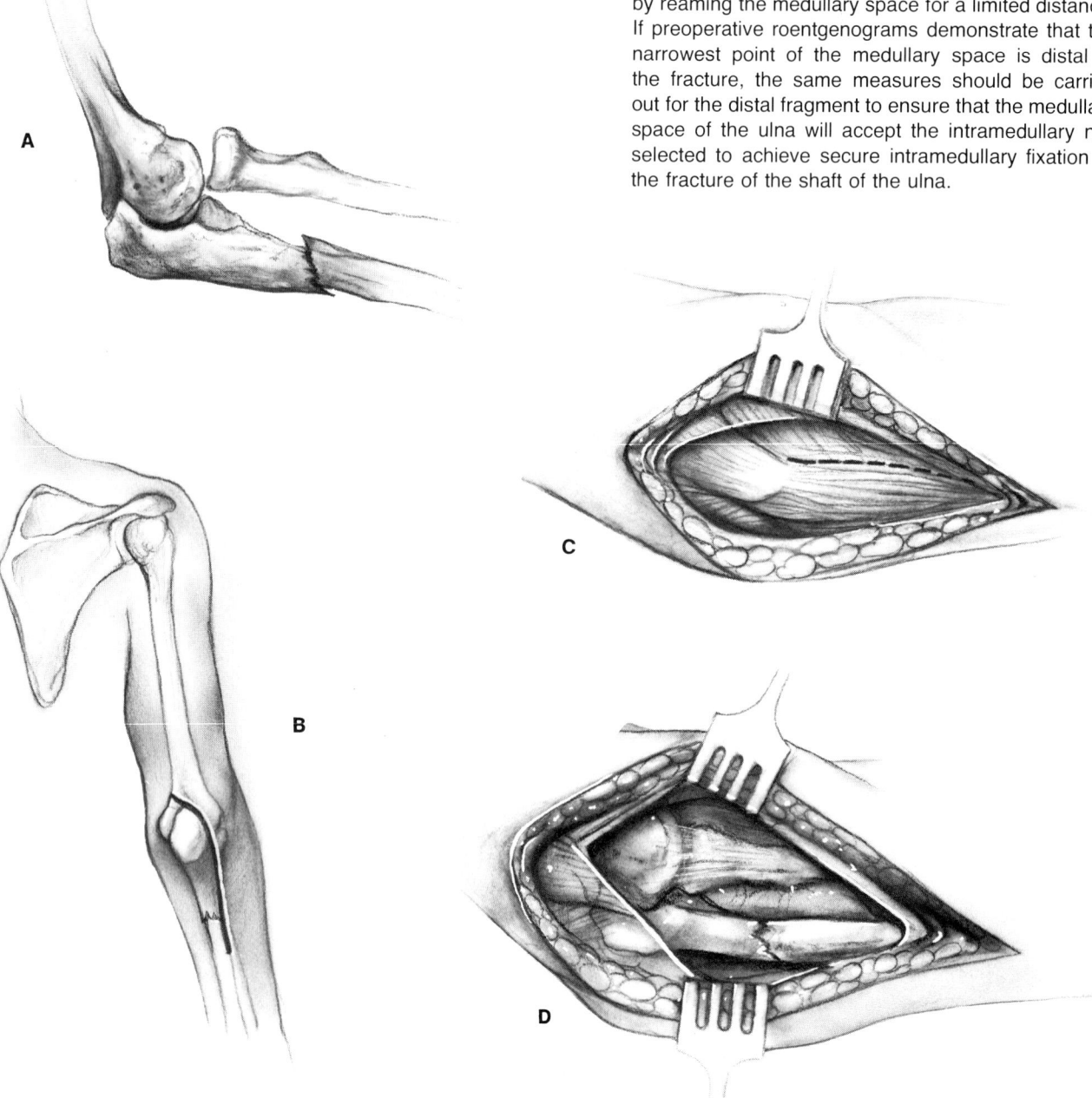

MEDULLARY FIXATION FOR FRACTURE OF SHAFT OF ULNA (INCLUDING MONTEGGIA FRACTURE-DISLOCATION) (Plate 3-7)

GENERAL DISCUSSION. In adults fractures of the shaft of the radius or ulna, or both, with angulation or displacement that cannot be satisfactorily realigned by closed manipulation are best treated by open reduction and internal fixation if the general condition of the patient and the local condition of the arm present no contraindication. Although the choice between a bone plate or a strong medullary nail may depend on several factors, intramedullary fixation is a satisfactory means for internal stabilization of a fracture of the shaft of the ulna.

DETAILS OF PROCEDURE. For a fracture of the proximal shaft, a single longitudinal incision is made along the subcutaneous border of the ulna, extending distally to a level approximately 3 cm beyond the level of the fracture. The incision curves in a medial direction at the proximal end to allow exposure of the posterior surface of the olecranon process (**A** and **B**). The fracture site is exposed (**C** and **D**). If there is any question about adequacy of the medullary space to accept the intramedullary nail, the proximal end of the fracture is delivered into the operative wound and the intramedullary nail is tented by tapping it into the proximal fragment in retrograde fashion. If the medullary canal is too small, it is enlarged at the narrowest point by reaming the medullary space for a limited distance. If preoperative roentgenograms demonstrate that the narrowest point of the medullary space is distal to the fracture, the same measures should be carried out for the distal fragment to ensure that the medullary space of the ulna will accept the intramedullary nail selected to achieve secure intramedullary fixation of the fracture of the shaft of the ulna.

(Plate 3-7) MEDULLARY FIXATION FOR FRACTURE OF SHAFT OF ULNA (INCLUDING MONTEGGIA FRACTURE-DISLOCATION)

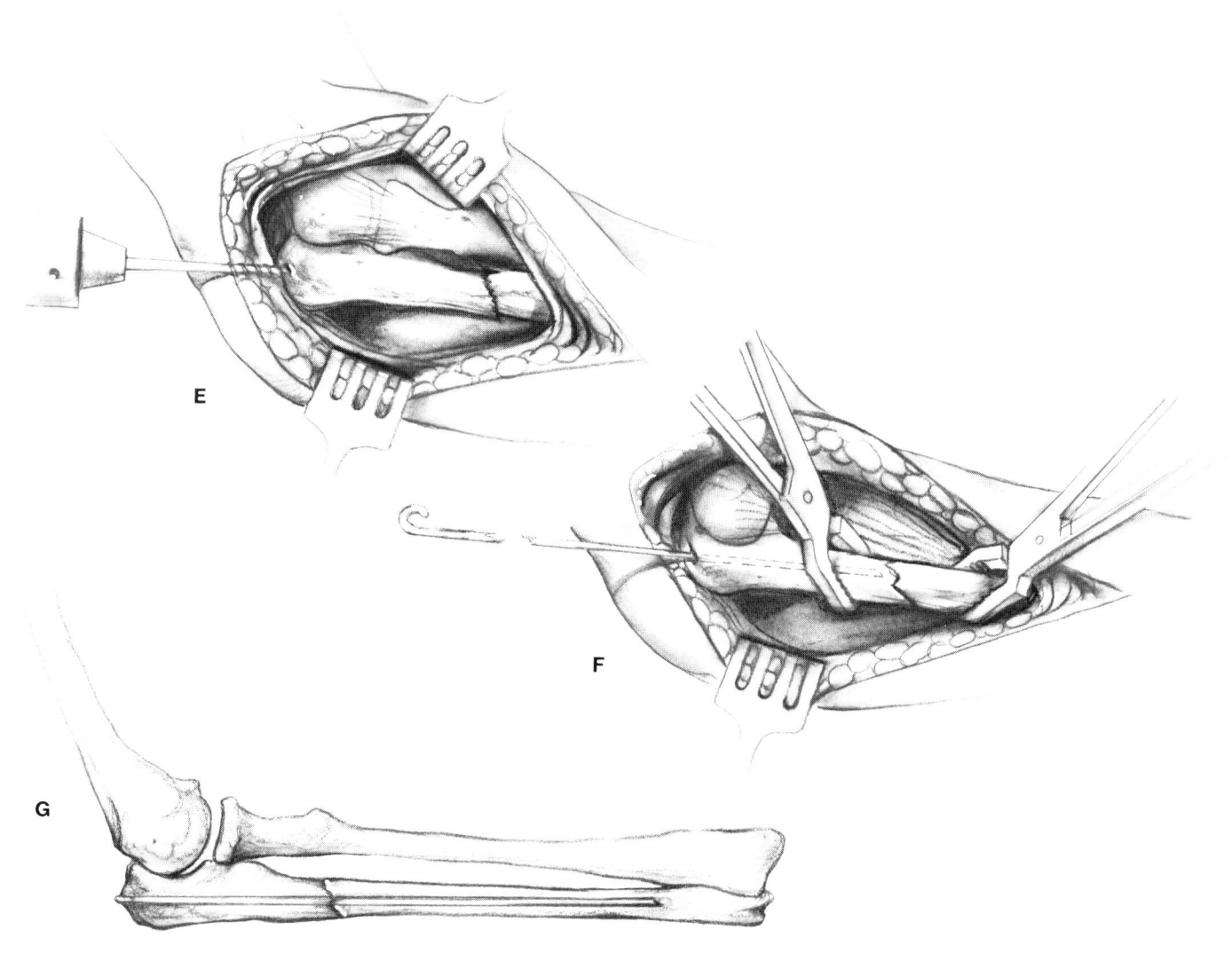

A small area on the posterior surface of the olecranon process is exposed through a short incision in the triceps insertion. The cortex of the posterior surface of the olecranon process is prepared with a drill hole, very slightly larger in diameter than the intended intramedullary nail (E). The intramedullary nail is inserted into the proximal fragment, and when the distal end of the nail reaches the fracture site, the fracture is reduced and held in anatomic apposition (F). The nail is driven across the fracture site into the medullary space of the distal fragment until its proximal end is essentially flush with the posterior cortex of the olecranon process (G). Secure fixation, good alignment, and good contact at the fracture site should be obtained. If there is any question about the position of the intramedullary nail in the distal portion of the ulna, roentgenograms should be obtained in the operating room prior to wound closure.

If there has been an associated dislocation of the radial head, that is, the Monteggia-type fracture-dislocation, reduction and internal fixation of the fracture of the proximal ulna often brings about simultaneous reduction and adequate stability of the associated dislocation of the radial head. However, when there is an associated disruption of the radial humeral joint, the reduction of the radial head into normal relationship with the capitulum of the humerus should be confirmed either by opening the capsule of the radiohumeral joint or with roentgenograms in two planes before wound closure.

The wound is closed with attention to suture of the triceps insertion over any minimal projecting prominence of the proximal end of the intramedullary nail. A long-arm cast is applied with the forearm in neutral position.

POSTOPERATIVE MANAGEMENT. Plaster immobilization is continued until there is roentgenographic evidence of satisfactory fracture healing, usually at about 10 weeks. In subsequent months, when the fracture of the ulna is solidly united, the intramedullary nail may be extracted electively if bothersome tenderness persists over the proximal end of the nail on the posterior surface of the olecranon process.

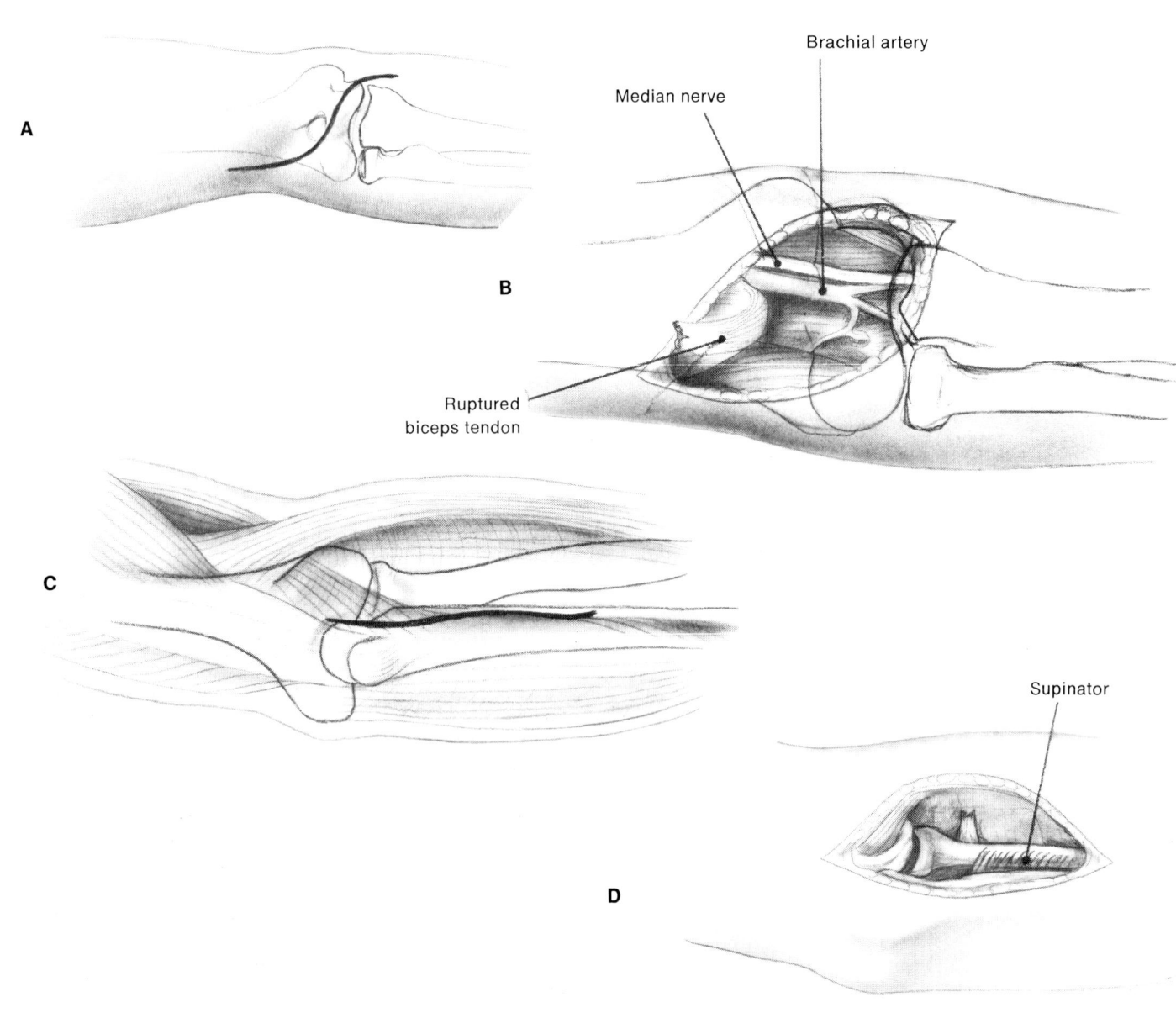

REPAIR OF RUPTURE OF DISTAL TENDON OF BICEPS BRACHII MUSCLE (Plate 3-8)

GENERAL DISCUSSION. Patients with rupture of the proximal portion of the biceps brachii muscle or the tendon of the long head of the biceps brachii muscle generally do not require operative treatment. Rupture of the distal tendon of the biceps muscle, however, is best treated by operative repair.

DETAILS OF PROCEDURE. The elbow and distal portion of the arm are approached initially through an anterior approach with an S-shaped incision **(A)**. The biceps tendon may have retracted 5 to 6 cm from the site of the tendon rupture, which is usually close to its insertion into the tuberosity of the radius. The median cubital vein is retracted or ligated and divided to facilitate adequate exposure. The lateral cutaneous nerve of the forearm should be protected during any subcutaneous dissection or retraction of the lateral portion of the wound. The brachial artery and median nerve are located immediately adjacent to and on the medial side of the distal tendon of the biceps and must be protected **(B)**. A Bunnell-type suture is placed in the end of the ruptured biceps tendon. A blunt instrument is used to locate the path through which the tendon will later be passed to reach the tuberosity of the radius. As this is done, the radial recurrent artery, which leaves the radial artery on its lateral side and is located in close proximity anterior to the normal location of the distal tendon of the biceps, must be kept in mind.

The elbow is not repositioned to expose the tuberosity of the radius through a posterolateral approach **(C)**. This is accomplished by reflecting the muscles off the lateral surface of the proximal ulna and following a plane along the interosseous membrane to reach the proximal radius. The posterior interosseous nerve should be protected within the substance of the supinator muscle **(D)**.

(Plate 3-8) REPAIR OF RUPTURE OF DISTAL TENDON OF BICEPS BRACHII MUSCLE

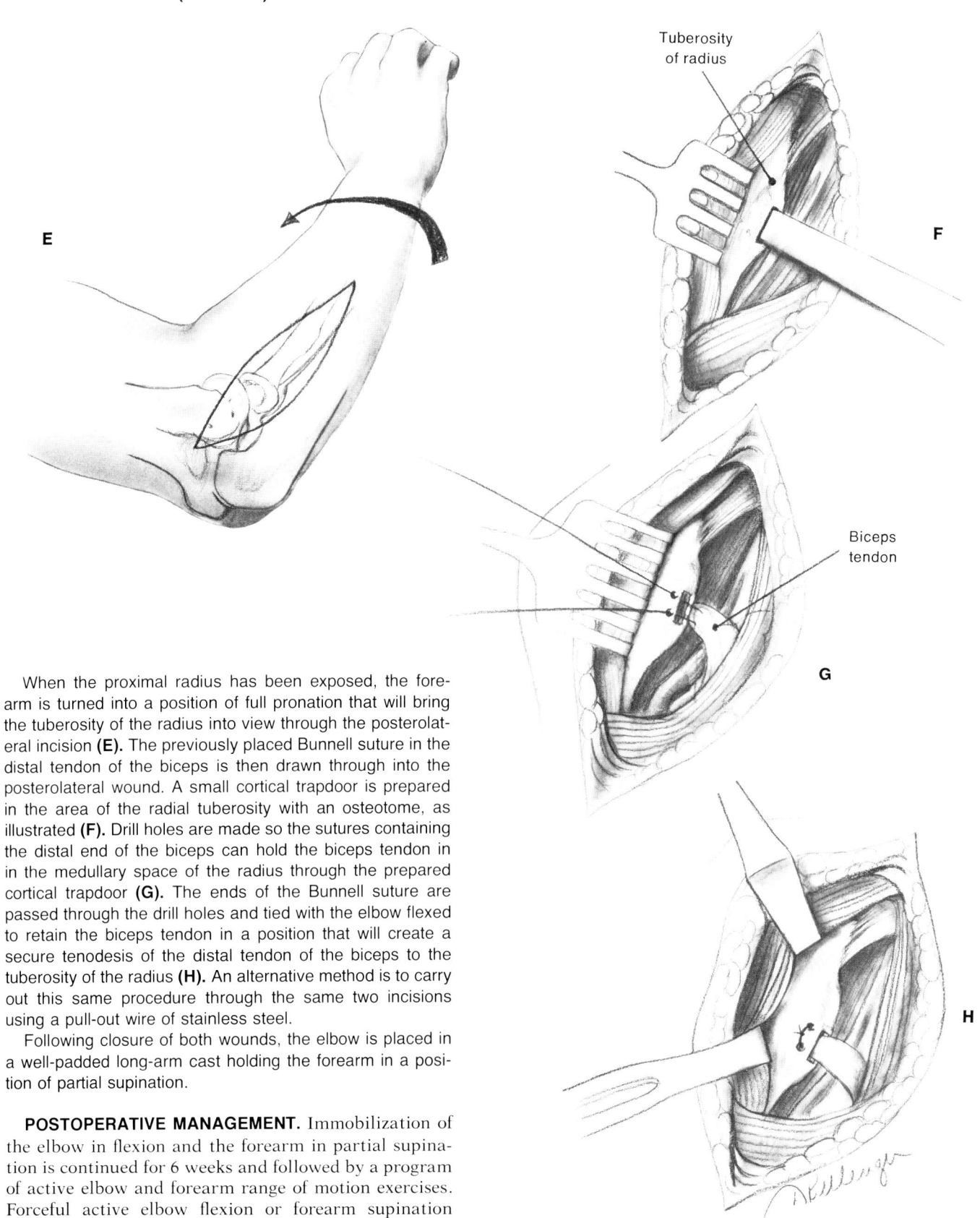

When the proximal radius has been exposed, the forearm is turned into a position of full pronation that will bring the tuberosity of the radius into view through the posterolateral incision **(E)**. The previously placed Bunnell suture in the distal tendon of the biceps is then drawn through into the posterolateral wound. A small cortical trapdoor is prepared in the area of the radial tuberosity with an osteotome, as illustrated **(F)**. Drill holes are made so the sutures containing the distal end of the biceps can hold the biceps tendon in in the medullary space of the radius through the prepared cortical trapdoor **(G)**. The ends of the Bunnell suture are passed through the drill holes and tied with the elbow flexed to retain the biceps tendon in a position that will create a secure tenodesis of the distal tendon of the biceps to the tuberosity of the radius **(H)**. An alternative method is to carry out this same procedure through the same two incisions using a pull-out wire of stainless steel.

Following closure of both wounds, the elbow is placed in a well-padded long-arm cast holding the forearm in a position of partial supination.

POSTOPERATIVE MANAGEMENT. Immobilization of the elbow in flexion and the forearm in partial supination is continued for 6 weeks and followed by a program of active elbow and forearm range of motion exercises. Forceful active elbow flexion or forearm supination against resistance is avoided for an additional 6 weeks.

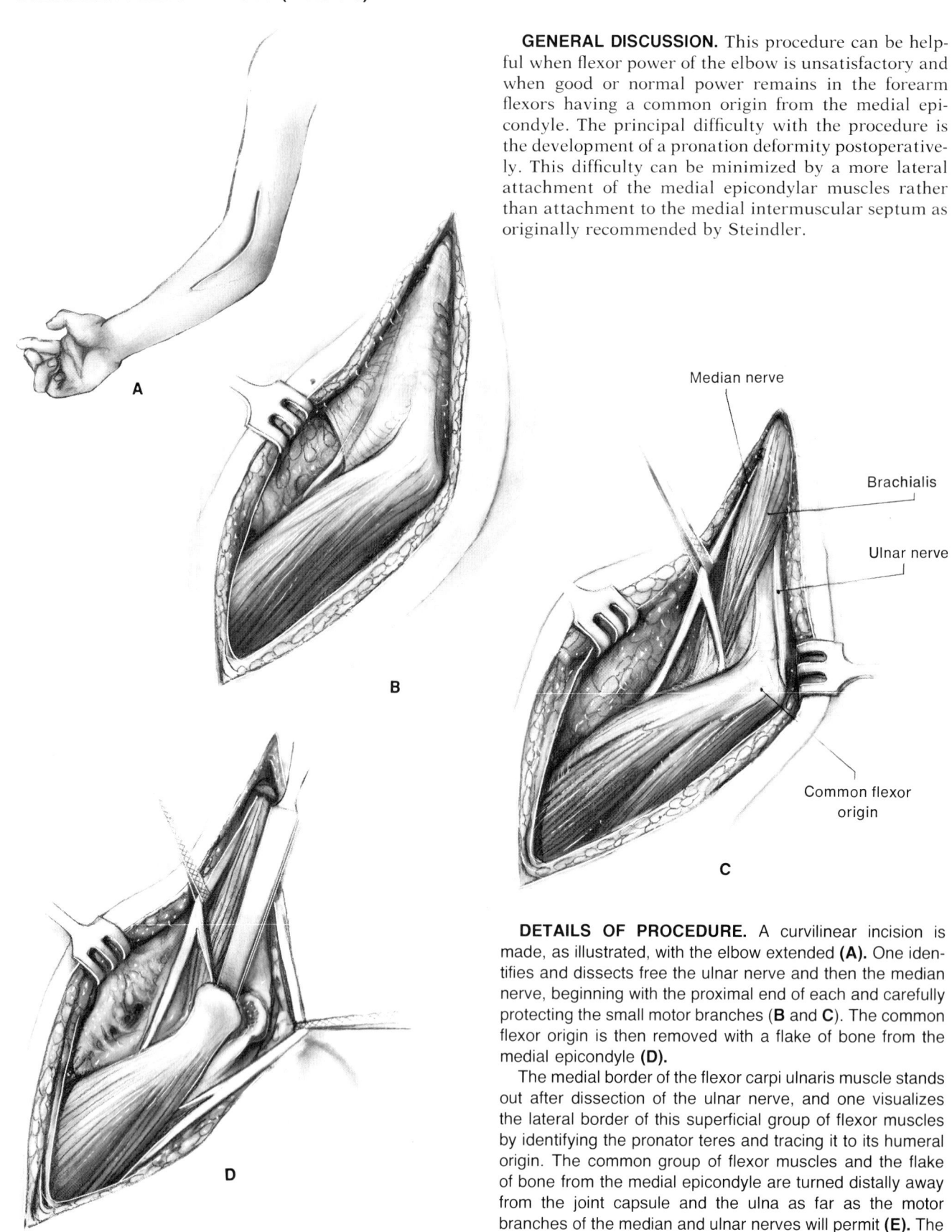

STEINDLER FLEXORPLASTY (Plate 3-9)

GENERAL DISCUSSION. This procedure can be helpful when flexor power of the elbow is unsatisfactory and when good or normal power remains in the forearm flexors having a common origin from the medial epicondyle. The principal difficulty with the procedure is the development of a pronation deformity postoperatively. This difficulty can be minimized by a more lateral attachment of the medial epicondylar muscles rather than attachment to the medial intermuscular septum as originally recommended by Steindler.

DETAILS OF PROCEDURE. A curvilinear incision is made, as illustrated, with the elbow extended **(A)**. One identifies and dissects free the ulnar nerve and then the median nerve, beginning with the proximal end of each and carefully protecting the small motor branches **(B** and **C)**. The common flexor origin is then removed with a flake of bone from the medial epicondyle **(D)**.

The medial border of the flexor carpi ulnaris muscle stands out after dissection of the ulnar nerve, and one visualizes the lateral border of this superficial group of flexor muscles by identifying the pronator teres and tracing it to its humeral origin. The common group of flexor muscles and the flake of bone from the medial epicondyle are turned distally away from the joint capsule and the ulna as far as the motor branches of the median and ulnar nerves will permit **(E)**. The

(Plate 3-9) STEINDLER FLEXORPLASTY

elbow is then flexed 135° to determine a level for insertion of the transplanted epicondyle group (usually 5 to 7 cm above the elbow) **(F)**. The median nerve, brachial vessels, and biceps muscle are retraced laterally, and the atrophied brachialis muscle is divided longitudinally to expose the anterior aspect of the humerus. The periosteum is reflected, and an opening is made in the anterior surface of the humerus sufficient to receive the transplanted epicondylar group. This is subsequently secured over a button posteriorly, as illustrated, and a pull-out suture exits anteriorly (**G** and **H**). It is helpful to close the distal part of the wound up to the flexion crease in the elbow before finally securing the transfer to the humerus.

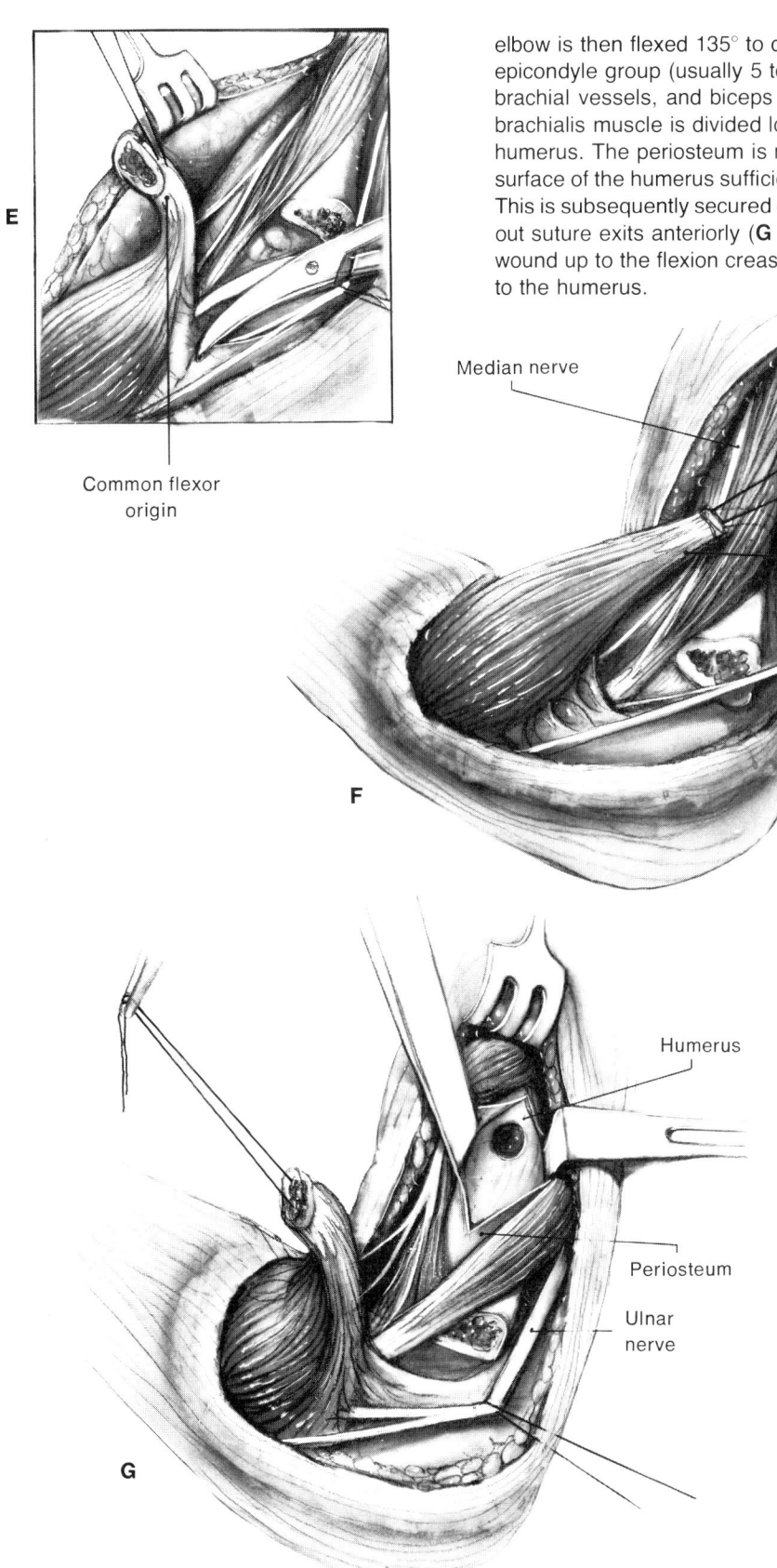

POSTOPERATIVE MANAGEMENT. Postoperatively a plaster cast that holds the elbow in 150° of flexion and the forearm in full supination is used for 3 weeks. A posterior splint is used for 2 more weeks, permitting movement of the arm for extension and supination exercises six times a day. If a severe flexion deformity is to be avoided, vigorous active elbow extension exercises must be started 3 weeks after surgery.

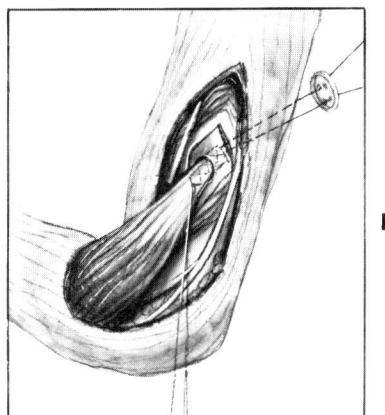

TRANSFER OF TRICEPS TENDON (Plate 3-10)

GENERAL DISCUSSION. Transfer of the triceps tendon may be indicated when the more universally accepted Steindler flexorplasty cannot be used because of paralysis or traumatic loss of effective function of the common flexor muscles arising from the medial epicondyle. Transfer of the triceps around the lateral aspect of the humerus to the radius as described by Carroll and Hill can restore active flexion to a paralyzed elbow. As with other muscle transfers, any partial transfer of a specific muscle cannot function effectively, and the entire triceps insertion should be transferred.

DETAILS OF PROCEDURE. The patient is placed in a lateral position lying on the unaffected side, and the involved arm is draped free to permit exposure of both the posterior and anterior aspects of the elbow and to allow free movement of the elbow and forearm during the procedure.

The posterior aspect of the arm is approached first to outline the distal portion of the triceps in the lower third of the arm. The incision is continued distally along the subcutaneous surface of the proximal ulna to a point several centimeters beyond the tip of the olecranon process **(A)**. Skin and subcutaneous tissues are reflected medially and laterally with care to protect the posterior cutaneous nerve of the forearm in the lateral aspect of the wound. The ulnar nerve is identified medially and is protected as a tail of periosteum 4 to 5 cm in length is reflected from the proximal ulna in continuity with the triceps insertion, while the muscle mass of the triceps is mobilized from the distal third of the shaft of the humerus **(B)**. The branches of the radial nerve providing motor innervation to the triceps muscle will be protected within the substance of the triceps muscle. The lower end of the muscle is then fashioned into the form of a tube to facilitate its subsequent transfer around the lateral aspect of the arm.

An anterior curvilinear incision is now made over the antecubital space **(C)** to expose the biceps tendon and to allow adequate exposure for the forward transfer of the triceps tendon. Intervening antecubital veins are retracted or ligated and divided, and, if necessary, the radial recurrent artery is ligated and divided. A subcutaneous tunnel is prepared between the anterior and posterior wounds along the lateral margin of the brachialis muscle so that the tube of triceps and extension of periosteum from the ulna in continuity with the triceps tendon can reach the biceps tendon close to its insertion into the tuberosity of the radius **(D)**.

With the elbow in 90° flexion and the forearm in full supination, the transferred triceps insertion is passed through and around the biceps tendon and sutured securely in that position with moderate tension on the triceps muscle. An alternative method could include extension of the triceps insertion with a free graft taken from fascia lata **(E)**. An alternative technique for anchoring the transferred triceps into the biceps tendon is the use of stainless steel wire and a pull-out suture to anchor the transferred tendon into the tuberosity of the radius. This is done by passing the wire suture through a drill hole in the opposite side of the proximal radius and out the posterior aspect of the proximal forearm to be tied over the well-padded button for tenodesis of the transferred triceps **(E)**.

Following closure of both wounds, the arm is placed in a well-padded long-arm cast with the elbow in 90° flexion and the forearm in full supination.

POSTOPERATIVE MANAGEMENT. Plaster immobilization with the elbow in 90° flexion and the forearm in supination is continued for 4 weeks. This is followed by active elbow exercise. Forceful or passive elbow extension is specifically avoided for an additional 6 weeks.

(Plate 3-10) TRANSFER OF TRICEPS TENDON

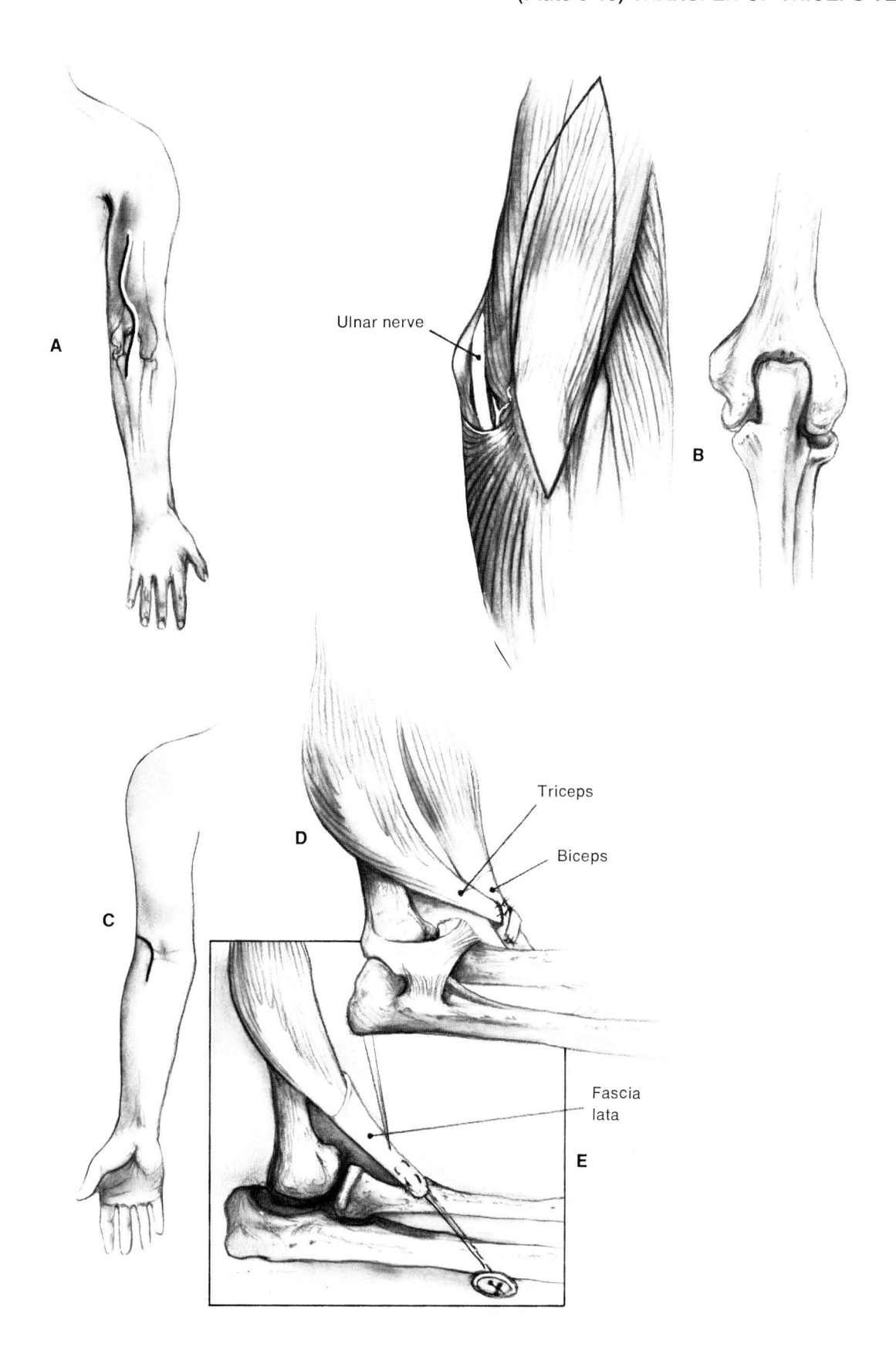

A

Ulnar nerve

B

C

D

Triceps

Biceps

Fascia lata

E

85

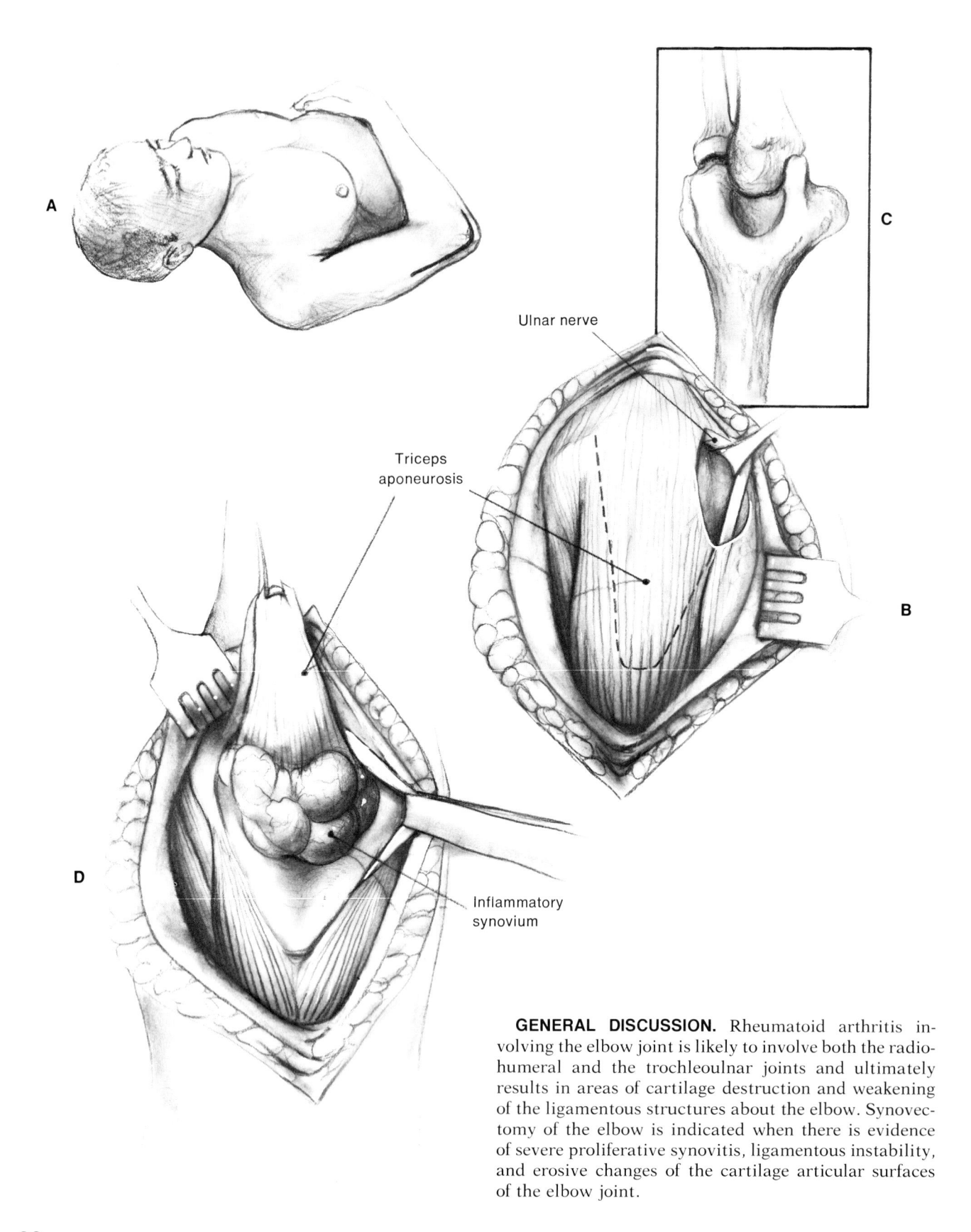

SYNOVECTOMY OF ELBOW (Plate 3-11)

Labels: Ulnar nerve; Triceps aponeurosis; Inflammatory synovium

GENERAL DISCUSSION. Rheumatoid arthritis involving the elbow joint is likely to involve both the radiohumeral and the trochleoulnar joints and ultimately results in areas of cartilage destruction and weakening of the ligamentous structures about the elbow. Synovectomy of the elbow is indicated when there is evidence of severe proliferative synovitis, ligamentous instability, and erosive changes of the cartilage articular surfaces of the elbow joint.

86

(Plate 3-11) SYNOVECTOMY OF ELBOW

DETAILS OF PROCEDURE. With the patient in the supine position and tilted slightly toward the opposite side, the arm is positioned in a flexed position for a posterior incision. The arm must be draped free. A pneumatic tourniquet is helpful.

A posterior longitudinal incision is made **(A)** crossing the posterior aspect of the elbow slightly on the radial side (a transolecranon approach is an optional alternative). The skin flaps are undermined and retracted medially and laterally. The medial flap will include the medial cutaneous nerve of the forearm, and the lateral flap will include the posterior cutaneous nerve of the forearm until the lateral condyle and medial epicondyle have both been exposed. The ulnar nerve is identified, carefully isolated, and gently retracted with a Penrose drain **(B)**. In the distal portion of the wound the anconeus is incised along its attachment to the lateral aspect of the proximal ulna and reflected anteriorly with the adjacent muscles originating from the common extensor origin on the lateral condyle of the humerus. These muscles are reflected anteriorly and laterally, exposing the radial humeral joint **(C)**. A tongue of the triceps aponeurosis is developed and reflected for exposure of the posterior portion of the joint **(D)**.

The synovium in the notch of the olecranon is removed. A pituitary rongeur may be helpful in separation and removal of the synovium from the elbow-joint capsule and from beneath the collateral ligaments. Removal of the head of the radius may be desirable for relief of pain and better exposure of the radiohumeral joint. All of the synovium should be removed from the radiohumeral joint and both sides of the trochleoulnar joint **(E)**. Any bony irregularities adjacent to the joint surfaces of the humerus and ulna should be removed with osteotome, rongeurs, or a bone file.

The ulnar nerve is replaced in its normal position, and the tongue of the triceps aponeurosis, which was reflected for exposure of the posterior portion of the joint, is sutured in its normal place **(F)**. Any subcutaneous nodules, common in the area of the olecranon and along the subcutaneous surface of the ulna, are removed prior to final wound closure if these are of sufficient size to warrant excision. Suction catheters may be placed for drainage of the wound. After wound closure a bulky compression dressing is applied, including a posterior plaster splint holding the elbow in 90° flexion and the forearm in neutral rotation.

POSTOPERATIVE MANAGEMENT. Any suction drains are removed on the first or second postoperative day. The bulky compression dressing is removed on the second postoperative day, and a graded program of active assistive flexion and extension exercises is started at that time. Between periods of exercise the patient keeps the elbow at rest in a new posterior molded splint for 2 to 3 weeks postoperatively.

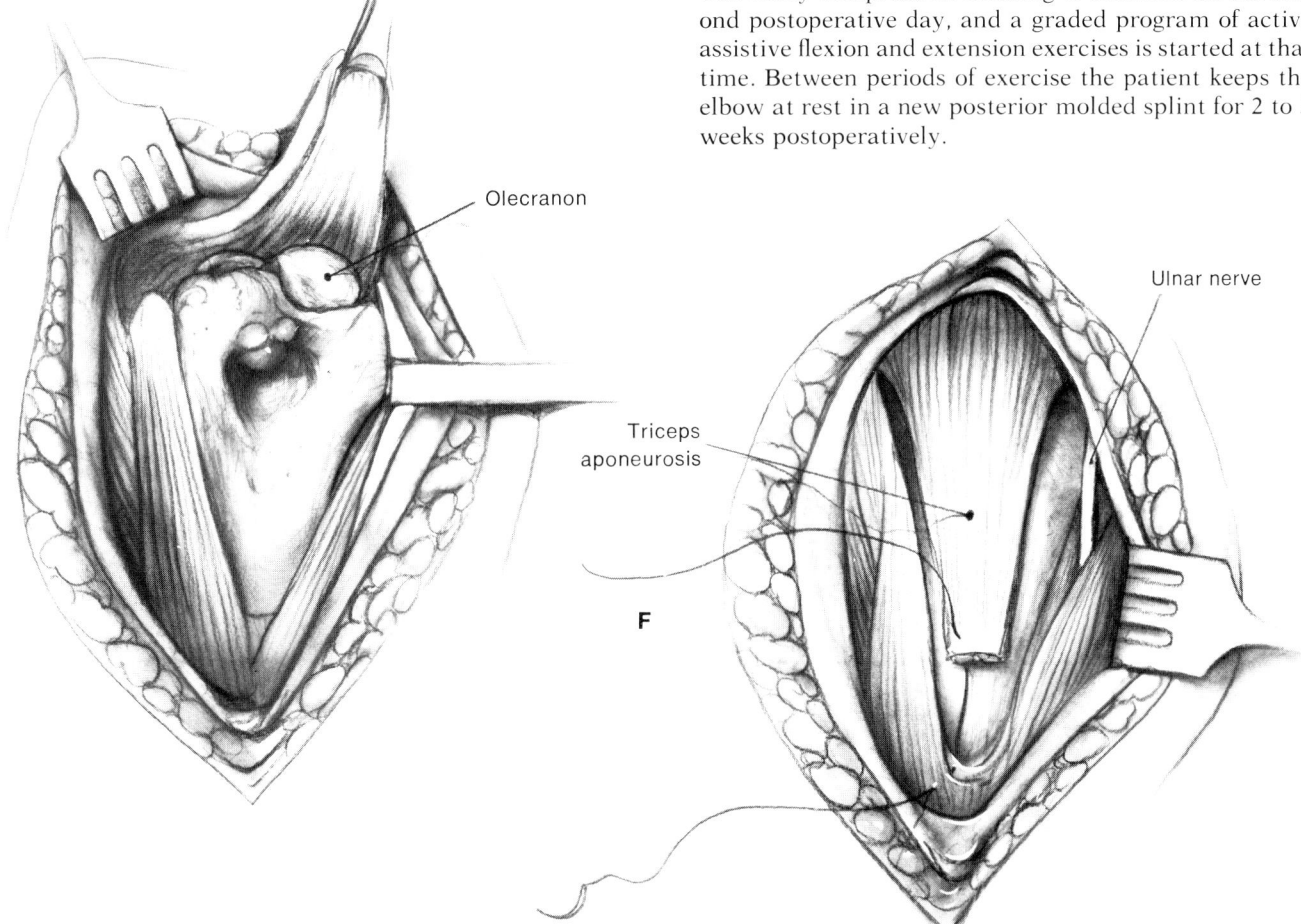

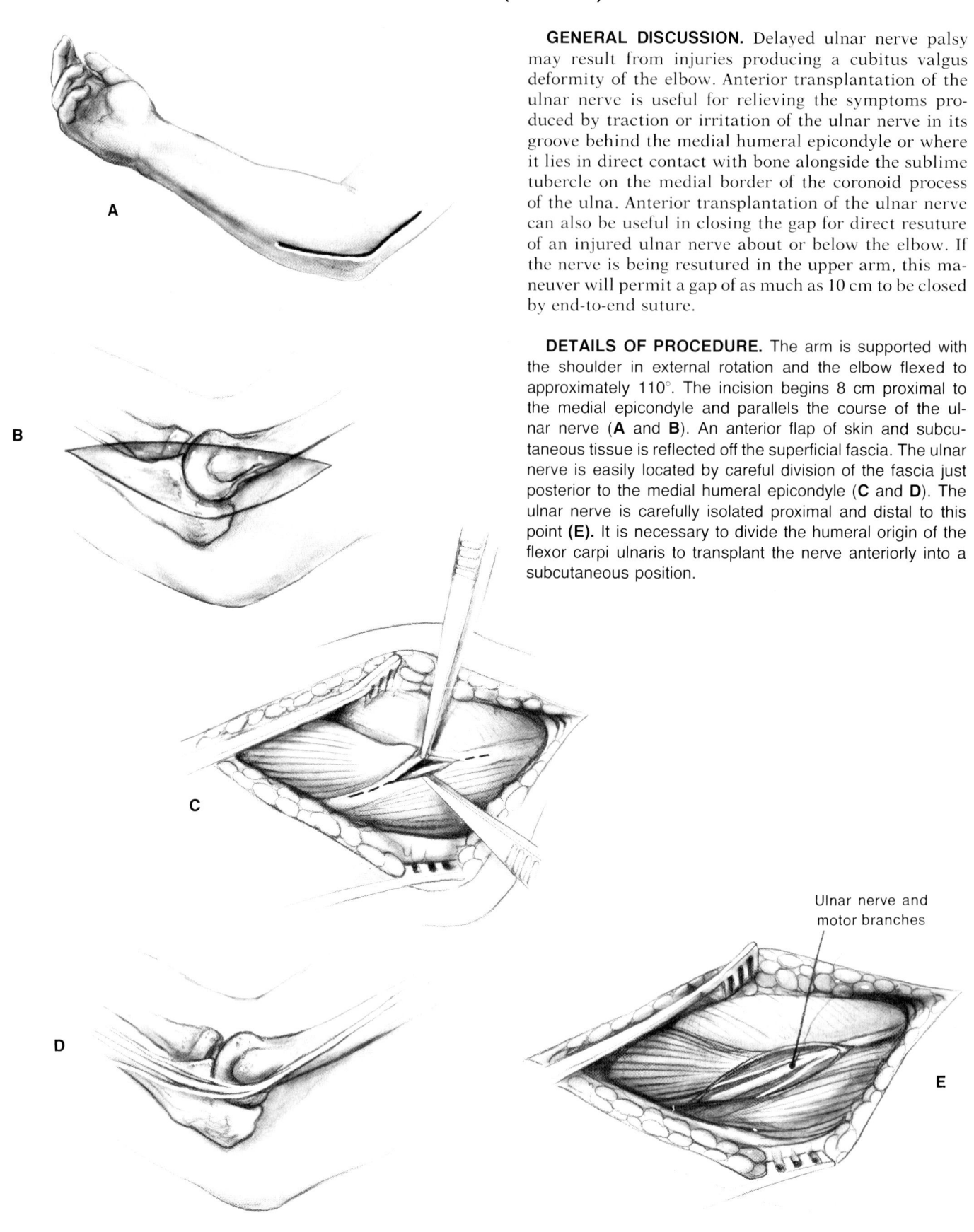

ANTERIOR TRANSPLANTATION OF ULNAR NERVE (Plate 3-12)

GENERAL DISCUSSION. Delayed ulnar nerve palsy may result from injuries producing a cubitus valgus deformity of the elbow. Anterior transplantation of the ulnar nerve is useful for relieving the symptoms produced by traction or irritation of the ulnar nerve in its groove behind the medial humeral epicondyle or where it lies in direct contact with bone alongside the sublime tubercle on the medial border of the coronoid process of the ulna. Anterior transplantation of the ulnar nerve can also be useful in closing the gap for direct resuture of an injured ulnar nerve about or below the elbow. If the nerve is being resutured in the upper arm, this maneuver will permit a gap of as much as 10 cm to be closed by end-to-end suture.

DETAILS OF PROCEDURE. The arm is supported with the shoulder in external rotation and the elbow flexed to approximately 110°. The incision begins 8 cm proximal to the medial epicondyle and parallels the course of the ulnar nerve (**A** and **B**). An anterior flap of skin and subcutaneous tissue is reflected off the superficial fascia. The ulnar nerve is easily located by careful division of the fascia just posterior to the medial humeral epicondyle (**C** and **D**). The ulnar nerve is carefully isolated proximal and distal to this point (**E**). It is necessary to divide the humeral origin of the flexor carpi ulnaris to transplant the nerve anteriorly into a subcutaneous position.

(Plate 3-12) ANTERIOR TRANSPLANTATION OF ULNAR NERVE

A sensory branch of the ulnar nerve to the elbow joint may come off the nerve as it lies in the groove behind the medial epicondyle, and this is necessarily sacrificed in the relocation of the nerve, but all other branches (including motor branches to the flexor carpi ulnaris and flexor digitorum profundus) must be carefully preserved. When the nerve is relocated to the anterior aspect of the elbow (**F**) on the surface of the fascia of the flexor pronator group of muscles, the new course of the nerve is inspected and any fascial or tendinous bands that might constrict or irritate the transplanted nerve are excised. Sutures are placed medial to the nerve in its new location (**G** and **H**), and subcutaneous tissue and the fascia are approximated to prevent the nerve from slipping back toward its original location.

POSTOPERATIVE MANAGEMENT. The elbow is supported in a sling for 2 to 3 weeks postoperatively and then mobilized progressively.

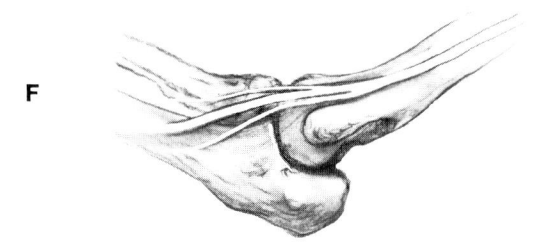

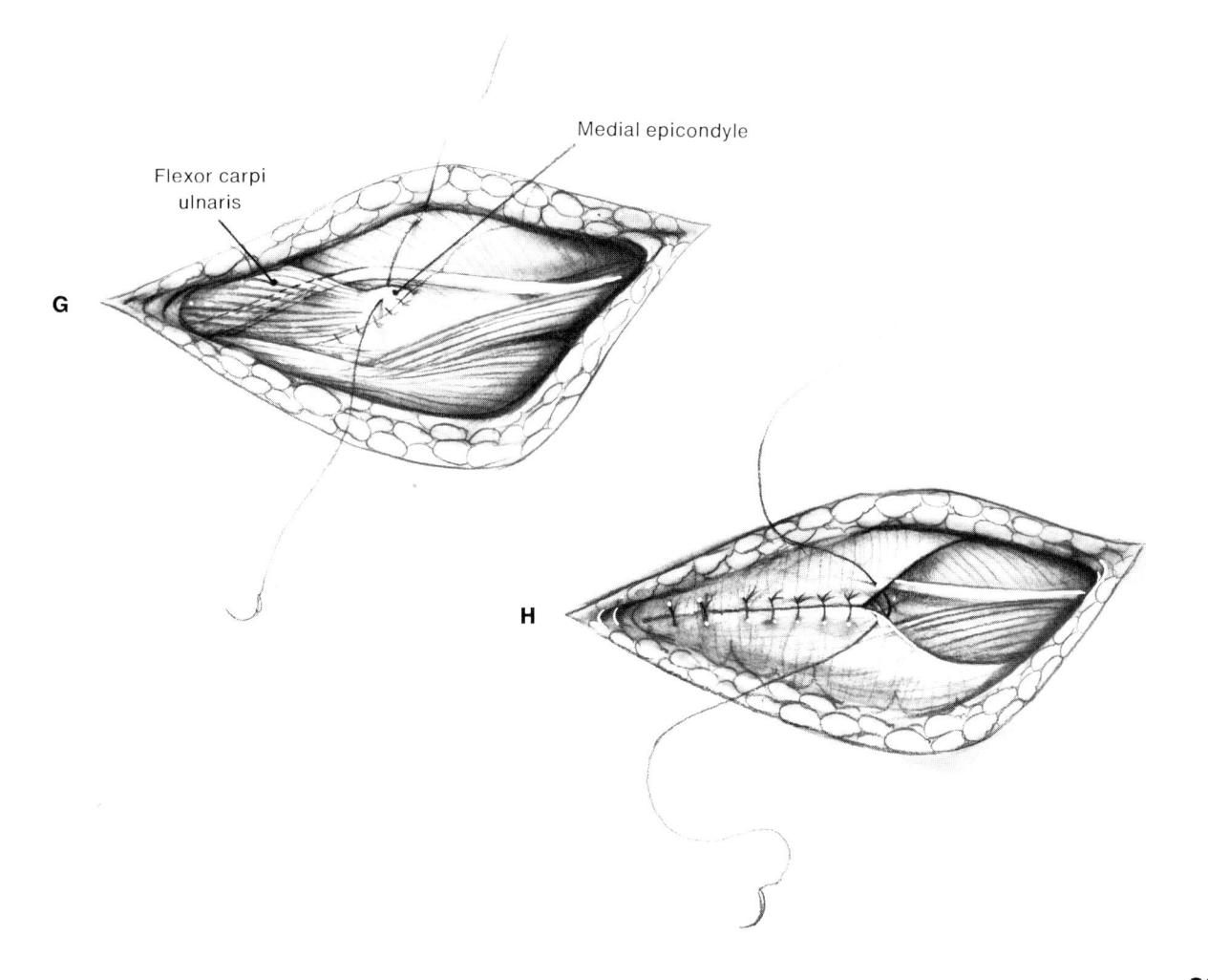

REFERENCES

Adler, S., Fay, G. F., and MacAusland, R.: Treatment of olecranon fractures—indications for excision of the olecranon fragment and repair of the triceps tendon, J. Trauma **2**:597, 1962.

Badger, F. G.: Fractures of the lateral condyle of the humerus, J. Bone Joint Surg. **36-B**:147, 1954.

Bado, J. L.: The Monteggia lesion, Clin. Orthop. **50**:71, 1967.

Barr, J. S., and Eaton, R. G.: Elbow reconstruction with a new prosthesis to replace the distal end of the humerus. A case report, J. Bone Joint Surg. **47-A**:1408, 1965.

Bell Tawse, A. J. S.: The treatment of malunited anterior Monteggia fractures in children, J. Bone Joint Surg. **47-B**:718, 1965.

Blount, W. P.: Fractures in children, Baltimore, 1955, The Williams & Wilkins Co.

Bost, F. C., Schottstaedt, E. R., Larsen, L. J., and Abbott, L. C.: Surgical approaches to the elbow joint, American Academy of Orthopaedic Surgeons Instructional Course Lectures, vol. 10, Ann Arbor, 1953, J. W. Edwards.

Boyd, H. B., and Anderson, L. D.: A method for reinsertion of the distal biceps brachii tendon, J. Bone Joint Surg. **43-A**:1041, 1961.

Boyd, H. B., and Boals, J. C.: The Monteggia lesion. A review of 159 cases, Clin. Orthop. **66**:94, 1969.

Brattstrom, H., and Alkhudairy, H.: Synovectomy of elbow in rheumatoid arthritis, Acta Orthop. Scand. **46**:744, 1975.

Brett, M. S.: Excision of the head of the radius. In Rob, C. and Smith, R., editors: Operative surgery, vol. 9, ed. 2, London, 1969, Butterworth & Co., Ltd.

Bunnell, S.: Restoring flexion to the paralytic elbow, J. Bone Joint Surg. **33-A**:565, 1951.

Bush, L. F., and McClain, E. J., Jr.: Operative treatment of fractures of the elbow in adults, American Academy of Orthopaedic Surgeons Instructional Course Lectures, vol. 16, St. Louis, 1959, The C. V. Mosby Co., p. 265.

Campbell, W. C.: Arthroplasty of the elbow, Ann. Surg. **76**:615, 1922.

Carroll, R. E.: Restoration of flexor power to the flail elbow by transplantation of the triceps tendon, Surg. Gynecol. Obstet. **95**:685, 1952.

Carroll, R. E., and Hill, N. A.: Triceps transfer to restore elbow flexion. A study of fifteen patients with paralytic lesions and arthrogryposis, J. Bone Joint Surg. **52-A**:239, 1970.

Chacha, P. B.: Fracture of the medial condyle of the humerus with rotational displacement. Report of two cases, J. Bone Joint Surg. **52-A**:1453, 1970.

Conner, A. N., and Smith, M. G. H.: Displaced fractures of the lateral humeral condyle in children. J. Bone Joint Surg. **52-B**:460, 1970.

Copeland, S. A., and Taylor, J. G.: Synovectomy of the elbow in rheumatoid arthritis, J. Bone Joint Surg. **61-B**:69, 1979.

Davidson, A. J., and Horwitz, M. T.: Late or tardy ulnar-nerve paralysis, J. Bone Joint Surg. **17**:844, 1935.

Davis, W. M., and Yassine, Z.: An etiological factor in tear of the distal tendon of the biceps brachii, J. Bone Joint Surg. **38-A**:1365, 1956.

Dobbie, R. P.: Avulsion of the lower biceps brachii tendon, analysis of fifty-one previously unreported cases, Am. J. Surg. **51**:662, 1941.

Dobyns, J. H., Bryan, R. S., Linscheid, R. L., and Peterson, L. F. A.: Special problems in total elbow arthroplasty, Geriatrics **31**:57, 1976.

Dunlop, J.: Transcondylar fractures of the humerus in childhood, J. Bone Joint Surg. **21**:59, 1939.

Dunn, A. W.: A distal humeral prosthesis, Clin. Orthop. **77**:199, 1971.

Evans, E. M.: Pronation injuries of forearm with special reference to anterior Monteggia fracture, J. Bone Joint Surg. **31-B**:578, 1949.

Fahey, J. J.: Fractures of the elbow in children, American Academy of Orthopaedic Surgeons Instructional Course Lectures, vol. 17, St. Louis, 1960, The C. V. Mosby Co., p. 13.

Fahey, J. J., and O'Brien, E. T.: Fracture-separation of the medial humeral condyle in a child confused with fracture of the medial epicondyle, J. Bone Joint Surg. **53-A**:1102, 1971.

Flynn, J. C., and Richards, J. F.: Non-union of minimally displaced fractures of the lateral condyle of the humerus in children, J. Bone Joint Surg. **53-A**:1096, 1971.

Gordon, M. L.: Monteggia fracture. A combined surgical approach employing a single lateral incision, Clin. Orthop. **50**:87, 1967.

Hardacre, J. A., Nahigian, S. H., Froimson, A. I., and Brown, J. E.: Fractures of the lateral condyle of the humerus in children, J. Bone Joint Surg. **53-A**:1083, 1971.

Harty, M., and Joyce, J. J., III: Surgical approaches to the elbow, J. Bone Joint Surg. **46-A**:1598, 1964.

Ingersoll, R. E.: Fractures of the humeral condyles in children, Clin. Orthop. **41**:32, 1965.

Inglis, A. E., Ranawat, C. S., and Straub, L. R.: Synovectomy and debridement of the elbow in rheumatoid arthritis, J. Bone Joint Surg. **53-A**:652, 1971.

Jessing, P.: Monteggia lesions and their complicating nerve damage, Acta Orthop. Scand. **46**:601, 1975.

Kaplan, S. S., and Reckling, F. W.: Fracture separation of the lower humeral epiphysis with medial displacement. Review of the literature and report of a case, J. Bone Joint Surg. **53-A**:1105, 1971.

Kettelkamp, D. B., and Larson, C. B.: Evaluation of the Steindler flexorplasty, J. Bone Joint Surg. **45-A**:513, 1963.

Key, J. A.: Treatment of fractures of the head and neck of the radius, J.A.M.A. **96**:101, 1931.

Kini, M. G.: Fractures of the lateral condyle of the lower end of the humerus with complications, J. Bone Joint Surg. **24**:270, 1942.

Knight, R. A.: The management of fractures about the elbow in adults, American Academy of Orthopaedic Surgeons Instructional Course Lectures, vol. 14, Ann Arbor, 1957, J. W. Edwards, p. 123.

Laine, V., and Vainio, K.: Synovectomy of the elbow. In Hijmans, W., Paul, W. D., and Herschel, H., editors: Early synovectomy in rheumatoid arthritis. Proceedings of the Symposium on Early Synovectomy in Rheumatoid Arthritis, Amsterdam, April 12-15, 1967. Amsterdam, 1969, Excerpta Medica Foundation.

Larmon, W. A., and Kurtz, J. F.: The surgical management of chronic tophaceous gout, J. Bone Joint Surg. **40-A**:743, 1958.

Linscheid, R. L.: Surgery for rheumatoid arthritis—timing and techniques: the upper extremity, J. Bone Joint Surg. **50-A**:605, 1968.

Livingstone, S. M.: Some arguments in favour of direct electric drive for an artificial elbow, J. Bone Joint Surg. **47-B**:453, 1965.

MacAusland, W. R.: Arthroplasty of the elbow, N. Engl. J. Med. **236**:97, 1947.

MacAusland, W. R.: Replacement of the lower end of the humerus with a prosthesis; report of four cases, West. J. Surg. **62:**557, 1954.

MacAusland, W. R.: Fracture of the medial epicondylar epiphysis of the humerus, Am. J. Surg. **104:**77, 1962.

Macnicol, M. F.: The results of operation for ulnar neuritis, J. Bone Joint Surg. **61-B:**159, 1979.

Mann, T. S.: Prognosis in supracondylar fractures, J. Bone Joint Surg. **45-B:**516, 1963.

Marmor, L.: Surgery of the rheumatoid elbow. Follow-up study on synovectomy combined with radial-head excision, J. Bone Joint Surg. **54-A:**573, 1972.

Matthewson, M. H., and McCreath, S. W.: Tension band wiring of olecranon fractures. In Proceedings of the British Orthopaedic Association, J. Bone Joint Surg. **57-B:**339, 1975.

Mayer, L., and Greene, W.: Experiences with the Steindler flexorplasty at the elbow, J. Bone Joint Surg. **36-A:**775, 1954.

Maylahn, D. J., and Fahey, J. J.: Fractures of the elbow in children: a review of 300 cases (in Proceedings of the American Medical Association Section on Orthopaedic Surgery), J. Bone Joint Surg. **40-A:**233, 1958.

McKeever, F. M., and Buck, R. M.: Fracture of the olecranon process of the ulna; treatment by excision of fragment and repair of triceps tendon, J.A.M.A. **135:**1, 1947.

McLearie, M., and Merson, R. D.: Injuries to the lateral condyle ephiphysis of the humerus in children, J. Bone Joint Surg. **36-B:**84, 1954,

Meyerding, H. W.: Volkmann's ischemic contracture associated with supracondylar fracture of the humerus, J.A.M.A. **106:**1139, 1936.

Millard, D. R., Jr., and Ortiz, A. C.: Correction of severe elbow contractures, J. Bone Joint Surg. **47-A:**1347, 1965.

Miller, W. E.: Comminuted fractures of the distal end of the humerus in the adult, J. Bone Joint Surg. **46-A:**644, 1964.

Mital, M. A.: Lengthening of the elbow flexors in cerebral palsy, J. Bone Joint Surg. **61-A:**515, 1979.

Mobley, J. E., and Janes, J. M.: Monteggia fractures, Proc. Staff Meet. Mayo Clin. **30:**497, 1955.

Monteggia, G. B.: Instituzioni chirurgiche, ed. 2, Milan, 1813-1815, G. Maspero. (Cited in J. Bone Joint Surg. **16:**354, 1934.)

Morrey, B. F., Chao, E. Y., and Hoi, F. C.: Biomechanical study of the elbow following excision of the radial head, J. Bone Joint Surg. **61-A:**63, 1979.

Nirschal, R. P., and Pettrone, F. A.: Tennis elbow. The surgical treatment of lateral epicondylitis, J. Bone Joint Surg. **61-A:**832, 1979.

Pankovich, A. M.: Anconeus approach to the elbow joint and the proximal part of the radius and ulna, J. Bone Joint Surg. **59-A:**124, 1977.

Penrose, J. H.: Monteggia fracture with posterior dislocation of the radial head, J. Bone Joint Surg. **33-B:**65, 1951.

Radin, E. L., and Riseborough, E. J.: Fractures of the radial head, J. Bone Joint Surg. **48-A:**1055, 1966.

Riseborough, E. J., and Radin, E. L.: Intercondylar T fractures of the humerus in the adult. A comparison of operative and nonoperative treatment in twenty-nine cases, J. Bone Joint Surg. **51-A:**130, 1969.

Roberts, J. B., and Pankratz, D. G.: The surgical treatment of heterotopic ossification at the elbow following long-term coma, J. Bone Joint Surg. **61-A:**760, 1979.

Smith, F. M.: Monteggia fractures. An analysis of twenty-five consecutive fresh injuries, Surg. Gynecol. Obstet. **85:**630, 1947.

Smith, F. M., and Joyce, J. J., III: Fractures of the lateral condyle of the humerus in children, Am. J. Surg. **87:**324, 1954.

Speed, J. S.: Surgical treatment of condylar fractures of the humerus, American Academy of Orthopaedic Surgeons Instructional Course Lectures, vol. 7, Ann Arbor, 1950, J. W. Edwards, p. 187.

Speed, J. S., and Boyd, H. B.: Treatment of fractures of ulna with dislocation of head of radius (Monteggia fractures), J.A.M.A. **115:**1699, 1940.

Speed, J. S., and Macey, H. B.: Fractures of the humeral condyle in children, J. Bone Joint Surg. **15:**903, 1933.

Staples, O. S.: Dislocation of the brachial artery. A complication of supracondylar fracture of the humerus in childhood, J. Bone Joint Surg. **47-A:**1525, 1965.

Steindler, A.: Operative treatment of paralytic conditions of the upper extremity, J. Orthop. Surg. **1:**608, 1919.

Steindler, A.: Tendon transplantations in the upper extremity, Am. J. Surg. **44:**260, 1939.

Steindler, A.: Orthopedic operations: indications, technic and end results, Springfield, Ill., 1940, Charles C Thomas, Publisher.

Steindler, A.: Muscle and tendon transplantation at the elbow, American Academy of Orthopaedic Surgeons Instructional Course Lectures, vol. 2, Ann Arbor, 1944, J. W. Edwards.

Strachan, J. C. H., and Ellis, B. W.: Vulnerability of the posterior interosseous nerve during radial head resection, J. Bone Joint Surg. **53-B:**320, 1971.

Todd, T. W.: Atlas of skeletal maturation (hand), St. Louis, 1937, The C. V. Mosby Co.

Tompkins, D. G.: The anterior Monteggia fracture. Observations on etiology and treatment, J. Bone Joint Surg. **53-A:**1109, 1971.

Torgerson, W. R., and Leach, R. E.: Synovectomy of the elbow in rheumatoid arthritis. Report of five cases, J. Bone Joint Surg. **52-A:**371, 1970.

Vanderpool, D. W., Chalmers, J., Lamb, D. W., and Whiston, T. B.: Peripheral compression lesions of the ulnar nerve, J. Bone Joint Surg. **50-B:**792, 1968.

Van Gorder, G. W.: Surgical approach in supracondylar "T" fractures of the humerus requiring open reduction, J. Bone Joint Surg. **22:**278, 1940.

Watson-Jones, R.: Primary nerve lesions in injuries of the elbow and wrist, J. Bone Joint Surg. **12:**121, 1930.

Weseley, M. S., Barenfeld, P. A., and Eisenstein, A. L.: The use of the Zuelzer hook plate in fixation of olecranon fractures, J. Bone Joint Surg. **58-A:**859, 1976.

Wiley, J. J., Pegington, J., and Horwich, J. P.: Traumatic dislocation of the radius at the elbow, J. Bone Joint Surg. **56-B:**501, 1974.

Wilson, J. N.: Fractures of the external condyle of the humerus in children, Br. J. Surg. **43:**88, 1955.

Wilson, P. D.: Fractures of the lateral condyle of the humerus in childhood, J. Bone Joint Surg. **18:**301, 1936.

4

FOREARM

RELEASE OF FLEXOR-PRONATOR ORIGIN (FOR CEREBRAL PALSY) (Plate 4-1)

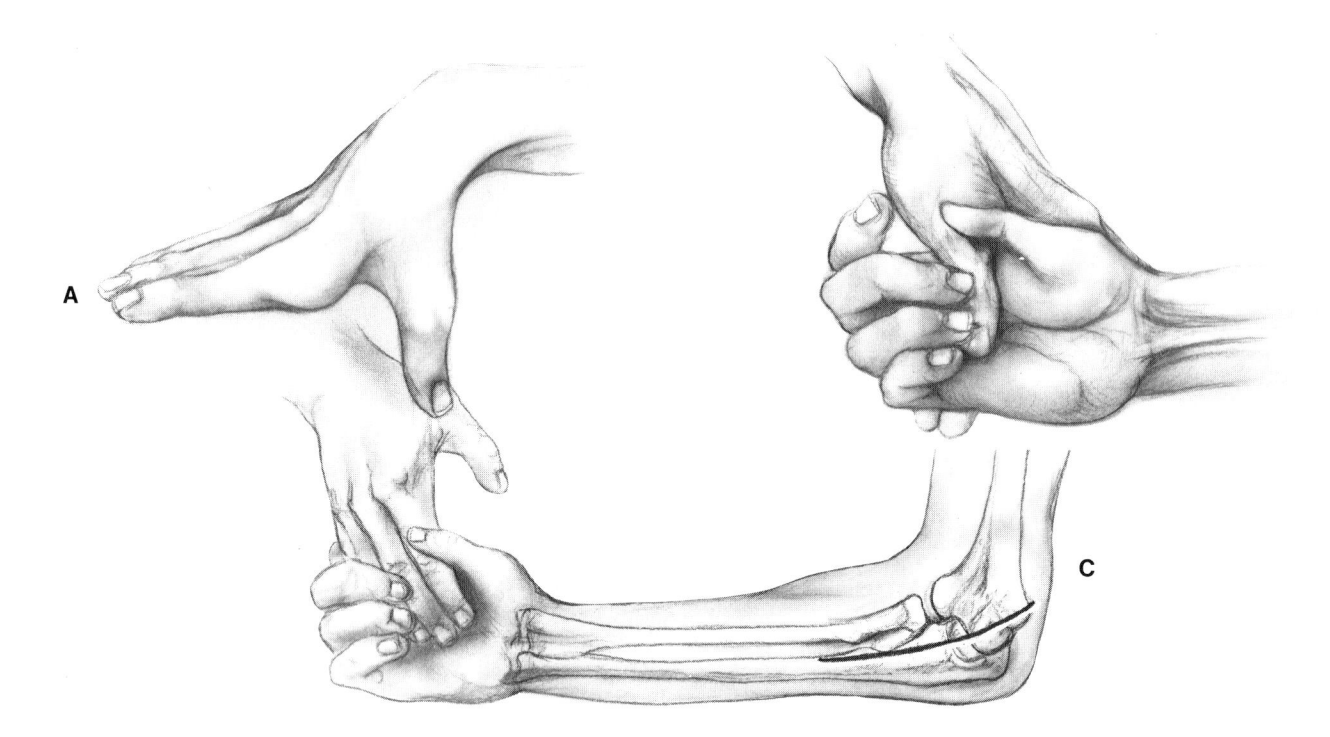

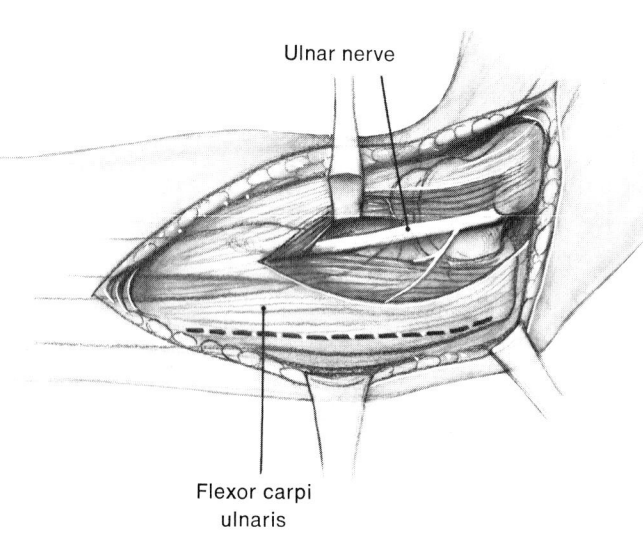

GENERAL DISCUSSION. Patients with spastic paralysis of the upper extremity frequently have some degree of disability resulting from flexion deformities of the wrist and fingers (**A** and **B**). Release of the flexor-pronator origin can produce improvement in control and function of the hand in many of these patients. The same procedure may at times be useful to produce some functional improvement in selected stroke patients.

DETAILS OF PROCEDURE. The patient is positioned supine with the elbow flexed and the arm supported in a position of maximum external rotation of the shoulder (or with the patient prone and the dorsal aspect of the patient's wrist placed over the midportion of the back in a position similar to that which may be used for open reduction of a displaced fracture of the medial epicondyle). The incision is made (**C**) over the distal portion of the upper arm medially and is extended along the subcutaneous border of the ulna. The wound edges containing skin and subcutaneous tissue are retracted. It may be necessary to ligate and divide the basilic vein in the distal portion of the wound. The medial cutaneous nerve of the forearm should be carefully protected. The ulnar nerve is identified in the proximal portion of the wound and isolated by careful dissection from proximal to distal until its branches to flexor carpi ulnaris and both heads of the flexor digitorum profundus have been identified (**D**). These motor nerves are protected as the flexor muscles are elevated from the anterior surface of the ulna beginning at the distal portion of the wound. Dissecting in a plane between the anterior surface of the ulna (an interosseous membrane) and the flexor muscles protects the ulnar artery along with the motor branches of the ulnar nerve.

(Plate 4-1) RELEASE OF FLEXOR-PRONATOR ORIGIN (FOR CEREBRAL PALSY)

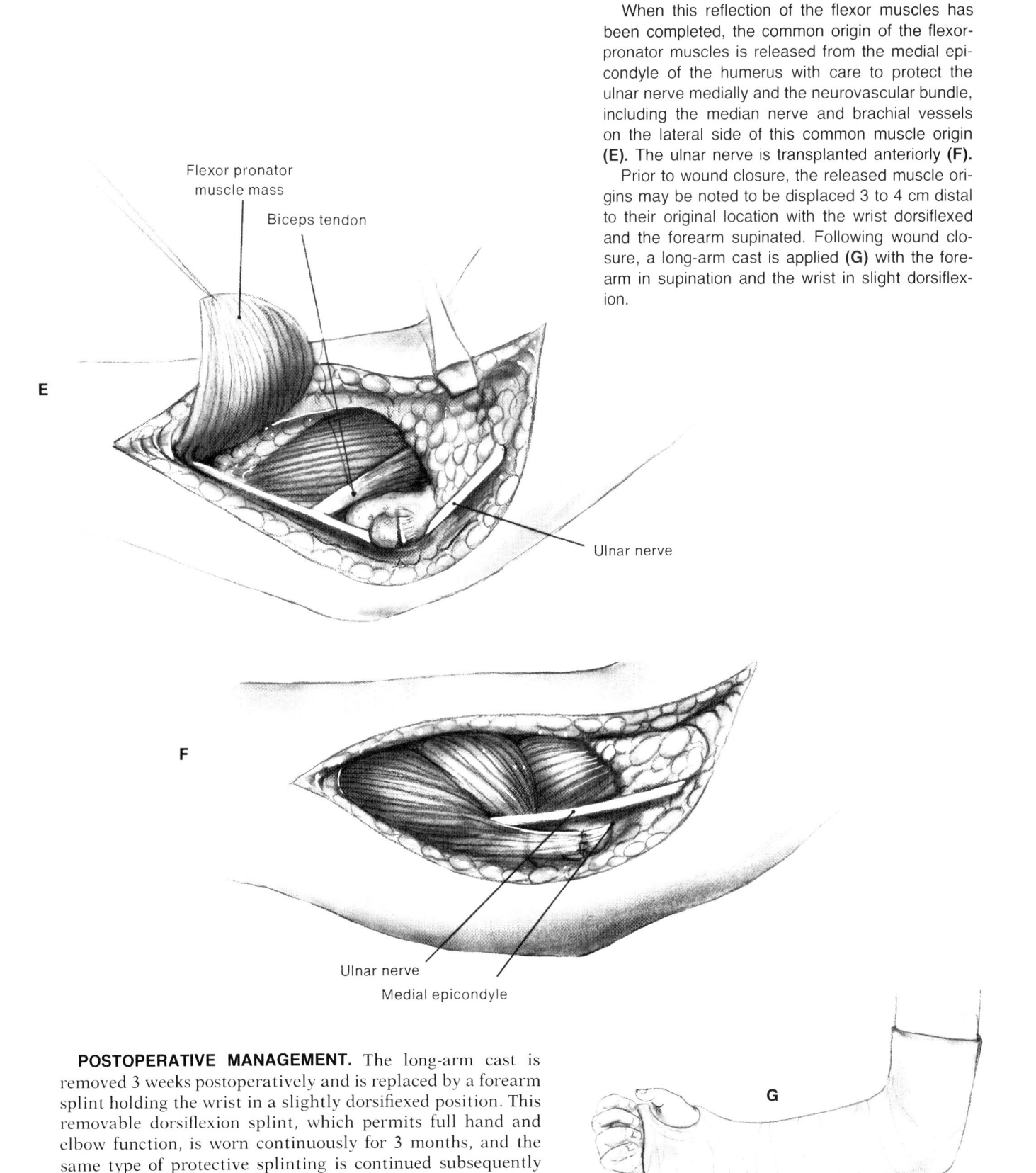

When this reflection of the flexor muscles has been completed, the common origin of the flexor-pronator muscles is released from the medial epicondyle of the humerus with care to protect the ulnar nerve medially and the neurovascular bundle, including the median nerve and brachial vessels on the lateral side of this common muscle origin **(E)**. The ulnar nerve is transplanted anteriorly **(F)**.

Prior to wound closure, the released muscle origins may be noted to be displaced 3 to 4 cm distal to their original location with the wrist dorsiflexed and the forearm supinated. Following wound closure, a long-arm cast is applied **(G)** with the forearm in supination and the wrist in slight dorsiflexion.

POSTOPERATIVE MANAGEMENT. The long-arm cast is removed 3 weeks postoperatively and is replaced by a forearm splint holding the wrist in a slightly dorsiflexed position. This removable dorsiflexion splint, which permits full hand and elbow function, is worn continuously for 3 months, and the same type of protective splinting is continued subsequently at night for an additional 3 or more months.

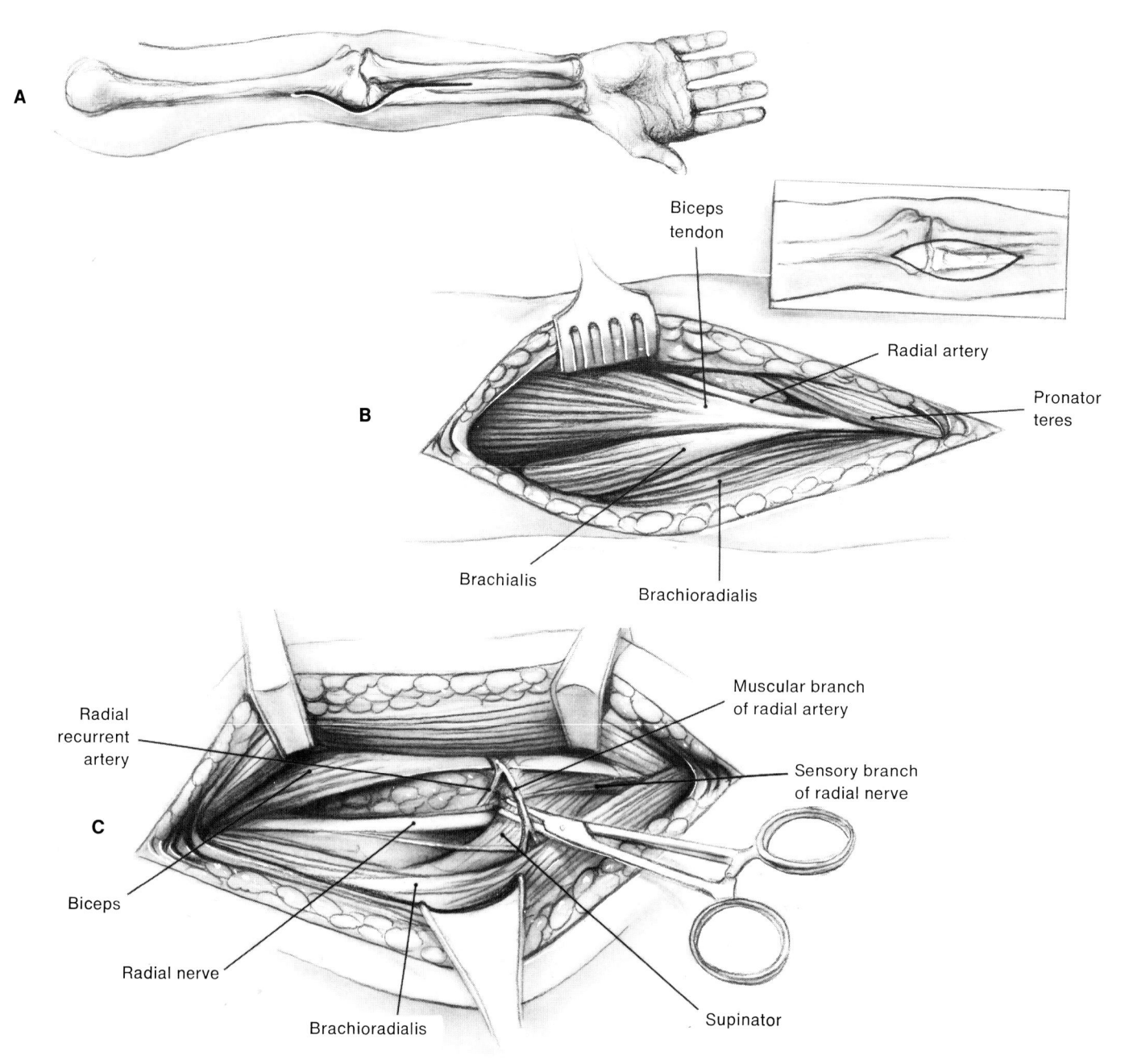

OPEN REDUCTION FOR FRACTURE OF PROXIMAL RADIUS (ANTERIOR EXPOSURE) (Plate 4-2)

GENERAL DISCUSSION. For open reduction and internal fixation of fractures involving the proximal shaft of the radius, exposure of the radius through an anterior approach will be most satisfactory. Specific care must be taken to protect the deep branch of the radial nerve. The radial recurrent artery and vein must be isolated and ligated. Flexing the elbow will allow more complete retraction of the brachioradialis and radial extensor muscles for improved exposure of the underlying supinator muscle and the shaft of the radius. For fractures of the proximal shaft of the radius, plate fixation is best applied to the posterior surface.

DETAILS OF PROCEDURE. With the patient's elbow extended and the forearm in supination, an incision is made (A) beginning proximally along the lateral aspect of the biceps muscle. After curving laterally in the midportion of the incision to specifically avoid a straight longitudinal incision across the flexor surface of the elbow, the incision extends distally along the medial border of the brachioradialis muscle to the midportion of the forearm. The biceps tendon is identified by palpation (B), and the fascia is incised along its lateral side. A retractor placed along the lateral aspect of the biceps tendon for medial retraction is helpful. The radial recurrent artery and veins must be specifically identified, doubly li-

(Plate 4-2) OPEN REDUCTION FOR FRACTURE OF PROXIMAL RADIUS (ANTERIOR EXPOSURE)

gated, and divided (**C**). Dissection is then continued down to the proximal radius.

With the forearm still in supination, the attachment of the supinator muscle to the proximal radius is reflected subperiosteally (**D**) in a lateral direction, and this is continued distally as the forearm is gradually pronated (**E**). In this manner the posterior interosseous nerve is protected within the sbustance of the supinator muscle. The brachial vessels and median nerve are protected by keeping the plane of dissection lateral to the biceps tendon within the antecubital space. Flexing the elbow will help to improve the exposure of the proximal radius (**F**) by relaxing the brachioradialis muscle, which is retracted laterally. The proximal two fifths of the radius can be exposed.

OPEN REDUCTION FOR FRACTURE OF PROXIMAL RADIUS (ANTERIOR EXPOSURE) (Plate 4-2)

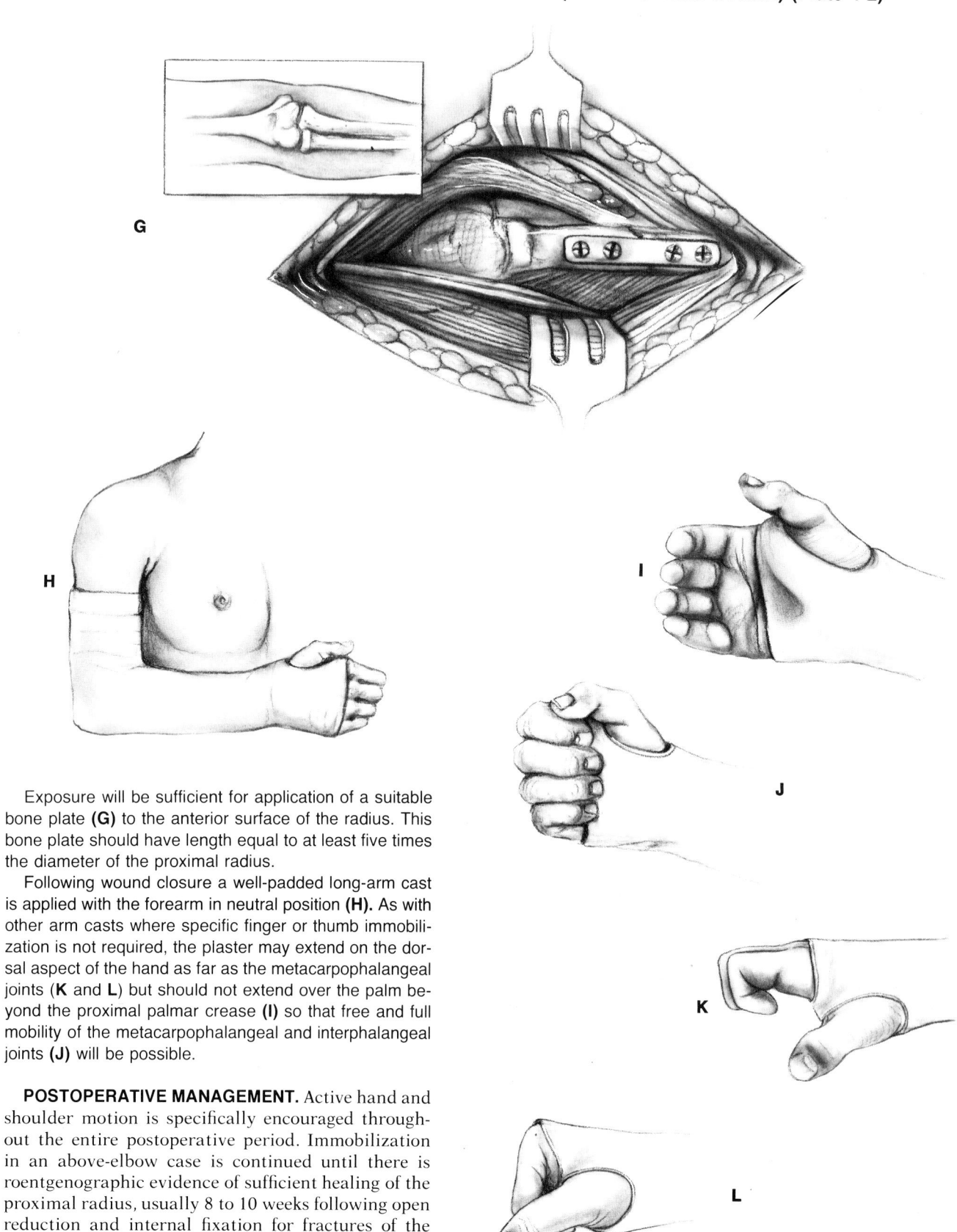

Exposure will be sufficient for application of a suitable bone plate **(G)** to the anterior surface of the radius. This bone plate should have length equal to at least five times the diameter of the proximal radius.

Following wound closure a well-padded long-arm cast is applied with the forearm in neutral position **(H)**. As with other arm casts where specific finger or thumb immobilization is not required, the plaster may extend on the dorsal aspect of the hand as far as the metacarpophalangeal joints **(K and L)** but should not extend over the palm beyond the proximal palmar crease **(I)** so that free and full mobility of the metacarpophalangeal and interphalangeal joints **(J)** will be possible.

POSTOPERATIVE MANAGEMENT. Active hand and shoulder motion is specifically encouraged throughout the entire postoperative period. Immobilization in an above-elbow case is continued until there is roentgenographic evidence of sufficient healing of the proximal radius, usually 8 to 10 weeks following open reduction and internal fixation for fractures of the proximal shaft of the radius.

98

(Plate 4-3) OPEN REDUCTION FOR MIDSHAFT FRACTURE OF RADIUS AND ULNA

GENERAL DISCUSSION. For open reduction of midshaft fractures of the radius and ulna in adults, plate fixation is a good means for providing internal stabilization of the reduced fracture. After open fractures, it is best to obtain good soft tissue coverage initially and then wait 1 to 3 weeks before open plating of forearm fractures. If the fracture involves the distal shaft of the radius, it will be best to apply the plate to the anterior surface, which is usually broad, flat, and smooth, and will be a better bed for placement of the bone plate than the posterior surface of the distal radius, which is slightly convex. For fractures of the proximal radius it is best to apply the plate to the posterior surface of the radius. For plate fixation of fractures of the ulnar shaft it is best to apply the plate to whichever surface seems to fit best. If comminution of midshaft forearm fractures is extensive, supplemental bone grafting should be considered.

DETAILS OF PROCEDURE. A longitudinal incision is made along the lateral aspect of the forearm, which is positioned in supination. The incision is centered at the level of the fracture in the mid or distal shaft of the radius **(A)**. The plane is developed between brachioradialis and flexor carpi radialis muscles **(B)**. The sensory branch of the radial nerve is identified and retracted posteriorly along with the brachioradialis muscle. The radial artery is retracted medially with the flexor carpi radialis muscle **(C)**.

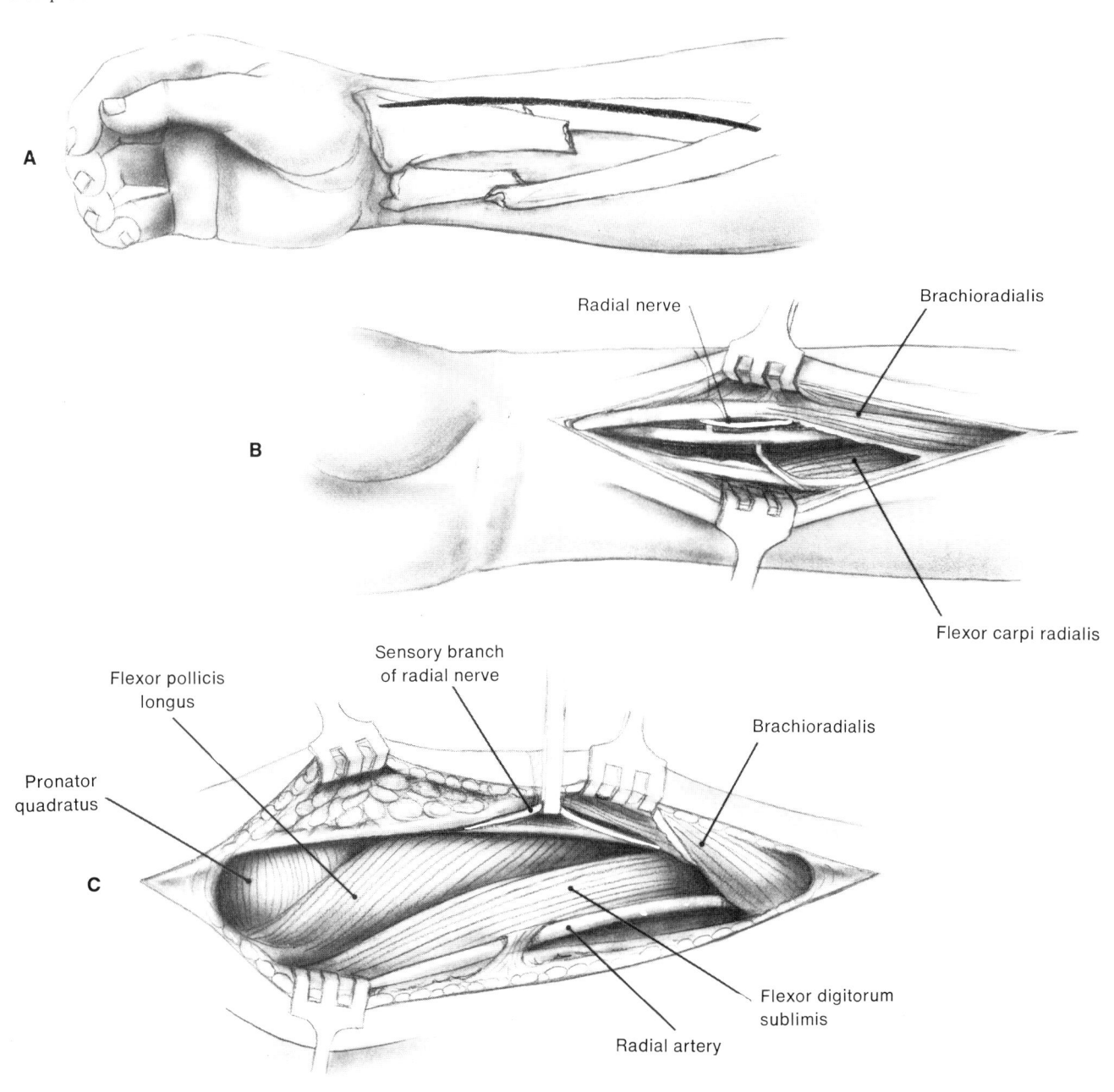

OPEN REDUCTION FOR MIDSHAFT FRACTURE OF RADIUS AND ULNA (Plate 4-3)

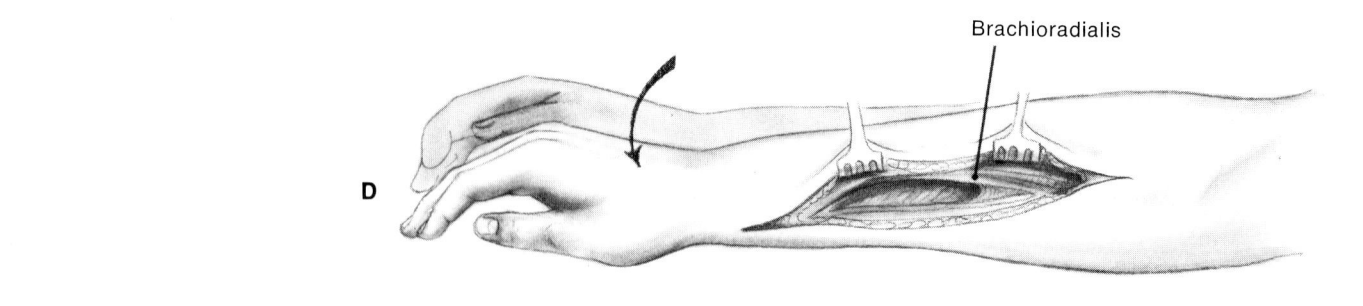

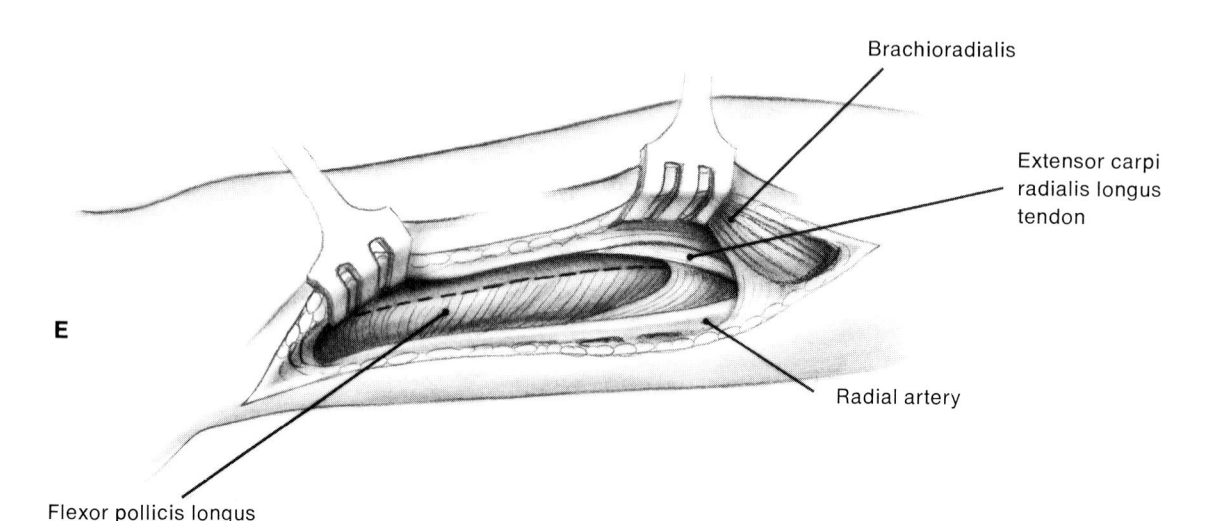

D

Brachioradialis

E

Brachioradialis

Extensor carpi radialis longus tendon

Radial artery

Flexor pollicis longus

The underlying attachments of flexor pollicis longus and pronator quadratus to the anterior surface of the radius are visualized. The origin of these muscles if reflected to expose the anterior surface of the radius. This is best carried out by pronating the forearm and beginning the reflection of these muscles on the lateral aspect of the anterior surface of the radius distal to the insertion of the pronator teres (**D** and **E**). Periosteal stripping should be avoided wherever possible.

After the fracture site and the adjacent anterior surface of the radius on each side of the fracture (**F**) are exposed, it should be possible to reduce the fracture and apply an appropriate plate. The plate is secured in place with transfixion screws. The length of the plate should be approximately five times the diameter of the bone, and there must be a minimum of two transfixion screws on each side of the fracture. A bone plate should adapt easily to the anterior surface of the radius, which is relatively flat. As the plate is applied, one should keep in mind that there is normally a slight radial bow of the radius as visualized from the anterior aspect. If a compression plate is selected for internal fixation, it is preferable, if possible, to place the compression device at the end of the plate nearest the middle of the bone. As the wound is closed, the muscles are replaced in their original position. If there is any question about increased tension on the deep fascia as it is reapproximated, it should be purposely left open to minimize the likelihood of postoperative ischemic muscle necrosis secondary to edema within a closed fascial compartment. Subcutaneous tissue and skin are closed in layers.

Any associated fracture of the ulna that requires open reduction is approached through a separate incision along the subcutaneous border of the ulna. Postoperatively a long-arm cast is applied, generally with the forearm in neutral rotation.

(Plate 4-3) OPEN REDUCTION FOR MIDSHAFT FRACTURE OF RADIUS AND ULNA

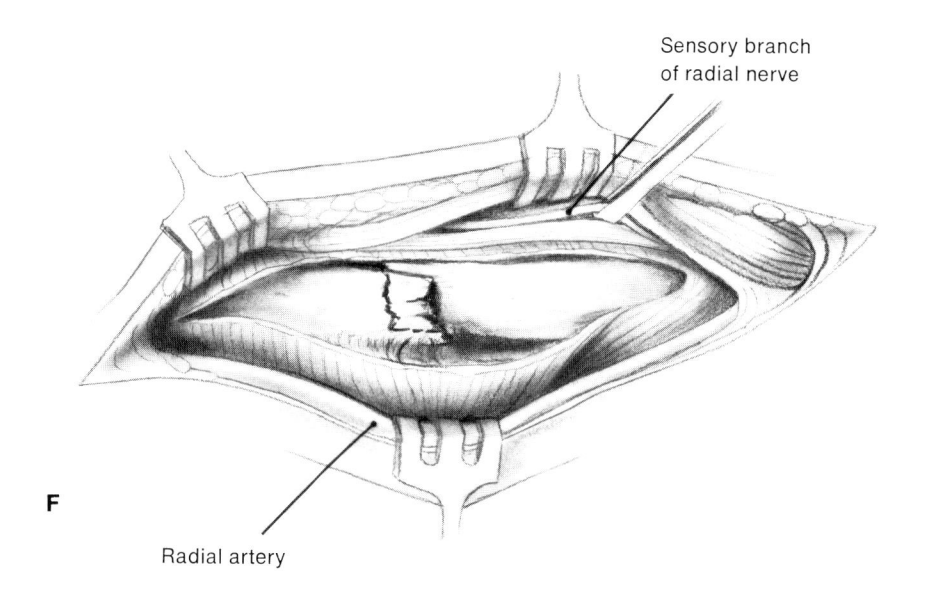

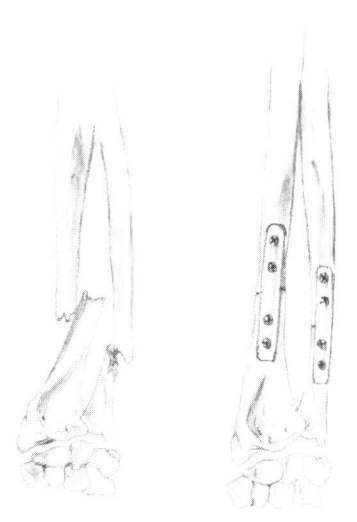

Sensory branch of radial nerve

F

Radial artery

POSTOPERATIVE MANAGEMENT. External plaster immobilization is continued in a long-arm cast until there is evidence of fracture healing, this period varying from 8 to 12 weeks as a rule depending on the nature of the fracture and the degree of stability obtained at the time of internal fixation. When a compression plate is applied securely, there will be little or no roentgenographic evidence of periosteal new bone formation about the fracture site to help in determining the duration of necessary external plaster immobilization. However, when secure internal fixation with compression has been applied, it should be possible to discontinue external plaster immobilization relatively early. Throughout the postoperative period of neccessary long arm plaster immobilization, the patient should be encouraged to maintain active mobility of all fingers and the shoulder of the involved extremity.

If an internal fixation plate is removed subsequently, it should not be done before 1 year (and preferably not before 18 months) following open reduction and internal fixation. The arm should be protected with a splint for 4 to 6 weeks after removal of forearm plates.

BELOW-ELBOW AMPUTATION (Plate 4-4)

INDICATIONS. Below-elbow amputation occasionally may be indicated for a diseased or severely injured limb.

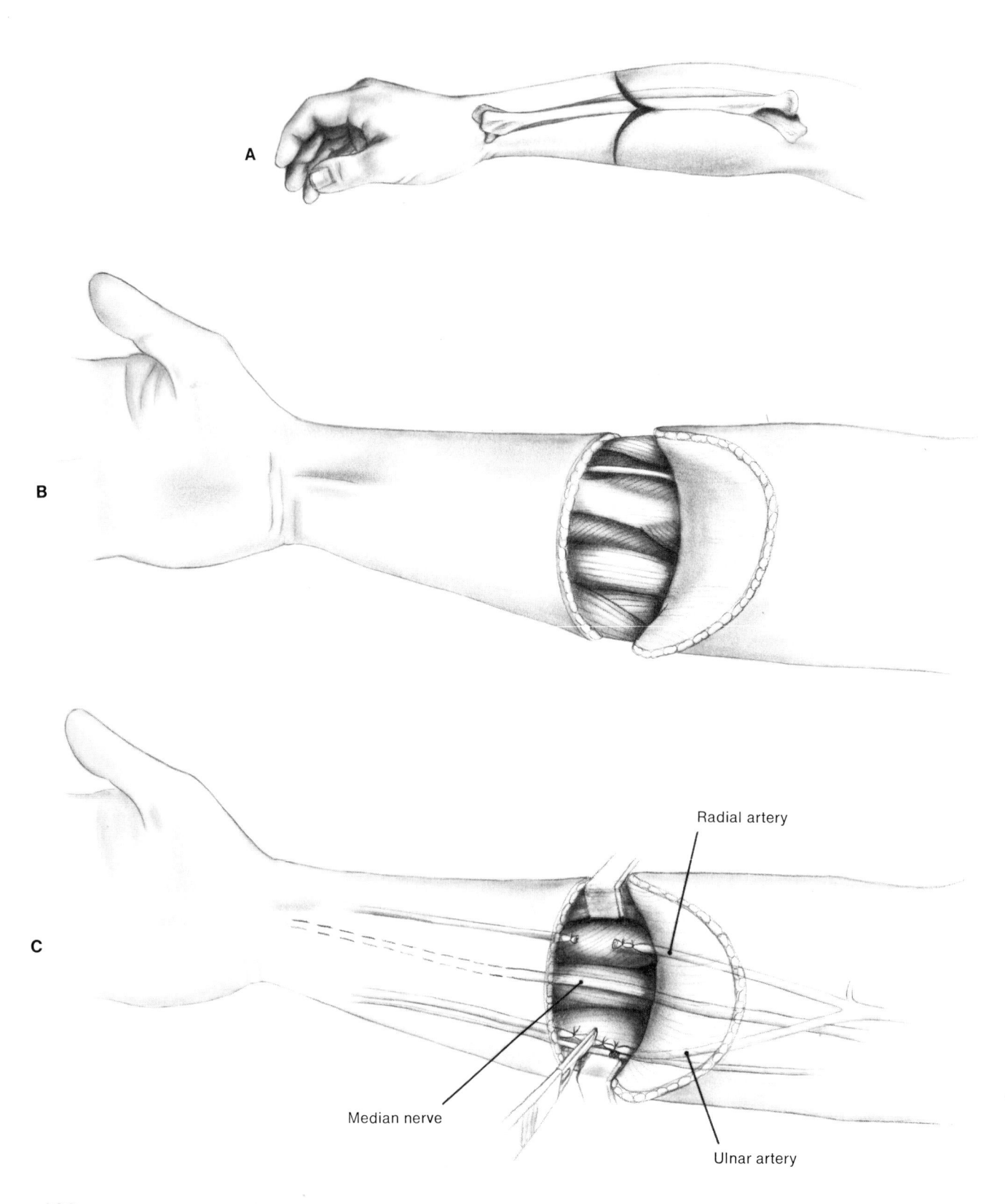

A

B

C

Radial artery

Median nerve

Ulnar artery

102

(Plate 4-4) BELOW-ELBOW AMPUTATION

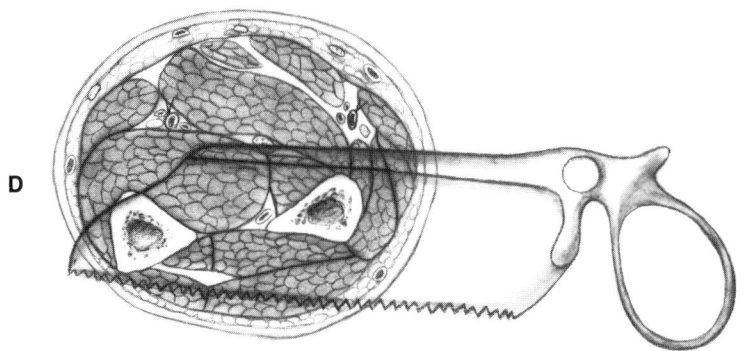

DETAILS OF PROCEDURE. Anterior and posterior flaps of equal size are mapped out, with the incision ending on the medial and lateral sides of the forearm at the level of the intended bone division **(A)**. The anterior and posterior flaps are developed with skin, subcutaneous tissue, and fascia in continuity **(B)**. The radial and ulnar arteries are identified, doubly ligated, and divided **(C)**. The median, radial and ulnar nerves are isolated individually, and each is drawn gently in a distal direction and then transected so that the end of each divided nerve will retract to a location well proximal to the ultimate closure of the amputation stump. The forearm muscles are incised transversely distal to the intended site of bone division and allowed to retract to that level.

The radius and ulna are divided transversely **(D)**, and any sharp bone edges are smoothed with a rasp **(E)**. The fascia of the anterior and posterior flaps is closed with interrupted absorbable sutures **(F)**. A Penrose drain may be left under the fascia to exit at one side of the stump closure **(G)**. Subcutaneous tissue is also reapproximated with interrupted absorbable sutures and the skin with interrupted nonabsorbable sutures. A bulky compression dressing is applied.

POSTOPERATIVE MANAGEMENT. The Penrose drain, when used, is generally removed 24 to 48 hours after surgery. A clean, evenly applied compression dressing is reapplied on a daily basis. Active elbow motion is encouraged as the wound discomfort subsides. Sutures are removed 2 weeks postoperatively. Early fabrication and use of an appropriate prosthetic device is desirable.

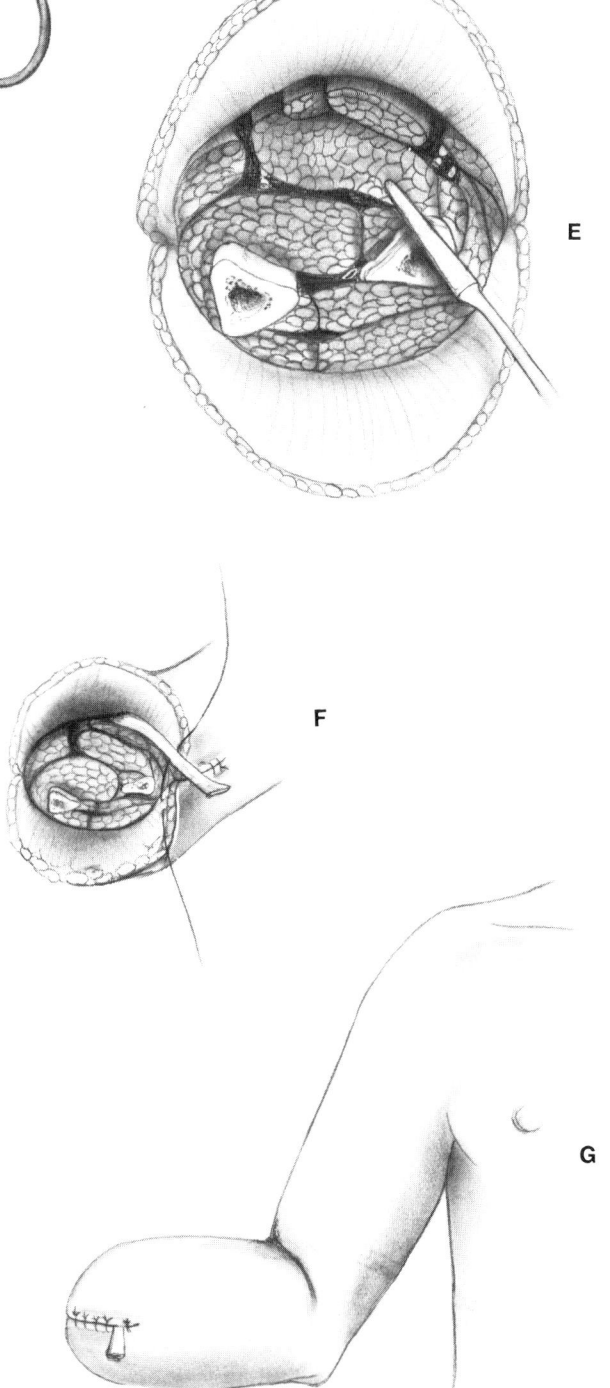

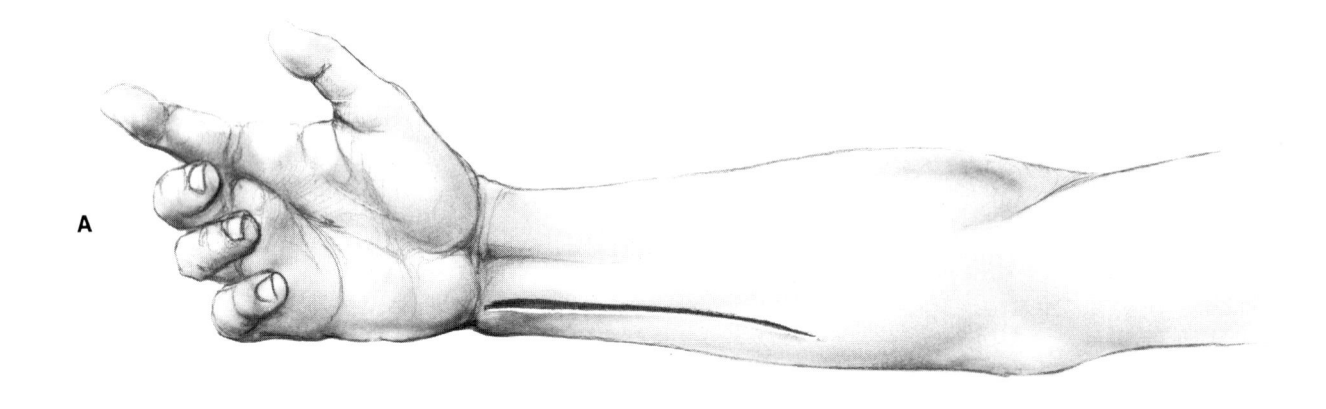

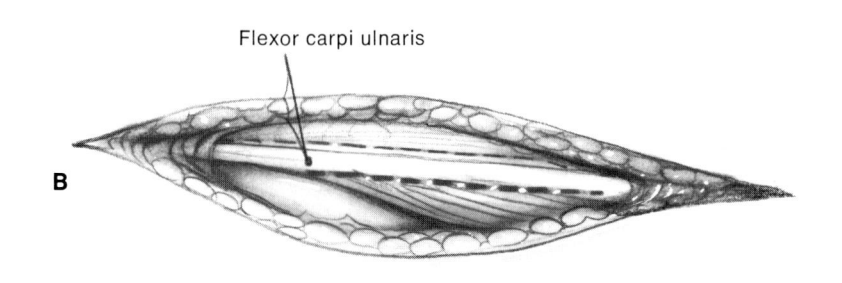

TENDON TRANSFERS FOR RADIAL NERVE PALSY (Plate 4-5)

GENERAL DISCUSSION. Restoration of function with radial nerve palsy requires a motor for dorsiflexion of the wrist, a motor for abduction and extension of the thumb, and a motor for extension of the fingers. A satisfactory plan is to transfer the insertion of the pronator teres to the extensor carpi radialis longus and brevis tendons, the flexor carpi ulnaris to the long finger extensors, and the palmaris longus to the extensor pollicis longus. The flexor carpi radialis and flexor digitorum sublimis to the middle or ring fingers are also potential motor muscles that have adequate power and amplitude if they are available and functioning.

DETAILS OF PROCEDURE. Three tendon transfers are carried out to restore finger extension, wrist extension, and thumb extension and abduction.

The flexor carpi ulnaris is exposed through a longitudinal incision over the anteromedial aspect of the forearm **(A)**. Insertion of this tendon is released near the pisiform bone as far distally as possible for transfer to the tendons of extensor digitorum longus on the dorsal aspect of the forearm. Sharp dissection is necessary to isolate the flexor carpi ulnaris from its long attachment to the subcutaneous surface of the ulna. It may be necessary to detach the central tendon from adjacent muscle fibers **(B)** in order to have a portion of tendon that will not be so bulky as to interfere with function in its subcutaneous position following transfer to the extensor digitorum communis tendons. Through a separate incision on the dorsal aspect of the distal forearm, the extensor digitorum communis tendons are exposed proximal to the dorsal carpal ligament. A wide subcutaneous tunnel is prepared around the ulnar aspect of the forearm to permit a straight line of pull for the flexor carpi ulnaris to the extensor digitorum communis tendons. The flexor carpi ulnaris tendon is passed through this tunnel **(C)**. A small longitudinal hole is created in each of the individual extensor digitorum communis tendons, creating an oblique path proximal to distal. The fingers are placed in functional position with successively less extension index to little fingers. The distal end of the flexor carpi ulnaris tendon is passed successively through each of these tendons and sutured to each tendon while the flexor carpi ulnaris tendon is held under moderate tension **(D)**.

Through a separate incision on the anterolateral aspect of the proximal forearm, the insertion of the pronator teres is identified and isolated with the forearm in supination **(E)**.

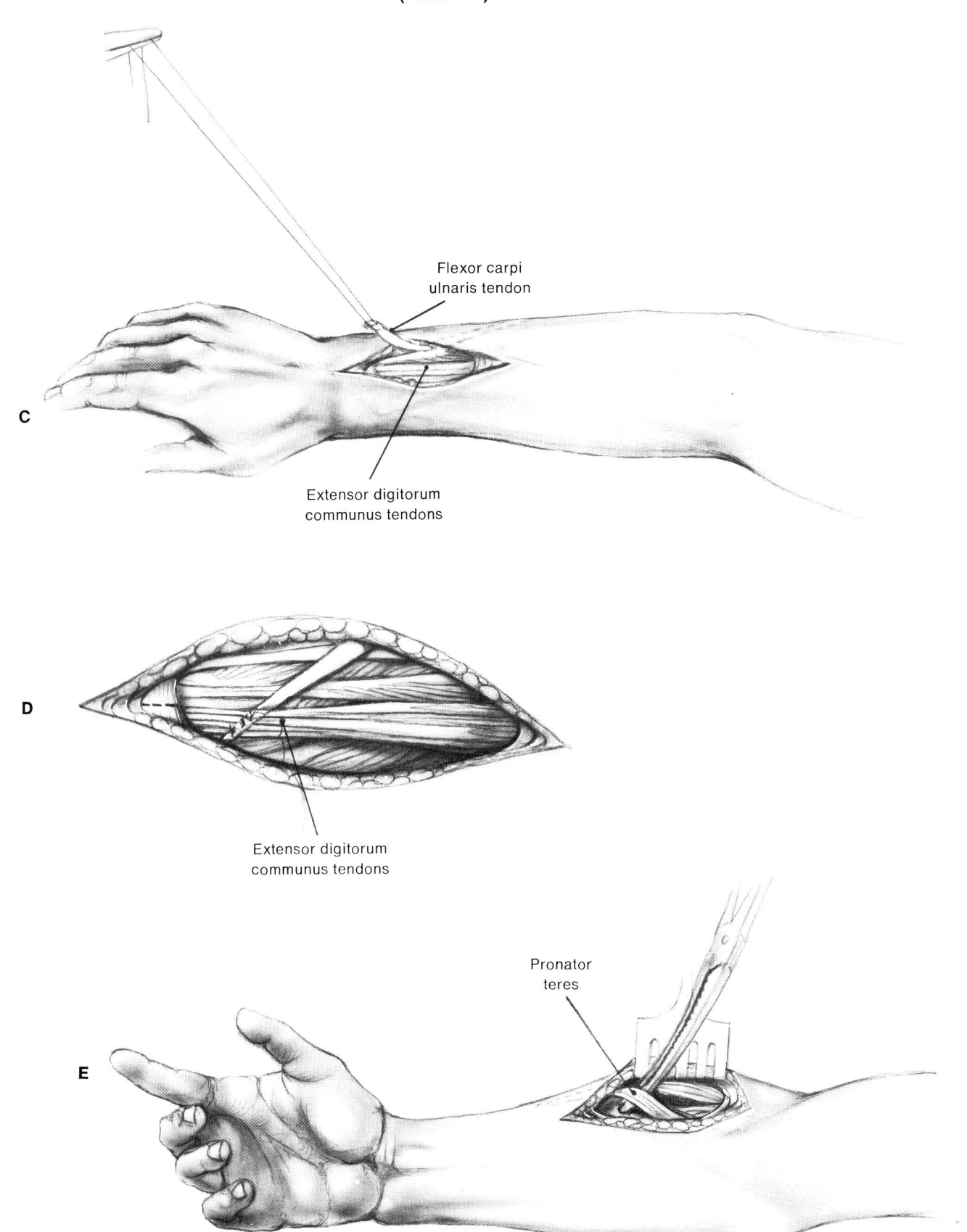

(Plate 4-5) TENDON TRANSFERS FOR RADIAL NERVE PALSY

C — Flexor carpi ulnaris tendon; Extensor digitorum communus tendons

D — Extensor digitorum communus tendons

E — Pronator teres

105

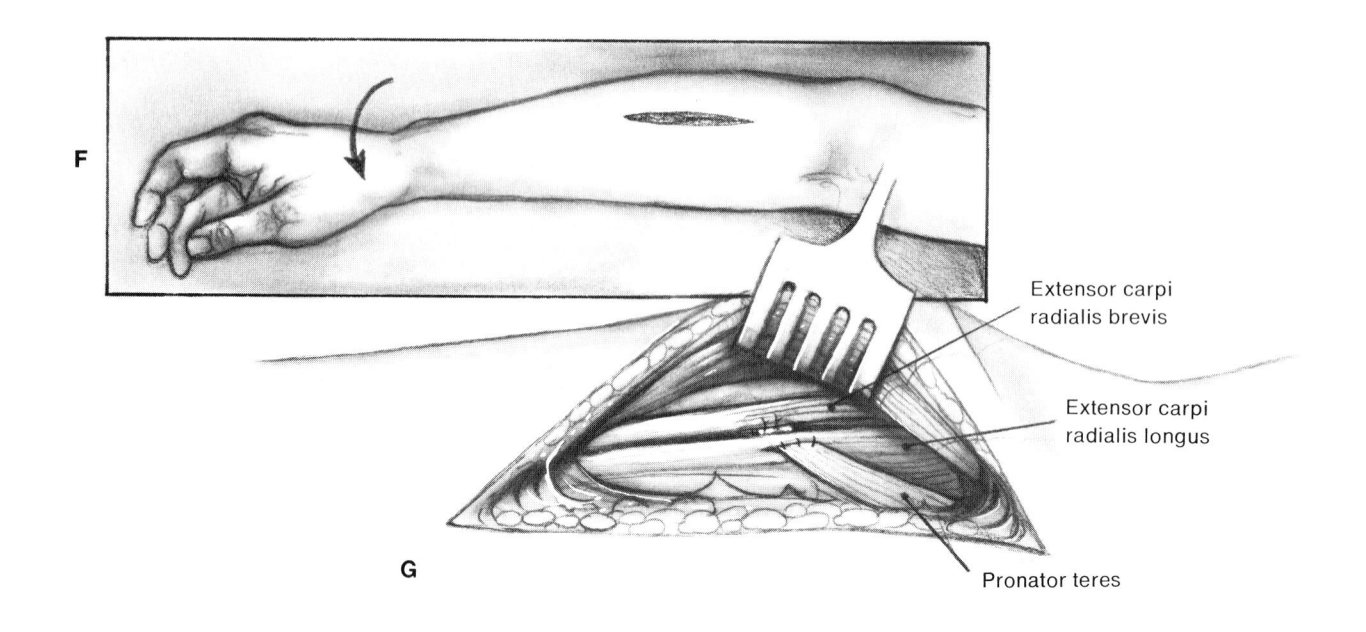

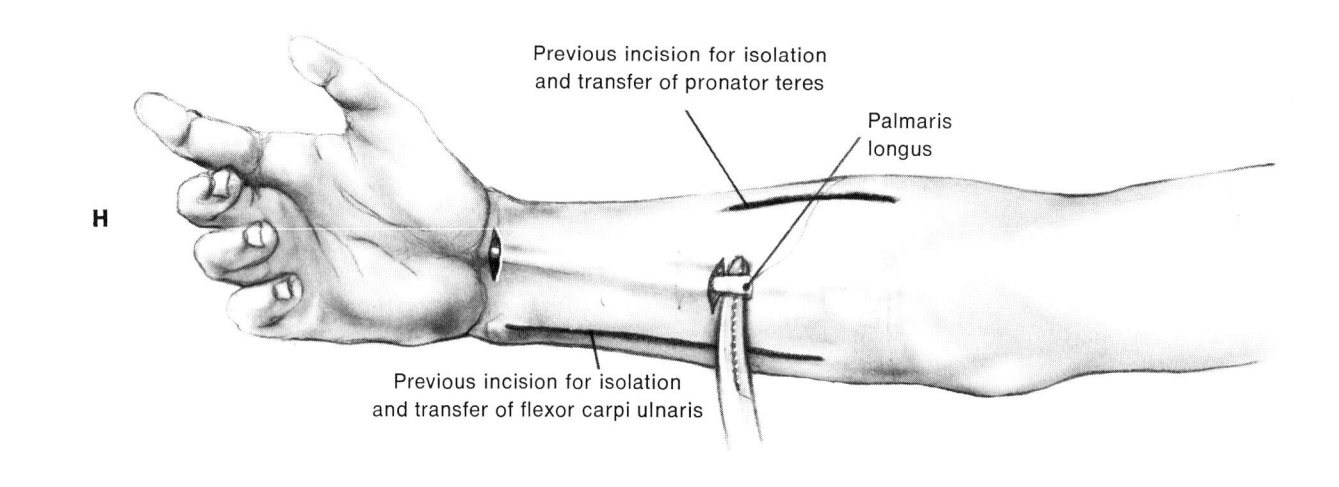

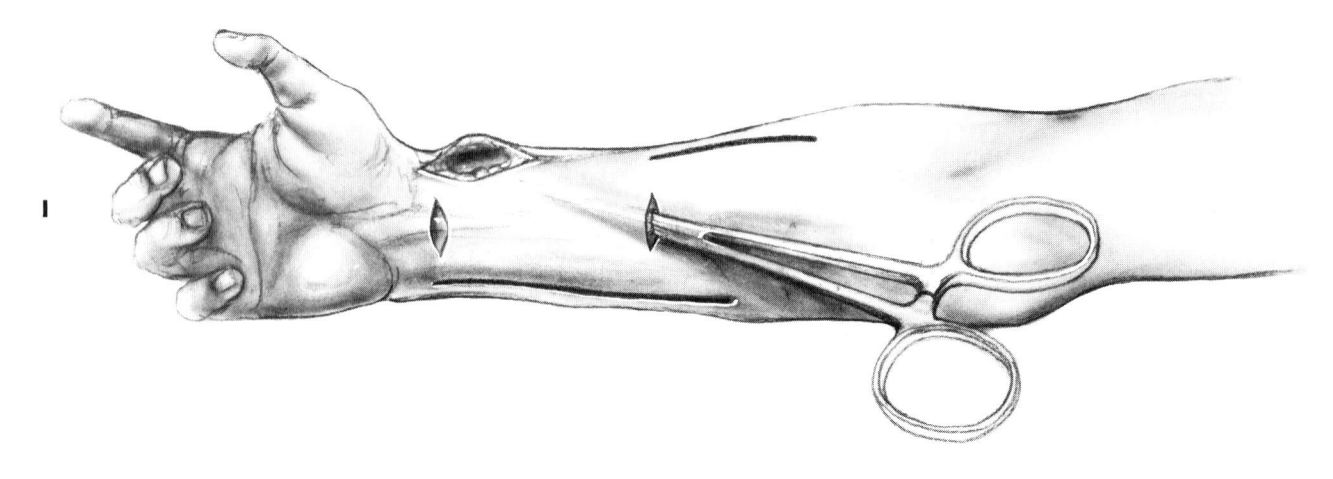

TENDON TRANSFERS FOR RADIAL NERVE PALSY (Plate 4-5)

F

G
- Extensor carpi radialis brevis
- Extensor carpi radialis longus
- Pronator teres

H
- Previous incision for isolation and transfer of pronator teres
- Palmaris longus
- Previous incision for isolation and transfer of flexor carpi ulnaris

I

106

(Plate 4-5) TENDON TRANSFERS FOR RADIAL NERVE PALSY

The pronator teres insertion to the lateral aspect of the anterior surface of the radius near the junction of the proximal and middle thirds of the radial shaft is divided at its attachment to the radius. White the fascia is retracted at the lateral edge of the wound, the forearm is pronated **(F)** to bring into view the extensor carpi radialis longus and extensor carpi radialis brevis muscles and their tendons. A longitudinal slit is created in these two tendons through which the tendon of pronator teres is passed and sutured under moderate tension with the wrist supported in moderate dorsiflexion **(G)**.

Next, the distal portion of the palmaris longus tendon is identified near the flexor crease of the wrist where it lies medial and adjacent to the median nerve. This tendon is isolated and divided just proximal to its insertion into the palmar fascia. Through a separate incision on the lateral aspect of the wrist, the tendon of extensor pollicis longus is identified. An additional incision is made on the anterior aspect of the forearm approximately 10 cm proximal to the wrist. Through this incision the palmaris longus will be withdrawn **(H)** and subsequently passed through a subcutaneous tunnel to the incision on the lateral aspect of the wrist **(I)**. The palmaris longus tendon is placed under moderate tension and divided transversely at a point that will ensure adequate length for end-to-end suture to the transposed extensor pollicis longus tendon **(J)**. If the length of the distal portion of the extensor pollicis longus tendon then appears to be excessive, additional length of the distal portion of extensor pollicis longus tendon can be resected to allow end-to-end suture with the palmaris longus under moderate tension for satisfactory active function of this tendon transfer postoperatively.

All wounds are closed and a well-padded short-arm cast is applied that holds the wrist in slight dorsiflexion. It extends onto the fingers to the level of the proximal phalanges to maintain the metacarpophalangeal joints in extension but permits full flexion of the proximal interphalangeal joints. The cast should likewise extend onto the thumb to maintain the thumb metacarpophalangeal joint in extension and permit free mobility of the interphalangeal joint of the thumb.

POSTOPERATIVE MANAGEMENT. The short-arm cast is bivalved at 3 weeks postoperatively, and skin sutures are removed at that time. A progressive program of active range of motion exercises for all joints involved is encouraged, but the anterior portion of the cast or a new splint holding the wrist and metacarpophalangeal joints in a similar position is continued for an additional 3 weeks except for periods of specific daily exercises. At 6 weeks after surgery all splinting is discontinued unless it seems desirable to continue with the anterior splint as a protective splint at bedtime.

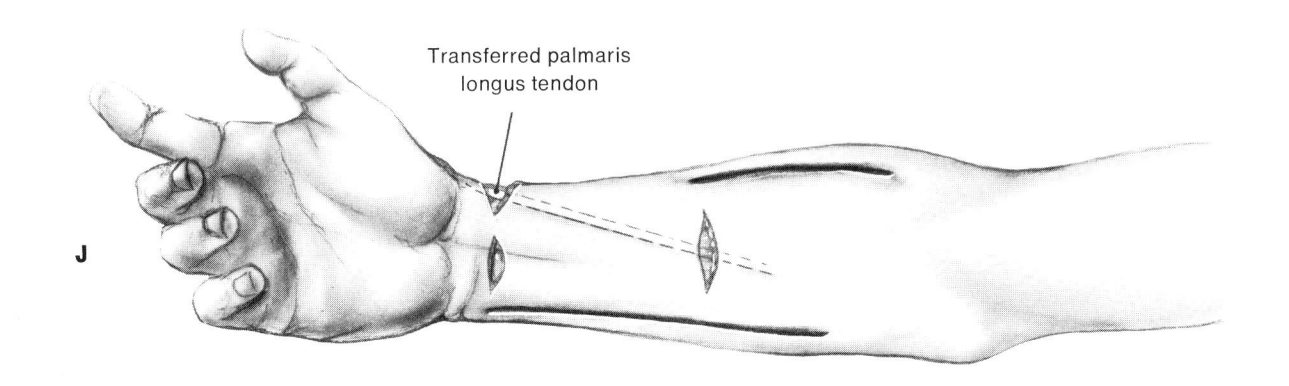

Transferred palmaris longus tendon

J

TRANSFER OF FLEXOR CARPI ULNARIS TO EXTENSOR CARPI RADIALIS BREVIS (Plate 4-6)

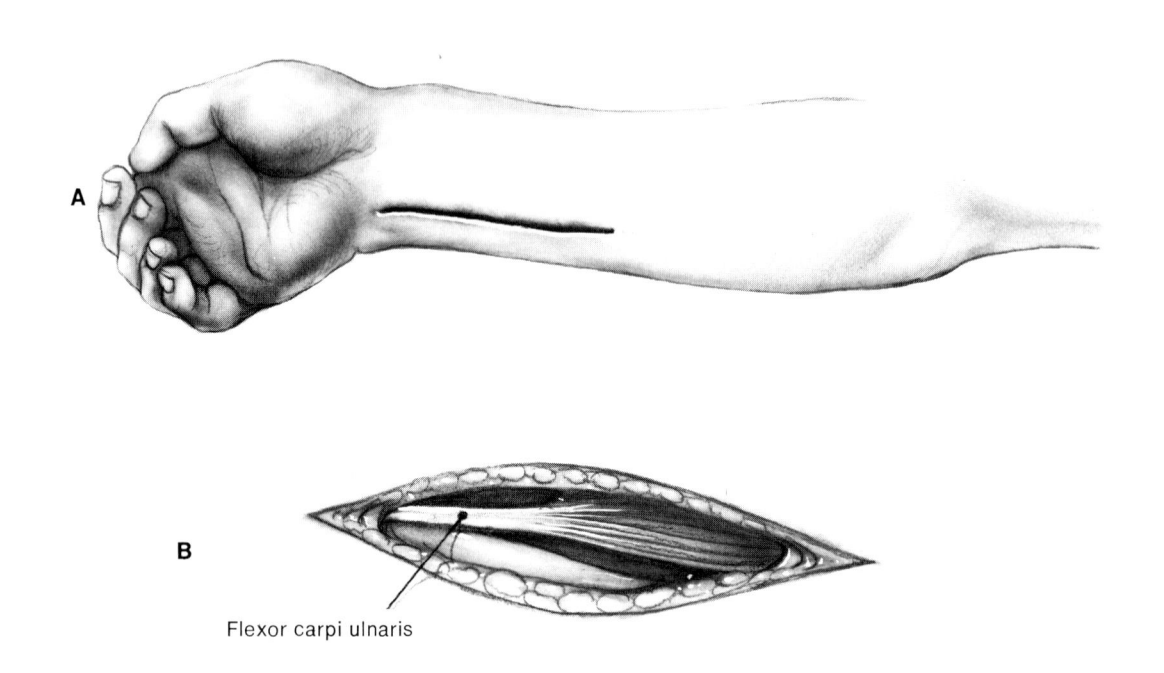

Flexor carpi ulnaris

GENERAL DISCUSSION. For the patient with a spastic wrist flexion deformity, transfer of the flexor carpi ulnaris around the ulnar aspect of the arm to the radial wrist extensor tendons can simultaneously remove a deforming force and provide active control for improved wrist extension and supination of the forearm. Any fixed deformity must be corrected preoperatively for this operation to be effective. There should be reasonable finger control in addition to passive mobility of the fingers, wrist, and forearm preoperatively.

DETAILS OF PROCEDURE. A longitudinal incision is made over the anteromedial aspect of the forearm extending proximally from the flexor crease of the wrist to expose the distal half of the flexor carpi ulnaris (**A** and **B**). This tendon is divided at its point of insertion into the pisiform bone. The tendon is tagged with a suture, and with longitudinal tension on the tendon in a distal direction, it is possible to outline and isolate the distal half of the flexor carpi ulnaris. This muscle takes origin from the subcutaneous border of the ulna throughout all but the last 5 to 7 cm of ulna, and sharp dissection will be required to free an adequate portion of this muscle for tendon transfer. Care must be taken to protect the branches of ulnar nerve providing motor innervation to this muscle. These motor nerve branches may be a factor in determining the limit to which the flexor carpi ulnaris can be isolated proximally.

(Plate 4-6) TRANSFER OF FLEXOR CARPI ULNARIS TO EXTENSOR CARPI RADIALIS BREVIS

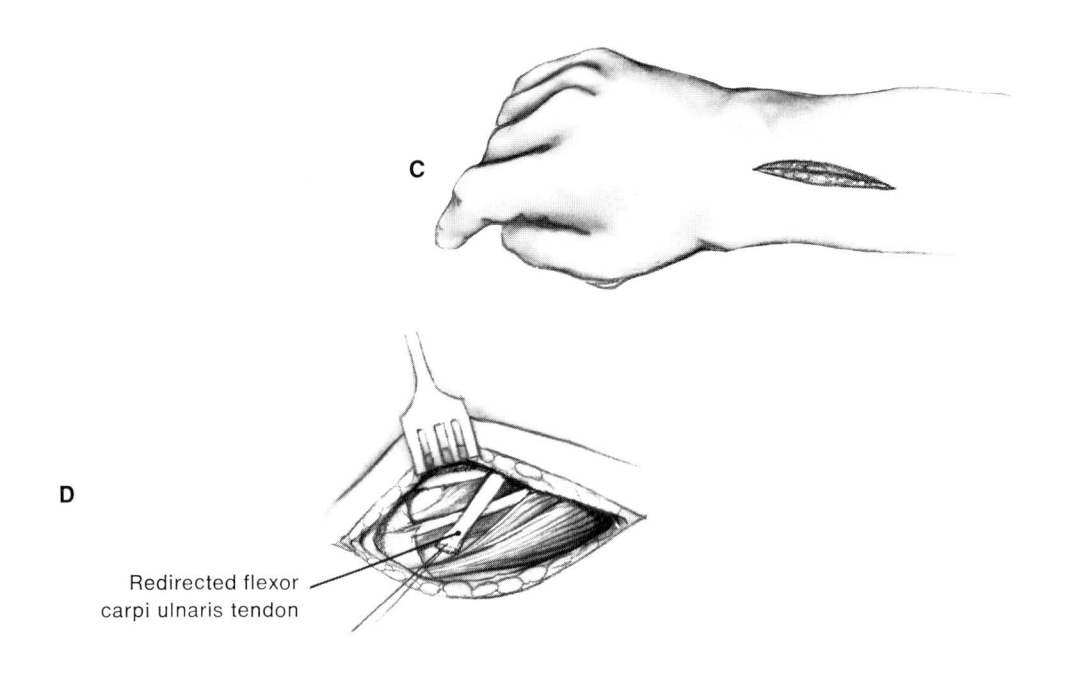

Through a separate incision on the dorsal aspect of the distal forearm **(C)** extending proximally from the area of Lister's tubercle on the dorsal aspect of the radius, tendons of the extensor carpi radialis longus and extensor carpi radialis brevis are identified proximal to the dorsal carpal ligament. Gentle retraction of the extensor pollicis brevis and abductor pollicis longus muscle toward the radial side of the forearm may help to allow improved visualization of the radial wrist extensor tendons as they pass over the distal radius toward their insertion into the base of the second and third metacarpals. The distal end of the flexor carpi ulnaris is passed around the ulnar aspect of the arm subcutaneously **(D)** in a tunnel prepared to allow a straight-line pull of the transferred tendon. A large window must be excised from the intermuscular septum to allow free muscle belly passage. Selection of the extensor carpi radialis brevis rather than the longus will provide more central and stronger wrist extension movement because of the point of insertion and mechanical advantage of the brevis.

A longitudinal opening is made in the recipient wrist extensor tendon. The flexor carpi ulnaris is passed through and sutured to the recipient tendon while moderate tension in maintained on the flexor carpi ulnaris **(E)** with the forearm in full supination and the wrist in 45° of extension. After wound closure, a long-arm cast is applied that holds the wrist and metacarpophalangeal joints in extension and the forearm in supination.

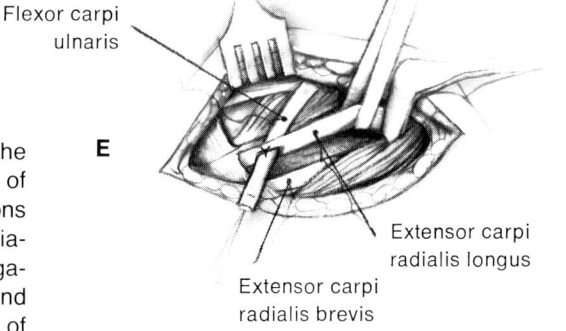

POSTOPERATIVE MANAGEMENT. The cast is bivalved 2 weeks postoperatively, and sutures are removed. A short-arm protective splint is continued between exercise periods for an additional 4 weeks and then at night for another 4 weeks to maintain the wrist in optimum position.

FOREARM DECOMPRESSION FOR IMPENDING VOLKMANN'S ISCHEMIC CONTRACTURE (Plate 4-7)

GENERAL DISCUSSION. Volkmann's ischemic contracture was first described in 1881. The classically described precipitating event is the supracondylar fracture. But many other causes may trigger the phenomenon: crush injury, overdose with compression secondary to the patient lying on the forearm for a long period of time, circumferential burns, arterial catheter studies, hemophilia with bleeding into a closed compartment, reflex arterial spasm from certain hand injuries, subfascial infiltration of intravenous fluid into the forearm of a young child, and others.

The pathomechanics of this condition have been the subject of considerable research. The final common pathway is probably increased intracompartmental pressure, which gradually decreases venous return, further increasing intracompartmental pressure and thus causing more muscle edema with progressively more histamine release. A vicious cycle is thus established, and the arterial inflow is shut off by the increasing intracompartmental pressure. The anoxic muscle then progresses to tissue necrosis. This necrotic muscle is gradually replaced by contracting fibrous tissue that causes (1) fixed flexion contractures of the wrist and finger joints, and (2) a "strangulation neuropathy" of median and ulnar nerves with the superimposed claw deformity and numbness seen in late Volkmann's contracture (**A**).

Early diagnosis is essential to prevent muscle damage. The traditional "four Ps," paralysis, pulselessness, pallor, and pain are misleading and dangerous. If the clinician waits for these to appear before initiating treatment, irreversible damage may occur.

The essential factor is early diagnosis based on a high index of suspicion, triggered by the history. The most reliable early sign of impending acute Volkmann's contracture is severe pain in the forearm, usually made much more severe by gentle passive extension of the index finger, long finger, or thumb.

A second early sign is that of paresthesia, which may be in the median nerve distribution, or occasionally also in the ulnar nerve distribution.

The hand may be cyanotic and cool but not necessarily pale. It should be noted that the anatomy of the deep compartment form is such that the anterior interosseous artery functions essentially as an end artery supplying all the muscles of the deep compartment, but can be completely occluded while still maintaining a relatively normal radial pulse at the wrist.

Techniques are now available to measure intracompartmental pressure if there is any question about the diagnosis.

Once the diagnosis of acute Volkmann's contracture is established, it is absolutely essential that the fascial compartments be *immediately* decompressed. This is one of the true emergencies in orthopaedic surgery.

"Subacute" Volkmann's contracture. As described by Eaton and Green, there is also a phenomenon of subacute Volkmann's contracture, which may have an insidious onset and may not be associated with pain. This usually develops within 3 to 6 weeks following injury and is manifest by progressive induration and fibrosis in the forearm with gradual loss of median and/or ulnar nerve function and gradual contracture of the extrinsic flexor musculature.

Late Volkmann's contracture. The treatment of the late established Volkmann's contracture (**A**) is a complex surgical challenge beyond the scope of this volume. In summary, the concepts of Seddon and of Littler are followed. The entire muscle infarct is excised, the median and ulnar nerves require extensive neurolysis, joint contractures are released, and tendon transfers are performed.

DETAILS OF PROCEDURE. As mentioned, if the awesome deformity of late established Volkmann's contracture (**A**) is to be avoided, it is essential that the decompression be done before muscle ischemia progresses to the point of muscle death, thus avoiding the fixed flexion contractures from the contracted extrinsic finger flexors and intrinsic minus hand.

The principles of the basic incision are outlined in **B**. The forearm is divided into thirds. The junction between the proximal and middle thirds is approximately that of the insertion of the pronator teres. The incision at the junction between the middle and distal thirds is then extended distally so as to easily become confluent with that used for carpal tunnel release.

Through this incision all the muscles of the forearm, median, and ulnar nerves, and radial and ulnar arteries can be exposed. Should subsequent tendon transfers be necessary, the same incision can be used again. Note that the median and ulnar nerves as well as the flexor muscles lie to the ulnar two thirds of the forearm, and the incision does not extend to the radial border.

As is seen in **C**, the fascia must be completely split the full length of the forearm. Furthermore, as recommended by Eaton and Green, it is advisable to perform an epimysiotomy of the individual facial coverings to each of the muscle bellies.

(Plate 4-7) FOREARM DECOMPRESSION FOR IMPENDING VOLKMANN'S ISCHEMIC CONTRACTURE

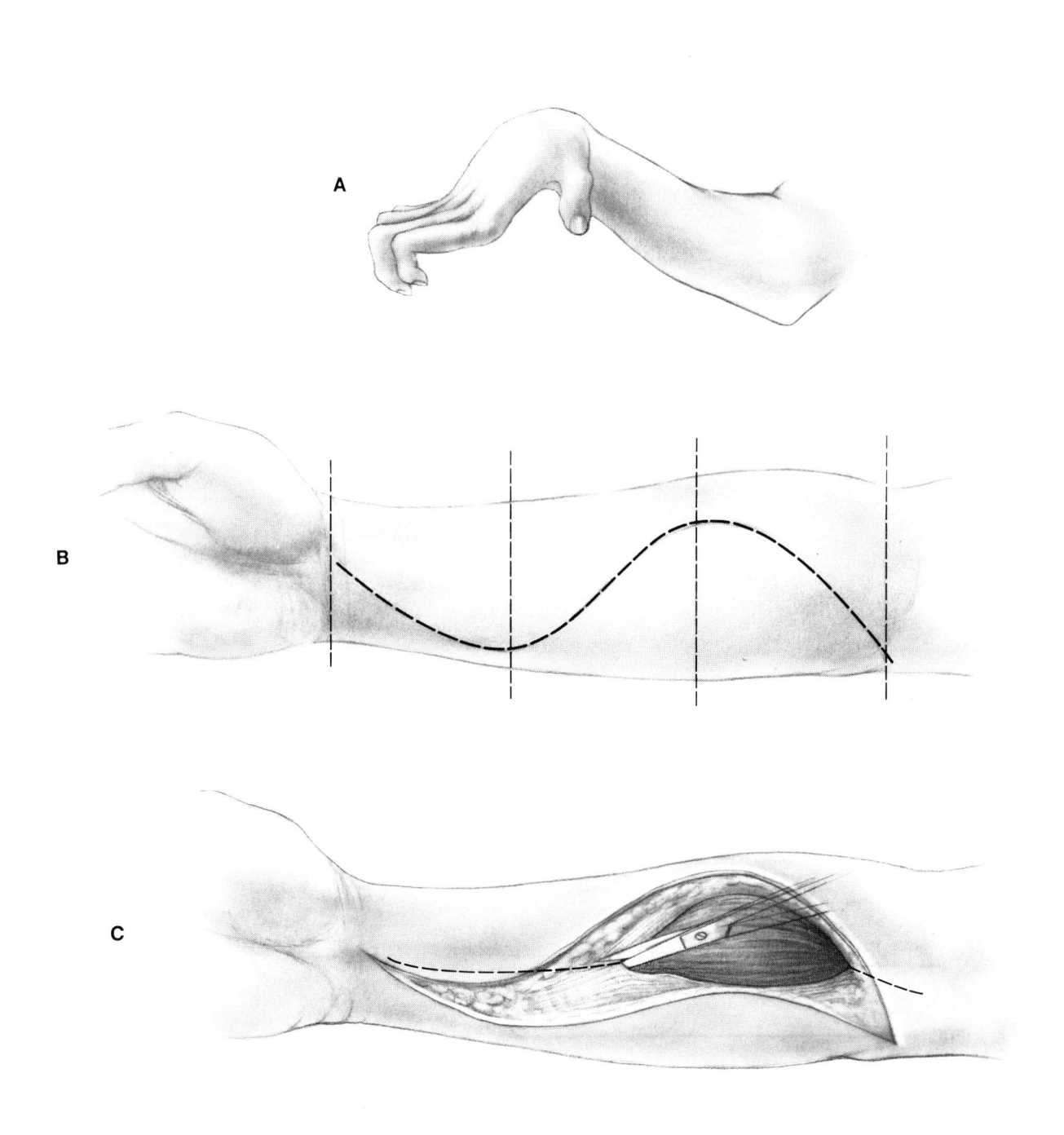

REFERENCES

Anderson, L. D.: Compression plate fixation and the effect of different types of internal fixation on fracture healing, J. Bone Joint Surg. **47-A:**191, 1965.

Anderson, L. D., Sisk, T. D., Tooms, R. E., and Park, W. I., III: Compression-plate fixation in acute diaphyseal fractures of the radius and ulna, J. Bone Joint Surg. **57-A:**287, 1975.

Boyd, H. B.: Surgical exposure of the ulna and proximal third of the radius through one incision, Surg. Gynecol. Obstet. **71:**86, 1940.

Braun, R. M., Mooney, V., and Nickel, V. L.: Flexor-origin release for pronation-flexion deformity of the forearm and hand in the stroke patient. An evaluation of the early results in eighteen patients, J. Bone Joint Surg. **52-A:**907, 1970.

Bruce, H. E., Harvey, J. P., Jr., and Wilson, J. C., Jr.: Monteggia fractures, J. Bone Joint Surg. **56-A:**1563, 1974.

Burkhalter, W. E., Mayfield, G., and Carmona, L. S.: The upper extremity amputee. Early and immediate post-surgical prosthetic fitting, J. Bone Joint Surg. **58-A:**46, 1976.

Burwell, H. N., and Charnley, A. D.: Treatment of forearm fractures in adults with particular reference to plate fixation, J. Bone Joint Surg. **46-B:**404, 1964.

Cooper, W., and Inglis, A. E.: Release of the flexor-pronator origin for flexion deformities of the hand and wrist in spastic paralysis, J. Bone Joint Surg. **48-A:**847, 1966.

Eaton, R. G., and Green, W. T.: Epimysiotomy and fasciotomy in the treatment of Volkmann's ischemic contracture, Orthop. Clin. North. Am. **3:**175-186, March, 1972.

Freehafer, A. A., and Mast, W. A.: Transfer of the brachioradialis to improve wrist extension in high spinal-cord injury, J. Bone Joint Surg. **49-A:**648, 1967.

Goldner, J. L.: Function of the hand following peripheral nerve injuries, American Academy of Orthopaedic Surgeons Instructional Course Lectures, vol. 10, Ann Arbor, 1953, J. W. Edwards, p. 268.

Green, W. T., and Banks, H. H.: The flexor carpi ulnaris transplant and its use in cerebral palsy, J. Bone Joint Surg. **44-A:**1343, 1962.

Green, W. T., and Mital, M. A.: Congenital radio-ulnar synostosis: surgical treatment, J. Bone Joint Surg. **61-A:**738, 1979.

Hall, C. B., and Bechtol, C. O.: Modern amputation technique in the upper extremity, J. Bone Joint Surg. **45-A:**1717, 1963.

Henry, A. K.: Extensile exposure applied to limb surgery, Baltimore, 1945, The Williams & Wilkins Co.

Henry, A. K.: Extensile exposure, ed. 2, Baltimore, 1957, The Williams & Wilkins Co.

Holden, C. E. A.: The pathology and prevention of Volkmann's ischaemic contracture, J. Bone Joint Surg. **61-B:**296, 1979.

Hughston, J. C.: Fractures of the forearm. Anatomical considerations, J. Bone Joint Surg. **44-A:**1664, 1962.

Jacobs, R. J., and Brady, W. M.: Early postsurgical fitting in upper extremity amputations, J. Trauma **15:**966, 1975.

Johnson, M., Zuck, F. N., and Wingate, K.: The motor age test: measurement of motor handicaps in children with neuromuscular disorders such as cerebral palsy, J. Bone Joint Surg. **33-A:**698, 1951.

Jones, R.: Tendon transplantation in cases of musculospiral injuries not amenable to suture, Am. J. Surg. **35:**333, 1921.

Jones, R.: Volkmann's ischaemic contracture, with special reference to treatment, Br. Med. J. **2:**639, 1928.

Kettelkamp, D. B., and Alexander, H.: Clinical review of radial nerve injury, J. Trauma **7:**424, 1967.

Knight, R. A., and Purvis, G. D.: Fractures of both bones of the forearm in adults, J. Bone Joint Surg. **31-A:**755, 1949.

Lam, S. J.: The place of delayed internal fixation in the treatment of fractures of the long bones, J. Bone Joint Surg. **46-B:**393, 1964.

Lichter, R. L., and Jacobsen, T.: Tardy palsy of the posterior interosseous nerve with a Monteggia fracture, J. Bone Joint Surg. **57-A:**124, 1975.

McCue, F. C., Honner, R., and Chapman, W. C.: Transfer of the brachioradialis for hands deformed by cerebral palsy, J. Bone Joint Surg. **52-A:**1171, 1970.

McKenzie, D. S.: The clinical application of externally powered artificial arms, J. Bone Joint Surg. **47-B:**399, 1965.

Mikic, Z.: Galeazzi fracture-dislocations, J. Bone Joint Surg. **57-A:**1071, 1975.

Milch, H.: Rotation osteotomy of the ulna for pronation contracture of the forearm, J. Bone Joint Surg. **25:**142, 1943.

Mubarak, S. J., and Carroll, N. C.: Volkmann's contracture in children: aetiology and prevention, J. Bone Joint Surg. **61-B:**285, 1979.

Naiman, P. T., Schein, A. J., and Siffert, R. S.: Use of ASIF compression plates in selected shaft fractures of the upper extremity. A preliminary report, Clin. Orthop. **71:**208, 1970.

Omer, G. E., Jr.: Evaluation and reconstruction of the forearm and hand after acute traumatic peripheral nerve injuries, J. Bone Joint Surg. **50-A:**1454, 1968.

Riordan, D. C.: Congenital absence of the radius, J. Bone Joint Surg. **37-A:**1129, 1955.

Rush, L. V., and Rush, H. L.: A technique for longitudinal pin fixation of certain fractures of the ulna and of the femur, J. Bone Joint Surg. **21:**619, 1939.

Sage, F. P.: Medullary fixation of fractures of the forearm. A study of the medullary canal of the radius and a report of fifty fractures of the radius treated with a prebent triangular nail, J. Bone Joint Surg. **41-A:**1489, 1959.

Sage, F. P.: Fractures of the shaft of the radius and ulna in the adult. In Adams, J. P., editor: Current practice in orthopaedic surgery, vol. 1, St. Louis, 1963, The C. V. Mosby Co.

Samilson, R. L., and Morris, J. M.: Surgical improvements of the cerebral-palsied upper limb. Electromyographic studies and results of 128 operations, J. Bone Joint Surg. **46-A:**1203, 1964.

Sargent, J. P., and Teipner, W. A.: Treatment of forearm shaft fractures by double-plating. A preliminary report, J. Bone Joint Surg. **47-A:**1475, 1965.

Schmidt, G. H., and Jaffe, S.: Restoration of supination in deep electrical burns of the wrist, Plast. Reconstr. Surg. **45:**555, 1970.

Scuderi, C. S.: Operative indications in fractures of both bones of the forearm, J. Bone Joint Surg. **44-A:**1671, 1962.

Skerik, S. K., and Flatt, A. E.: The anatomy of congenital radial dysplasia. Its surgical and functional implications, Clin. Orthop. **66:**125, 1969.

Slocum, D. B.: Amputations of the hand and forearm, American Academy of Orthopaedic Surgeons Instructional Course Lectures, vol. 7, Ann Arbor, 1951, J. W. Edwards.

Smith, H., and Sage, F. P.: Medullary fixation of forearm fractures, J. Bone Joint Surg. **39-A:**91, 1957.

Swanson, A. B.: The Krukenberg procedure in the juvenile amputee, J. Bone Joint Surg. **46-A:**1540, 1964.

Swanson, A. B.: Surgery of the hand in cerebral palsy and muscle origin release procedures, Surg. Clin. North Am. **48:**1129, 1968.

Zachary, R. B.: Tendon transplantation for radial paralysis, Br. J. Surg. **33:**358, 1946.

Zancolli, E. A.: Paralytic supination contracture of the forearm, J. Bone Joint Surg. **49-A:**1275, 1967.

5

WRIST

TENOLYSIS FOR de QUERVAIN'S TENOSYNOVITIS (Plate 5-1)

GENERAL DISCUSSION. Symptomatic constrictive tenosynovitis of the abductor pollicis longus and extensor pollicis brevis tendons is encountered typically between the ages of 30 and 50 years and most frequently among women. There may be some predisposing occupational cause, and it may be associated with rheumatoid arthritis. The symptoms and findings may closely mimic those of carpometacarpal arthritis of the thumb, from which it must be carefully distinguished. Presenting symptoms are pain and tenderness in the area of the radial styloid along the course of these tendons. Often there is a palpable thickening of the fibrous sheath. With the patient's thumb in the adducted position, any passive ulnar deviation of the wrist will rapidly reproduce discomfort in the area of the radial styloid. When symptoms persist in spite of conservative measures, tenolysis of the tendon sheath of the extensor pollicis brevis and abductor pollicis longus is indicated. Among these patients, one or more aberrant tendons (especially of the abductor pollicis longus) are frequently encountered within the same tendon sheath, and all should be decompressed.

DETAILS OF PROCEDURE. A transverse incision is made at the level of the radial styloid on the lateral aspect of the wrist, crossing the area of maximum preoperative tenderness **(A)**. The transverse skin incision should be made with great care to avoid any possible injury to the superficial branch of the radial nerve. The course of the nerve can be varied, and it may have several branches in this area. Division of even a small branch may result in a painful scar more incapacitating than the original tenosynovitis. The skin edges and sensory branches of the radial nerve are gently retracted. All subsequent dissection should be in a longitudinal direction. The tendon sheath of the extensor pollicis brevis and abductor pollicis longus is located, and a short initial longitudinal incision is made to open the tendon sheath **(B)**, preferably on the dorsal side of the extensor pollicis brevis (to minimize the likelihood of any difficulty with volar subluxation of these tendons postoperatively). The thickened portion of the tendon sheath is opened with small blunt scissors proximally and distally for the full length of tendon sheath **(C)**. The thickened or stenosed portion of the tendon sheath may extend for a distance of 1 to 2 cm. It is important to be sure that the entire length of the tendon sheath has been released. This must be ascertained by direct vision, not blindly. The tendons of the extensor pollicis brevis and abductor pollicis longus should be identified **(D)**. Only subcutaneous tissue and skin are closed. A supportive compression dressing is applied, with a splint to hold the wrist in 10° of extension.

POSTOPERATIVE MANAGEMENT. Active motion of the thumb and fingers is encouraged beginning on the day of the operation and subsequently as symptoms permit. The patient is weaned from the wrist splint at 2 weeks as wrist motion is started.

(Plate 5-1) TENOLYSIS FOR de QUERVAIN'S TENOSYNOVITIS

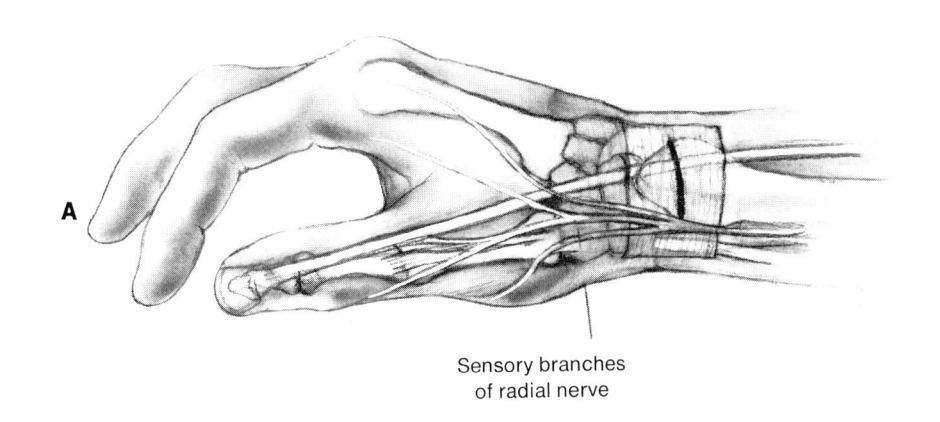

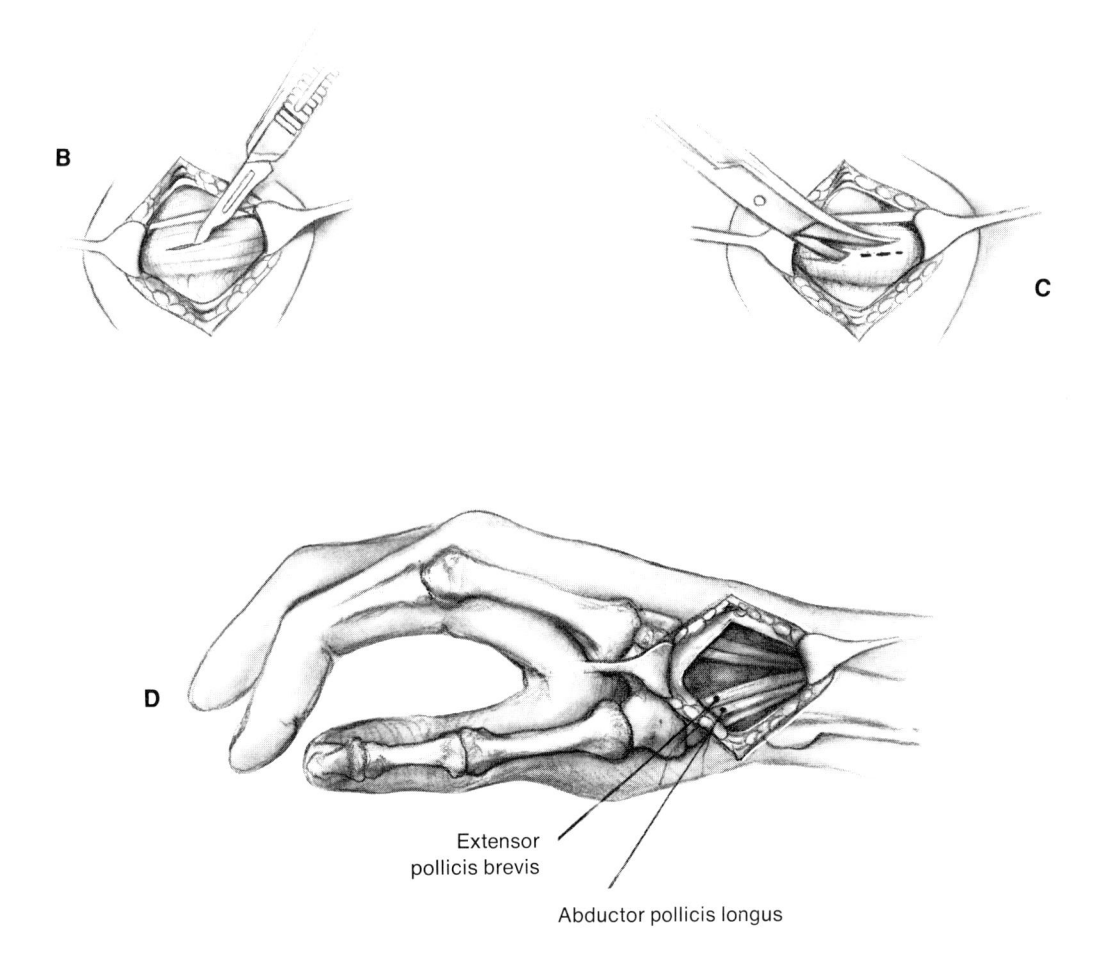

A

Sensory branches of radial nerve

B

C

D

Extensor pollicis brevis

Abductor pollicis longus

115

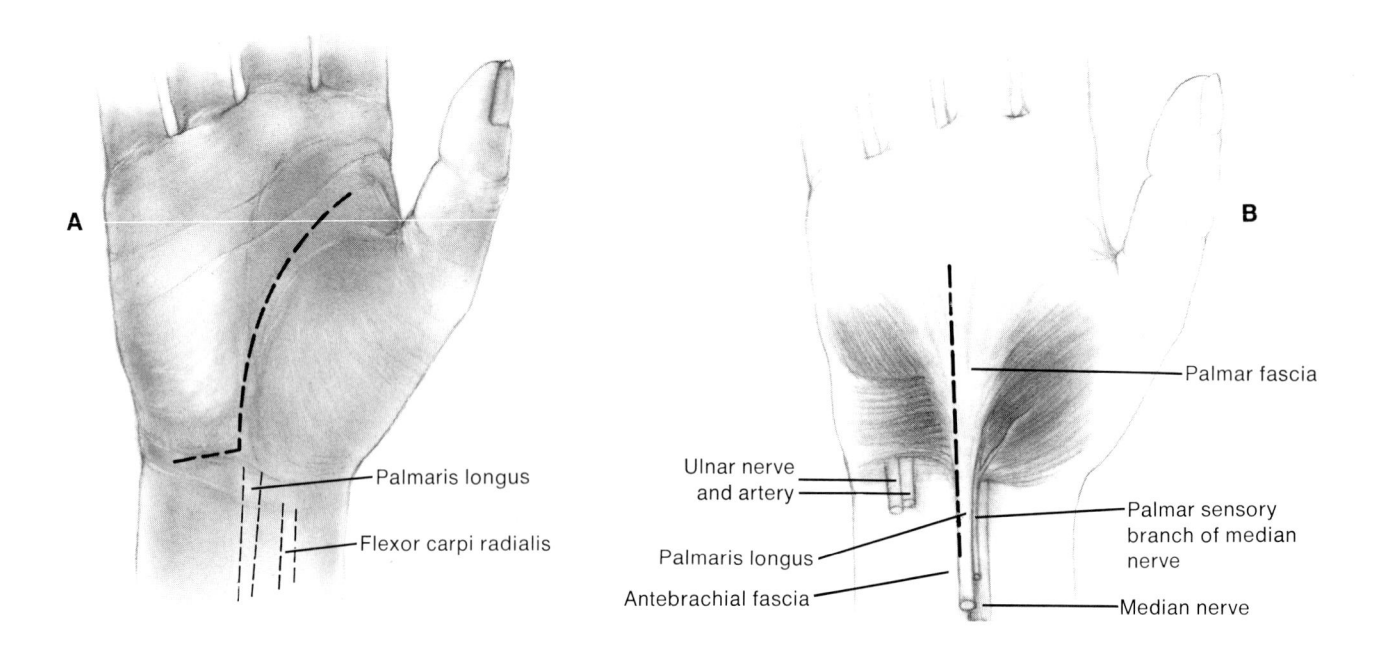

RELEASE OF TRANSVERSE CARPAL LIGAMENT FOR CARPAL TUNNEL SYNDROME (Plate 5-2)

GENERAL DISCUSSION. Compression of the median nerve within the osseous-ligamentous carpal tunnel may produce a varied clinical picture of symptoms and findings in the hand. The problem is often that of being certain of the diagnosis, that symptoms are being caused by compression neuropathy of the median nerve at the wrist level rather than other conditions of the cervical spine, thoracic outlet, or upper extremity, which may produce somewhat similar symptoms. Pain, numbness, and tingling over distribution of the median nerve in the hand (often particularly distressing at night) and Tinel's sign (distal sensory symptoms produced by tapping the median nerve at the wrist) are characteristic of the carpal tunnel syndrome. Demonstration of delayed median nerve conduction time across the wrist can be a valuable aid in the diagnosis. In long-standing cases, isolated atrophy of the abductor pollicis brevis and opponens muscles may be noted. Simultaneous compression syndrome of the ulnar nerve in its separate ulnar tunnel also at the wrist (under the *volar* carpal ligament) is not infrequent.

The ligamentous roof of the carpal tunnel is the transverse carpal ligament, in the same plane as the antebrachial fascia. This ligament is a distinctly localized fibrous thickening transversely covering the concavity on the anterior surface of the carpal bones through which the long flexor tendons and the median nerve pass. It is attached ulnarly to the hook of the hamate bone and radially to the tuberosity of the scaphoid and the ridge of the trapezium. The palmar cutaneous branch of the median nerve passes over the central portion of the transverse carpal ligament, usually in close proximity to the radial side of the palmaris longus tendon.

DETAILS OF PROCEDURE. Although it is possible to divide the transverse carpal ligament (TCL) through a transverse incision, this is to be condemned for several reasons. (1) There is an unacceptable risk of damage to the motor branch of the median nerve, which does not always arise from the radial aspect of the median nerve and, indeed, may even arise occasionally from the ulnar border. (2) The superficial transverse arterial arch is often very close to the distal margin of the TCL. (3) There is no way specifically to decompress the motor branch that passes through the fascia, to do an epineurotomy of the median nerve, or to perform an adequate flexor tenosynovectomy, if these are indicated, depending on the operative findings.

An incision is made parallel to and just to the ulnar side of the base of the thenar eminence **(A)**. At the level of the wrist it is extended toward the ulna and slightly proximally. Note that this proximal corner is to the ulnar side of the palmaris longus (PL) to minimize the risk of damage to the palmar sensory branch of the median nerve, which almost always passes to the radial side of that tendon. Dissection is extended to the level of the palmar fascia, but care must be taken to avoid recurrent branches of the palmar sensory nerve, which may pass in an ulnar direction across the incision.

The antebrachial fascia, which is deep to the PL tendon, is in the same plane as the TCL. The palmar fascia, which is in the same plane as the PL, is incised throughout its exposed portion **(B)**, and then the antebrachial fascia is incised in the distal 2 cm of the forearm. Dissection is carried distally in that same plane, and the TCL completely released **(C)**. Essential for this dissection is an understanding of the relationships between the volar carpal ligament, the transverse

(Plate 5-2) RELEASE OF TRANSVERSE CARPAL LIGAMENT FOR CARPAL TUNNEL SYNDROME

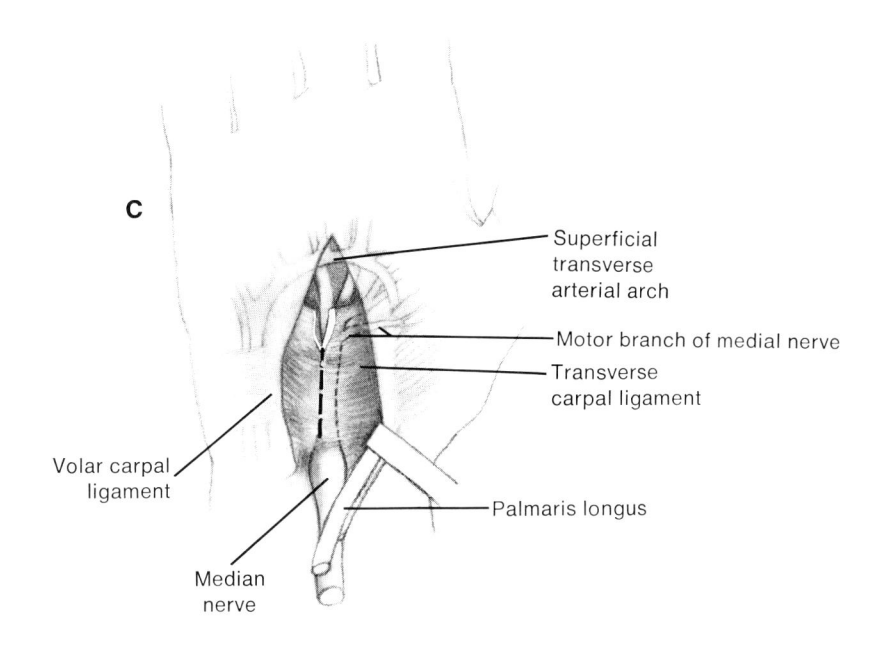

carpal ligament, the ulnar nerve and artery, and the median nerve (**D**).

The flexor tendon synovium is biopsied.

With skin hooks placed on the radial incised margin of the TCL, and retracting straight anteriorly, the motor branch is carefully explored. Magnification and fine instruments are essential for this. Not infrequently the motor branch itself passes through the fascia into the thenar musculature, rather than distal to the fascia. If the former be the case, it is necessary to decompress this motor branch separately if optimal postoperative thenar muscle function is to recover.

If the epineurium is thickened or the nerve constricted with proximal pseudoneuroma formation, an epineurotomy is indicated. Using magnification and very fine instruments with a small sharp scalpel blade, the epineurotomy is done throughout the exposed portion of the median nerve (**E**). It is important that this extend proximally through the area of pseudoneuroma formation. The skin is then closed with vertical mattress sutures.

POSTOPERATIVE MANAGEMENT. A supportive hand dressing is applied with an overlying plaster shell or incorporating a splint. The purpose of this is to maintain the wrist in 10° of extension for approximately 2 weeks. This avoids the risk of tendon and nerve prolapse against the wound with wrist flexion during the initial healing phase. The sutures and dressing can be removed at 2 to 3 weeks and an exercise program commenced.

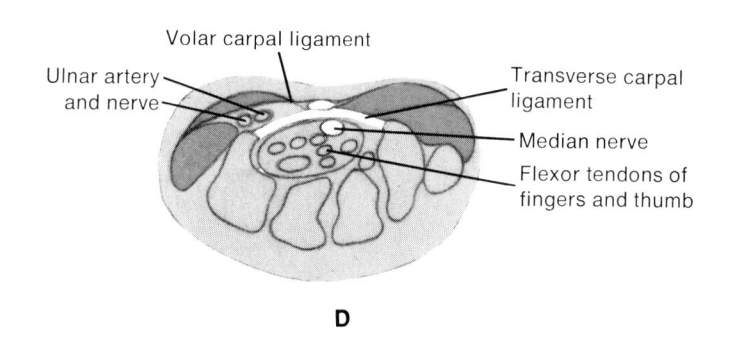

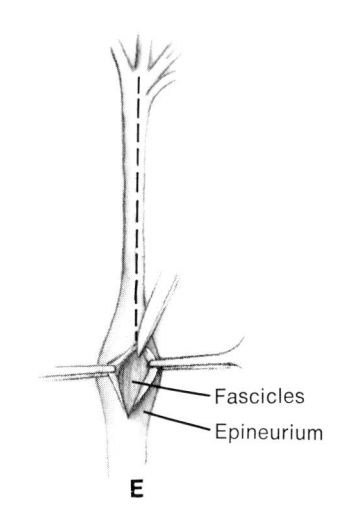

EXCISION OF DISTAL ULNA (DARRACH PROCEDURE) (Plate 5-3)

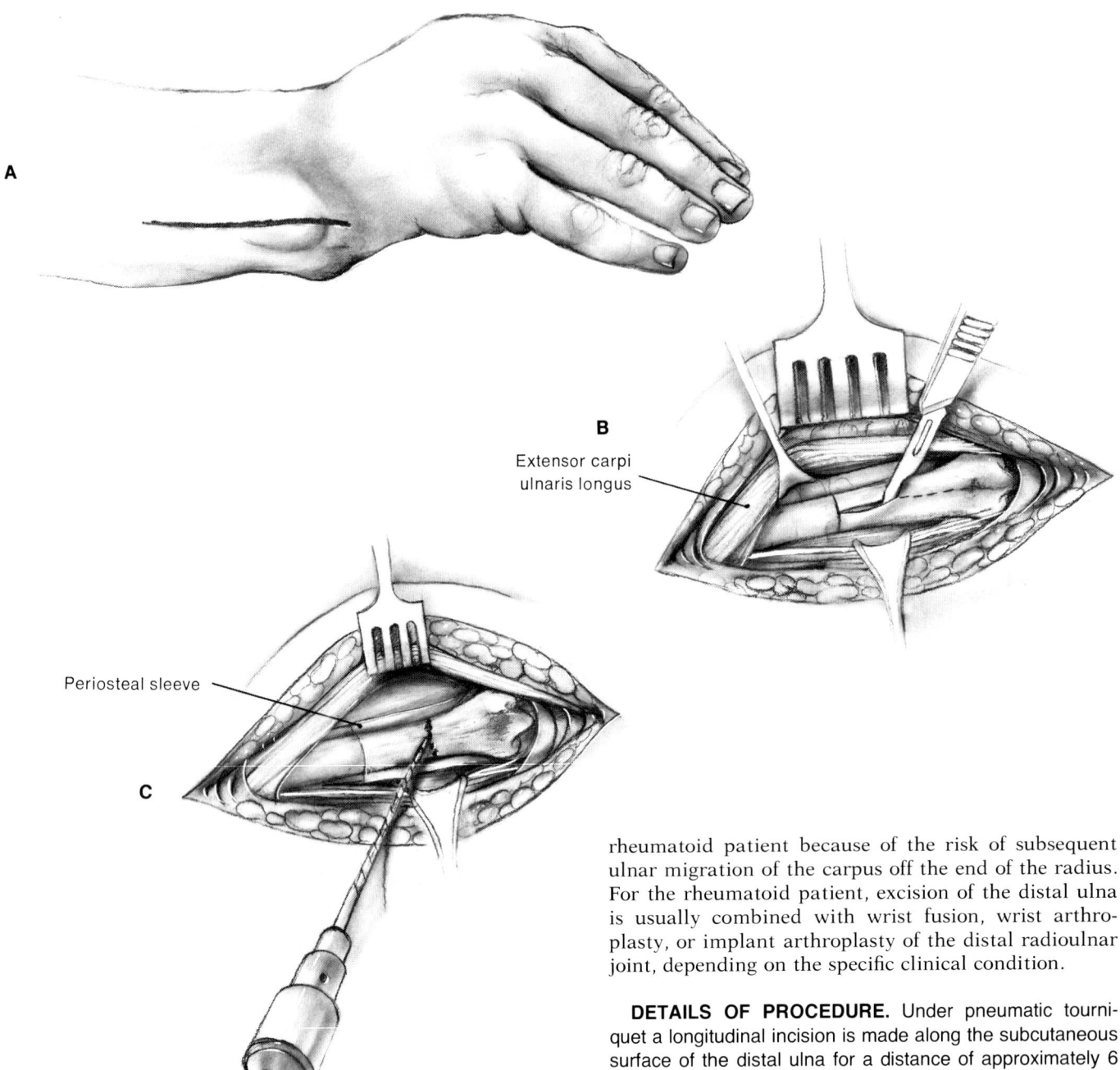

A

B Extensor carpi ulnaris longus

C Periosteal sleeve

GENERAL DISCUSSION. Among the indications for excision of the distal ulna, the most common is for malunion of a Colles' fracture with limited pronation and supination. This procedure is useful for many disruptions of the distal radioulnar articulation, producing significant symptoms from limitation of forearm rotation. This procedure is seldom indicated by itself in the rheumatoid patient because of the risk of subsequent ulnar migration of the carpus off the end of the radius. For the rheumatoid patient, excision of the distal ulna is usually combined with wrist fusion, wrist arthroplasty, or implant arthroplasty of the distal radioulnar joint, depending on the specific clinical condition.

DETAILS OF PROCEDURE. Under pneumatic tourniquet a longitudinal incision is made along the subcutaneous surface of the distal ulna for a distance of approximately 6 cm ending 1 cm distal to the ulnar styloid **(A)**. Along the posteromedial aspect of the distal ulna, the extensor carpi ulnaris musculotendinous unit is encountered and should be retracted dorsally. A longitudinal incision is made through the periosteum on the ulnar aspect of the distal ulna **(B)**. The periosteum is reflected to expose the distal 4 cm of ulna. The distal 1.5 to 2 cm of ulna should be removed. Some attachment of the pronator quadratus to the remaining shaft of the ulna is retained to avoid troublesome dorsal subluxation of the remaining ulna with forearm pronation postoperatively. Multiple drill holes are made through both cortices of the ulna at a level 2 cm from the ulnar styloid **(C)**.

(Plate 5-3) EXCISION OF DISTAL ULNA (DARRACH PROCEDURE)

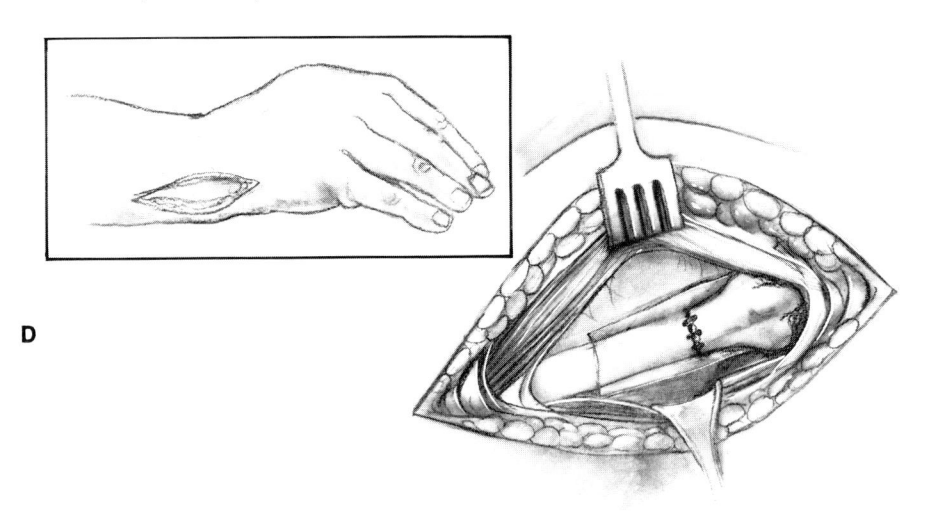

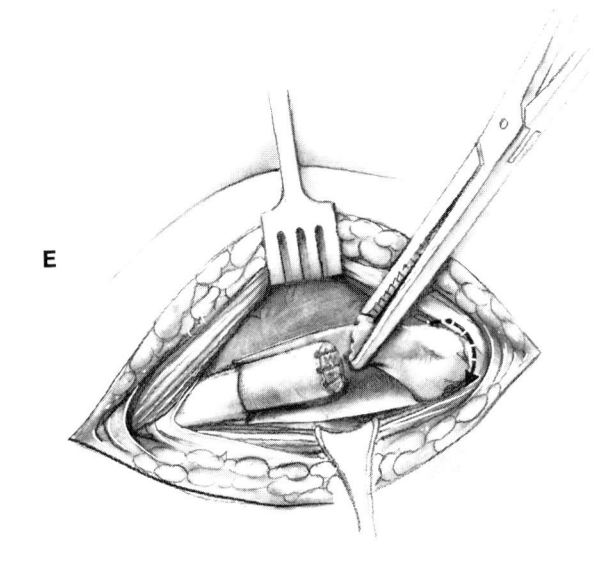

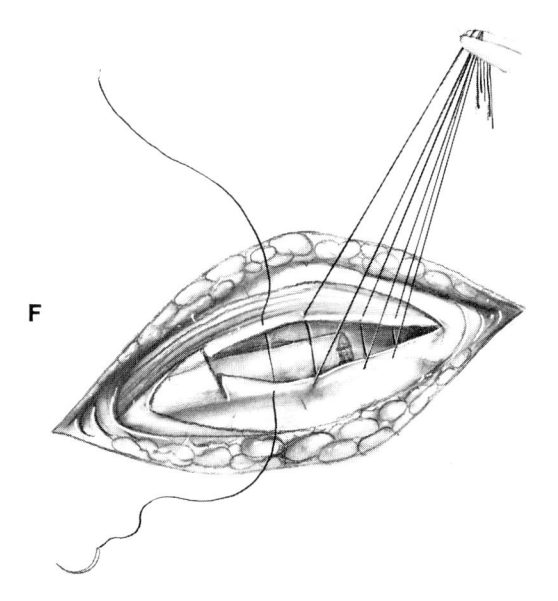

The ulna is divided with bone cutters at this level (**D**). The fragment of distal ulna is rotated out of its periosteal sleeve (**E**). The periosteum is more densely adherent to the distal centimeter of ulna as a rule and may require sharp dissection in this area. The tip of the ulnar styloid is divided transversely with bone cutters and left in place as the distal 1.5 to 2 cm of ulna is removed. The reflected periosteum is reconstituted with interrupted sutures (**F**). After wound closure, a soft dressing bandage is applied with plaster immobilization to support the wrist in 10° of extension.

POSTOPERATIVE MANAGEMENT. Active forearm pronation and supination are encouraged in the immediate postoperative period. The sutures are removed at 2 weeks, and at 3 weeks a program of wrist flexion-extension exercises is added to those of forearm rotation. The splint is continued between exercises for 6 weeks after surgery.

OSTEOTOMY OF DISTAL RADIUS (FOR CORRECTION OF MALUNION) (Plate 5-4)

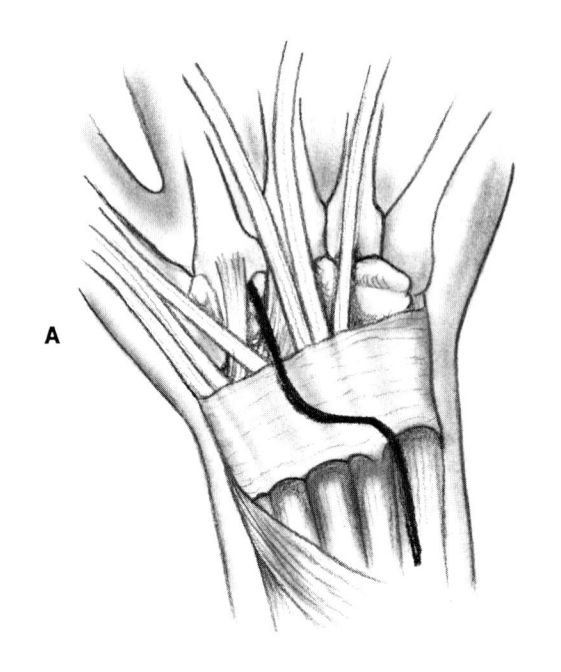

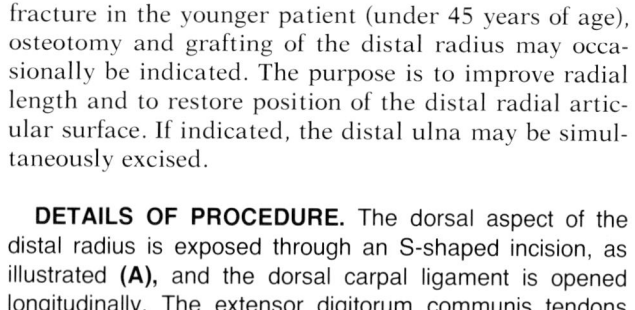

GENERAL DISCUSSION. For the malunited Colles' fracture in the younger patient (under 45 years of age), osteotomy and grafting of the distal radius may occasionally be indicated. The purpose is to improve radial length and to restore position of the distal radial articular surface. If indicated, the distal ulna may be simultaneously excised.

DETAILS OF PROCEDURE. The dorsal aspect of the distal radius is exposed through an S-shaped incision, as illustrated **(A)**, and the dorsal carpal ligament is opened longitudinally. The extensor digitorum communis tendons over the dorsal aspect of the distal radius are reflected toward the ulna. The extensor pollicis longus is retracted toward the radius along with tendons of extensor carpi radialis longus and brevis. The distal radius is osteotomized (**B** and **C**) to correct the existing malunion. The opening wedge is held open with a bone graft taken from the distal ulna through a separate longitudinal incision along the medial aspect of the distal ulna (**D** and **E**). The distal ulna is exposed between tendons of the extensor carpi ulnaris and flexor carpi ulnaris to permit removal of a segment of cortical and cancellous bone graft, as illustrated, leaving the ulnar styloid intact. Kirshner wire fixation may be necessary to secure the osteotomy and graft. The iliac crest can be used for the donor bone graft if preferred.

POSTOPERATIVE MANAGEMENT. External plaster immobilization is continued until there is roentgenographic evidence of good bony union at the osteotomy site in the distal radius.

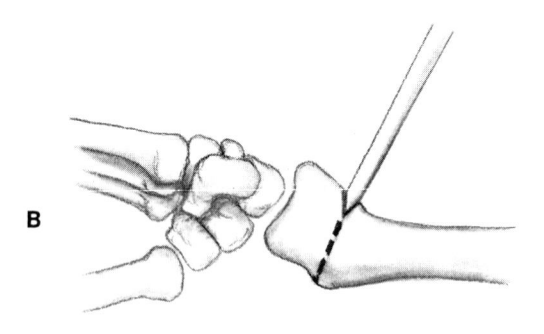

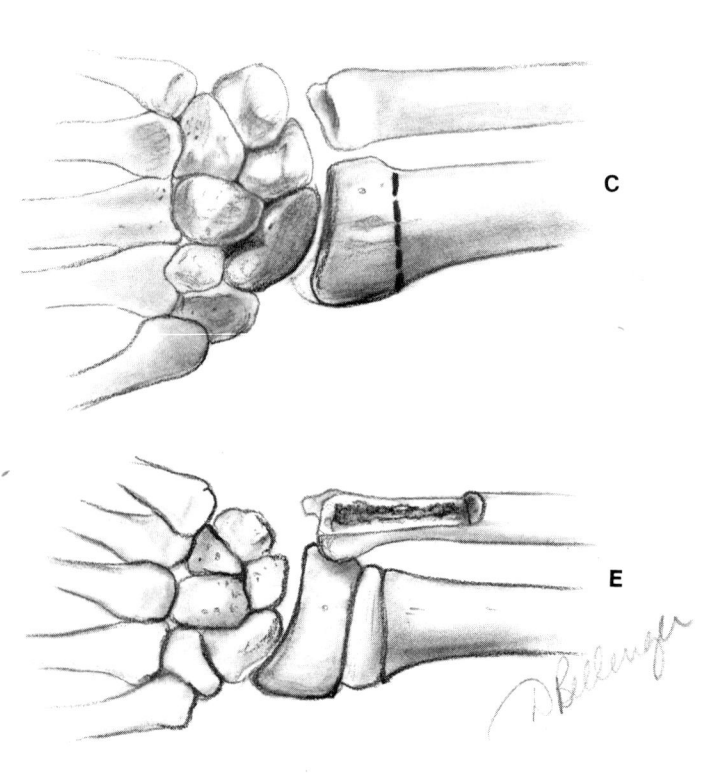

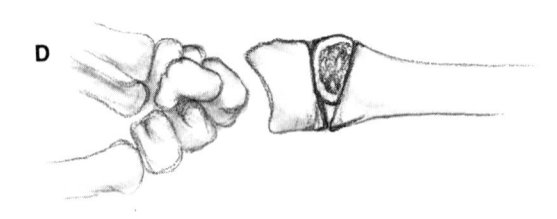

(Plate 5-5) OPEN REDUCTION AND BONE GRAFT FOR FRACTURE OF SCAPHOID: ANTERIOR APPROACH

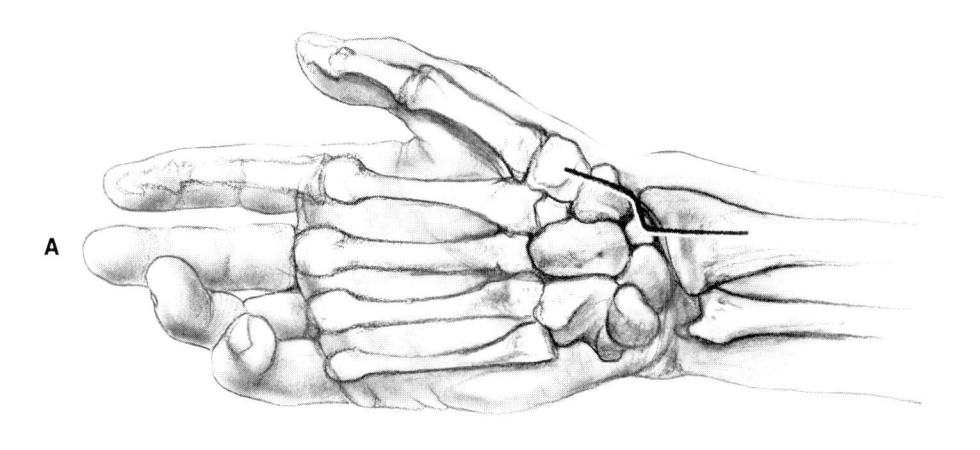

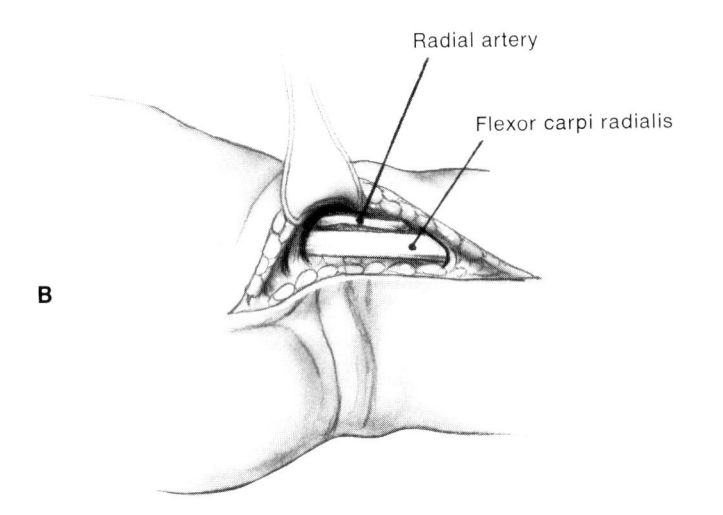

GENERAL DISCUSSION. Open reduction for a fracture of the scaphoid may occasionally be indicated immediately for the acute fracture that cannot be reduced satisfactorily, or later for those nonunions which fail to respond to prolonged effective immobilization. A nonunion of fracture of the scaphoid can be effectively exposed for bone grafting through an anterior approach.

DETAILS OF PROCEDURE. The incision is made approximately 4 cm in length over the anterolateral aspect of the wrist as illustrated (**A** and **B**). The tendon of the flexor carpi radialis is identified and retracted to the ulnar side. The radial artery is retracted radially toward the tendon of the abductor pollicis longus. A longitudinal incision is made in the capsule of the wrist joint over the scaphoid. The capsular margins are carefully tagged to facilitate subsequent accurate and firm repair (**C**). Visualization of the scaphoid is improved by extending the wrist. The fracture site is identified (**D**). Any dead sclerotic bone or fibrous tissue between the fracture fragments is excised.

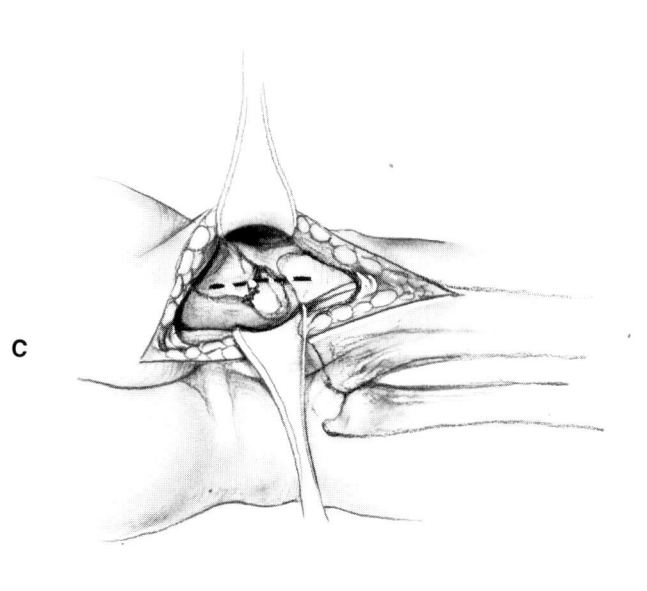

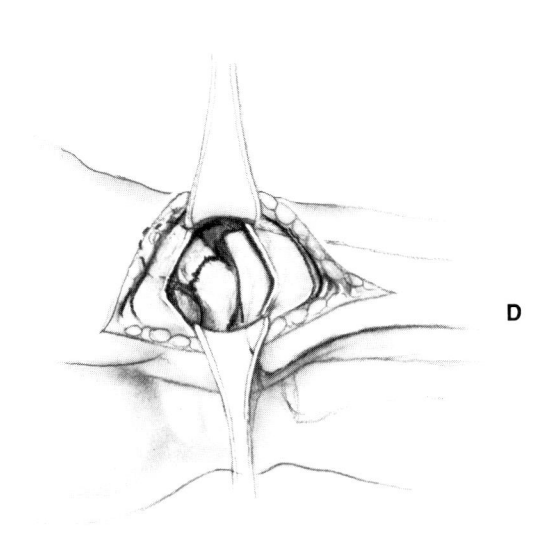

OPEN REDUCTION AND BONE GRAFT FOR FRACTURE OF SCAPHOID: ANTERIOR APPROACH (Plate 5-5)

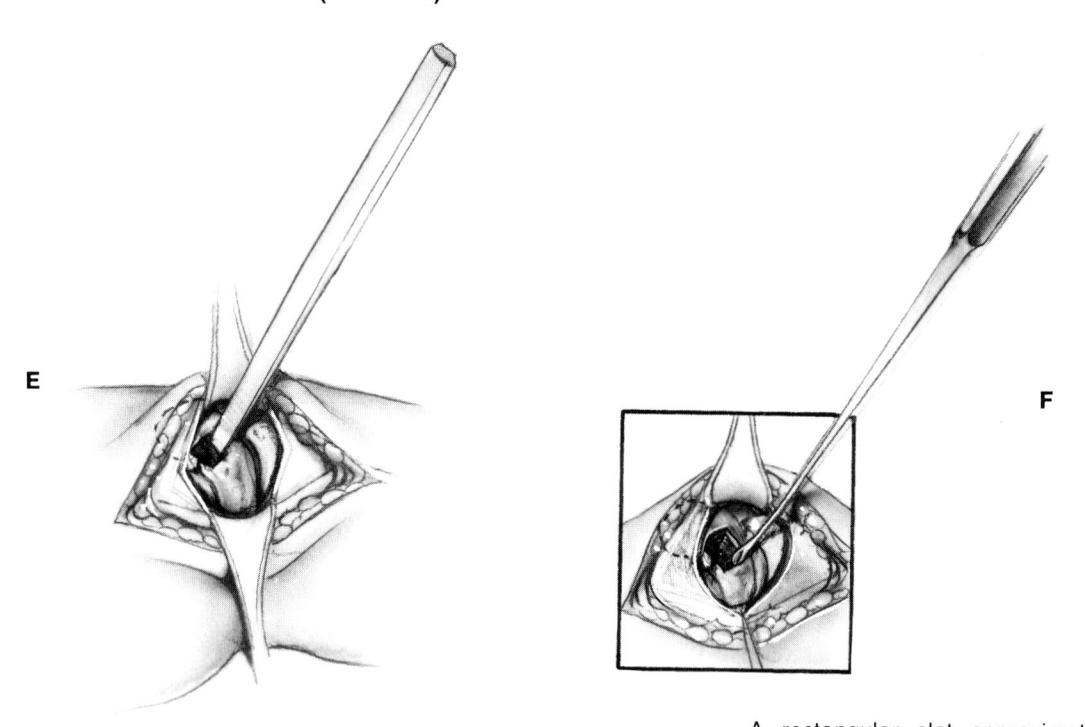

A rectangular slot approximately 4 × 14 mm that bridges both fragments of the scaphoid is developed with a small hand osteotome and curet (**E** and **F**). The curet is used to hollow out the scaphoid by removing the sclerotic and cystic bone. A corticocancellous graft from iliac crest or the distal radius is fashioned to fit securely into this rectangular slot, extending into both proximal and distal scaphoid fragments. The slot is deepened if necessary with a small curet. An alternative and often preferred technique is to countersink a series of parallel longitudinal corticocancellous strips inside the scaphoid spanning the nonunion, regaining scaphoid length and providing stability. The remainder of the hollowed scaphoid is packed tightly with medullary chips. With either technique, after the corticocancellous graft is in place, the anterior surface of the graft should be flush with adjacent anterior surfaces of both the proximal and distal fragments of the scaphoid (**G**). It should be properly fitted so as to provide a degree of stability for the two separate fragments of the scaphoid. Following wound closure, a long-arm cast is applied extending to the interphalangeal joint of the thumb, which is maintained in a functional position.

POSTOPERATIVE MANAGEMENT. The long-arm cast is replaced by a snug short-arm cast 6 weeks postoperatively, and the short-arm cast is continued until there is roentgenographic evidence of bony union between the two fragments of the scaphoid.

OPEN REDUCTION FOR FRACTURE OF THE SCAPHOID

GENERAL DISCUSSION. Open reduction and internal fixation for acute fractures of the scaphoid may occasionally be necessary when the fracture fragments are not anatomically reduced. Frequently these injuries are associated with, or are a variant of, transscaphoid perilunate dislocations of the wrist.

DETAILS OF PROCEDURE. Wide exposure is necessary and may require both dorsal and volar approaches. Frequently, however, a posterior approach alone is adequate. The incision is essentially as that on Plate 5-5 except that the horizontal limb is centered over the proximal carpal row.

The fracture of the scaphoid is reduced under direct vision and fixed with a percutaneous Kirschner pin. This pin frequently needs to be extended across both segments of the scaphoid and into the lunate. This is required to stabilize the relationship between the scaphoid and the lunate. Any intercarpal ligamentous tears that occurred at the time of scaphoid fracture must also be repaired at that time.

POSTOPERATIVE MANAGEMENT. Postoperatively the patient is immobilized in a long-arm thumb spica-type cast, as would be used for the bone graft of a nonunion fractured scaphoid. This immobilization is continued until there is evidence for bony union.

RADIAL STYLOIDECTOMY (Plate 5-6)

GENERAL DISCUSSION. Radial styloidectomy may occasionally be utilized as a separate procedure to bring about relief of symptoms and possible improvement in wrist function with established nonunion of a scaphoid fracture or in the presence of traumatic arthritic changes involving the joint between distal radius and scaphoid.

This procedure should never be done if there is the future possibility of a scaphoid prosthesis implant arthroplasty. Styloidectomy will destroy the seating for such an implant and render it unstable.

DETAILS OF PROCEDURE. The lateral longitudinal incision approximately 3 cm in length is centered over the radial styloid if excision of the radial styloid is to be carried out as an isolated procedure. **(A).** After the skin incision is made, there must be care to protect the superficial sensory branches of the radial nerve **(B)**. The extensor pollicis longus tendon is retracted dorsally. The radial artery, extensor pollicis brevis, and abductor pollicis longus are retracted anteriorly. A longitudinal incision is made over the lateral aspect of the wrist capsule and is extended proximally along the lateral aspect of the distal radius. The wrist capsule is opened sufficiently to visualize the anteroposterior ridge on the distal articular surface of the radius that separates the contiguous portions of the articular surface of the distal radius that articulate with the scaphoid and the lunate. The periosteum is reflected from the distal radius.

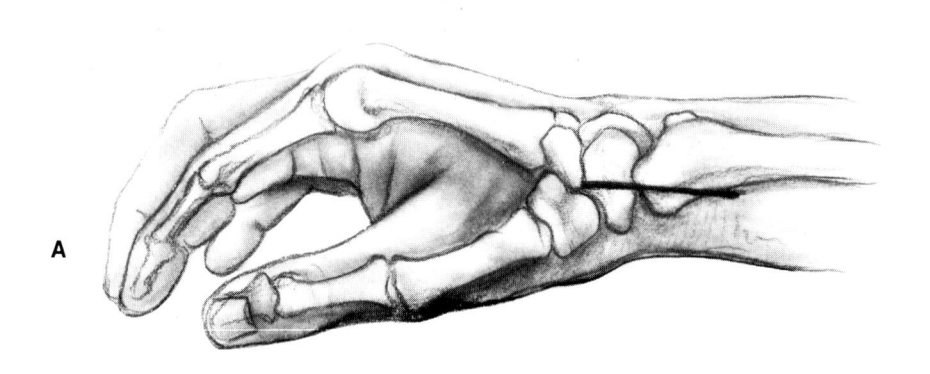

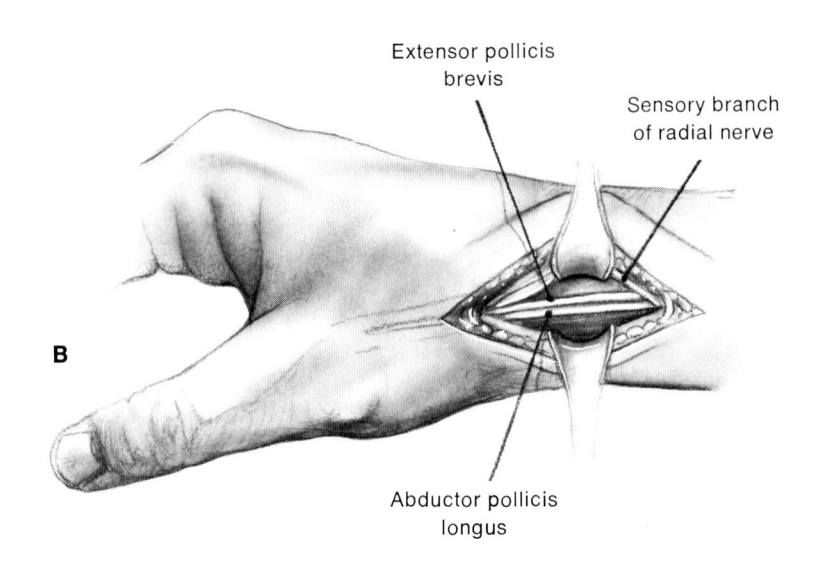

(Plate 5-6) RADIAL STYLOIDECTOMY

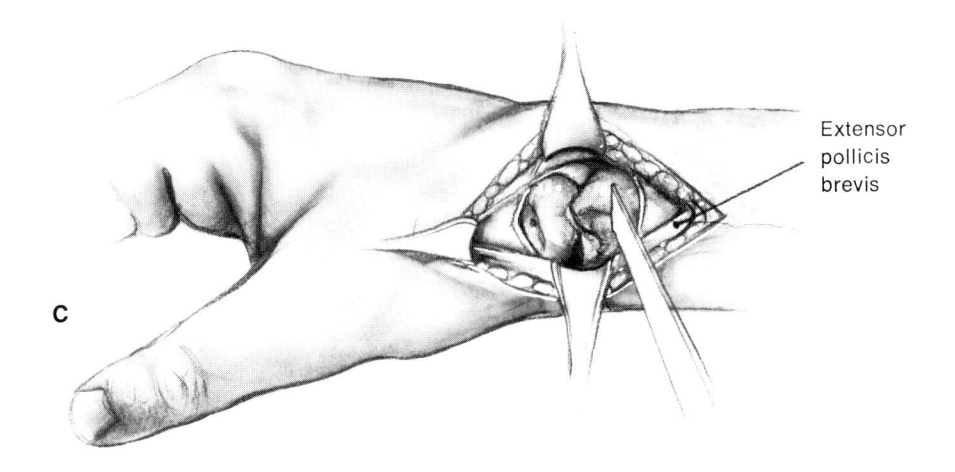

Extensor pollicis brevis

C

The radial styloid is separated with an osteotome perpendicularly to the shaft of the radius from the lateral cortex of the radius to remove the entire surface of the radius that articulates specifically with the navicular (**C** to **E**). The articular surface between radius and lunate should not be disturbed. The wrist should be moved passively to be sure there are no irregularities that will subsequently interfere with active wrist movement. As the wound is closed in layers including the joint capsule, subcutaneous tissue, and skin, care must be continued to protect the superficial sensory branch of the radial nerve in addition to the radial artery and thumb extensor tendons. A well-padded short-arm cast is applied holding the wrist in slight dorsiflexion and the thumb in slight abduction. The cast extends onto the thumb to the level of the interphalangeal joint.

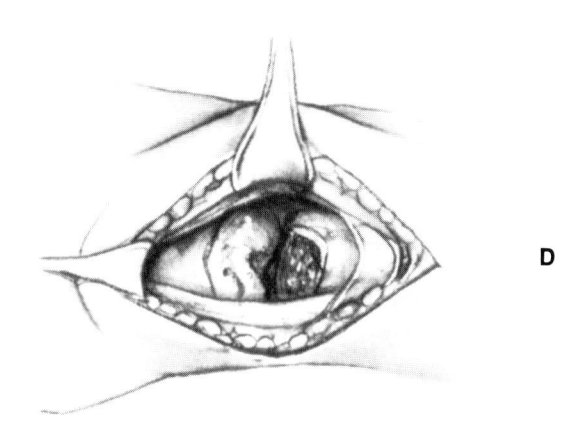

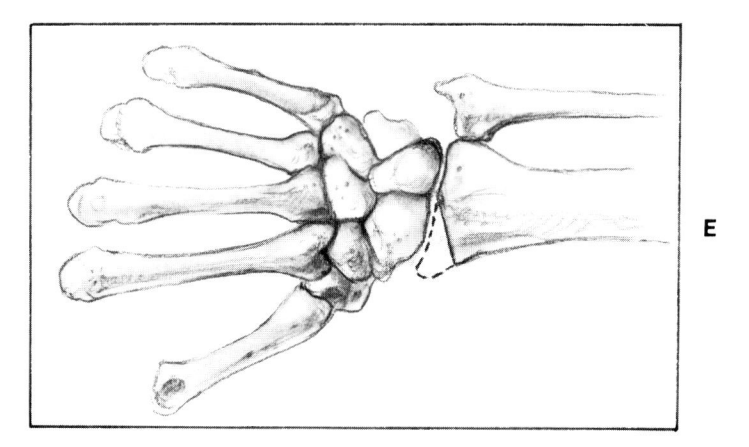

D

E

POSTOPERATIVE MANAGEMENT. The plaster immobilization is removed 3 weeks postoperatively. Progressive motion and active use of the wrist are encouraged thereafter.

125

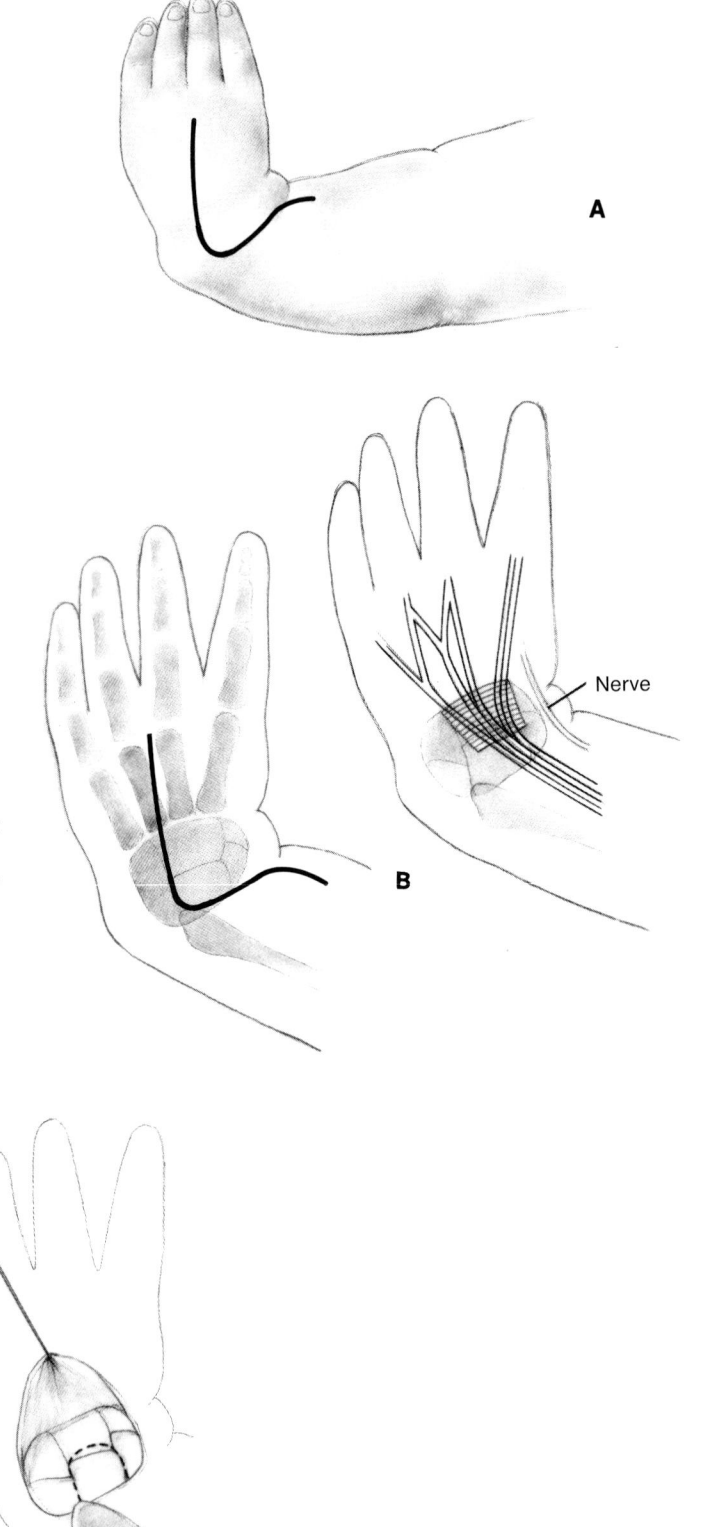

SURGICAL CORRECTION OF RADIAL CLUBHAND (Plate 5-7)

GENERAL DISCUSSION. For the child born with radial clubhand, treatment must start at the time of delivery. Beginning in the newborn nursery, the nurses and then the parents should be instructed on an exercise program that may be combined with either serial splints or castings to correct the deformity as much as possible. This is analogous to the early treatment rendered to the child with the clubfoot deformity.

Ideally between the ages of 6 and 12 months a surgical procedure can be performed if necessary to centralize the carpal bones on the distal ulna. Various bone graft techniques have been attempted to create a new radial strut, but these have generally either absorbed or failed to grow with the child. It may be that in the future vascularized bone grafts utilizing microsurgical techniques will provide this radial bone graft with adequate epiphyseal growth.

DETAILS OF PROCEDURE. A curved incision is made over the dorsal aspect of the wrist as indicated **(A)**. All the extensor tendons are mobilized sufficiently to permit their relocation in a more centralized position relative to the axis of wrist motion after the hand has been repositioned over the distal end of the ulna **(B)**.

Great caution must be exercised, since frequently the tethering structure on the radial border of the wrist may represent the congenitally abnormal median-radial sensory nerve composite that supplies sensibility to the radial border of this hand. This must be carefully distinguished from the radial anlage, which is a heavy fibrocartilaginous band that tethers the clubhand in its deformed position. This anlage, if present, must be excised over a distance of approximately 3 cm.

(Plate 5-7) SURGICAL CORRECTION OF RADIAL CLUBHAND

With the tendons thus retracted, a distally based capsular flap is raised. The carpal bone, which probably represents the lunate, is removed, and a portion of the capitate must also sometimes be taken. It is important to realize that the depths of the socket created in the carpal bones must be equal to the width of the distal ulna if the centralization of the ulna into the carpus is to be stable **(C)**.

A Steinmann pin is then driven down the shaft of either the ring or long metacarpal, the wrist is reduced, and this pin is driven down the shaft of the ulna. If possible, it should be passed through the very center of the ulna epiphysis, since it has been well shown that this is less apt to damage future epiphyseal growth than is a pin that passes down the periphery of the epiphysis. Note that the ulna is frequently bowed, and it may not be possible to tap the Steinmann pin as far down the shaft of the ulna as is shown in **D**.

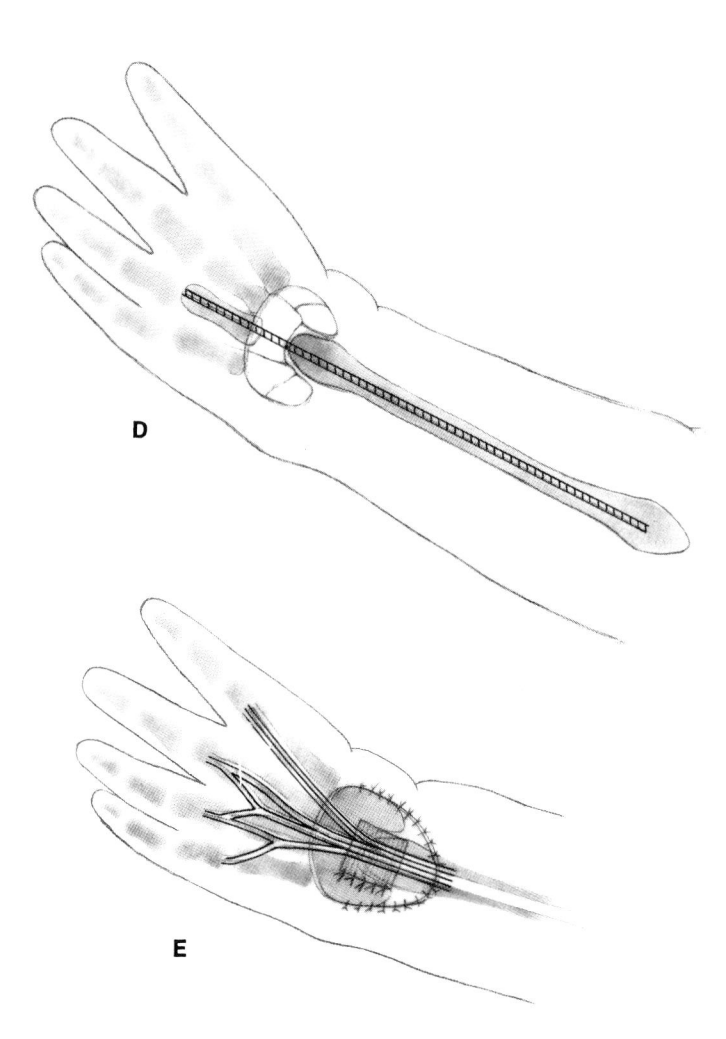

If this is the situation, it is sometimes necessary to combine the above procedure with an osteotomy of the ulna to correct forearm alignment. This osteotomy of the ulna may be done at the same time as the procedure just described or as a second stage.

The dorsally and distally based capsule or flap is then repaired to the deeper structures overlying the distal radius to facilitate maintenance of the hand in the reduced position **(E)**. The extensor tendons at this point should be centralized over the future center of rotation.

It is important that the appropriate tendon transfers be done to maintain, if possible, active muscle balance across the newly created wrist joint. These transfers may be done at the time of the initial procedure or as a second-stage procedure, as suggested by Bora, Nicholson, and Cheena. One such transfer is the use of the flexidigitorum superficialis tendon of either the middle or ring finger. The digit must be carefully examined before surgery to be certain that the profundus tendon is also functioning, and that the superficial flexor is of sufficient strength that the child can actively flex the proximal interphalangeal joint of that involved finger with force while the distal joint is retained in extension.

The two tendons that have been divided at the proximal interphalangeal level are withdrawn into the proximal forearm and then routed around the subcutaneous ulna border of the forearm to be inserted into the index finger metacarpal. The long finger metacarpal should be the insertion if future index finger pollicization is planned. The tendon is passed extraperiosteally around the metacarpal, deep to the extensor tendons, interossei, and flexor tendons, and then sutured to itself.

POSTOPERATIVE MANAGEMENT. One end or the other of the Steinmann pin may be left subcutaneously so that it can be removed about 2 to 3 months after surgery, when the child is started on a gentle exercise program, combined with splinting to control wrist position. This splinting usually is needed until growth is complete, especially at night. Frequently the splints are hinged at the wrist level. An alternative possibility is the continuation of the long-term transepiphyseal rod fixation during childhood growth (in the manner described by Delorme).

SYNOVECTOMY OF TENDONS AT WRIST

GENERAL DISCUSSION. Rheumatoid arthritis of the wrist often results in dorsal subluxation of the distal ulna, laxity of the radiocarpal joint secondary to capsular stretching, and loss of articular cartilage, in addition to synovitis of the tendon sheaths and tendons crossing the wrist. If there are roentgenographic changes within the wrist joints, synovectomy of the tendons must be combined with either wrist fusion or arthroplasty.

Before bony changes occur, if significant extensor tenosynovitis has been present for 6 months in spite of good medical management, synovectomy of the extensor tendons can be helpful in preserving function, preventing tendon rupture, and relieving symptoms.

DETAILS OF PROCEDURE. This procedure is done with the same technique as the first steps of a wrist fusion, Plate 5-8, **A** to **D**. Lister's tubercle is excised, and the extensor retinaculum is repaired deep to the extensor tendons (Plate 5-8, **I** and **J**), thus transposing these tendons into a subcutaneous plane.

(Plate 5-8) ARTHRODESIS OF THE WRIST

GENERAL DISCUSSION. There are several different indications for arthrodesis of the wrist, the most common probably being the painful or unstable wrist in the patient with rheumatoid arthritis who is not suitable for arthroplasty. This is particularly the situation if the patient does require crutches for assistance in ambulation. Other indications occasionally include traumatic arthritis and tuberculosis. In certain selected situations it may be advisable in paralytic or spastic conditions. However, tendon transfers are usually more effective in the presence of a functioning wrist, and therefore arthrodesis is usually avoided in these conditions.

The optimal position for wrist arthrodesis is with the wrist in a neutral position with the axis of the index—long metacarpal shafts, a continuation of that of the radius.

DETAILS OF PROCEDURE. Arthrodesis of the wrist can be performed with the insertion of a large cortical cancellous block graft that is inset into a trough in the dorsal two thirds of the distal 3 cm of the radius, slotted across the dorsal two thirds of the intervening carpal bones, and set into the dorsal half of the index and long metacarpal bases. This is a technique that can be used in the osteoarthritic wrist (not illustrated). Since wrist arthrodesis is now most commonly done for rheumatoid arthritis, the technique described here is that recommended for such a rheumatoid patient.

A dorsal midline longitudinal incision is made, centered over the wrist **(A)**. It is essential that curvilinear and bayonet incisions *not* be used in the dorsum of the rheumatoid wrist because of the significant risk of slough of the wound margins on the distal based flap so created. Dissection is carried down through the superficial tissues to the extensor retinaculum. Great care must be taken during this portion of the dissection to avoid damage to the dorsal sensory branches of the radial nerve and the ulnar sensory nerve.

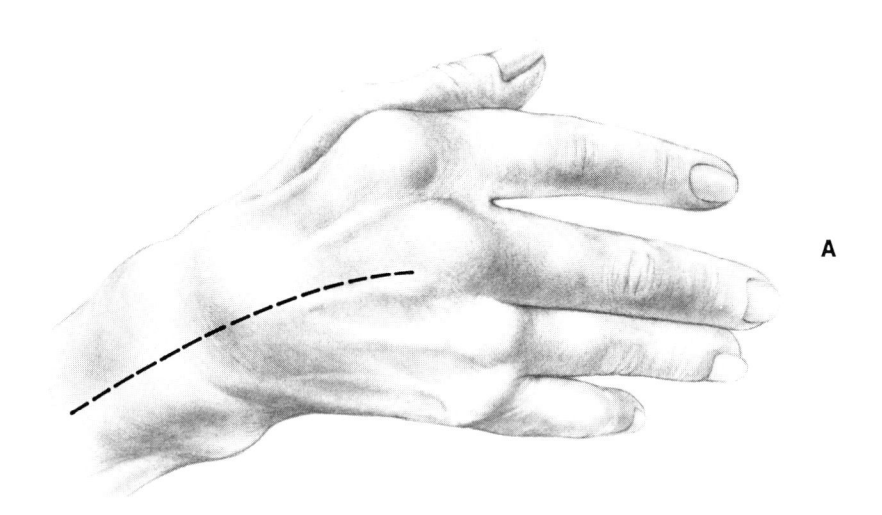

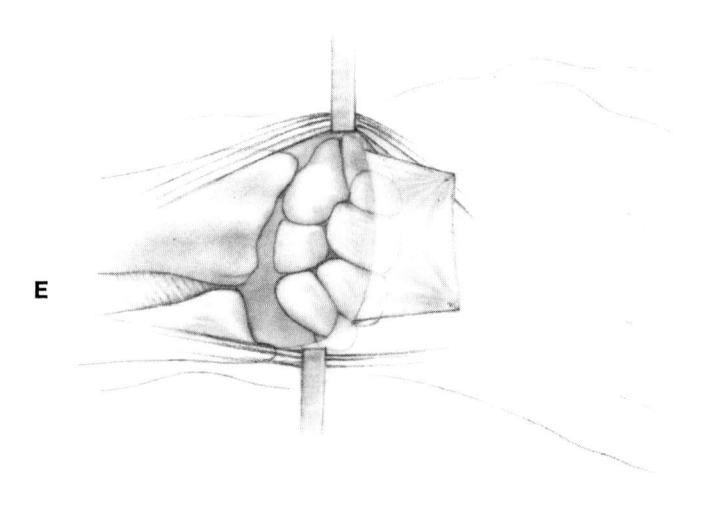

ARTHRODESIS OF THE WRIST (Plate 5-8)

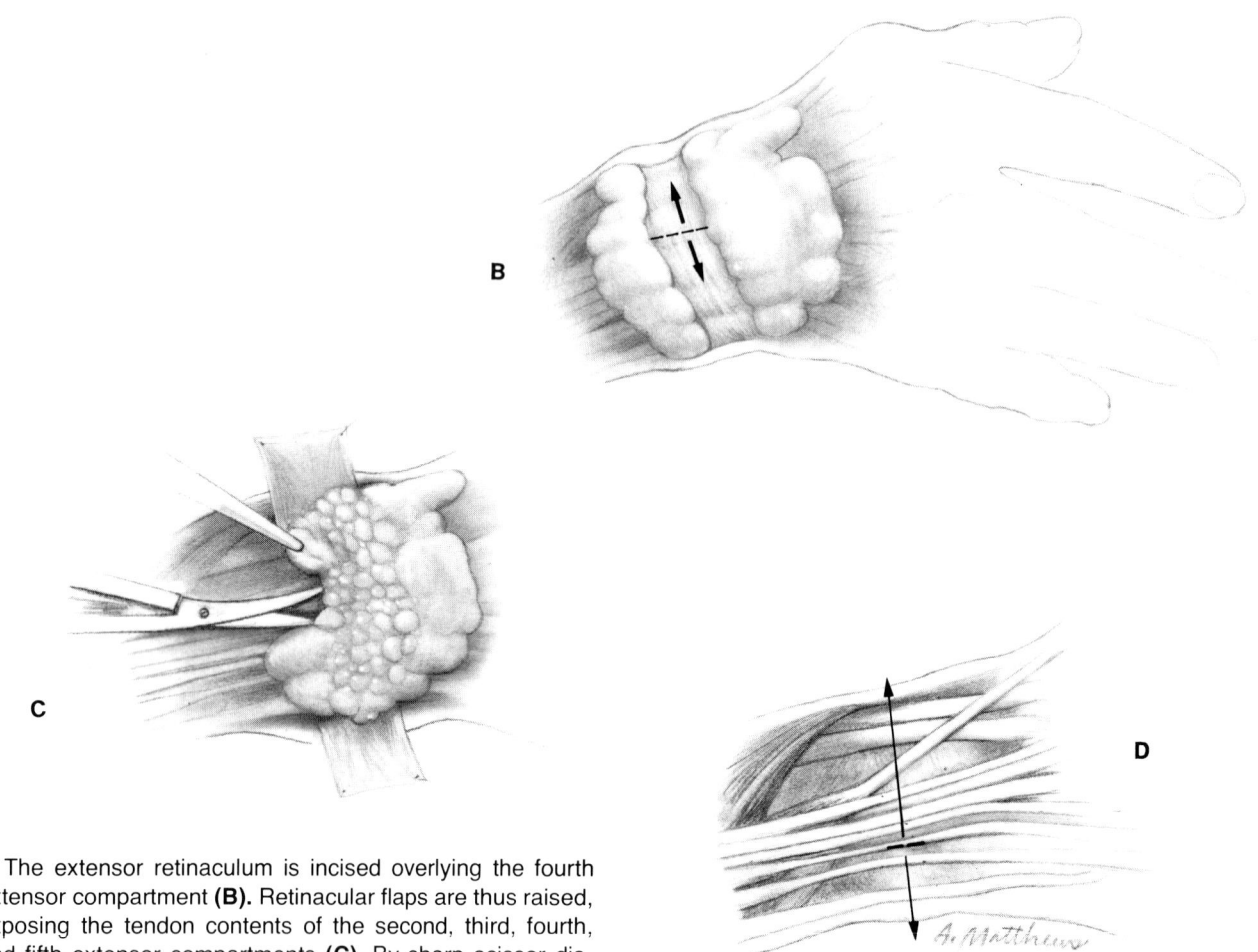

The extensor retinaculum is incised overlying the fourth extensor compartment (**B**). Retinacular flaps are thus raised, exposing the tendon contents of the second, third, fourth, and fifth extensor compartments (**C**). By sharp scissor dissection, a meticulous dorsal tenosynovectomy is then performed of all the tendons in these compartments (**C**).

Some of the extensor tendons are then retracted to the radial side and some to the ulnar side, with the interval usually being between the fourth and fifth extensor compartments (**D**). A distally based rectangular flap is then raised from the dorsal wrist capsule (**E**).

(Plate 5-8) ARTHRODESIS OF THE WRIST

Lister's tubercle is then excised. Ronguers are used to remove the subcortical bone and whatever cartilage remains from the articular surface of the distal radius, as well as from all the intercarpal joints **(F)**. The incision in the capsule is then extended proximally along the ulnar margin. The distal ulna is exposed, and 1 to 1.5 cm of the distal ulna is removed. All cancellous bone removed from the distal radius and ulna is saved for subsequent local bone grafting.

A large Steinmann pin is then driven distally with a power drill through the base of the capitate and down the interval between the index and long metacarpal. The arthrodesis site is then accurately aligned, and this pin is tapped in a retrograde fashion down the shaft of the radius **(G)**.

All the medullary bone that has been removed from the distal ulna and from the distal radius is then packed into the interstices of the arthrodesis site. The arthrodesis site is then tightly impacted, and the Steinmann pin is driven down so that its distal end is proximal to the metacarpal heads of the index and long rays **(H)**. If necessary, a staple or smaller oblique pin may be placed across the fusion to maintain firm coaptation. The rectangular capsular flap is sutured to the distal radius **(H)**.

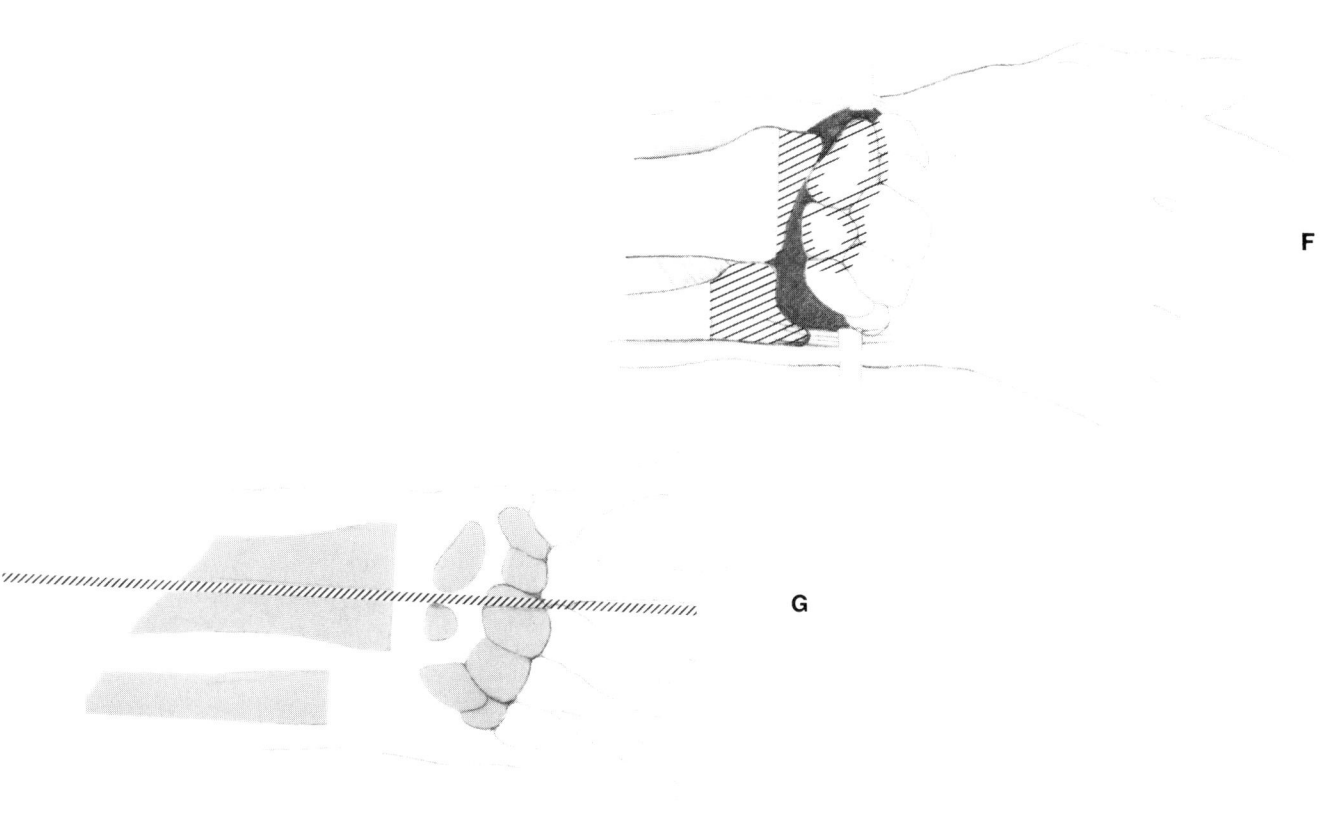

F

G

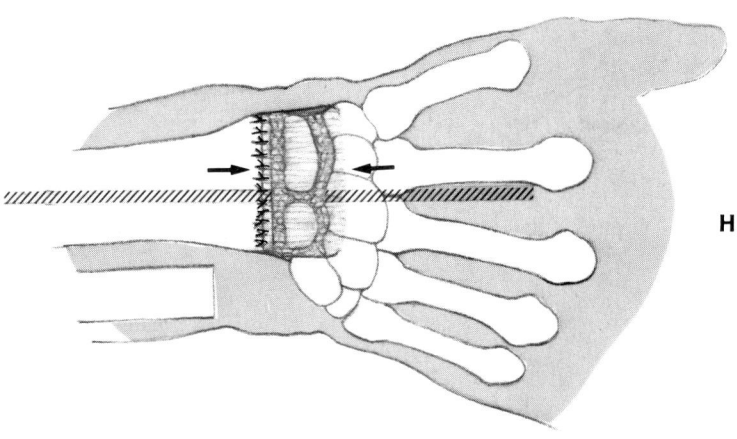

H

ARTHRODESIS OF THE WRIST (Plate 5-8)

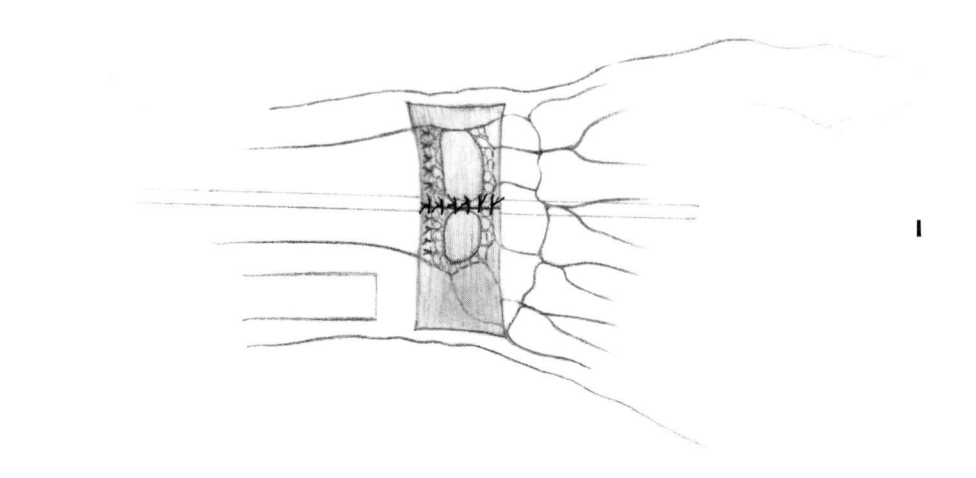

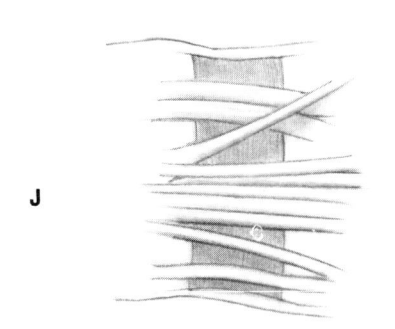

I

J

The extensor retinacular flaps are then transposed deep to the extensor tendons and sutured each to the other. This forms a smooth floor for extrinsic extensor tendon excursion, and transposes the tendons into a subcutaneous plane, thus minimizing the risk of subsequent extensor tendon rupture (**I** and **J**).

It is important that meticulous hemostasis be obtained throughout the procedure. A suction drain is used.

If digital extensor tendon ruptures are encountered, transfers will be necessary, either simultaneously with the fusion or as a second procedure (p. 160, Plate 6-12).

POSTOPERATIVE MANAGEMENT. The appropriate soft tissue dressing is applied with a voluminous overlying supportive fluff gauze or Dacron batting with overlying gauze, splint, and plaster shell. The suction drain is removed after 24 to 48 hours. If indicated, the bulky dressing can be removed at 2 weeks and the patient placed in a short-arm cast, which is worn for a total of 4 to 6 weeks following surgery.

This cast must be designed to allow full finger and thumb mobility, and the patient is encouraged in an active program of finger and thumb exercises. Obviously this program has to be modified if simultaneous tendon transfers are performed.

REFERENCES
General

Brewerton, D. A.: Hand deformities in rheumatoid disease, Ann. Rheum. Dis. **16:**183, 1957.

Bunnell, S.: Surgery of the rheumatic hand. J. Bone Joint Surg. **37-A:**759, 1955.

Burton, R. I.: Introduction, arthroplasty in the hand, Orthop. Clin. North Am. **4:**313, 1973.

Campbell, R. D., Jr., and Straub, L. R.: Surgical consideration for rheumatoid diseases in the forearm and wrist, Am. J. Surg. **109:**361, 1965.

Clayton, M. L.: Surgery of the rheumatoid hand, Clin. Orthop. **36:**47, 1964.

Cregan, J. C. F.: Indications for surgical intervention in rheumatoid arthritis of the wrist and hand, Ann. Rheum. Dis. **18:**29, 1959.

Entin, M. A.: Surgical treatment of rheumatoid arthritis, Surg. Clin. North Am. **44:**1081, 1964.

Eyler, D. L., and Markee, J. E.: The anatomy and function of the intrinsic musculature of the fingers. J. Bone Joint Surg. **36-A:**1, 18, 1954.

Flatt, A. E.: Surgical rehabilitation of arthritic hand, Arthritis Rheum. **2:**278, 1959.

Flatt, A. E.: Reclamation of the rheumatoid hand, Lancet **1:**1136, 1961.

Flatt, A. E.: The care of the rheumatoid hand, St. Louis, 1974, The C. V. Mosby Co.

Garner, R. W., Mowat, A. G., and Hazelman, B. L.: Wound healing after operations on patients with rheumatoid arthritis, J. Bone Joint Surg. **55-B:**134, 1973.

Goldner, J. L.: Upper extremity reconstructive surgery in cerebral palsy or similar conditions, American Academy of Orthopaedic Surgeons Instructional Course Lectures, vol. 18, St. Louis, 1961, The C. V. Mosby Co., p. 169.

Henderson, E. D., and Lipscomb, P. R.: Surgical treatment of the rheumatoid hand, J.A.M.A. **175:**431, 1961.

Kampner, S. L., and Ferguson, A. B., Jr.: Efficacy of synovectomy in juvenile rheumatoid arthritis, Clin. Orthop. **88:**94, 1972.

Landsmeer, J. M. F.: A report of the coordination of the interphalangeal joints of the human finger and its disturbances, Acta Morphol. Neerl. Scand. **2:**59, 1959.

Last, R. J.: Specimens from the Hunterian collection. The ligaments of the tarsus. The interosseous ligaments of the wrist, J. Bone Joint Surg. **33-B:**114, 1951.

Linscheid, R. L.: Surgery for rheumatoid arthritis—timing and techniques: the upper extremity, J. Bone Joint Surg. **50-A:**605, 1968.

Lipscomb, P. R.: Surgery of rheumatoid arthritis–timing and techniques: summary, J. Bone Joint Surg. **50-A:**614, 1968.

McEwen, C.: Early synovectomy in the treatment of rheumatoid arthritis, N. Engl. J. Med. **279:**420, 1968.

Millender, L. H., and Nalebuff, E. A.: Evaluation and treatment of early rheumatoid hand involvement, Orthop. Clin. North Am. **6:**697, 1975.

Millender, L. H., and Nalebuff, E. A.: Reconstructive surgery in the rheumatoid hand. Orthop. Clin. North Am. **6:**709, 1975.

Millender, L. H., Nalebuff, E. A., and Holdsworth, D. E.: Posterior interosseous nerve syndrome secondary to rheumatoid synovitis, J. Bone Joint Surg. **55-A:**753, 1973.

Moberg, E.: Cartilage lesions. In Hijmans, W., Paul, W. D., and Herschel, H., editors: Symposium on Early Synovectomy in Rheumatoid Arthritis, Amsterdam, 1969, Excerpta Medica Foundation.

Nalebuff, E. A.: Hand surgery and the rheumatoid patient, Surg. Clin. North Am. **49:**787, 1969.

Pulkki, T.: Rheumatoid deformities of the hand, Acta Rheumatol. Scand. **7:**85, 1961.

Riordan, D. C., and Fowler, S. B.: Surgical treatment of rheumatoid deformities of the hand, J. Bone Joint Surg. **40-A:**1431, 1958.

Slocum, D. B.: Amputations of the hand and forearm, American Academy of Orthopaedic Surgeons Instructional Course Lectures, vol. 8, Ann Arbor, 1951, J. W. Edwards, p. 235.

Sones, D. A.: Surgery for rheumatoid arthritis—timing and techniques: general and medical aspects. J. Bone Joint Surg. **50-A:**576, 1968.

Stelling, F. H.: Surgery of the hand in the child, American Academy of Orthopaedic Surgeons Instructional Course Lectures, vol. 15, Ann Arbor, 1958, J. W. Edwards, p. 172.

Straub, L. R.: The rheumatoid hand, Clin. Orthop. **15:**127, 1959.

Swanson, A. B.: The need for early treatment of the rheumatoid hand, J. Mich. State Med. Soc. **60:**348, 1961.

Swanson, A. B.: Silicone rubber implants for replacement for arthritis or destroyed joints in the hand, Surg. Clin. North Am. **48:**1113, 1968.

Swanson, A. B.: Flexible implant resection arthroplasty in the hand and extremities, St. Louis, 1973, The C. V. Mosby Co.

Vaughan-Jackson, O. J.: Rheumatoid hand deformities considered in the light of tendon imbalance, J. Bone Joint Surg. **44-B:**764, 1962.

Vesely, D. G.: The distal radio-ulnar joint, Clin. Orthop. **51:**75, 1967.

Fractures and dislocations

Agerholm, J. C., and Lee, M. L. H.: The acrylic scaphoid prosthesis in the treatment of the ununited carpal scaphoid fracture, Acta Orthop. Scand. **37:**67, 1966.

Albert, S. M., Wohl, M. A., and Rechtman, A. M.: Treatment of the disrupted radioulnar joint, J. Bone Joint Surg. **45-A:**1373, 1963.

Barnard, L., and Stubbins, S. G.: Styloidectomy of the radius in the surgical treatment of non-union of the carpal navicular. A preliminary report, J. Bone Joint Surg. **30-A:**98, 1948.

Barr, J. S., Elliston, W. A., Musnick, H., Delorme, T. L., Hanelin, J., and Thibodeau, A. A.: Fracture of the carpal navicular (scaphoid) bone. An end-result study in military personnel, J. Bone Joint Surg. **35-A:**609, 1953.

Barton, J. R.: Views and treatment of an important injury of the wrist, Med. Examiner **1:**365, 1838.

Campbell, R. D., Jr., Lance, E. M., and Yeoh, C. B.: Lunate and perilunate dislocations, J. Bone Joint Surg. **46-B:**55, 1964.

Campbell, R. D., Jr., Thompson, T. C., Lance, E. M., and Adler, J. B.: Indications for open reduction of lunate and perilunate dislocations of the carpal bones, J. Bone Joint Surg. **47-A:**915, 1965.

Cave, E. F.: The carpus, with reference to the fractured navicular bone, Arch. Surg. **40:**54, 1940.

Cave, E. F.: Retrolunar dislocation of the capitate with fracture or subluxation of the navicular bone, J. Bone Joint Surg. **23:**830, 1941.

Cole, J. M., and Obletz, B. E.: Comminuted fractures of the distal end of the radius treated by skeletal transfixion in plaster cast. An end-result study of thirty-three cases, J. Bone Joint Surg. **48-A:**931, 1966.

Darrach, W.: Anterior dislocation of the head of the ulna, Ann. Surg. **56**:802, 1912.

Darrach, W.: Habitual forward dislocation of the head of the ulna, Ann. Surg. **57**:928, 1913.

Decoulx, P., Hamon, G., Decoulx, J., Duquennoy, A., and Duport, M.: Traitement des fractures récentes du scaphoide carpien par vissage, Rev. Chir. Orthop. **52**:51, 1966.

Dingman, P. V. C.: Resection of the distal end of the ulna (Darrach operation). An end-result study of twenty-four cases, J. Bone Joint Surg. **34-A**:893, 1952.

Dooley, B. J.: Inlay bone grafting for non-union of the scaphoid bone by the anterior approach, J. Bone Joint Surg. **50-B**:102, 1968.

Ellis, J.: Smith's and Barton's fractures. A method of treatment, J. Bone Joint Surg. **47-B**:724, 1965.

Graner, O., Lopes, E. I., Carvalho, B. C., and Atlas, S.: Arthrodesis of the carpal bones in the treatment of Kienböck's disease, painful ununited fractures of the navicular and lunate bones with avascular necrosis, and old fracture-dislocations of carpal bones, J. Bone Joint Surg. **48-A**:767, 1966.

Green, D. P.: Pins and plaster treatment of comminuted fractures of the distal end of the radius, J. Bone Joint Surg. **57-A**:304, 1975.

Kienböck, R.: Über traumatische Malazie des Mondbeins und über Folgezustande, Fortschr. Geb. Röntgenstr. **14**:77, 1910-11.

Lugnegård, H.: Resection of the head of the ulna in post-traumatic dysfunction of the distal radioulnar joint, Scand. J. Plast. Reconstr. Surg. **3**:65, 1969.

MacAusland, W. R.: Perilunar dislocation of the carpal bones and dislocation of the lunate, Surg. Gynecol. Obstet. **79**:256, 1944.

Mazet, R., Jr., and Hohl, M.: Radial styloidectomy and styloidectomy plus bone graft in the treatment of old ununited carpal scaphoid fractures, Ann. Surg. **152**:296, 1960.

Mazet, R., Jr., and Hohl, M.: Fractures of the carpal navicular. Analysis of ninety-one cases and review of the literature, J. Bone Joint Surg. **45-A**:82, 1963.

McLaughlin, H. L.: Fracture of the carpal navicular (scaphoid) bone; some observations based on treatment by open reduction and internal fixation, J. Bone Joint Surg. **36-A**:765, 1954.

Milch, H.: Cuff resection of the ulna for malunited Colles' fracture, J. Bone Joint Surg. **23**:311, 1941.

Milch, H.: So-called dislocation of the lower end of the ulna, Ann. Surg. **116**:282, 1942.

Mulder, J. D.: The results of 100 cases of pseudarthrosis in the scaphoid bone treated by the Matti-Russe operation, J. Bone Joint Surg. **50-B**:110, 1968.

Murray, G.: End results of bone-grafting for non-union of the carpal navicular, J. Bone Joint Surg. **28**:749, 1946.

Russe, O.: Fracture of the carpal navicular. Diagnosis, nonoperative treatment, and operative treatment, J. Bone Joint Surg. **42-A**:759, 1960.

Smith, H.: Malunited fractures of the wrist, American Academy of Orthopaedic Surgeons Instructional Course Lectures, vol. 6, Ann Arbor, 1949, J. W. Edwards, p. 48.

Smith, L., and Friedman, B.: Treatment of ununited fracture of the carpal navicular by styloidectomy of the radius, J. Bone Joint Surg. **38-A**:368, 1956.

Smith, R. W.: A treatise on fractures in the vicinity of joints, and on certain forms of accidental and congenital dislocations, Dublin, 1847, Hodges & Smith.

Soto-Hall, R., and Haldeman, K. O.: The conservative and operative treatment of fractures of the carpal scaphoid (navicular), J. Bone Joint Surg. **23**:841, 1941.

Speed, J. S., and Knight, R. A.: The treatment of malunited Colles' fractures, J. Bone Joint Surg. **27**:361, 1945.

Sprague, B., and Justis, E. J., Jr.: Nonunion of carpal navicular: modes of treatment, Arch. Surg. **108**:692, 1974.

Stewart, M. J.: Fractures of the carpal navicular (scaphoid), J. Bone Joint Surg. **36-A**:998, 1954.

Stewart, M. J.: Treatment of fracture of the carpal navicular—conservative versus surgical (with review of 697 cases), J. Bone Joint Surg. **48-A**:1025, 1966.

Stewart, M., and Cross, H.: The management of injuries of the carpal lunate with a review of sixty cases, J. Bone Joint Surg. **50-A**:1489, 1968.

Taleisnik, J., and Kelly, P. J.: Extraosseous and intraosseous blood supply of the scaphoid bone, J. Bone Joint Surg. **48-A**:1125, 1966.

Arthritis

Abernathy, P. J., and Dennyson, W. G.: Decompression of the extensor tendons at the wrist in rheumatoid arthritis, J. Bone Joint Surg. **61-B**:64, 1979.

Albright, J. A., and Chase, R. A.: Palmar-shelf arthroplasty of the wrist in rheumatoid arthritis. A report of nine cases, J. Bone Joint Surg. **52-A**:896, 1970.

Backdahl, M.: The caput ulnae syndrome in rheumatoid arthritis. A study of the morphology, abnormal anatomy and clinical picture, Acta Rheumatol. Scand. (Supp.)**5**:1, 1963.

Beckenbaugh, R. D., and Linscheid, R. L.: Total wrist arthroplasty: preliminary report, J. Hand Surg. **2**:337, 1977.

Brånemark, P.-I., Ekholm, R., Goldie, I., and Lindström, J.: Synovectomy in rheumatoid arthritis. Experimental, biological and clinical aspects, Acta Rheum. Scand. **13**:161, 1967.

Burton, R. I.: The rheumatoid hand. In Kilgore, E. S., and Graham, W. P., editors: The hand: surgical and nonsurgical management, Philadelphia, 1977, Lea & Febiger.

Campbell, C. J., and Keokarn, T.: Total and subtotal arthrodesis of the wrist, J. Bone Joint Surg. **46-A**:1520, 1964.

Campbell, R. D., Jr., and Straub, L. R.: Surgical considerations for rheumatoid disease in the forearm and wrist, Am. J. Surg. **109**:361, 1965.

Carroll, R. E., and Kick, H. M.: Arthodesis of the wrist for rheumatoid arthritis, J. Bone Joint Surg. **53-A**:1365, 1971.

Clayton, M. L.: Surgical treatment at the wrist in rheumatoid arthritis: a review of thirty-seven patients, J. Bone Joint Surg. **47-A**:741, 1965.

Dupont, M., and Vainio, K.: Arthrodesis of the wrist in rheumatoid arthritis. A study of 140 cases, Ann. Chir. Gynaecol. Fenn. **57**:513, 1968.

Fink, C. W., Baum, J., Paradies, L. H., and Carrell, B. C.: Synovectomy in juvenile rheumatoid arthritis, Ann. Rheum. Dis. **28**:612, 1969.

Haddad, R. J., Jr., and Riordan, D. C.: Arthrodesis of the wrist. A surgical technique. J. Bone Joint Surg. **49-A**:950, 1967.

Hastings, D. E., Evans, J. A., and Hewitson, W. A.: Rheumatoid wrist deformities and their relation to ulnar drift, J. Bone Joint Surg. **54-A**:1797, 1972.

Kessler, I., and Vainio, K.: Posterior (dorsal) synovectomy for rheumatoid involvement of the hand and wrist. A follow-up study of sixty-six procedures, J. Bone Joint Surg. **48-A**:1085, 1966.

Linscheid, R. L., and Beckenbaugh, R. D.: Total arthroplasty

of the wrist to relieve pain and increase motion, Geriatrics **31:**48, 1976.
Lipscomb, P. R.: Synovectomy of the wrist for rheumatoid arthritis, J.A.M.A. **194:**655, 1965.
Lipscomb, P. R.: Surgery for rheumatoid arthritis—timing and techniques: summary, J. Bone Joint Surg. **50-A:**614, 1968.
Mannerfelt, L., and Malmstem, M.: Arthrodesis of the wrist in rheumatoid arthritis. A technique without external fixation, Scand. J. Plast. Reconstr. Surg. **5:**124, 1971.
Mannerfelt, L., and Norman, O.: Attrition ruptures of flexor tendons in rheumatoid arthritis caused by bony spurs in the carpal tunnel. A clinical and radiological study, J. Bone Joint Surg. **51-B:**270, 1969.
McEwen, C.: Early synovectomy in the treatment of rheumatoid arthritis, N. Engl. J. Med. **279:**420, 1968.
Millender, L. H., and Nalebuff, E. A.: Arthrodesis of the rheumatoid wrist. An evaluation of sixty patients and a description of a different surgical technique, J. Bone Joint Surg. **55-A:**1026, 1973.
Mitchell, N. S., and Cruess, R. L.: Synovial regeneration after synovectomy, Can. J. Surg. **10:**234, 1967.
Pahle, J. A., and Raunio, P.: The influence of wrist position on finger deviation in the rheumatoid hand. A clinical and radiological study, J. Bone Joint Surg. **51-B:**664, 1969.
Peterson, H. A., and Lipscomb, P. R.: Intercarpal arthrodesis, Arch. Surg. **95:**127, 1967.
Ranawat, C. S., and Straub, L. R.: Volar tenosynovitis of wrist in rheumatoid arthritis, Arthritis Rheum. **13:**112, 1970
Shapiro, J. S.: The etiology of ulnar drift: a new factor, J. Bone Joint Surg. **50-A:**634, 1968.
Shapiro, J. S.: A new factor in the etiology of ulnar drift, Clin. Orthop. **68:**32, 1970.
Smith-Petersen, M. N., Aufranc, O. E., and Larson, C. B.: Useful surgical procedures for rheumatoid arthritis involving joints of the upper extremity, Arch. Surg. **46:**764, 1943.
Stack, H. G., and Vaughan-Jackson, O. J.: The zig-zag deformity in the rheumatoid hand, Hand **3:**62, 1971.
Stein, I.: Gill turnabout radial graft for wrist arthrodesis, Surg. Gynecol. Obstet. **106:**231, 1958.
Steindler, A.: Arthritic deformities of the wrist and fingers, J. Bone Joint Surg. **33-A:**849, 1951.
Straub, L. R., and Ranawat, C. S.: The wrist in rheumatoid arthritis. Surgical treatment and results, J. Bone Joint Surg. **51-A:**1, 1969.
Swanson, A. B.: The ulnar head syndrome and its treatment by implant resection arthroplasty, J. Bone Joint Surg. **54-A:**906, 1972.
Swanson, A. B.: Flexible implant arthroplasty for arthritis disabilities of the radio-carpal joint. A silicone rubber intramedullary stemmed flexible hinge implant for the wrist joint, Orthop. Clin. North Am. **4:**383, 1973.
Swanson, A. B.: Implant arthroplasty for disabilities of the distal radio-ulnar joint. Use of a silicone rubber capping implant following resection of the ulnar head, Orthop. Clin. North Am. **4:**373, 1973.
Vesely, D. G.: The distal radio-ulnar joint, Clin. Orthop. **51:**75, 1967.

Nerve

Abbott, L. C., and Saunders, J. B. deC. M.: Injuries of the median nerve in fractures of the lower end of the radius, Surg. Gynecol. Obstet. **57:**507, 1933.
Ariyan, S., and Watson, H. K.: Palmar approach for visualization and release of the carpal tunnel: analysis of 429 cases, Plast. Reconstr. Surg. **60:**539, 1977.
Brain, W. R., Wright, A. D., and Wilkinson, M.: Spontaneous compression of both median nerves in the carpal tunnel. Six cases treated surgically, Lancet **1:**277, 1947.
Burton, R. I., and Littler, J. W.: Carpal tunnel syndrome. In Ravitch, M., editor: Current problems in surgery, Chicago, 1975, Year Book Medical Publishers, Inc.
Camitz, H.: Surgical treatment of paralysis of opponens muscle of the thumb, Acta Chir. Scand. **65:**77, 1929.
Cannon, B. W., and Love, J. G.: Tardy median palsy: median neuritis: median thenar neuritis amenable to surgery, Surgery **20:**210, 1946.
Cseuz, K. A., Thomas, J. E., Lambert, E. H., Love, J. G., and Lipscomb, P. R.: Long-term results of operation for carpal-tunnel syndrome, Mayo Clin. Proc. **41:**232, 1966.
Curtis, R. M., and Eversmann, W. W.: Internal neurolysis as an adjunct to the treatment of carpal tunnel syndrome, J. Bone Joint Surg. **55-A:**753, 1973.
Dupont, C., Cloutier, G. E., Prevost, Y., and Dion, M. A.: Ulnar-tunnel syndrome at the wrist. A report of four cases of ulnar-nerve compression at the wrist, J. Bone Joint Surg. **47-A:**757, 1965.
Eaton, R. G., and Morris, J. de L. S.: What's new with bones In Littler, J. W., Cramer, L. M., and Smith, J. W., editors: Symposium on Reconstructive Hand Surgery, St. Louis, 1974, The C. V. Mosby Co., pp. 274-278.
Frymoyer, J. W., and Bland, J.: Carpal tunnel syndrome in patients with myxedematous arthroplasty, J. Bone Joint Surg. **55-A:**78, 1973.
Fullerton, P. M.: The effect of ischemia on nerve conduction in the carpal tunnel syndrome, J. Neurol. Neurosurg. Psychiatry **26:**385, 1963.
Grantham, S. A.: Ulnar compression in the loge de Guyon, J.A.M.A. **197:**509, 1966.
Harris, C. M., Tanner, E., Goldstein, M. N., and Pettee, D. S.: The surgical treatment of the carpal-tunnel syndrome correlated with preoperative nerve conduction studies, J. Bone Joint Surg. **61-A:**93, 1979.
Hayden, J. W.: Median neuropathy in the carpal tunnel caused by spontaneous intraneural hemorrhage, J. Bone Joint Surg. **46-A:**1242, 1964.
Herndon, J. H., Eaton, R. G., and Littler, J. W.: Carpal tunnel syndrome. An unusual presentation of osteoid osteomas of the capitate, J. Bone Joint Surg. **56-A:**1715, 1974.
Howard, F. M.: Ulnar-nerve palsy in wrist fractures, J. Bone Joint Surg. **43-A:**1197, 1961.
Hybbinette, C-H., and Mannerfelt, L.: Carpal tunnel syndrome: Retrospective study of 400 operated patients, Acta Orthop. Scand. **46:**610, 1975.
Kopell, H. P., and Goodgold, J.: Clinical and electrodiagnostic features of carpal tunnel syndrome, Arch. Phys. Med. Rehabil. **49:**371, 1968.
Kleinert, H. F., and Hayes, J. R.: The ulnar tunnel syndrome, Plast. Reconstr. Surg. **47:**21, 1971.
Lewis, M. H.: Median nerve decompression after Colles's fracture, J. Bone Joint Surg. **60-B:**195, 1978.
Lipscomb, P. R.: Tenosynovitis of the hand and the wrist: Carpal tunnel syndrome, de Quervain's disease, trigger digit, Clin. Orthop. **13:**164, 1959.
Littler, J. W., and Li, C. S.: Primary restoration of thumb opposition with median nerve decompression, Plast. Reconstr. Surg. **39:**74, 1967.

Lynch, A. C., and Lipscomb, P. R.: The carpal tunnel syndrome and Colles' fractures, J.A.M.A. **185**:363, 1963.

Marie, P., and Foix, C.: Atrophie isolée de l'éminence thénar d'origine névritique. Rôle du ligament annulaire antérieur du carpe dans la pathogénie de la lésion, Rev. Neurol. **26**:647, 1913.

McCormack, R. M.: Carpal tunnel syndrome, Surg. Clin. North Am. **40**:517, 1960.

O'Hara, L. J., and Levin, M.: Carpal tunnel syndrome and gout, Arch. Int. Med. **120**:180, 1967.

Omer, G. E., and Spinner, M.: Management of peripheral nerve problems, Philadelphia, 1980, W. B. Saunders Co.

Omerod, J. A.: On a peculiar numbness and paresis of the hands, St. Bart's Hosp. Rep. **19**:17, 1883.

Paget, J.: Lectures on surgical pathology, Philadelphia, 1854, Lindsay and Blakiston.

Phalen, G. S.: Spontaneous compression of the median nerve at the wrist, J.A.M.A. **145**:1128, 1951.

Phalen, G. S.: The carpal tunnel syndrome, American Academy of Orthopaedic Surgeons Instructional Course Lectures, vol. 14, Ann Arbor, 1957, J. W. Edwards, p. 142.

Phalen, G. S.: The carpal-tunnel syndrome. Seventeen years' experience in diagnosis and treatment of six hundred fifty-four hands, J. Bone Joint Surg. **48-A**:211, 1966.

Phalen, G. S.: Reflections on 21 years experience with the carpal tunnel syndrome, J.A.M.A. **212**:1365, 1970.

Phalen, G. S., Gardner, W. J., and LaLonde, A. A.: Neuropathy of the median nerve due to compression beneath the transverse carpal ligament, J. Bone Joint Surg. **32-A**:109, 1950.

Phalen, G. S., and Kendrick, J. I.: Compression neuropathy of the median nerve in the carpal tunnel, J.A.M.A. **164**:524, 1957.

Robbins, H.: Anatomical study of the median nerve in the carpal tunnel and etiologies of the carpal-tunnel syndrome, J. Bone Joint Surg. **45-A**:953, 1963.

Seddon, H. J.: Carpal ganglion as a cause of paralysis of the deep branch of the ulnar nerve, J. Bone Joint Surg. **34-B**:386, 1952.

Semple, J. C., and Cargill, A. O.: Carpal-tunnel syndrome. Results of surgical decompression, Lancet **1**:918, 1969.

Shea, J. D., and McClain, E. J.: Ulnar nerve compression syndromes at and below the wrist, J. Bone Joint Surg. **51-A**:1095, 1969.

Spinner, M.: Injuries to the major branches of peripheral nerves of the forearm, Philadelphia, 1980, W. B. Saunders Co.

Tanzer, R. C.: The carpal tunnel syndrome. A clinical and anatomical study, J. Bone Joint Surg. **41-A**:626, 1959.

Uriburu, I. J. F., Morchio, F. J., and Marin, J. C.: Compression syndrome of the deep motor branch of the ulnar nerve (Pisohamate Hiatus syndrome), J. Bone Joint Surg. **58-A**:145, 1976.

Vanderpool, D. W., Chalmers, J., Lamb, D. W., and Whiston, T. B.: Peripheral compression lesions of the ulnar nerve, J. Bone Joint Surg. **50-B**:792, 1968.

Woltman, H. W.: Neuritis associated with acromegaly, Arch. Neurol. Psychiat. **45**:680, 1941.

Congenital

Blockey, N. J.: Observations on the fate of fibular transplants for congenital absence of the radius, J. Bone Joint Surg. **49-B**:762, 1967.

Bora, F. W., Jr., Nicholson, J. T., and Cheema, H. M.: Radial meromelia. The deformity and its treatment, J. Bone Joint Surg. **52-A**:966, 1970.

Delorme, T. L.: Treatment of congenital absence of the radius by transepiphyseal fixation, J. Bone Joint Surg. **51-A**:117, 1969.

Lamb, D. W.: Radial club hand. A continuing study of sixty-eight patients with one hundred and seventeen hands, J. Bone Joint Surg. **59-A**:1, 1977.

Madelung, O. W.: Die spontane luxation der hand, Arch. Klin. Chir. **23**:395, 1879.

Meyerding, H. W.: Correction of congenital deformities of the hand, Am. J. Surg. **44**:218, 1939.

Ranawat, C. S., DeFiore, J. D., and Straub, L. R.: Madelung's deformity. An end-result study of surgical treatment, J. Bone Joint Surg. **57-A**:772, 1975.

Riordan, D. C.: Congenital absence of the radius, J. Bone Joint Surg. **37-A**:1129, 1955.

Miscellaneous

Agerholm, J. C., and Goodfellow, J. W.: Avascular necrosis of the lunate bone treated by excision and prosthetic replacement, J. Bone Joint Surg. **45-A**:110, 1963.

Boyd, H. B., and Stone, M. M.: Resection of the distal end of the ulna, J. Bone Joint Surg. **26**:313, 1944.

Finkelstein, H.: Stenosing tendovaginitis at the radial styloid process, J. Bone Joint Surg. **12**:509, 1930.

Lacey, T., III, Goldstein, L. A., and Tobin, C. E.: Anatomical and clinical study of the variations in the insertions of the abductor pollicis longus tendon associated with stenosing tendovaginitis, J. Bone Joint Surg. **33-A**:347, 1951.

Lichtman, D. M.: Kienbock's disease: the role of silicone replacement arthroplasty, J. Bone Joint Surg. **59-A**:899, 1977.

Lipscomb, P. R.: Stenosing tenosynovitis at the radial styloid process, Ann. Surg. **134**:110, 1951.

Reid, S. F.: Tenovaginitis stenosans at the carpal tunnel, Aust. N. Z. J. Surg. **25**:204, 1956.

Roca, J., Beltran, J. E., Fairen, M. F., and Alvarez, A.: Treatment of Kienbock's disease using a silicone rubber implant, J. Bone Joint Surg. **58-A**:373, 1976.

Stack, J. K.: End results of excision of the carpal bones, Arch. Surg. **57**:245, 1948.

6
HAND

INCISIONS (Plate 6-1)

GENERAL DISCUSSION. Incisions in the hand can be varied and complex. They must be placed accurately. It is distressing that so many hands are needlessly compromised by inappropriate incisions made electively or to enlarge existing wounds. Any incision in the hand must be so conceived and designed that it can be extended if unexpected findings are encountered at surgery.

DETAILS OF PROCEDURE. Palmar incisions should be made, whenever possible, parallel to the palmar creases **(A)**.

Digital incisions must follow two principles. First, incisions on the side of a digit should be midaxial, not midlateral (index finger, **A**). The abrupt change in the normal character of dorsal and volar skin should be noted. It is better to err to the dorsal rather than to the volar aspect in the placement of incisions on the side of a digit, especially in children; digital incisions in children tend to migrate anteriorly with growth.

Second, incisions that transgress onto the flexor side of a digit must avoid the shaded areas shown on the index finger **(A)**. These shaded contiguous diamonds are formed by the midaxial points lateral to each joint and the anterior points at the middle of each digital segment. Skin in these shaded areas has maximum mobility with digital flexion and extension, and any longitudinal or oblique scars here are predisposed to contracture with resultant jeopardized function.

Note the great variety of incisions that are thus possible in the fingers, a few of which are shown on the index, long, and ring fingers.

Design of combined incisions for the palm and digit is simply a matter of coordinating these principles for palmar and digital incisions, as is seen for the long finger **(A)**. It is helpful to recall that an imaginary line drawn from the intereminential point to the cleft will overlie the lumbrical muscle and the common digital artery and nerve, whereas the line passing to the base of the digit will overlie the extrinsic flexor tendons passing to that digit.

Dorsal incisions can be equally varied. The multiple possibilities on the digits are illustrated **(B)**. Note that for surgery of the rheumatoid wrist, the dorsal incision should be straight or minimally curved. A bayonet incision, which is otherwise best for dorsal wrist exposure, may lead to slough of the distal based flap in the rheumatoid patient, thus making an abdominal pedicle flap necessary for closure.

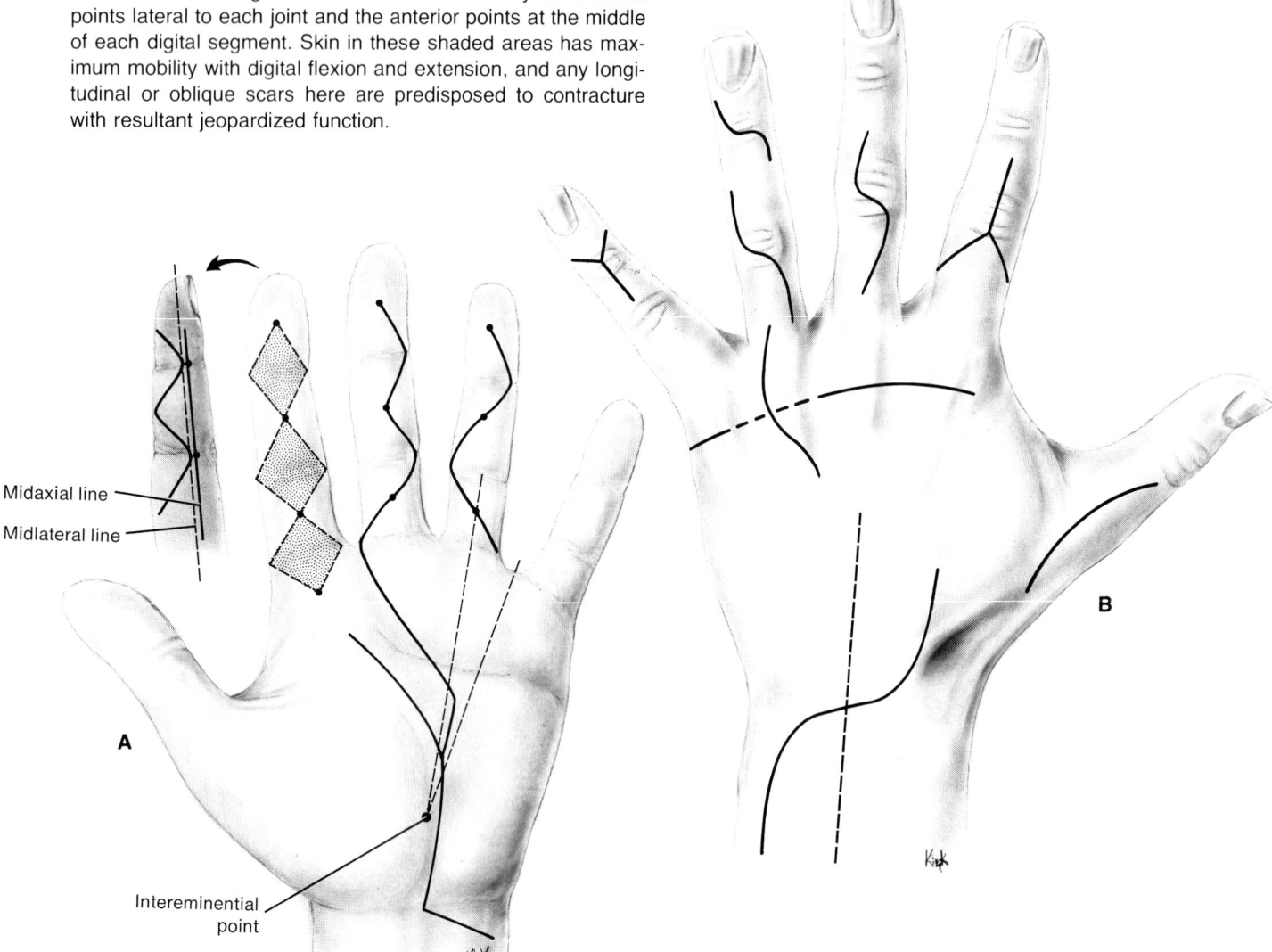

138

BASIC PRINCIPLES OF HAND DRESSINGS

The hand dressing is an integral part of the surgical procedure. It is not to be relegated to a junior member of the surgical team. An ill-conceived or poorly applied hand dressing will negate the purpose of the surgical procedure and indeed may leave the patient more compromised than if no procedure had been undertaken at all.

The layer applied directly to the wound should be conforming and absorptive. It should *not* be occlusive; the use of Telfa or Vaseline gauze is contraindicated. A well-contoured, moistened, smooth gauze sponge, or a single layer of Xeroform is excellent for this first layer. Subsequent layers of the dressing should be soft, supportive, and absorptive, such as gauze sponges (*never* with paper or fiber filling) fully opened and carefully applied to the contours of the hand resting in the so-called "safe position." This safe position is with the wrist in 20° to 30° of extension, the metacarpophalangeal joints in 60° to 90° of flexion, the interphalangeal joints extended, and the thumb extending from the hand in the first projection (the projection that the metacarpal shaft of the thumb takes from the remainder of the hand when a fist is made).

These are held in place with a Kling type gauze bandage. It is essential that this Kling roller bandage be applied in such a fashion that the wound is supported, but *not compressed.*

A Webril layer is then applied followed by a plaster external immobilization. This may take the form of anterior and/or posterior plaster splints that are held in place with either a Kling type of bandage or a roll of plaster. It is important that no pressure be applied over the dorsum of the wrist, since this will decrease the venous drainage from the hand.

The uninjured and/or unoperated on portions of the hand should be left free from the immobilization. It is absolutely essential that the patient keep the hand elevated at all times following surgery. The simplest way of accomplishing this is for the patient to elevate the arm on pillows while recumbent, keep elbows on the table while eating and whenever sitting at a desk or table, and to ambulate like the "Statue of Liberty." A sling is to be discouraged except in young children, since it does not hold the hand elevated and it tends to stiffen the shoulder.

TOURNIQUET USE IN UPPER EXTREMITY SURGERY

The use of a tourniquet to ensure a bloodless field is essential in hand surgery. According to Sterling Burnell's often quoted observation, "A watch maker cannot repair a watch at the bottom of an inkwell." Certain points in the use of a tourniquet merit emphasis:

1. The "on-off" type tourniquets that are powered by small canisters of compressed gas can be unreliable and deliver varying amounts of pressure even during the same tourniquet time without any indicated change on the gauge. It is urged that a reliable tourniquet gauge be used that connects to a central pressure source or large tanks. Prior to each day's surgery the accuracy of the pressure gauge in the tourniquet box should be checked by a responsible member of the operating room staff with the separate pressure manometer that is supplied with the tourniquet regulator.

2. The tourniquet should be applied over Webril padding, which is smoothly rolled onto the surface of the upper arm without wrinkle. The tourniquet itself should be of the proper length; a tourniquet designed for the leg, requiring wrapping of the cuff several times around the upper extremity should never be used. An 18-inch tourniquet length is usually best except in children and in adults with very heavy arms. Special pediatric size cuffs are available for small children and infants.

3. The tourniquet should be applied as far proximal on the upper arm as possible to avoid the slow filling of the extremity through collateral blood flow via the humeral shaft.

4. A limb should be well exsanguinated prior to tourniquet inflation. The more avascular the extremity, the better the tourniquet will be tolerated by the patient.

5. Under no circumstances should the tourniquet be allowed to remain inflated for more than 2 hours. For adults 275 mm Hg is adequate (unless the patient is hypertensive), and 200 mm Hg is adequate for children.

6. Should the tourniquet need to be released, or should it be necessary to do the procedure under two separate tourniquet times, if possible the tourniquet and Webril should be released while the tourniquet is deflated, *or* the hand should be supported with a general supportive dressing with gentle external pressure with the arm elevated. These two safeguards are to allow adequate perfusion of the extremity during the tourniquet "down time" but to minimize edema in the soft tissues being perfused.

OPPONENS TRANSFER FOR MEDIAN PALSY (Plate 6-2)

GENERAL DISCUSSION. The prehensile function of the human hand is predicated on the ability of the person to abduct and pronate the thumb into a position where it can oppose either the individual finger in pinch or the combined flexion force of all the digits in the combined pinch or the grasp position. Loss of the median and ulnar nerves will denervate all the thenar muscles and thus make it impossible for the patient to position the thumb in palmar abduction, and markedly weaken the thumb in pinch. Loss of the median function alone will weaken palmar abduction, and loss of ulnar function alone will weaken thumb adduction. Various types and combinations of transfers are available. The choice of the best type of opponensplasty transfer or transfers depends on the details of a careful assessment of the patient's overall hand function. Absolute prerequisites are a mobile thumb web space with a supple but stable carpometacarpal joint, relatively good motion of interphalangeal joint, and stability of the metacarpophalangeal joint. If more than 30° of motion of the metacarpophalangeal joint is present, or the metacarpophalangeal joint is unstable, it may be necessary to arthrodese this joint.

The most common opponensplasty is that to replace a pure median nerve motor loss, that is, loss of palmar abduction and pronation. If the median nerve lesion has occurred at the wrist level, the flexor digitorum superficialis for the ring or the long finger is suitable as a motor unit. Obviously if the median nerve lesion is at the elbow level or proximal, the superficialis muscles will also be denervated. The superficialis should never be used as a motor unit if the profundus musculotendinous unit to that digit is weak. Other possible choices for opponensplasty motor unit include the extensor indicis proprius, extensor digiti quinti, extensor carpi ulnaris, flexor carpi ulnaris, palmaris longus, or the abductor digiti quinti (Huber procedure).

The most common transfer is that of the flexor digitorum superficialis of the ring finger, which is passed either around the flexor carpi ulnaris or through a pulley of the flexor carpi ulnaris at the wrist level, across the subcutaneous plane of the palm, and inserted at the metacarpophalangeal joint level of the thumb into the tendon of the abductor pollicis brevis. Following is a description of this procedure.

DETAILS OF PROCEDURE. Under pneumatic tourniquet each of the two slips of the flexor digitorum superficialis to the middle phalanx of the ring finger is identified through an incision on the anterior aspect of the ring finger (**A** and **B**). The two slips of the tendon are divided, and then a second incision is made longitudinally over the course of the flexor carpi ulnaris, extending to the flexion crease at the wrist. A third incision is made over the volar radial aspect of the thumb metacarpophalangeal joint, exposing the distal muscle and tendon of the abductor pollicis brevis.

The superficialis tendon to the ring finger is identified at the wrist and pulled into the proximal wound. A loop is created by longitudinally dividing the distal 6 cm of the flexor carpi ulnaris tendon, leaving both portions attached distally, and passing the ulnar half of the tendon through a slit in the radial half to form a pulley at the wrist (**C**). The superficialis tendon to the ring finger is passed through the pulley and a subcutaneous tunnel over the thenar eminence. As an alternative, the superficialis tendon may be passed around the flexor carpi ulnaris, and thence subcutaneously to the point of new insertion (**D**).

The intact flexor pollicis longus and the extensor pollicis longus tendons adequately control the interphalangeal joint. If the metacarpophalangeal joint is stable and does not have more than a 30° arc of motion, the transfer is inserted as described below. If the metacarpophalangeal joint has a greater arc of flexion extension, it should be arthrodesed at this time in 10° flexion to prevent the distal two segments of the thumb acting as a crankshaft in forceful tip to side pinch. Such a crankshaft will obviate the purpose of the transfer as the thumb is forced into supination in pinch.

The distal portion of the transferred tendon is split. Each half of the split distal portion of the flexor digitorum superficialis is passed in an opposite direction through a split in the tendon of the abductor pollicis brevis. These two tails are then pulled until sufficient tone is present on the transfer so that with the wrist in 40° to 45° of extension the thumb is tenodesed into a fully opposed position. These two superficialis tendon strips are then interwoven each through the other and through the parent tendon, and secured with horizontal mattress sutures.

After the wounds are closed, a bulky supportive dressing is applied with an overlying plaster shell that holds the wrist in 30° of flexion, and with the thumb in the opposed position with the distal joints supported.

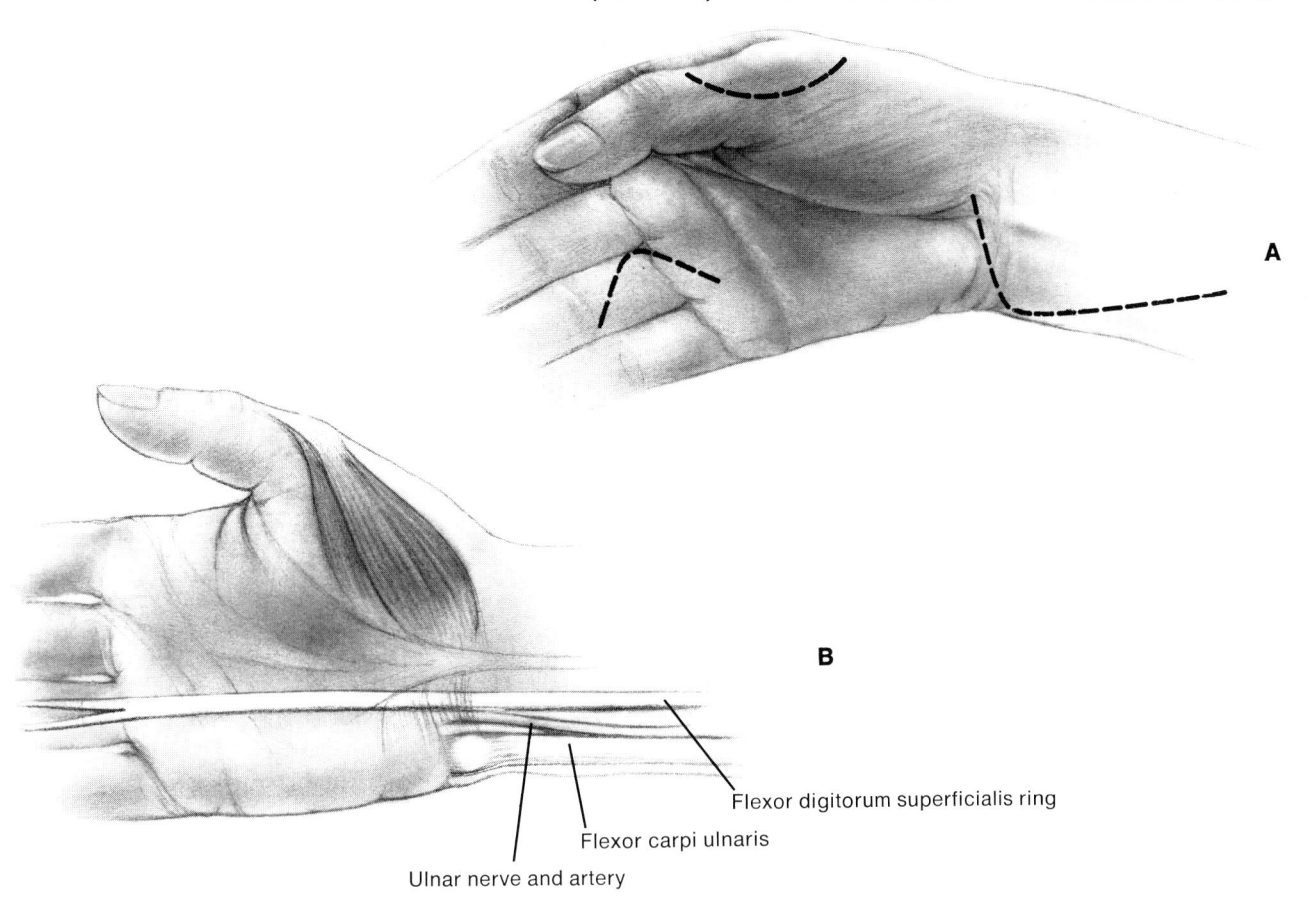

(Plate 6-2) OPPONENS TRANSFER FOR MEDIAN PALSY

A

B

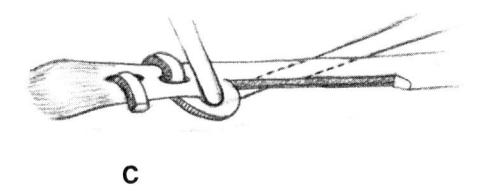

Flexor digitorum superficialis ring
Flexor carpi ulnaris
Ulnar nerve and artery

C

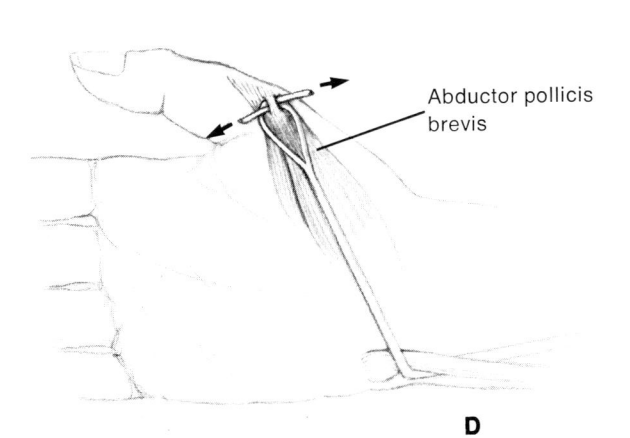

Abductor pollicis brevis

D

POSTOPERATIVE MANAGEMENT. The dressing and splints are removed at 4 weeks, and the patient is started on a hand therapy program. The splinting is continued between the exercise programs for an additional 3 weeks in an isoprene splint. Transfer training is continued as long as is necessary.

TENDON TRANSFERS FOR CLAWING OF FINGERS (SECONDARY TO ULNAR NERVE PALSY) (Plate 6-3)

GENERAL DISCUSSION. When clawing of the fingers develops following paralysis of the ulnar innervated intrinsics, the involved digits assume the posture of hyperextension at the metacarpophalangeal joints and flexion at the interphalangeal joints when the patient attempts active digital extension. In the pathomechanics of this condition, the extrinsic finger extensors are unable to effectively extend the interphalangeal joints because the metacarpophalangeal joints are hyperextended. The basis for reconstructive surgery of this condition is to prevent hyperextension of these metacarpophalangeal joints.

There are two basic types of surgical procedures for this. One is a static tenodesis of the volar plate mechanism of these metacarpophalangeal joints in flexion such that the extrinsic extensors can then extend the interphalangeal joints. Unfortunately, these tenodeses tend to stretch out.

The most effective procedures for the claw hand involve the use of active tendon transfers. Any functioning musculotendinous unit can be used for these transfers providing that (1) the donor motor musculotendinous unit is expendable in its present location and is not required for another transfer; (2) it has adequate power; and (3) the path of the transfer is anterior to the deep transverse metacarpal ligament (intervolar plate ligament), such that its active contraction causes metacarpophalangeal flexion primarily. The two most commonly used motor units are the extensor indicis proprius or the flexor digitorum superficialis of the ring finger. However, the former donor may be needed as a transfer to restore index finger abduction (Plate 6-4).

If the extensor indicis proprius is used, the donor tendon is divided over the dorsum of the hand at a level just proximal to the metacarpophalangeal joint, is rerouted through the substance of the hand between the ring and little metacarpals to pass anterior to the intervolar plate ligament, and thence is inserted into either the base of the proximal phalanx or the flexor sheath, as is illustrated later for the flexor digitorum superficialis. The use of the extensor indicis proprius is particularly helpful in patients with a high ulnar nerve lesion that causes the flexor digitorum profundus of the ring finger to be either weak or absent, thus preventing the superficial flexor to that digit being used as a donor motor unit.

The alternative surgical procedure is the use of the flexor digitorum superficialis, particularly in ulnar nerve lesions at the wrist level.

DETAILS OF PROCEDURE. The flexor aspects of the proximal phalanges of the ring and little fingers are exposed in accordance with the principles of incisions for the hand (see Plate 6-1). The flexor digitorum superficialis to the ring finger is transected at the level of the distal end of the proximal phalanx. The superficial flexor of the ring finger is preferred to that of the little, since the latter unit is often small and weak.

The tendon is then drawn into the palmar incision (**A** and **B**). The decussation is extended proximally so that the length of each tail is sufficient to be inserted as a primary metacarpophalangeal joint flexor with a good line of pull.

The insertion may be passed through the substance of the bone of the proximal phalanx, or may be passed through a window of the flexor sheath and sutured back to itself, as illustrated for the ring and little fingers, respectively (**C**). If there is adequate tendon length, the insertion into bone is preferred. It may be drawn through the substance of the phalanx and attached to a pull-out button suture on the opposite side of the digit. Great care must be taken to avoid damage to the adjacent neurovascular bundles. The tension on the transfer when the wrist is in 20° of extension should hold the metacarpophalangeal joints in at least 45° of flexion, but not more than 60°.

Following the wound closure the wrist and fingers are immobilized, the wrist held in 45° of extension and the metacarpophalangeal joints flexed 70°, with the interphalangeal joints at 0°.

(Plate 6-3) TENDON TRANSFERS FOR CLAWING OF FINGERS (SECONDARY TO ULNAR NERVE PALSY)

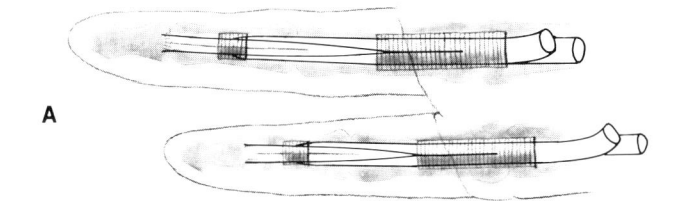

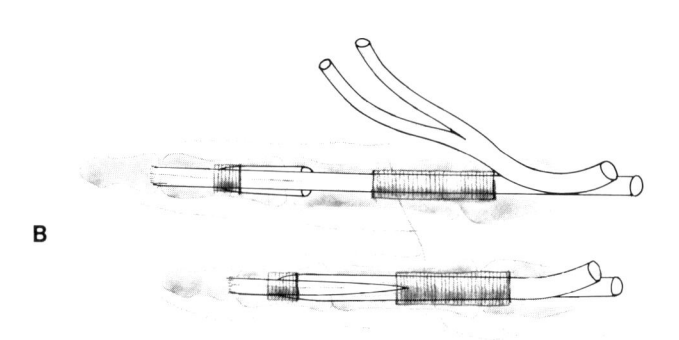

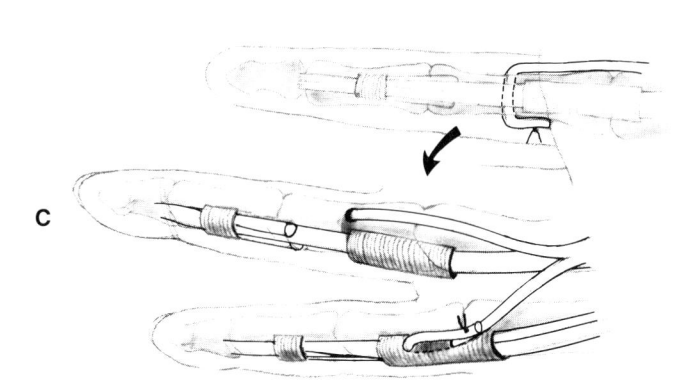

POSTOPERATIVE MANAGEMENT. The external immobilization is removed at 3 to 4 weeks postoperatively. It is essential that the patient be protected with a splint that prevents metacarpophalangeal joint extension past the point of 10° flexion for at least an additional 2 months. The patient does require an exercise program to regain full digital mobility with strength. Care must be taken to regain full flexion of the donor digit.

Note that these transfers are contraindicated in the patient with a claw deformity should the hyperextension of the metacarpophalangeal joint *or* the flexion deformity interphalangeal joints be fixed. A full range of passive mobility must be present prior to these tendon transfers.

143

TENDON TRANSFERS FOR WEAK OR ABSENT FIRST DORSAL INTEROSSEOUS (Plate 6-4)

GENERAL DISCUSSION. In patients with permanent loss of ulnar nerve function there are three basic deficiencies of the hand that may be significantly helped by transfers. A modified opponens transfer (Plate 6-2), with a pulley of a different type located near the midpalm to change the vector of force and which is inserted through the adductor tendon rather than the abductor, is used to reestablish more power to the thumb in pinch. The second type of transfer is that to correct the claw deformity by reestablishing active metacarpophalangeal finger flexion (Plate 6-3). The third deficiency of the ulnar palsied hand that may be helped by tendon transfer is that of lateral instability/weakness of index finger abduction because of weakness or absence of first interosseous function. In many types of pinch activities the patient can be taught to first make a fist, thereby using the ulnar three fingers in the fist position to buttress the index finger in pinch function. Should a transfer procedure still be necessary, there are two alternatives.

If the extensor indicis proprius has not been used for previous transfers, and if the extensor digitorum communis is functioning normally, the proprius tendon can be inserted into the tendon of the first dorsal interosseous. Another alternative is the use of one slip of the abductor pollicis longus tendon, extended with a tendon graft, in a subcutaneous plane paralleling the normal course of the first dorsal interosseous muscle and inserting into the tendon of that muscle at the metacarpophalangeal level. This latter procedure has proved effective and is well described by Neviaser. Following is a description of the technique for transfer of the extensor indicis proprius.

DETAILS OF PROCEDURE. Through an S-shaped incision **(A)** centered over the dorsal aspect of the metacarpophalangeal joint of the index finger, the tendons of the extensor indicis proprius and the extensor digitorum communis to the index finger are identified. The tendon of the extensor indicis proprius lying on the ulnar side of the extensor communis tendon is isolated **(B)**. The mobilized tendon is then passed deep to the tendon of the extensor digitorum communis to be sutured to the tendon of the first dorsal interosseus on the radial side of the proximal phalanx of the index finger **(C)**. As an alternative, it may be passed through the recipient tendon and then sutured back to itself. Following wound closure, a protective hand dressing is applied with the index finger in a functional position and with care to avoid any ulnar deviation of the index finger.

POSTOPERATIVE MANAGEMENT. At 4 weeks the protective dressing is removed and active exercise is begun. The protective splint is continued at night for an additional 3 weeks.

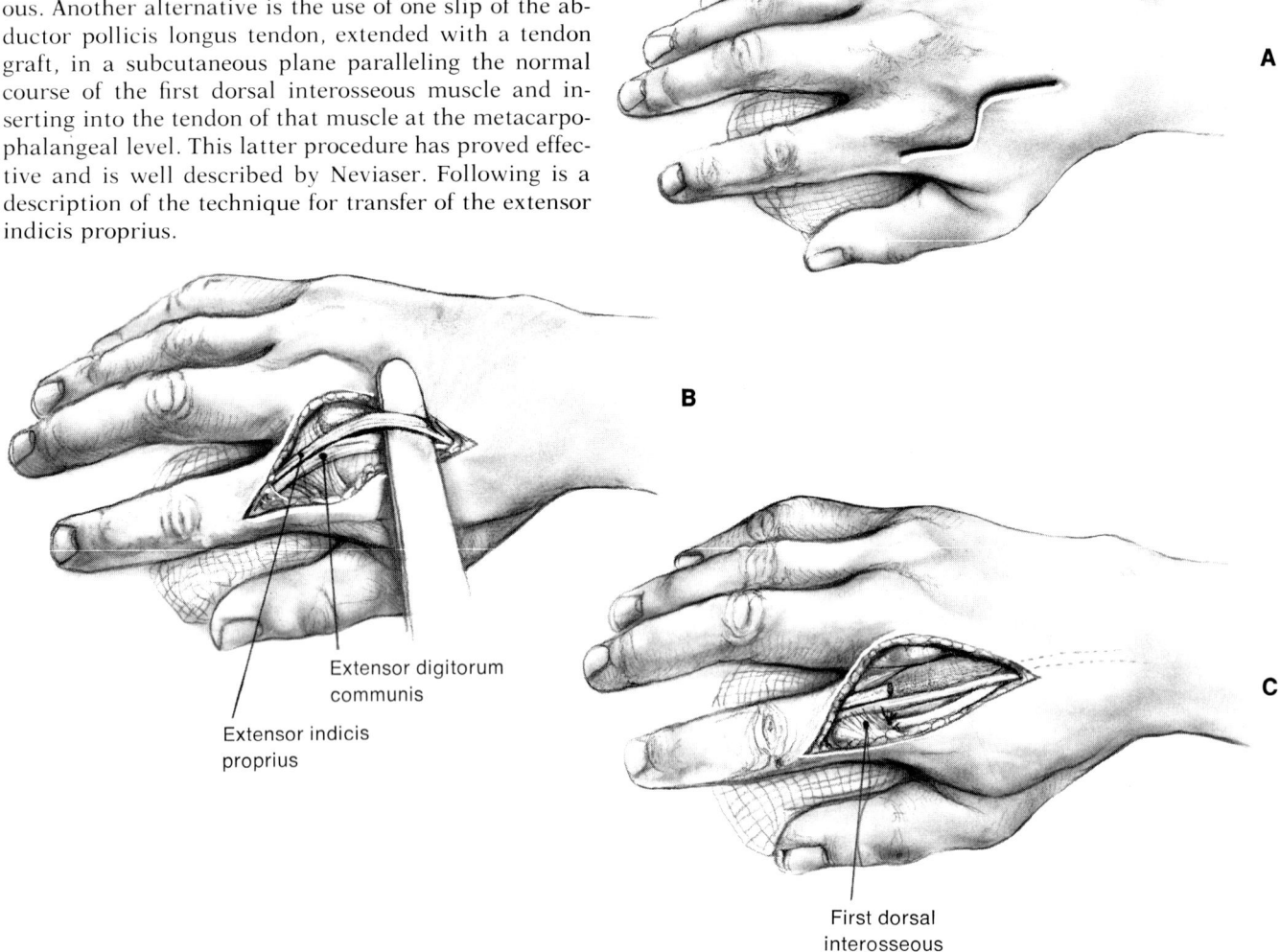

A

B

Extensor digitorum communis
Extensor indicis proprius

C

First dorsal interosseous

(Plate 6-5) HINGED HAND (FLEXOR OR EXTENSOR TENODESIS)

GENERAL DISCUSSION. Secondary to injuries of the cervical spine or to neurologic disorders such as poliomyelitis, patients may have good active wrist extension, but absent finger flexors or extensors. These patients' hands are postured (**A** and **B**), and although they can actively place the hand because of good elbow and shoulder control and good wrist extension, overall hand function is limited by the flaccidity of the digits.

The several types of tendon transfer available to power actively portions of thumb or finger function obviously vary with the level of the cervical lesion and the graded strength of the retained musculotendinous units. A detailed discussion of these various possibilities is beyond the scope of this text. As a generality, it is usually contraindicated to fuse the wrist, but far better to maintain active wrist control and provide tenodesis control of the fingers. Any additional transfers that are available are used to power the thumb.

The bone block fusion between the thumb and index metacarpals to fix rigidly the thumb in the opposed-abducted position is no longer thought to be advisable. To position the thumb rigidly interferes significantly with the ability of the patient to transfer from bed to chair and to manipulate a wheelchair.

Any attempt to create this type of functional hand with selected transfers obviously is predicated on the simplification of the multiarticulated system. Accordingly, it is often necessary to combine the tendon transfers or flexor/extensor hinge tenodeses with specific small joint fusions (see Plate 6-20). The most common arthrodeses indicated are those of the metacarpophalangeal joint of the thumb when combined with abduction-extension and/or flexion-opposition transfers, and arthrodesis of the proximal interphalangeal joints of the index and long fingers.

Control of the metacarpophalangeal joint of the fingers is provided by a tenodesis of the flexor or extensor tendons to the distal radius, passively powered by the patient's active wrist control.

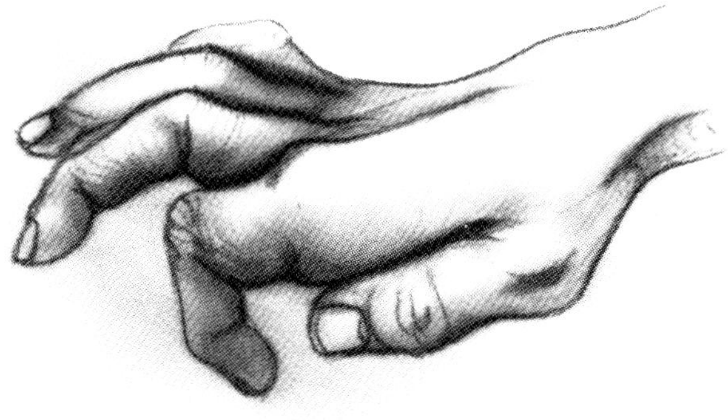

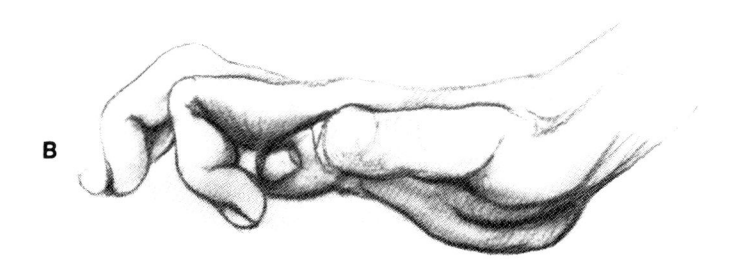

HINGED HAND (FLEXOR OR EXTENSOR TENODESIS) (Plate 6-5)

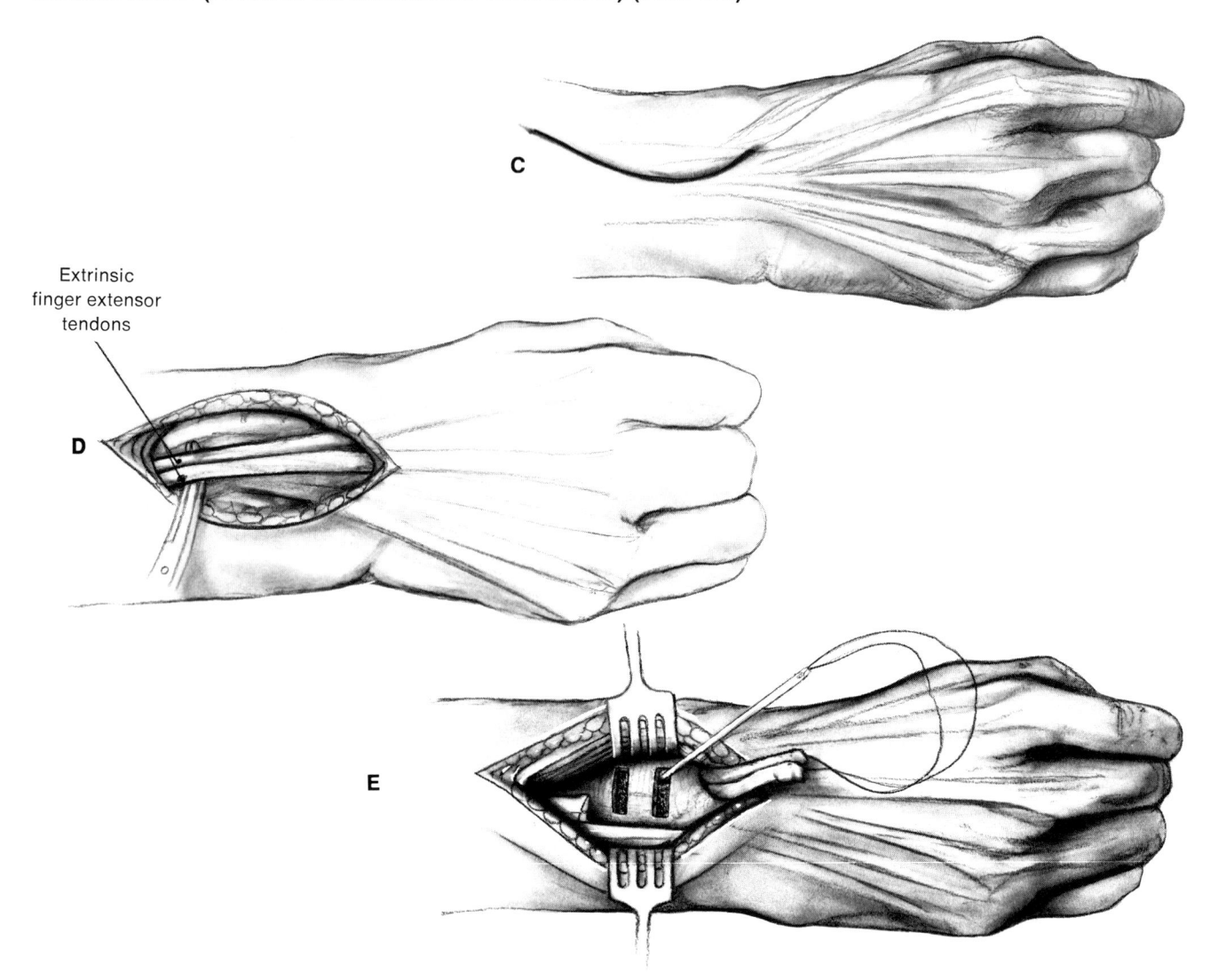

DETAILS OF PROCEDURE. Should the patient require a tenodesis of the flexor tendons, they are exposed at the wrist level with care taken to protect median and ulnar nerves. The terminal phalangeal flexors of the fingers to be tenodesed (usually all four) are identified in the depths of the wound.

A window (1½ × 1.5 cm) is placed in the anterior surface of the distal radius approximately 2.5 cm proximal to the wrist. A similar second window is placed 1 cm more proximal. A crisscross type of suture (Plate 6-7, A) is passed through all four flexor digitorum profundi tendons side to side, the tendon is transected just proximal to this suture, and then the tendons are drawn into the more distal hole, through the medullary canal, and out the proximal hole, and then sutured back to themselves.

The tension on the tenodesis is adjusted so that with the wrist in extension the fingers are flexed into the palm, and with the wrist in flexion the fingers can extend through the passive dorsal tenodesis of tension on the extrinsic extensors.

Conversely to the described type of patient with no active flexor function, a patient may have a residual of some intact active flexor function but lack active extrinsic extensors. In this situation, an analogous dorsal tenodesis is performed of the extrinsic tendons through similar cortical windows (**C** to **E**). The tension on this is adjusted so that with the wrist in extension, full passive digital flexion is possible, and when the wrist flexes, the fingers tenodese into extension at the metacarpophalangeal joint level.

POSTOPERATIVE MANAGEMENT. The patient's hand is immobilized following the tenodesis with the wrist in 5° to 10° of extension (flexor tenodesis) or 40° to 50° of extension (extensor tenodesis), and with the metacarpophalangeal joints flexed with the interphalangeal joints extended. Immobilization must be provided for 4 to 6 weeks in this fashion. The patient's plaster dressing is then removed and the exercise program instituted. It is essential that these tenodeses be protected with a removable splint for at least 3 to 4 additional months between the periods of exercise.

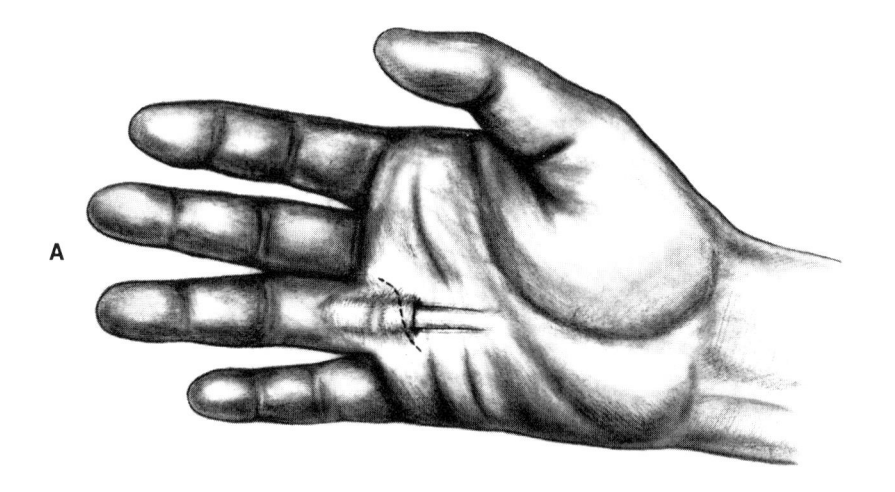

(Plate 6-6) TENOLYSIS FOR SNAPPING FINGER (OR THUMB)

GENERAL DISCUSSION. Stenosing tenosynovitis may develop with the flexor tendon sheath to any finger but most commonly involves the middle or ring finger and produces the snapping, catching, or locking of the so-called trigger finger. Constrictive tenosynovitis of the flexor tendon sheath of the thumb may be congenital (in which case the interphalangeal joint will be locked in flexion), or it may develop in later years. When symptoms or limitation of motion persists in spite of conservative measures, release of the proximal collar of the involved flexor sheath is indicated.

DETAILS OF PROCEDURE. Except in the young, the procedure can be carried out under local or wrist block anesthesia so that the patient may actively flex and extend the involved digit. A palpable and slightly tender nodular swelling is usually present along the course of the flexor tendon at the level of the base of the proximal phalanx.

A 2 to 3 cm gently curved incision is made over the proximal end of the fibro-osseous tunnel at the base of the involved digit **(A)**. Note that the base of the proximal phalanx and thus the proximal end of the fibro-osseous tunnel is at the level of the distal plamar crease. After the skin has been incised, the remainder of the dissection is done in a longitudinal plane by blunt scissor dissection directly over the anterior aspect of the flexor sheath. The adjacent digital nerves should be carefully identified and retracted. The proximal end of the fibro-osseous tunnel and the two flexor tendons are then easily identified. The flexor tendons are easier to visualize just proximal to this collar (**B** and **C**).

The proximal end of this fibro-osseous tunnel is released (**C** and **D**) under direct vision in increments of approximately 2 mm. Gradually increasing portions of the collar are incised, with the patient being asked to actively flex and extend the digit. This is done to demonstrate actively that the "trigger" phenomenon is no longer present and that adequate decompression has occurred. It is essential that no more of the sheath than necessary be released to prevent bowstringing, for to completely release the pulley will squander effective extrinsic flexor tendon excursion in prolapse and thus significantly diminish active interphalangeal joint flexion. The wound is closed with vertical sutures in the skin.

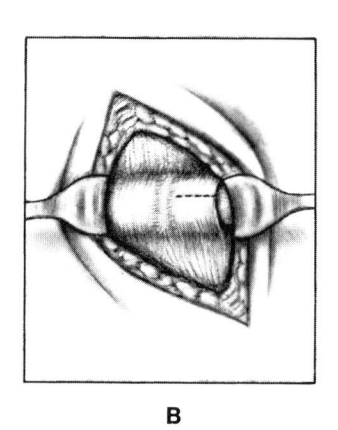

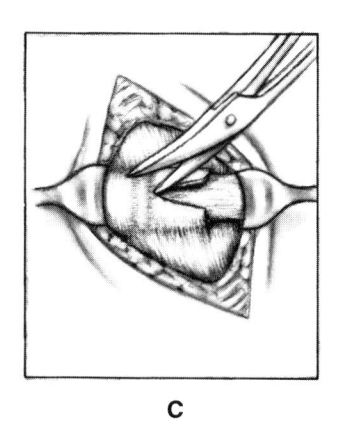

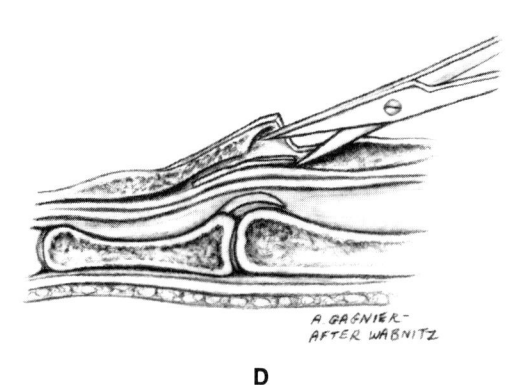

TENOLYSIS FOR SNAPPING FINGER (OR THUMB) (Plate 6-6)

The same principles apply in the decompression of the flexor pollicis longus tendon for the "trigger thumb." The incision is of a similar gently curved oblique nature over the proximal end of the fibro-osseous tunnel (**E**). Note that the digital nerves are much closer to the pulley mechanism in the thumb than in the fingers, and that indeed the radial one passes obliquely across the proximal end of the sheath itself (**F** and **G**). The decompression is done in an identical fashion (**G**). Should the trigger thumb be of a congenital type, it is helpful to close the skin with a 6-0 ophthalmic plain so that suture removal in a very young child will not be necessary in the office.

POSTOPERATIVE MANAGEMENT. A small, dry sterile dressing is required. Sutures are removed at 10 days after surgery. Note that frequently these patients will lose the last few degrees of extension of the proximal interphalangeal joint unless specifically and carefully started on an active assisted exercise program for that joint. These exercises should be started approximately 24 to 48 hours after surgery and continued until full active digital motion has returned both in the flexion and the extension arcs.

After decompression of the flexor pollicis longus tendon for "trigger thumb" in the infant, the only dressing that can actually be kept in place in infants for 10 days must be incorporated in a well-padded long-arm cast.

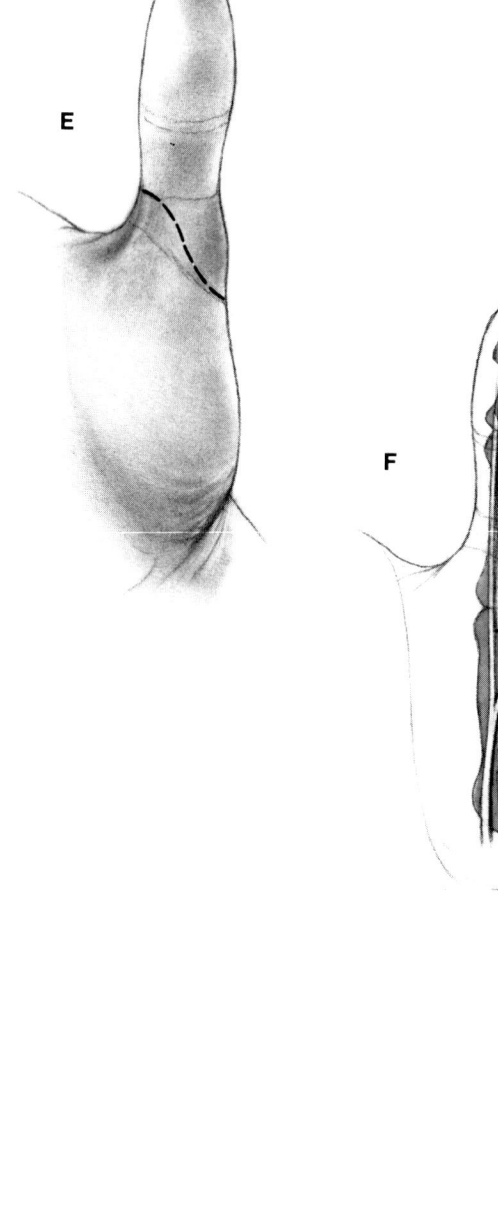

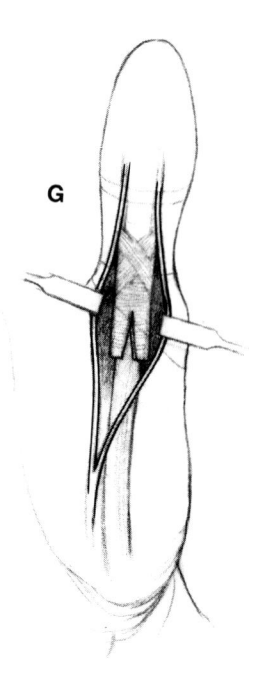

(Plate 6-7) TENDON REPAIR OF THE HAND

GENERAL DISCUSSION. The need for repair of flexor or extensor tendons in the hand occurs most frequently after lacerations, sometimes following avulsion or crush injuries, and not infrequently in association with other conditions such as fractures or rheumatoid arthritis. Detailed discussion of all the factors involved in the choices and alternatives of various surgical procedures and their techniques at each of the several levels of flexor and extensor tendon injury is beyond the scope of this text. The following is an attempt to give certain guidelines.

Note that the level of tendon laceration need not correspond to that of the skin laceration, depending on whether the tendon was cut with the fingers in extension or in maximum forced flexion. The level of laceration in the following discussion of the procedure refers to that of the tendon itself and not the skin.

Flexor tendon injuries can be divided into those which occur at five different zones. First, for tendons lacerated distal to the pulley at the midportion of the middle phalanx, primary repair is often possible and may yield favorable results. Second, lacerations of the tendons that occur in the zone between the distal palmar crease and the pulley at the midportion of the middle phalanx are an area (so-called no-man's-land) in which it is difficult to obtain predictably good results from surgery either with primary repair or with flexor tendon graft. Surgery on flexor tendons in this area should be performed only by those well trained and experienced in hand surgery.

Injuries at the three more proximal zones—midpalm, carpal tunnel, and wrist/forearm—are best repaired within a few hours, or at the 7- to 10-day interval following injury before myostatic contractures occur. The technical aspects of repairing a given flexor tendon in the hand may not be difficult in these areas, but obtaining a good functional end result may be extremely difficult. If at all possible, the surgery should be done by those experienced in these techniques.

There are many possible alternatives is choosing the best treatment of lacerations of flexor tendons. These include primary repair within the first few hours, delayed primary repair at 5 to 7 days, secondary repair at 10 days to 3 weeks, primary flexor tendon grafts, secondary flexor tendon grafts, two-stage flexor tendon grafts with the use of a silicone spacer rod as a first stage, tendon transfers, and in certain circumstances either arthrodesis or tenodesis of a distal joint. Primary flexor tendon repair is *not* the "easy way out" to avoid the need for later tendon graft. To obtain a good functional result is technically as difficult as the graft, and should be done only by surgeons well trained in these specific techniques.

Lacerations of extensor tendons are also divided into zones. Lacerations over the dorsum of the digits distal to the metacarpophalangeal joints can usually be treated by proper splinting rather than open tendon repair, since the fixed points of the extensor tendon mechanism distal to the metacarpophalangeal joint will prevent proximal tendon retraction. The splints should be made to support the appropriate interphalangeal joint in 0° of extension. The splint must be worn for approximately 2 months, and then the patient weaned from the splint as the joint is mobilized.

Lacerations of the extensor mechanism over the metacarpophalangeal joints of the fingers should be considered human bites until proved otherwise. A tooth laceration over the knuckle that has transected an extensor tendon almost invariably has extended into the joint, and frequently the organisms have been innoculated into the metacarpal head as well. These injuries need to be treated vigorously with local wound care and antibiotics. The laceration should never be sutured.

Lacerations of the extrinsic extensor tendons over the dorsum of the hand, at the wrist level, or in the forearm level are best treated by primary tendon repair.

Certain aspects of the examination of the lacerated hand merit emphasis. The wound itself should not be explored to determine what has been lacerated. The location of the wound should be carefully noted, and a careful history taken that includes when the injury occurred, where it happened and under what conditions, the exact mechanism of injury, whether the fingers were flexed or extended, whether previous treatment has been rendered, whether the patient has a history of injury to this area, and the patient's handedness, occupation, and avocations. The wound itself can then be gently covered. The most important part of the examination is that of the hand *distal* to the site of laceration. This must include a meticulous sensory examination (using light touch or two-point discrimination) to detect an associated nerve injury and then a careful examination for specific tendon systems. When there is a question of the division of a profundus tendon, the examiner should stabilize the patient's proximal interphalangeal joint and then ask the patient to actively flex the distal joint. When a conscientious and cooperative patient is unable to do so, the flexor digitorum profundus tendon has probably been divided. If the profundus tendon is intact and there is a question as to the continuity of the flexor digitorum superficialis, the examiner should stabilize all the other digits in neutral extension and then ask the patient to independently and actively flex the finger in question. The intercommunications between the profundus tendons at the wrist level will prevent the intact profundus tendon from flexing the free finger, and thus active flexion of the free finger at the proximal interphalangeal joint requires the intact flexor digitorum superficialis function. If a patient seems to have an excessive amount of discomfort while attempting any of these maneuvers, this may indicate an incomplete tendon laceration and be indication for exploration of the wound in the operating room. When there has been a laceration to the extensor surface of the wrist or hand, the extensor mechanism can be presumed divided if the patient is unable to extend the metacarpophalangeal joint.

Note that just as the intrinsic system flexes the metacarpophalangeal joint, it extends the interphalangeal

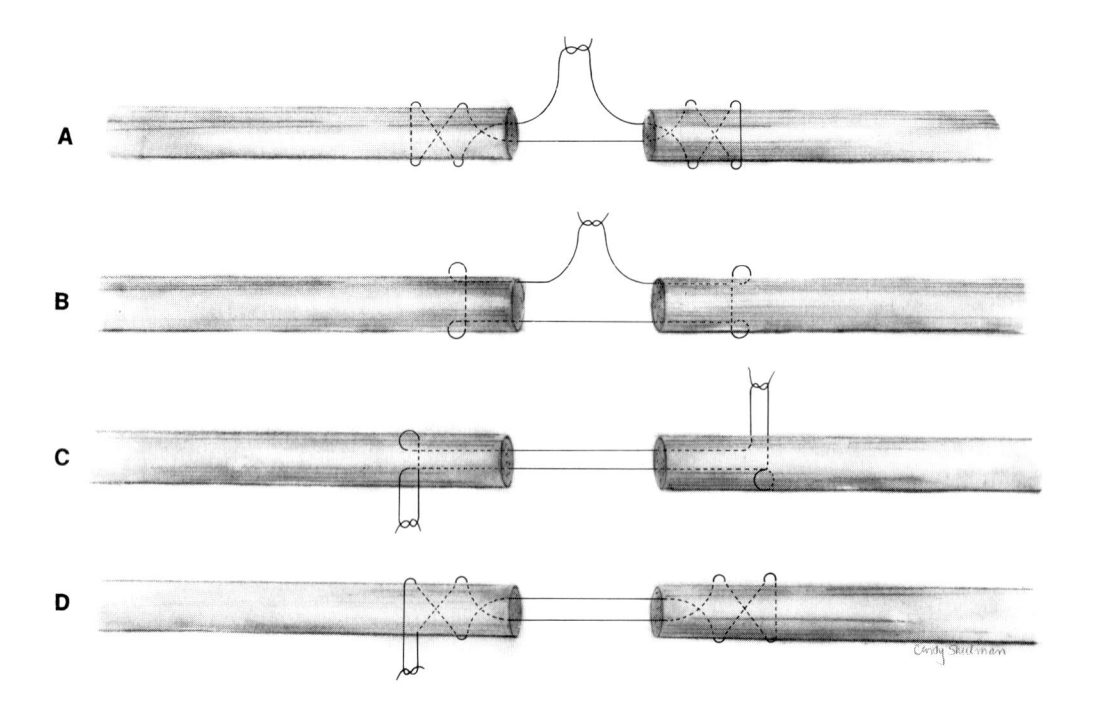

TENDON REPAIR OF THE HAND (Plate 6-7)

joint. This anatomic fact must be remembered if the examiner is not to be misled in assessing the patient with lacerations of the wrist and hand.

In evaluating the extensor tendon mechanism of the thumb, one must keep in mind the fact that the extensions of the intrinsic muscles into the extensor pollicis longus tendon over the dorsal aspect of the proximal phalanx will provide some active extension of the interphalangeal joint of the thumb, even if the extensor pollicis longus tendon has been divided or ruptured over the proximal hand or wrist.

If there is any question as to the presence of a tendon or nerve laceration, either flexor or extensor, the wound should be explored in the operating room.

DETAILS OF PROCEDURE. The goal of tendon surgery in the hand is to place a minimally traumatized tendon in the most benign bed possible. Every place where the tendon is touched with an instrument or where a suture has passed through the tendon is a point of tendon adhesion. There should be constant awareness that eventual function will depend on the ease of gliding of these tendons.

The laceration should be extended in accordance with the standard principles of hand incisions (Plate 6-1). Tendon repair can be done by one of several techniques. Tendon lacerations are usually repaired with a modification of the Kessler stitch (**B** or **C**) or Bunnell stitch (**A** or **D**). The Pulvertaft technique (**E**) is reserved for tendons of unequal size, such as a palmaris tendon graft to a profundus. The interweaving repair (**F**) is helpful in tendon transfers.

Two other conditions of the extensor mechanism that merit mention are intrinsic and extrinsic tightness. On occasion the intrinsic musculotendinous unit scars and contracts, leading to intrinsic tightness. This most frequently occurs following either crush injuries of the hand or as a consequence of rheumatoid arthritis. The diagnosis is made on physical examination; when the metacarpophalangeal joint is passively brought into full extension by the examiner, the proximal interphalangeal joint is tenodesed into extension, and passive flexion of the proximal interphalangeal joint is limited. The finger with intrinsic tightness frequently responds to an appropriate exercise program. If it does not, this condition can be treated by excision of the wing tendon from the involved extensor mechanism (**G** and **H**). This is *not* an operation for correction of the swan neck deformity.

(Plate 6-7) TENDON REPAIR OF THE HAND

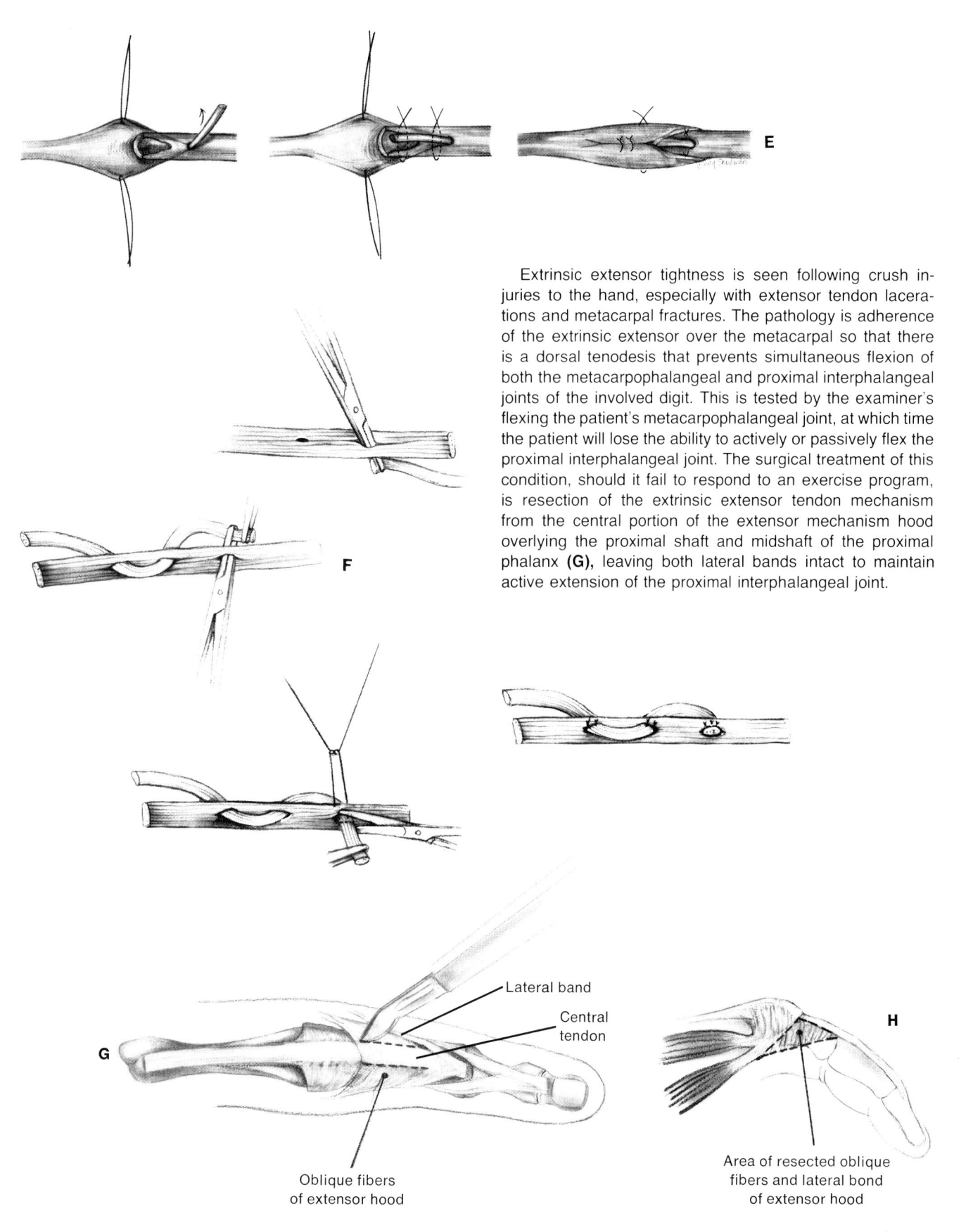

Extrinsic extensor tightness is seen following crush injuries to the hand, especially with extensor tendon lacerations and metacarpal fractures. The pathology is adherence of the extrinsic extensor over the metacarpal so that there is a dorsal tenodesis that prevents simultaneous flexion of both the metacarpophalangeal and proximal interphalangeal joints of the involved digit. This is tested by the examiner's flexing the patient's metacarpophalangeal joint, at which time the patient will lose the ability to actively or passively flex the proximal interphalangeal joint. The surgical treatment of this condition, should it fail to respond to an exercise program, is resection of the extrinsic extensor tendon mechanism from the central portion of the extensor mechanism hood overlying the proximal shaft and midshaft of the proximal phalanx **(G)**, leaving both lateral bands intact to maintain active extension of the proximal interphalangeal joint.

151

REMOVAL OF DONOR TENDON FOR TENDON GRAFTING (Plate 6-8)

GENERAL DISCUSSION. When there is loss of tendon substance, significant damage to or shortening of an existing tendon, or need to lengthen a tendon that is to be transferred as an active power unit, a tendon graft may be considered. If a palmaris longus tendon is present, this would ordinarily be the first choice for a donor tendon for tendon grafting. The palmaris longus is adequate in caliber and 10 to 14 cm in length. Other possibilities for a donor tendon source for tendon grafting may be a plantaris tendon, a long extensor tendon to one of the toes, the extensor indicis proprius tendon, or the extensor digiti quinti tendon.

In addition to a satisfactory bed for tendon gliding, the ultimate function of a tendon graft will also be dependent on correct placement of the graft for proper mechanics, a good muscle motor unit, and unrestricted joint motion. Any previous soft tissue injury or fracture should be well healed before tendon grafting is carried out. Any deep scar tissue must be adequately excised and the tendon graft handled with care at all times when any tendon graft procedure is carried out.

The donor tendon itself must be kept moist, must not be allowed to dry in the operating room lights, must not be handled with instruments on its gliding surface but only at the cut ends, and must not be rubbed with sponges (moist or dry).

DETAILS OF PROCEDURE. If the palmaris longus tendon is to be selected for tendon grafting, it is important to determine preoperatively whether this tendon is present. This may be done by asking the patient to oppose the tips of the thumb and little finger while flexing the wrist slightly; if a palmaris longus is present, its tendon will stand out prominently superficial to, and on the ulnar side of, the flexor carpi radialis tendon **(A)**. Reported to be present bilaterally in approximately 70% of people and present unilaterally in half of the remaining 30% of people, this tendon has good length and strength, and may be removed without producing any functional loss.

An incision is made near the flexion crease of the wrist to isolate the palmaris longus tendon just proximal to its insertion into the palmar fascia, as illustrated. Great care must be taken to avoid damage to the palmar sensory branch of the median nerve, which is located just to the radial side of the palmaris longus tendon. After a retention suture is placed in the palmaris longus tendon, it should be divided just distal to the suture. Then, when traction is applied distally with the retention suture, the outline of the palmaris longus in the forearm is visualized. A proximal transverse incision over the tendon at the junction of the middle and proximal thirds of the forearm (and, if necessary, intervening short transverse incisions) makes it possible to withdraw the palmaris longus tendon **(B)**.

The plantaris tendon (reportedly present in 93% of persons) may be small in caliber, but a segment as long as 25 cm can be obtained. This tendon is isolated anteromedial to the tendo Achillis near the heel, and the tendon is removed by proximal dissection. Although tedious, the procedure is best done using successive multiple short incisions after isolating the tendon near its insertion into the calcaneus **(C*)**. If a tendon stripper is used, the divided plantaris tendon should be held taut after it has been divided near the calcaneus and passed through the loop of the tendon stripper. The patient's knee should be kept in extension as the loop of the tendon stripper is passed proximally to a level near or just above the midportion of the calf, where a second incision is then made over the palpated loop of the tendon stripper for division. The stripper must be used cautiously and gently *without* force. Failure to do so will cause damage to the tendon surface and most assuredly cause functional failure of a tendon graft. The gastrocnemius muscle is retracted in the proximal wound to allow division of the plantaris tendon under direct vision in the midcalf area. Both plantaris tendon and the tendon stripper are then removed through the initial incision near the heel.

For removal of the tendon of the extensor indicis proprius or extensor digiti quinti two short transverse incisions are used, one near its insertion into the extensor hood and the other near the musculotendinous junction. The remaining distal portion of the extensor should be sutured to the tendon of the extensor digitorum communis, which lies adjacent to and on the radial side of the resected tendon.

*From White, W. L.: Surg. Clin. North Am. **41**:403, 1960.

(Plate 6-8) REMOVAL OF DONOR TENDON FOR TENDON GRAFTING

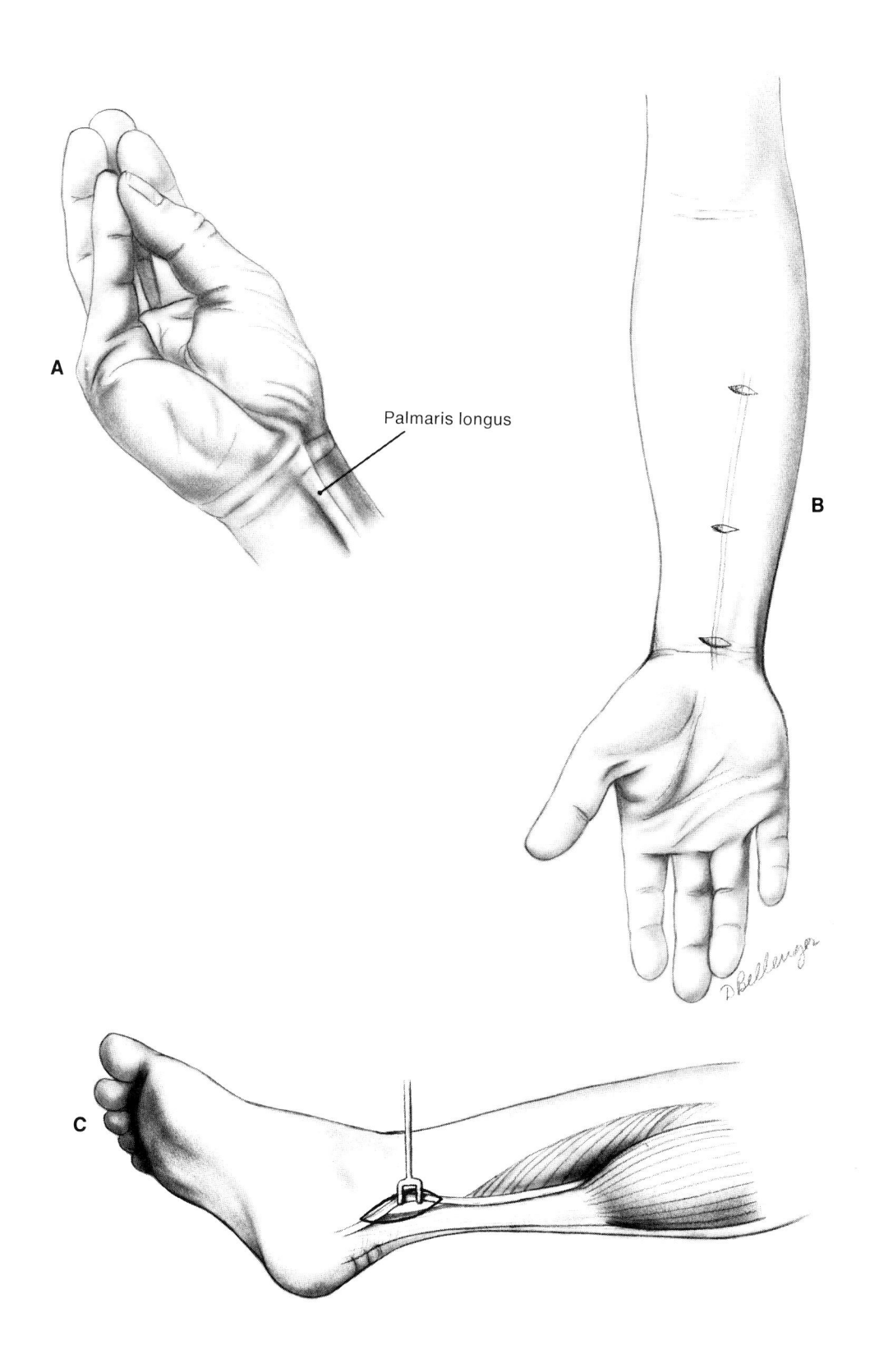

Palmaris longus

A

B

C

153

FASCIECTOMY FOR DUPUYTREN'S CONTRACTURE (Plate 6-9)

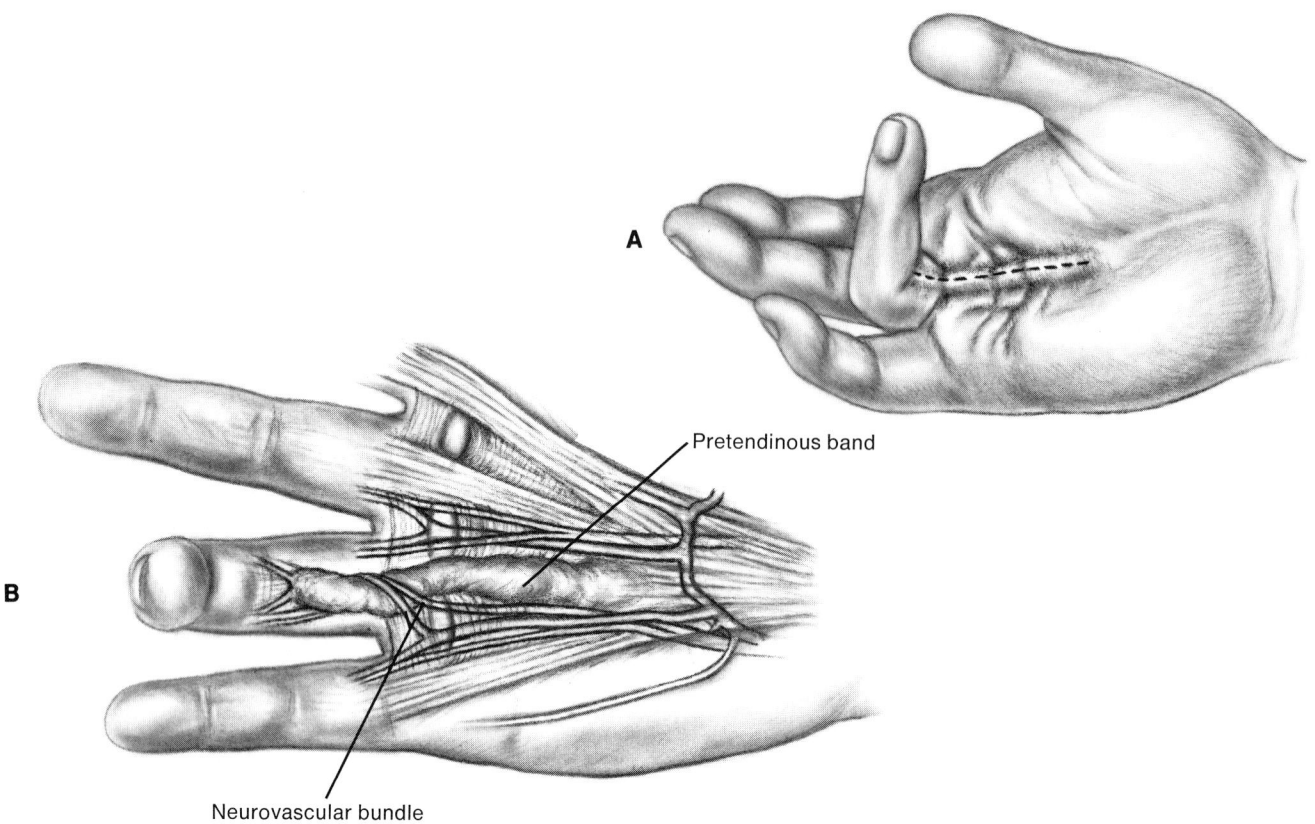

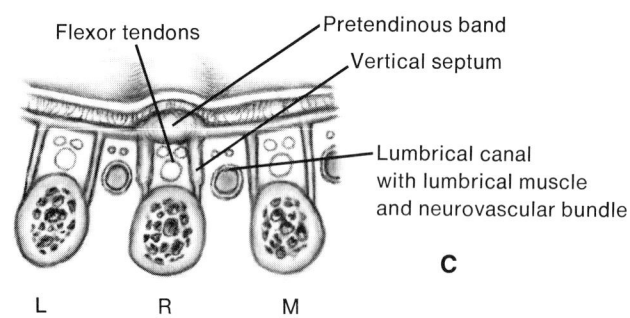

GENERAL DISCUSSION. Complete fasciectomy is less commonly done than in the past, most surgeons preferring to take a more conservative approach with excisions of the contracted tissue only in the involved rays, a subtotal fasciectomy.

The palmar fascial involvement in Dupuytren's contracture most commonly involves the ring and/or the little rays. In some patients it may involve the radial side of the palm and even the thumb web space, with or without involvement of the ulnar border of the hand. Indications for surgical intervention primarily are those of progressive contractures of the joints of the involved fingers, particularly if there is progressive contracture of the proximal interphalangeal joint. The major complications that occur from this surgery are recurrence and wound slough. The recurrence is sometimes a more rapidly contracting process than the original Dupuytren's disorder. The younger the patient, the more likely is a recurrence, especially if there are knuckle pads present. Women are also much more likely to have a recurrence than are men.

Since the process does involve the small fascial fibers that run between the palmar fascia and the skin, in some patients the skin is integrally involved in the process. In these situations the skin that remains after the dissection may be only thin epidermis without blood supply. Any wound necrosis that takes place will prolong convalescence significantly and potentially may lead to scars and predisposal to recurrence. For these reasons skin grafting is sometimes advisable at the time of the original procedure in patients with extensive dermal involvement. Any delay in the wound healing process that necessitates more prolonged immobilization or causes hand edema definitely will predispose the patient to small joint stiffness of the hand.

The partial or subtotal fasciectomy is the procedure of choice when only one or two digits are involved. In hands in which the wound heals per primum, good correction of the contractures at the level of metacarpophalangeal joints can be anticipated, but in patients with progressive preoperative fixed flexion deformities of the proximal interphalangeal joint, recovery of full extension at that level is less likely to occur. In patients with the fascial involvement extending dorsally to the level of the lateral bands, there may be a coexistent boutonniere deformity.

(Plate 6-9) FASCIECTOMY FOR DUPUYTREN'S CONTRACTURE

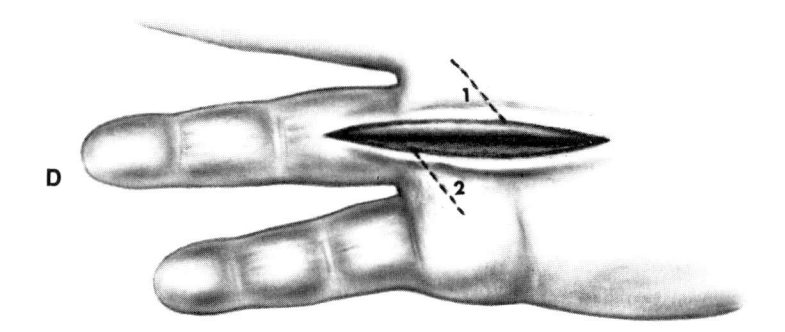

DETAILS OF PROCEDURE. A typical patient has the appearance seen in **A**. The goal of surgery is to remove the longitudinal pretendinous bands that run from the intereminential area (Plate 6-1) to the level of the proximal interphalangeal joint **(B)**. It is also important to remove the vertical extensions down the substance of the vertical septae to the metacarpal level **(C)**. It is essential to note that frequently the digital artery and nerve may spiral around this pretendinous band and/or may pass through it **(B)**. Either the radial or ulnar digital nerves, or occasionally both, may be so involved. For these reasons, the dissection of this pretendinous hand becomes in fact a neurolysis of these digital nerves. As the vertical septae pass to either side of the flexor mechanism **(C)**, it is important in dissecting that portion of the pretendinous bands and the vertical septi not to violate the flexor tendon sheath, which may be directly adjacent to the undersurface of the pretendinous band at the level of the distal palmar crease.

The incision can be one of three types. A straight transverse incision across the palm is possible if the goal of surgery is only to remove localized palmar fascia at the level of the incision. It may not be possible to remove significant longitudinal components through a transverse incision, and with correction of a significant deformity, wound closure may be difficult. Some surgeons advocate open treatment of these wounds.

A second alternative is a longitudinal zigzag incision. However, wound closure may be difficult if significant correction is obtained of the deformities, and the apices of the flaps raised will be based on the very thin subcutaneous tissue that overlies this band itself. On many occasions it is advisable to use a straight incision **(D)**. This gives excellent exposure of the pretendinous band. Through this incision it is relatively easy to identify the nerves in the proximal palm, and then they can be carefully separated from the pretendinous band as the dissection proceeds, including removal of the vertical septi. The linear longitudinal nature of this incision can be broken up with Z-plasties that are based on more normal tissue. The flaps are then transposed and the wound closed **(E)**. A single Z-plasty may be done, or frequently small multiple Z-plasties are more suitable, depending on the nature of the wound. Regardless of the type of incision(s), all the vertical blood supply to the palmar skin must be protected.

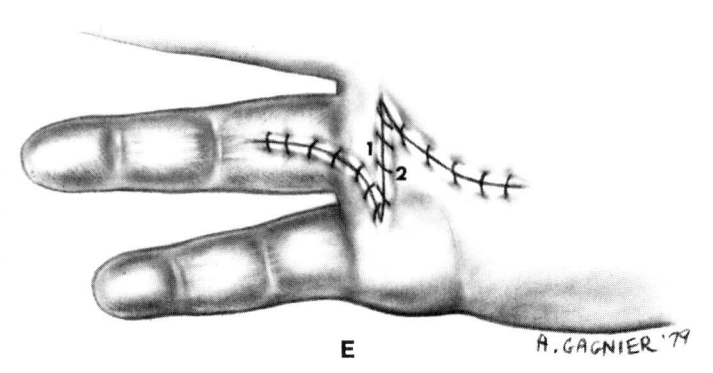

Should the patient have a significant contracture of the proximal interphalangeal joint that does not correct with excision of the pretendinous band and the involved vertical septi, it may be necessary to explore the volar plate and collateral ligament mechanism of this joint and selectively release these involved structures.

Meticulous hemostasis is essential. Dissection technique and preventing hematoma are the two most important precautions that the surgeon can take to prevent loss of the flaps. Should a hematoma occur, it must be promptly recognized and evacuated if unnecessary scarring is to be avoided and flap viability preserved.

POSTOPERATIVE MANAGEMENT. Superb dressing technique is essential. The wound must be adequately and firmly supported, without compression. The patient must keep the hand elevated at all times for the first 2 weeks. Gentle digital mobility at the proximal interphalangeal joint level may be encouraged early in the postoperative course if such mobility is free of pain. These exercises must be active and not passive. The dressing and sutures are removed at approximately 3 weeks. The patient must be advised against holding the hand in any dependent position or immersing it in warm water. An active exercise program is important in regaining full digital flexion and strength, and maintaining maximum possible extension. This is encouraged after the second week, but may be necessary for many weeks thereafter.

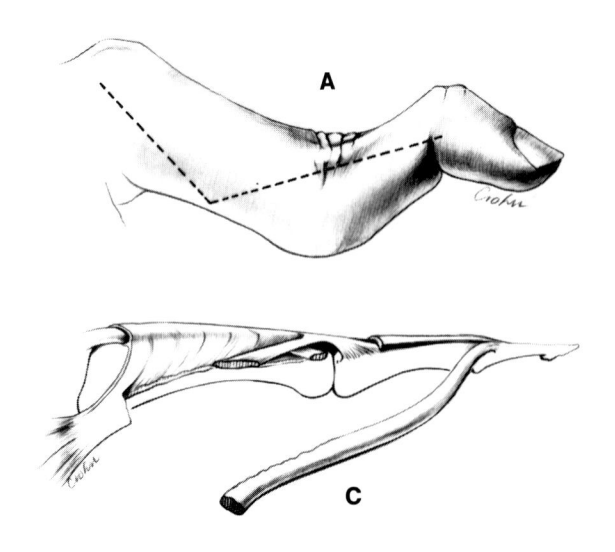

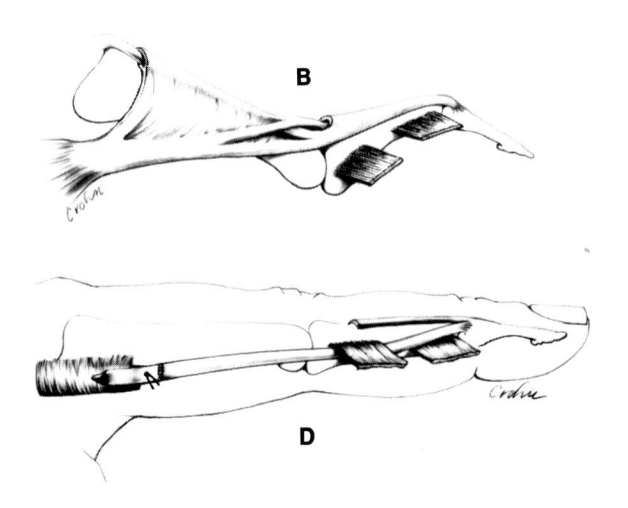

REPAIR OF SWAN NECK DEFORMITY (Plate 6-10)

GENERAL DISCUSSION. The swan neck deformity is one in which the proximal interphalangeal joint is hyperextended and the distal interphalangeal joint flexed when the patient attempts maximum active digital extension (**A** and **E**). This dynamic finger imbalance can progress to fixed deformity. Swan neck is commonly seen in rheumatoid arthritis, but it also is seen (1) in spastic conditions, (2) secondary to trauma with fractures of the middle phalanx, (3) in injuries to the volar plate mechanism at the proximal interphalangeal joint, (4) secondary to mallet deformities at the distal interphalangeal joints when there is coexistent volar plate laxity at the proximal interphalangeal joint, and (5) in some people with joint laxity at the proximal joint as part of a generalized systemic ligamentous laxity.

Furthermore, patients with these deformities can be subdivided into those of fixed deformity with secondary joint changes and contractures, and those with full active proximal interphalangeal joint flexion but simply a dynamic imbalance of the extensor mechanism.

In the patient with rheumatoid arthritis it is absolutely essential to correct any tendon imbalance or flexion contractures at the metacarpophalangeal joint before evaluating and treating a swan neck deformity. Failure to correct the more proximal metacarpophalangeal flexion deformity or imbalance will predetermine failure of the attempt at swan neck reconstruction in the rheumatoid hand.

Patients with swan neck deformity frequently have intrinsic tightness. But correction of the intrinsic tightness will *not* correct swan neck deformity unless something is done simultaneously to eliminate the volar plate laxity at the proximal interphalangeal joint and the droop of the extensor mechanism at the distal interphalangeal joint.

In deciding the most appropriate treatment for swan neck deformity, the function of the entire hand must be evaluated. As mentioned earlier, should the deformity be secondary to metacarpophalangeal joint pathology in the rheumatoid hand, this pathology at the more proximal level must be corrected first. If the swan neck deformity is secondary to a malunion of a fracture of the middle phalanx in hyperextension, correction of this bony malalignment is the best treatment for the deformity.

Should it be secondary to spasticity, the tenodesis using the flexor digitorum superficialis is recommended. In patients with fixed swan neck deformities or with marked limitation of active or passive proximal interphalangeal joint flexion, it will be necessary to combine the extensor mechanism reconstruction with either arthrodesis or arthroplasty of the proximal interphalangeal joint.

If the swan neck deformity is a matter of extensor tendon mechanism imbalance with coexistent incompetence of the volar plate at the proximal interphalangeal joint without joint contractures, there are two commonly used methods of reconstruction: (1) the superficialis tenodesis at the proximal interphalangeal joint, and (2) oblique retinacular ligament reconstruction. Each of these procedures is described.

DETAILS OF PROCEDURE. The oblique retinacular ligament reconstruction as originally described by Littler must be done in the digit without fixed deformities. The exposure is through a long hockey-stick type of incision (**A**). The lateral band is left attached distally and divided at its musculotendinous junction (**B** and **C**). It is then rerouted volar to Cleland's ligaments and either passed through a window in the proximal flexor tendon sheath and sutured back to itself, or passed transversely through a hole in the substance of the proximal phalanx (**D**). The tension on this should be adjusted so that the proximal interphalangeal joint rests in approximately 20° of flexion with the distal joint at neutral.

An alternative technique that has been described more recently by Littler and Eaton involves the use of a free palmaris longus tendon graft that is passed from volar to dorsal

(Plate 6-10) REPAIR OF SWAN NECK DEFORMITY

through the substance of the base of the distal phalanx and is then spiraled around the digit in a subcutaneous plane deep to the neurovascular bundles and passed through a transverse drill hole placed in the base of the proximal phalanx. The tension on this tenodesis is adjusted by sliding the graft through its distal insertion until the proximal interphalangeal joint rests in approximately 20° of flexion.

The tenodesis using a slip of the flexor digitorum superficialis as described by Swanson, is a stout tenodesis at the proximal interphalangeal joint, but does not rebalance the extensor mechanism at the distal joint and may not be as effective in correcting the distal joint extensor lag. The exposure is made through an anterior incision of the Bruner type **(F)**, usually requiring only the limbs of the incision over the proximal and middle phalanges, but may occasionally need to be extended proximally and distally to get adequate exposure.

The sheath is resected directly anterior to the proximal interphalangeal joint, with care taken not to violate pulleys at the midportion of the middle phalanx or the base of the proximal phalanx **(G)**. One slip of the flexor digitorum superficialis is transected at a point distal to the proximal phalangeal pulley **(G** and **H)**. This slip is then passed through a drill hole from a volar to dorsal direction through the neck of the proximal phalanx and sutured to a button over the dorsum **(I** and **J)**. The joint is then stabilized in a position of 20° of flexion with a percutaneous Kirschner pin **(K)**.

POSTOPERATIVE MANAGEMENT. The protective dressing is removed 4 weeks after surgery and the remainder of the hand mobilized while the involved digits are protected with a splint for an additional 2 weeks. At approximately 6 weeks the percutaneous Kirschner pin is removed. A removable splint is applied, and the patient is carefully started on a flexion and extension exercise program with the splint used as a "backstop" to block active extension at a position of 20° flexion. This protective splint is gradually straightened to the neutral position over the following month. Carefully supervised exercises may be necessary for several months.

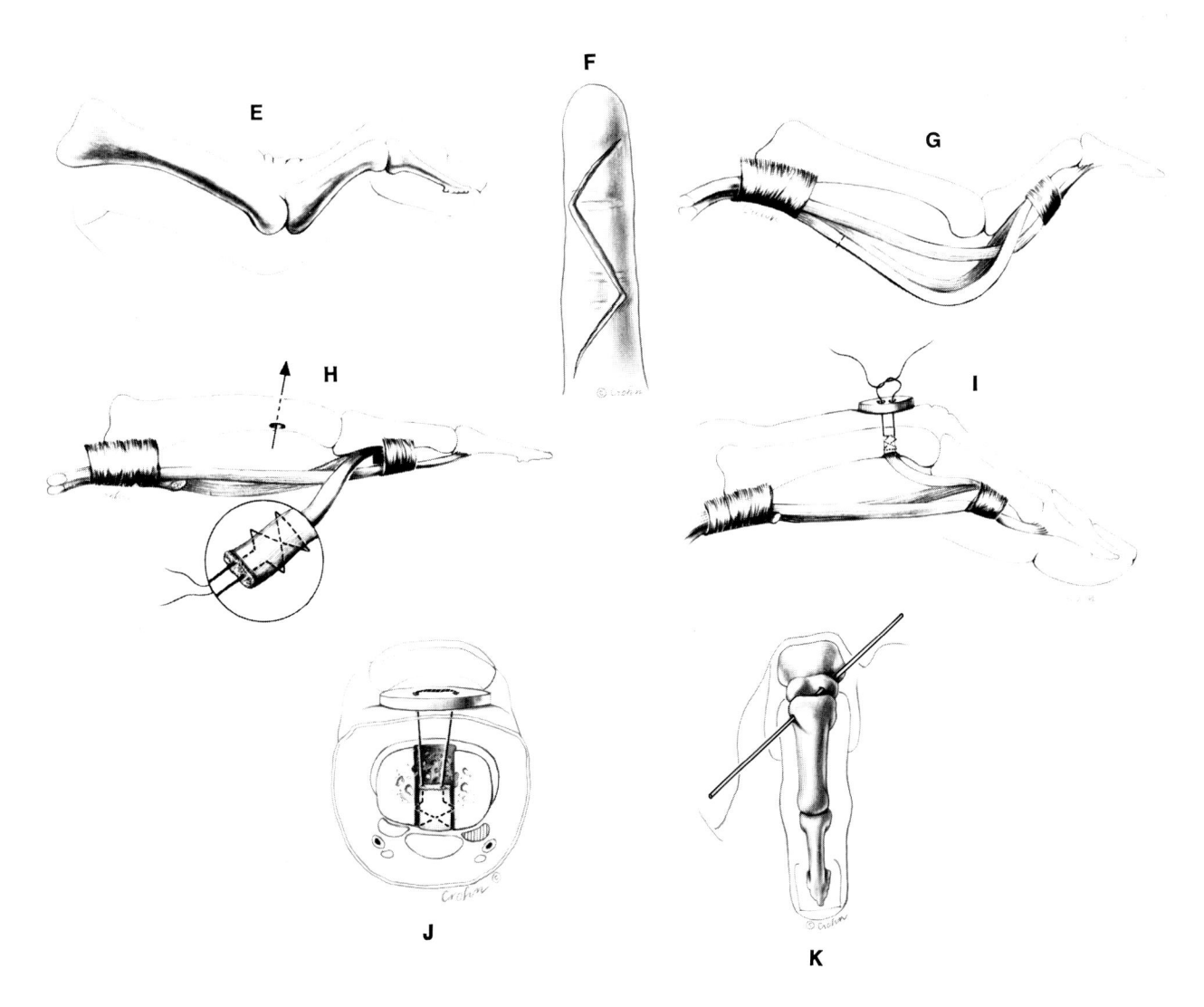

REPAIR OF BOUTONNIERE DEFORMITY OF FINGER (Plate 6-11)

GENERAL DISCUSSION. Boutonniere deformity, a common deformity of the digit, which may be secondary to trauma with avulsion of the central tendon or from various types of arthritis, involves the positioning of the finger as is seen in **A**. The proximal interphalangeal joint is flexed, and the distal joint hyperextended. This may be a fixed deformity, in which case there are fixed joint contractures in this posture, or may involve a dynamic imbalance of the extensor mechanism with good passive joint motion. In this situation there is positioning of the finger in this posture with attempted active extension, although passively the joints are supple.

The basic pathomechanics of this condition involve (1) an attenuation of the central tendon with (2) a prolapse of the lateral bands anterior to the axis of motion at the proximal interphalangeal joint so that the patient has no active extensors that can accomplish full active proximal interphalangeal joint extension (**B**).

Frequently the boutonniere deformity can be treated with a specific exercise and splinting program, with a result equal to or exceeding that possible from surgery. The exercises involve a two-step maneuver. The first is an active assisted proximal interphalangeal joint extension. The second is an active flexion of the distal joint while the proximal interphalangeal joint is held at 0° (or as close to that as it can be passively supported gently). The splinting involves a combination of active and static splints in the daytime and static splints at night. The splints involve only the proximal joint and proximal and middle phalanges, leaving the metacarpophalangeal joint and the distal joint free. The exercise and splinting program usually must be maintained for 2 to 3 months after acute injury and much longer in old injuries or arthritic processes.

The surgical procedures described for this condition are many but essentially involve a rebalancing of the extensor mechanism. It is absolutely essential that no tendon procedures be done to reestablish balance in the extensor mechanism until the joint contractures have completely resolved, either with a therapy program or with open joint release.

DETAILS OF PROCEDURE. The operative procedure basically involves a rebalancing of the extensor mechanism to decrease the tone at the distal joint and increase it at the proximal joint. These procedures are technically demanding and deceptively difficult, and should not be done by the surgeon who only occasionally operates on the hand. The most reliable procedure is that currently advocated by Littler and Eaton. This involves the division of the extensor mechanism over the junction of the mid and proximal thirds of the middle phalanx, allowing the central tendons and lateral bands to slide proximally. This increases the tone at the proximal interphalangeal joint and yet releases the excess extensor tone at the distal joint. The basic pathology of the initial lesion is shown in **B**, and the plane of release in **C**. The amount of proximal tendon slide involves only 1 to 3 mm and is indicated in **D**.

Following this procedure the patient is treated with a light dressing and started on an early exercise program. It is essential that the patient use a splint holding the proximal interphalangeal joint at 0° between the periods of exercise. The exercise and splinting program will be necessary for many months if recurrence is to be avoided.

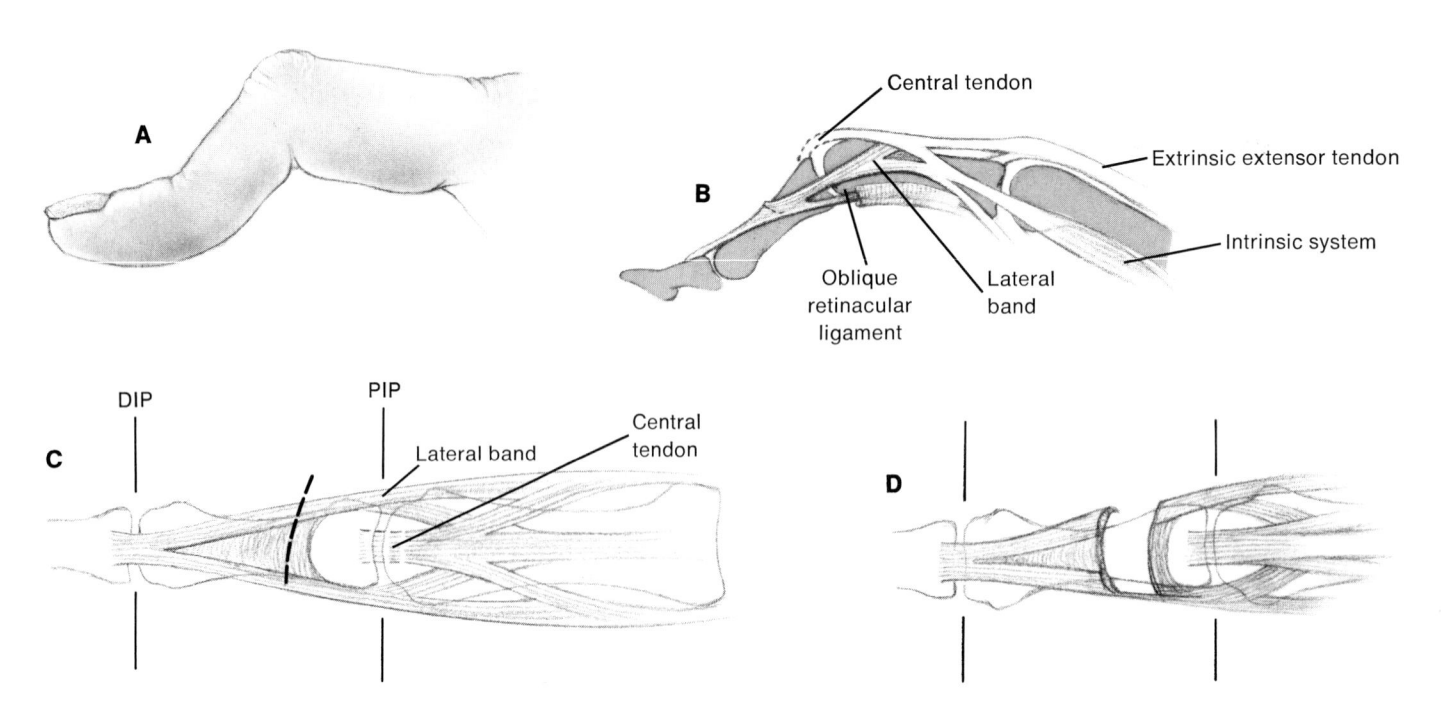

(Plate 6-12) REPAIR OF RUPTURED EXTENSOR TENDONS BY TENDON TRANSFER

GENERAL DISCUSSION. Rupture of the extrinsic extensor tendons frequently occurs in the rheumatoid hand. This rupture most commonly occurs over the dorsal aspect of the wrist. The most common tendons to rupture are the extensor digiti quinti and the extensor digitorum communis tendons to the ring and little fingers. The next most common tendon to rupture is the extensor pollicis longus at Lister's tubercle. It should be noted that the extensor tendons in the hand of the rheumatoid patient may rupture in a great variety of possible combinations.

Tendon transfers frequently are required to reestablish active digital extension. It is rare that repair by direct suture is either possible or advisable, for the tendons are usually softened from synovial infiltration, frayed, and attenuated from the attritional changes that occur from rubbing over the bony prominences of the wrist. Except in unusual circumstances it is not advisable to do only a tendon transfer to reestablish digital extension in the rheumatoid hand. It is usually necessary to do other procedures at the wrist level at the same time to try to prevent future tendon ruptures either of the transferred tendons or of previously intact motor units.

These simultaneous possible other procedures are varied and have specific indications. Tenosynovectomy with transposition of the extensor tendons into a subcutaneous plane is possible if there are no arthritic bony changes in the wrist joint itself and the ulnar head is not prominent. If the ulnar head has subluxed dorsally and is prominent (the so-called caput ulnae syndrome) it may be necessary to resect the head of the ulna and do some type of arthroplasty of this joint, frequently using a silicone rubber implant. If there are extensive changes within the wrist joint itself with the tendency for wrist subluxation anteriorly with secondary prominence of the distal radius dorsally, it may be necessary to combine these tendon transfers with either wrist fusion or total wrist replacement. The techniques and alternative techniques of total wrist replacement are beyond the scope of this text. The techniques for wrist arthrodesis are described elsewhere (see Plate 5-8).

The choice of the best tendon for transfer depends on the combination of tendons ruptured and the condition of the tendons that remain. The extensor indicis proprius is the most favorable donor to be used for isolated ruptures of the extensor pollicis longus, or of the extensor digiti quinti and the extensor digitorum communis of the little finger. Should both the extensor tendons to the ring and little fingers be ruptured, the extensor indicis proprius can be transferred to both tendons distally, or transferred just to the tendons of the little finger, with the extensor tendon to the ring finger distally being repaired side to side to that of the long.

Occasionally, if all the finger extensor tendons are ruptured at the wrist level, it may be necessary to transfer two of the flexor digitorum superficialis tendons around the radial subcutaneous border of the forearm and repair them to the distal ruptured tendons, one to the index extensors, and one to the extensors of the other three fingers. As another alternative, should the patient have the need for simultaneous wrist fusion, those wrist extensor tendons which remain in good condition can be transferred to the digital extensors. Note that finger flexor tendons used as transfers to reestablish digital extension are out of phase and are more difficult for the patient to master. The disadvantage of transferring wrist extensor tendons when combined with wrist fusion is their relatively limited excursion compared to those of the normal extrinsic digital extensor musculotendinous units.

REPAIR OF RUPTURED EXTENSOR TENDONS BY TENDON TRANSFER (Plate 6-12)

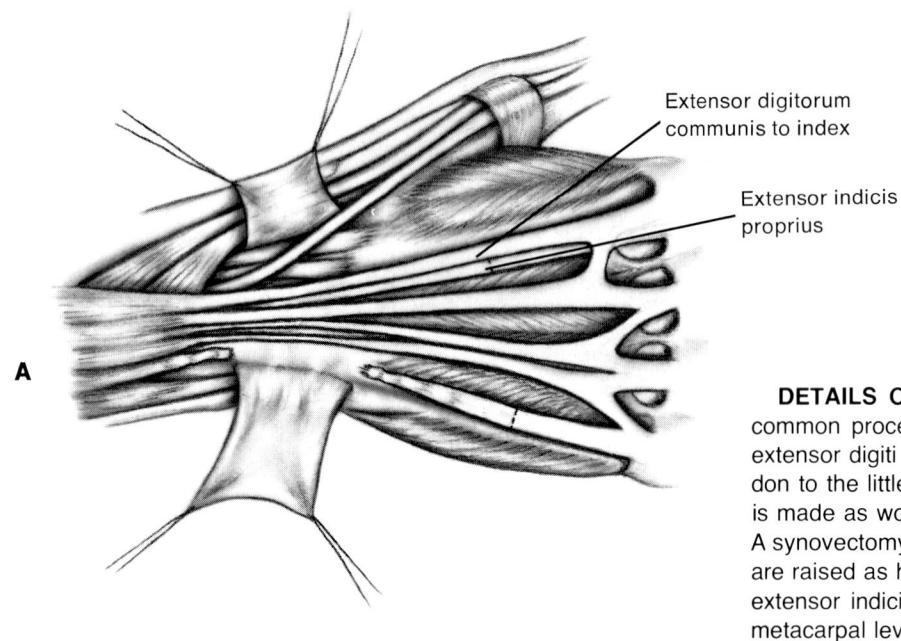

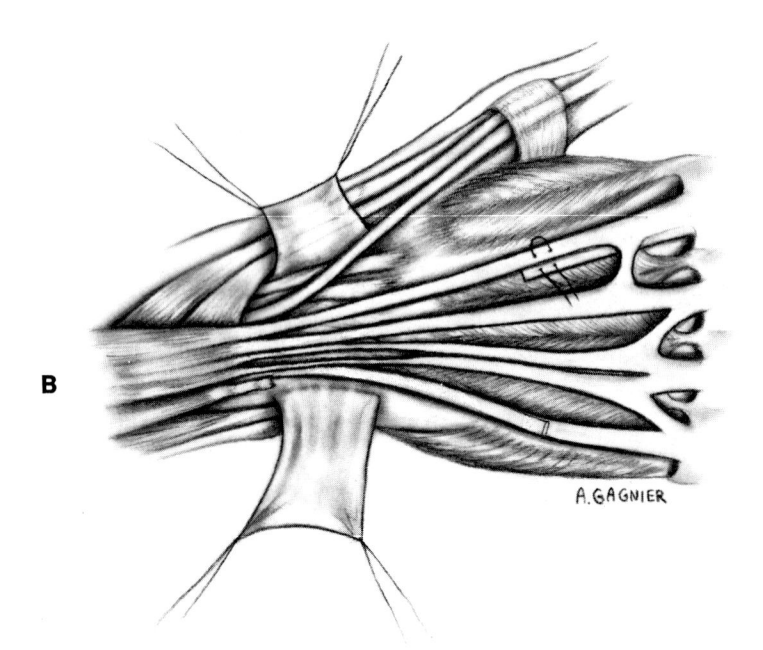

Extensor digitorum communis to index

Extensor indicis proprius

DETAILS OF PROCEDURE. As an example, the most common procedure is illustrated—that is, a rupture of the extensor digiti quinti and extensor digitorum communis tendon to the little finger. A dorsal midline longitudinal incision is made as would be made for a wrist fusion (Plate 5-8, *A*). A synovectomy is performed, and the dorsal retinacular flaps are raised as has been illustrated (Plate 5-8, *B* and *C*). The extensor indicis proprius tendon is transected at the distal metacarpal level, and the distal tendon sutured side to side to the extensor communis **(A)**. The extensor indicis proprius tendon is then translocated across the dorsum of the wrist and repaired to the distal little finger extensor tendon under normal tension **(B)**, relatively easy to judge if the level of its original transection is carefully noted. The technique of tendon repair can be either end to end or interweaving (see Plate 6-7). Most often the extensor tendons on the dorsum of the hand are somewhat flat in cross section, and the interweaving repair more secure than the end to end.

The extensor retinacular flaps are then transposed deep to all the extensor tendons as would be done at the time of wrist fusion, thus rerouting the extensor tendons into the subcutaneous plane (Plate 5-8, *I* and *J*).

POSTOPERATIVE MANAGEMENT. As in all dorsal wrist wounds in a rheumatoid patient, suction drainage is essential. A supportive hand dressing with overlying plaster splint or shell is applied that holds the wrist at a neutral or slightly extended position and the metacarpophalangeal joints of the fingers in extension. Obviously in the rheumatoid patient it is not advisable to leave these joints immobilized for a long period of time, and therefore at approximately 10 days following surgery, it is important to start a carefully regulated exercise program with a dynamic extension splinting to protect the tendon transfer and yet allow early digital mobility. Static splinting must be maintained between the exercise programs for a total of approximately 2 months following surgery.

(Plate 6-13) REPLACEMENT ARTHROPLASTY OF THE METACARPOPHALANGEAL JOINT

GENERAL DISCUSSION. The metacarpophalangeal joints are commonly involved in the rheumatoid hand. A rather complex derangement of the anatomy occurs secondary to abnormal musculotendinous pull, ligamentous laxity, and deforming forces in the patterns of hand use. As a result, the metacarpophalangeal joints dislocate anteriorly, the metacarpal heads become prominent, and tightness of the volar plate and ulnar collateral ligaments develop. Ulnar intrinsic tightness occurs. The dorsal joint capsule becomes attenuated. The extrinsic extensor tendons dislocate off the apex of the metacarpal head and become adherent in the valley between the appropriate metacarpal head and the next most ulnar metacarpal head.

The technique of implant arthroplasty most commonly used has been developed and perfected by Swanson. The implant functions as a spacer and is basically a refinement of resectional arthroplasty. Good function of the rheumatoid hand following reconstruction at the metacarpophalangeal joint level is contingent on careful patient selection, meticulous surgical technique, accurate rebalancing of tendon forces, patient motivation and cooperation, and a carefully structured and regulated postoperative program of exercises combined with static and dynamic splinting.

DETAILS OF PROCEDURE. All four fingers are usually involved **(A)**. As mentioned, the underlying anatomy is distorted. A transverse incision is made across the dorsum of the hand at the level of the metacarpal necks **(B)**. The subcutaneous skin is often very thin, and care must be taken not to damage the underlying extrinsic extensor tendons. The dorsal veins and nerves must be carefully maintained and protected, and usually can be dissected free to rest between the metacarpal heads.

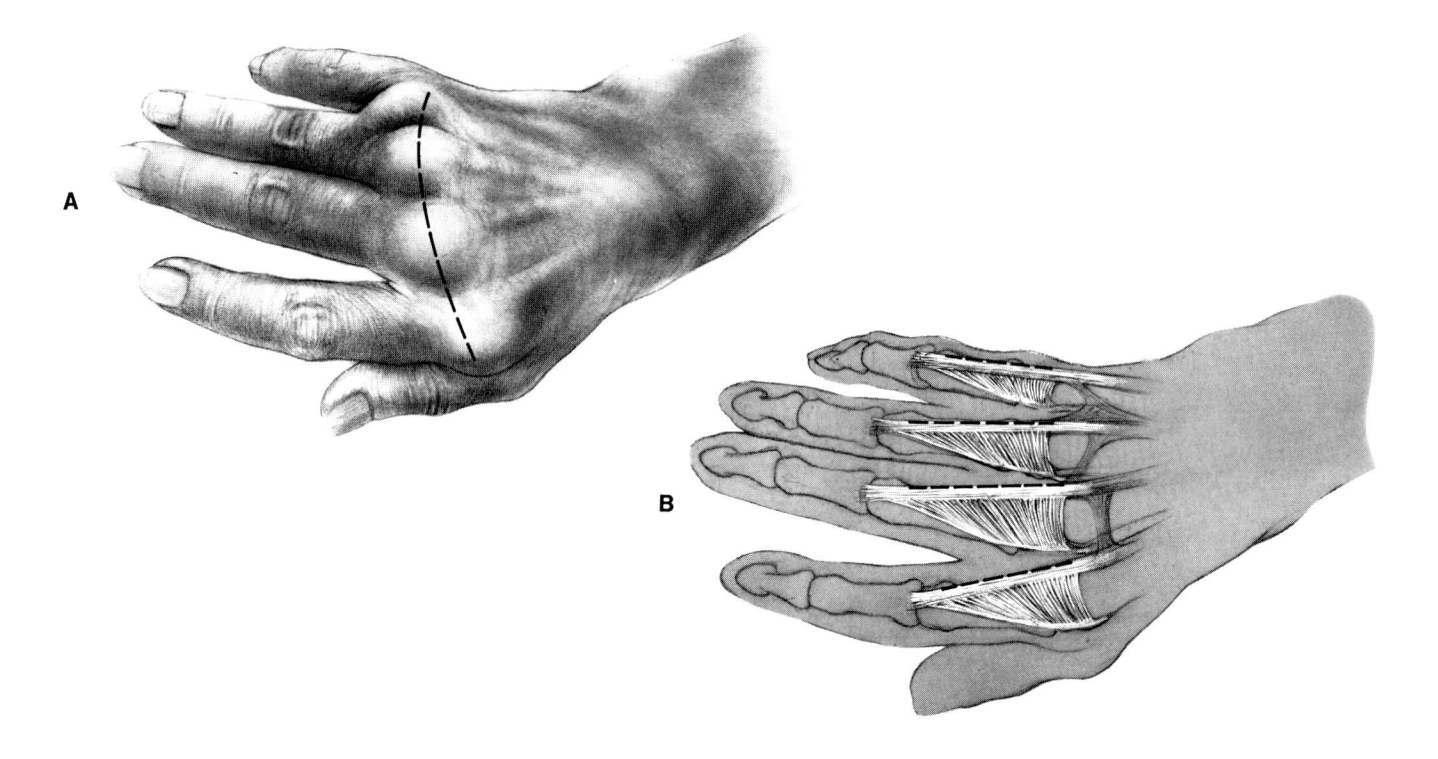

REPLACEMENT ARTHROPLASTY OF THE METACARPOPHALANGEAL JOINT (Plate 6-13)

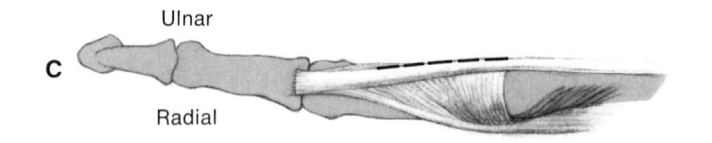

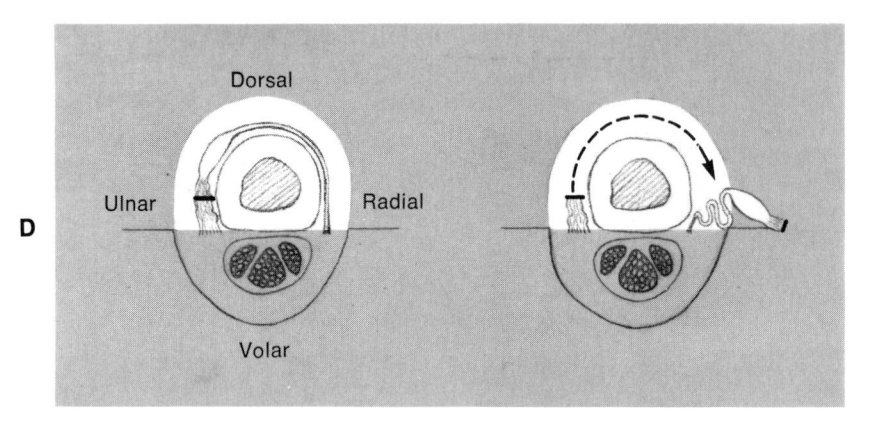

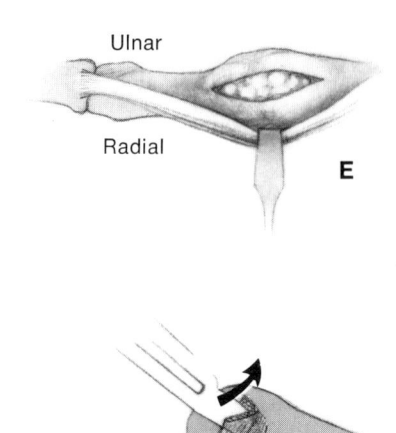

The sagittal bands, which are foreshortened on the ulnar border of the extrinsic extensor tendon, are incised from that extrinsic extensor tendon (**B** and **C**). As is demonstrated in **D**, the extrinsic extensor tendon that has then been released from its tether on the ulnar border, can be dissected free from the capsule and reduced to the radial side of the metacarpal head in a plane external to the capsule. The radial shroud fibers must be carefully protected (**D**).

A longitudinal incision is made in the dorsal capsule of the joint (**E**). A synovectomy of the joint is performed.

The collateral ligaments are released from their proximal attachments (**F**). If possible, the radial collateral ligament on the index metacarpophalangeal joint should be retained for stability in pinch. This may not be possible if the ligament is excessively foreshortened because of the preexistent contracture.

Osteotomes can be used to remove the metacarpal head (**G** and **H**). If there is gross deformity at the base of the proximal phalanx, it also needs to be partially removed either with an osteotome or rongeurs to create a flush surface into which the implant may be subsequently inserted.

At this point the synovectomy of the joint can then be completed. It may be necessary to release the volar plate from the volar base of the proximal phalanx to reduce the anterior dislocation.

The ulnar intrinsic tendon is released either at its musculotendinous junction or at the level of the wing tendon, depending on the amount of preoperative deformity.

Powered drills are used to ream the canal of the metacarpal and the proximal phalanx (**I** and **J**). Various implant sizers are then tested and the appropriate one selected. The wounds should be copiously irrigated, first with a sterile Ringer solution and then with an antibiotic solution.

The implant is then inserted with a no-touch technique using instruments (**K**). The prosthesis will pick up lint from gloves and drapes, and therefore this contact must be avoided.

After the implant has been inserted (**K** and **L**), the reconstruction continues as follows. The dorsal capsule is reapproximated, bringing the distal capsule radially to the ulnar capsule proximally, thus tending to supinate the finger and correct the preoperative pronation deformity that usually existed (**M**).

To rebalance the extrinsic extensor tendon over the dorsum of the implant, the radial shroud fibers are imbricated (**N** and **O**).

An identical procedure is carried out on each involved metacarpophalangeal joint.

Suction drainage is used. The skin is accurately closed with vertical mattress sutures of a 5-0 nonreactive suture (nylon).

An absorptive overlying hand dressing is then applied with an external plaster splint and shell to maintain the metacarpophalangeal joints in 0° of extension, in slight radial alignment, and with slight supination rotation toward the thumb.

POSTOPERATIVE MANAGEMENT. The suction drainage is removed at 24 to 48 hours. The supportive hand dressing is left in place for approximately 4 to 7 days. It is essential the hand remain elevated during this time.

Thereafter a smaller supportive soft hand dressing is applied to the area of the wound, and the patient is fitted with static splints and subsequently dynamic splints. A carefully regulated and graduated exercise program is then commenced and followed for approximately 6 months.

(Plate 6-13) REPLACEMENT ARTHROPLASTY OF THE METACARPOPHALANGEAL JOINT

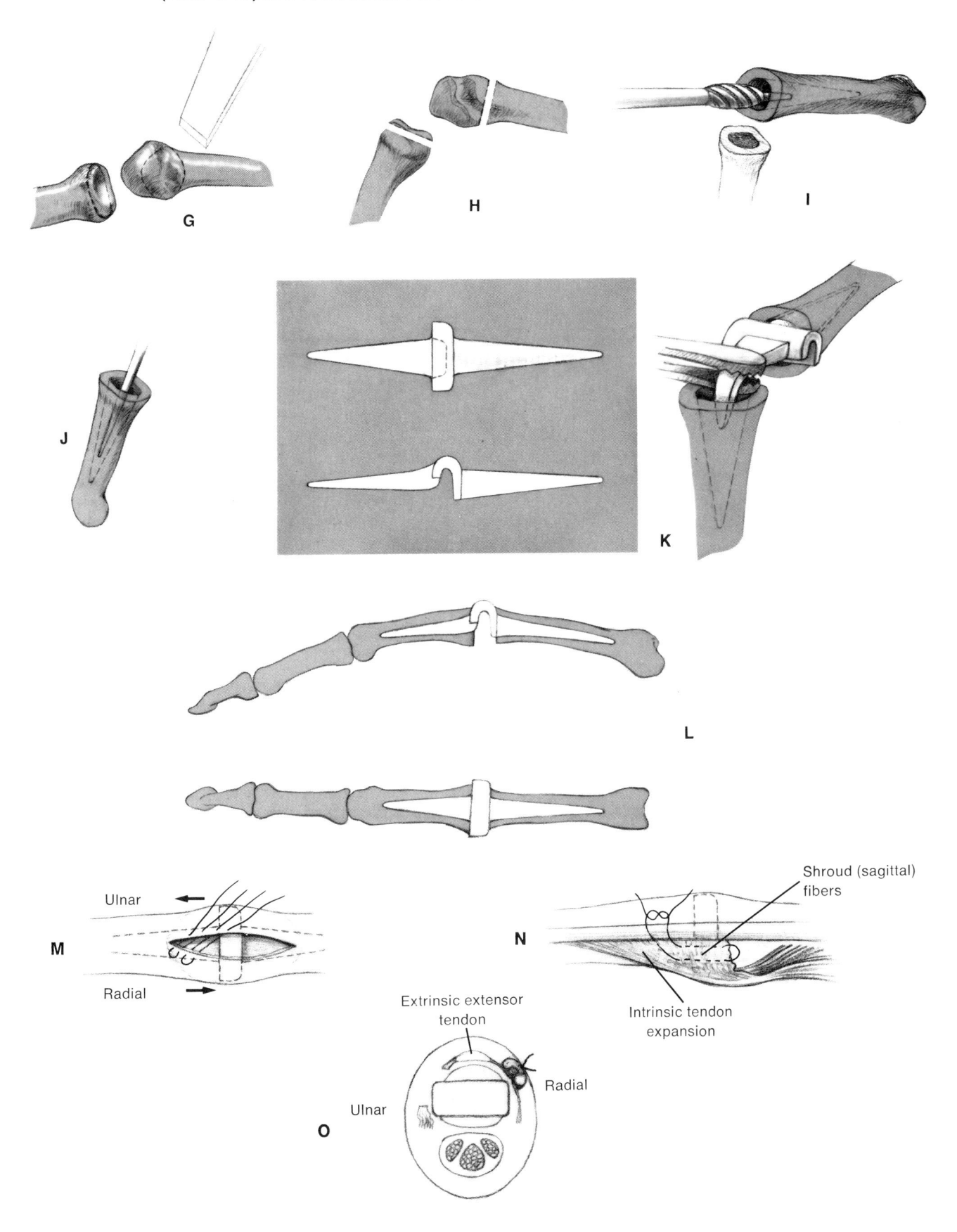

G

H

I

J

K

L

M
Ulnar
Radial

N
Shroud (sagittal) fibers
Intrinsic tendon expansion

O
Extrinsic extensor tendon
Radial
Ulnar

163

RELEASE OF THUMB ADDUCTION CONTRACTURE (Plate 6-14)

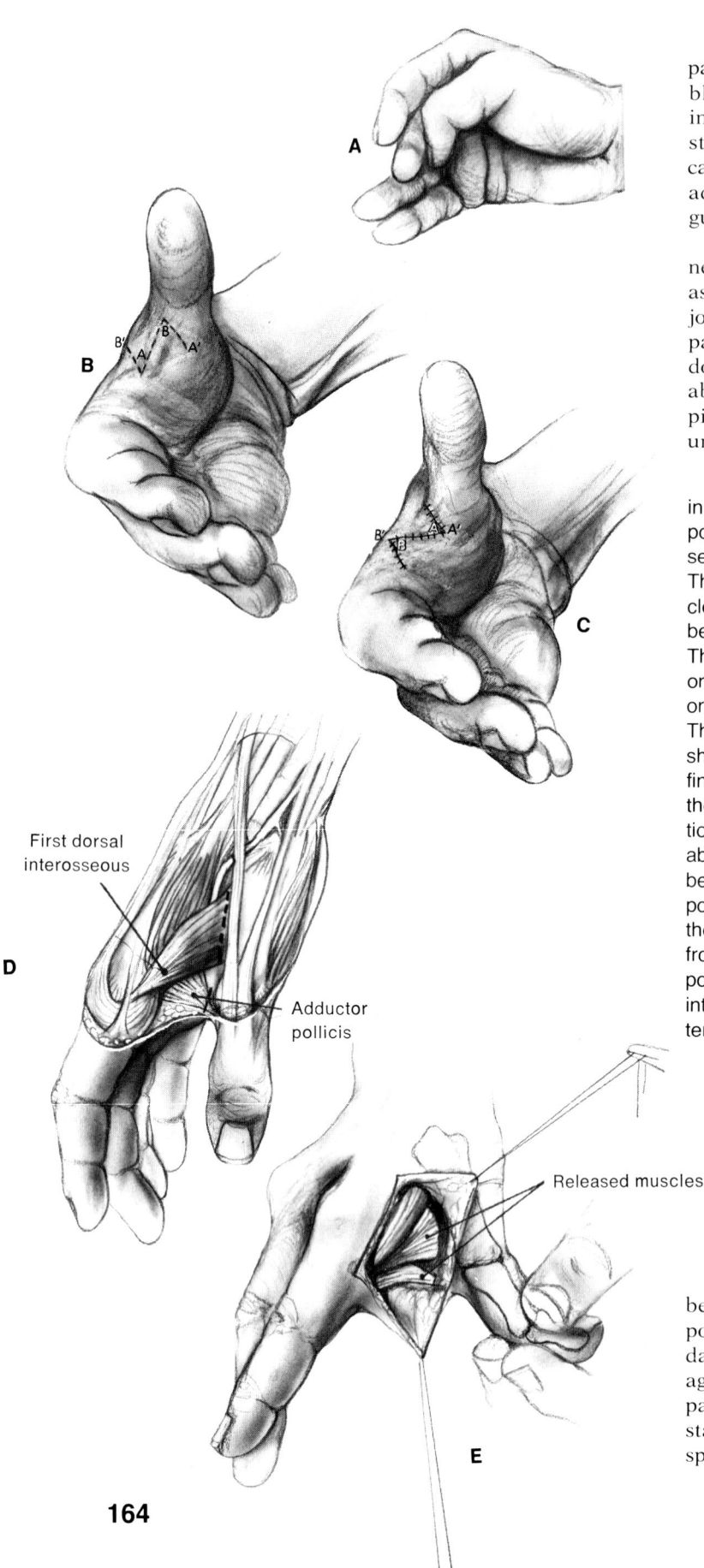

GENERAL DISCUSSION. In the patient with cerebral palsy, the thumb-in-palm deformity (**A**) may be a troublesome handicap that interferes with grasp. This thumb-in-palm deformity in the spastic hand can be relieved by stripping the first dorsal interosseous from the first metacarpal. It may be necessary to release the tendon of the adductor pollicis. Lengthening of the flexor pollicis longus may also occasionally be necessary.

Good abductor power of the thumb metacarpal is necessary for opposition, pinch, and grasp. If there is associated abduction weakness at the carpometacarpal joint of the thumb following release of the thumb-in-palm deformity, transfer of the flexor carpi radialis tendon or the brachioradialis tendon to the tendon of the abductor pollicis longus can aid in regaining function of pinch. If the metacarpophalangeal joint of the thumb is unstable, the joint should be fused.

DETAILS OF PROCEDURE. A Z-plasty incision is made in the first web space (**B** and **C**). The insertion of the adductor pollicis is identified and divided at its attachment to the ulnar sesamoid at the metacarpophalangeal joint of the thumb. The two heads of origin of the first dorsal interosseous muscle are identified, and the radial artery that passes proximally between the two heads of origin of this muscle is protected. The portion of the first dorsal interosseus muscle that takes origin from the thumb metacarpal is released, leaving the origin from the second metacarpal bone intact (**D** and **E**). The remaining portion of the first dorsal interosseus muscle should continue to assist flexion and abduction of the index finger. The wound is closed by reversing the skin flaps of the Z-plasty. The hand is splinted with the thumb in abduction. If the thumb requires transfers to strengthen metacarpal abduction, the flexor carpal radialis or brachioradialis may be used. If the latter tendon is used, it is necessary to expose the musculotendinous unit to the midproximal third of the forearm to free the brachial radialis tendon and muscle from its surrounding fascial attachments and gain maximum possible tendon excursion. The repair of the transfer tendon into the abductor pollicis longus is best done using the interweaving technique (Plate 6-7).

POSTOPERATIVE MANAGEMENT. If no transfers have been done, the dressing and splint are removed 2 weeks postoperatively. Active motion combined with gentle daily active assisted abduction of the thumb is encouraged subsequently. If transfers were necessary (spastic patient), splinting is continuous and exercises are not started for 6 weeks. The spastic patient may need night splints for 1 year.

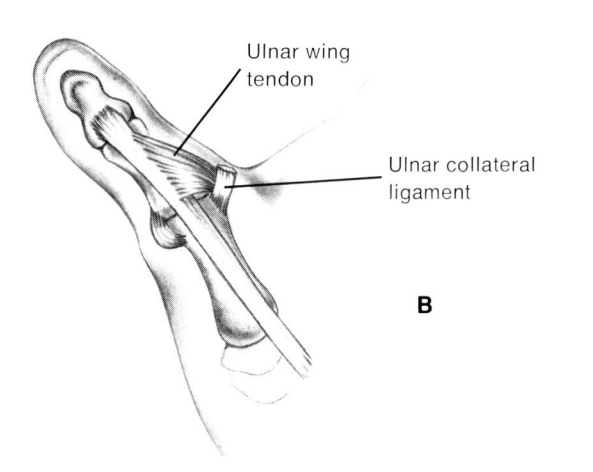

(Plate 6-15) REPAIR OF COLLATERAL LIGAMENT OF METACARPOPHALANGEAL JOINT OF THUMB

GENERAL DISCUSSION. Sprain or incomplete rupture of the ulnar collateral ligament of the metacarpophalangeal joint of the thumb is a frequent injury and requires 3 weeks of splinting for protection. Complete rupture of the ulnar collateral ligament of the thumb can be a disabling injury leaving the patient with ineffective pinch. Complete rupture of the ulnar collateral ligament of the thumb can be determined clinically if the stability of the injured thumb is compared with that of the opposite thumb.

A stress test is best done with the metacarpophalangeal joint at both 0° and 30° of flexion. If there is more than 15° to 20° of difference between the injured and the normal thumb, the ligament should be explored. The normal anatomy is such that the intact ligament is covered by the ulnar wing tendon of the intrinsic mechanism of the thumb (**A**). With complete tear of the ligament, in a high percentage of cases (as has been pointed out by Stener) the proximal end of the torn ligament comes to lie superficial to the wing tendon (**B**). Thus no amount of immobilization will provide good ligament healing and joint stability unless the ligament is surgically reduced and repaired. The lateral x-ray picture may frequently show anterior subluxation of the proximal phalanx on the metacarpal. In this situation the dorsal capsule should be repaired as well.

Rupture of the ulnar collateral ligament may occur at any point in the ligament but will usually occur near its distal insertion into the base of the proximal phalanx of the thumb. If complete rupture of the ulnar collateral ligament of the thumb is recognized and repaired within 10 days, a direct reconstitution of the ligament may be accomplished. However, if the diagnosis is delayed for a longer period of time, fibrosis will probably make repair of the ligament almost impossible and a graft may be necessary to accomplish an effective repair.

DETAILS OF PROCEDURE. A conventional dorsal ulnar incision is made (see Plate 6-1). The ulnar wing tendon is incised from its margin of insertion into the extensor pollicis longus, exposing the pathologic condition (**C**). As mentioned, the dorsal capsule may or may not be torn, and if it is, it should be repaired. In the ligament, one of three lesions will be found. The first is that of a mid or distal substance tear (**C** and **D**). In this situation a direct repair of the ligament with a horizontal mattress suture (3-0, nonabsorbable) is usually adequate.

A second pathologic lesion that may be encountered is an avulsion of the ligament from its bony insertion on the proximal phalanx (**E**).

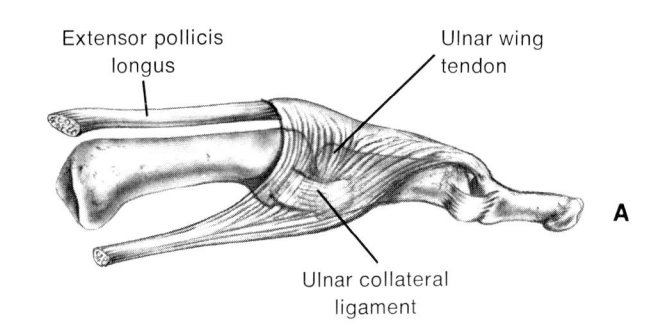

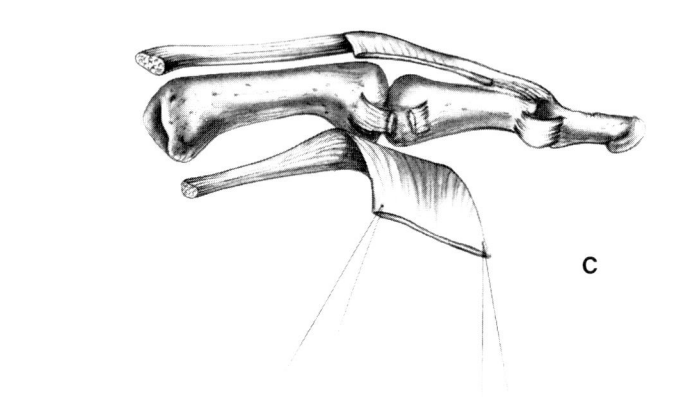

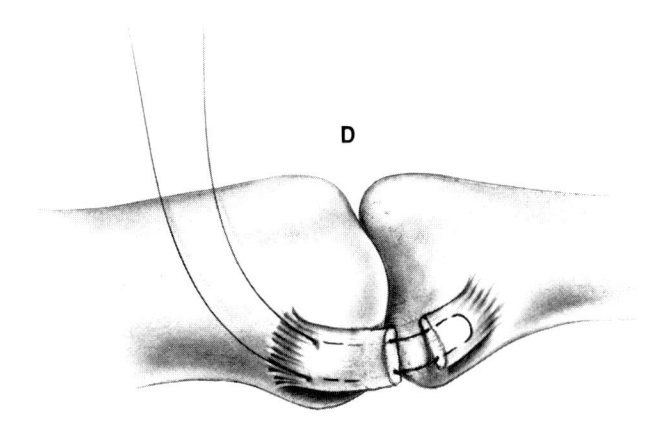

REPAIR OF COLLATERAL LIGAMENT OF METACARPOPHALANGEAL JOINT OF THUMB (Plate 6-15)

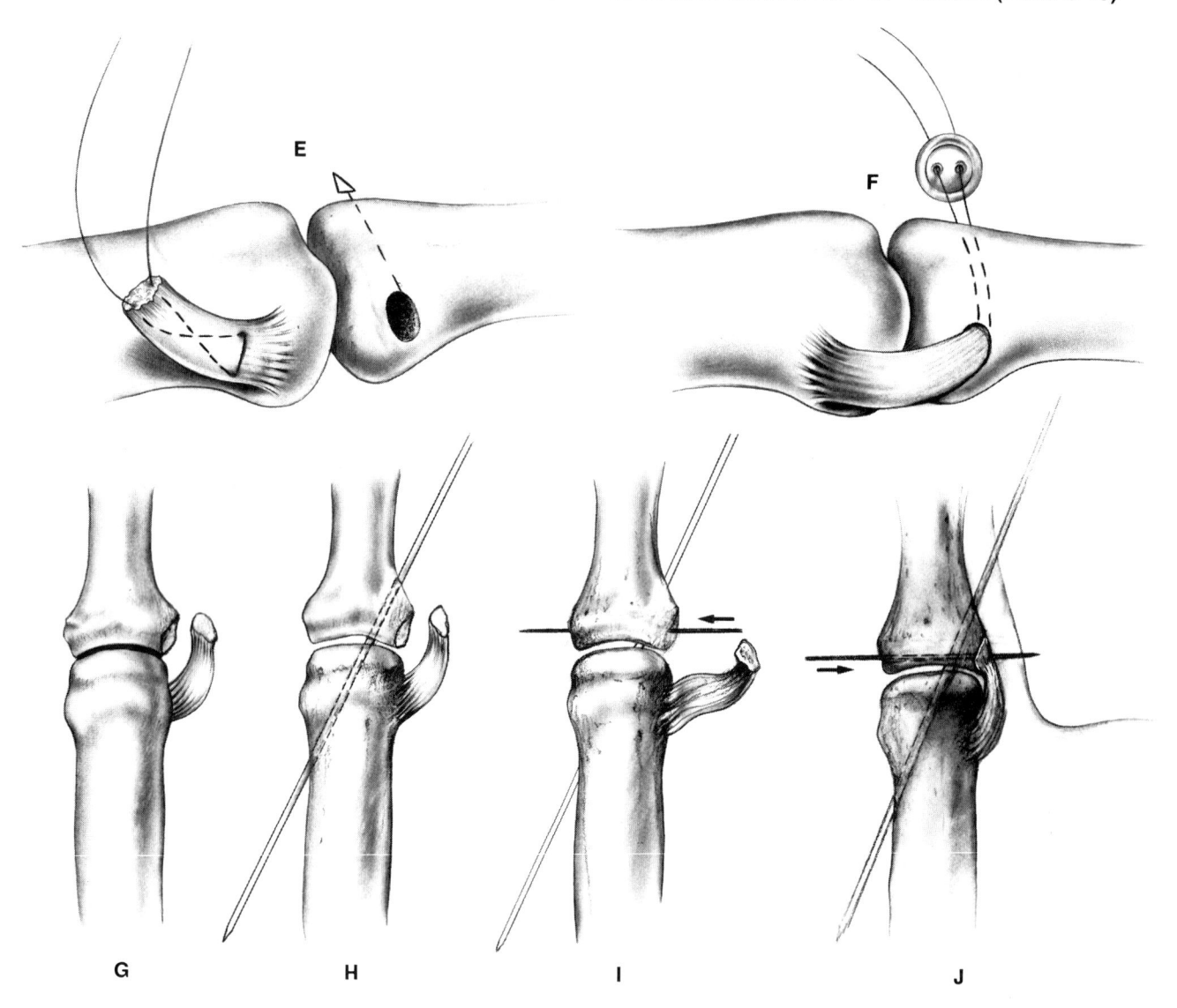

In this situation a modified pull-out suture may be inserted (3-0, nonabsorbable), a drill hole placed transversely through the base of the proximal phalanx, and the avulsed ligament drawn into the drill hole by the pull-out wire attached to a button on the opposite side of the thumb (**E** and **F**).

The third pathologic lesion is that of an avulsion fracture from the base of the proximal phalanx. If the fracture is a small fleck, it is treated as in **E** and **F**. Should the fracture fragment be large (**G**), it requires reduction and internal fixation to provide stability and restore the joint surface. The joint is first stabilized in neutral alignment with an oblique Kirschner pin placed with a power drill (**H**).

A 0.028 Kirschner pin, double ended, is then driven transversely across the base of the proximal phalanx parallel to the articular surface through the center of the bony defect created by the fracture (**I**). The fracture fragment is anatomically reduced, and the transverse pin then driven in a retrograde fashion to secure the fragment and maintain the reduction (**J**).

During the course of the procedure it is important to avoid injury to cutaneous branches of the radial nerve, which may be somewhat concealed by the hematoma in the subcutaneous tissues.

After repair of the collateral ligament, the adductor aponeurosis is carefully resutured. Following wound closure, a short-arm cast is applied extending to the tip of the thumb and to the distal palmar crease. As the cast is made, care should be taken to avoid molding it in any way that might produce ulnar deviation of the first metacarpal and indirectly produce abduction at the metacarpophalangeal joint of the thumb.

POSTOPERATIVE MANAGEMENT. The protective cast and pins are removed 6 weeks postoperatively. Active motion is started at that time, but activities are adjusted to minimize the likelihood of any forceful abduction stress at the metacarpophalangeal joint for at least an additional 6 weeks.

(Plate 6-16) VOLAR PLATE ADVANCEMENT FOR DORSAL FRACTURE-DISLOCATIONS OF THE PROXIMAL INTERPHALANGEAL JOINT

GENERAL DISCUSSION. A dorsal type dislocation of the proximal interphalangeal joint with no avulsion fracture from the volar base of the middle phalanx shown on a lateral x-ray picture is commonly stable once reduced. Reduction, splinting in 30° flexion for 3 weeks, and then a careful exercise program will usually result in a stable joint with good mobility.

However, the dorsal fracture-dislocation in which the fracture constitutes more than one fourth to one third of the articular surface from the volar base of the middle phalanx is an unstable lesion **(A)**. The collateral ligaments remain attached to the volar fracture fragment, and thus there are no ligament attachments left to maintain stability between the proximal and middle phalanges. This is best treated by surgical correction utilizing the volar plate advancement described by Eaton.

DETAILS OF PROCEDURE. The exposure is best done through an anterior incision, much like that used for the superficialis tenodesis in swan neck deformity (see Plate 16-10, F).

The flexor sheath is excised between the pulley at the midportion of the middle phalanx and the midshaft of the proximal phalanx. The flexor tendons are carefully retracted, exposing the volar plate and the avulsed fragment **(B)**.

The fracture fragment is excised **(C)**. If the lesion is a recent one (within 1 week), it will not be necessary to resect the collateral ligaments. Should the fracture-dislocation be older than 3 weeks, it is usually necessary to resect the majority of the collateral ligaments.

In either the fresh or old fracture-dislocation, two parallel drill holes are then placed in the margins of the defect created by the fracture **(D)**. Pull-out sutures are then carefully placed in the corners of the volar plate, drawn through the two drill holes, and passed through the holes of a button on the dorsum of the finger. The joint is then accurately reduced, and an oblique Kirschner pin is passed through the joint to maintain the proximal and middle phalanges in an accurately reduced position. The volar plate is then drawn into the defect, and the suture is tied over the button on the dorsum of the middle phalanx **(E** and **F)**.

POSTOPERATIVE MANAGEMENT. The oblique Kirschner pin and pull-out sutures are removed at 4 to 5 weeks. A dorsal splint that prevents extension of the joint past a position of 20° flexion is used for an additional 2 weeks. The patient is started on a flexion and extension exercise program with this extension stop splint as soon as the Kirschner pin has been removed. This dorsal splint can be discontinued at 6 to 7 weeks following surgery. It will be necessary to continue the exercise program for several months thereafter.

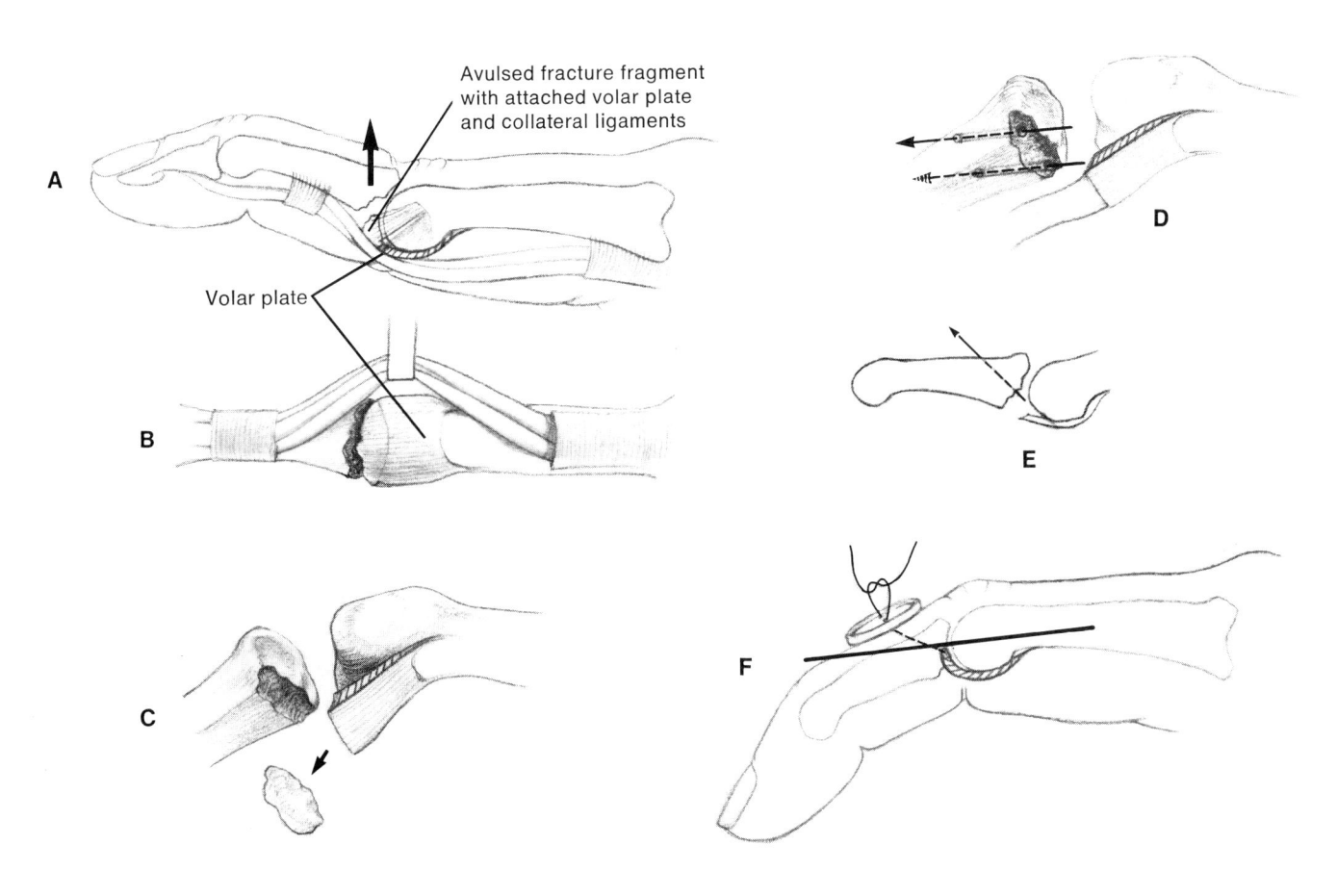

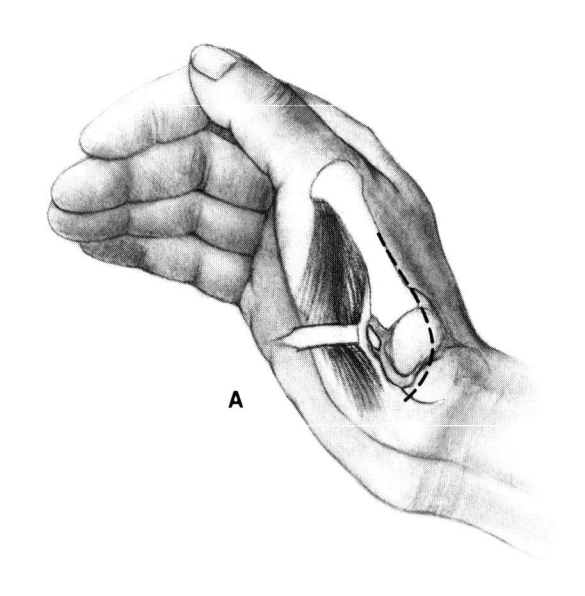

OPEN REDUCTION AND INTERNAL FIXATION FOR FRACTURE OF BASE OF THUMB METACARPAL (BENNETT'S FRACTURE) (Plate 6-17)

GENERAL DISCUSSION. Intra-articular fracture through the base of the thumb metacarpal, described by Bennet (an Irish surgeon) in 1881, is characteristically associated with lateral displacement of the shaft of the thumb metacarpal produced by the pull of the abductor pollicis longus while the proximal fragment remains in place or slightly rotated **(A)**. In the acute injury, reduction is easily accomplished, but maintenance of the reduction is difficult.

This reduction must be accurate because (1) this is an intra-articular fracture and joint congruity must be restored and (2) accurate reduction is necessary for joint stability. This accurate reduction can be maintained with either percutaneous fixation or open reduction and internal fixation.

DETAILS OF PROCEDURE. The carpometacarpal joint of the thumb is a particularly mobile joint that necessitates accurate restoration of the articular surface to provide optimum function of the thumb and hand in future years. Closed reduction, including percutaneous pinning with a Kirschner pin, may be done. This pin passes from the thumb metacarpal shaft into the carpus and does not attempt to transfix the small fracture fragment. To do so might well distract and displace the small fragment. This small fragment is usually held in good position by the ligaments to which it is attached, and the purpose of reduction is to realign the main portion of the metacarpal with the trapezium. Usually two percutaneous Kirschner pins are more secure. If anatomic reduction is not accomplished, open reduction is advisable unless there is some contraindication.

The incision is made along the radial aspect of the thumb metacarpal, curving medially at the wrist crease **(A)**. The soft tissues, including the abductor pollicis brevis muscle and a portion of the opponens pollicis muscle, are reflected from the proximal end of the metacarpal to expose the fracture **(B)**. The carpometacarpal joint is opened. With distal traction on the thumb, the articular surface of the larger fragment should be aligned with the smaller fragment.

(Plate 6-17) OPEN REDUCTION AND INTERNAL FIXATION FOR FRACTURE OF BASE OF THUMB METACARPAL (BENNETT'S FRACTURE)

The technique of Gedda and Moberg is often helpful. Under direct vision a 0.028 Kirschner pin is driven with a power drill through the small fracture fragment and out through the ulnar border of the thenar eminence **(B)**. A small loop of No. 30 wire is passed around this Kirschner pin just to the ulnar border of this fracture fragment. Using the Kirschner pin and this wire loop **(C)**, and with appropriate manipulation of the main thumb metacarpal fragment, it is usually possible to manipulate these two pieces into an anatomic reduction. The pin is driven with the power drill into the main metacarpal fragment **(D)**. The wire loop is easily withdrawn.

Usually one or two additional 0.045 Kirschner pins are then driven with a power drill from the main metacarpal fragment into the trapezium to maintain alignment of the metacarpal shaft to the trapezium. The purpose of the first small Kirschner pin is merely to stabilize and align the small fragment relative to the main metacarpal shaft with accurate restoration of the joint surface. The constant deforming pull of the abductor pollicis longus is countered by the two larger Kirschner pins.

POSTOPERATIVE MANAGEMENT. The patient's thumb is placed in a thumb spica type cast holding the wrist in 20° of extension and the thumb in the abducted position, and extending to the proximal forearm. The cast is changed at 3 weeks, and the sutures are removed. A similar cast is reapplied and continued until x-ray pictures demonstrate healing of the fracture, at which time the Kirschner pins are removed, a splint is applied, and a gradually increasing exercise program is instituted.

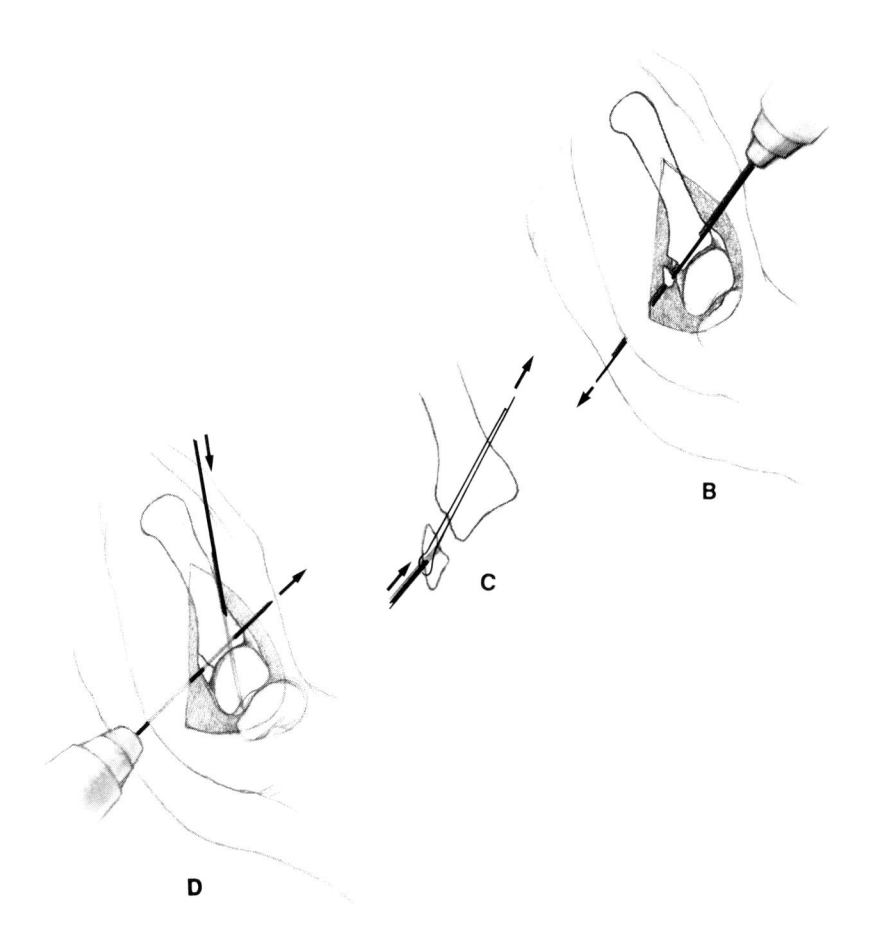

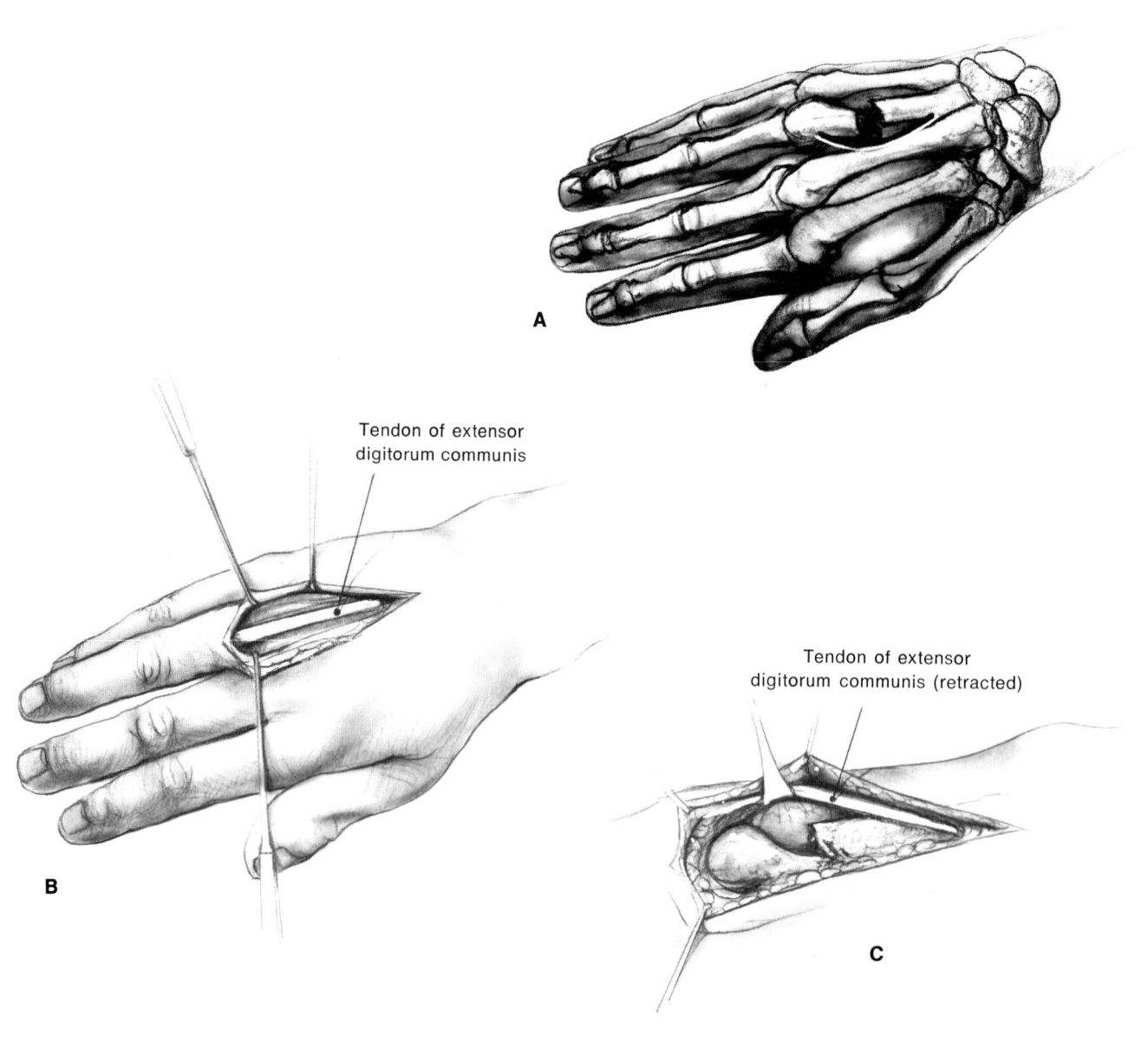

OPEN REDUCTION AND INTERNAL FIXATION FOR FRACTURE OF METACARPAL SHAFT (Plate 6-18)

GENERAL DISCUSSION. Open reduction and internal fixation for fracture of the shaft of a metacarpal may be indicated when displacement of the fracture is so great that soft tissue interposition appears likely, or if the fracture cannot be held in a satisfactory position once reduced.

It is frequently possible to reduce metacarpal fractures by closed means, but the reduction cannot be maintained with a simple splinting or cast technique. Percutaneous internal fixation is helpful in these conditions. Once the fracture has been reduced, in an operating room environment a longitudinal Kirschner pin can be placed with a power drill down the shaft of the metacarpal. A small stab wound is placed just to one side or the other of the extensor tendon at the metacarpophalangeal joint level, and the pin is placed with a power drill down the shaft of the distal fragment, across the fracture site, and into the proximal fragment. If such internal fixation is used percutaneously, it is absolutely essential that it be recognized that this is merely an adjunct to the external immobilization with a plaster cast, which should extend from the proximal forearm to the proximal interphalangeal joint level of the involved digit and its next most ulnar digit. It is particularly important that metacarpal fractures be accurately aligned in rotation, and this must be carefully checked. Note that in long spiral oblique fractures of the metacarpal, any shortening is usually accompanied by some malrotation.

(Plate 6-18) OPEN REDUCTION AND INTERNAL FIXATION FOR FRACTURE OF METACARPAL SHAFT

DETAILS OF PROCEDURE. Should open reduction be necessary, the fracture is exposed through a gently curved dorsal incision (**A**). An incision is then made in the fascia overlying the interosseous muscle (**B**). Dissection is carried directly to the fracture site, and the rest of the surgery is done in a subperiosteal plane (**C**). This leaves some fascia and interosseous musculature between the extrinsic extensor tendon and the fracture site. Thus at the time of closure, soft tissue can be interposed, and the risk of extrinsic extensor tendon tightness thereby diminished.

A Kirschner wire is introduced into the proximal portion of the distal metacarpal fragment at the fracture site and drilled out through the skin at the metacarpal head (**D**). The fracture is reduced, and the Kirschner wire is drilled in retrograde fashion into the proximal fragment (**E**).

As with percutaneous internal fixation, it is absolutely essential to realize that this type of internal fixation is an adjunct to the external immobilization. A plaster cast or splint must be used to hold the wrist in 20° of extension and the involved fingers in the "safe position" with the metacarpophalangeal joints flexed 45° to 60° and the interphalangeal joints straight.

POSTOPERATIVE MANAGEMENT. The internal fixation is removed at 4 weeks. Usually external plaster support for an additional 2 weeks is advisable before starting the exercise program.

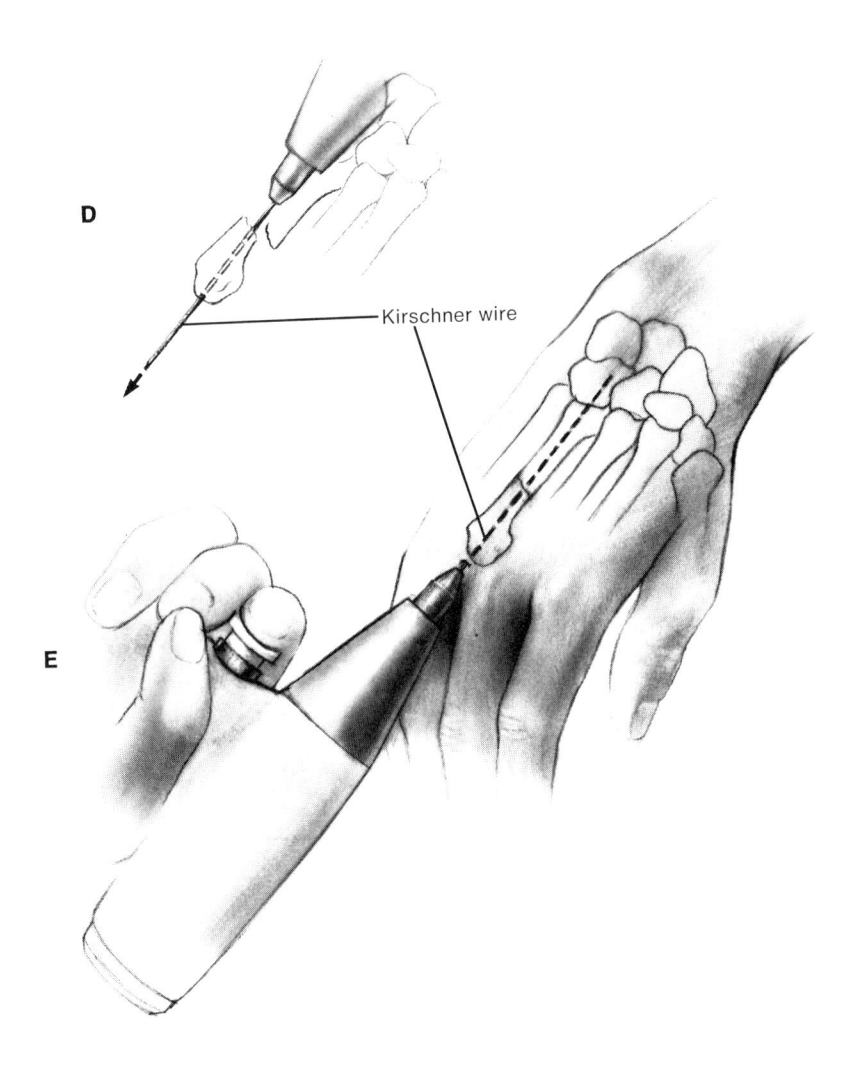

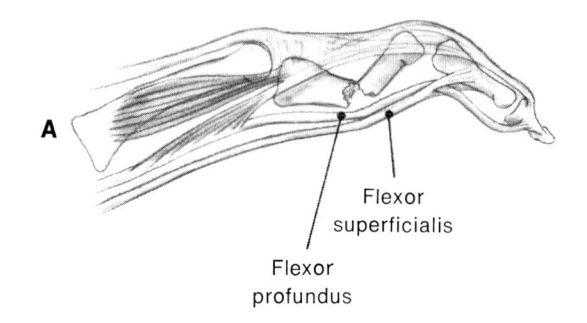

OPEN REDUCTION AND INTERNAL FIXATION FOR PHALANGEAL SHAFT FRACTURE (Plate 6-19)

GENERAL DISCUSSION. Most fractures of the proximal or middle phalanx are best treated by closed means, but open reduction and internal fixation are occasionally necessary to obtain the best end result.

As for the fractures of the metacarpal, frequently accurate closed reduction of fractures of the proximal phalangeal shaft can be obtained, but it is difficult to control the fragments with external support only. Often anatomic reduction can be maintained by percutaneous internal fixation. As for metacarpal fractures, this should be done in an operating room setting, and external support is mandatory until the pins have been removed. It is essential that fractures of the proximal phalanx be immobilized with the digits in the so-called safe position. If fractures are unstable in that position, either percutaneous internal fixation or open reduction and internal fixation are advisable. If technically feasible, percutaneous internal fixation is usually preferable.

Fractures of the shaft of the proximal or middle phalanx often angulate toward the palm (**A**), causing the fingers to assume a claw position. Open reduction and internal fixation is indicated when a fragment of an intra-articular fracture is too small to manipulate and accurate reduction is necessary for good joint function, when satisfactory realignment cannot be obtained because of probability of soft tissue interposition, when there are multiple fractures in the hand that cannot be held in the correct position without internal fixation, or when the fracture is open (compound) and proper dressing of the hand is not possible without internal fixation.

(Plate 6-19) OPEN REDUCTION AND INTERNAL FIXATION FOR PHALANGEAL SHAFT FRACTURE

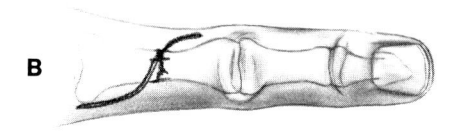

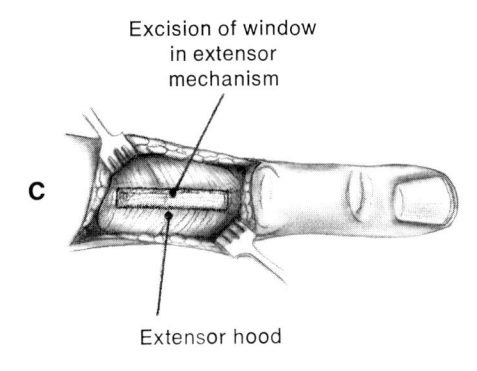

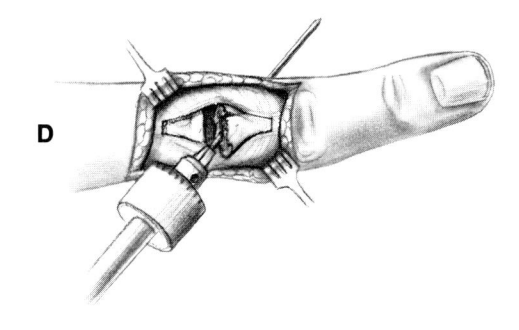

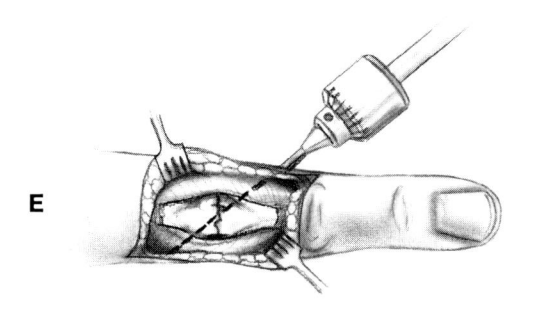

DETAILS OF PROCEDURE. A midshaft fracture of the proximal phalanx is exposed through a dorsal approach with an S-shaped skin incision as illustrated (**B**). A window is then removed from the extensor mechanism. This may either be the extrinsic extensor tendon as is illustrated in **C** or one of the lateral bands and wing tendons as would be done for an intrinsic extensor tendon release (see Plate 6-7, *H*). It is not advisable to incise the extensor mechanism and then repair it, since this predisposes to scarring of the extensor mechanism to the underlying fracture site. If at all possible, the periosteum should be carefully preserved so that it may be carefully closed with inverted sutures over the fracture site once it has been reduced, similarly with the intent to decrease the tendency for scarring of the extensor mechanism to the underlying fracture. A Kirschner wire is drilled obliquely into the distal fragment (**D**). After the fracture is reduced with particular attention to correction of any rotational deformity, the Kirschner wire is drilled retrograde across the fracture site into the proximal fragment (**E** and **F**). The Kirschner wire is cut off outside the skin. Following wound closure, the finger is splinted in a position of function.

POSTOPERATIVE MANAGEMENT. The hand, including one adjacent finger, is immobilized with a cast in the "safe position" (see p. 171) for 3 to 4 weeks. The Kirschner wire is removed when there is roentgenographic evidence that the fracture of the phalanx is starting to heal. If the fracture site is nontender and early healing is seen on x-ray examination, usually at 3 to 4 weeks after surgery, the internal fixation should be removed. External splinting is then absolutely necessary, but can be removed for a carefully instituted program of exercises to reestablish gliding of the extensor mechanism past the proximal phalangeal level. The external splinting is then maintained between the periods of exercise until there is roentgenographic evidence of more mature fracture healing.

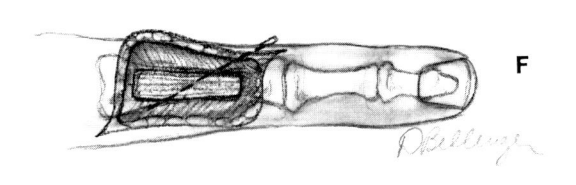

OSTEOTOMY OF PHALANX (FOR ROTATIONAL DEFORMITY) (Plate 6-20)

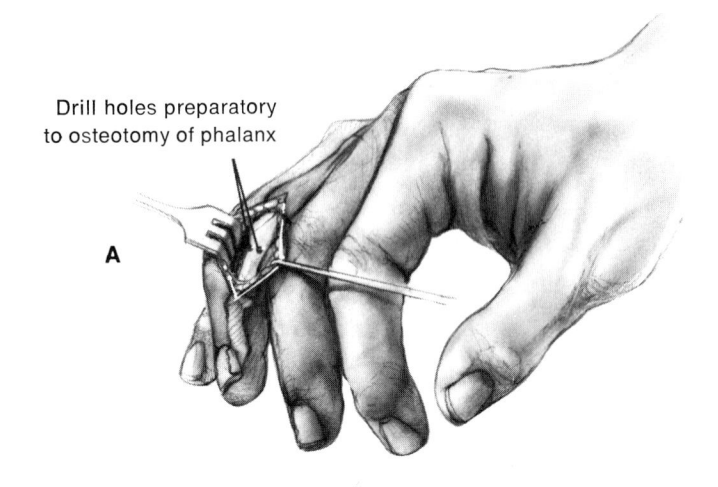

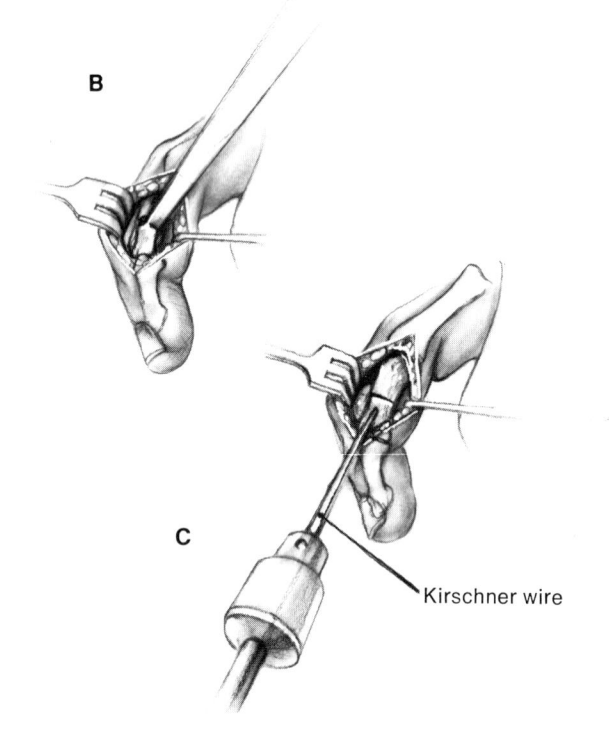

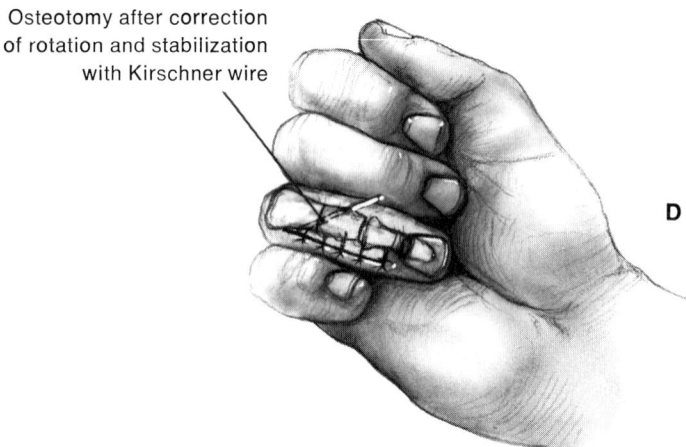

Drill holes preparatory to osteotomy of phalanx

Kirschner wire

Osteotomy after correction of rotation and stabilization with Kirschner wire

GENERAL DISCUSSION. When a fracture of the metacarpal or proximal or middle phalanx has healed with less than perfect rotation at the fracture site, one finger may overlap another when the fingers are fully flexed. There may be an apparent difference in the plane of the fingernails when all fingers are fully extended. If the degree of rotational change is distressing to the patient, rotational osteotomy for correction of the finger may be indicated.

DETAILS OF PROCEDURE. For malunions of fractures of the metacarpal or proximal phalanx, osteotomy of that bone is advisable, usually through the broad metaphyseal portion. The exposure and the internal fixation are identical in principal to that illustrated in Plates 6-18 and 6-19. The procedure for osteotomy of the middle phalanx is as follows.

A lateral approach is best **(A)**. The fracture site is exposed and osteotomized transversely **(B)**. The rotational change is corrected with attention to the alignment of the fingernails and the position of the finger in relation to the adjacent fingers when the interphalangeal joints are flexed. With the bone fragments in the correct rotational position and in firm apposition, a Kirschner wire is drilled obliquely in a proximal direction across the osteotomy site **(C)** to maintain the fragments securely in the corrected position. The Kirschner wire is cut off outside the skin **(D)**. Following wound closure, the finger is splinted with the interphalangeal joints in extension.

POSTOPERATIVE MANAGEMENT. The finger is splinted for a minimum of 6 weeks postoperatively. The Kirschner wire is removed when there is clinical evidence that the phalangeal osteotomy has united. There is usually clinical evidence of bony union with stability and loss of tenderness, considerably before the osteotomy site is obliterated on x-ray examination. Usually the Kirschner wire can be removed and the exercise program started approximately 6 weeks after surgery, although it may be 3 to 4 months before the osteotomy line has been completely obliterated by roentgenogram.

(Plate 6-21) ARTHRODESIS OF CARPOMETACARPAL JOINT OF THUMB

GENERAL DISCUSSION. Degenerative arthritis at the carpometacarpal joint of the thumb is a common cause of discomfort in the hand. In some patients symptoms at the carpometacarpal joint of the thumb may be severe enough to require arthrodesis or arthroplasty. Pinching and grasping aggravate the discomfort, and effective rest of the thumb relieves these symptoms. If conservative rest and protection of the thumb fail to relieve distressing and localized symptoms at the carpometacarpal joint, arthrodesis of this joint can achieve stability and comfort and restore good thumb function.

There is wide individual variation in the normal mobility of the metacarpophalangeal joint and interphalangeal joint of the thumb. At the interphalangeal joint, full motion may range from 50° of hyperextension to 95° of flexion. The metacarpophalangeal joint may normally flex to as little as 30° or as much as 100°. There may be concern that arthrodesis of the carpometacarpal joint of the thumb will take away needed thumb mobility. However, opposition and abduction are not excessively decreased by arthrodesis of the carpometacarpal joint in a good position. Abduction radially away from the second metacarpal shaft or span of the hand will be decreased (a loss that might be of importance to a pianist). Opposition to the index, long, and ring fingers is usually possible but not to the little. If motion of the metacarpophalangeal joint and interphalangeal joint of the thumb are adequate, arthrodesis of the carpometacarpal joint of the thumb can result in good thumb motion and function.

In children, fusion of the carpometacarpal joint of the thumb is only occasionally indicated, primarily to stabilize a joint that is subluxed in a paralytic hand. The procedure may be one part of a combined tendon transfer–joint stabilization–physical restoration program for a paralytic hand disability.

Arthrodesis of the carpometacarpal joint of the thumb is most commonly indicated in the osteoarthritic thumb. It occasionally is a very valuable procedure in the reconstruction of the rheumatoid thumb.

Arthroplasty of the carpometacarpal area is also an excellent procedure. There are several types available. These include a simple excisional arthroplasty, fascial interposition arthroplasty, resection arthroplasty with silicone implant with capsular reconstruction, silicone implant with a core hole for simultaneous ligament reconstruction, implant arthroplasty with Dacron mesh to increase stability, prosthesis with Proplast resurfacing to enhance stability, resurfacing arthroplasties of the base of the thumb metacarpal, resurfacing arthroplasties of the trapezium, and ball and socket type metal high-density polyethylene implants that are cemented into the proximal trapezium and metacarpal. A detailed discussion of each of these arthroplasty techniques and their various indications is beyond the scope of this text.

DETAILS OF PROCEDURE. An incision is made over the base of the thumb metacarpal (**A**). The sensory branches of the radial nerve that cross the incision are identified, mobilized, and retracted. A linear incision is made in the joint capsule, starting over the base of the thumb metacarpal and extending proximally, thereby exposing the base of the first metacarpal and the trapezium (**B** and **C**).

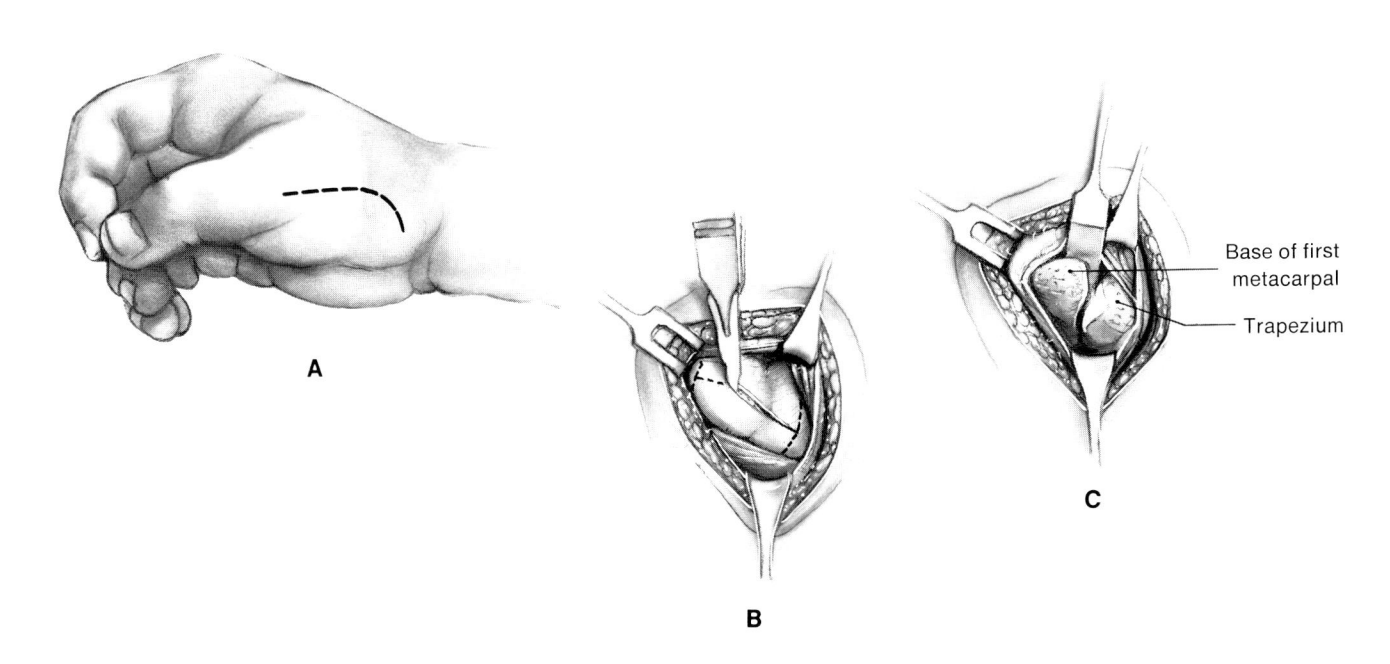

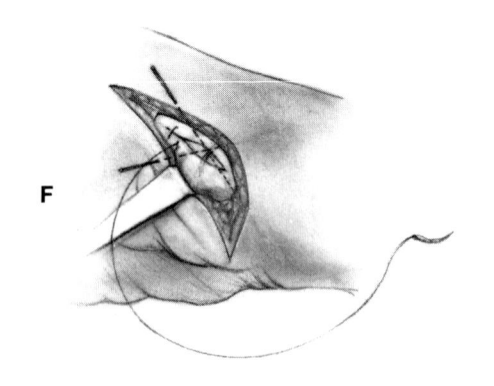

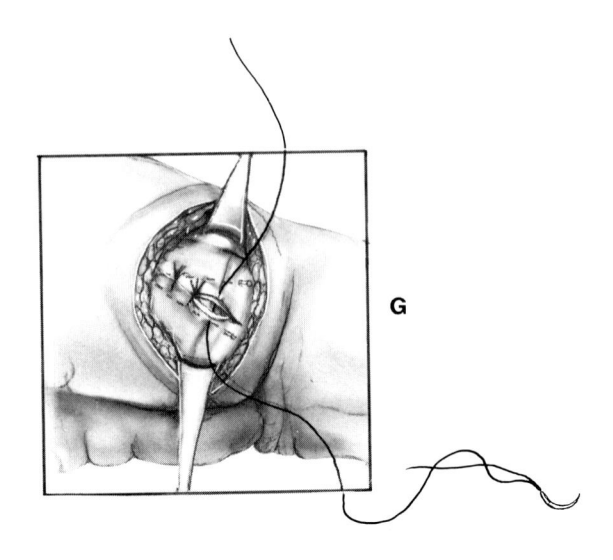

ARTHRODESIS OF CARPOMETACARPAL JOINT OF THUMB (Plate 6-21)

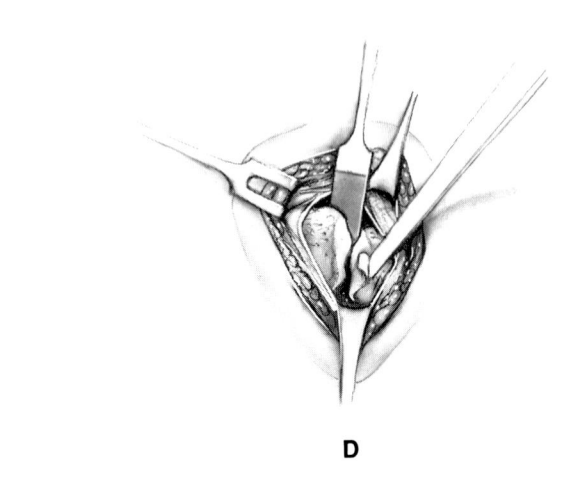

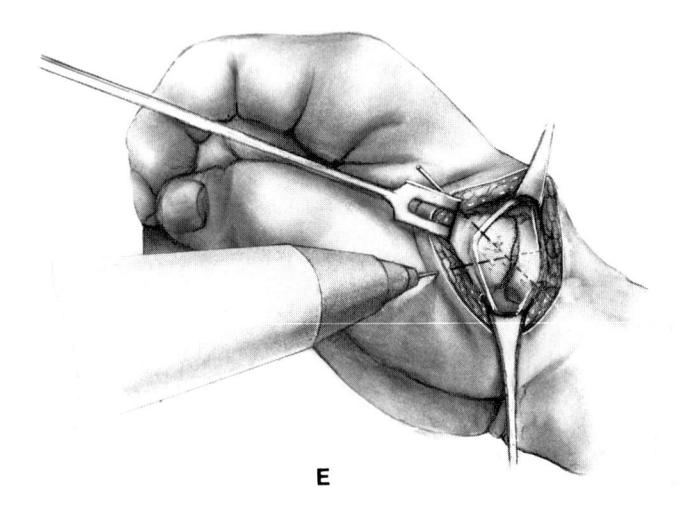

The linear capsular incision can be converted to an H by short, perpendicular cuts at either end to provide adequate exposure of the joint and its articular surfaces if necessary. The cartilaginous surface of the contiguous bones is excised to cancellous bone (D).

The thumb metacarpal is carefully put in "the fist projection." Osteotomes and rongeurs are used to create two parallel surfaces at the base of the thumb metacarpal and in the surface of the trapezium with the thumb in this fist position. Care must be taken to remove the frequently occurring bony osteophyte at the ulnar base of the thumb metacarpal so that it will not impinge on the base of the index metacarpal. After the fusion has healed, compensatory motion will occur in the joints between the scaphoid and the trapezium, and between the trapezium and the trapezoid. This osteophyte on the ulnar base of the thumb metacarpal will, unless removed, become painful as it moves across the surface of the radial base of the index metacarpal with thumb function. With the resected joint surfaces well apposed, the joint is transfixed with two crossed Kirschner wires (E and F). The capsule is sutured, and the wound is closed (G). The ends of the Kirschner wires remain percutaneous. The wrist and thumb are immobilized in a well-padded short-arm cast extending to the tip of the thumb.

POSTOPERATIVE MANAGEMENT. The gauntlet cast to the interphalangeal joint of the thumb is continued until the fusion is solid (approximately 8 to 12 weeks), and the wires are removed.

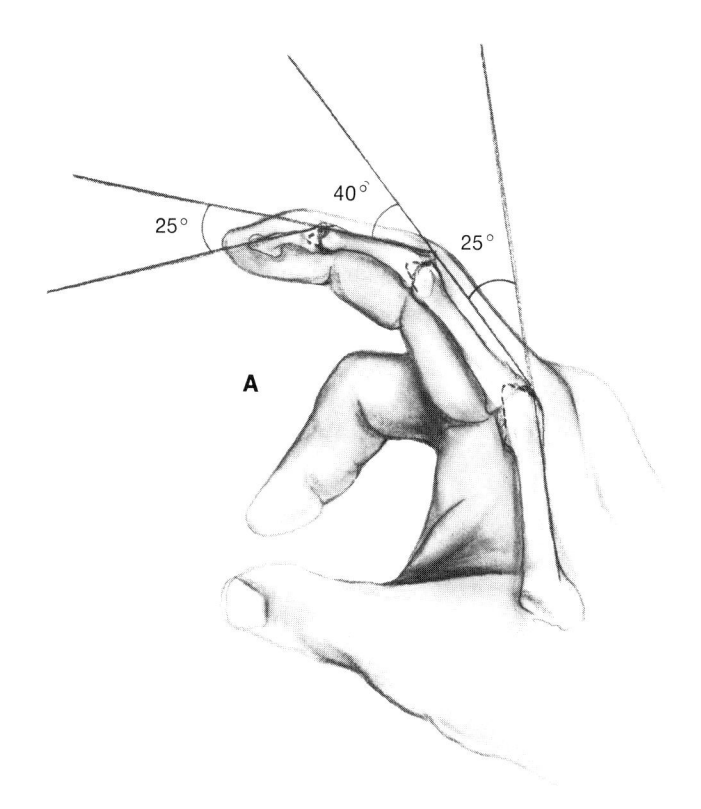

(Plate 6-22) ARTHRODESIS OF SMALL JOINTS

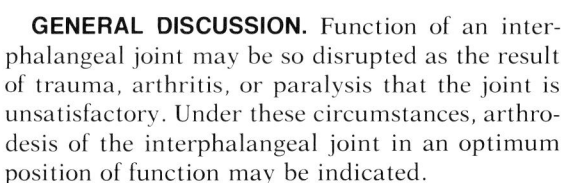

GENERAL DISCUSSION. Function of an interphalangeal joint may be so disrupted as the result of trauma, arthritis, or paralysis that the joint is unsatisfactory. Under these circumstances, arthrodesis of the interphalangeal joint in an optimum position of function may be indicated.

The recommended position for arthrodesis of individual joints in the fingers or thumb is illustrated in **A** and **B**. These generally optimal positions for arthrodesis are not meant to be arbitrary. The best angle for each joint will be that which permits optimum function of the hand. The distal interphalangeal joint is generally arthrodesed at 25° flexion, the proximal interphalangeal joint at 30° to 40° flexion, and the metacarpophalangeal joint at 25° to 30° flexion. The proximal interphalangeal joints of the ring and little fingers should be flexed slightly more than that of the index finger. In the thumb, function usually will be best if the interphalangeal joint is arthrodesed in a position of 15° flexion. If metacarpophalangeal arthrodesis of the thumb should be required, 15° to 20° flexion is usually the most functional position.

In one technique for arthrodesis of small joints (as recommended by Carroll and Hill), cartilage and cancellous bone can be removed from contiguous joint surfaces to create reciprocally fitting cone-shaped surfaces (**C** to **E**).

Another technique is illustrated in more detail in **F** to **Q**.

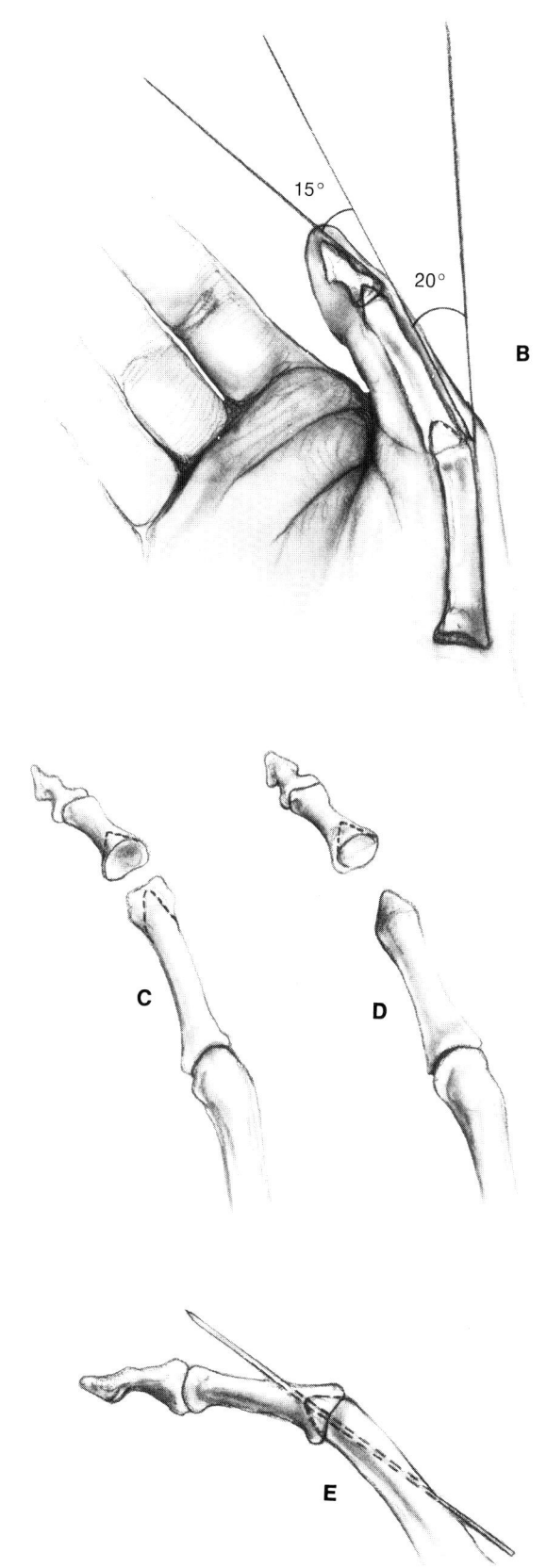

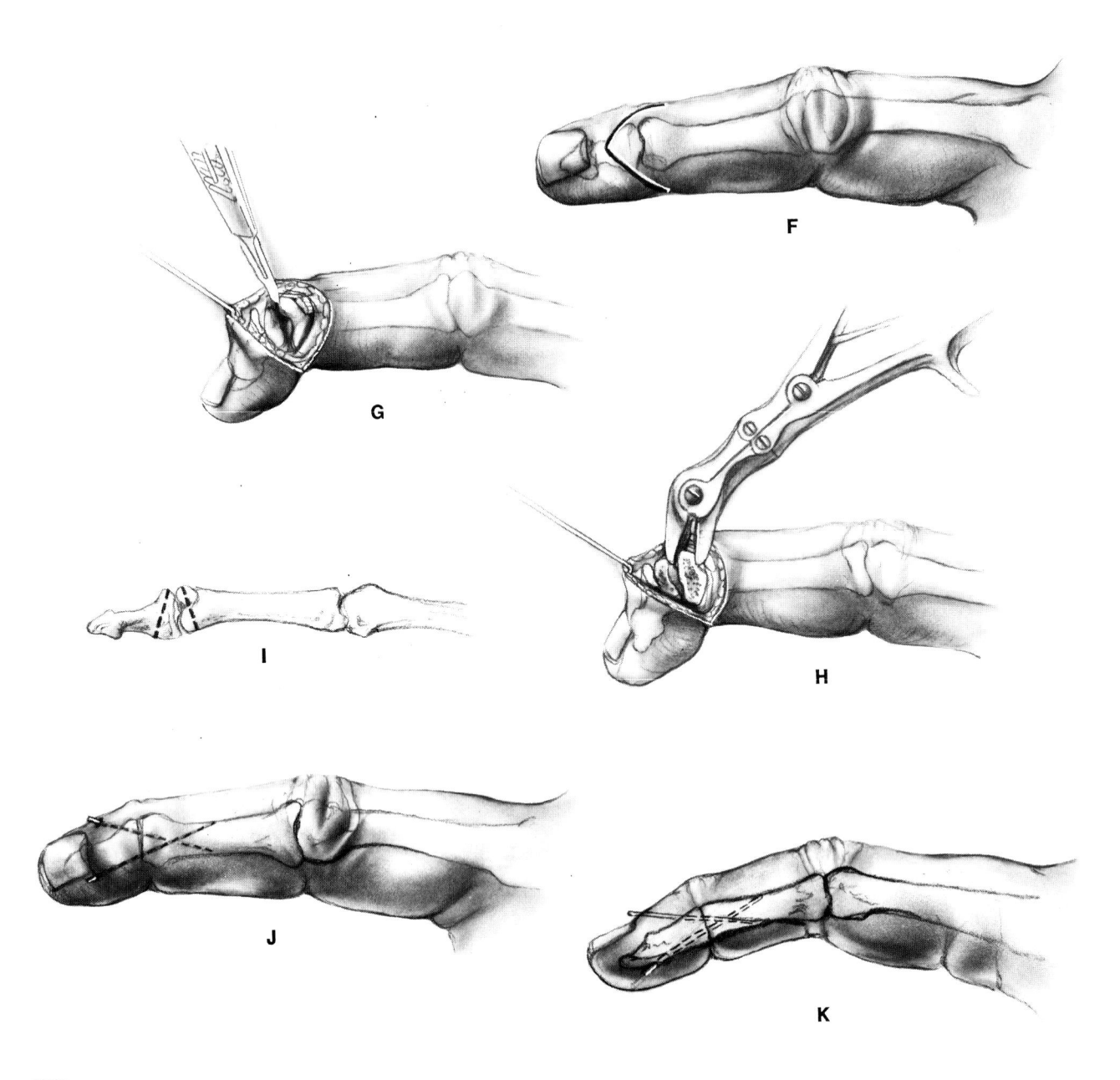

ARTHRODESIS OF SMALL JOINTS (Plate 6-22)

DETAILS OF PROCEDURE. For the distal joint, a dorsal incision is used **(F)** (see also Plate 6-1). The interphalangeal joint is opened **(G)**. A small hand osteotome and/or rongeurs are used to remove the articular cartilage and subchondral bone from the opposing surfaces of the interphalangeal joint and to shape the remaining surfaces until the desired angle for arthrodesis is obtained **(H** and **I)**. A dental burr may facilitate removal of articular surfaces. The prepared cancellous surfaces of the two phalanges are held compressed as Kirschner wires are inserted in crisscross fashion from each side of the finger to stabilize the two phalanges in the planned position **(J** and **K)**. Any small fragments of resected bone may be helpful as small grafts about the joint. The Kirschner wires are cut off outside the skin. Following wound closure, the finger is splinted to protect the arthrodesis.

(Plate 6-22) ARTHRODESIS OF SMALL JOINTS

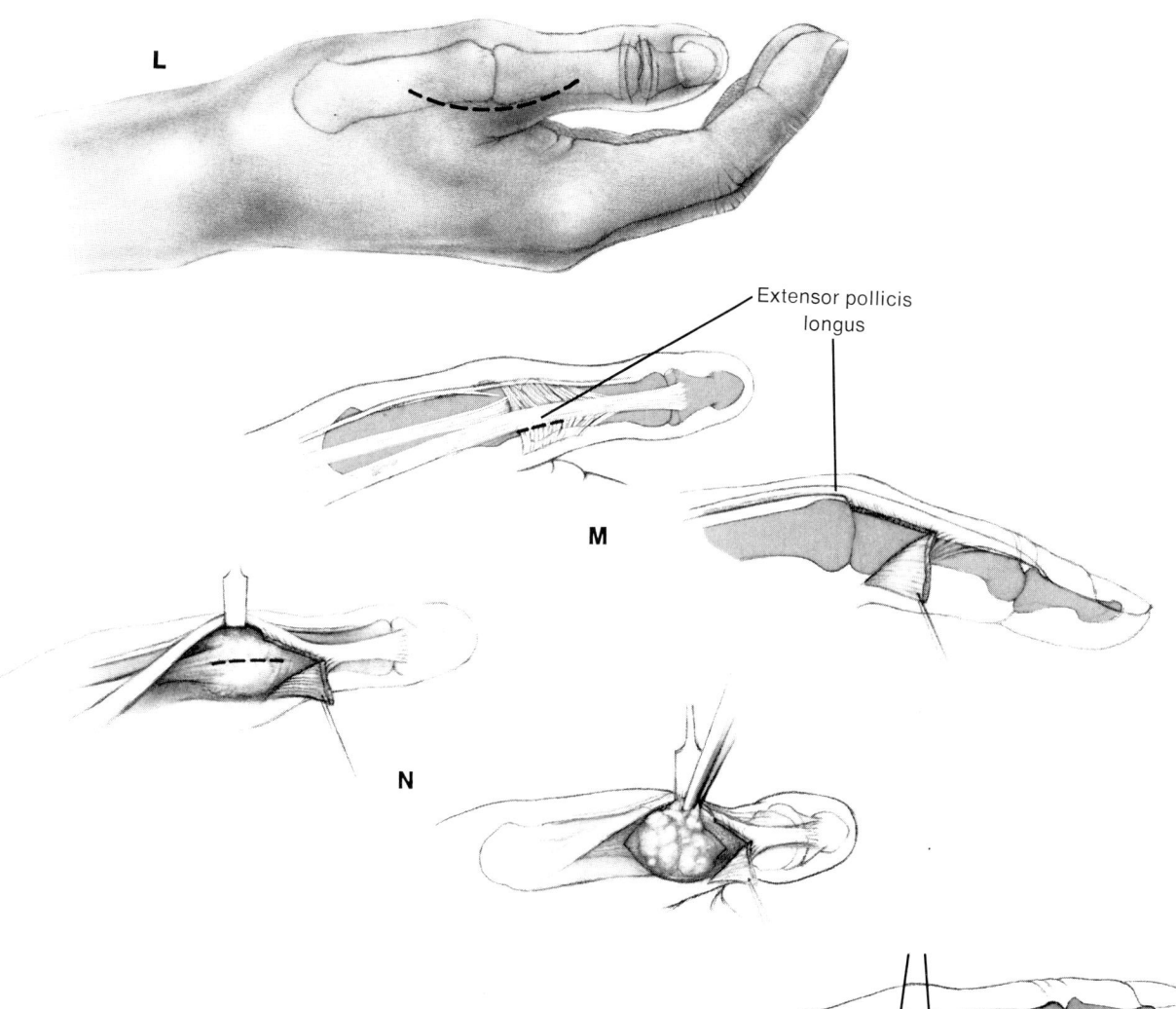

A similar procedure is used to arthrodese the proximal interphalangeal joint of the finger. Parallel cuts are placed through the head of the proximal phalanx and base of the middle phalanx so that when the surfaces are accurately opposed, the proposed arthrodesis site rests in the desired amount of flexion. It is similarly stabilized with crossed Kirschner pins. The easiest access to this joint for that procedure is by a longitudinal incision placed through the extensor mechanism over the central dorsum of the joint.

The metacarpophalangeal joint of the thumb not infrequently requires arthrodesis in the rheumatoid patient. The exposure is through a dorsal-ulnar gently curved longitudinal incision (**L**). The ulnar wing tendon is incised from the extensor pollicis longus (**M**). A dorsal incision is made in the joint capsule, and a synovectomy performed if the patient is rheumatoid (**N**). A similar fusion technique is used (**O** to **Q**).

POSTOPERATIVE MANAGEMENT. The Kirschner wires are removed 4 to 6 weeks postoperatively. The site of arthrodesis is protected with subsequent splinting until there is roentgenographic evidence of solid fusion.

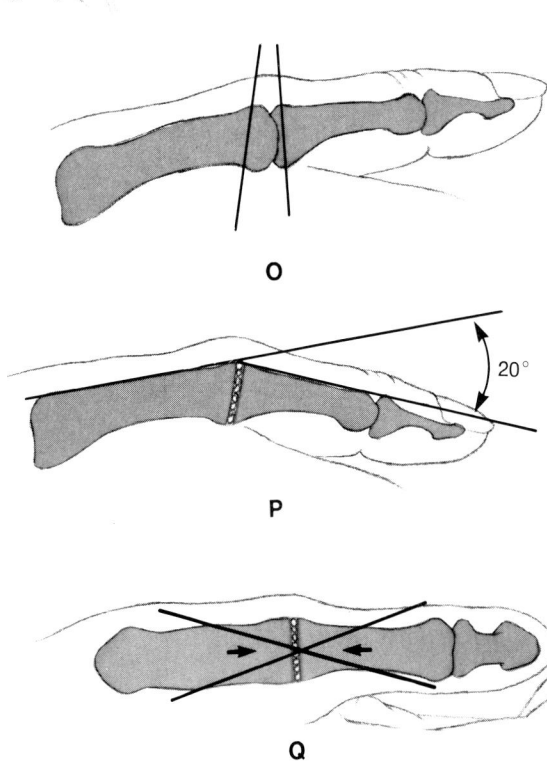

179

REPAIR OF SYNDACTYLY (Plate 6-23)

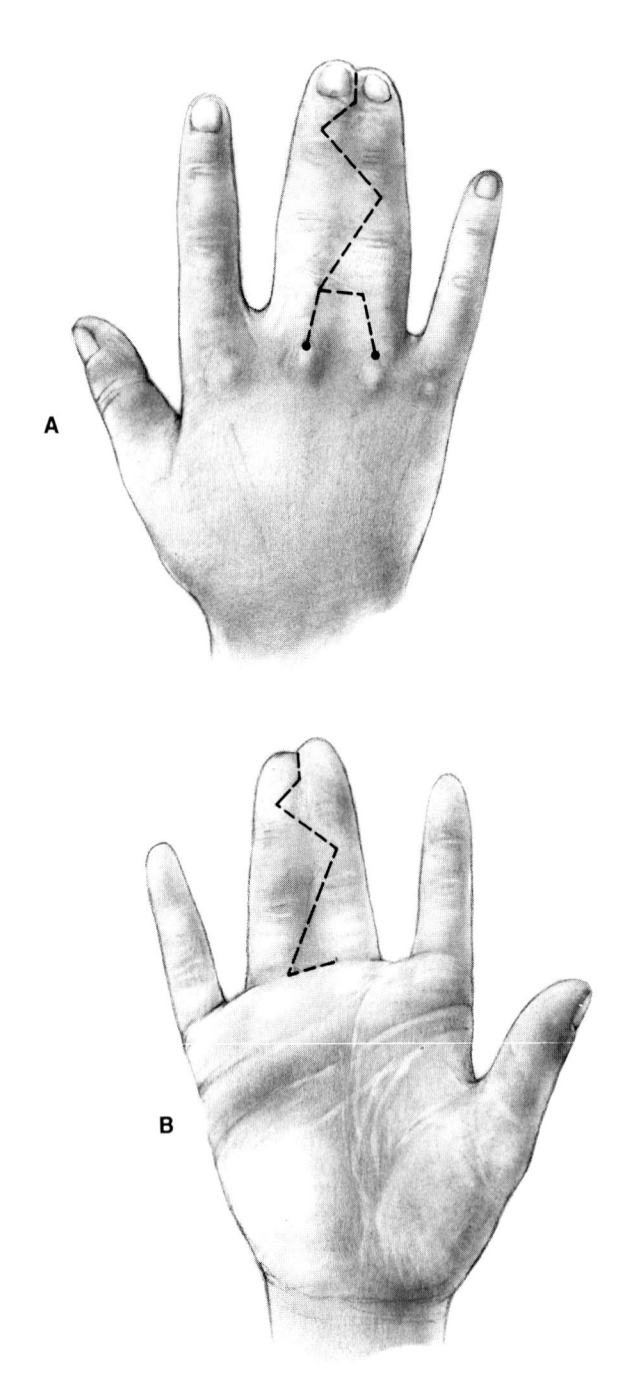

GENERAL DISCUSSION. Syndactyly is a relatively common congenital deformity in the hand. Often hereditary and more frequent among males, syndactyly may involve any two digits or all (although infrequently the thumb). The most commonly involved digits are the middle and ring fingers (**A**). In almost half of these patients, this condition is symmetric bilaterally. It may occur in the toes also. There also may be defects elsewhere in the body.

The fingers may be joined by any degree of length or thickness of the web. This may involve the tendons or digital nerves and sometimes may extend proximally to the metacarpals and even the carpal bones. In some cases there is a common broad distal phalanx. When the nails are joined, they are broad and there will be a groove between the two parts. In rare circumstances, only the ends of the fingers are joined.

When the deformity is severe with multiple fingers involved, surgery may be indicated as early as 12 to 18 months of age. If a common distal phalanx or nail is causing progressive deformity of digits with growth of one finger faster than another, surgery should be done at that time. Otherwise, surgery is probably best delayed until the age of approximately 3 to 5 years.

In the correction of syndactylism, the skin is always deficient, and additional skin should be planned so as not to impair motion or cause secondary deformity during growth.

(Plate 6-23) REPAIR OF SYNDACTYLY

DETAILS OF PROCEDURE. A dorsal trapezoidal flap is designed to reconstitute the web space **(A)**. The normal web is an inclined plane on its dorsal surface, and the length of this trapezoidal flap can be judged by measuring the length of the inclined plane of the adjacent web spaces. The base of the trapezoid is marked with a dot placed over each metacarpal head. The distal incision dorsally is made in a zigzag fashion with a matching mirror image zigzag design on the flexor aspect (**A** and **B**). On the palmar surface a transverse incision connects to this zigzag at the level of the web space, this level being judged by that of the adjacent finger web spaces (**A** and **B**). The skin flaps are then carefully raised (**C** and **D**). It is of critical importance to identify the neurovascular bundles in the web space and to protect these. In some cases it may be necessary to defat the flaps that have been raised and also to defat the excess subcutaneous tissue from the digit itself. Obviously great care must be taken not to damage the neurovascular bundles if defatting is required.

The flaps are then transposed and closed **(E)**. The shaded areas indicate those which will be without flap coverage and will require skin grafts. Full-thickness skin grafts are used and are best taken from the groin. These should be taken well laterally from the groin in an area that is not anticipated to be hair bearing after puberty.

It is advisable to suture these flaps and grafts in place with a 6-0 ophthalmic absorbable suture (plain is excellent for this purpose). This absorbable suture eliminates the necessity for traumatizing the child in the office in an attempt to remove the stitches.

The dressing must be carefully conformed to support the flaps and grafts. Stents may be used on the grafts if desired. Over these initial layers, the usual type of hand dressing is applied with an overlying well-padded long-arm cast to maintain the dressing securely in position.

POSTOPERATIVE MANAGEMENT. The hand must remain elevated for approximately 72 hours after surgery. If the child is comfortable and the dressing without odor or stain, it is first changed at 3½ to 4 weeks after surgery. Usually the wounds are benign and healed at that point, and the child can be allowed to resume activities.

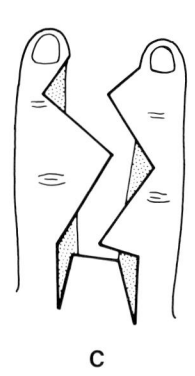

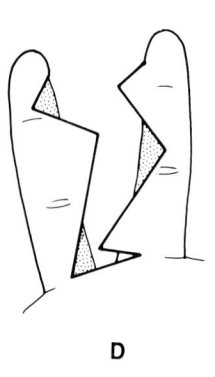

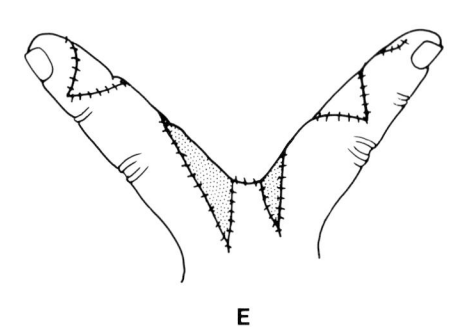

DRAINAGE OF PARONYCHIA (Plate 6-24)

GENERAL DISCUSSION. The paronychia is usually a staphylococcus infection beginning at one corner under the nail and spreading under the eponychium toward the other side. If the abscess underlies one corner of the nail root, it is best to remove that corner. Sometimes, separation of the fold from the nail or a small incision to the depth of the infection that lets out a small amount of purulent material may be adequate to resolve the situation.

It should be noted that the early paronychia appear as a cellulitis. At this stage, treatment is best with oral antibiotics and soaks. Drainage is not necessary unless pus is present under the eponychium or under the nail.

DETAILS OF PROCEDURE. A longitudinal incision is made on the medial and/or lateral side of the base of the fingernail as illustrated (**A**). The scalpel blade should be angled away from the nail to avoid cutting the nail bed. Unless the infection is localized on one side only, incisions will be necessary medially and laterally at the base of the nail. After the second incision is made, the skin should be folded back proximally and the proximal one third of the nail is excised at its base (**B** and **C**). The wound is held open with a sheet of Xeroform.

POSTOPERATIVE MANAGEMENT. The packing placed beneath the proximal skin flap is removed 48 hours postoperatively. Elevation, warm soaks, and antibiotics based on cultures taken at the time of the operative incision and drainage are continued as necessary depending on the individual circumstances.

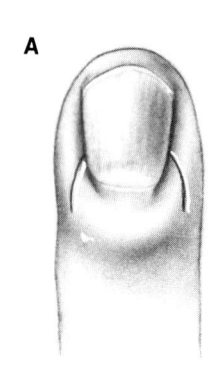

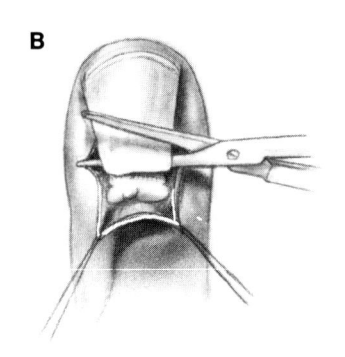

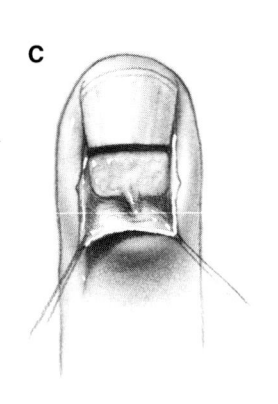

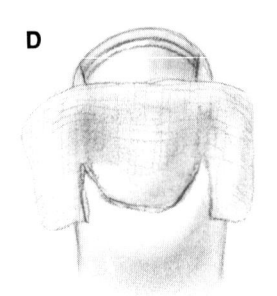

(Plate 6-25) DRAINAGE OF FELON

GENERAL DISCUSSION. When the pulp of the terminal portion of a digit becomes involved with an infection, severe throbbing discomfort with a swollen indurated distal pulp of the finger may require prompt treatment **(A)**.

If there is an abscess in the pulp of the digit under pressure, it is essential that drainage be done promptly if avascularity and resultant slough of the fingertip are to be prevented. Furthermore, long-standing undrained infection in this area will lead to osteomyelitis of the distal phalanx, or may occasionally rupture into the flexor tendon sheath.

The distal pulp of the finger is divided into compartments of strong fibrous septa traversing skin to bone **(B)**. As a result of these septa, any swelling or distension causes immediate discomfort from increased pressure.

DETAILS OF PROCEDURE. The incision should be made as illustrated **(A)**. It should be just at the leading margin of the nail, and may be J-shaped or along the entire nail margin. The fish-mouth type of incision well anterior to the nail margin is to be avoided. All septa in the pulp of the fingertip must be divided **(B)**. Care must be taken not to cut through into the flexor tendon sheath in the proximal portion of the incision. If there is a sequestrum present, this is removed. Cultures are taken, and the wound is left open with a small rubber drain in the open wound after all the vertical septa from skin to periosteum have been divided **(C)**.

POSTOPERATIVE MANAGEMENT. The drain is removed 48 hours postoperatively. Elevation, warm soaks, and appropriate antibiotics are continued.

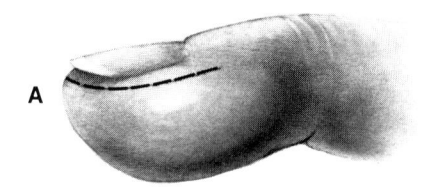

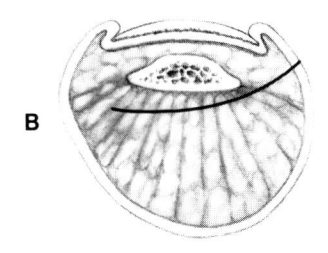

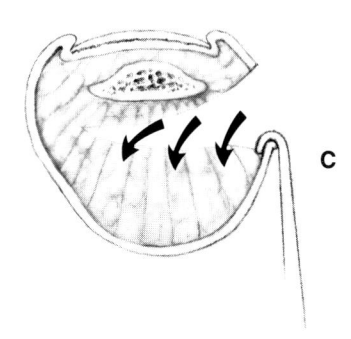

REFERENCES
General

American Society for Surgery of the Hand: The hand: examination and diagnosis, Edinburgh, 1981, Churchill Livingstone.

Boyes, J. H.: Bunnell's surgery of the hand, ed. 5, Philadelphia, 1970, J. B. Lippincott Co.

Bruner, J. M.: Safety factors in the use of the pneumatic tourniquet for hemostasis in surgery of the hand, J. Bone Joint Surg. **33-A:**221, 1951.

Bunnell, S.: Reconstructive surgery of the hand, Surg. Gynecol. Obstet. **39:**259, 1924.

Burton, R. I., and Littler, J. W.: Soft tissue afflictions of the hand, Curr. Probl. Surg., July, 1975.

Capener, N.: The hand in surgery, J. Bone Joint Surg. **38-B:**128, 1956.

Conway, H., and Stark, R. B.: Arterial vascularization of the soft tissue of the hand, J. Bone Joint Surg. **36-A:**1238, 1954.

Flatt, A. E.: Minor hand injuries, J. Bone Joint Surg. **37-B:**117, 1955.

Flatt, A. E.: The care of the rheumatoid hand, ed. 3, St. Louis, 1974, The C. V. Mosby Co.

Flatt, A. E.: The care of congenital hand anomalies, St. Louis, 1977, The C. V. Mosby Co.

Flynn, J. E., editor: Hand surgery, Baltimore, 1966, The Williams & Wilkins Co.

Furlong, R.: Injuries of the hand, Boston, 1957, Little, Brown & Co.

Grant, J. C. B.: An atlas of anatomy, ed. 5, Baltimore, 1962, The Williams & Wilkins Co.

Kaplan, E. B.: Functional and surgical anatomy of the hand, ed. 2, Philadelphia, 1965, J. B. Lippincott Co.

Lipscomb, P. R.: Surgery of the arthritic hand. Sterling Bunnell Memorial Lecture, Mayo Clin. Proc. **40:**132, 1965.

Littler, J. W.: Basic principles of reconstructive surgery of the hand, Surg. Clin. North Am. **40:**383, 1960.

Littler, J. W.: The hand and upper extremity, vol. 6. Converse, J. M.: Reconstructive plastic surgery, Philadelphia, 1977, W. B. Saunders Co.

Mason, M. L.: Fifty years' progress in surgery of the hand, Surg. Gynecol. Obstet. **101:**541, 1955.

Mason, M. L., and Bell, J. L.: The treatment of open injuries to the hand, Surg. Clin. North Am. **36:**1337, 1956.

Mayer, L.: The physiological method of tendon transplantation, Surg. Gynecol. Obstet. **22:**298, 1916.

McCormack, R. M.: Reconstructive surgery and the immediate care of the severely injured hand, Clin. Orthop. **13:**75, 1959.

McCormack, R. M.: Primary reconstruction in acute hand injuries, Surg. Clin. North Am. **40:**337, 1960.

Milford, L.: Resurfacing hand defects by using deboned useless fingers, Am. Surg. **32:**196, 1966.

Milford, L.: The hand. In Crenshaw, A. H., editor: Campbell's operative orthopaedics, vol. 1, ed. 5, St. Louis, 1971, The C. V. Mosby Co.

Nagel, D. A., Albright, J. A., Southwick, W. O., and Chase, R. A.: The use of bone grafts in the reconstruction of the bony architecture of the wrist and hand, Surg. Gynecol. Obstet. **122:**55, 1966.

Peacock, E. E., Jr.: Dynamic splinting for the prevention and correction of hand deformities. A simple and inexpensive method, J. Bone Joint Surg. **34-A:**789, 1952.

Rank, B. K., and Wakefield, A. R.: Surgery of repair as applied to hand injuries, Baltimore, 1960, The Williams & Wilkins Co.

Robins, R. H. C.: The primary reconstruction of the injured hand, Ann. R. Coll. Surg. Engl. **14:**355, 1954.

Stelling, F. H.: Surgery of the hand in the child, J. Bone Joint Surg. **45-A:**623, 1963.

Sudeck, P.: Akute und chronische entzuendliche Knochenatropie, Arch. Klin. Chir. **191:**180, 1938.

Swanson, A. B.: Flexible implant resection arthroplasty in the hand and extremities, St. Louis, 1973, The C. V. Mosby Co.

Verdan, C. E.: Basic principles in surgery of the hand, Surg. Clin. North Am. **47:**355, 1967.

Wakefield, A. R.: Hand injuries in children, J. Bone Joint Surg. **46-A:**1226, 1964.

Zancolli, E. A.: Structural and dynamic bases of hand surgery, Philadelphia, 1968, J. B. Lippincott Co.

Congenital problems

Bora, F. W., Nicholson, J. T., and Cheema, H. M.: Radial meromelia. The deformity and its treatment, J. Bone Joint Surg. **52-A:**966, 1970.

Eaton, R. G.: Hand problems in children; a timetable for management, Pediatr. Clin. North Am. **14:**643, 1967.

Flatt, A. E.: Treatment of syndactylism, Plast. Reconstr. Surg. **29:**336, 1962.

Goldner, J. L., and Clippinger, F. W.: Excision of the greater multangular bone as an adjuvant to mobilization of the thumb, J. Bone Joint Surg. **41-A:**609, 1959.

Kelikian, H.: Congenital deformities of the hand and forearm, Philadelphia, 1974, W. B. Saunders Co.

Kettelkamp, D. B., and Flatt, A. E.: An evaluation of syndactylia repair, Surg. Gynecol. Obstet. **113:**471, 1961.

Maisels, D. O.: Lobster-claw deformities of the hand and feet, Br. J. Plast. Surg. **23:**269, 1970.

Sayre, R. H.: A contribution to the study of club-hand, Trans. Am. Orthop. Ass. **6:**208, 1893.

Watson, H. K., and Boyes, J. H.: Congenital angular deformity of the digits, J. Bone Joint Surg. **49-A:**333, 1967.

Weckesser, E. C., Reed, J. R., and Heiple, K. G.: Congenital clapsed thumb (congenital flexion-adduction deformity of the thumb). A syndrome, not a specific entity, J. Bone Joint Surg. **50-A:**1417, 1968.

Fractures and joint injuries

Alldred, A. J.: Rupture of the collateral ligament of the metacarpo-phalangeal joint of the thumb, J. Bone Joint Surg. **37-B:**443, 1955.

Bennett, E. H.: Fractures of the metacarpal bones, Dublin J. Med. Sci. **73:**72, 1882.

Burton, R. I.: Acute joint injuries. In Wolfort, F. G., editor: Acute hand injuries, a multispecialty approach, Boston, 1980, Little, Brown & Co.

Burton, R. I., and Eaton, R. G.: Common hand injuries in the athlete, Orthop. Clin. North Am. **4:**809, 1973.

Campbell, C. S.: Gamekeeper's thumb, J. Bone Joint Surg. **37-B:**148, 1955.

Coonrad, R. W., and Goldner, J. L.: A study of the pathological findings and treatment in soft-tissue injury of the thumb metacarpophalangeal joint. With a clinical study of the normal range of motion in one thousand thumbs and a study of post mortem findings of ligamentous structures in relation to function, J. Bone Joint Surg. **50-A:**439, 1968.

Coonrad, R. W., and Pohlman, M. H.: Impacted fractures in the proximal portion of the proximal phalanx of the finger, J. Bone Joint Surg. **51-A**:1291, 1969.

Curtis, R. M.: Capsulectomy of the interphalangeal joints of the fingers, J. Bone Joint Surg. **36-A**:1219, 1954.

Curtis, R. M.: Treatment of injuries of proximal interphalangeal joints of fingers. In Adams, J. P., editor: Current practice in orthopaedic surgery, vol. 2, St. Louis, 1964, The C. V. Mosby Co.

Eaton, R. G.: Joint injuries in the hand, Springfield, Ill., 1971, Charles C Thomas, Publisher.

Eaton, R. G., and Burton, R. I.: Fractures of the hand. In Kilgore, E. S., and Graham, W. P., editors: The hand, surgical and nonsurgical management, Philadelphia, 1977, Lea & Febiger, pp. 121-142.

Flatt, A. E.: Closed and open fractures of the hand. Fundamentals of management, Postgrad. Med. **39**:17, 1966.

Gedda, K.-O., and Moberg, E.: Open reduction and osteosynthesis of the so-called Bennett's fracture in the carpometacarpal joint of the thumb, Acta Orthop. Scand. **22**:249-257, 1953.

Gedda, K.-O.: Studies on Bennett's fracture. Anatomy, roentgenology, and therapy, Acta Chir. Scand. (Suppl.) 193, 1954, p. 1-114.

Griffiths, J. C.: Fractures at the base of the first metacarpal bone, J. Bone Joint Surg. **46-B**:712, 1964.

Kaplan, E. B.: Dorsal dislocation of the metacarpophalangeal joint of the index finger, J. Bone Joint Surg. **39-A**:1081, 1957.

Kaplan, E. B.: The pathology and treatment of radial subluxation of the thumb with ulnar displacement of the head of the first metacarpal, J. Bone Joint Surg. **43-A**:541, 1961.

Kessler, I.: Chronic subluxation of the metacarpophalangeal joint of the thumb, J. Bone Joint Surg. **45-B**:805, 1963.

Lee, M. L. H.: Intra-articular and peri-articular fractures of the phalanges, J. Bone Joint Surg. **45B**:103, 1963.

Littler, J. W.: Metacarpal reconstruction, J. Bone Joint Surg. **29**:723, 1947.

Moberg, E.: Fractures and ligamentous injuries of the thumb and fingers, Surg. Clin. North Am. **40**:297, 1960.

Moberg, E., and Stener, B.: Injuries to the ligaments of the thumb and fingers. Diagnosis, treatment and prognosis, Acta Chir. Scand. **106**:166, 1953.

Murphy, A. F., and Stark, H. H.: Closed dislocation of the metacarpophalangeal joint of the index finger, J. Bone Joint Surg. **49-A**:1579, 1967.

Neviaser, R. J., Wilson, J. N., and Lievano, A.: Rupture of the ulnar collateral ligament of the thumb (gamekeeper's thumb). Correction by dynamic repair, J. Bone Joint Surg. **53-A**:1357, 1971.

Sakellarides, H. T., and DeWeese, J. W.: Instability of the metacarpophalangeal joint of the thumb. Reconstruction of the collateral ligaments using the extensor pollicis brevis tendon, J. Bone Joint Surg. **58-A**:106, 1976.

Schultz, R. T., and Fox, J. M.: Gamekeeper's thumb. Result of skiing injuries, N.Y. State J. Med. **73**:2329, 1973.

Skoog, T.: Syndactyly. A clinical report on repair, Acta Chir. Scand. **130**:537, 1965.

Smith, R. J.: Post-traumatic instability of the metacarpophalangeal joint of the thumb, J. Bone Joint Surg. **59-A**:14, 1977.

Spinner, M., and Choi, B. Y.: Anterior dislocation of the proximal interphalangeal joint. A cause of rupture of the central slip of the extensor mechanism, J. Bone Joint Surg. **52-A**:1329, 1970.

Stark, H. H.: Troublesome fractures and dislocations of the hand, American Academy of Orthopaedic Surgeons Instructional Course Lectures, vol. 19, St. Louis, 1970, The C. V. Mosby Co., p. 130.

Stener, B.: Displacement of the ruptured ulnar collateral ligament of the metacarpophalangeal joint of the thumb. A clinical and anatomical study, J. Bone Joint Surg. **44-B**:869, 1962.

Sutro, C. J.: Fracture of the metacarpal bones and proximal manual phalanges. Treatment with emphasis on the prevention of rotational deformities, Am. J. Surg. **81**:327, 1951.

Swanson, A. B.: Flexible implant resection arthroplasty in the hand and extremities, St. Louis, 1973, The C. V. Mosby Co.

Wagner, C. S.: Method treatment of Bennett's fracture dislocation, Am. J. Surg. **80**:230, 1950.

Weckesser, E. C.: Rotational osteotomy of the metacarpal for overlapping fingers, J. Bone Joint Surg. **47-A**:751, 1965.

Wilson, J. N., and Rowland, S. A.: Fracture-dislocation of the proximal interphalangeal joint of the finger. Treatment by open reduction and internal fixation, J. Bone Joint Surg. **48-A**:493, 1966.

Wright, T. A.: Early mobilization in fractures of the metacarpals and phalanges, Can. J. Surg. **11**:491, 1968.

Tendon injuries

Allen, H. S.: Primary and delayed tendon repair to the hand, American Academy of Orthopaedic Surgeons Instructional Course Lectures, vol. 8, Ann Arbor, Mich., 1951, J. W. Edwards, p. 223.

Brand, P. W.: Tendon grafting, J. Bone Joint Surg. **43-B**:444, 1961.

Bell, J. L., Mason, M. L., Koch, S. L., and Stromberg, W. B., Jr.: Injuries to flexor tendons of the hand in children, J. Bone Joint Surg. **40-A**:1220, 1958.

Boyes, J. H.: Operative technique of digital flexor tendon grafts, American Academy of Orthopaedic Surgeons Instructional Course Lectures, vol. 10, Ann Arbor, Mich., 1953, J. W. Edwards, p. 263.

Boyes, J. H.: Evaluation of results of digital flexor tendon grafts, Am. J. Surg. **89**:1116, 1955.

Boyes, J. H., Wilson, J. N., and Smith, J. W.: Flexor-tendon ruptures in the forearm and hand, J. Bone Joint Surg. **42-A**:637, 1960.

Boyes, J. H., and Stark, H. H.: Flexor-tendon grafts in the fingers and thumb. A study of factors influencing results in 1000 cases, J. Bone Joint Surg. **53-A**:1332, 1971.

Bunnell, S.: Suturing tendons, American Academy of Orthopaedic Surgeons Instructional Course Lectures, vol. 1, Ann Arbor, Mich., 1943, J. W. Edwards, p. 1.

Burton, R. I.: Severed flexor tendons distal to metacarpophalangeal joint. In Littler, J. W., Cramer, L. M., and Smith, J. W., editors: Symposium on reconstructive hand surgery, vol. 9, St. Louis, 1974, The C. V. Mosby Co.

Burton, R. I., Littler, J. W., and Eaton, R. G.: Sound/slide program: the finger flexor mechanism and its restoration by tendon grafting, no. 423, Part I (The history of flexor tendon surgery; the dynamic anatomy of the finger flexor system), no. 424, Part II (The technique of tendon graft), no. 425, Part III (The complications of flexor tendon surgery), American Academy of Orthopaedic Surgeons, 1973.

Carter, S. J., and Mersheimer, W. L.: Deferred primary tendon repair. Result in 27 cases, Ann. Surg. **164**:913, 1966.

Colville, J., Callison, J. R., and White, W. L.: Role of mesotenon in tendon blood supply, Plast. Reconstr. Surg. **43:**53, 1969.

Dargan, E. L.: Management of extensor tendon injuries of the hand, Surg. Gynecol. Obstet. **128:**1269, 1969.

Entin, M. A.: Repair of extensor mechanism of the hand, Surg. Clin. North Am. **40:**275, 1960.

Fetrow, K. O.: Tenolysis in the hand and wrist. A clinical evaluation of 220 flexor and extensor tenolyses, J. Bone Joint Surg. **49-A:**667, 1967.

Flynn, J. E., and Graham, J. H.: Healing following tendon suture and tendon transplants, Surg. Gynecol. Obstet. **115:**467, 1962.

Forward, A. D., and Cowan, R. J.: Tendon suture to bone. An experimental investigation in rabbits, J. Bone Joint Surg. **45-A:**807, 1963.

Goldner, J. L., and Coonrad, R. W.: Tendon grafting of the flexor profundus in the presence of a completely or partially intact flexor sublimis, J. Bone Joint Surg. **51-A:**527, 1969.

Hallberg, D., and Lindholm, A.: Subcutaneous rupture of the extensor tendon of the distal phalanx of the finger; "mallet finger," Acta Chir. Scand. **119:**260, 1960.

Harrison, S. H.: Delayed primary flexor tendon grafts of the fingers. A comparison of results with primary and secondary tendon grafts, Plast. Reconstr. Surg. **43:**366, 1969.

Howard, N. J.: Pathological changes induced in tendons through trauma and their accompanying clinical phenomena, Am. J. Surg. **51:**689, 1941.

Hunter, J. M.: Artificial tendons, J. Bone Joint Surg. **4-A:**631, 1965.

Hunter, J. M., and Salisbury, R. E.: Flexor-tendon reconstruction in severely damaged hands. A two-stage procedure using a silicone-Dacron reinforced gliding prosthesis prior to tendon grafting, J. Bone Joint Surg. **53-A:**829, 1971.

Jaffe, S., and Weckesser, E.: Profundus tendon grafting with the sublimis intact. An end-result study of 30 patients, J. Bone Joint Surg. **49-A:**1298, 1967.

Kelly, A. P., Jr.: Primary tendon repairs: a study of 789 consecutive tendon severances, J. Bone Joint Surg. **41-A:**581, 1959.

Kleinert, H. E., Kutz, J. E., Ashbell, T. S., and Martinez, E.: Primary repair of lacerated flexor tendons in "no-man's land," J. Bone Joint Surg. **49-A:**577, 1967.

Koch, S. L.: Division of flexor tendons within digital sheath, Surg. Gynecol. Obstet. **78:**9, 1944.

Leffert, R. D., Weiss, C., and Athanasoulis, C. A.: The vincula. With particular reference to their vessels and nerves, J. Bone Joint Surg. **56-A:**1191, 1974.

Lindsay, W. K., and McDougall, E. P.: Direct digital flexor tendon repair, Plast. Reconstr. Surg. **26:**613, 1960.

Littler, J. W.: Free tendon grafts in secondary flexor tendon repair, Am. J. Surg. **74:**315, 1947.

Littler, J. W.: The severed flexor tendon, Surg. Clin. North Am. **39:**435, 1959.

Littler, J. W.: The finger extensor mechanism, Surg. Clin. North Am. **47:**415, 1967.

Littler, J. W.: The digital extensor-flexor system. In Converse, J. W., editor: Reconstructive plastic surgery, vol. 6, Philadelphia, 1977, W. B. Saunders Co.

Littler, J. W., Burton, R. I., and Eaton, R. G.: Sound/slide program: The dynamics of finger extension, no. 467, Part I; no. 468, Part II, American Academy of Orthopaedic Surgeons.

Madsen, E.: Delayed primary suture of flexor tendons cut in the digital sheath, J. Bone Joint Surg. **52-B:**264, 1970.

Mason, M. L., and Allen, H. S.: The rate of healing of tendons— an experimental study of tensile strength, Ann. Surg. **113:**424, 1941.

McCormack, R. M., Demuth, R. J., and Kindling, P. H.: Flexor tendon grafts in the less-than-optimum situation, J. Bone Joint Surg. **44-A:**1360, 1962.

McFarlane, R. M., and Hampole, M. K.: Treatment of extensor tendon injuries of the hand, Can. J. Surg. **16:**1-10, 1973.

Peacock, E. E., Jr.: Some technical aspects and results of flexor tendon repair, Surgery, **58:**330, 1965.

Potenza, A. D.: Healing of autogenous tendon grafts within the flexor digital sheath in dogs, J. Bone Joint Surg. **46-A:**1462, 1964.

Pulvertaft, R. G.: Tendon grafts for flexor tendon injuries in the fingers and thumb, J. Bone Joint Surg. **38-B:**175, 1956.

Pulvertaft, R. G.: Treatment of flexor tendon injuries in the hand; discussion, J. Bone Joint Surg. **43-B:**403, 1961.

Pulvertaft, R. G.: Problems of flexor-tendon surgery of the hand, J. Bone Joint Surg. **47-A:**123, 1965.

Rank, B. K., and Wakefield, A. R.: The repair of flexor tendons in the hand, Br. J. Plast. Surg. **4:**244, 1952.

Riddell, D. M.: Spontaneous rupture of the extensor pollicis longus; the results of tendon transfer, J. Bone Joint Surg. **45-B:**506, 1963.

Shaw, P. C.: A method of flexor tendon suture, J. Bone Joint Surg. **50-B:**578, 1968.

Tubiana, R.: Incisions and technics in tendon grafting, Am. Surg. **109:**339, 1965.

Urbaniak, J. R., and Goldner, J. L.: Laceration of the flexor pollicis longus tendon: delayed repair by advancement, free graft or direct suture. A clinical and experimental study, J. Bone Joint Surg. **55-A:**1123, 1973.

Urbaniak, J. R., Bright, D. S., Gill, L. H., and Goldner, J. L.: Vascularization and the gliding mechanism of free flexor-tendon grafts inserted by the silicone-rod method, J. Bone Joint Surg. **56-A:**473, 1974.

Verdan, C. E.: Primary repair of flexor tendons, J. Bone Joint Surg. **42-A:**647, 1960.

Verdan, C. E.: Practical considerations for primary and secondary repair in flexor tendon injuries, Surg. Clin. North Am. **44:**951, 1964.

Verdan, C. E.: Half a century of flexor-tendon surgery, J. Bone Joint Surg., **54-A:**472, 1972.

Nerve injuries

Omer, G. E., Jr.: Evaluation and reconstruction of the forearm and hand after acute traumatic peripheral nerve injuries, J. Bone Joint Surg. **50-A:**1454, 1968.

Omer, G. E., and Spinner, M.: Management of peripheral nerve problems, Philadelphia, 1980, W. B. Saunders Co.

Spinner, M.: Injuries to the major branches of peripheral nerves of the forearm, Philadelphia, 1978, W. B. Saunders Co.

Tendon transfers (in paralytic and spastic condition)

Brand, P. W.: Paralytic claw hand. With special reference to paralysis in leprosy and treatment by the sublimis transfer of Stiles and Bunnell, J. Bone Joint Surg. **40-B:**618, 1958.

Brown, P. W.: Zancolli capsulorrhaphy for ulnar claw hand. Appraisal of forty-four cases, J. Bone Joint Surg. **52-A:**868, 1970.

Bunnell, S.: Opposition of the thumb, J. Bone Joint Surg. **20:**269, 1938.

Bunnell, S.: Tendon transfers in the hand and forearm,

American Academy of Orthopaedic Surgeons Instructional Course Lectures, vol. 6, Ann Arbor, Mich., 1949, J. W. Edwards.

Camitz, H.: Surgical treatment of paralysis of opponens muscle of the thumb, Acta Chir. Scand. **65**:77, 1929.

Cooley, S. G. E., and Littler, J. W.: Opposition of thumb and its restoration by abduction digiti quinti transfer, J. Bone Joint Surg. **45-A**:1389, 1963.

Goldner, J. L.: Reconstructive surgery of the hand in cerebral palsy and spastic paralysis resulting from injury to the spinal cord, J. Bone Joint Surg. **37-A**:1141, 1955.

Goldner, J. L.: Upper extremity reconstructive surgery in cerebral palsy or similar conditions, American Academy of Orthopaedic Surgeons Instructional Course Lectures, vol. 18, St. Louis, 1961, The C. V. Mosby Co., p. 169.

Huber, E.: Hilfsoperation bei medianuslähmung, Dtsch. Z. Chir. **162**:271, 1921.

Inglis, A. E., and Cooper, W.: Release of the flexor-pronator origin for flexion deformities of the hand and wrist in spastic paralysis. A study of the eighteen cases, J. Bone Joint Surg. **48-A**:847, 1966.

Inglis, A. E., Cooper, W., and Bruton, W.: Surgical correction of thumb deformities in spastic paralysis, J. Bone Joint Surg. **52-A**:253, 1970.

Keats, S.: Surgical treatment of the hand in cerebral palsy: correction of thumb-in-palm and other deformities. Report of nineteen cases, J. Bone Joint Surg. **47-A**:274, 1965.

Kessler, I.: Transfer of extensor carpi ulnaris to tendon of extensor pollicis brevis for opponensplasty, J. Bone Joint Surg. **51-A**:1303, 1969.

Lam, S. J.: The operative correction of severe spastic "thumb-in-palm" deformity, Guys Hosp. Rep. **115**:27, 1966.

Littler, J. W.: Tendon transfers and arthrodeses in combined median and ulnar nerve paralysis, J. Bone Joint Surg. **31-A**:225, 1949.

Littler, J. W., and Cooley, S. G. E.: Opposition of the thumb and its restoration by abductor digiti quinti transfer, J. Bone Joint Surg. **45-A**:1389, 1963.

Littler, J. W., and Li, C. S.: Primary restoration of thumb opposition with median nerve decompression, Plast. Reconstr. Surg. **39**:74, 1967.

Matev, I.: Surgical treatment of spastic "thumb-in-palm" deformity, J. Bone Joint Surg. **45-B**:703, 1963.

Mortens, J.: Surgery of the hand in cerebral palsy, Acta Orthop. Scand. **36**:441, 1965.

Mulder, J. D., and Landsmeer, J. M. F.: The mechanism of claw finger, J. Bone Joint Surg. **50-B**:664, 1968.

Nickel, V. L.: The flexor-hinge hand (in Proceedings of the American Society for Surgery of the Hand), J. Bone Joint Surg. **46-A**:914, 1964.

Nickel, V. L., Perry, J., and Garrett, A. L.: Development of useful function in the severely paralyzed hand, J. Bone Joint Surg. **45-A**:933, 1963.

Ramselaar, J. M.: Tendon transfers to restore opposition of the thumb, Leiden, 1970, H. E. Stenfert Kroese N. V.

Riordan, D. C.: Tendon transplantations in median nerve and ulnar nerve paralysis, J. Bone Joint Surg. **35-A**:312, 1953.

Riordan, D. C.: Surgery of the paralytic hand, American Academy of Orthopaedic Surgeons Instructional Course Lectures, vol. 16, St. Louis, 1959, The C. V. Mosby Co., p. 79.

Royle, N. D.: An operation for paralysis of the intrinsic muscles of the thumb, J.A.M.A. **111**:612, 1938.

Sakellarides, H. T.: Modified pulley for opponens tendon transfer, J. Bone Joint Surg. **52-A**:178, 1970.

Samilson, R. L., and Morris, J. M.: Surgical improvement of the cerebral-palsied upper limb, J. Bone Joint Surg. **46-A**:1203, 1964.

Schneider, L. H.: Opponensplasty using the extensor digiti minimi, J. Bone Joint Surg. **51-A**:1297, 1969.

Swanson, A. B.: Surgery of the hand in cerebral palsy with muscle origin release procedures, Surg. Clin. North Am. **48**:1129, 1968.

Thompson, T. C.: Modified operation for opponens paralysis, J. Bone Joint Surg. **24**:632, 1942.

Tubiana, R.: Anatomic and physiologic basis for the surgical treatment of paralyses of the hand, J. Bone Joint Surg. **51-A**:643, 1969.

Williams, R., and Haddad, R. J.: Release of flexor origin for spastic deformities of the wrist and hand, South. Med. J. **60**:1033, 1967.

Zancolli, E. A.: Claw-hand caused by paralysis of the intrinsic muscles. A simple surgical procedure for its correction, J. Bone Joint Surg. **39-A**:1076, 1957.

Extensor mechanism (including swan neck, boutonnière, intrinsic tightness)

Dolphin, J. A.: Extensor tenotomy for chronic boutonnière deformity of the finger. Report of two cases, J. Bone Joint Surg. **47-A**:161, 1965.

Goldner, J. L.: Deformities of the hand incidental to pathological changes of the extensor and intrinsic muscle mechanisms, J. Bone Joint Surg. **35-A**:115, 1953.

Harris, C., Jr., and Riordan, D. C.: Intrinsic contracture in the hand and its surgical treatment, J. Bone Joint Surg. **36-A**:10, 1954.

Heywood, A. W. B.: Correction of the rheumatoid boutonnière deformity, J. Bone Joint Surg. **51-A**:1309, 1969.

Kaplan, E. B.: Anatomy, injuries and treatment of the extensor apparatus of the hand and the digits, Clin. Orthop. **13**:24, 1959.

Littler, J. W.: Quoted by Harris, C., and Riordan, D. C.: Intrinsic contracture in the hand and its surgical treatment, J. Bone Joint Surg. **36-A**:10, 1954.

Littler, J. W.: Restoration of the oblique retinacular ligament for correction of hyperextension-deformity of the proximal interphalangeal joint. In Fourniee, A., editor: La Main Rheumatismale, Paris, 1966, Expansion Scientifique Française.

Littler, J. W.: The finger extensor mechanism, Surg. Clin. North Am. **47**:415-432, 1967.

Littler, J. W., and Cooley, S. G. E.: Restoration of the retinacular system in hyperextension deformity of the interphalangeal joint (in Proceedings of the American Society for Surgery of the Hand), J. Bone Joint Surg. **47-A**:637, 1965.

Littler, J. W., and Eaton, R. G.: Redistribution of forces in the correction of the boutonniere deformity, J. Bone Joint Surg. **49-A**:1267, 1967.

Nalebuff, E. A., and Millender, L. H.: Surgical treatment of the swan-neck deformity in rheumatoid arthritis, Orthop. Clin. North Am. **6**:733, 1975.

Nalebuff, E. A., and Millender, L. H.: Surgical treatment of the boutonniere deformity in rheumatoid arthritis, Orthop. Clin. North Am. **6**:753, 1975.

Schenck, R.: Variations of the extensor tendons of the fingers—surgical significance, J. Bone Joint Surg. **46-A**:103, 1964.

Souter, W. A.: The boutonniere deformity. A review of 101 patients with division of the central slip of the extensor expansion of the fingers, J. Bone Joint Surg. **49-B**:710, 1967.

Swanson, A. B.: Surgery of the hand in cerebral palsy and the swan-neck deformity, J. Bone Joint Surg. **42-A**:951, 1960.

Tubiana, R., and Valentin, P.: The physiology of the extension of the fingers, Surg. Clin. North Am. **44**:909, 1964.

Dupuytren's contracture

Boyes, J. H., and Jones, F. E.: Dupuytren's disease involving the volar aspect of the wrist, Plast. Reconstr. Surg. **41**:204, 1968.

Browne, W. E.: Dupuytren's contracture. A report of surgical correction in 83 cases (1945-1957), Clin. Orthop. **13**:255, 1959.

Burton, R. I., and Littler, J. W.: Dupuytren's contracture, Curr. Probl. Surg., pp. 44-51, July, 1975.

Conway, H.: Dupuytren's contracture, Am. J. Surg. **87**:101, 1954.

Dupuytren, G.: Permanent retraction of the fingers produced by an affection of the palmar fascia, Lancet **2**:222, 1834.

Freehafer, A. A., and Strong, J. M.: The treatment of Dupuytren's contracture by partial fasciectomy, J. Bone Joint Surg. **45-A**:1207, 1963.

Heuston, J. T.: Limited fasciectomy for Dupuytren's contracture, Plast. Reconstr. Surg., **27**:569, 1961.

Heuston, J. T.: Dupuytren's contracture, Edinburgh, 1963, E & S Livingstone, Ltd.

Honner, R., Lamb, D. W., and James, J. I. P.: Dupuytren's contracture. Long term results after fasciectomy, J. Bone Joint Surg. **53-B**:240, 1971.

Howard, L. D., Jr.: Dupuytren's contracture; a guide for management, Clin. Orthop. **15**:118, 1959.

Kanavel, A. B., Koch, S. L., and Mason, M. L.: Dupuytren's contracture with a description of the palmar fascia. A review of the literature and a report of 29 surgically treated cases, Surg. Gynecol. Obstet. **48**:145, 1929.

Kaplan, E. B.: Palmar fascia in connection with Dupuytren's contracture, Surgery **4**:415, 1938.

Larsen, R. D., and Posch, J. L.: Dupuytren's contracture, Int. Abstr. Surg. **115**:1, 1962. In Surg. Gynecol. Obstet. **115(1)**, 1962.

Luck, J. V.: Dupuytren's contracture: a new concept of the pathogenesis correlated with surgical management, J. Bone Joint Surg. **41-A**:635, 1959.

MacCallum, P., and Hueston, J. T.: The pathology of Dupuytren's contracture, Aust. N. Z. J. Surg. **31**:241, 1962.

Madden, J.: On "the contractile fibroblast," editorial, Plast. Reconstr. Surg. **52**:291, 1973.

McCash, C. R.: The open palm technique in Dupuytren's contracture, Br. J. Plast. Surg. **17**:271, 1964.

McFarland, R. M.: Patterns of the disease fascia in the fingers in Dupuytren's contracture. Displacement of the neurovascular bundle, Plast. Reconstr. Surg. **54**:31, 1974.

McFarland, R. M., and Jamieson, W. G.: Dupuytren's contracture. The management of 100 patients, J. Bone Joint Surg. **48-A**:1095, 1966.

Meyerding, H. W., Black, J. R., and Broders, A. C.: The etiology and pathology of Dupuytren's contracture, Surg. Gynecol. Obstet. **72**:582, 1941.

Riordan, D. C.: Dupuytren's contracture, South. Med. J. **54**:1391, 1961.

Rodrigo, J. J., Niebauer, J. J., Brown, R. L., and Doyle, J. R.: Treatment of Dupuytren's contracture. Long term results after fasciotomy and fascial excision, J. Bone Joint Surg. **58-A**:380, 1976.

Skoog, T.: Dupuytren's contraction, Acta Chir. Scand. (Suppl.) **139**:9, 1948.

Skoog, T.: Dupuytren's contracture: pathogenesis and surgical treatment, Surg. Clin. North Am. **47**:433, 1967.

Stack, H. G.: The palmar fascia, Edinburgh, 1973, Churchill Livingstone.

Tubiana, R.: Limited and extensive operation in Dupuytren's contracture, Surg. Clin. North Am. **44**:1071, 1964.

Tubiana, R., and Heuston, J. T.: La maladie de Dupuytren, monographies du groupe d'étude de la main, Paris, 1972, L'Expansion Scientifique Française.

Arthritis—general

Bunnell, S.: Surgery of the rheumatic hand, J. Bone Joint Surg. **37-A**:759, 1955.

Burton, R. I.: Other arthritides. In Kilgore, E. S., and Graham, W. P., editors: The hand, surgical and nonsurgical management, Philadelphia, 1977, Lea & Febiger.

Burton, R. I.: The rheumatoid hand, In Kilgore, E. S., and Graham, W. P., editors: The hand, surgical and nonsurgical management, Philadelphia, 1977, Lea & Febiger, pp. 388-428.

Clayton, M. L.: Surgery of the rheumatoid hand, Clin. Orthop. **36**:47, 1964.

Henderson, E. W., and Lipscomb, P. R.: Surgical tretament of the rheumatoid hand, J.A.M.A. **175**:431, 1961.

Laine, V. A., Sairanin, E., and Vainio, K.: Finger deformities caused by rheumatoid arthritis, J. Bone Joint Surg. **39-A**:527, 1957.

Linscheid, R. L.: Surgery for rheumatoid arthritis—timing and techniques: the upper extremity, J. Bone Joint Surg. **50-A**:605, 1968.

Lipscomb, P. R.: Surgery for rheumatoid arthritis—timing and techniques; summary, J. Bone Joint Surg. **50-A**:614, 1968.

Marmor, L.: The role of hand surgery in rheumatoid arthritis, Surg. Gynecol. Obstet. **116**:335, 1963.

Riordan, D. C., and Fowler, S. B.: Surgical treatment of rheumatoid deformity of the hand, J. Bone Joint Surg. **40-A**:1431, 1958.

Straub, L. R.: The rheumatoid hand, Clin. Orthop. **15**:127, 1959.

Arthritis—joints

Beckenbaugh, R. D., Dobyns, J. H., Linscheid, R. L., and Bryan, R. S.: Review and analysis of silicone-rubber metacarpophalangeal implants, J. Bone Joint Surg. **58-A**:483, 1976.

Brannon, E. W.: Replacement arthroplasty in military patients, Milit. Med. **121**:325, 1957.

Brewerton, D. A.: Pathological anatomy of rheumatoid finger joints. Hand, **3**:121, 1971.

Burton, R. I.: Small joint arthrodesis in the hand, In Kilgore, E. S., and Graham, W. P., editors: The hand, surgical and nonsurgical management, Philadelphia, 1977, Lea & Febiger, pp. 155-162.

Carroll, R. E.: Small joint arthrodesis in hand reconstruction, J. Bone Joint Surg. **51-A**:1219, 1969.

Carroll, R. W., and Hill, N. A.: Small joint arthrodesis in hand reconstruction, J. Bone Joint Surg. **51-A**:1219, 1969.

Carroll, R. E., and Taber, T. H.: Digital arthroplasty of the proximal interphalangeal joint, J. Bone Joint Surg. **36-A:**912, 1954.

Ellison, M. R., Kelly, K. J., and Flatt, A. E.: The results of surgical synovectomy of the digital joints in rheumatoid disease, J. Bone Joint Surg. **53-A:**1041, 1971.

Flatt, A. E.: Restoration of rheumatoid finger joint function: interim report on trial of prosthetic replacement, J. Bone Joint Surg. **43-A:**753, 1961.

Flatt, A. E.: Restoration of rheumatoid finger-joint function, J. Bone Joint Surg. **45-A:**1101, 1963.

Flatt, A. E.: Prosthetic substitution for theumatoid finger joints, Plast. Reconstr. Surg. **40:**565, 1967.

Flatt, A. E.: Prosthetic replacement of joints in the rheumatoid hand. In Tubiana, R., editor: La Main Rheumatoide, Paris, 1969, L'Expansion Scientifique Française.

Flatt, A. E.: Studies in finger joint replacement. A review of the present position, Arch. Surg. **107:**437, 1973.

Flatt, A. E., and Ellison, M. R.: Restoration of rheumatoid finger joint function. III. A follow up note after fourteen years of experience with a metallic-hinge implant, J. Bone Joint Surg. **54-A:**1317, 1972.

Fowler, S. B.: Arthroplasty of the metacarpophalangeal joint in rheumatoid arthritis, J. Bone Joint Surg. **44-A:**1037, 1962.

Girzadas, D. V., and Clayton, M. D.: Limitations of the use of metallic prosthesis in the rheumatoid hand, Clin. Orthop. **67:**127, 1969.

Goldner, J. L., Gould, J. S., Urbaniak, J. R., and McCollum, D. E.: Metacarpophalangeal joint arthroplasty with silicone-Dacron prostheses (Niebauer type): six and a half years' experience, J. Hand Surg. **2:**200, 1977.

Granowitz, S., and Vainio, K.: Proximal interphalangeal joint arthrodesis in rheumatoid arthritis. A follow up study of 122 operations, Acta Orthop. Scand. **37:**301, 1966.

Hakstian, R. W., and Tubiana, R.: Ulnar deviation of the fingers. The role of joint structure and function, J. Bone Joint Surg. **49-A:**299, 1967.

Kettelkamp, D. B., Alexander, H. H., and Dolan, J.: A comparison of experimental arthroplasty and metacarpal head replacement, J. Bone Joint Surg. **50-A:**1564, 1968.

Kuczynski, K.: The synovial structures of the normal and rheumatoid digital joints, Hand **3:**41, 1971.

Laine, V. A. I., Sairanen, E., and Vainio, K.: Finger deformities caused by rheumatoid arthritis, J. Bone Joint Surg. **39-A:**527, 1957.

Lipscomb, P. R.: Synovectomy of the distal two joints of the thumb and fingers in rheumatoid arthritis, J. Bone Joint Surg. **49-A:**1135, 1967.

Mannerfelt, L., and Andersson, K.: Silastic arthroplasty of the metacarpophalangeal joints in rheumatoid arthritis. Long-term results, J. Bone Joint Surg. **57-A:**484, 1975.

McMaster, M.: The natural history of the rheumatoid metacarpophalangeal joint, J. Bone Joint Surg. **54-B:**687, 1972.

Millender, L. H., and Nalebuff, E. A.: Metacarpophalangeal joint arthroplasty utilizing the silicone rubber prosthesis, Orthop. Clin. North Am. **4:**349, 1973.

Nalebuff, E. A.: Surgical treatment of finger deformities in the rheumatoid hand. Surg. Clin. North Am. **49:**833, 1969.

Niebauer, J. J., and Landry, R. M.: Dacron-silicone prosthesis for the metacarpophalangeal joints, Hand **3:**55, 1971.

Niebauer, J. J., Shaw, J. L., and Doren, W. W.: The silicone-Dacron hinge prosthesis: design, evaluation and application, J. Bone Joint Surg. **50-A:**634, 1968.

Shapiro, J. S.: The etiology of ulnar drift, J. Bone Joint Surg. **50-A:**634, 1968.

Smith, R. J., and Kaplan, E. B.: Rheumatoid deformities at the metacarpophalangeal joints of the fingers. A correlative study of anatomy and pathology, J. Bone Joint Surg. **49-A:**31, 1967.

Smith, R. J., and Kaplan, E. B.: Rheumatoid deformities at the metacarpophalangeal joints of the fingers, J. Bone Joint Surg. **49-A:**31, 1967.

Swanson, A. B.: Surgery of the hand in cerebral palsy and the swanneck deformity, J. Bone Joint Surg. **42-A:**951, 1960.

Swanson, A. B.: A flexible implant for replacement of arthritic or destroyed joints in the hand, New York Univ. Post-Grad. Med. Sch. Inter-Clin. Inform. Bull. **6:**16, 1966.

Swanson, A. B.: Silicone rubber implants for replacement of arthritis or destroyed joints in the hand, Surg. Clin. North Am. **48:**1113, 1968.

Swanson, A. B.: Finger joint replacement by silicone rubber implants and the concept of implant fixation by encapsulation, International Workshop on Artificial Finger Joints. Ann. Rheum. Dis. (Suppl.) **28:**47, 1969.

Swanson, A. B.: Flexible implant arthroplasty for arthritic finger joints. Rationale, technique and results of treatment, J. Bone Joint Surg. **54-A:**435, 1972.

Swanson, A. B.: Flexible implant resection arthroplasty, Hand, **4:**119, 1972.

Swanson, A. B. et al.: Durability of silicone implants—an in vivo study, Orthop. Clin. North Am. **4:**1097, 1973.

Vainio, K., and Oka, M.: Ulnar deviation of the fingers, Ann. Rheum. Dis. **12:**122, 1953.

Vainio, K., Reiman, I., and Pulkki, T.: Results of arthroplasty of the metacarpophalangeal joints in rheumatoid arthritis, Trauma, **9:**1, 1967.

Weeks, P. M.: Volar approach for metacarpophalangeal joint capsulotomy, Plast. Reconstr. Surg. **46:**473, 1970.

Arthritis—thumb

Aune, S. L.: Osteoarthritis in first carpo-metacarpal joint. An investigation of 22 cases, Acta Clin. Scand. **109:**449, 1955.

Burton, R. I.: Basal joint arthrosis of the thumb, Orthop. Clin. North Am. **4:**331, 1973.

Carroll, R. E., and Hill, N. A.: Carpo-metacarpal arthrodesis of the thumb: a clinical and cineroentgenographic study, presented at 27th Annual Meeting of the American Society for Surgery of the Hand, Washington, Jan., 1972.

Carroll, R. E., and Hill, N. A.: Arthrodesis of the carpometacarpal joint of the thumb, J. Bone Joint Surg. **55-B:**292, 1973.

Carstam, N., Fiken, O., and Andren, L.: Osteoarthritis of the trapezio-scaphoid joint, Acta Orthop. Scand. **39:**354, 1968.

Clayton, M. L.: Surgery of the thumb in rheumatoid arthritis, J. Bone Joint Surg. **44-A:**1376, 1962.

Eaton, R. G.: Joint Injuries of the Hand, Springfield, Ill., 1971, Charles C Thomas Publisher.

Eaton, R. G.: Replacement of the trapezium for arthritis of the basal articulations. A new technique with stabilization by tenodesis, J. Bone Joint Surg. **61-A:**76, 1979.

Eaton, R. G., and Littler, J. W.: A study of the basal joint of the thumb. Treatment of its disabilities by fusion, J. Bone Joint Surg. **51-A:**661, 1969.

Eaton, R. G., and Littler, J. W.: Ligament reconstruction for the painful thumb carpometacarpal joint, J. Bone Joint Surg. **55-A:**1655, 1973.

Froimson, A. I.: Tendon arthroplasty of the trapeziometacarpal joint, Clin. Orthop. **70**:191, 1970.

Gervis, W. H.: Excision of the trapezium for osteoarthritis of the trapeziometacarpal joint, J. Bone Joint Surg. **31-B**:537, 1949.

Goldner, J. L., and Clippinger, F. W.: Excision of the greater multangular bone as an adjunct to mobilization of the thumb, J. Bone Joint Surg. **41-A**:609, 1959.

Howard, L. D., Jr.: Contracture of the thumb web, J. Bone Joint Surg. **32-A**:267, 1950.

Inglis, A. E., Hamlin, C., Sengelmann, R. P., and Straub, L. R.: Reconstruction of the metacarpophalangeal joint of the thumb in rheumatoid arthritis, J. Bone Joint Surg. **54-A**:704, 1972.

Lasserre, C., Pauzat, D., and Derennes, R.: Osteoarthritis of the trapeziometacarpal joint, J. Bone Joint Surg. **31-B**:534, 1949.

Leach, R. E., and Bolton, P. E.: Arthritis of carpometacarpal joint of thumb: results of arthrodesis, J. Bone Joint Surg. **50-A**:1171, 1968.

Littler, J. W.: The prevention and the correction of adduction contractures of the thumb, Clin. Orthop. **13**:182, 1959.

McFarlane, R. M.: Observations on the functional anatomy of the intrinsic muscles of the thumb, J. Bone Joint Surg. **44-A**:1013, 1962.

Muller, G. M.: Arthrodesis of the trapezio-metacarpal joint for osteoarthritis, J. Bone Joint Surg. **31-B**:540, 1949.

Murley, A. H. G.: Excision of the trapezium in osteoarthritis of the first carpo-metacarpal joint, J. Bone Joint Surg. **42-B**:502, 1960.

Nalebuff, E. A.: Diagnosis, classification and management of rheumatoid thumb deformities, Bull. Hosp. Joint Dis. **29**:119, 1968.

Napier, J. R.: The form and function of the carpometacarpal joint of the thumb, J. Anat. **89**:362, 1955.

Stark, H. H., Moore, J. F., Ashworth, C. R., and Boyes, J. H.: Fusion of the first metacarpotrapezial joint for degenerative arthritis, J. Bone Joint Surg. **59-A**:22, 1977.

Swanson, A. B.: Disabling arthritis at the base of the thumb. Treatment by resection of the trapezium and flexible (silicone) implant arthroplasty, J. Bone Joint Surg. **54-A**:456, 1972.

Swanson, A. B., and Herndon, J. H.: Flexible (silicone) implant arthroplasty of the metacarpophalangeal joint of the thumb, J. Bone Joint Surg. **59-A**:362, 1977.

Thompson, T. C.: Discussion of paper by Goldner and Clippinger, J. Bone Joint Surg. **41-A**:625, 1959.

Arthritis—tendon systems

Backhouse, K. M.: Rheumatoid tenosynovial involvement in the hand, Hand **1**:7, 1969.

Ehrlich, G. E., Peterson, L. T., Sokoloff, L., and Bunin, J. J.: Pathogenesis of rupture of the extensor tendons at the wrist in rheumatoid arthritis, Arthritis Rheum. **2**:332, 1959.

Ellison, M. R., Flatt, A. E., and Kelly, K. J.: Ulnar drift of the fingers in rheumatoid disease. Treatment by crossed intrinsic tendon transfer, J. Bone Joint Surg. **53-A**:1061, 1971.

Kellgren, J. H., and Ball, J.: Tendon lesions in rheumatoid arthritis: clinico-pathological study, Ann. Rheum. Dis. **9**:48, 1950.

Laine, V. A. I., and Vaino, K. J.: Spontaneous ruptures of tendons in rheumatoid arthritis, Acta Orthop. Scand. **24**:250, 1955.

Littler, J. W., Burton, R. I., and Eaton, R. G.: The dynamics of finger extension, Am. Acad Orthop. Surg. Sound Slide Program #467, 468, 1976.

Mannerfelt, L., and Norman, O.: Attrition ruptures of flexor tendons in rheumatoid arthritis caused by bony spurs in the carpal tunnel; a clinical and radiological study, J. Bone Joint Surg. **51-B**:270, 1969.

Millender, L. H., and Nalebuff, E. A.: Preventive surgery—tenosynovectomy and synovectomy, Orthop. Clin. North Am. **6**:765, 1975.

Nalebuff, E. A.: Surgical treatment of rheumatoid tenosynovitis in the hand, Surg. Clin. North Am. **49**:799, 1969.

Nalebuff, E. A.: Surgical treatment of tendon rupture in the rheumatoid hand, Surg. Clin. North Am. **49**:811, 1969.

Nalebuff, E. A., and Potter, R. A.: Rheumatoid involvement of tendon and tendon sheaths in the hand, Clin. Orthop. **59**:147, 1968.

Potter, T. A., and Kuhns, J. G.: Rheumatoid tenosynovitis. Diagnosis and treatment, J. Bone Joint Surg. **40-A**:1230, 1958.

Stellbrink, G.: Trigger finger syndrome in rheumatoid arthritis not caused by flexor tendon nodules, Hand **3**:76, 1971.

Straub, L. R., and Wilson, E. H.: Spontaneous rupture of extensor tendons in the hand associated with rheumatoid arthritis, J. Bone Joint Surg. **38-A**:1208, 1956.

Stuart, D.: Duration of splinting after repair of extensor tendons in the hand. A clinical study, J. Bone Joint Surg. **47-B**:72, 1965.

Vainio, K.: Carpal canal syndrome caused by tenosynovitis, Acta Rheumatol. Scand. **4**:22, 1957.

Vaughan-Jackson, O. J.: Rupture of extensor tendons by attrition at the inferior radio-ulnar joint. Report of two cases, J. Bone Joint Surg. **30-B**:528, 1948.

Vaughan-Jackson, O. J.: Attrition ruptures of tendons in the rheumatoid hand, J. Bone Joint Surg. **40-A**:1431, 1958.

Wissinger, A.: Digital flexor lag in rheumatoid arthritis, Plast. Reconstr. Surg. **47**:465, 1971.

Infections

Flynn, J. E.: Clinical and anatomic investigations of deep fascial space infections, Am. J. Surg. **55**:467, 1942.

Kanavel, A. B.: Infections of the hand. A guide to the surgical treatment of acute and chronic suppurative processes in the fingers, hand and forearm, ed. 6, Philadelphia, 1933, Lea & Febiger.

Miscellaneous conditions

Fahey, J. J., and Bollinger, J. A.: Trigger-finger in adults and children, J. Bone Joint Surg. **36-A**:1200, 1954.

Flynn, J. E.: Adduction contracture of the thumb, N. Engl. J. Med. **254**:677, 1956.

Lapidus, P. W., and Fenton, R.: Stenosing tenovaginitis at the wrist and fingers, Arch. Surg. **64**:475, 1952.

Littler, J. W.: The prevention and the correction of adduction contracture of the thumb, Clin. Orthop. **13**:182, 1959.

Littler, J. W.: The craft of surgery. In Cooper, P., editor: The hand, ed. 2, Boston, 1971, Little, Brown & Co.

Sprecher, E. E.: Trigger thumb in infants, J. Bone Joint Surg. **31-A**:672, 1949.

7

NECK AND CERVICAL SPINE

RELEASE OF STERNOCLEIDOMASTOID FOR TORTICOLLIS (Plate 7-1)

GENERAL DISCUSSION. Congenital torticollis that is evident shortly after birth and is unrelated to underlying cervical spine or visual disturbances will vary considerably in the degree of severity. Some of the patients require surgical treatment if the associated deformities of neglected torticollis are to be prevented.

The majority of the deformities will resolve with conservative management. Operative treatment is indicated occasionally in infants or young children who have persistent deformity caused by unrelieved contracture of the sternocleidomastoid muscle.

DETAILS OF PROCEDURE. A transverse incision is made just above the clavicle (**A**). The underlying platysma is cut in line with the skin incision to expose the tumor (**B**). If there is a tumor, it and both portions of the sternocleidomastoid insertion are carefully isolated. The sternal and clavicular attachments of the muscle are identified, isolated, and sectioned, and the tumor, if present, is excised (**C** and **D**). Care must be taken to protect the spinal accessory nerve, which pierces the sternocleidomastoid muscle in its upper portion to innervate this muscle. (The remainder of this nerve emerges beneath the posterior border of the sternocleidomastoid muscle at the junction of its upper and middle thirds, and passes almost vertically downward to disappear beneath the anterior border of the trapezius muscle.) The external jugular vein is encountered at the posterior border of the muscle. The wound is closed with a few interrupted sutures for subcutaneous tissue and skin.

POSTOPERATIVE MANAGEMENT. No immobilization is used immediately postoperatively, but a modified Minerva jacket is applied with the head held in the overcorrected position (**E**) 5 to 7 days after surgery. The Minerva jacket is maintained for 6 weeks. In the older child the sternocleidomastoid muscle is sectioned proximally in addition to the division of the sternal and clavicular attachments distally, but the postoperative management is the same. In all cases, exercises are performed for several months after the cast is removed.

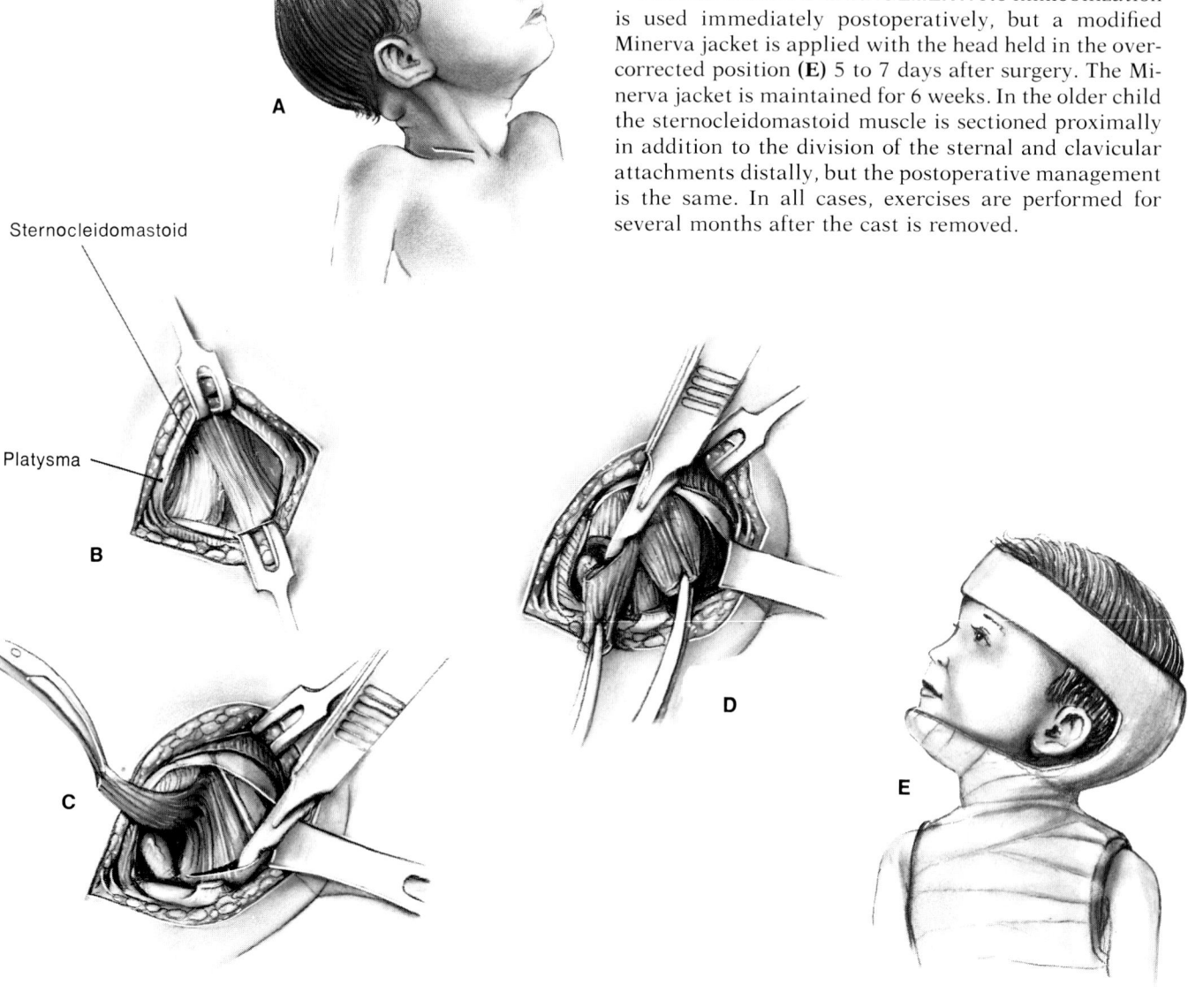

(Plate 7-2) RELEASE OF SCALENUS ANTERIOR MUSCLE

GENERAL DISCUSSION. Irritation or compression of the nerves and the blood supply to the arm may occur at a number of sites in the base of the neck and may be due to a variety of causes. Conditions in the neck producing neurovascular symptoms are sometimes lumped together as "thoracic outlet syndrome."

An anatomic anomaly producing compression may be a cervical rib or an elongated transverse process of the seventh cervical vertebra. The next most frequent anomaly may be compression of the neurovascular bundle by the anterior scalene muscle, the medial scalene muscle, or fibrous bands. At the distal end of the subclavian region the pectoralis minor muscle or an anomalous coracoid process may rarely also compress the neurovascular bundle.

In spite of the attractiveness of simplification afforded by assigning the first rib as a common denominator for all neurovascular compression syndromes involving the upper extremity, the surgeon should make every effort to determine the exact site of compression. The operative procedure is then determined accordingly. Unfortunately, the symptoms produced by irritation or compression at the various potential sites are usually neither uniquely characteristic nor diagnostic of the underlying pathology. The majority of these patients will have a positive Adson sign, a few will have diminution or absence of peripheral pulse, and even fewer will have evidence of venous obstruction.

Surgical correction is indicated only after a trial of nonoperative treatment, and then only if there are objective findings of vascular and/or nerve trunk irritation.

DETAILS OF PROCEDURE. A transverse skin incision is made over the supraclavicular fossa **(A)**. The sternocleidomastoid muscle can usually be retracted medially (**B** and **C**). The external jugular vein is ligated and divided.

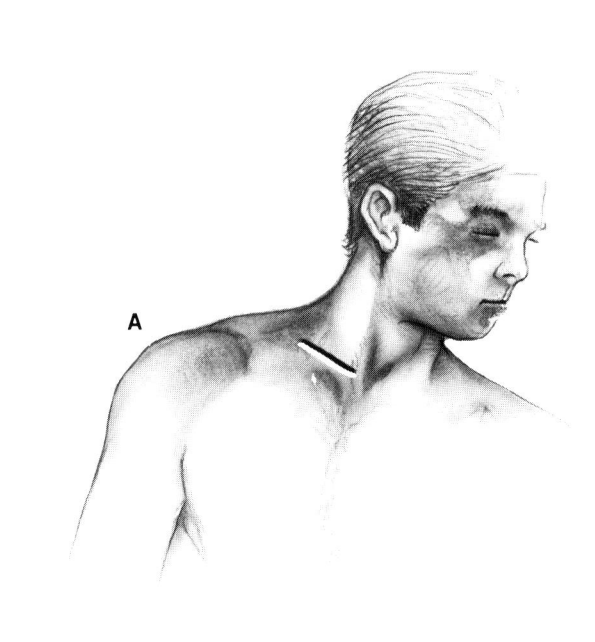

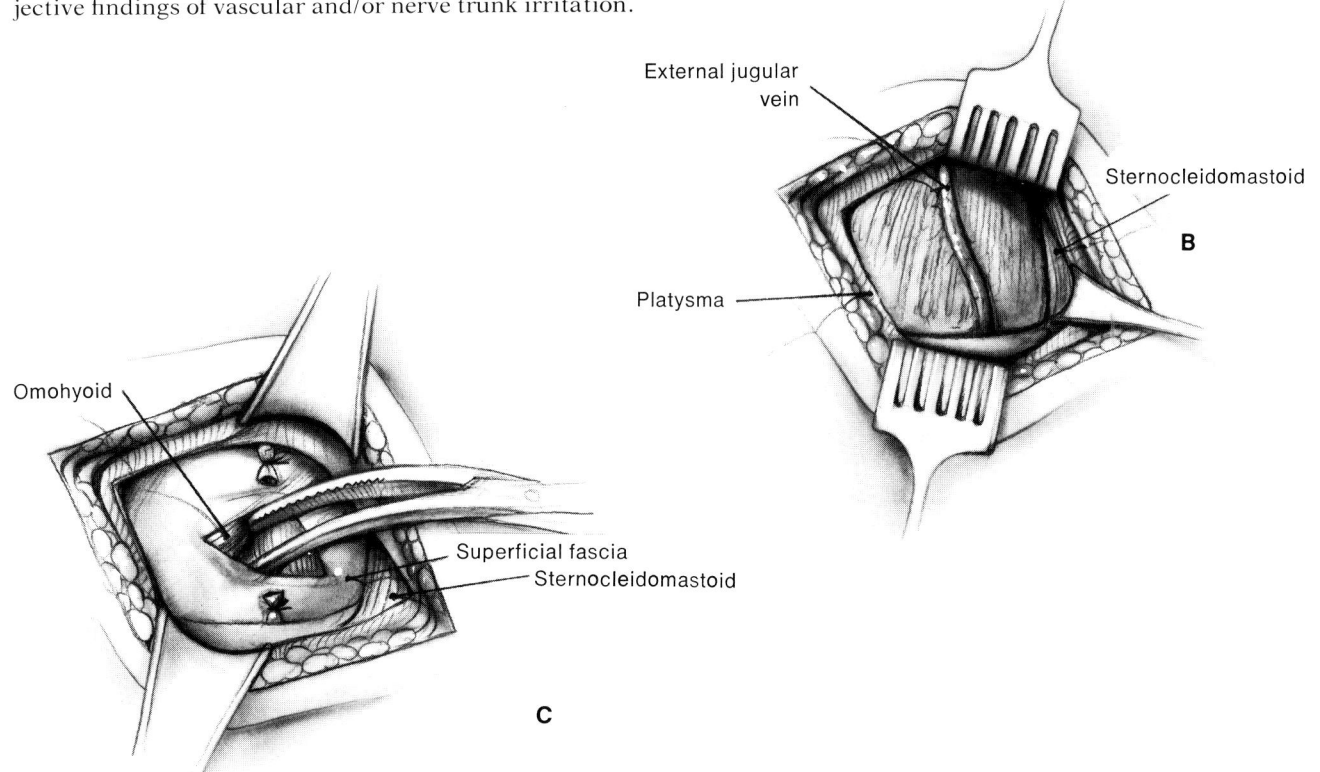

RELEASE OF SCALENUS ANTERIOR MUSCLE (Plate 7-2)

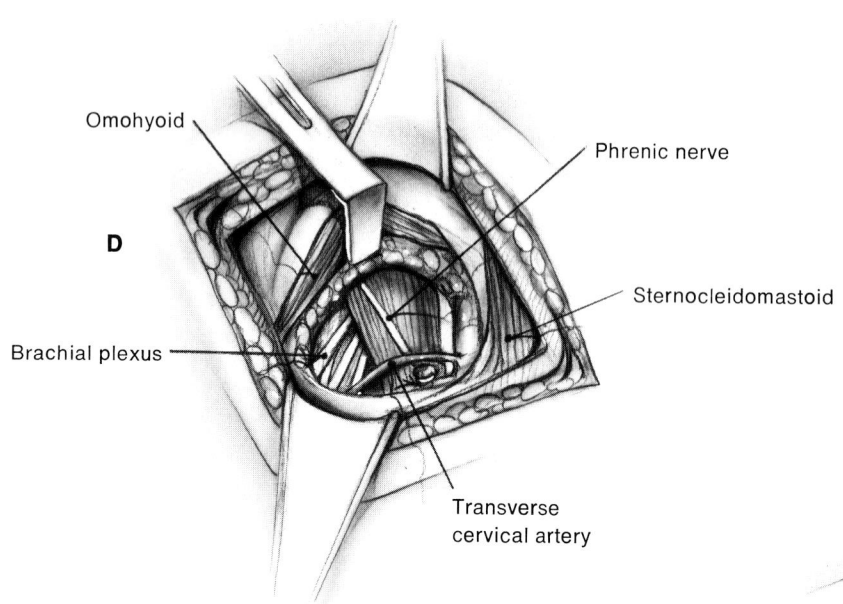

The transverse cervical artery and the transverse scapular artery lie anterior to the anterior scalene muscle, and, if necessary, these are ligated and divided. The inferior portion of the omohyoid muscle crosses the field obliquely immediately above the transverse cervical artery. The omohyoid muscle can usually be retracted superiorly and laterally out of the way, but may be divided if necessary **(D)**. The phrenic nerve descends downward along the anterior border of the anterior scalene muscle and must be isolated and gently retracted **(E)**. With care to protect the subclavian artery, which is posterior to the anterior scalene, and the branches of the brachial plexus between the anterior scalene muscle and the medial scalene, the anterior scalene muscle is transected just above its attachment to the first rib **(F)**. The anterior scalene muscle usually inserts onto the anterior portion of the first thoracic rib, but if a cervical rib is present, it occasionally inserts on the cervical rib. If no cervical rib is present, the trunks of the brachial plexus should be inspected to be sure they are free of restriction by any fibrous bands, aberrant scalene muscles, or elongated transverse process of the seventh cervical vertebra. Particular attention to good hemostasis is important. Following wound closure, a small dressing is applied and the arm is protected in a sling.

POSTOPERATIVE MANAGEMENT. Protection of the arm in a sling is continued for 5 to 7 days postoperatively. Active rotation of the head toward the involved side is encouraged as the wound discomfort subsides.

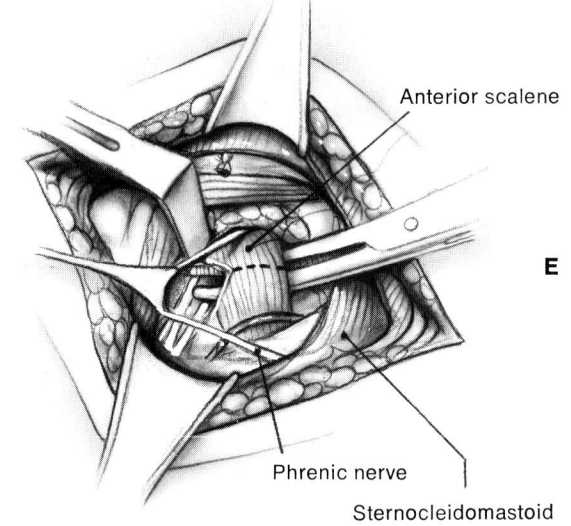

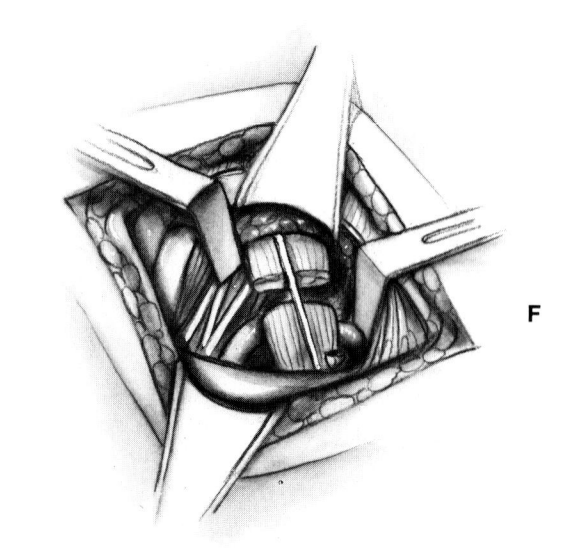

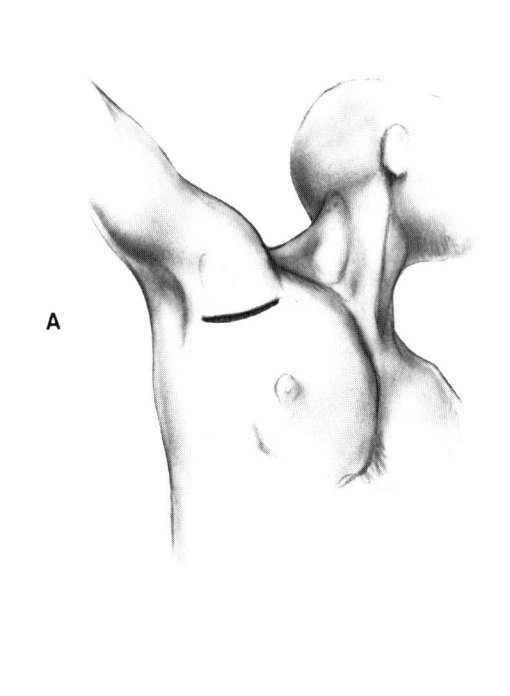

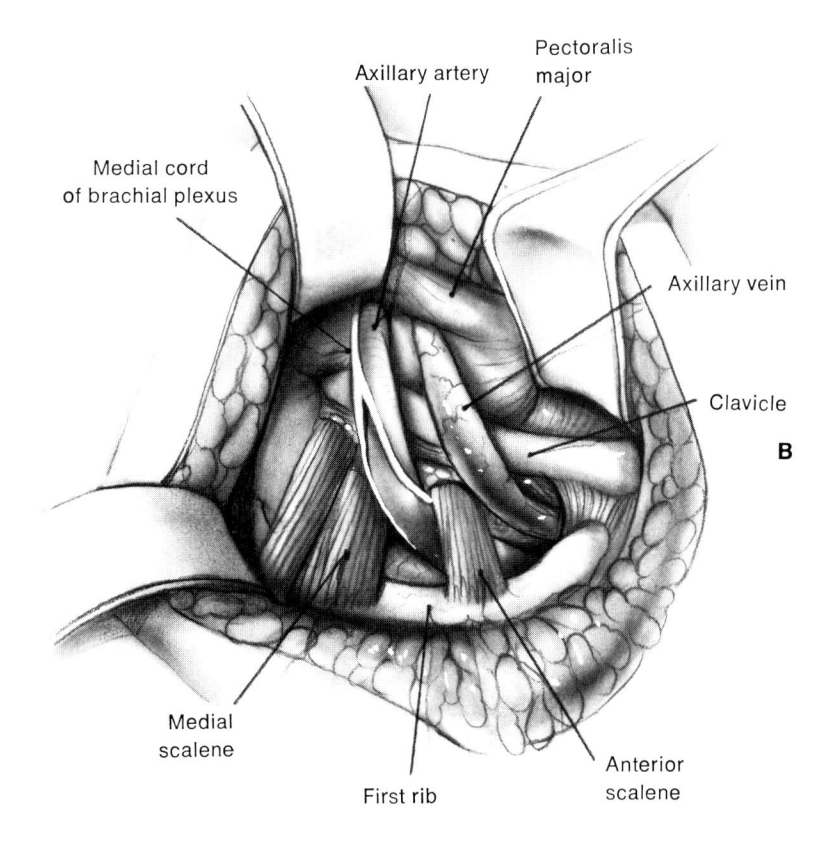

(Plate 7-3) RESECTION OF FIRST RIB (AXILLARY APPROACH)

GENERAL DISCUSSION. Symptoms of a thoracic outlet syndrome may be caused by neurovascular compression due to a decrease in the size of the opening between the clavicle and the first rib. This may be postural or secondary to space-occupying lesions, including malunion or pseudarthrosis of clavicular fractures or tumors of the clavicle or first rib. The presence of a cervical rib may also contribute to encroachment on the thoracic outlet.

The diagnosis of costoclavicular compression syndrome should be considered when obliteration or diminution of the radial pulse occurs with abduction of the shoulder beyond 90° to 100°. False positive obliteration of the radial pulse can be produced by abducting and extending the shoulder, and it can also occur in asymptomatic individuals. There may be a bruit, best heard below the clavicle. Before considering operation, other causes of cervicobrachial pain should be ruled out. When there is conclusive evidence of costoclavicular compression syndrome and conservative efforts to relieve symptoms with postural exercises to elevate the shoulder girdle have failed, operative removal of the first rib may be indicated.

For those few cases requiring excision of the first rib, resection of the first rib through the transaxillary approach as described by Roos has the following advantages. The operation is technically easier and shorter through the transaxillary approach, which permits safer and clearer exposure of the entire first rib, major vessels, and nerves. There is little blood loss through this approach, and there are no major muscles to divide or repair. Complete rib resection can be carried out under direct vision. There is good proximal control in case of major vessel injury. Closure of the wound is simple and quick. Postoperative shoulder disability is minimal, and the postoperative axillary scar is small and inconspicuous.

DETAILS OF PROCEDURE. The patient is placed in a lateral position on the unaffected side. The entire upper extremity, the chest, and the base of the neck are prepped so that the arm can be completely elevated and manipulated by an assistant. With the arm fully abducted a transverse incision is made in the inferior portion of the axilla **(A)**. The dissection is continued directly toward the thorax paralleling the third rib. When the plane of loose areolar tissue is reached on the surface of the rib cage and the serratus anterior muscle, the dissection is redirected superiorly in this plane deep to the axillary fascia to expose the first rib **(B)**. The intercostobrachial cutaneous nerve, which courses from the second intercostal space to the axilla, is isolated and retracted.

195

(Plate 7-3) RESECTION OF FIRST RIB (AXILLARY APPROACH)

With the shoulder abducted and the elbow flexed 90°, an assistant should exert traction on the limb directly toward the ceiling. This will open the thoracic outlet and expose the important structures that cross over the first rib. During the subsequent dissection, the limb should be retained in this position except for lowering it occasionally to temporarily relieve tension on the muscles and the brachial plexus. Care must be taken to avoid any excessive traction on the brachial plexus or the cervical nerve roots. The areolar tissue is removed from the first rib by blunt dissection. The brachial plexus should be identified posteriorly, the sbuclavian vein anteriorly, and the subclavian artery and scalenus anterior muscle in the middle of the wound. The pectoralis major muscle is retracted anteriorly and the latissimus dorsi muscle posteriorly to improve the exposure. The insertions of the subclavius, scalenus anterior **(C),** and the scalenus medius muscles are isolated and carefully divided at their insertions onto the first rib.

Over the superior surface of the first rib the periosteum is incised in line with the rib and is carefully elevated **(D).** Care must be taken to avoid damage to the parietal pleura. With the subclavian vein and brachial plexus in view, the first rib is divided anteriorly through its costal cartilage **(E)** and then posteriorly at its junction with the transverse process. If a cervical rib is present, it should be resected as far posteriorly as the transverse process in addition to resection of any fibrous band attached to it.

Before the wound is closed, the pleura should be inspected. If the pleura is opened inadvertently, it can be closed about an inserted catheter, which is then attached to a water-seal drainage system for a few hours to ensure expansion of the lung. The wound is closed by suturing the subcutaneous fascia and skin.

C

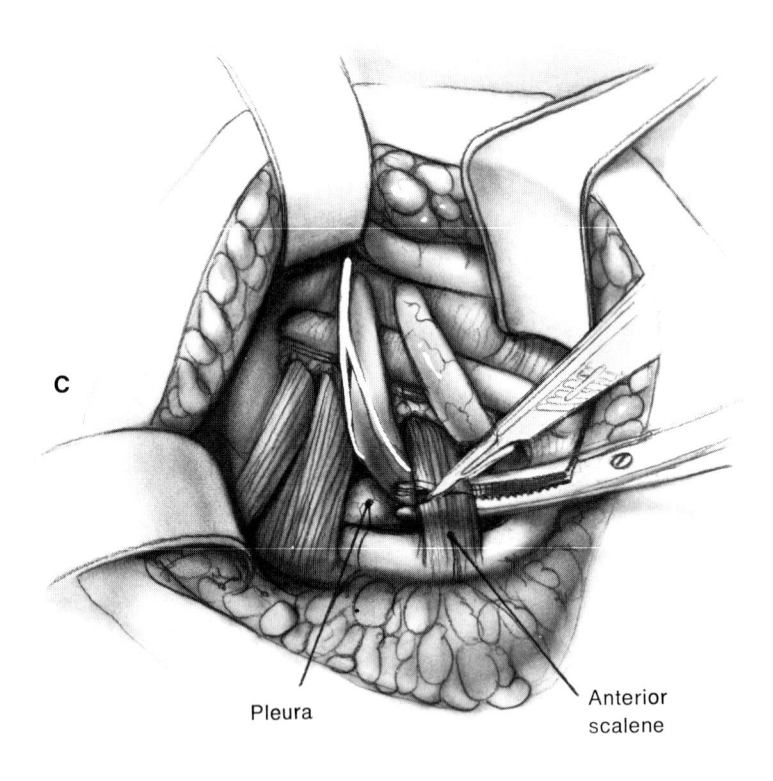

Pleura

Anterior scalene

RESECTION OF FIRST RIB (AXILLARY APPROACH) (Plate 7-3)

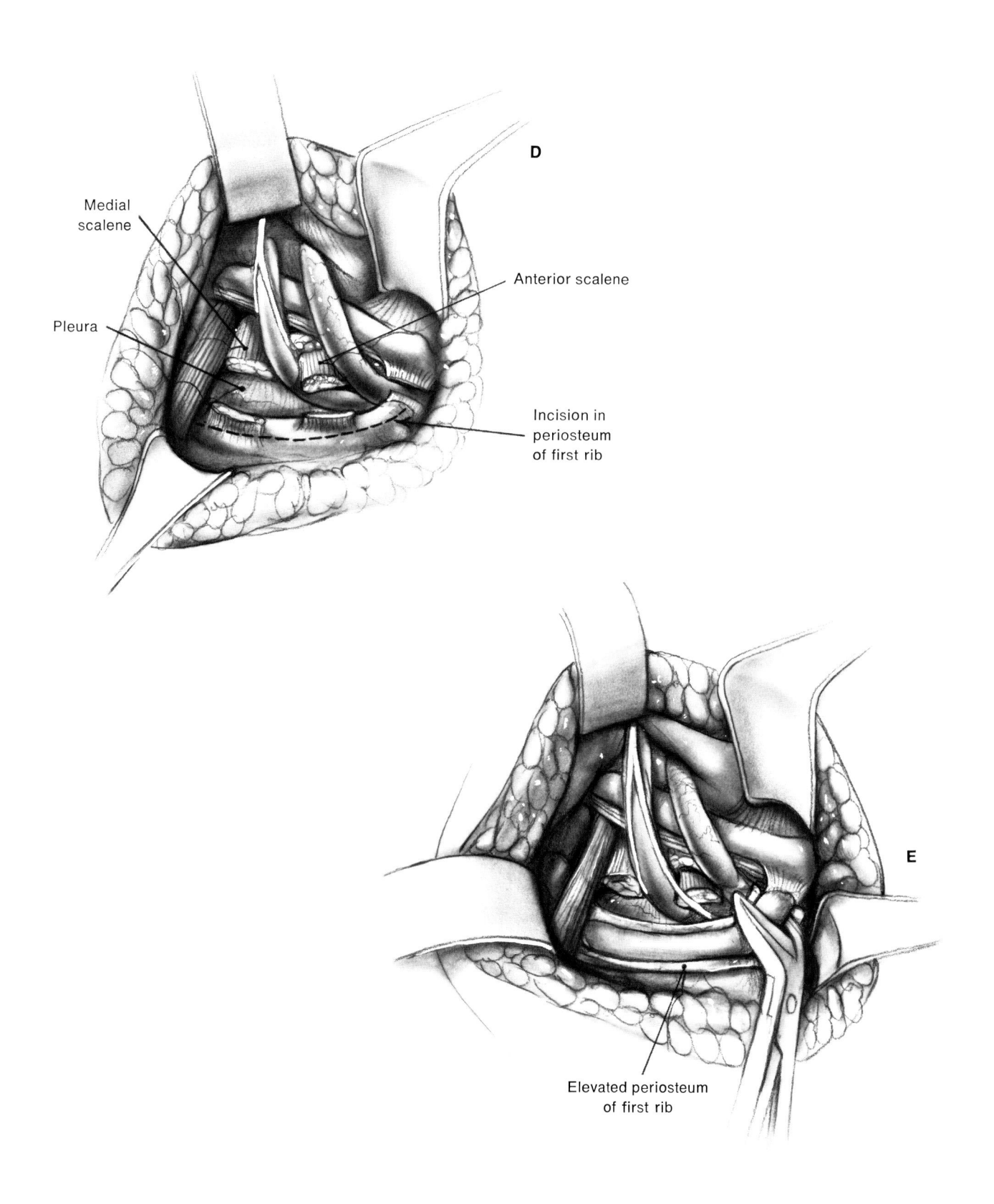

D

Medial scalene

Pleura

Anterior scalene

Incision in periosteum of first rib

E

Elevated periosteum of first rib

197

POSTERIOR CERVICAL SPINE FUSION

GENERAL DISCUSSION. Posterior cervical spine fusion may be performed when there is instability of the cervical spine. The instability may be at the occipito-atlantal, atlantoaxial, or lower cervical spine. The instability may be due to a variety of causes, such as congenital anomaly, trauma, neoplasia, rheumatoid arthritis, or extensive laminectomy.

DETAILS OF PROCEDURE. When posterior spine fusion is indicated, the patient's cervical spine is immobilized initially with either the halocast or halojacket. The latter is preferred when the patient is a quadriplegic or an elderly rheumatoid. This form of immobilization is effective because it allows for (1) preoperative alignment of the spine, (2) support during nasotracheal intubation and turning under anesthesia, (3) support of the unstable spine during the operative procedure, and (4) continued external immobilization after surgery until fusion is solid, usually in 12 weeks. Internal fixation with wire is used to hold the bone graft in place and also to help in stabilizing the spine.

Autogenous iliac bone graft is used whenever possible. Decortication of the spinous processes, laminae, and facets in an unstable cervical spine can be hazardous when a gouge and mallet are used. Decortication should be performed with a power burr followed by use of rongeurs.

(Plate 7-4) OCCIPITOCERVICAL FUSION

GENERAL DISCUSSION. Occipitocervical fusion is indicated for instability of the occipitoatlantal articulation due to rheumatoid arthritis, trauma, congenital anomaly, and other causes.

DETAILS OF PROCEDURE. The patient is already immobilized in either a halovest or a halocast. Endotracheal intubation is carried out. The patient is turned onto a spine frame. The posterior half of the vest is removed, with the uprights attached to the anterior half of the vest still supporting the cervical spine (**A** to **C**). When the halocast is used, the two posterior uprights are removed, leaving the two anterior upright bars connected to the halocast for support of the cervical spine. With the halovest, there is enough room to allow for draping of the posterior ilium for harvesting of bone graft.

To make it possible to harvest bone in a patient with a halocast, the cast must be cut out appropriately over the posterior ilium on one side. This is done before the patient is anesthetized. The neck and the iliac donor sites are prepared and draped. A midline incision is made from the occiput to the midcervical level. The incision is carried deeper through the ligamentum nuchae, and the paracervical muscles are held retracted with self-retaining retractors. Staying in the midline will cause less bleeding. The spinous process of the C2 vertebra, which is usually very prominent, is easily palpable and identified. The posterior arch of the atlas is at a deeper level and may not be readily palpable until sharp dissection of the musculotendinous attachments to the spinous process of C2 has been carried out. The occiput is exposed subperiosteally approximately 2.5 cm to each side of the midline (**D**). The arch of C1 is exposed subperiosteally no more than 2 cm to each side of the midline to avoid injury to the vertebral arteries and veins.

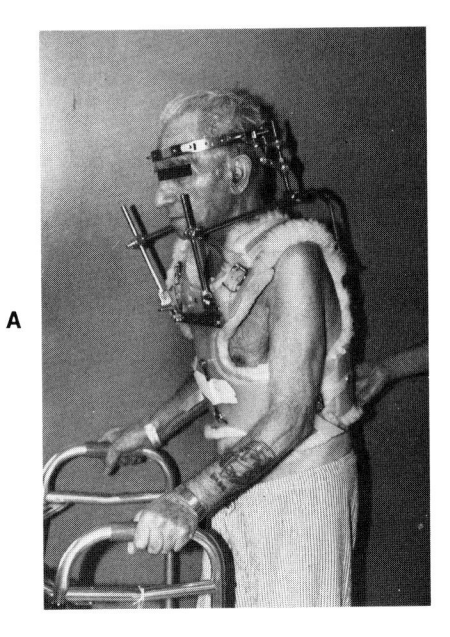

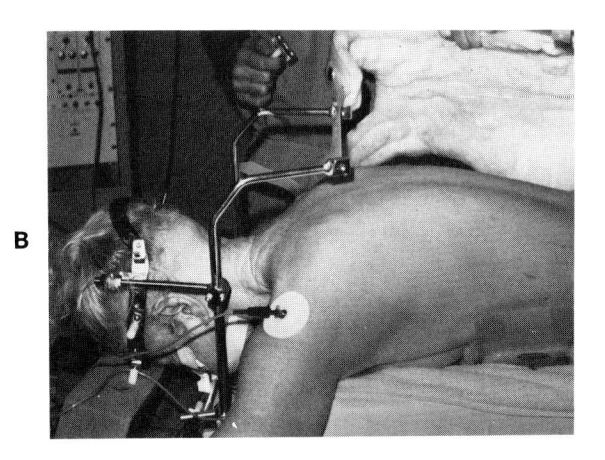

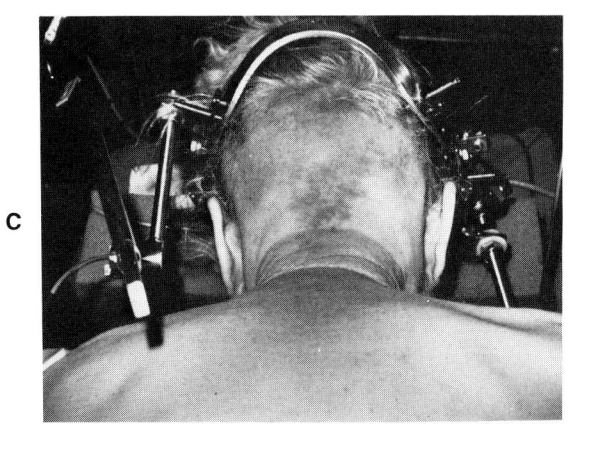

199

OCCIPITOCERVICAL FUSION (Plate 7-4)

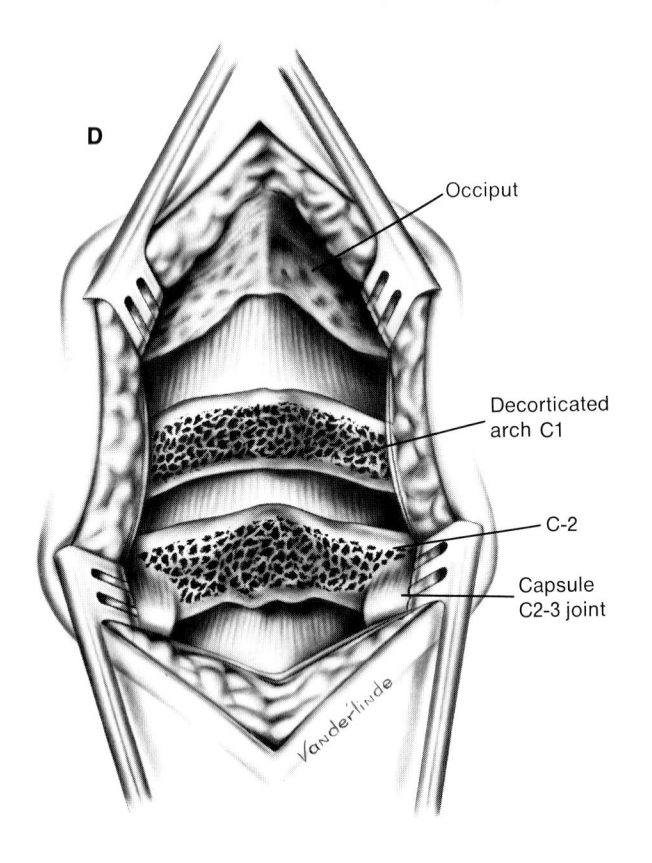

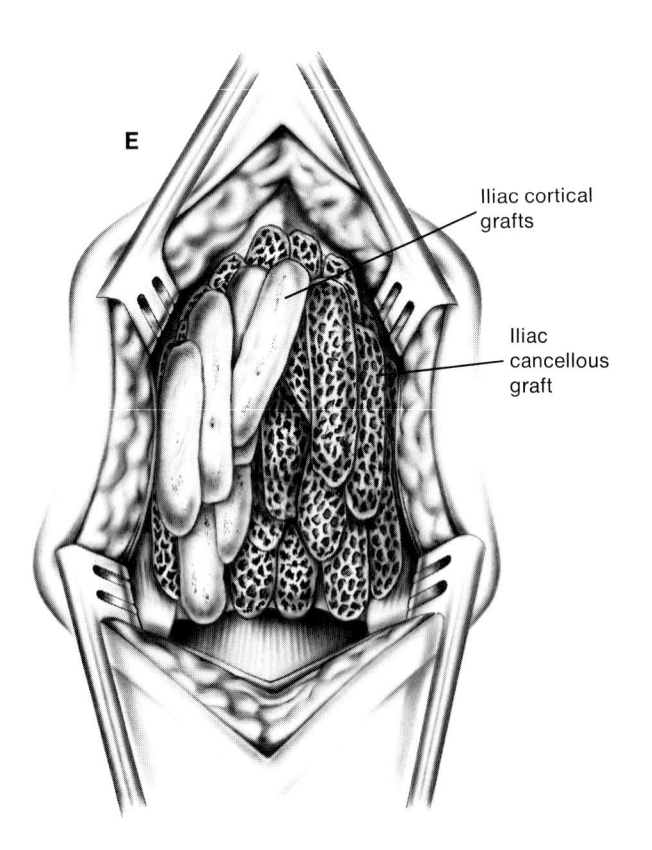

The lamina of C2 is exposed to the lateral facets, leaving the capsule of C2-3 intact **(D)**. Fixation with 20-gauge wire when desired (not illustrated), may be performed from the occiput to the base of the spinous process of C2. With a small burr, two outer cortical holes are made in the occiput, 0.5 cm on each side of the midline, and below the superior nuchal line. These two cortical holes can then be connected by using a towel clip or a nerve hook. The 20-gauge wire is passed through these holes and through a hole made through the base of the spinous process of C2. The two ends of the wire are twisted until the desired tension is obtained.

The surface of the occiput is roughened with a power burr. The C1 arch and C2 laminae are decorticated with the burr and rongeurs. Iliac bone graft is harvested through a straight oblique incision just lateral and inferior to the posterior superior iliac spine (see Plate 9-1). Autogenous iliac cancellous bone grafts cut to size are placed on each side extending from the occiput to the C2 laminae. Iliac corticocancellous strips are placed over the cancellous graft **(E)**.

When wiring is performed, the wire serves to hold down the bone graft on the fusion bed. The cortical graft is placed transversely between the wire and the cancellous graft as illustrated in Plate 7-6, *D*.) The muscle layer is closed over the graft, and the remaining wound closed in layers. The posterior half of the vest is reapplied, and the patient turned onto a regular bed.

POSTOPERATIVE MANAGEMENT. The patient is allowed to sit on the second or third day. When the patient is comfortable and able, ambulation with a walker is encouraged. The halovest or cast is worn for 12 weeks, followed by collar support for another 12 weeks.

(Plate 7-5) ATLANTOAXIAL SPINE FUSION

GENERAL DISCUSSION. Atlantoaxial spine fusion is indicated when there is instability due to trauma, rheumatoid arthritis, or congenital anomalies.

DETAILS OF PROCEDURE. The procedure is performed with the patient in a halovest or halocast. The positioning of the patient and preparation and draping of the operative field are described in the procedure for occipitocervical fusion (Plate 7-4, B and C).

A midline incision is made from the occipital protuberance to the midcervical spine. The dissection is carried through the ligamentum nuchae exposing the tips of the spinous process. The C2 spinous process is usually most easily identified by palpation.

The firmly attached musculotendinous structures to the bifid spinous process of C2 are divided circumferentially with a scalpel. These muscles are retracted by deeper placement of the self-retaining retractors. This facilitates subperiosteal exposure of the spinous process. The self-retaining retractor is placed more deeply, allowing subperiosteal exposure of the arch of the atlas. Careful exposure of the arch, 1.5 to 2 cm to each side of the midline is performed with a Cobb elevator. Extreme care during this maneuver is essential to avoid injury to the vertebral arteries. Maintaining meticulous subperiosteal stripping will prevent troublesome and difficult-to-control venous bleeding as one approaches the lateral limits of the exposure of C1 and C2. Lateral exposure of C2 is carried out to the facet joint capsule of C2-3 **(A)**. The capsule is left intact to avoid subsequent arthrosis or spontaneous fusion of C2-3. The soft tissue attachments to the posterior elements of C3 should also be left intact, as should the soft tissue attachments of the occiput.

Subperiosteal exposure of the midportion of the anterior surface of the C1 arch is initiated lateral to the midline with a small, sharp periosteal elevator. The firmly attached ligamentous fibers above and below the arch in the midline often require division with a scalpel. This allows further subperiosteal reflection of the anterior surface. A 20-gauge wire loop is passed under the arch of C1 from below **(A)**. Placement of this loop may be facilitated by passing a heavy silk suture tied to the wire loop, which allows easier and safe passage of the loop under the arch.

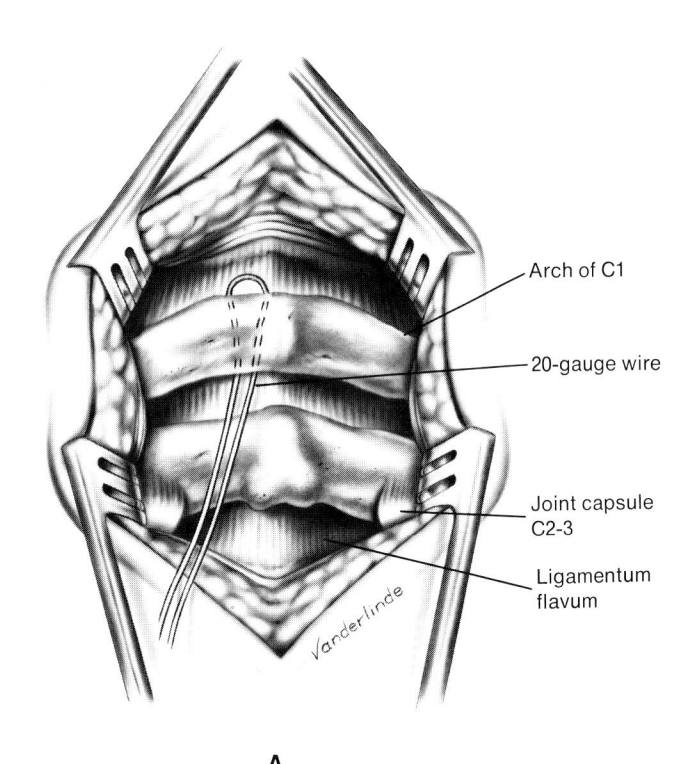

A

ATLANTOAXIAL SPINE FUSION (Plate 7-5)

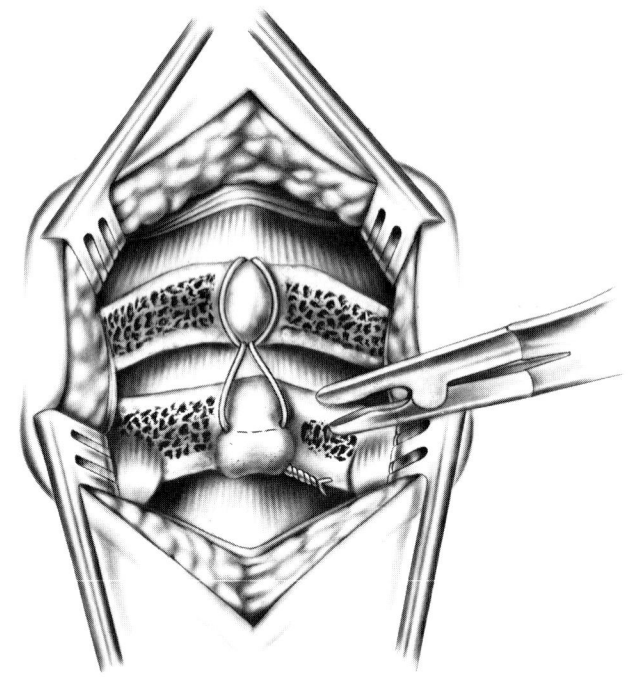

A towel clip is used to make a transverse hole through the base of the spinous process of C2. The wire fixation is carried out as illustrated **(B)**. Decortication is accomplished with the use of a power burr and rongeurs (see Plate 7-6, *A*).

Autogenous cancellous iliac bone is placed over the decorticated area. Corticocancellous bone is laid transversely between the wire and the cancellous graft **(C)**. The paraspinal muscles are grasped on each side while the self-retaining retractors are removed. The graft is held down as the muscles are approximated to avoid displacement of the laterally placed grafts toward the midline.

The wound is closed in layers. The removed portion of the halovest or cast is reapplied and the patient turned safely onto the hospital bed.

POSTOPERATIVE MANAGEMENT. The care following atlantoaxial spine fusion is the same as outlined for occipitocervical fusion (Plate 7-4).

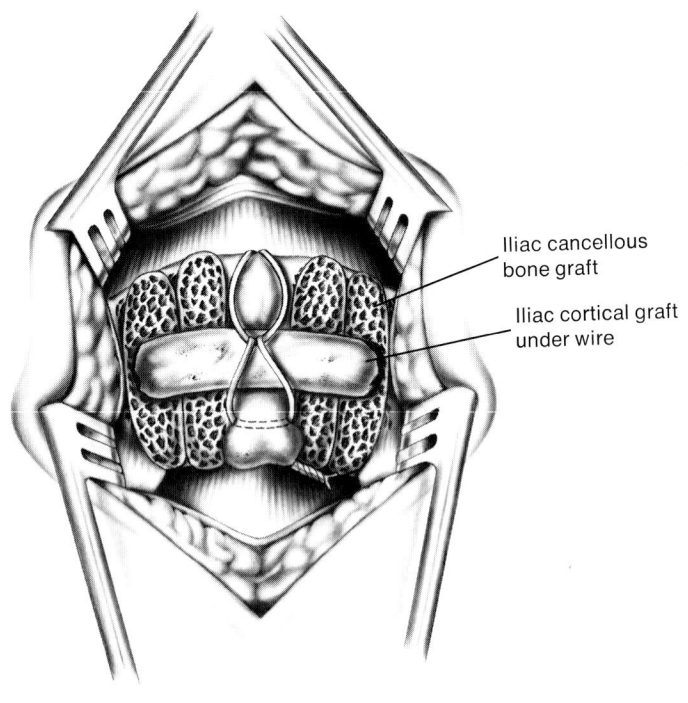

B

Iliac cancellous bone graft
Iliac cortical graft under wire

C

(Plate 7-6) POSTERIOR CERVICAL FUSION (C3 AND BELOW)

GENERAL DISCUSSION. Indications for posterior cervical fusion are the following:
1. Fracture or fracture/dislocations of the lower cervical spine (C3 to C7) with failure of reduction or failure to maintain reduction with halo traction and halo vest or cast immobilization
2. Late traumatic instability
3. Status post-multiple level wide laminectomy usually performed for tumor removal or spinal cord decompression
4. Instability caused by rheumatoid arthritis
5. Progressive kyphosis following radiation therapy
6. Delayed treatment of infections involving multiple levels with advanced destruction of vertebral bodies, instability, and progressive deformity (may require anterior fusion with supplementary posterior fusion)

It should be noted that adequate treatment of infections of the vertebral bodies with prompt anterior debridement, interbody fusion, antibiotics, and halovest or cast immobilization usually results in healing and stability.

DETAILS OF PROCEDURE. Preparation and positioning of the patient are similar to the procedures described for the upper cervical spine fusion (Plate 7-4). A midline skin incision is made. The dissection is carried through the ligamentum nuchae. Self-retaining retractors placed at either angle of the wound allow for ready palpation of the spinous processes. The musculotendinous attachments are divided from a spinous process, and a towel clip is placed into the spinous process. A cross-table lateral roentgenogram is made to identify accurately the vertebral level. The spinous processes and laminae of the segments to be fused are exposed subperiosteally as described for the upper cervical spine (Plate 7-5). Decortication is carried out with a power burr and rongeurs **(A)**. The spinous processes to be wired are not decorticated **(A** and **B)**. A narrow margin of cortical bone at the base of these spinous processes is left as the laminae and facets are decorticated **(B)**. The spinous processes between those wired are excised at the bases, and the usual decortication is carried out **(B)**. A hole is made with a towel clip in the base of the two spinous processes to be wired. A 20-gauge wire is passed through the hole in

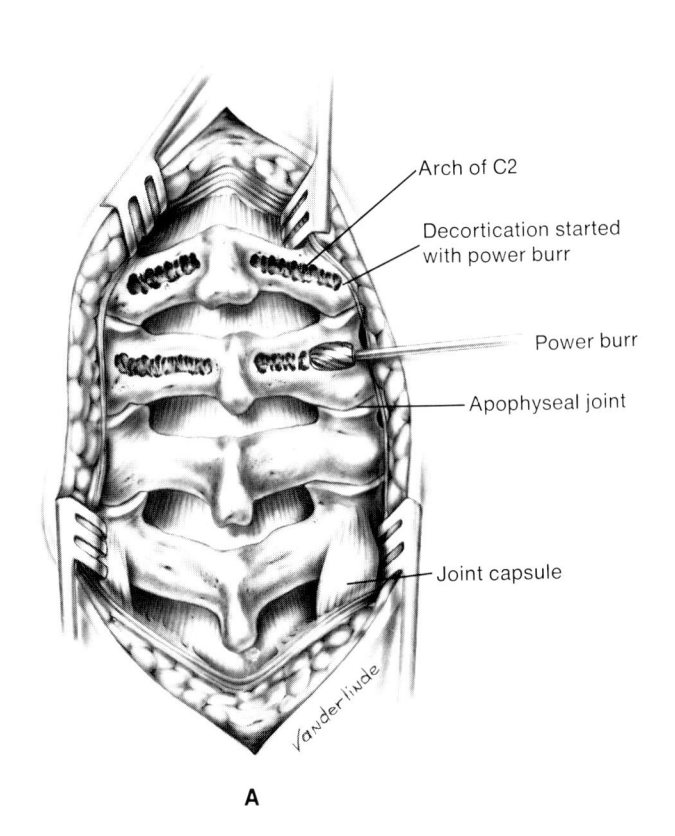

A

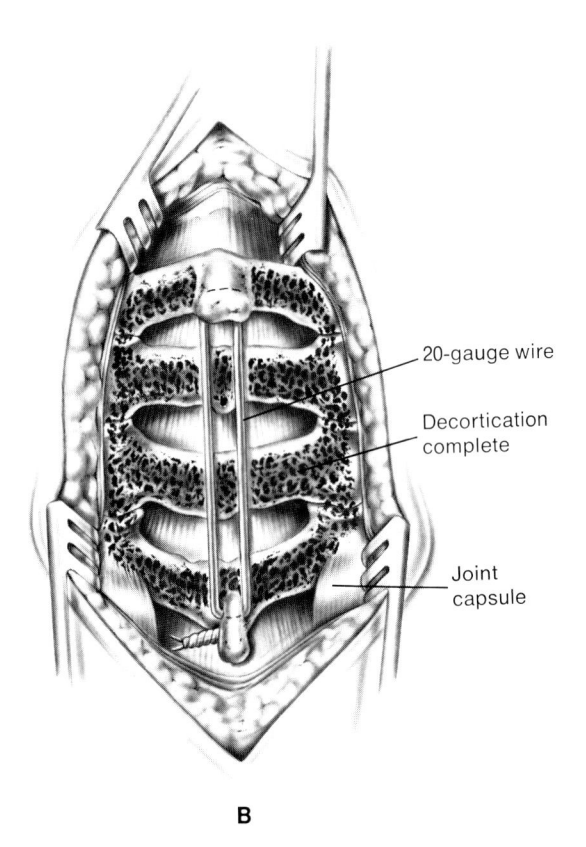

B

203

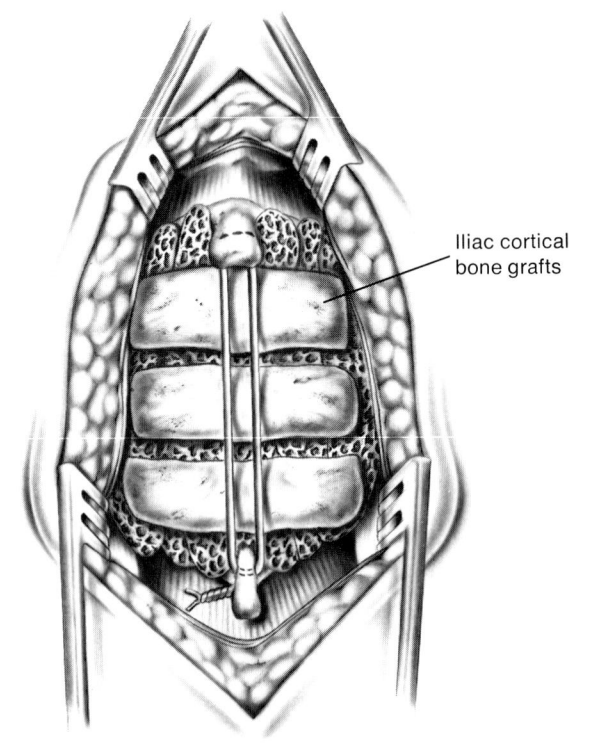

POSTERIOR CERVICAL FUSION (C3 AND BELOW) (Plate 7-6)

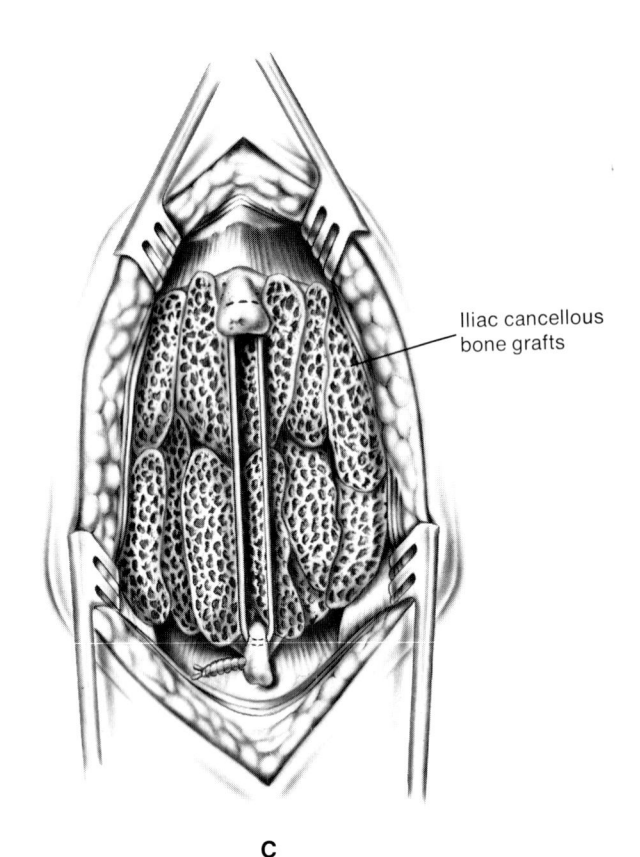

the upper spinous process and the lower one. The ends are twisted until the "loop" is taut, but approximation of the two spinous processes is avoided (B). A variety of wiring techniques may be used, but light-gauge wire and excessive tensioning should be avoided. The major function of the wiring is to retain the grafts in place. A generous amount of fresh autogenous iliac cancellous bone graft is laid over the entire decorticated area (C). Iliac cortical bone slabs are placed transversely over the bed of cancellous graft and under the wire "loop" (D). The wound is closed in layers.

When posterior fusion is performed immediately following laminectomy, the exposed dura is covered with a layer of Gelfoam. The facets on each side of the laminectomy defect are decorticated as well as one or two intact laminae above and below. Iliac cancellous and cortical grafts are laid over the entire decorticated area and over the Gelfoam-protected dura. In a late fusion following laminectomy the dura is protected by dense scar tissue.

POSTOPERATIVE MANAGEMENT. Postoperative care is the same as that for occipitocervical fusion (Plate 7-4).

(Plate 7-7) ANTERIOR CERVICAL SPINE FUSION

GENERAL DISCUSSION. The anterior approach is indicated under the following conditions:

1. For diagnosis and/or treatment of diseases of the cervical vertebral bodies or discs, such as infections or neoplasms, anterior fusion is advantageous.

2. Single- or two-level involvement in cervical spondylosis with intractable nerve root signs and symptoms may be treated by anterior interbody fusion when adequate nonoperative management has failed to relieve the symptoms.

3. Kyphotic deformity following extensive laminectomy requires anterior and posterior fusion to stabilize the cervical spine. Early stabilization by posterior facet fusion with autogenous iliac bone graft will prevent the complications of progressive kyphosis.

DETAILS OF PROCEDURE. In cervical spondylosis, where instability is not a problem, surgery is performed under general anesthesia and endotracheal intubation. The neck is supported by a roll, and the head is turned away from the side of the incision. No preoperative external immobilization is used.

When surgery is being performed in the presence of cervical instability or kyphosis, the patient is immobilized in a halojacket (Plate 7-4, *A* to *C*) or halocast (Plate 7-8) preoperatively. This permits preoperative correction of the deformity and stabilization of the cervical spine during the operation. In these instances nasotracheal intubation is used.

The usual exposure is through a transverse incision **(A)**. When the upper cervical spine is to be exposed or an extensive cervical fusion is to be performed, an incision along the anterior border of the sternocleidomastoid muscle is made **(A)**. The plane of approach to the vertebral bodies is between the thyroid gland and the carotid sheath **(B,** *B1* **)**.

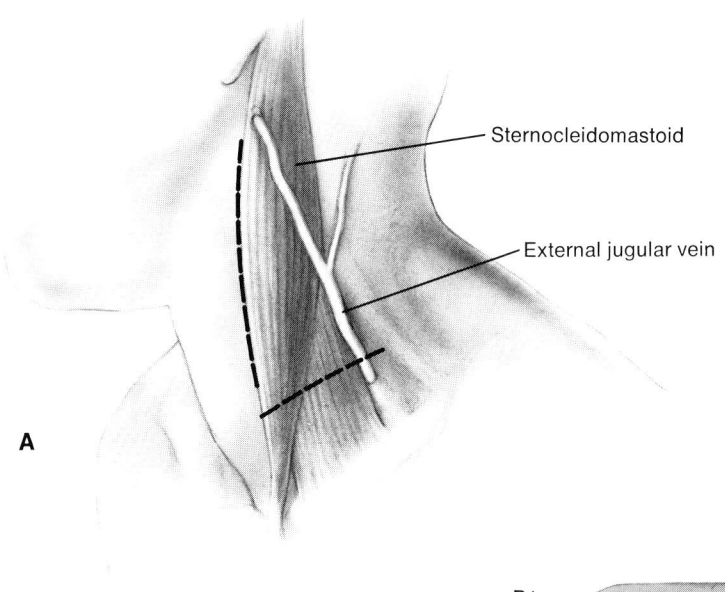

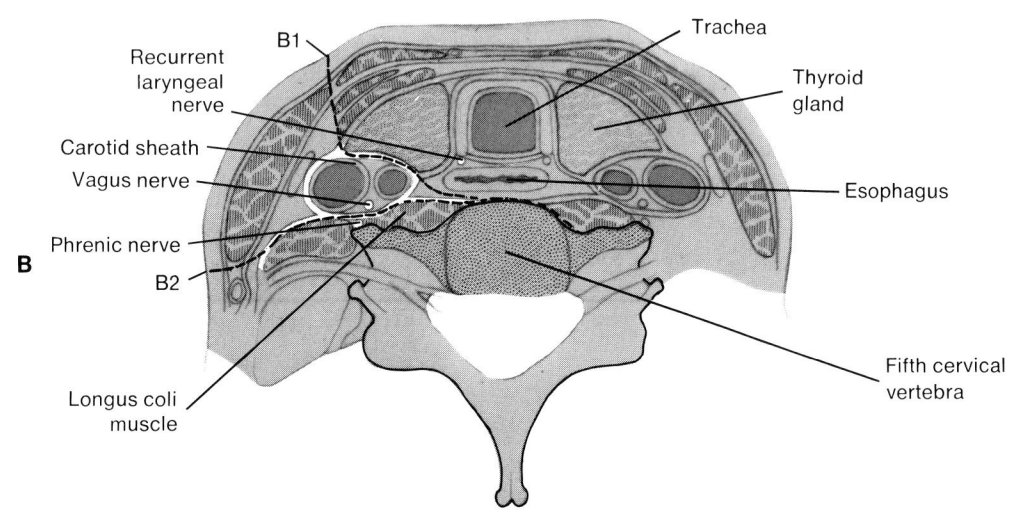

ANTERIOR CERVICAL SPINE FUSION (Plate 7-7)

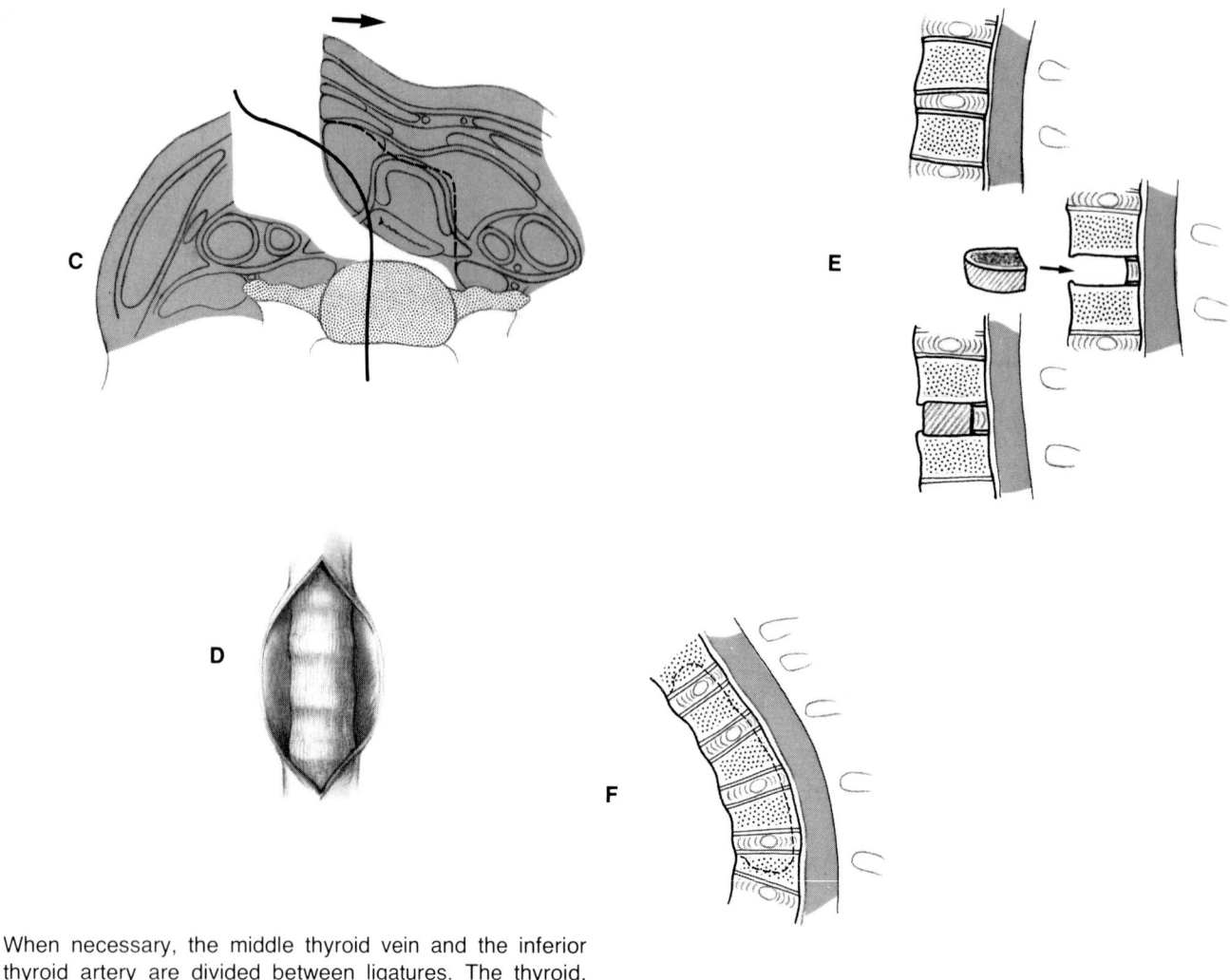

When necessary, the middle thyroid vein and the inferior thyroid artery are divided between ligatures. The thyroid, trachea, recurrent laryngeal nerve, and esophagus are gently retracted medially. The carotid sheath and its contents are retracted laterally. The prevertebral fascia is incised and easily stripped from the anterior aspect of the vertebral column. The longus coli muscles on each side of the vertebral bodies are reflected to allow adequate exposure of the bodies and discs (**C** and **D**). An alternative plane of approach suitable for surgery of the lower cervical spine is through the posterior triangle (**B**, *B2*). In this approach the sternocleidomastoid muscle and the carotid sheath and its contents are retracted anteriorly and medially.

When interbody fusion is being performed, the disc is excised and the end-plates are osteotomized down to cancellous bone. The posterior annulus and posterior longitudinal ligament are left intact. The vertebral bodies are spread, and a full-thickness bicortical iliac bone graft of appropriate height and size is gently countersunk into the intervertebral space (**E**).

In an extensive fusion for a kyphotic deformity, a trough is prepared in the vertebral bodies over the extent of the fusion (**F**). A matching full-thickness iliac graft is countersunk into the trough (**G**). The wound is closed in layers.

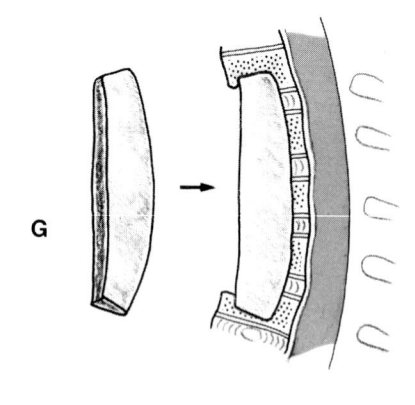

POSTOPERATIVE MANAGEMENT. When fusion is performed for cervical spondylosis, a cervical collar is worn for 6 to 8 weeks. Patients in whom fusion is done for cervical spine instability, kyphosis, or decompression and fusion for trauma, infection, or tumor, wear the halo jacket or halo cast for 3 months.

(Plate 7-8) APPLICATION OF CRANIAL HALO

GENERAL DISCUSSION. Preoperative or posttraumatic immobilization of the cervical spine may be achieved by a plaster cast, the traction sling, the cervical collar or brace, or by skeletal traction to the skull by tongs or wires. Discomfort, inadequate fixation, or other complications are frequent with these methods, particularly when used for long periods of time. An alternative method for immobilization of the cervical spine for the severely crippled patient to ensure adequate respiratory function is occasionally necessary. The following conditions may be needed: precise positional control in all three planes, progressive adjustable longitudinal traction, rigid stabilization, simple application, freedom from complications during the prolonged use (potentially including that necessary for bone fusion), and minimum patient discomfort.

The cranial halo traction apparatus meets these requirements. It consists of a skeletal traction device attached to the skull and connected to a plaster body cast (or to a pelvic halo) by an adjustable steel frame. Four threaded traction rods connect the headring to the horizontal attachment sleeves of the suspension assembly. To the well-molded body cast (or pelvic halo) are attached the adjustable mounting brackets that accept the main support rods of the steel frame.

DETAILS OF PROCEDURE. The apparatus includes a headring, mounting bracket, overhead support, suspension assembly, and skull pins with a locking nut and Allen screw (**A** and **B**).

As recommended by Nickel et al., the cranial halo apparatus is applied in two stages. First the headring is attached to the skull. Then the body cast (or pelvic halo) and suspension assembly are added (**C** and **D**). The sequence and timing depend on the circumstances. Either local or general anesthesia can be used for application of the ring depending on the patient's tolerance for the procedure. If a general anesthetic is necessary, it is best to wait 1 or 2 days before applying the cast (or pelvic halo) and suspension assembly. When a patient can tolerate application of the cranial halo under local anesthesia (and most will), the body cast (or pelvic halo) and suspension assembly can be attached at the same time.

A

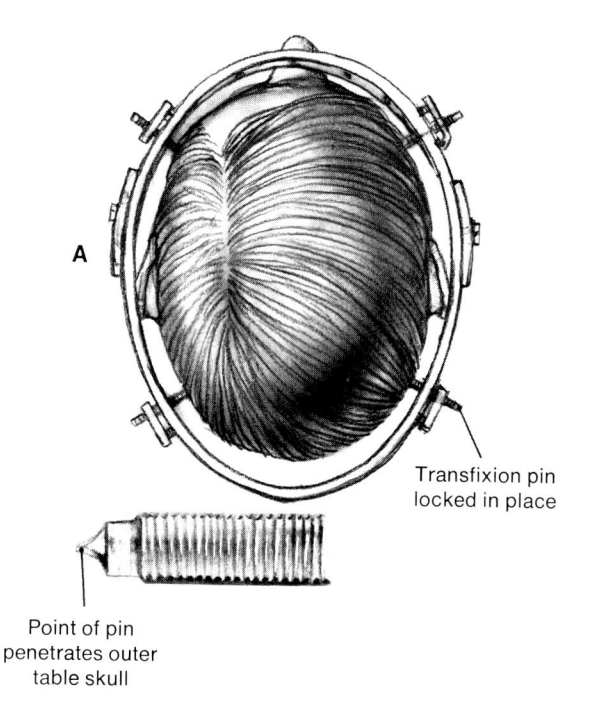

Transfixion pin locked in place

Point of pin penetrates outer table skull

B

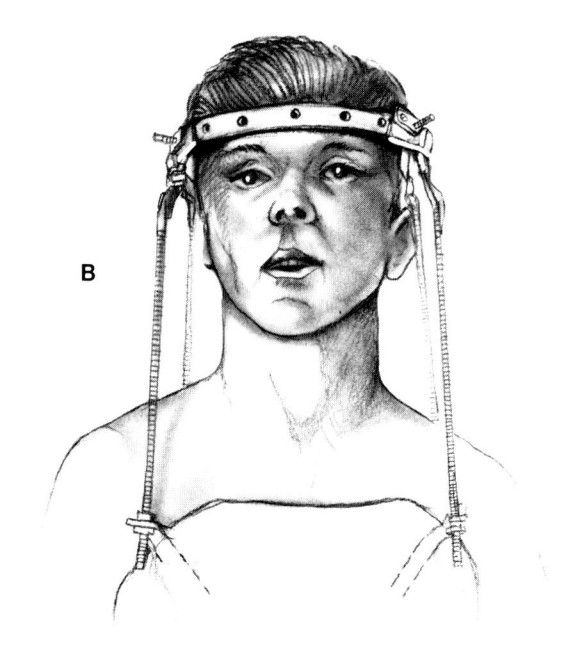

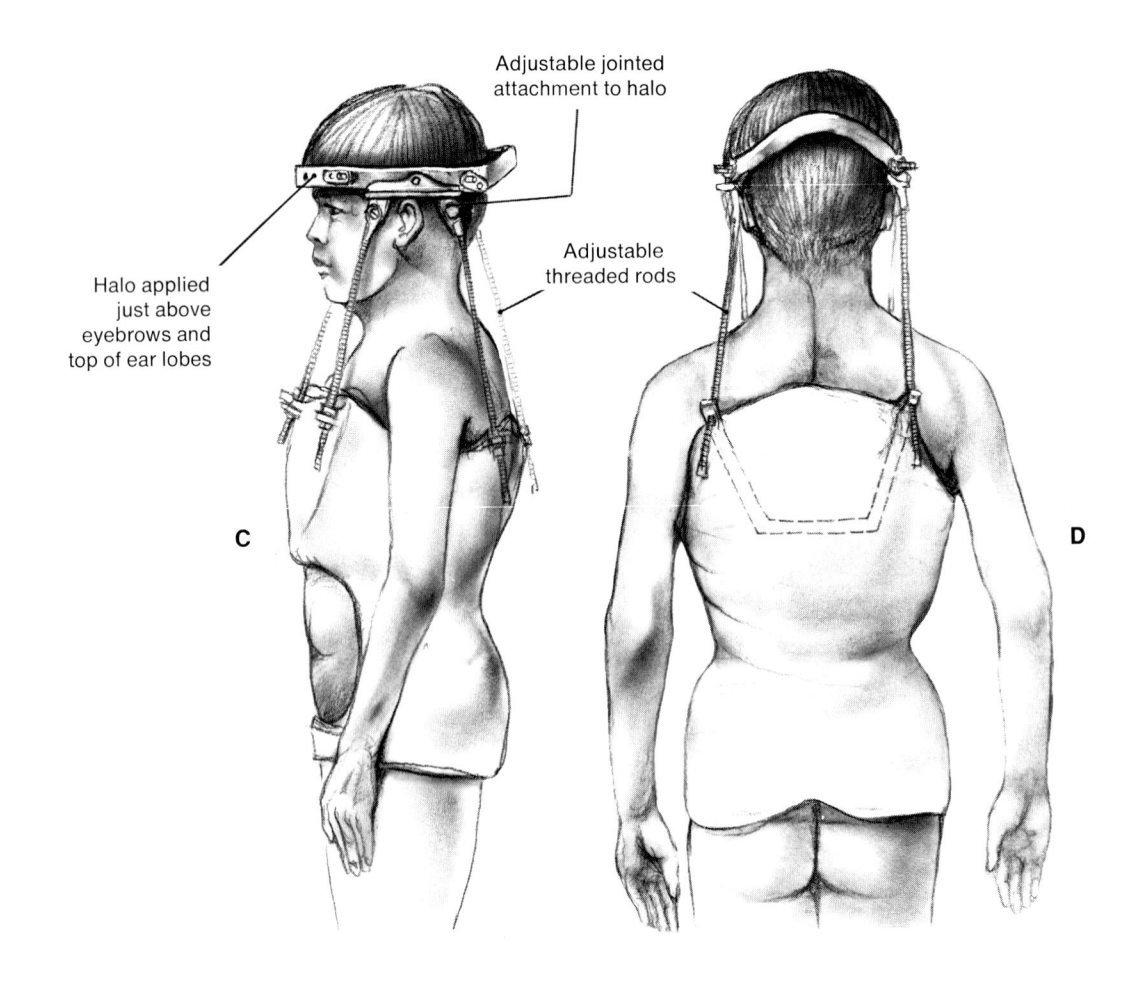

APPLICATION OF CRANIAL HALO (Plate 7-8)

Headrings are made in four sizes, and a ring about 1 to 1.5 cm larger than the circumference of the patient's head is best. To determine the correct size, the circumference of the head is measured 1.25 cm (½ inch) above the ears and just above the eyebrow. This measurement is then used to select the size. A table (furnished by the manufacturer) designated halo size for various circumference measurements. The final size is selected by inspecting the halo around the head to be certain of proper distance from the skin.

It is best to apply the headring with the patient in a semi-sitting position, but it can be done with the patient supine. The patient's head is supported posteriorly by a 7 cm wide metal or wood strip placed between the back and the operating table. The patient's head is shaved for a distance of approximately 5 cm around each pin site, and these areas are scrubbed. If the patient will be in the cranial halo a long time, routine cleaning of the pin sites will be easier if the patient's hair is short and if the shaved areas are made continuous.

The headring, pins, and locking assembly having been autoclaved previously, the headring is positioned on the head with four positioning pins and plates. In adults the headring is fixed to the skull with six threaded pins. These pins have small, sharp points that rapidly flare onto a broad shoulder, creating a large area of contact against the skull with a minimum of penetration **(A)**. Each of the six pin-insertion areas on the headring contain three alternative threaded holes. These provide a selection of insertion sites and permit new pin placement if one site becomes inflamed. The pins are then locked in place by threading the locking plate on the pin and tightening the lock screw with the Allen wrench. This secures the pin in place so that it cannot loosen. The headring also has alternative areas of attachment for each vertical traction rod.

No unusual equipment is needed to apply the cranial halo except two torque screwdrivers used to tighten the skull pin onto the cranium. A torque force of 5½ inch-pounds provides good fixation without complications. Thirty minutes after the pins are torqued, they will be found to have loosened slightly and should be again torqued to 5½ inch-pounds before the locking device is tightened. If torque screwdrivers are not available, a short screwdriver will serve if no greater than fingertip grasp is used when tightening. This furnishes the approximate amount of force desired.

Horizontally, the lower margin of the ring should be just above the ears and about 0.5 cm above the eyebrows. This usually places the anterior pin in the shallow groove on the

(Plate 7-8) APPLICATION OF CRANIAL HALO

forehead between the supraorbital ridges and the frontal protuberances. If the anterior pins are in this groove, chances of the halo slipping are minimized. Optimum sites for the initial skull-pin placement are usually the second or third holes from the front and the second from the rear. When six pins are used, one pin is located equidistant from the front and rear pins.

With an assistant holding the ring in its proper place, the surgeon either inserts the pins directly in the holes or uses stabilizer plates for trial alignment. The stabilizer plates are flat and snap on the rounded end of a threaded bolt. The bolt is placed at four diagonal positions in the halo; those to be used for the fixation pins are avoided. After the bolts are threaded through the ring, the plates are snapped on and the bolts are screwed in so the halo is located to provide proper clearance and location on the head.

When the headring is correctly positioned, local anesthesia, if used, is injected. The skull pins are then inserted in the headring. No scalp incisions are needed, since the pins easily penetrate through the soft tissues. To avoid side-to-side drifting, it is important to tighten diagonally opposite pins simultaneously. After all four pins are screwed in with maximum finger tolerance, the stabilizer plates are removed and all diagonally opposite pins are further tightened simultaneously to 5½ inch-pounds of torque.

If a body cast is planned, the patient is placed on a modified Risser localizer table and the body cast is applied. The cast is carefully molded over the iliac crests and over all other body prominences. The mounting brackets and suspension rods are then placed on the cast in trial alignment. The position of the mounting brackets is such that the distance between the supports in all directions is greater at the cast than the halo attachments so that a truncated pyramid is formed for stability. The lower supports are positioned so the threaded rod supports do not require bending. The four rods are fixed to right-angle plates which in turn are bolted to the halo ring. After all the necessary adjustments are completed, the mounting brackets are plastered to the body cast. All nuts and setscrews are tightened after the head is placed in the final position. The orthopaedic surgeon must not let the head fall back, extending the neck and creating or aggravating any swallowing or breathing difficulties.

If the patient is to be managed supine with traction on the cranial halo, a modified type of cranial halo (with posterior rollers) is used **(E)**.

Five days after application of the halo the fixation pins are tightened once to 5½ inch-pounds of torque. After this adjustment no further tightening should be performed.

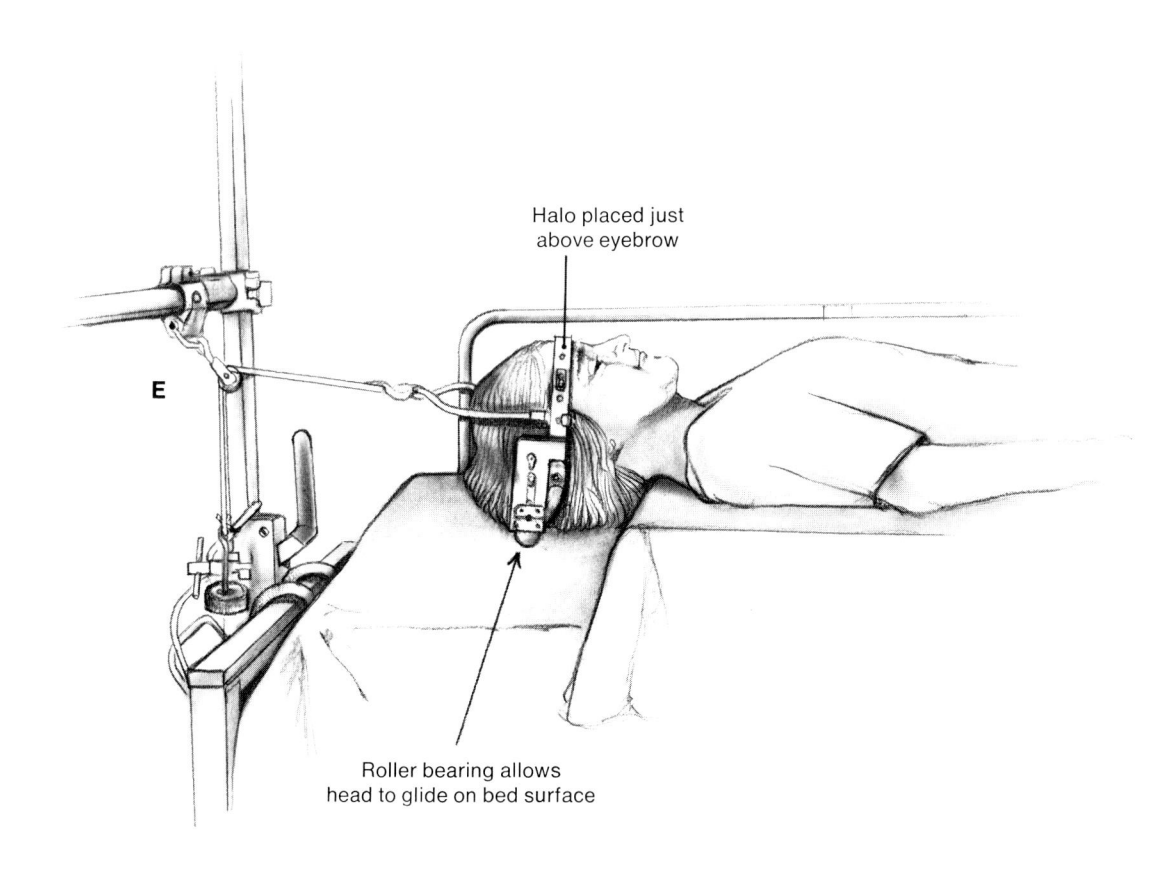

E

Halo placed just above eyebrow

Roller bearing allows head to glide on bed surface

APPLICATION OF PELVIC HOOP (Plate 7-9)

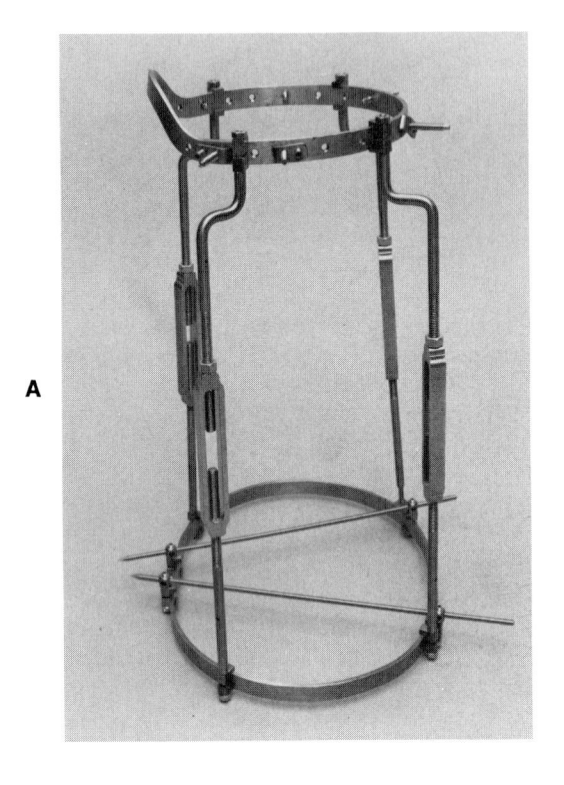

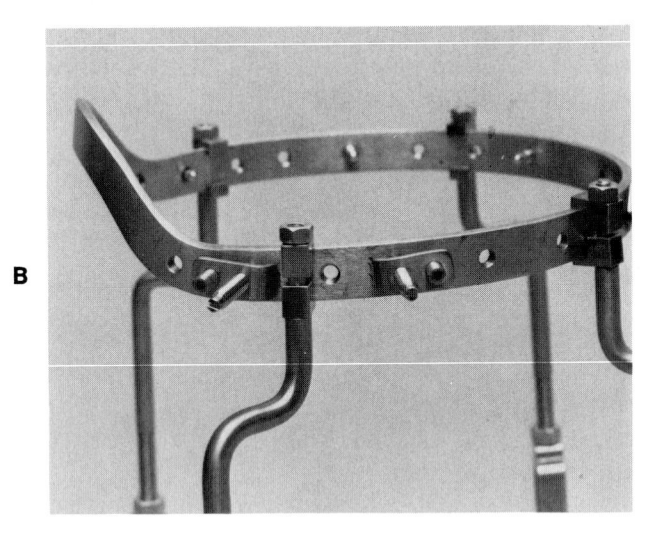

GENERAL DISCUSSION. The halo-pelvic hoop apparatus can be useful in treating severe scoliosis. As reported by Dewald and Ray, the potential advantages of this method are elimination of plaster cast that may decrease pulmonary vital capacity, control of the pelvis (decompensation of the spine can be eliminated and pelvic obliquity or rotation corrected), gradual correction of the scoliosis with the patient ambulatory, no undetected pressure sores as may happen beneath a cast, and ease of surgical access (the apparatus permits both anterior and posterior surgical approaches).

The pelvic hoop is a stainless steel band that is manufactured in several sizes. The proper size is selected by first measuring the anteroposterior and the transverse diameter of the pelvic area at the level of the anterosuperior iliac spines. These measurements are then applied to the available sizes of hoops, and one is selected that will provide 2.5 to 5 cm of clearance between the inside of the hoop and the skin. The pelvic hoop is attached to heavy threaded pins inserted through the pelvic wings by special locking plates that may be adjusted to fit any location on the hoop (**A** and **B**). The pelvic hoop is then attached to the halo by four turnbuckles. The turnbuckles are attached to the halo and pelvic hoop by sliding clips that can be adjusted to any portion on the halo and pelvic hoop (**A** to **C**). The length of the turnbuckles is determined by measuring the distance between the eyebrow and the anterosuperior iliac spines. Two sizes of turnbuckles are available. Occasionally special sizes of turnbuckles must be obtained preoperatively.

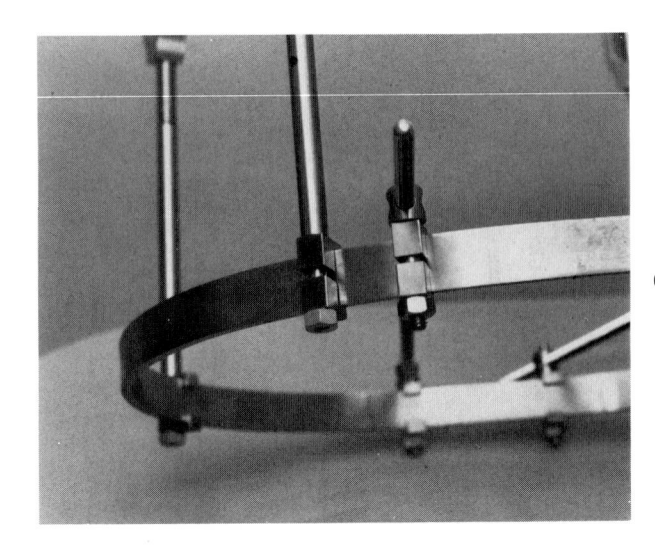

(Plate 7-9) APPLICATION OF PELVIC HOOP

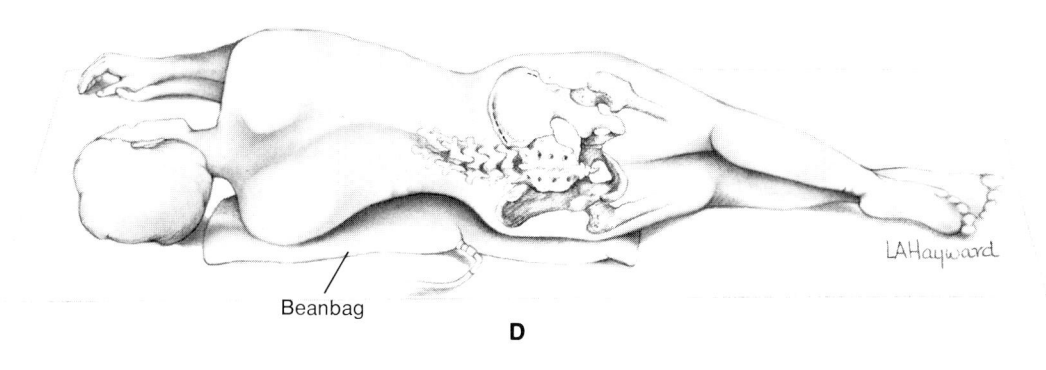

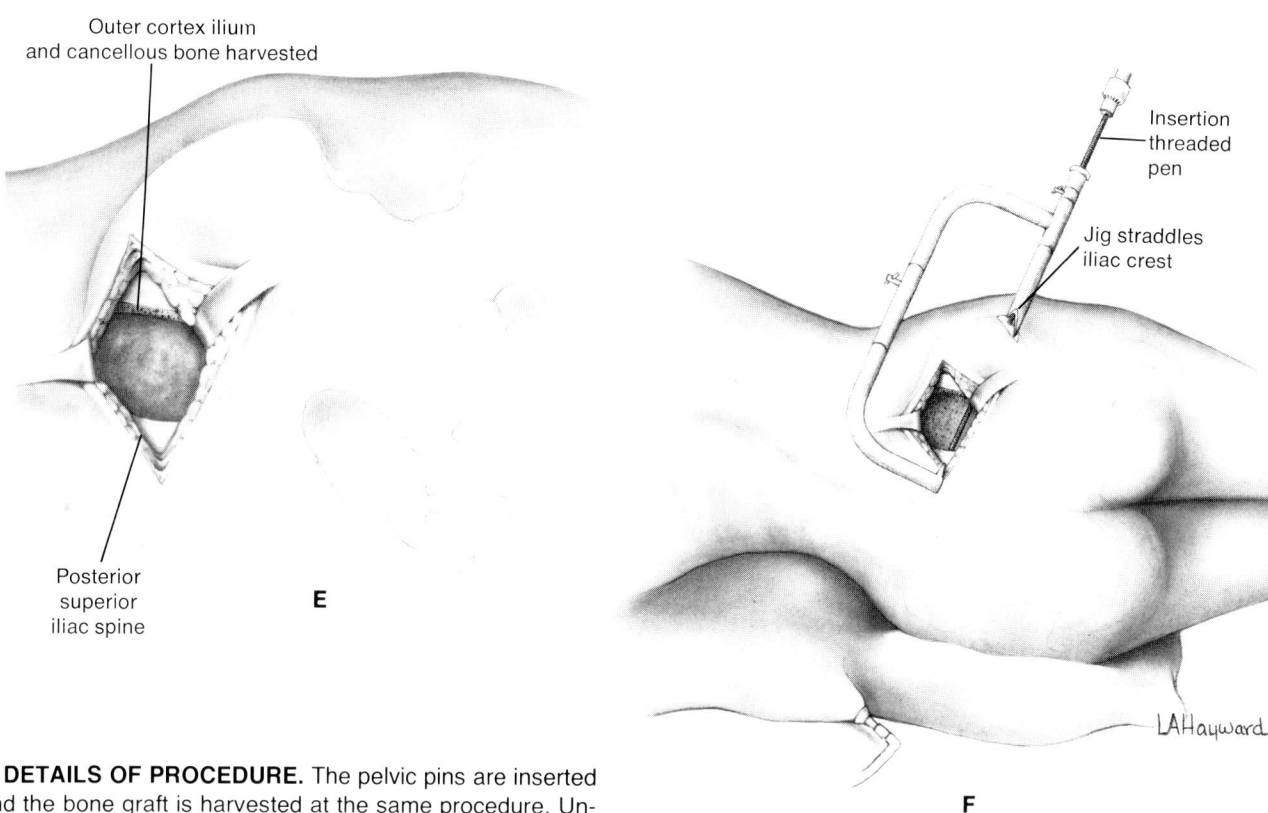

Beanbag

D

Outer cortex ilium and cancellous bone harvested

Posterior superior iliac spine

E

Insertion threaded pen

Jig straddles iliac crest

F

DETAILS OF PROCEDURE. The pelvic pins are inserted and the bone graft is harvested at the same procedure. Under general anesthesia the patient is placed in the lateral decubitus position **(D)**, and the usual surgical preparation and draping are carried out to allow access to the anterior and posterior ilium. A curved incision is made beginning at the posterosuperior iliac spine and following the iliac crest **(D)**. The bone graft is harvested as described in Chapter 9, but the cortex and cancellous bone of the posteriosuperior iliac spine are not removed. This provides adequate structural strength for the posterior fixation of the pelvic pin **(E)**. After cancellous bone has been removed, a short incision is made proximal and lateral to the anterosuperior iliac spine. The exposure is made to allow access to the tubercle of the crest. This widened part of the crest is the desirable entrance point of the pin. The jig **(F)** is then inserted so that the V-shaped notch straddles the crest in the front, and the sharp point is placed in a hole made with an awl in the posterosuperior iliac spine. The threaded pin is then inserted anteriorly in the jig. The power drill is used at low speed to insert the pin through the iliac wing. The first half of its insertion is blind, and care must be taken to ensure its proper course. Occasionally, if the iliac wall is thin, the pin will penetrate the inner wall. This is suspected when, with each revolution of the pin, a tic is felt through the handle of the power drill. If this occurs, the pin must be withdrawn and advanced several times slowly to allow the cutting edge to cut through the bone. If it is not withdrawn and advanced, it may follow the inner table, which is slightly curved, and the exit point will be malpositioned. It may be desirable at this point to palpate the inner wall with the gloved finger. When the pin is seen in the space left by harvesting of the graft, its proper placement can be evaluated. It the course is proper, it is drilled through the posterosuperior iliac spine **(F)**, and just before it exits,

211

APPLICATION OF PELVIC HOOP (Plate 7-9)

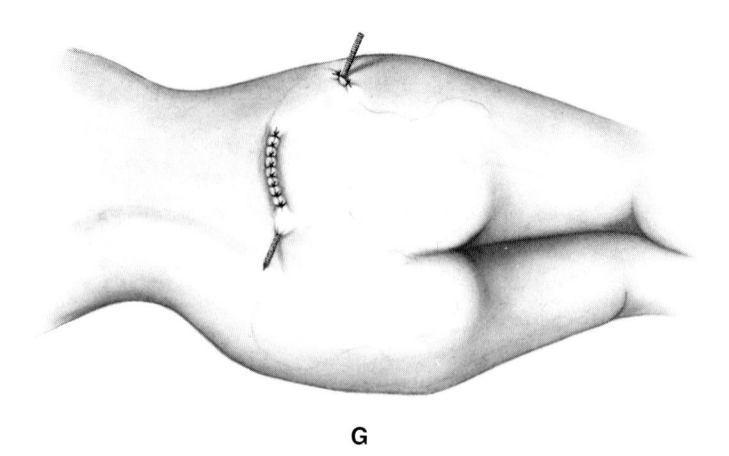

G

the jig is disassembled and removed. The surgeon continues to drill the pin through and makes a separate stab wound over the tip of the pin. The pin is in the proper place when there is an equal length protruding anteriorly and posteriorly **(G)**. The wounds are closed in the standard fashion, and the patient turned on the opposite side to repeat the procedure.

With both pins in place, the patient is turned supine and supported above and below the pins so that the pelvic hoop may be applied. The four fixation plates and sleeves are attached to the pins first and then fixed to the pelvic hoop. The hoop is adjusted for adequate clearance from the skin, and the setscrews and nuts are tightened. Four turnbuckles are then applied to the halo and pelvic hoop **(H)**. No immediate correction is attempted.

The patient is allowed to adjust to the cranial pelvic hoop apparatus for a day or two before gradually starting the turnbuckle correction (**B** to **D**).

POSTOPERATIVE MANAGEMENT. The turnbuckles are lengthened an average of 2 mm each day for 2 weeks and then 1 mm daily. The patient is observed for any abnormal neurologic findings or complaint of pain in the neck. During the process of correction with the distraction forces, the more mobile cervical segments may be excessively distracted. Subluxation and dislocation of the cervical spine have occurred. The appearance of neurologic deficit, subjective neurologic complaint, or pain in the neck demands immediate release of some of the distraction forces. During the process of correction, roentgenograms of the entire spine, including the cervical segment, should be obtained.

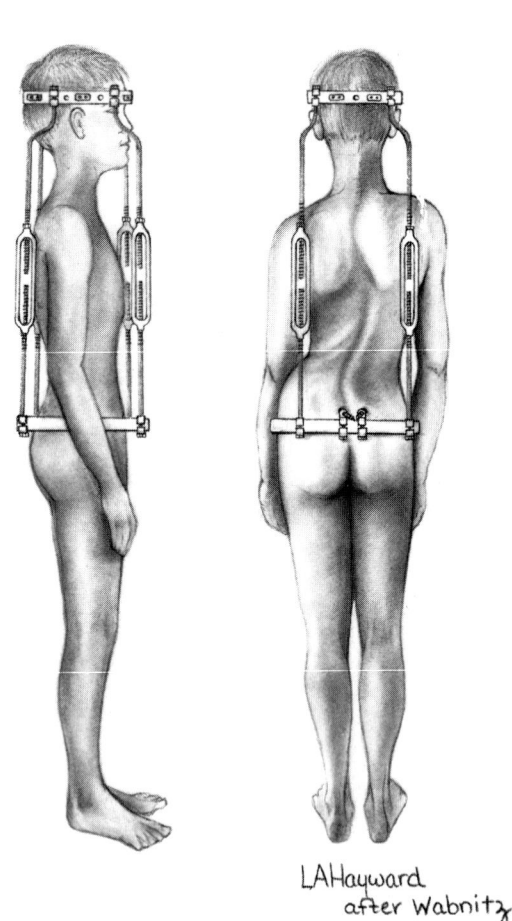

LAHayward
after Wabnitz

H

REFERENCES

Althoff, B., and Goldie, I. F.: The arterial supply of the odontoid process of the axis, Acta Orthop. Scand. **48**:622, 1977.

Anderson, L. D., and D'Alonzo, R. T.: Fractures of the odontoid process of the axis, J. Bone Joint Surg. **56-A**:1663, 1974.

Apuzzo, M. L. J., Heitn, J. S., Weiss, N. H., Ackerson, T. T., Harvey, J. P., and Kurze, T.: Acute fractures of the odontoid process. An analysis of 45 cases, J. Neurosurg. **48**:85, 1978.

Beighton, P., and Craig, J.: Atlanto-axial subluxation in the Morquio syndrome. Report of a case, J. Bone Joint Surg. **55-B**:478, 1973.

Bell, G. D., and Bailey, S. I.: Anterior cervical fusion for trauma, Corr. **128**:155, 1977.

Böhler, J.: Fractures of the odontoid process, J. Trauma **5**:386, 1965.

Brooks, A. L., and Jenkins, A. W.: Atlanto-axial arthrodesis by the Wedge compression method, J. Bone Joint Surg. **60-A**:279, 1978.

Buck, C. A., Dameron, F. D., Dow, N. J., and Skownund, H. H. V.: Study of normal range of motion in the neck utilizing a bubble Goniometer, Arch. Phys. Med. Rehab. **40**:390, 1959.

Cattell, H. S., and Clark, G. L. Jr.: Cervical kyphosis and instability following multiple laminectomies in children, J. Bone Joint Surg. **49-A**:713, 1967.

Cooper, P. R., Maravilla, K. R., Sklar, F. H., Moody, S. F., and Clark, W. K.: Halo immobilization of cervical spine fractures: indications and results, Orthop. Trans. **3**:126, 1979.

Dawson, E. G., and Smith, L.: Atlanto-axial subluxation in children due to vertebral anomalies, J. Bone Joint Surg. **61-A**:582, 1979.

Dewald, R. L., and Ray, R. D.: Skeletal traction for the treatment of severe scoliosis, The University of Illinois halo-hoop apparatus, J. Bone Joint Surg. **52-A**:233, 1970.

Dunn, E. J., and Anas, P. P.: The management of tumors of the upper cervical spine, Orthop. Clin. North Am. **9**:1065, 1978.

Evarts, C. M.: Traumatic occipito-atlantal dislocation. Report of a case with survival, J. Bone Joint Surg. **52-A**:1653, 1970.

Ewald, F. C.: Fracture of the odontoid process in a 17-month-old infant treated with a halo. A case report and discussion of the injury under the age of three, J. Bone Joint Surg. **53-A**:1635, 1971.

Fielding, J. W.: Cineroentgenography of the normal cervical spine, J. Bone Joint Surg. **39-A**:1280, 1957.

Fielding, J. W.: Normal and selected abnormal motion of the cervical spine from the second cervical vertebra to the seventh cervical vertebra based on cineroentgenography, J. Bone Joint Surg. **46-A**:1779, 1964.

Fielding, J. W., Burstem, A. A., and Frankel, B. A.: The nuchal ligament, Spine **1**:3, 1976.

Fielding, J. W., Hawkins, J. R., Hensinger, R. N., and Francis, W. R.: Atlantoaxial rotary deformities, Orthop. Clin. North Am. **9**:955, 1978.

Fielding, J. W., Hawkins, R. J., and Retzan, S. A.: Spine fusion for atlantoaxial instability, J. Bone Joint Surg. **58-A**:400, 1976.

Forsythe, M., and Rothman, R. H.: New concepts in the diagnosis and treatment of infections of the cervical spine. Orthop. Clin. North Am. **9**:1039, 1978.

Gabrielsen, T. O., and Maxwell, J. A.: Traumatic atlanto-occipital dislocation. With report of a patient who survived, Ann. J. Roentgenol. **97**:624, 1966.

Griffiths, S. C.: Fracture of odontoid process in children, J. Pediatr. Surg. **7**:680, 1972.

Griswold, D. M., Albright, J. A., Schiffman, E., Johnson, R., and Southwick, W. O.: Atlantoaxial fusion for instability, J. Bone Joint Surg. **60-A**:285, 1978.

Hahns, S. Y., Witten, D. M., and Mussleman, J. P.: Jefferson fracture of the atlas. Report of six cases. J. Neurosurg. **44**:368, 1976.

Hartman, J. T., Palumbo, F., and Hill, B. J.: Cineradiography of the braced normal cervical spine. A comparative study of five commonly used cervical orthoses, Clin. Orthop. **109**:97, 1975.

Herron, L. D., Westin, G. W., and Dawson, E. G.: Scoliosis in arthrogryposis multiplex Congenita, J. Bone Joint Surg. **60-A**:293, 1978.

Holmes, J. C., and Hall, J. E.: Fusion for instability and potential instability of the cervical spine in children and adolescents, Orthop. Clin. North Am. **9**:923, 1978.

Johnson, R. M., Hart, D. L., Simmons, E. F., Ramsby, G. R., and Southwick, W. O.: Cervical orthoses. A study comparing their effectiveness in restricting cervical motion in normal subjects, J. Bone Joint Surg. **59-A**:332, 1977.

Kalamchi, A., Yau, A. C. M. C., O'Brien, J. P., and Hodgson, A.: Halo pelvic distraction apparatus, J. Bone Joint Surg. **58-A**:1119, 1976.

Kopits, S. E., and Steingass, N. H.: Experience with the "halo-cast" in small children, Surg. Clin. North Am. **50**:935, 1970.

Lipson, S. J.: Dysplasia of the odontoid process in Morquio's syndrome causing quadriparesis, J. Bone Joint Surg. **59-A**:340, 1977.

Martell, W.: The occipital-atlanto-axial joints in rheumatoid arthritis and ankylosing spondylitis, Am. J. Roentgenol. **86**:223, 1961.

Martell, W., and Page, P. W.: Cervical vertebral erosions and subluxations in rheumatoid arthritis and ankylosing spondylitis, Arthrit. Rheum. **3**:546, 1960.

McJeraw, R. W., and Rusch, R. M.: Atlantoaxial arthrodesis, J. Bone Joint Surg. **55-B**:482, 1973.

McPhee, I. D., and O'Brien, J. P.: Reduction of severe spondylolisthesis. A preliminary report, Spine **4**:430, 1979.

Murphy, M. J., Wu, J. T., and Southwick, W. O.: Orthop. Trans. **3**:126, 1979.

Newman, P. H., Sweetnan, R.: Occipito-cervical fusion. An operative technique and its indications, J. Bone Joint Surg. **51-B**:423, 1969.

Nickel, V. L., Perry, J., Garrett, A., and Heppenstall, M.: The halo, J. Bone Joint Surg. **50-A**:1400, 1968.

O'Brien, J. P.: The halo pelvic apparatus, Acta Orthop. Scand. (Suppl.) **163**:79, 1975.

O'Brien, J. P., Yau, A. C., Smith, T. K., and Hodgson, A. R.: Halo pelvic traction. A preliminary report on the method of external skeletal fixation for correcting deformities and maintaining fixation of the spine, J. Bone Joint Surg. **53-B**:217, 1971.

Pierce, D. S., and Barr, J. S.: Use of the halo and cervical spine problems, Orthop. Trans. **3**:125, 1979.

Rana, N. A., Hancock, D. O., Taylor, A. R., and Hill, A. G. S.: Atlantoaxial subluxation in rheumatoid arthritis, J. Bone Joint Surg. **55-B**:458, 1973.

Ransford, A. O., and Manning, C. W. S. F.: Halo-pelvic apparatus: peritoneal penetration by pelvic pins, J. Bone Joint Surg. **60-B**:404, 1978.

Rogers, W. A.: Treatment of fracture-dislocations of the cervical spine, J. Bone Joint Surg. **24**:245, 1942.

Rogers, W. A.: Fractures and dislocations of the cervical spine. An end result study, J. Bone Joint Surg. **39-A**:341, 1957.

Russin, L. D., and Guinto, F. C., Jr.: Multidirectional tomography in cervical spine injury, J. Neurosurg. **45**:9, 1976.

Schweigel, J. F.: Halo-thoracic brace in the management of adontoid fractures, Orthop. Trans. **3**:126, 1979.

Sherk, H. H.: Fractures of the atlas and odontoid process, Orthop. Clin. North Am. **9**:973, 1978.

Sherk, H. H., Nicholson, J. D., and Chung, S. M. K.: Fractures of the odontoid process in young children, J. Bone Joint Surg. **60-A**:921, 1978.

Sherk, H. H., and Snyder, B.: Posterior fusions of the upper cervical spine: indications, techniques, and prognosis, Orthop. Clin. North. Am. **9**:1091, 1978.

Tredwell, S. J., O'Brien, J. T.: Apophyseal joint degeneration in the cervical spine following halo-pelvic distraction, presented at the Tenth Annual Meeting of the Scoliosis Research Society, Louisville, Ky., Sept., 1975.

Washington, E. R.: Non-traumatic atlanto-occipital and atlanto-axial dislocation. A case report. J. Bone Joint Surg. **41-A**:341, 1959.

White, A. A., III, Johnson, R. M., Panjabi, M. M., and Southwick, W. O.: Biomechanical analysis of clinical stability in the cervical spine, Clin. Orthop. **109**:85, 1975.

White, A. A., III, and Panjabi, M. M.: The clinical biomechanics of the occipitoatlantoaxial complex, Orthop. Clin. North Am. **9**:867, 1978.

Wiesal, S., Kraus, D., and Rothman, R. H.: Atlanto-occipital hypermobility, Orthop. Clin. North Am. **9**:969, 1978.

8

THORACOLUMBAR SPINE

SCOLIOSIS—GENERAL CONSIDERATIONS

It is not the purpose of this volume to discuss the details of all techniques for the correction of all types of spine deformities but rather to set forth the broad basic principles for management of the patient with spine deformity. Eighty-five percent of the scoliosis patients who appear for treatment are in the idiopathic group. Details of the management of the patient with idiopathic scoliosis will be described. The orthopaedic surgeon involved in the treatment of scoliosis should demonstrate competence in the management of the uncomplicated idiopathic curve before undertaking the more difficult techniques necessary for the correction and stabilization involved in the management of patients with congenital scoliosis, severe neglected deformities associated with cardiorespiratory dysfunction, and certain other deformities such as severe kyphotic and scoliotic deformities requiring a combination of anterior and posterior approaches for satisfactory correction and stabilization.

CLASSIFICATION OF SPINE DEFORMITY

I. Idiopathic scoliosis

Idiopathic scoliosis represents about 85% of the patients with scoliosis who appear for treatment. The etiology is unknown, but it is now recognized that there is definite familial tendency. Three groups are identified according to age of the patient at time of recognition.

A. *Infantile* occurs under 4 years of age. The infantile idiopathic curves are usually thoracic, with convexity to the left, and with a higher incidence in boys than girls. There are two types of infantile idiopathic scoliosis.
  1. Resolving. A rare curve pattern in the United States, more common in Great Britain and on the continent. The curves always spontaneously resolve without treatment.
  2. Progressive. This is a curve of poor prognosis that always increases to a severe deformity unless aggressive treatment with the Milwaukee brace is initiated early in the evolution of the curve.

B. *Juvenile* occurs from 4 to 10 years of age.

C. *Adolescent* occurs between 11 years and skeletal maturity. This curve pattern is the most common. It has the most favorable prognosis and occurs most frequently in girls, and the most common pattern is right thoracic.

II. Congenital spine deformity

Failure of normal development of the structures in the midline dorsum of the embryo in the fourth to seventh week results in abnormalities of the spine and neural structures. MacEwen's unpublished classification is based on segmentation defects subsequently enlarged on and clarified by Winter and others.

A. Deformity caused by abnormal bone development
  1. Congenital scoliosis
    a. Failure of formation
      (1) Complete unilateral (hemivertebra)
      (2) Partial unilateral (wedge)
    b. Failure of segmentation
      (1) Partial or unilateral (bar)
      (2) Complete or bilateral block)
    c. Mixed
  2. Congenital kyphosis
    a. Failure of formation
    b. Failure of segmentation
    c. Mixed
  3. Congenital lordosis
B. Deformity caused by abnormal spinal cord development
  1. Myelodysplasia scoliosis
  2. Myelodysplasia kyphosis
  3. Myelodysplasia lordosis
C. Deformity due to mixed causes; bony abnormality plus paralysis (relevant to congenital spine deformity is the term "spinal dysraphism," which is a failure of closure of the neural tube in the midline; the extent of this failure may be mild, moderate, or severe; myelomeningocele is the most common overt lesion)

III. Neuromuscular spine deformity
A. Neuropathic
  1. Lower motor neuron (e.g., poliomyelitis)
  2. Upper motor neuron (e.g., cerebral palsy)
  3. Others (e.g., syringomyelia)
B. Myopathic
  1. Progressive (e.g., muscular dystrophy)
  2. Static (e.g., amytonia)
  3. Others (e.g., Friedreich's ataxia)
  4. Unilateral amelia

IV. Deformity associated with neurofibromatosis

V. Mesenchymal disorders
A. Congenital (e.g., Marfan's syndrome, Morquio's syndrome, miscellaneous dysplasias, arthrogryposis)
B. Acquired (e.g., rheumatoid arthritis)
C. Others (e.g., juvenile apophysitis)

VI. Trauma
A. Vertebral (e.g., fracture, radiation, surgery)
B. Extravertebral (e.g., burns, thoracoplasty)

VII. Deformity secondary to irritative phenomena (transient structural curvatures; e.g., spinal cord tumor, osteoid osteoma, nerve root irritation)

VIII. Others (e.g., metabolic, nutritional, endocrine)

IDIOPATHIC SCOLIOSIS—INDICATIONS FOR OPERATION

1. Patients who are seen too late for Milwaukee brace treatment, including girls of more than 15 years of bone age and boys 17 years or more with thoracicurvatures over 50° and unacceptable clinical deformity, and unbalanced thoracolumbar and lumbar curves over 40°.

2. Failure of Milwaukee brace treatment to control the curve.

3. Patients with thoracic curvature greater than 60°, even though the deformity is cosmetically acceptable to the patient. There is increased morbidity and mortality associated with a thoracic curvature of 60° or greater. Collis and Ponseti reported increase in the angle of the curve, even after completion of vertebral growth, as well as a greater than 60% incidence of diminished vital capacity in patients with curvatures over 60°. Nachemson reported a twofold increase in mortality in scoliotic patients as compared with the general population. Sixty percent died of cardiac or pulmonary disease. Of living scoliotic patients 47% were receiving disability pensions. Surgical treatment in these patients for correction and stabilization of the curve is therefore indicated, both for cosmetic improvement and to stabilize or improve pulmonary function.

4. Pain.

5. Another indication for surgical treatment that is more difficult to define and evaluate is the psychologic reaction of the patient to the scoliotic deformity. To evaluate the full impact of the scoliotic deformity on the adult requires psychologic examination in depth. It is true that most adults accommodate to and accept their deformity, but who knows what compromises in ambition, career, choice of mate, etc., were made along the way? The psychologic response of the adolescent patient to good correction that is maintained is most gratifying. More adults are requesting treatment for scoliosis-related disabilities than ever before. Many patients would be better off and lead happier and healthier lives had successful treatment been accomplished in adolescence.

In the following discussion on the management of idiopathic scoliosis the *selection of the fusion area* is considered first, followed by *spine instrumentation and fusion techniques* and *preoperative and postoperative plaster techniques.*

SELECTION OF THE FUSION AREA

In this discussion of the selection of the fusion area, all illustrative radiographs are viewed from the back. The right side of each illustration is the right side of the patient.

The curve is measured by the Cobb method. The end vertebrae of a structural curve tilt maximally into the concavity of the curve. Vertebral rotation is determined by Moe's method, which depends on the relationship of the oval shadows of the pedicles to the lateral margins of the vertebral body. When the pedicle is further away from the lateral margin of the vertebral body, that vertebra is rotated to that side. When the pedicles are equidistant to the lateral margins of the vertebral body, the vertebra is in neutral rotation. The end vertebra is not necessarily a neutral vertebra. Moe has pointed out that all vertebrae rotated into the convexity of the major curve must be included in the fusion area, and preferably the fusion should extend from neutral vertebra above to neutral vertebra below. Short fusions are responsible for recurrent deformity. The minimum fusion area has been defined as that area of the spine including all vertebrae within the major curve. However, if the *minimum fusion area* in a particular patient is defined as that *area of the spine requiring stabilization to maintain correction,* then vertebral rotation must be taken into account. When preoperative correction is obtained either by traction or cast, the final decision about the extent of the fusion may be made after the correction because one or two vertebrae may be derotated and the fusion area may be shortened. Under any circumstances the fusion must always include at least all the vertebrae in the major curve.

To determine the fusion area, one defines whether there is (1) a single major curve, (2) a double curve pattern, (3) vertebral rotation beyond the major curve, and (4) the presence or absence of lumbosacral anomalies, particularly spondylolisthesis.

The guidelines we have used in the selection of the fusion area in the various curve patterns follow.

THORACIC CURVE PATTERNS. The several variations of this curve pattern may be classified as follows:

1. Single major thoracic curve with compensatory nonstructural or minimally structural upper thoracic and lumbar curves
2. Major thoracic curve with compensatory structural upper thoracic and compensatory nonstructural or mild structural lumbar curve
3. Major thoracic curve with compensatory significantly structural lumbar curve
4. Double major thoracic curve (Moe)

The single major thoracic curve (Fig. 1) requires fusion of the major curve alone and any vertebrae distal to the curve rotated into the convexity of the major curve. There is a difference of opinion regarding the fusion area required for the most satisfactory results in the variations of the thoracic curve patterns listed in numbers 2 and 3 above. The treatment of these curve patterns will be discussed later. The double major thoracic curve described by Moe (Fig. 11) requires fusion of both the upper and lower thoracic curves.

Single major thoracic curve pattern. When the end vertebrae are neutral, one should fuse all vertebrae in the curve and one vertebra proximal and one distal to the major curve (Fig. 1). Although fusion of the major curve alone is permissible in this situation, experience has shown that there may be lengthening of the curve with some recurrent deformity after immobilization is discontinued. Including one vertebra distal to the major curve in the fusion minimizes this complication.

When one or more vertebrae distal to the end vertebra are rotated into the convexity of the major curve, fuse the major curve and all vertebrae rotated into the major curve and preferably from neutral vertebra above to neutral vertebra below. If preoperative correction is obtained, the final decision on the length of the fusion may be made after localizer or traction correction. One or two vertebrae may be derotated during correction,

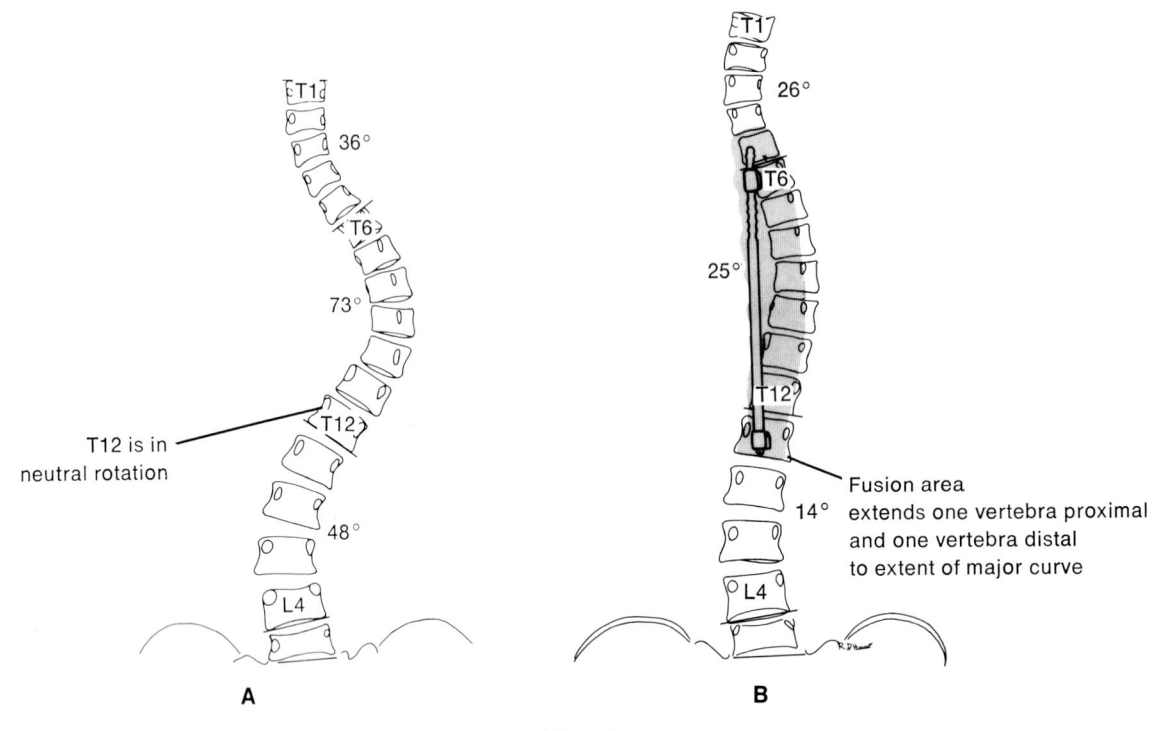

Fig. 1

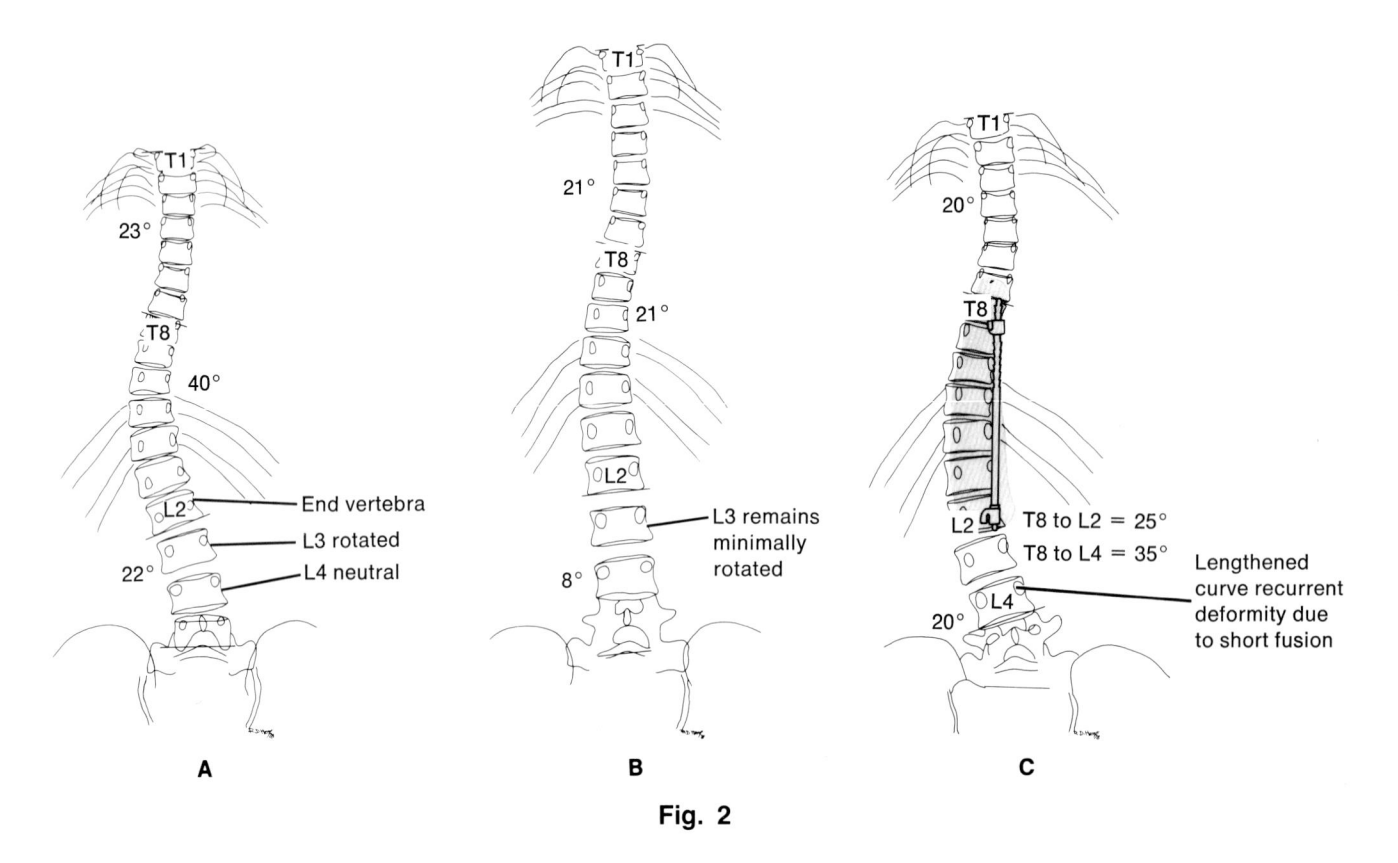

A
- 36°
- T1
- T6
- 73°
- T12 is in neutral rotation
- T12
- 48°
- L4

B
- T1
- 26°
- T6
- 25°
- T12
- 14°
- L4
- Fusion area extends one vertebra proximal and one vertebra distal to extent of major curve

Fig. 2

A
- T1
- 23°
- T8
- 40°
- L2 — End vertebra
- L3 rotated
- L4 neutral
- 22°

B
- T1
- 21°
- T8
- 21°
- L2
- L3 remains minimally rotated
- 8°

C
- T1
- 20°
- T8
- L2
- L4
- 20°
- T8 to L2 = 25°
- T8 to L4 = 35°
- Lengthened curve recurrent deformity due to short fusion

218

Fig. 3

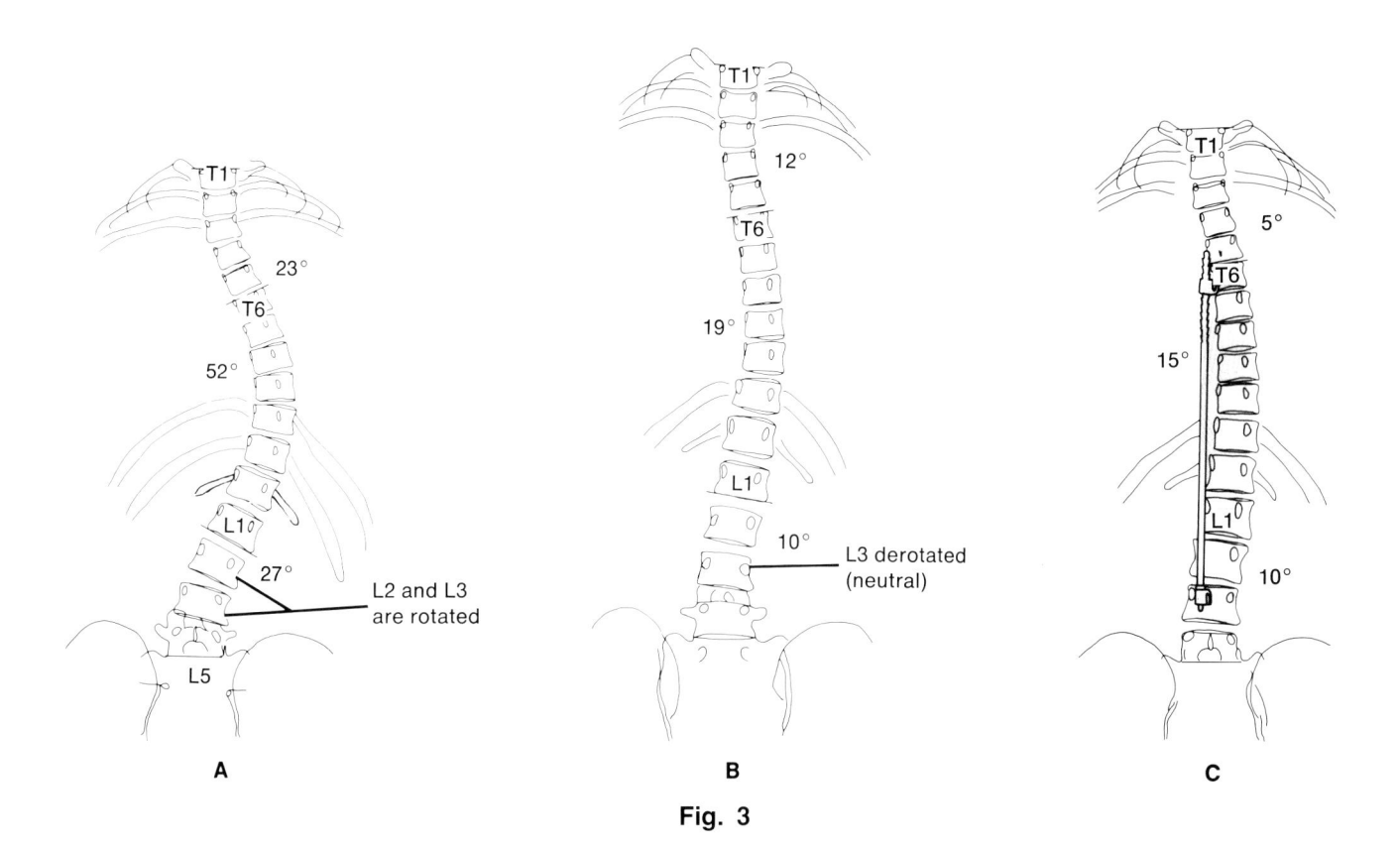

thus permitting shortening of the proposed fusion area.

Fig. 2 illustrates the importance of rotation of vertebrae distal to the major curve into the convexity of the curve in the selection of the fusion area. In Fig. 2, *A*, the major curve is T8 to L2, with L3 rotated into the convexity of the major curve, and L4 is neutral. The radiographic tracing after localizer cast correction in Fig. 2, *B*, shows L3 remains rotated into the convexity of the curve. Treatment was by surgery in the cast and instrumentation from T8 to L2 with spine fusion from T7 to L2. The fusion was too short. It did not include all the vertebrae rotated into the convexity of the curve preoperatively, and as a result the curve lengthened postoperatively. Fig. 2, *C*, shows maintenance of correction of the fused curve at 25°, with lengthening of the curve to include L4. The lengthened curve T8 to L4 is 35°, 10° more than the fused major curve. The lengthened curve compromised the cosmetic result. The proper fusion area in this patient should have included L3.

Fig. 3, *A*, shows the radiographic tracing of a major thoracic curve T6 to L1 measuring 52°. L2 and L3 are rotated into the convexity of the major curve; L4 is neutral. Unsegmented L5 is part of the sacrum. After preoperative localizer cast correction the major curve is reduced to 19°. L2 remained rotated into the convexity of the curve. L3 was derotated and is now neutral. The fusion area required to stabilize this curve and maintain correction is from T6 to L3. We prefer to fuse one vertebra proximal to the top end vertebra (see p. 239) of the curve. This was done, and fusion was from T5 to L3. Fig. 3, *C*, shows the result 6 years postoperatively.

When there is marked displacement of the thorax toward the convexity of the curve with the end vertebra neutral, at least two vertebrae distal to the major curve are included in the fusion. If preoperative correction by traction or localizer cast is accomplished, another useful guideline is to fuse to a level vertebra distally as determined on the preoperative correction radiograph. Fig. 4 shows a T4 to T12 curve measuring 77°, with marked displacement of the torso toward the convexity of the curve. T12 is neutral. L1 is slightly rotated into the lumbar curve below. Surgical instrumentation and fusion was performed without preliminary preoperative correction. Fusion extended from T4 to L1. The status at 6 days after surgery is seen in Fig. 4, *B*. At 9 years after surgery, in Fig. 4, *C*, correction within the fused major curve was maintained at 28°, but the curve is lengthened to include L2, with acute angulation between L1 and L2 and a 14° recurrent deformity caused by too short a fusion. In this patient the fusion should have extended to include at least L2. If there is doubt, it should extend to L3. The use of preliminary preoperative correction prior to instrumentation and fusion is helpful in the selection of the proper fusion area.

Fig. 5, *A*, is an example of a single major thoracic curve with neutral distal end vertebra, L1, and severe displacement of the torso toward the convexity of the major curve. The thoracic curve, T5 to L1, 78°, was treated by preoperative localizer cast correction (Fig. 5, *B*) and surgery in the cast, Harrington distraction instrumentation from T5 to L3, and spine fusion from T4 to L3. The fusion extended two vertebrae distal to the end vertebra, a parallel vertebra. Fig. 5, *C*, shows maintenance of correction with a balanced torso 7 years after surgery.

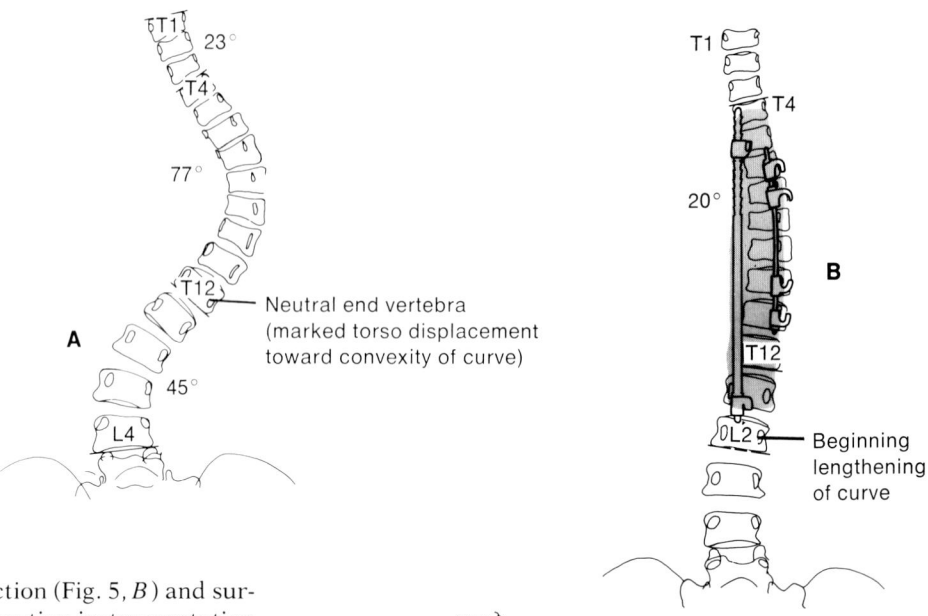

When recurrent deformity is the result of too short a fusion, the proper treatment is recorrection of the deformity, osteotomy of the fusion area if necessary, and extension of the fusion distally (and proximally as well, if necessary) sufficient to give a stable well-balanced spine.

Major thoracic curve with compensatory structural upper thoracic and compensatory nonstructural or mild structural lumbar curve. In this curve pattern, bend radiographs show the upper thoracic curve more highly structural than the lower thoracic curve. These patients often present a dilemma as to whether to include the upper thoracic curve in the fusion area. The criteria we have used to determine when to include the upper thoracic curve in the fusion are the following:

1. Clinical examination reveals a fullness of the trapezius outline on the side of the convexity of the upper thoracic curve with or without elevation of the shoulder girdle.
2. Radiographs show a positive obliquity of the first thoracic vertebra (Fig. 6, *A*), elevation of the first rib on the convex side of the upper thoracic curve, and significant structural change demonstrated on side-bending radiograph.

The sign and degree of obliquity of the first thoracic vertebra is measured and its relationship correlated with the patient's clinical appearance. This was determined on a roentgenogram of the spine made in erect posture (Fig. 6). The angle formed by the intersection of two reference lines is measured. This angle with its positive or negative sign is designated the obliquity of the T1 vertebra.

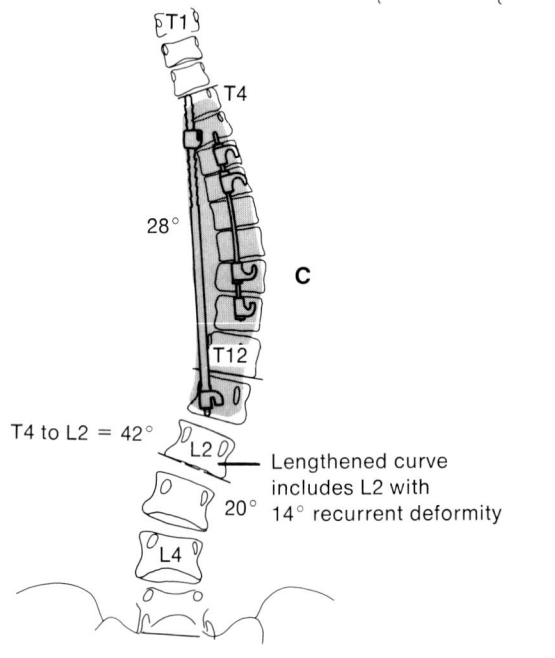

Fig. 4

The long edge of the film is perpendicular to the floor and is used as a line of reference to determine the obliquity of T1. The first line is drawn to the top of the pedicles or the superior cortical plate of the first thoracic vertebra. A second line is drawn perpendicular to the edge of the film intersecting the first at the top of the right pedicle of T1 in the left upper thoracic curve. The angle in degrees subtended by these two lines is the degree of obliquity. The acute angle formed above the horizontal is designated positive (Fig. 6, *A*). The acute angle formed below the horizontal is designated negative (Fig. 6, *B*).

Fig. 5

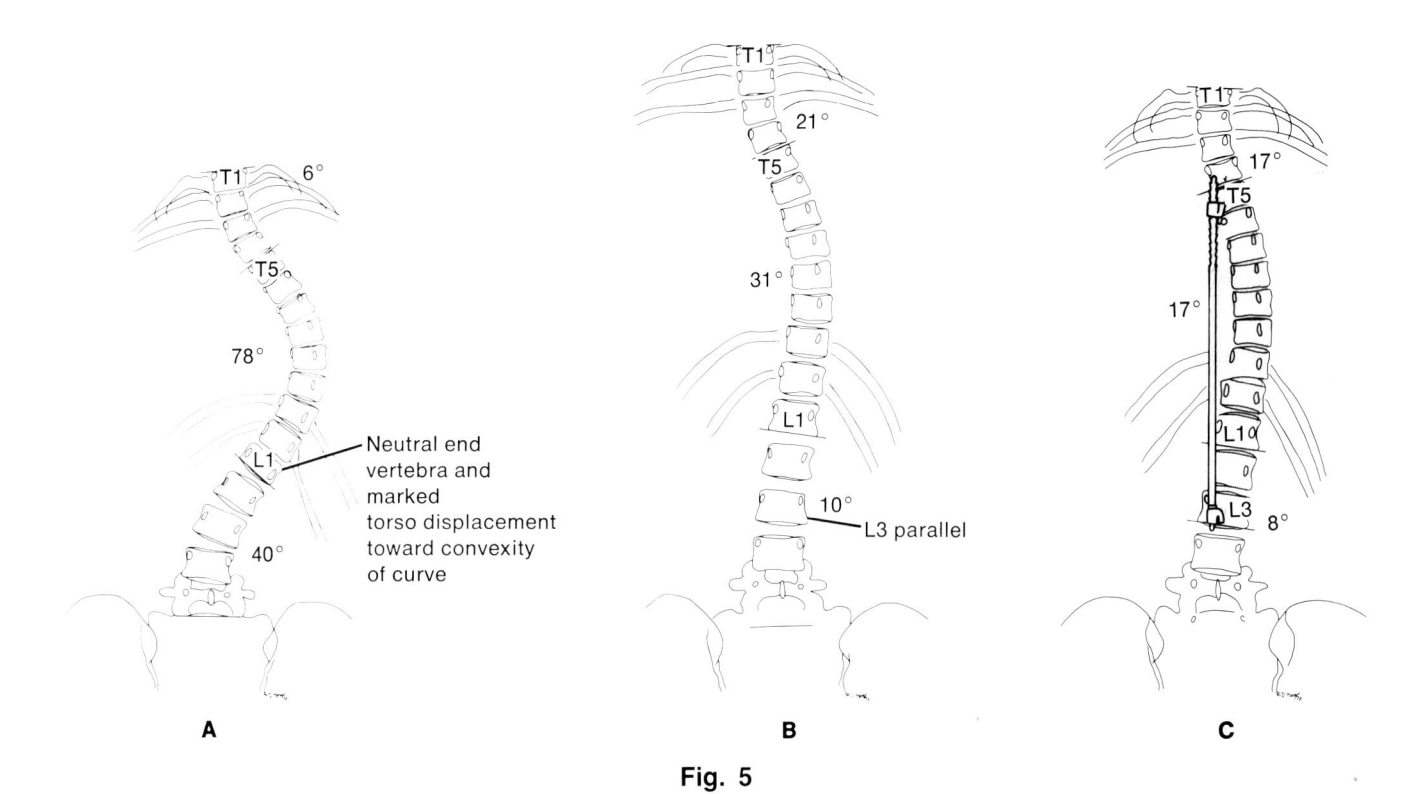

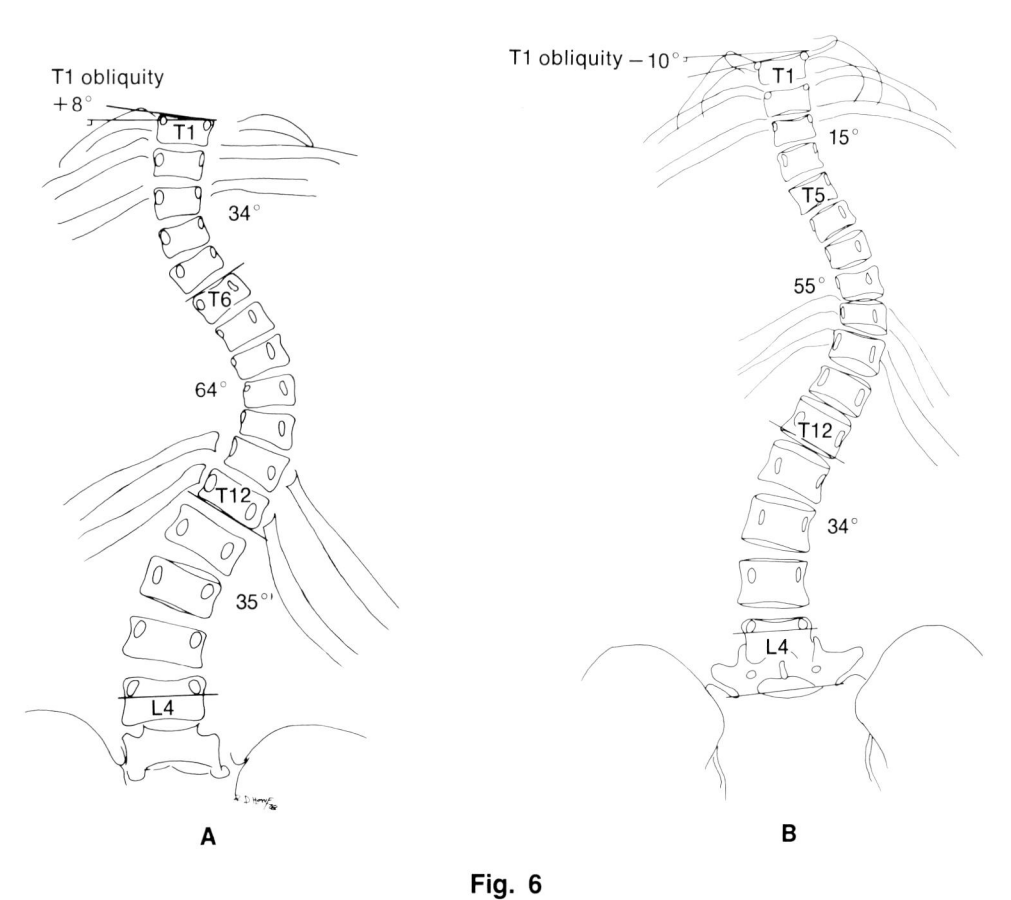

Fig. 6

Fig. 7, *A*, shows a patient with this curve pattern with an upper thoracic curve, T1 to T5, measuring 33°, and lower thoracic curve, T5 to L1, measuring 59°. The obliquity of T1 is +5° with elevation of the left first rib. The upper thoracic curve corrected only 23% as compared to 58% for the lower thoracic; this is indicative of the greater rigidity of the upper curve. Treatment was surgery in the cast with instrumentation from T5 to L2 and spine fusion from T4 to L2. Fig. 7, *C*, shows the postoperative result: T1 to T5, 27°, T5 to L1, 24°. The obliquity of T1 is +10° with elevation of the left first rib that is greater than in the precorrection radiograph. Postoperatively this patient showed elevation of the left shoulder, fullness of the left trapezius, and an unsatisfactory result cosmetically. The proper treatment in this patient would have been instrumentation from T2 to L2 and fusion from T1 to L2.

Fig. 8 shows a patient with the same curve pattern in whom both curves were instrumented and fused with an excellent postoperative result.

Indications for inclusion of the upper thoracic curve in the fusion area are the following:

1. The clinical finding of fullness of the trapezius outline on the convex side of the upper thoracic curve
2. The radiographic findings of a positive obliquity of T1, a greater degree of structural change in the upper thoracic than in the lower thoracic curve, and elevation of the first rib on the convex side of the upper curve

Major thoracic curve with compensatory significantly structural lumbar curve (bend radiographs show persistence of vertebral rotation as well as lateral angulation). In this curve pattern there are two options in selection of the fusion area:

1. Fuse the thoracic curve alone if bend radiographs indicate the potential of the lumbar curve to compensate for the correction of the thoracic curve and result in a balanced torso. If the spine is immature, it may be necessary to protect the lumbar curve in a Milwaukee brace postoperatively to skeletal maturity. Fig. 9 *A*, shows a 78° thoracic curve, T6 to T12, associated with a highly structural lumbar curve, T12 to L4, measuring 58°. The clinical picture was that of a major thoracic curve pattern with displacement of the torso toward the right. In Fig. 9, *B*, the preoperative localizer cast correction shows the thoracic curve at 38° and the lumbar curve at 31°. It was elected to instrument and fuse the thoracic curve alone, T5 to L1. In this instance in Fig. 9, *C*, the result at 5 years after surgery is seen. Good correction and a balanced torso are maintained.

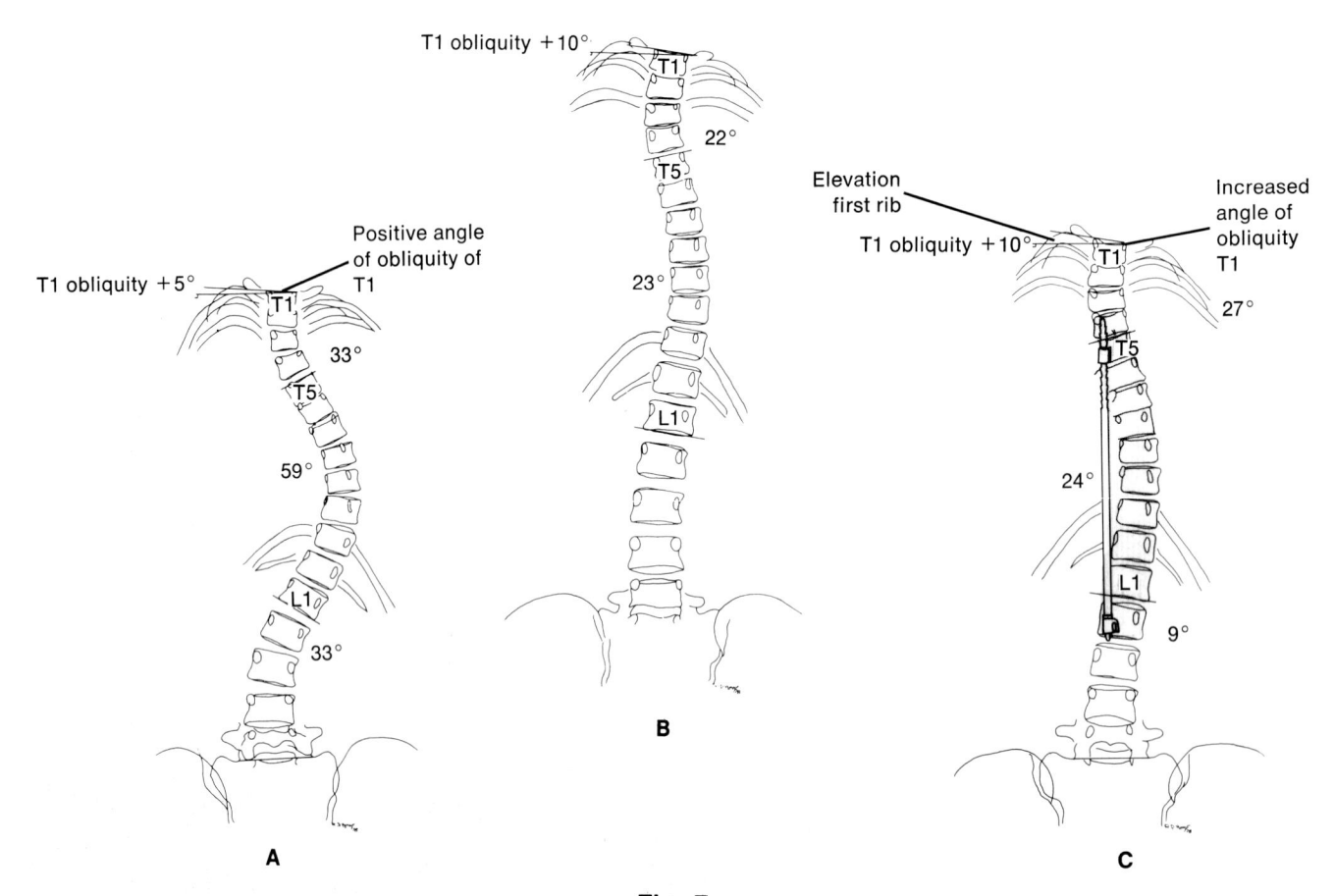

Fig. 7

Fig. 8

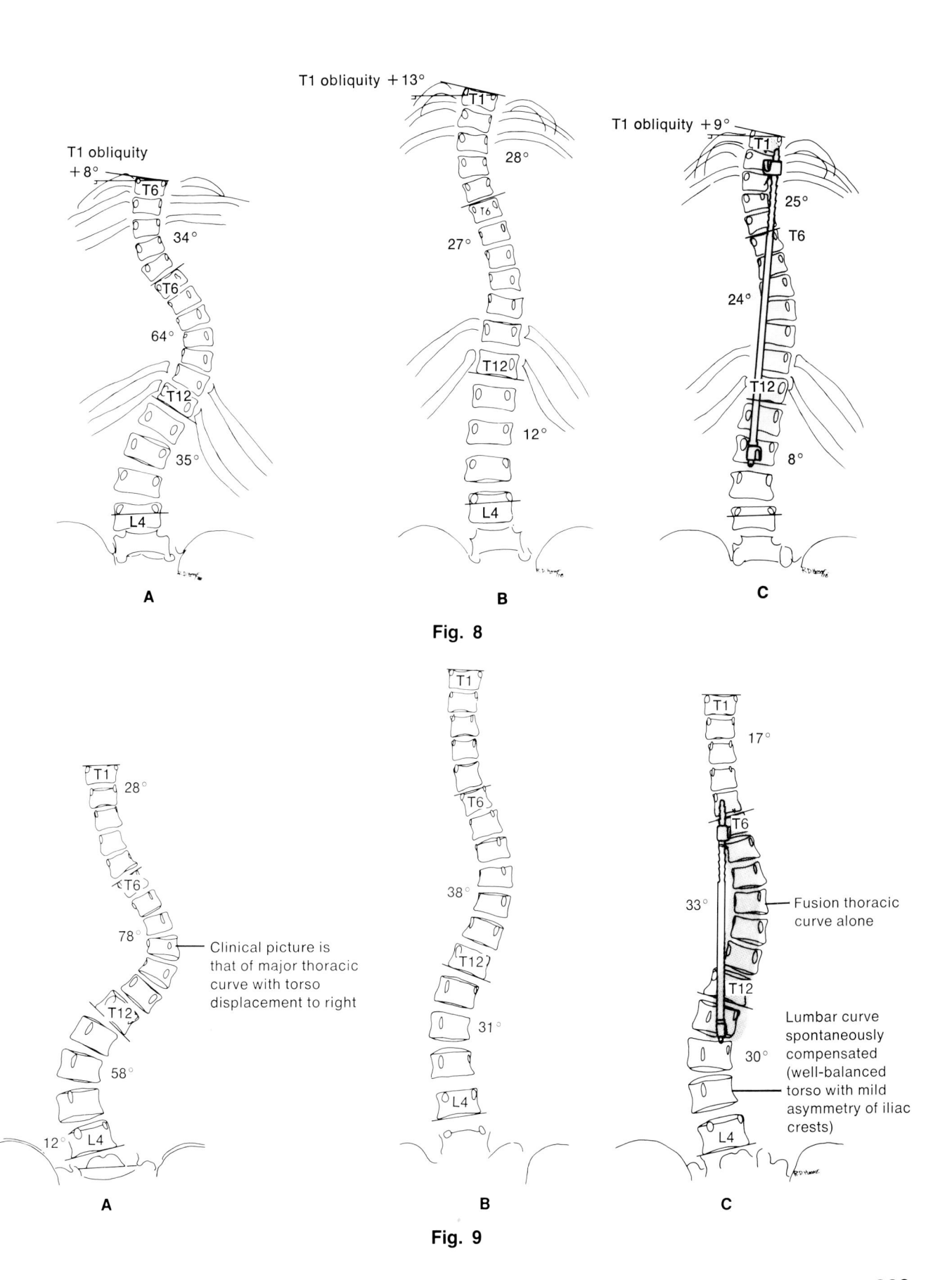

Fig. 9

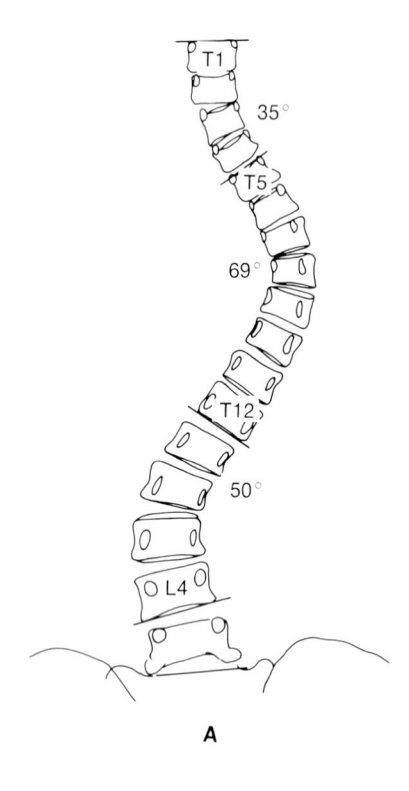

2. Fuse both curves, as in the double major curve pattern. Fig. 10, *A*, demonstrates a similar situation with a right T5 to T12 curve of 69° associated with a 50° left lumbar curve. Fig. 10, *B*, shows the preoperative localizer cast correction. In this patient, it was elected to instrument and fuse both curves, T5 to L4. Fig. 10, *C*, shows the result at 4 years after surgery with a well-corrected and perfectly balanced torso.

Double major thoracic curve pattern. This curve is characterized by structural upper and lower thoracic curves of about equal angulation. Fig. 11, *A*, shows a double major thoracic curve: T1 to T7, 60°, T7 to T12, 58°. Both curves require correction and stabilization. The precorrection radiograph shows an upper thoracic curve with a positive obliquity of T1 (Fig. 11, *A*) and elevation of the first rib. Treatment of this patient was by preoperative localizer cast correction (Fig. 11, *B*), surgery in the cast with instrumentation from T2 to L1 with the distraction rod spanning the concavity of both thoracic curves, and fusion from T1 to L1. Fig. 11, *C*, shows the postoperative result with slight residual elevation of the left first rib. Clinically the shoulders are level, and there is minimal fullness of the left trapezius and a balanced torso. If the lower thoracic curve alone is corrected and fused, the result is gross asymmetry of the shoulder girdles, high left side, and increased fullness of the left trapezius outline.

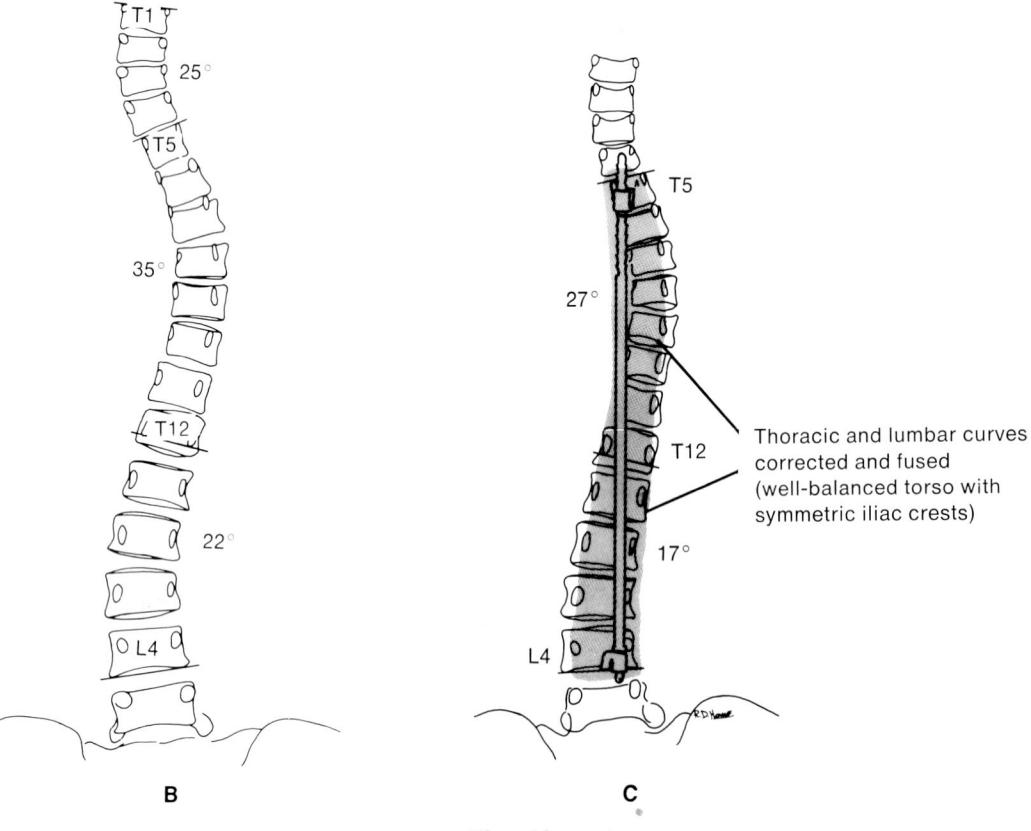

Fig. 10

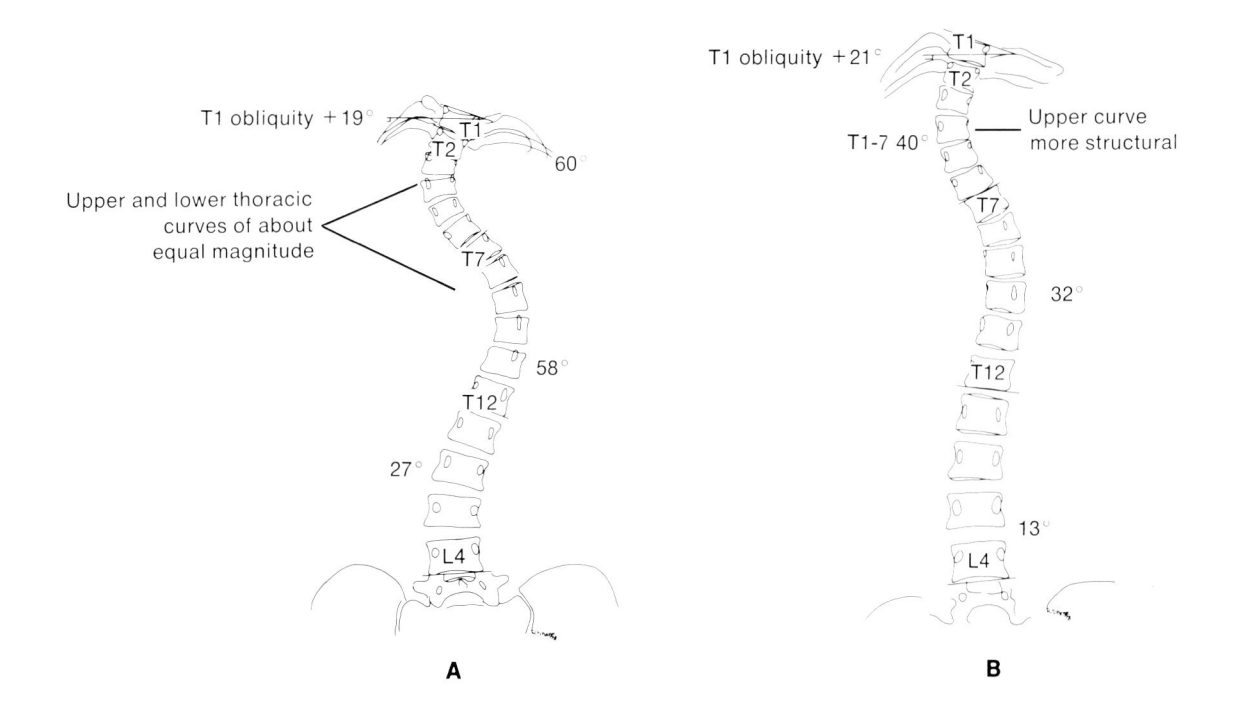

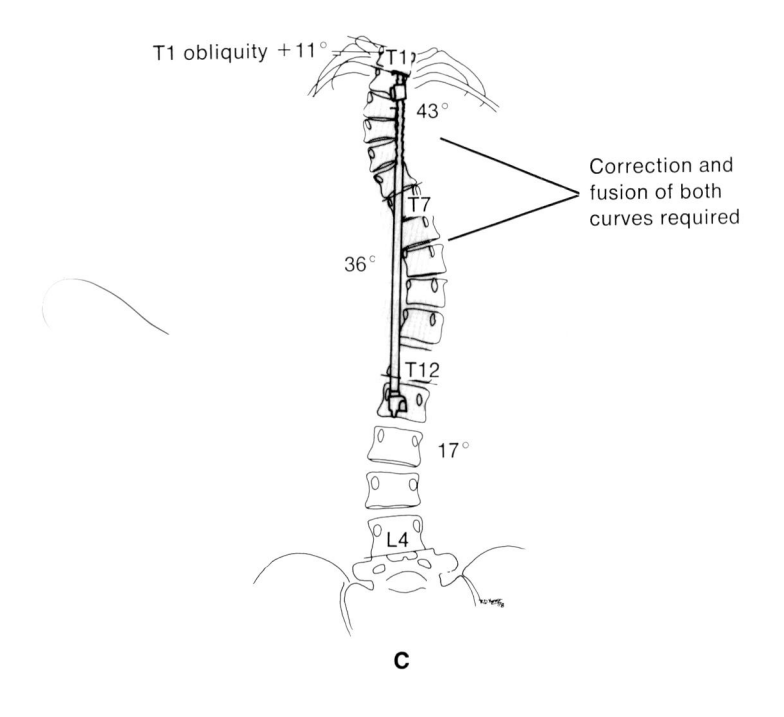

Fig. 11

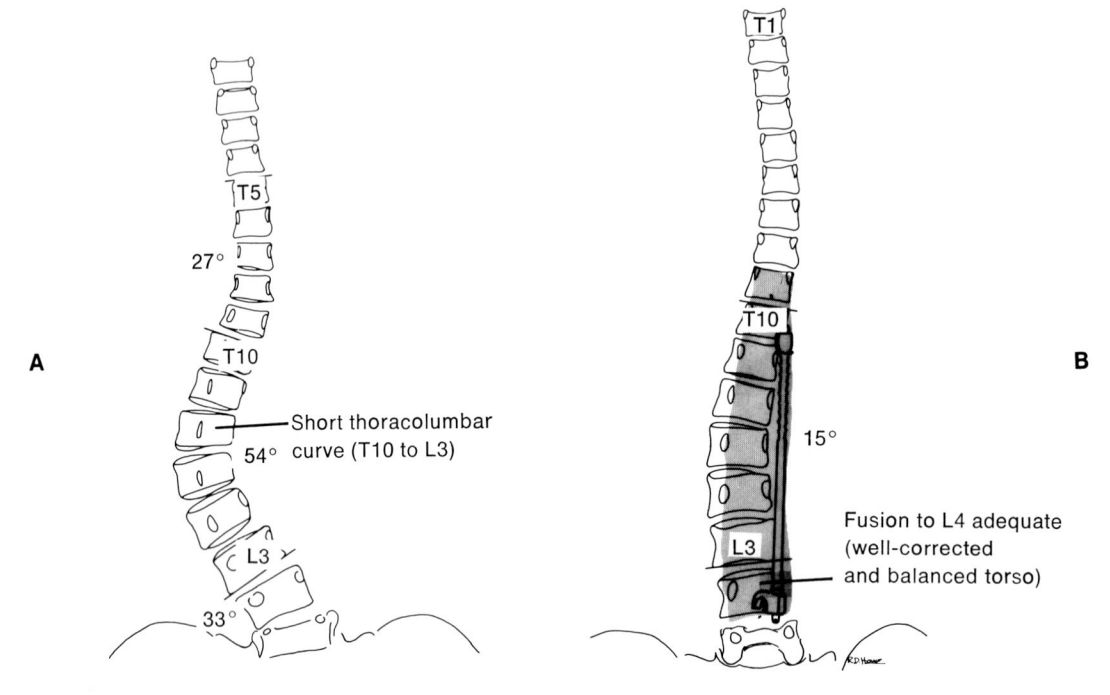

Fig. 12

- 27°
- T5
- T10
- 54° Short thoracolumbar curve (T10 to L3)
- L3
- 33°
- 15°
- T10
- L3
- Fusion to L4 adequate (well-corrected and balanced torso)

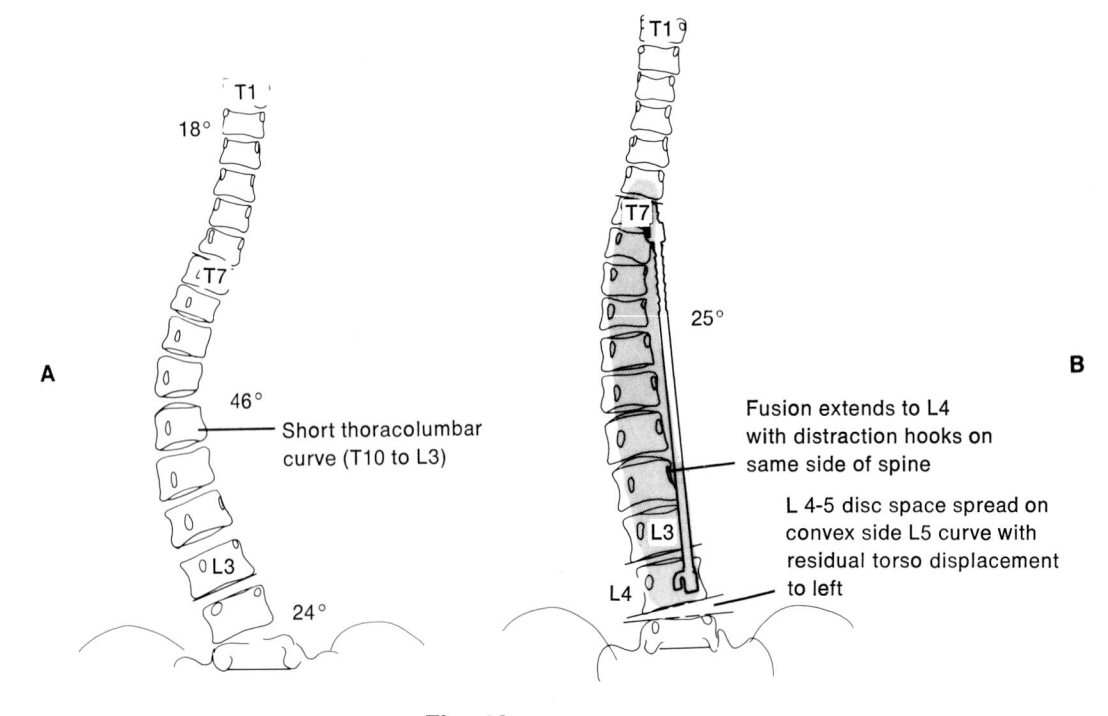

Fig. 13

- T1
- 18°
- T7
- 46° Short thoracolumbar curve (T10 to L3)
- L3
- 24°
- T1
- T7
- 25°
- L3
- L4
- Fusion extends to L4 with distraction hooks on same side of spine
- L 4-5 disc space spread on convex side L5 curve with residual torso displacement to left

THORACOLUMBAR AND LUMBAR CURVES. The distal end vertebra is usually L3. With a short thoracolumbar curve, T10 or T11 to L3, fusion to the fourth lumbar vertebra is adequate. Fig. 12, *A*, shows a short thoracolumbar curve, T10 to L3, measuring 54°. Fig. 12, *B*, illustrates the postoperative result, which shows maintenance of good correction with a well-balanced torso at 4 years 6 months after surgery, with instrumentation from T10 to L4 and fusion from T9 to L4. The fusion must extend to the fifth lumbar vertebra when there is marked displacement of the thorax or with a long thoracolumbar curve, T7, T8, or T9 to L3. In these circumstances it is also important to properly place the distraction hooks. The inferior distraction hook is placed over the lamina of L5 on the concave side of the lumbosacral curve, and the superior distraction hook is placed on the concave side of the curve above. The distraction rod will span the concavity of both curves. This prevents the L4 to L5 disc space from opening up on the convex side of the lumbosacral curve and ensures good torso balance. These principles are illustrated in Figs. 13 to 15. Fusion to the sacrum is not indicated in the absence of lumbosacral anomalies.

Fig. 13, *A*, shows a long thoracolumbar curve, T7 to L3, measuring 46°. This patient was treated with instrumentation, T7 to L4, and fusion, T6 to L4. Fig. 13, *B*, shows the postoperative result at 2 years 6 months after surgery. There is some residual displacement of the torso toward the convexity of the corrected curve caused by opening up of the L4 to L5 disc space on the convex (right) side of the lumbosacral curve. The proper fusion area in this patient was T6 to L5, with the inferior distraction hook placed over the lamina on the concave (left) side of the lumbosacral curve so that the distraction rod would span the concavity of both curves.

Fig. 14, *A*, shows a short thoracolumbar curve, T11 to L3, with marked displacement of the torso toward the convexity of the curve. Fig. 14, *B*, is a left bend radiograph showing structural change in the thoracolumbar curve. Fig. 14, *C*, is a right bend radiograph showing structural change in the concavity of the lumbosacral curve. This patient was treated with preoperative lo-

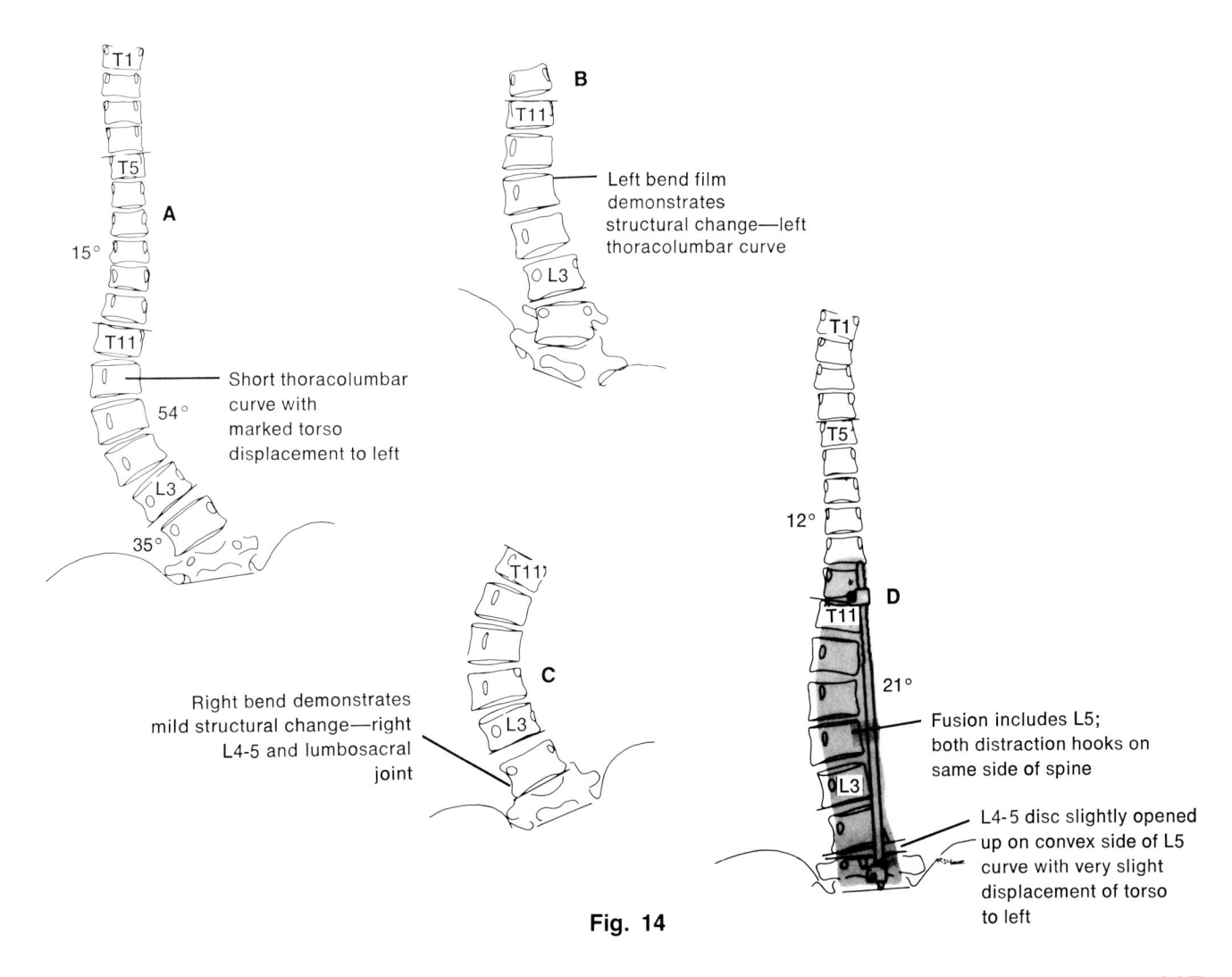

Fig. 14

Fig. 15

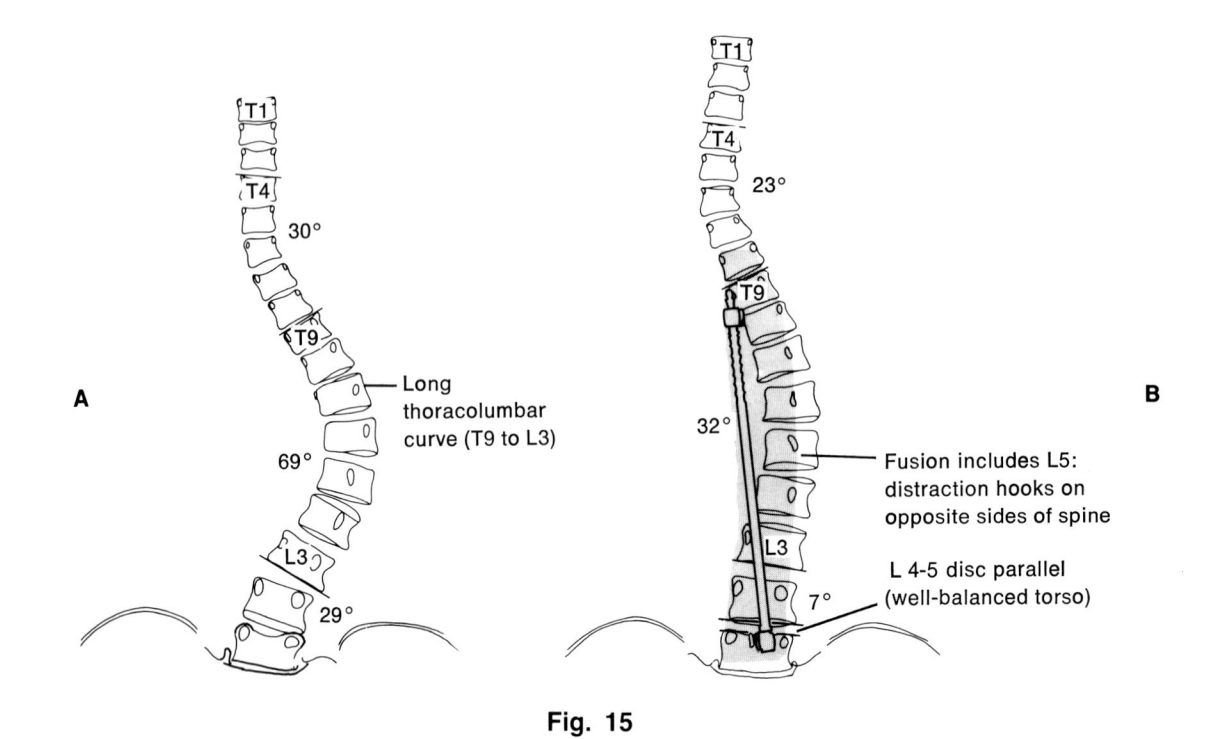

Fig. 16

calizer cast correction and surgery in the cast. Instrumentation was performed from T10 to L5 and fusion from T9 to L5. Fig. 14, *D*, demonstrates the postoperative results at 3 years. Note that the inferior and superior distraction hooks are both on the same side of the spine and there is a slight opening up of the L4 to L5 disc space on the convex (right) side of the lumbosacral curve. There was mild residual displacement of the torso toward the left. The fusion area is correct, but the inferior distraction hook should have been placed over the lamina of L5 on the left side rather than on the right side. During correction by distraction, the right side of the disc space between L4 and L5 opened up slightly. Placing the hook on the left side on the lamina would prevent this and maintain a symmetric disc space (Fig. 15, *B*).

Fig. 15 illustrates the proper fusion area and correct placement of the distraction hooks and distraction rod. Fig. 15, *A*, shows a T9 to L3 curve measuring 69°. Treatment was by preoperative localizer cast correction and surgery in the cast, instrumentation, T9 to L5, with the distraction hooks placed on opposite sides of the spine so that the distraction rod spanned the concavity of both curves. Fusion was from T8 to L5. Note that the L4 to L5 disc space is parallel. A well-balanced torso resulted (Fig. 15, *B*).

These guidelines for the inclusion of L5 in the fusion area and placement of the distraction hooks on opposite sides of the spine in the treatment of certain thoracolumbar and lumbar curves give more assurance of a balanced torso postoperatively. When the fusion is stopped at L4, as in the patient in Fig. 13, the opening up postoperatively of the disc space at L4-5 cannot always be predicted on preoperative analysis, even with the aid of bend radiographs. This phenomenon probably is related to instability of the disc at L4-5. Disc instability is still a mystery and probably plays a part in behavior of the unfused portion of the spine distal to the fusion and varies in individual patients.

DOUBLE MAJOR CURVE PATTERN. When there is a *double major curve*—either a combined thoracic and lumbar or a combined thoracic and thoracolumbar curve—both curves must be fused. Fig. 16, *A*, shows a combined thoracic and lumbar double major curve pattern. Fig. 16, *B*, demonstrates the correction obtained in the preoperative localizer cast. Treatment was by instrumentation and fusion in the cast of both curves. Fig. 16, *C*, shows the postoperative result at 4 years 5 months after surgery. Correction is maintained with a well-balanced torso.

SCOLIOSIS WITH LUMBOSACRAL SPONDYLOLISTHESIS. Anomalous development of the lumbosacral joint may be associated with various curve patterns in the anatomically normal vertebrae above. Routine scoliosis radiographs include a lateral of the lumbosacral joint. If there is evidence of anomalous development, a more complete study, including oblique and side-bending views of the lumbosacral spine, is indicated. When there is spondylolisthesis, its relationship, if any, to scoliosis must be defined and the proper treatment planned.

If the spondylolisthesis, associated with a thoracic curve, is of mild degree and asymptomatic, it requires no treatment. If it is severe, symptomatic, or associated with a thoracolumbar or lumbar curve, stabilization of the lumbosacral joint is indicated in the overall treatment.

The following situations have been experienced. A *structural thoracic curve* may be associated with a lumbosacral spondylolisthesis and a nonstructural lumbar curve. In this situation, the thoracic curve is corrected and fused. If the spondylolisthesis is severe or symptomatic, the lumbosacral level is stabilized, usually L4 to sacrum, leaving the joints of the lumbar spine between the two fusions open. Fig. 17, *A*, shows a major right thoracic structural curve, T6 to T12, measuring 67°, associated with a nonstructural left lumbar curve and a fourth-degree spondylolisthesis at the lumbosacral level. Treatment was by instrumentation and fusion of the thoracic curve followed 2 weeks later by the stabilization of the lumbosacral level with fusion of L3 to the sacrum, leaving the lumbar joints in between open. Fusion of L4 to the sacrum would have been adequate. Fig. 17, *B*, demonstrates the postoperative result at 5 years with solid fusion at both levels, a well-balanced torso, and relief of lumbosacral symptoms. Fig. 17, *C*, shows a lateral view of the spine with the two fusion areas.

Reduction of severe spondylolisthesis associated with scoliosis. The treatment described is a modified Harrington technique. The loose posterior arch of L5 is removed from adherent dura, which is tightly stretched over the sacrum. The fibrocartilaginous tissue in the pars defect is excised. Instrumentation is from L1 or L2 to the sacrum using special sacral hooks over the ala of the sacrum, and 1252 hooks are seated on the inferior surface of the lamina of L1 or L2 (Fig. 18, *C*). Gradual partial reduction is accomplished with two Harrington distraction rods. The dura becomes lax during the distraction process as the body of L5 moves cephalad and posterior toward reduction. A lateral radiograph is made on the operating table. A Stagnara "wake-up test" is performed after distraction to determine if there is neurologic deficit. The distraction relieves tension on the neural structures. Spine fusion including the transverse processes is performed from L1 or L2 (the level of the proximal distraction hooks) to the sacrum protecting the exposed dura. (See Plate 8-1, *E* to *G*). After the patient is on a turning frame for 2 weeks, a pantaloon localizer cast is applied. At 3 months after surgery an ambulatory localizer cast is applied and worn for 5 months. When indicated, a Milwaukee brace is worn for control of the thoracic curve. If the scoliosis is of sufficient severity, instrumentation and fusion of the thoracic curve is performed as a second-stage procedure. Fig. 18, *D*, shows about 50% reduction of L5. If more complete reduction of the spondylolisthesis is obtained, square-ended bent Harrington rods with square-hole sacral hooks are used to prevent rotation of the bent rods and to retain some lumbar lordosis. Operative re-

Fig. 17

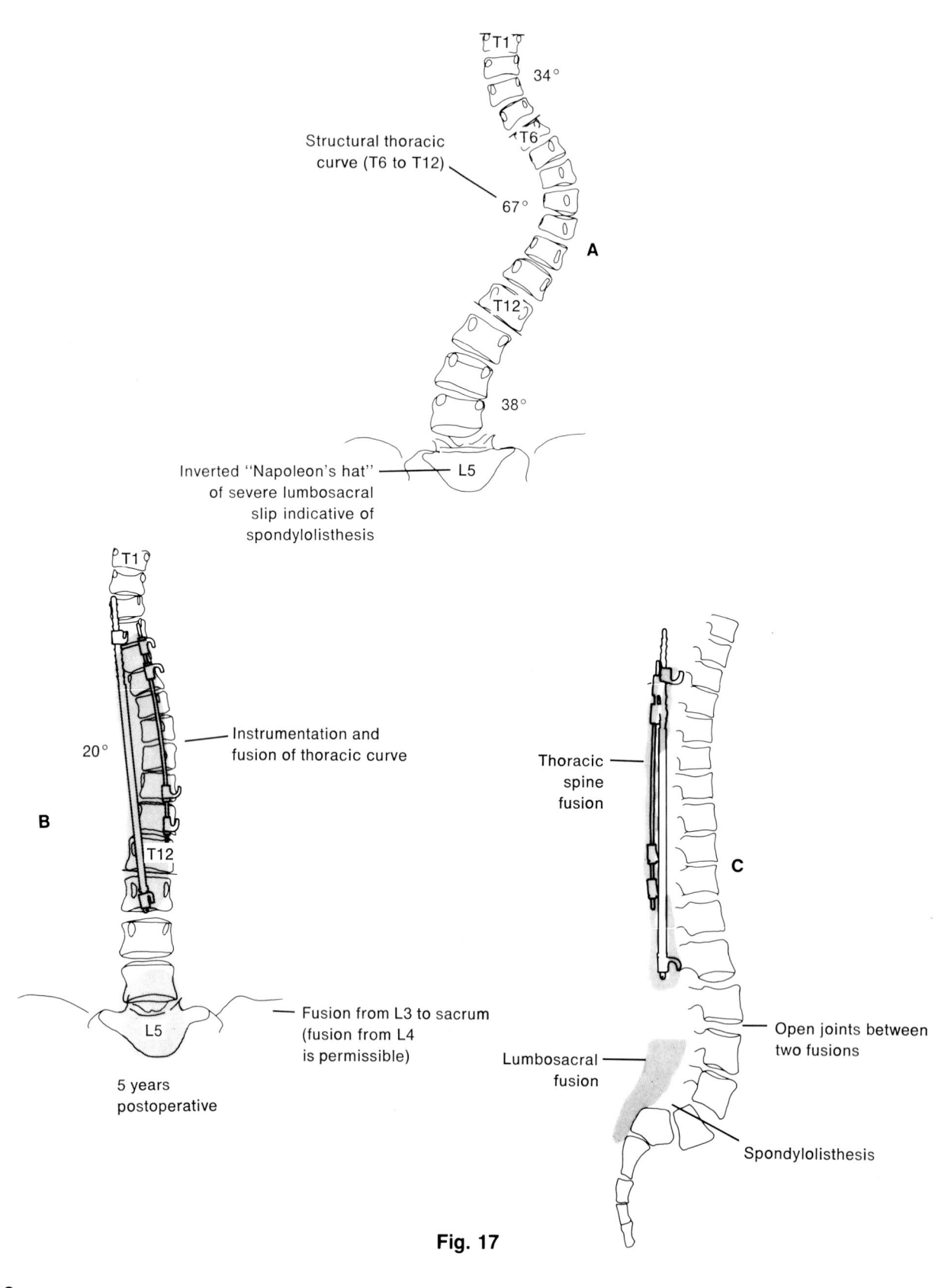

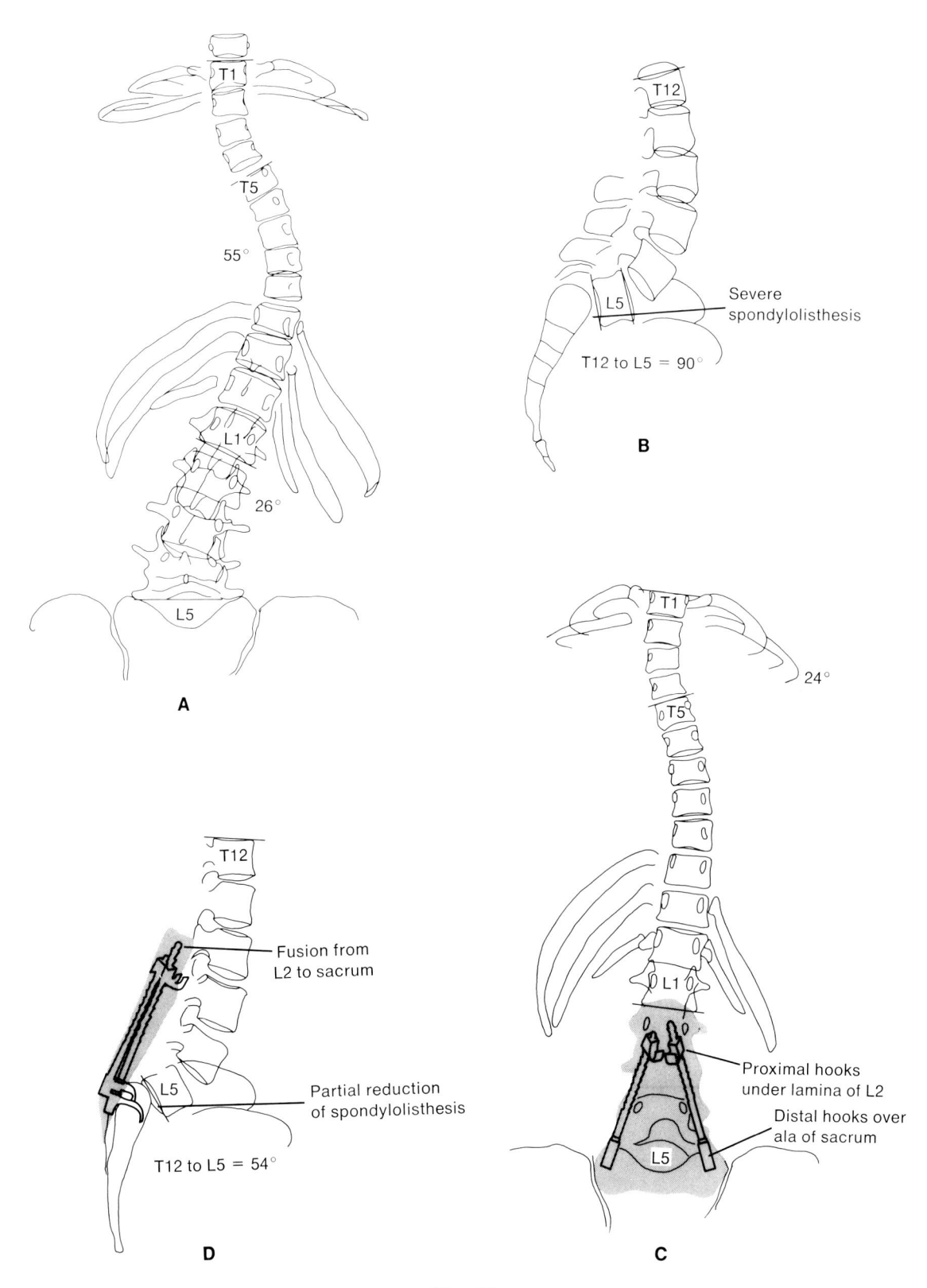

Fig. 18

duction of spondylolisthesis requires the expertise of a skilled spine surgeon.

In a *thoracolumbar nonstructural scoliosis* associated with spondylolisthesis, on bend radiograph the thoracolumbar curve completely corrects. In this circumstance the lumbosacral level can be stabilized by fusion with the lumbar curve corrected. One should not stabilize the lumbosacral level with L4 tilted and fuse the deformity in situ. The thoracolumbar curve should therefore first be corrected in a localizer cast, and it is best to perform the fusion in the cast, being certain that the fourth lumbar vertebra is fused to the sacrum in a corrected position. Fig. 19, *A*, shows a thoracolumbar curve, T 9 to L2, measuring 44° associated with a fourth-degree lumbosacral spondylolisthesis. Bend radiograph (not illustrated) showed the T9 to L2 curve to be nonstructural. Treatment was preoperative correction in a localizer cast and fusion of L2 to the sacrum. Fig. 19, *B*, shows the postoperative result at 7 years. The nonstructural curve above spontaneously corrected. The torso is well balanced. Fusion of L3 to the sacrum would have been adequate.

Fig. 19, *C*, shows a lateral view of the fusion mass.

In a *structural thoracolumbar or lumbar scoliosis associated with spondylolisthesis*, if the curve is severe enough to warrant surgical treatment, fusion would include the curvature and extend to the sacrum. The top vertebra in the fusion must be centered over the midline sacrum to ensure a balanced torso postoperatively. Fig. 20, *A*, shows a structural left lumbar curve, T11 to L4, measuring 37°, associated with a grade 1 spondylolisthesis (Fig. 20, *B*), with 2 cm displacement of the torso toward the left. The patient was 16 years of age and did not benefit by 1 year of treatment in Milwaukee brace. Treatment is by preoperative localizer cast correction (Fig. 20, *B*) with surgery in the cast and instrumentation from the right side of T11 to the left sacral ala. Spine fusion extended from T10 to the sacrum (Fig. 20, *C* and *D*). The Harrington distraction rod is bent to retain some lordosis (Fig. 20, *D*). A square-ended rod and square-hole sacral ala hook were used to prevent rotation of the distraction rod.

In the presence of asymptomatic spondylolisthesis or mild (grade 1) spondylolisthesis, spine fusion to L4 rather than to the sacrum is an option. With spine fusion to L4, the patient and family should be informed of the risk factor of developing lumbosacral symptoms in later years.

A combined thoracic and lumbar structural curve associated with a fractional lumbosacral structural curve and a spondylolisthesis is corrected as follows. The short lumbosacral curve is corrected in a localizer

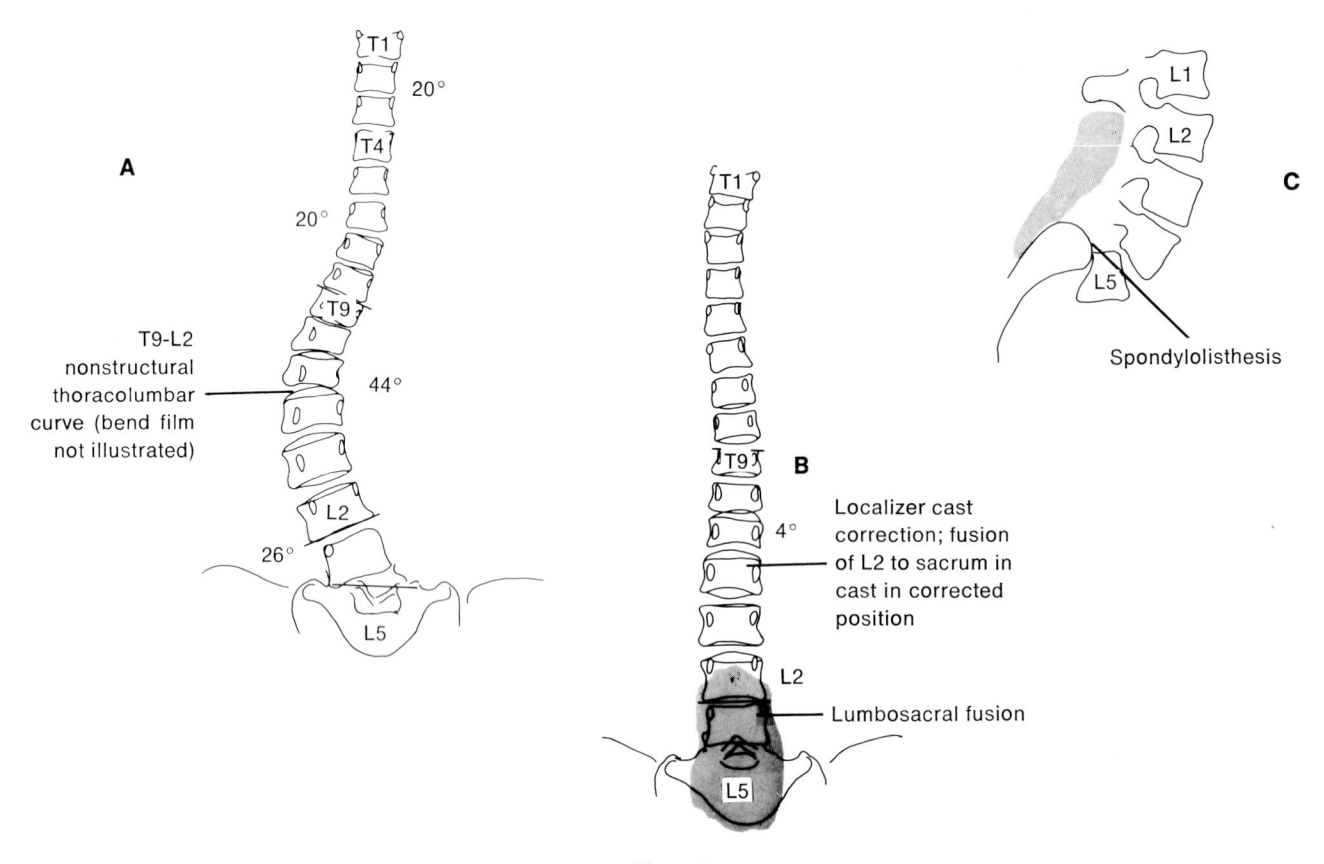

Fig. 19

cast, bringing L4 as near level to the pelvis as possible, and L4 is fused to the sacrum. If the patient's age and degree of the curves above are within the Milwaukee brace treatment range, then the curves above are treated in a Milwaukee brace after the fusion is solid, usually 6 months. If the brace does not control the deformity, the two structural curves must be corrected and fused in continuity with the lumbosacral fusion with the torso in balance. Fig. 21, A, shows a double structural lower thoracic and lumbar curve associated with a structural fractional lumbosacral curve and a first-degree lumbosacral spondylolisthesis. Initial treatment, stage 1, was by preoperative localizer cast correction, getting L4 as nearly centered and parallel over the sacrum as possible. Fusion was then performed in the cast, L4 to S2. After 6 months' recumbency in a localizer cast including thigh pantaloons, the patient was treated in a Milwaukee brace. Fig. 21, B, shows the situation at 6 months after surgery. Fig. 21, C, is 1 year following the lumbosacral fusion. The Milwaukee brace failed to control the structural lower thoracic and lumbar curves, which had progressed to 45° and 60°, respectively. These curves were then recorrected in a localizer cast. Instrumentation was from T7 to L3, and fusion from T7 to the lumbosacral first-stage fusion with the torso in good balance. Fig. 21, D, shows 3-year postoperative radiographic tracing with maintenance of correction and balanced torso.

If the pretreatment decision is made that the thoracic and lumbar curves require surgical treatment as well as the lumbosacral spondylolisthesis, an alternative approach would be a one-stage operative procedure with Harrington instrumentation and fusion from T7 to the sacrum. In retrospect, the severity of the lumbar curve and the lateral listhesis of L3 on L4 were adequate indications for surgical treatment in this patient. The curves are corrected in a preoperative pantaloon localizer cast centering T7 over the midline sacrum. A one-stage operation is performed with one distraction rod from the left sacral ala to the concave (left) side of T7 or T8 and fusion from T7 to the sacrum. If the postoperative radiograph shows T7 off center, adjustment must be made by cast wedging, even with the instruments in place (not illustrated).

One must be ever cautious *not* to stabilize the lumbosacral level for a symptomatic spondylolisthesis when there is associated scoliosis above *without analyzing* and correcting the curves above, balancing the torso, and fusing L4 to the sarcum in as near a balanced and corrected position as possible. Otherwise, a built-in deformed base on which the spine above rests will be created, and it will be impossible subsequently to correct the deformity adequately.

When the sacrum is included in the fusion, thigh pantaloons are always added to the localizer cast and the patient is treated supine for 3 to 4 months.

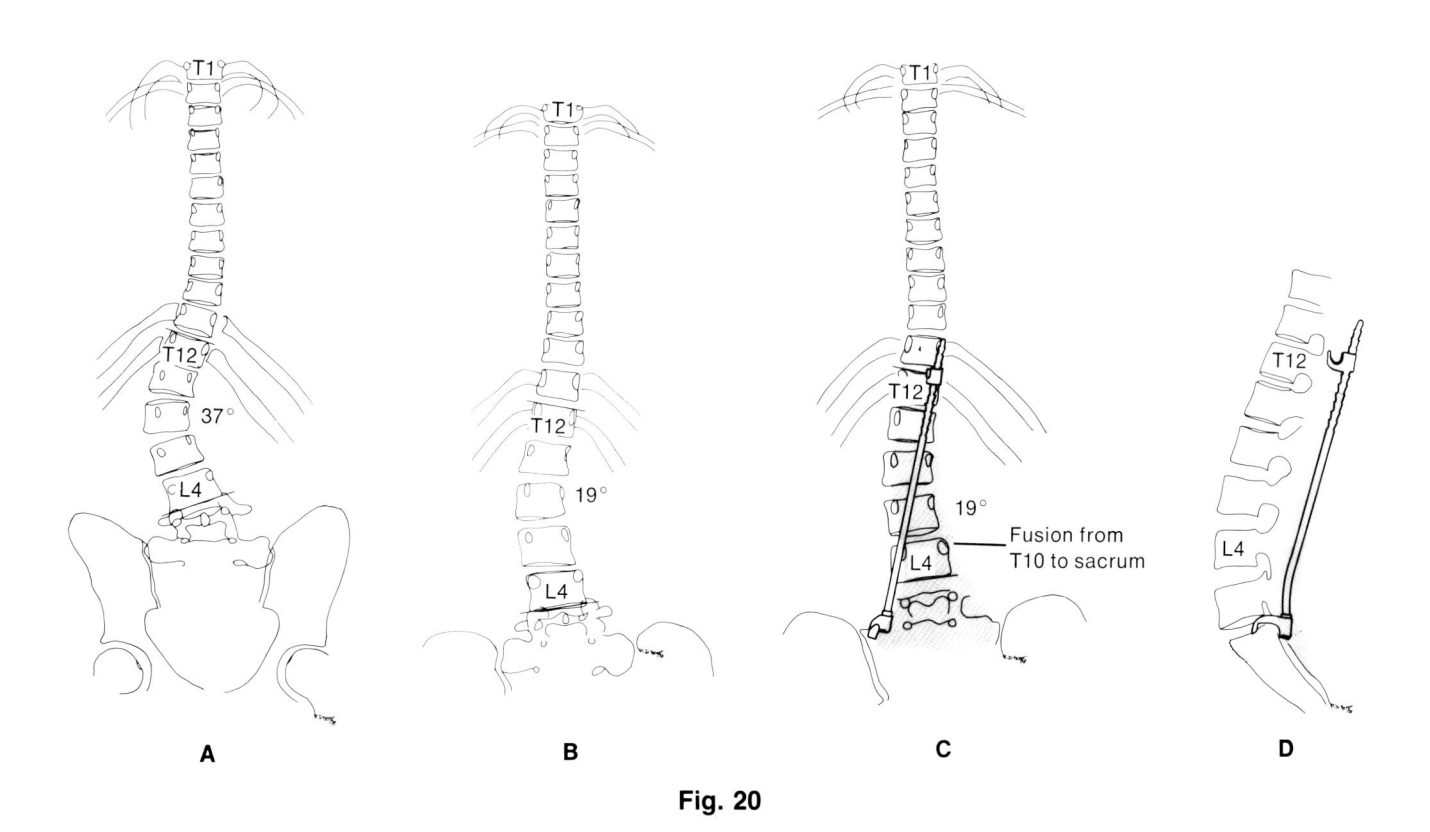

Fig. 20

METHODS OF CORRECTION OF SCOLIOSIS

The usual methods of correction for idiopathic scoliosis are nonskeletal (Cotrel) traction, skeletal traction for the more rigid curves, particularly those over 90°, and use of a preoperative localizer cast. Preoperative localizer cast correction is used most commonly. Most of our patients are operated on in the preoperative localizer cast (Fig. 23).

LOCALIZER CAST TECHNIQUE. Application of a corrective cast requires experience. One cannot delegate this task to inexperienced staff. The Risser localizer table has been modified to allow application of a Risser-Cotrel type of localizer cast (Fig. 22, A). An ordinary traction frame is attached to the Risser table. A ratchet is fixed to an overhead bar. The 15 cm–wide canvas is suspended from the ratchet. Three sizes of removable plywood sacral rests fit into a cross-bar, which is attached to the Risser frame with two C clamps. The patient's pelvis is supported on the sacral rest, and the shoulders are on the proximal crossbar of the Risser frame, thus eliminating the need for a supporting sling and allowing the application of a total body contact cast (Fig. 22, B). The degree of hip flexion is controlled either with a large linen roll or a padded leg rest. A soft felt pad is used over the sacral rest under the shoulders, back of the neck, and occiput. A foam-rubber pad is also placed over the sacrum and behind the occiput. Double stockinette is applied to the body, single stockinette over the head. Webril used for padding is applied firmly to the contours of the torso, reinforced with thin, soft, felt pads over the iliac crests, and a felt pad is contoured to the chin and anterior neck. The preoperative cast is more

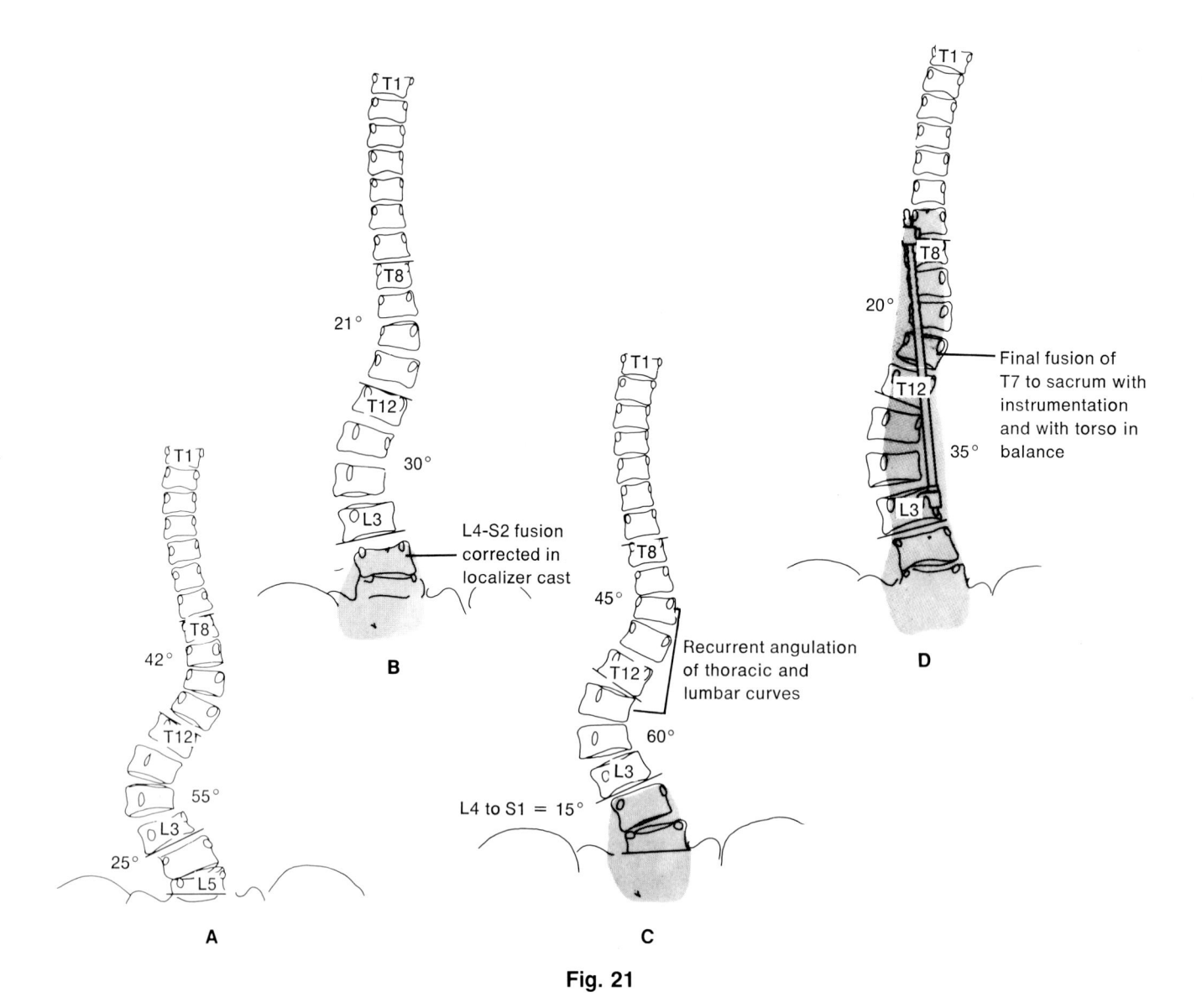

Fig. 21

heavily padded and not as severely molded as the postoperative cast. A large felt pad is placed over the anterior chest in the preoperative cast. After the patient is placed on the localizer table, gradually increasing distraction forces to patient tolerance are applied with crossed 2.5 cm webbing straps to the pelvis and to a disposable head halter (Fig. 22, B).

In the preoperative cast, localizers are used for the thoracic and lumbar spine as indicated (Fig. 22, A). For a right thoracic curve the right shoulder is tied down to the shoulder bar with a length of stockinette. This prevents torso rotation when the thoracic localizer is applied with anterolateral force directed over the rib prominence (Fig. 22, B). As the distraction forces are increased, the localizers are gradually adjusted as tolerated by the patient. The plaster rolls are soaked in cold water to slow the setting. Application is started around the pelvis; rolls are molded well over the iliac crest. The plaster is applied very rapidly. A trapezoid-shaped block is strapped to the cast just proximal to the pubis to get a closer fit of the plaster suprapubically. Webbing straps are secured with the block and drawn tightly above the iliac crests, completing the molding of the plaster into the soft parts above the crests (Fig. 24, A). The application of plaster is continued rapidly over the thorax and molded well under the chin and occiput.

The preoperative localizer cast has a large anterior window cut out (Fig. 23, A), which extends to the suprapubic area and exposes the abdomen and the lower two thirds of the anterior chest. This allows access to the chest during surgery if necessary and reduces pressure on abdominal structures when the patient is prone on the spine operation frame for surgery. The anterior neck

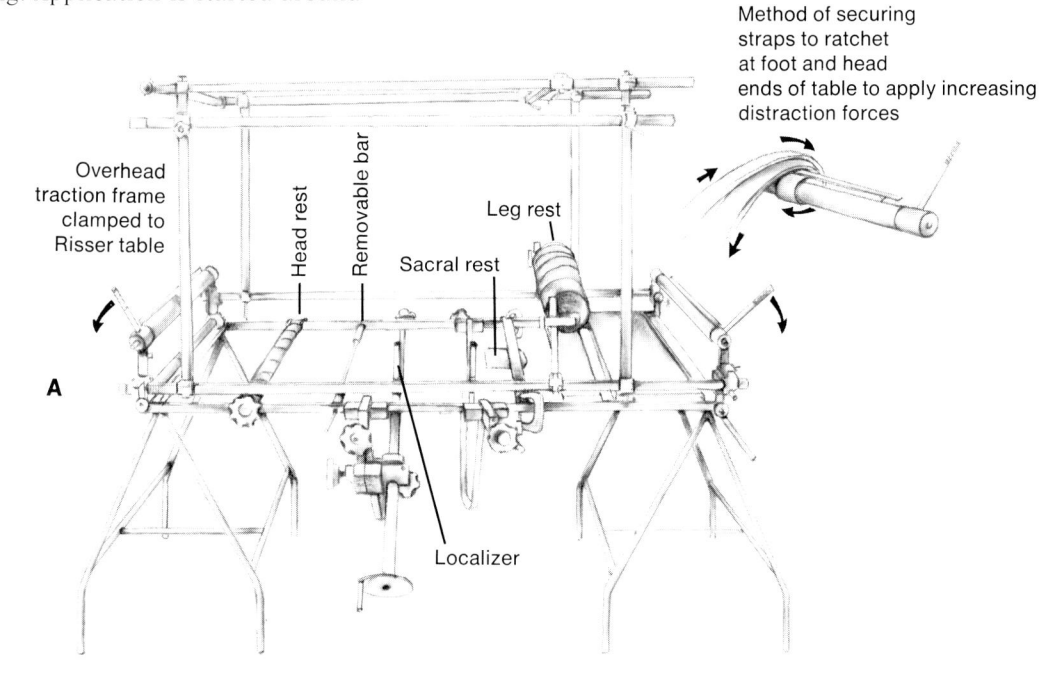

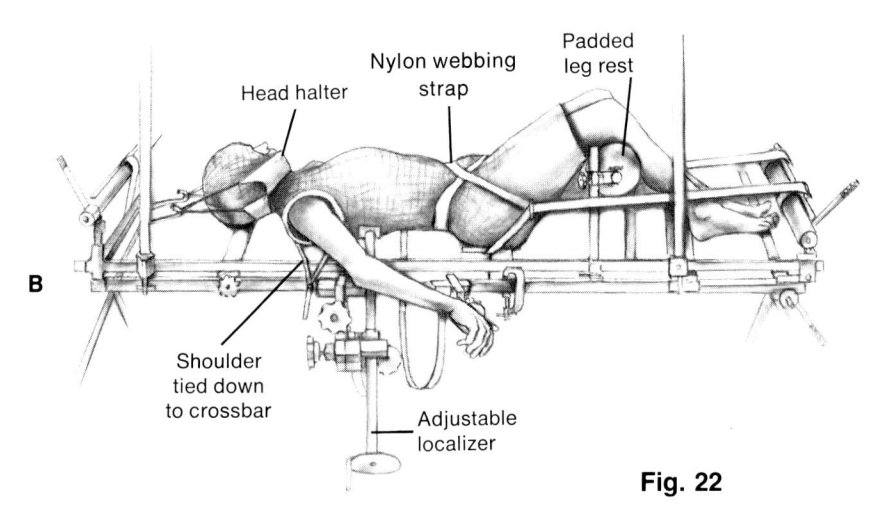

Fig. 22

235

Fig. 23

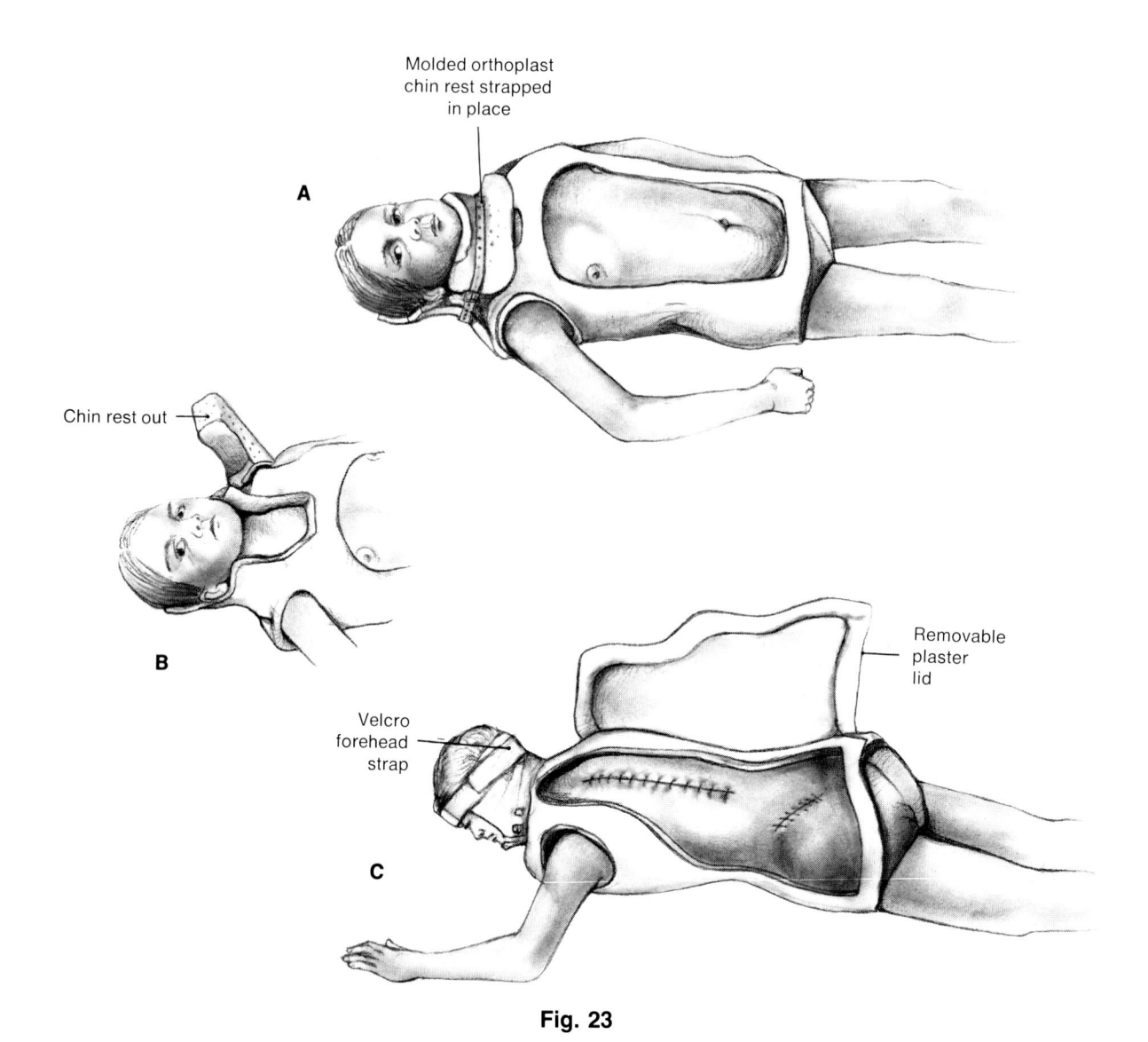

and chin are also widely cut out so that there is no pressure against the cervical vascular structures while the patient is prone under anesthesia. The plaster cutout is replaced by a molded Orthoplast chin rest (Fig. 23, B), which is removed to allow direct laryngoscopy for intubation during anesthesia. The chin rest is strapped in place before the patient is turned. Two days after application of the cast, a very large posterior window is cut out, allowing adequate exposure of the area of the spine to be fused and also wide exposure of one ilium for bone graft (Fig. 23, C). A plaster lid with an overhang is fashioned over a layer of 1.3 cm foam rubber. This fits securely into the large posterior window. It may be removed when the patient is prone and is strapped in place securely when the patient is supine. The sacral bar of the cast is cut out when necessary the morning of the operation to allow better preparation of the operative field.

At 12 days after surgery, the postoperative localizer cast is applied under full distraction forces. No localizer lateral pressure is used. The Cotrel derotation strap is used for thoracic scoliosis for further correction of the convex rib hump (Fig. 24, A). At the time of spine fusion, osteotomy at the base of the convex transverse processes in a thoracic curve is performed (Fig. 29). This allows further correction of the rib hump at the time of application of the postoperative cast. The principle of osteotomy of the convex transverse processes in correction of the convex rib hump as advocated by Yves Cotrel is illustrated in Fig. 24, B. The pressure of the strap against the plaster over the convex rib hump causes the ribs to pivot at the costovertebral joints, carrying the transverse processes along with them and reducing the rib hump without influencing the rotation of the vertebral segments. The postoperative localizer cast (Fig. 25) is more lightly padded and more severely molded, particularly

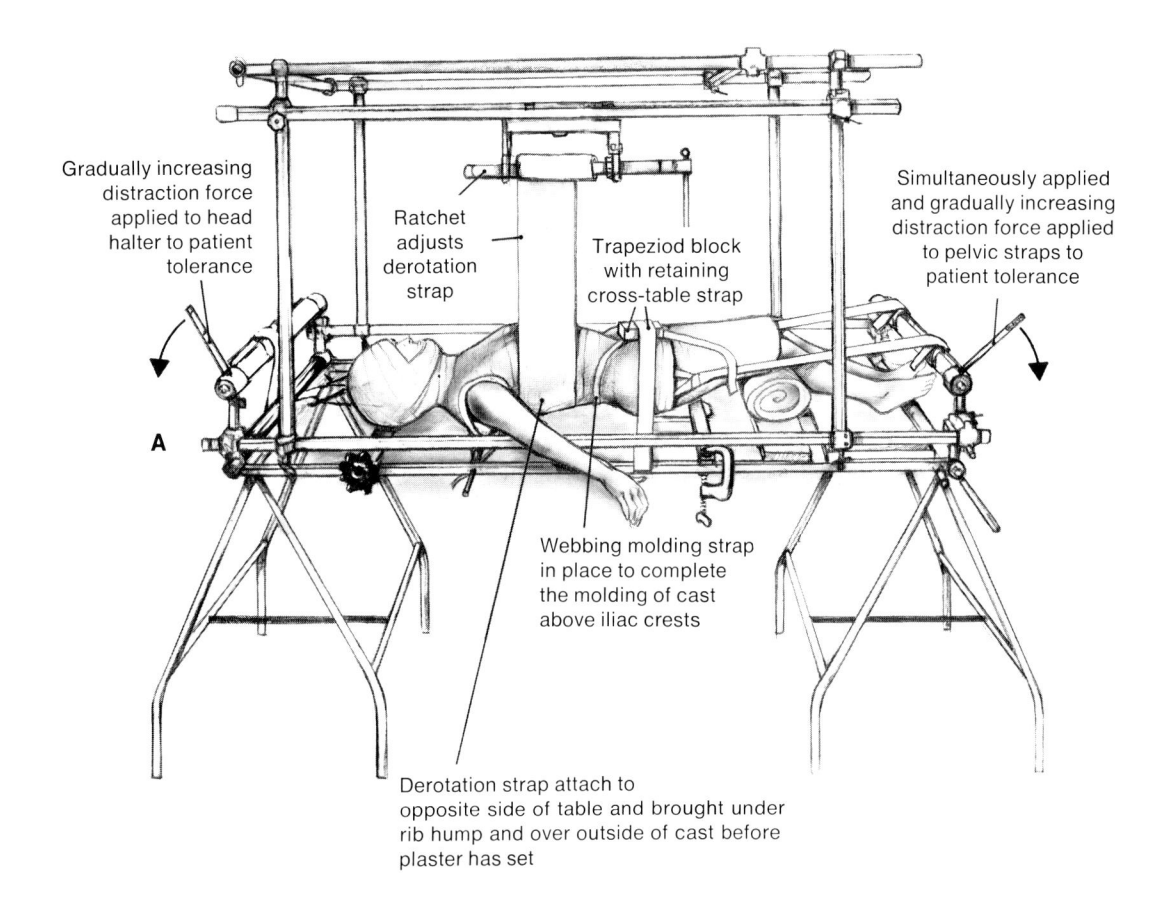

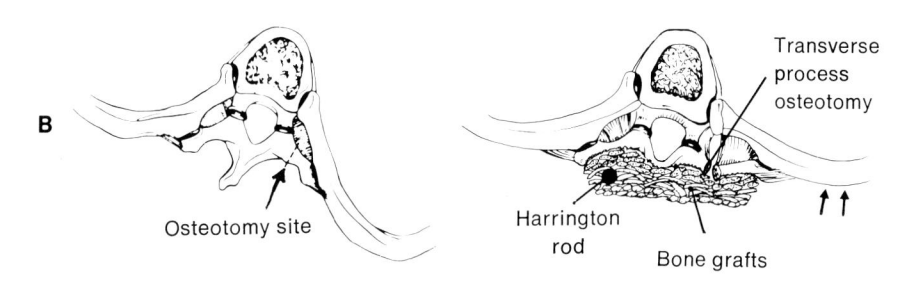

Fig. 24

above the iliac crests, than the preoperative cast. A narrow V cutout is made under the chin and over the anterior neck. A large anterior window is cut out over the thorax. With right thoracic curves, the left lower anterior ribs are usually more prominent so that the anterior window is made asymmetric to allow for pressure over the left lower anterior ribs. This favorably influences the restoration of better rib cage symmetry during the postoperative convalescent period in the cast with breathing exercises, particularly in young patients. A window is cut posteriorly on the concave side of the curve to allow expansion of the depressed concave ribs (Fig. 25). The patient is allowed to walk the day following application of the postoperative localizer cast except when the fusion extends into the sacrum.

POSTERIOR SPINE FUSION AND HARRINGTON INSTRUMENTATION

Details of procedure. The spine fusion requires precise technique. The exposure is wide, out to the tips of the transverse processes in the thoracic and lumbar spine. Wide, deep decortication is performed. A large amount of fresh autogenous iliac bone creates a favorable environment for the prompt formation, organization, and incorporation of a massive bone graft. The proper fusion area includes accurate localization of a level at the time of surgery and determination of the area of the spine requiring stabilization to maintain correction. Blood loss is measured, recorded, and replaced as it occurs. The extent of the fusion will have been determined preoperatively. The widely cut-out chin and anterior neck allow direct laryngoscopy for intubation for anes-

Narrow V cut anteriorly and plaster edges posterior to mandible

Posterior window over concave ribs

Asymmetric anterior window

A

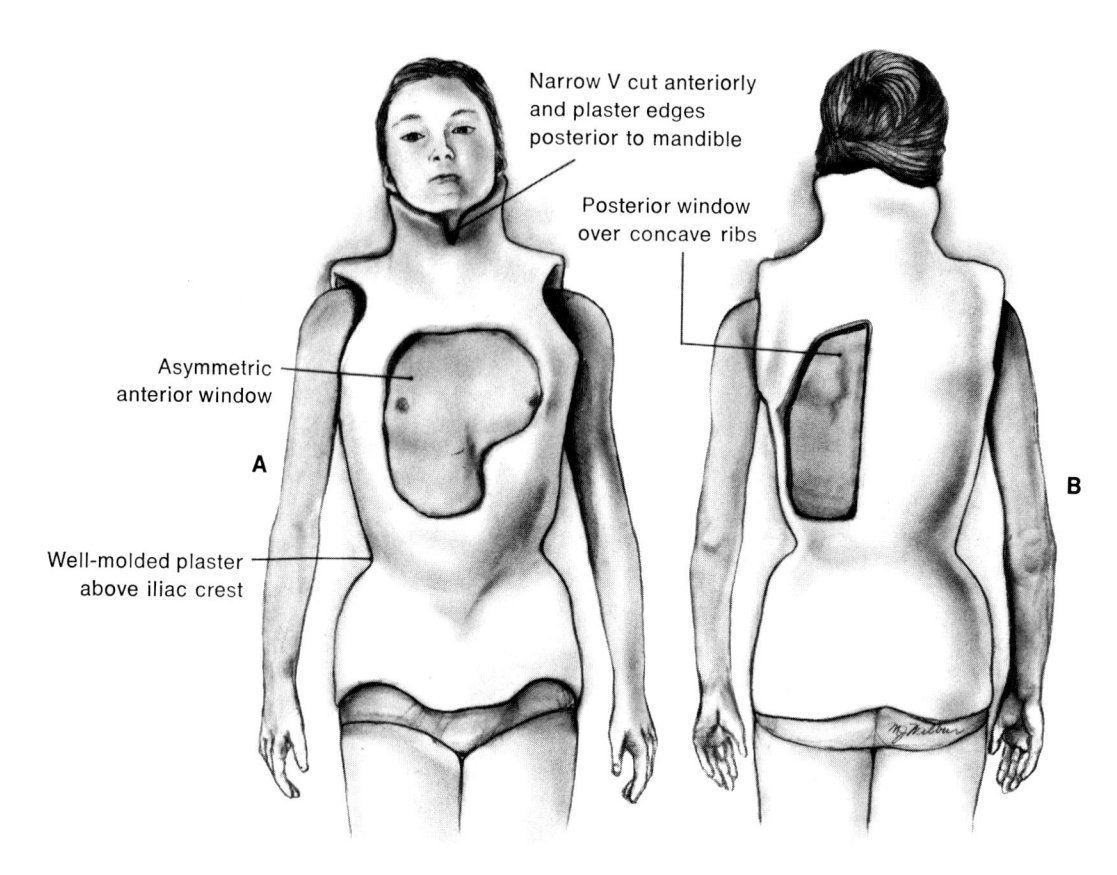

B

Well-molded plaster above iliac crest

Fig. 25

thesia. Before the patient is turned, a padded Velcro forehead strap fixes the head to the plaster. The Orthoplast molded chin rest is strapped in place. The patient is turned and supported on the MacKay spine operation frame so that the abdomen hangs free from pressure against the table. Fig. 26 shows the adjustable MacKay frame, which allows control of lordosis of the spine when the patient is operated on out of the cast. The frame can be used with the patient in or out of the localizer cast. Two electrocauteries are hooked up for the two assistants to use in controlling bleeding during the operation.

Exposure technique of spine fusion. Because of the obliquity of the thoracic spinous process, the upper end of the straight skin incision extends two vertebrae proximal to the proposed level of fusion to allow adequate exposure. Incision is made through the subcutaneous tissues, exposing the tips of the spinous processes in line with the curve in the midline (Fig. 27). Wheatlander retractors provide helpful wide retraction of the wound.

The deep exposure is started distally. The supraspinous ligament and cartilaginous tip of a spinous process are sharply incised down to bone while an assistant placed the tissues under tension with a partially opened Kelly clamp, the prongs pressing down on either side of the spinous process (Fig. 27, *A*). With a periosteal elevator, the cartilaginous tip and periosteum are reflected off the spinous process. This is repeated at each level in the fusion area, exposing just the most posterior portion of the spinous process in this initial step. Starting back at the distal end of the wound, a meticulous subperiosteal exposure is carried out with sharp periosteal elevators, scraping the joint capsules cleanly off their bony attachments. The capsules can be incised with the elevator at strategic points to facilitate the clean reflection of the capsule. The wound is packed as dissection progresses. In the lumbar spine the reflection is continued out over the lateral aspects of the superior articular process to the tip of the transverse process. In the thoracic spine the exposure is performed in similar fashion. The periosteal elevator is run carefully along the inferior margin of the lamina and inferior articular process, perpendicular to the articular process, cutting the capsule from the distal margin of the inferior articular process. Then with the elevator against the superior articular process, the capsule is reflected cleanly off bone and the reflection continued out to the tip of the transverse process. This allows clean reflection of the tissues in one thick layer. The exposure is wide on both sides of the spine, extending out to the tips of the transverse processes (Fig. 27, *B*). The ligamentous attachments of the short paraspinal muscles to the tips of the transverse process are left intact. The costotransverse joints are not en-

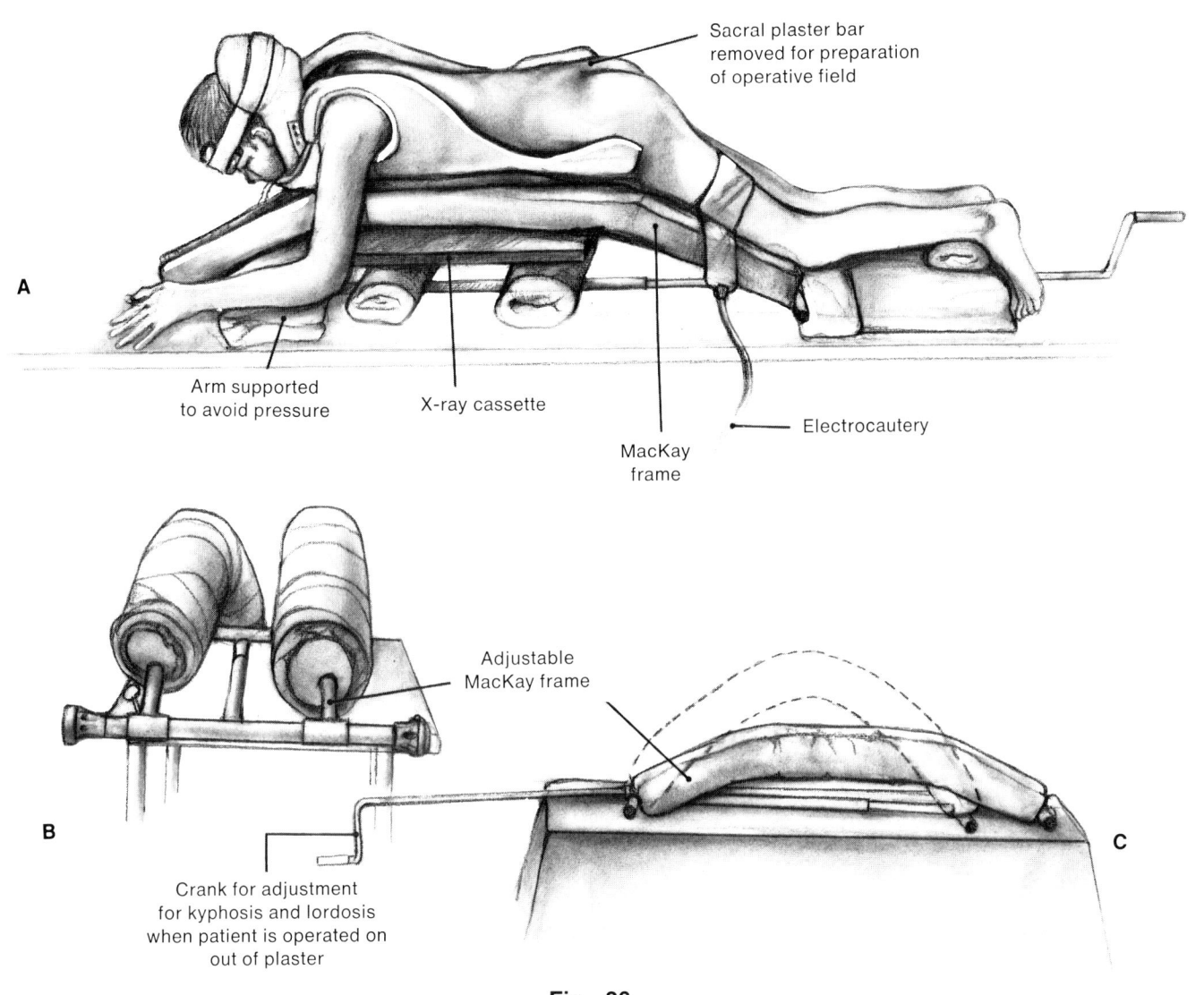

Fig. 26

tered to avoid postoperative joint stiffness and limited chest expansion. The wound is thoroughly irrigated during and after completion of the exposure of the posterior elements of the spine with a 2% neomycin solution.

Preparation of sites for hook seatings. The superior distraction hook is seated in a facet joint. The joint is tapped with a narrow periosteal elevator to define precisely its direction. A blunt-ended 1253 Harrington hook is inserted into the facet joint (Fig. 27, C). If the articular process is broad and relatively horizontal, the hook seating will be stable. However, if the articular process is somewhat oblique, a more stable seating is created by osteotomizing and removing the distal margin of the inferior articular process (Fig. 27, C). The hook is then seated. After this trial with a blunt-ended 1253 hook, the 1251 hook (Fig. 27, D and E), which has a sharp leading edge, is inserted into the joint and gently tapped in place so that the leading edge impales the base of the pedicle (Fig. 27, E). The hook is then removed. The proximal portion of the wound is packed. Attention is then directed to the distal end vertebra. The distal distraction hook is always placed on the most distal vertebra to be included in the fusion area. One vertebra proximal to the proximal distraction hook is included in the fusion (Fig. 30, A and B). As the graft organizes and incorporates, it further stabilizes this hook, which is the weakest link in the distraction system. The seating for the inferior distraction hook is made over the superior border of the lamina of a lumbar vertebra (Fig. 27, F and G). With a narrow, sharp elevator, the ligamentum flavum is gently reflected off the superior border of the lamina until the bluish epidural space comes into view. The natural elasticity of the ligamentum flavum retracts itself as it is freed from the lamina and excised. With a very sharp, solid-handle curet, slivers of bone are then removed from the superior border of the lamina

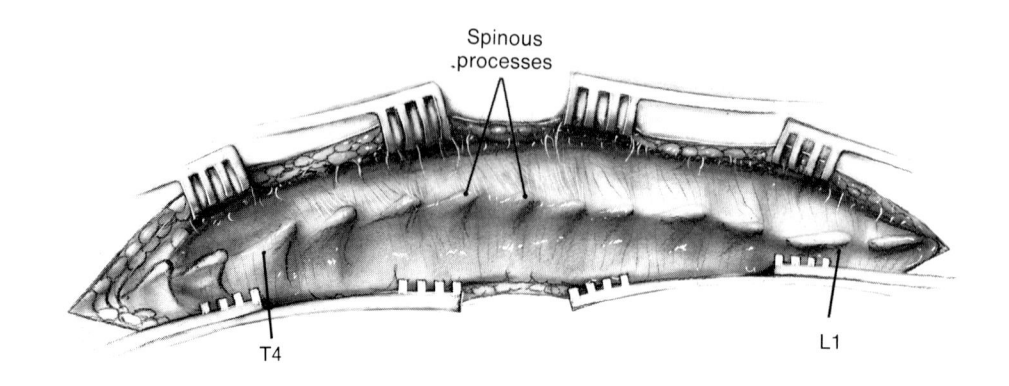

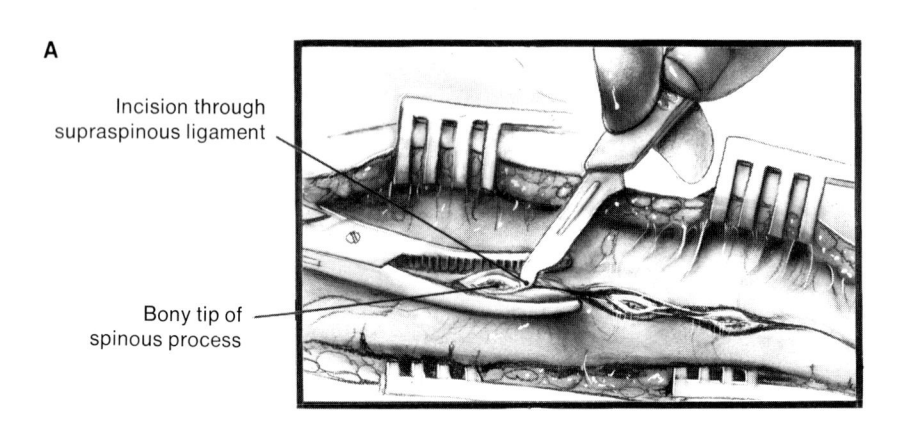

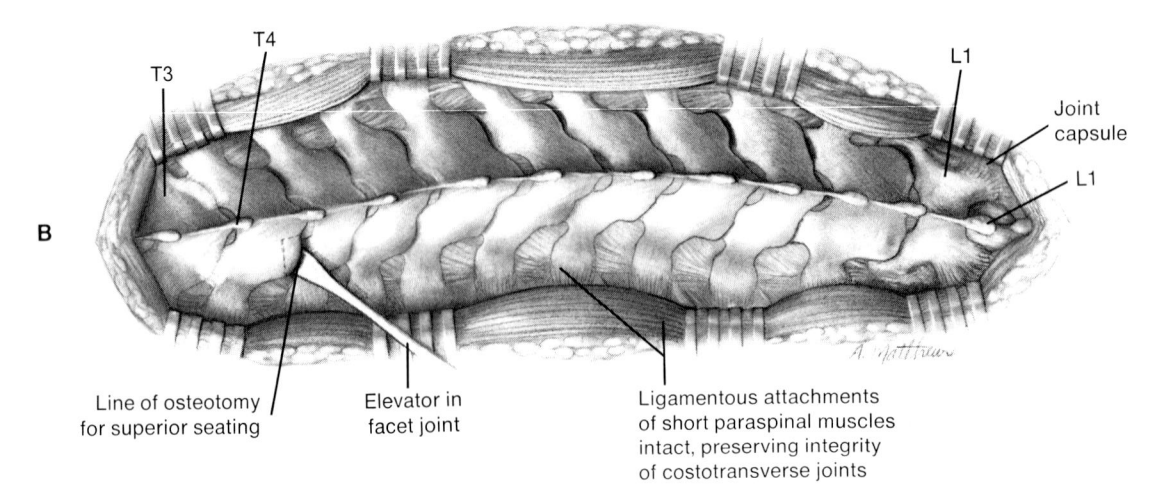

Fig. 27

240

to enlarge the hole of the interlaminar space. If necessary, a Kerrison rongeur may be used to osteotomize the superior border of the lamina. If the interlaminar space is still too narrow, the lamina immediately adjacent proximally is osteotomized to enlarge the opening and allow easy seating of a 1254 hook (Fig. 27, F and G). One can use either a 1253 or 1254 hook; however, the smaller 1254 hook is preferred.

The compression system is applied on the convex side of the curve when there is an increased thoracic kyphosis. When the compression system is used, the convex transverse processes are not osteotomized. A thoracic lordosis is a contraindication because the compression force increases the lordosis. Trial seatings of the 1259 hooks are made over the convex transverse process. Usually two hooks are placed proximal to the apex of the curve and two hooks distal to the apex. The proximal hooks are seated over the superior surface of the transverse process and the distal hooks over the inferior surface (Figs. 27, D, and 30, B and C). The hooks are temporarily removed. The spinal wound is packed with 2% neomycin solution–soaked sponges, and attention is directed to the donor iliac site.

Obtaining the iliac bone graft. The method of obtaining iliac bone is described in detail in Chapter 9 (p. 282).

Decortication of the posterior elements of the spine. Complete decortication is performed except of the posterior elements on which the hooks are to be seated. The spinous processes are split with a thin osteotome and excised at their base. In the lumbar spine (Fig. 28) the posterior two thirds of the facet joints are excised. Cancellous bone is packed into each facet joint as it is resected. Decortication of the lamina and the lateral aspect of the superior articular process, continuing out over the transverse process to its tip on both sides, is performed. The wound is packed as the decortication proceeds. If bleeding is excessive from the decorticated bone, the placement of cancellous grafts immediately or of Gelfoam will facilitate control of the bleeding.

In the thoracic spine, after the spinous process is excised, the distal third of the inferior articular process is excised, exposing the distal half of the superior articular facet at each level on each side of the spine (Fig. 29, A and B). The decortication includes lamina out to the tip of the transverse process and the exposed portion of the superior articular process. This destroys the distal half of the facet joint (Fig. 29, B). The concave side of the thoracic vertebra on which the superior hook is seated is not decorticated. On the convex side of this vertebra the inferior articular process is excised and the lamina and transverse process are decorticated. The

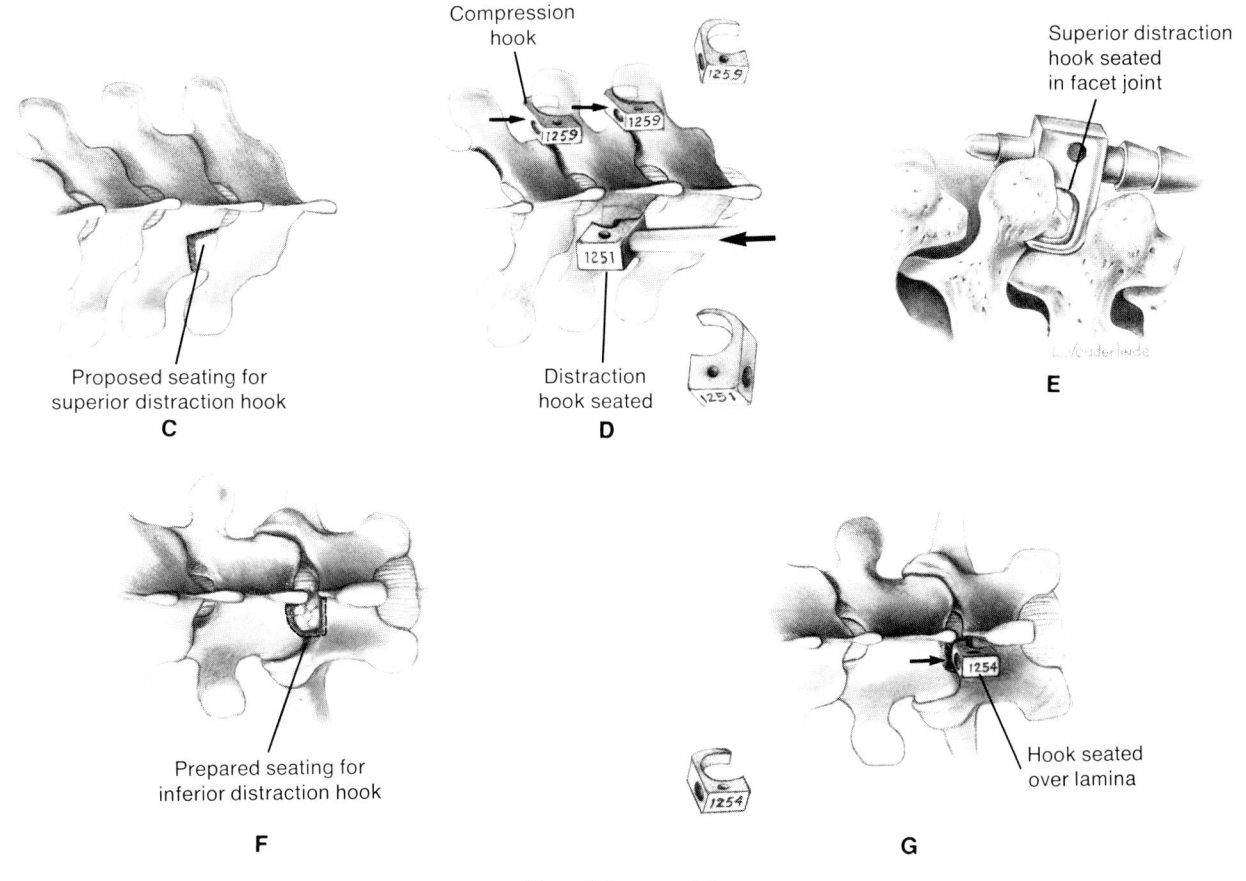

Fig. 27, cont'd

A
- Deep decortication of lamina, articular processes, and transverse processes
- Partial excision of facet joint
- Ligamentum flavum
- Excision of spinous process

B
- First layer of cancellous bone slivers in and over facet joint and transverse process

C
- Cancellous bone grafts
- Layers of cancellous bone grafts cover decorticated surfaces

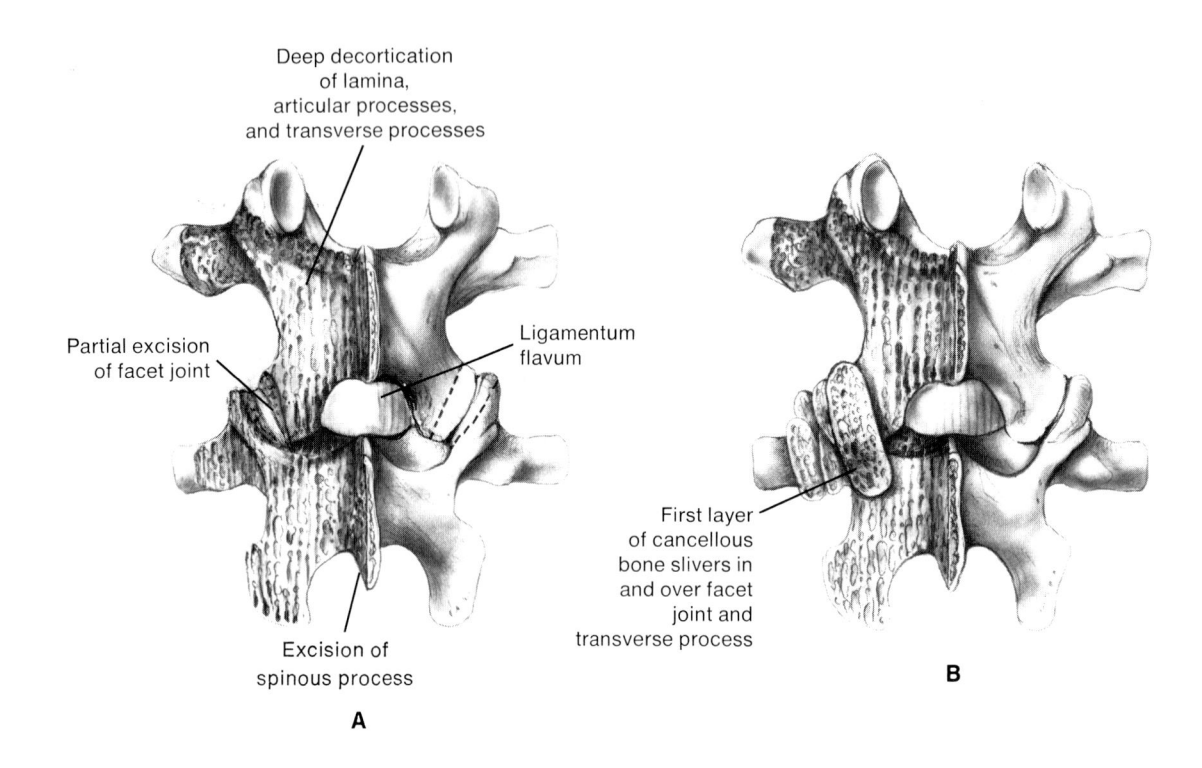

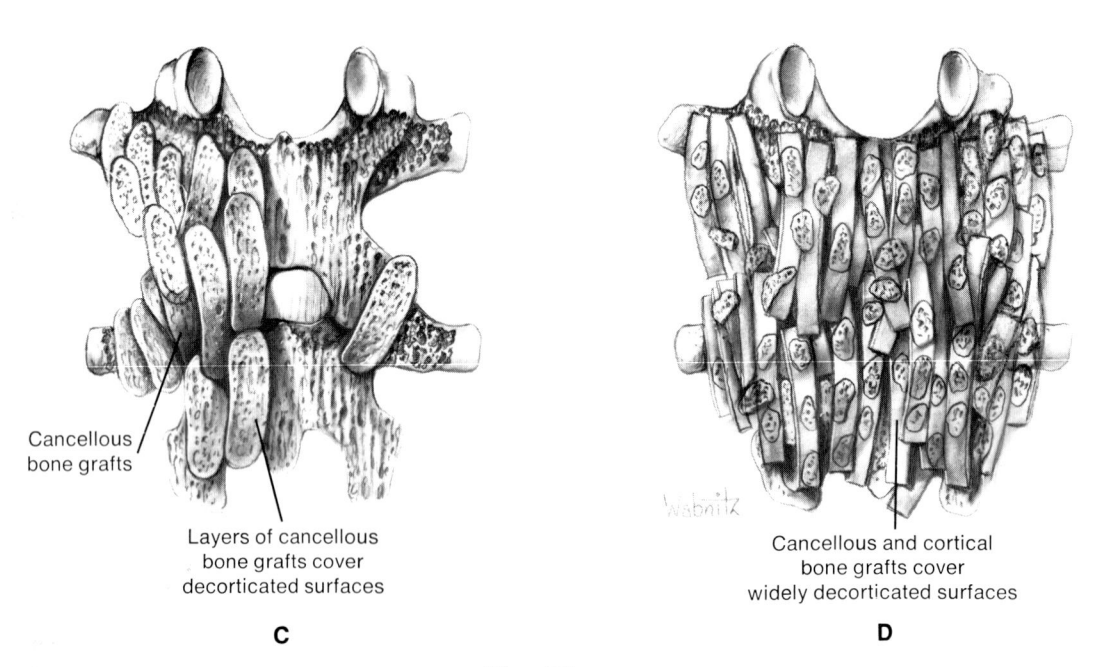

D
- Cancellous and cortical bone grafts cover widely decorticated surfaces

Fig. 28

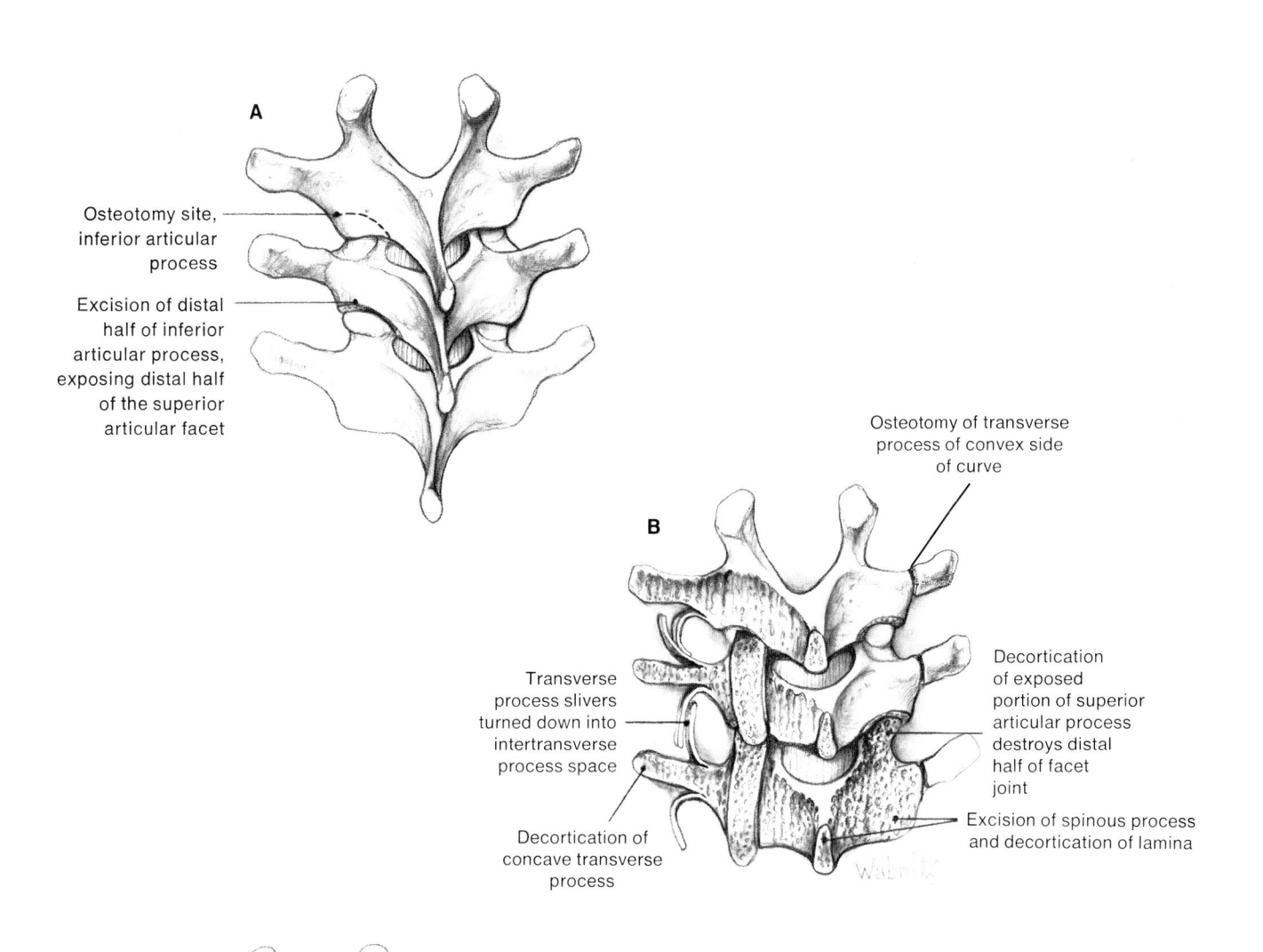

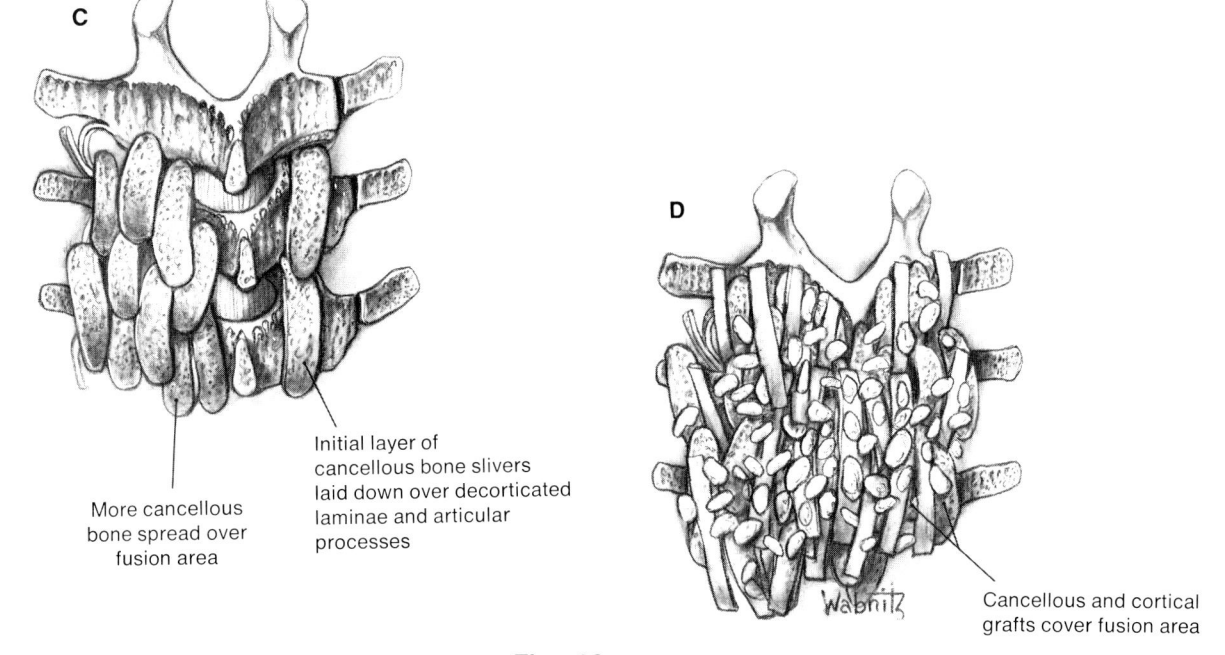

Fig. 29

vertebra proximal to the hook seating is completely decorticated (Fig. 30, *A*). The inferior and superior margins of the transverse processes on the concave side of the curve are reflected as thin slivers into the intertransverse process spaces (Fig. 31, *A*).

Osteotomy of convex transverse processes (thoracic). The transverse processes on the convex side of a thoracic curve are osteotomized at their base with a bone cutter and mobilized with an elevator at each level in the fusion area (Figs. 29, *B* and *C* and 31, *A*). When the postoperative localizer cast is applied, the ribs pivot at the costal vertebral joints as the Cotrel derotation strap is tightened over the convex rib hump, carrying the osteotomized transverse processes with them; this reduces the rib hump without influencing rotation of the vertebrae (Fig. 24, *B*).

Placement of bone grafts and instrumentation. Cancellous bone strips are laid down over the decorticated surfaces on the concave side of the curve before the distraction rod is inserted (Fig. 30, *A*). This ensures at least a single layer of cancellous bone covering the decorticated surfaces under the rod. In the lumbar spine the cancellous strips are laid down in and over the facet joints along the lateral aspect of the decorticated superior articular processes and out over the transverse processes (Fig. 28, *B*, and *C*). On the concave side of the thoracic curve the strips of cancellous bone are tucked into the resected portion of the facet joints and overlapped in shingle fashion, running from distal to proximal (Figs. 29, *B*, and 30, *A* and *C*). The 1251 hook is inserted into the prepared proximal seating. An assistant maintains the hook in position, being careful to avoid a

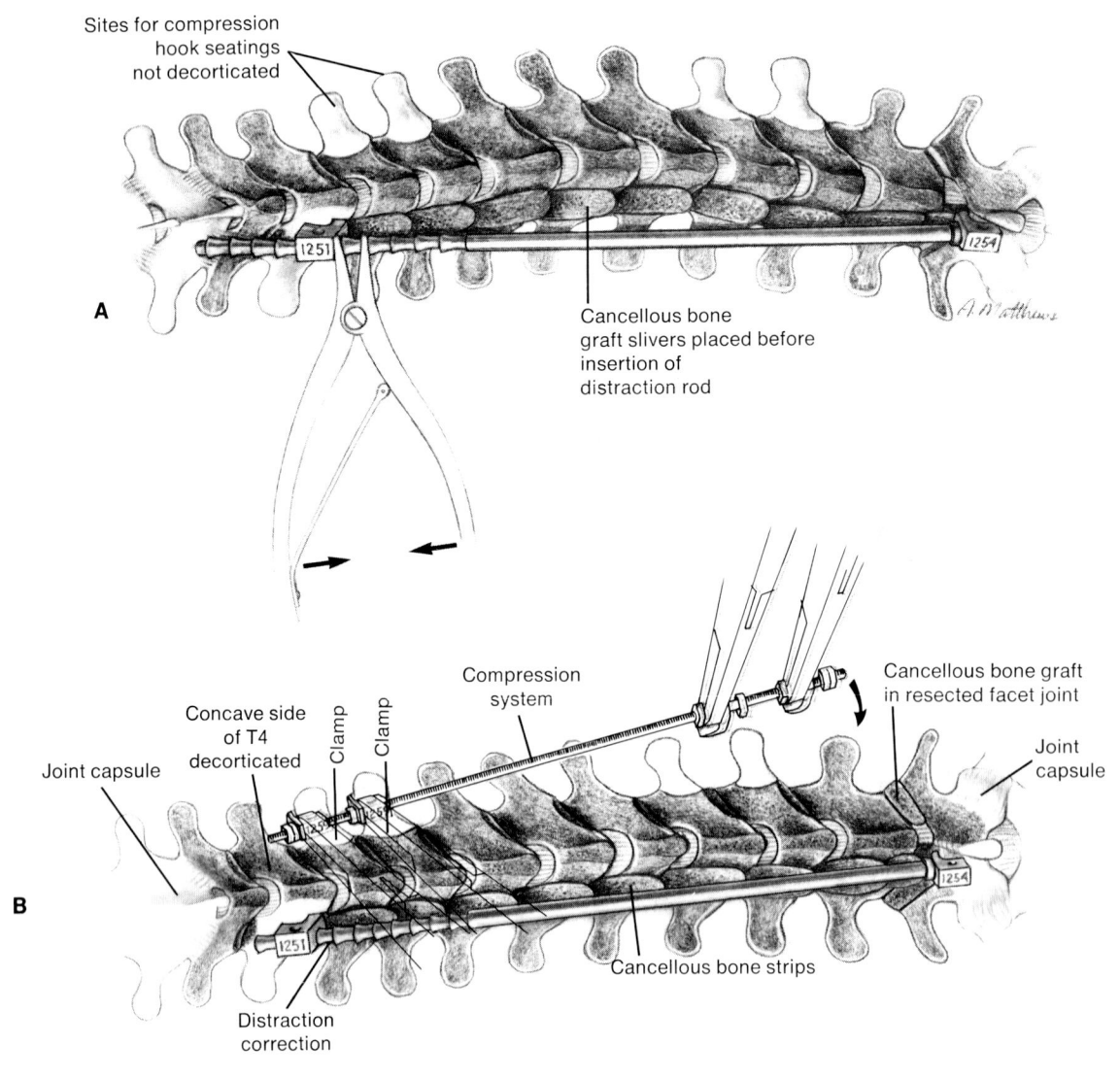

Fig. 30

change of position, particularly externally rotating the hook out of the facet joint. The handle of the hook clamp is held down against the side of the wound to be sure that the shoe of the hook points slightly medially. This is important to maintain a stable seating and prevent the hook from sliding or rotating out of the facet joint. The 1254 hook is seated distally over the lumbar lamina and held by a second assistant. The distraction rod is then placed; it is first inserted in the proximal hook far enough to allow the distal end to be slipped into the distal distraction hook. Correction is obtained gradually, with the distraction instrument lengthening the distance notch by notch (Fig. 30, A and B). The full correction possible is not made initially. The tissues under stretch in the concavity of the curve will allow further correction with less pressure on the distraction hooks if given 10 to 15 minutes to fatigue before further distraction is attempted.

After distraction is complete, a wire is slipped around the rod just distal to the superior distraction hook and twisted snugly in place to prevent slippage of the hook on the rod. When convex compression is used, osteotomy of the convex transverse processes is not performed. The appropriate number of 1259 hooks and hex nuts are assembled on the threaded rod. The proximal hooks are first seated over the superior margin of the transverse processes (Fig. 30, B), held in place by an assistant with hook clamps. The distal hooks are brought in position and securely seated around the inferior borders of the transverse processes. Care is taken so that the hooks do not cut into bone but pass around the ante-

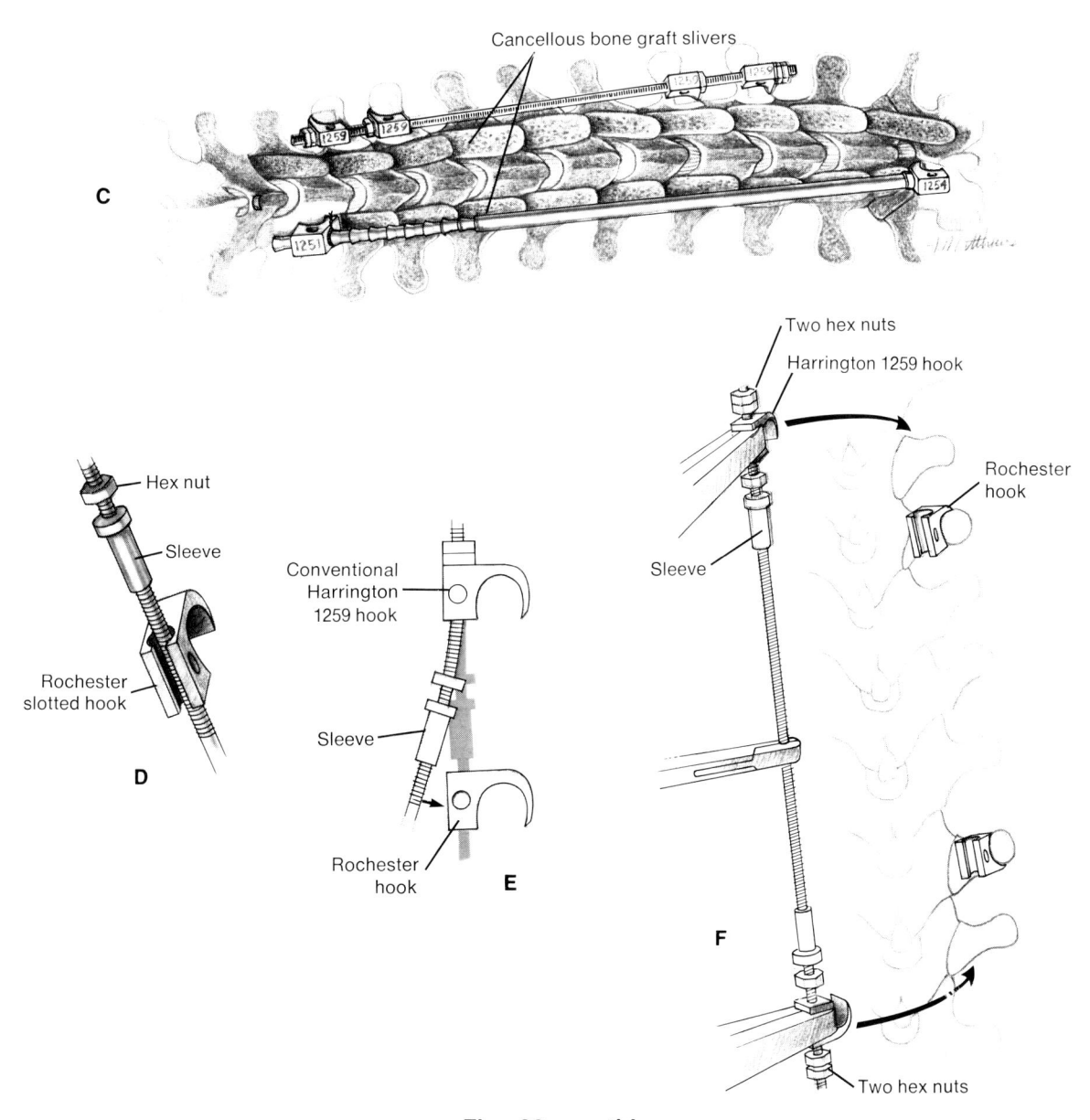

Fig. 30, cont'd

245

rior surface of the transverse process. The hex nuts are tightened to get the desired compression force (Fig. 30, C). The rod is crimped adjacent to the single nut, securing the middle hooks, and at each end two nuts are used to lock the system in place.

A modification of the Harrington 1259 compression hook, the "Rochester" hook (Fig. 30, D) facilitates application of the compression system. The design allows the hooks to be seated unassembled. The top of the body of the hook is slotted, and an unthreaded sleeve slips into the slot that accommodates the rod (Fig. 30, E). In applying this system, a standard compression rod of appropriate length is selected. As standard Harrington 1259 compression hooks are used at the proximal and distal ends, the number of special sleeves and hex nuts that need to be assembled on the rod corresponds to the number of hooks needed between the end hooks (Fig. 30, F). The slotted hooks are placed. The standard 1259 end hooks mounted on the assembled rods are then inserted. The rod is placed into the slotted hooks, and the sleeves are slid over the rod and seated in the hooks. The hex nuts are tightened down, and compression is carried out as usual (Fig. 30, G). The "Rochester" hook may be used for the entire compression system instead of the standard 1259 hook at each end.

The rest of the cancellous bone strips are laid down over the fusion area (Fig. 31). The grafts are brought well down on the convex side of the distal vertebra included in the fusion, as well as over the convex side of the proximal vertebra, which has the superior distraction hook, and over the decorticated vertebra proximal to this distraction hook (Fig. 31, B). The grafts are brought around the superior hook. As the bone grafts organize and incorporate, the superior hook seating becomes more secure. This is desirable because the superior hook is the weakest link in the distraction system. The rectangles of iliac cortex have been cut into slivers. These are laid down over the fusion area, followed by the laminar bone, which has been cut into small chips. The bone grafts are gently packed down with a flat retractor. At the conclusion of the operation, several layers of bone grafts cover widely decorticated bone base to the tips of the transverse processes. The bone grafts usually cover the distraction rod and the hooks almost completely (Fig. 31, B).

Wound closure. The two halves of the supraspinous liagment and the adjacent muscle structures are securely approximated with deeply placed No. 1 chromic catgut figure-of-eight sutures. The subcutaneous tissues are closed with

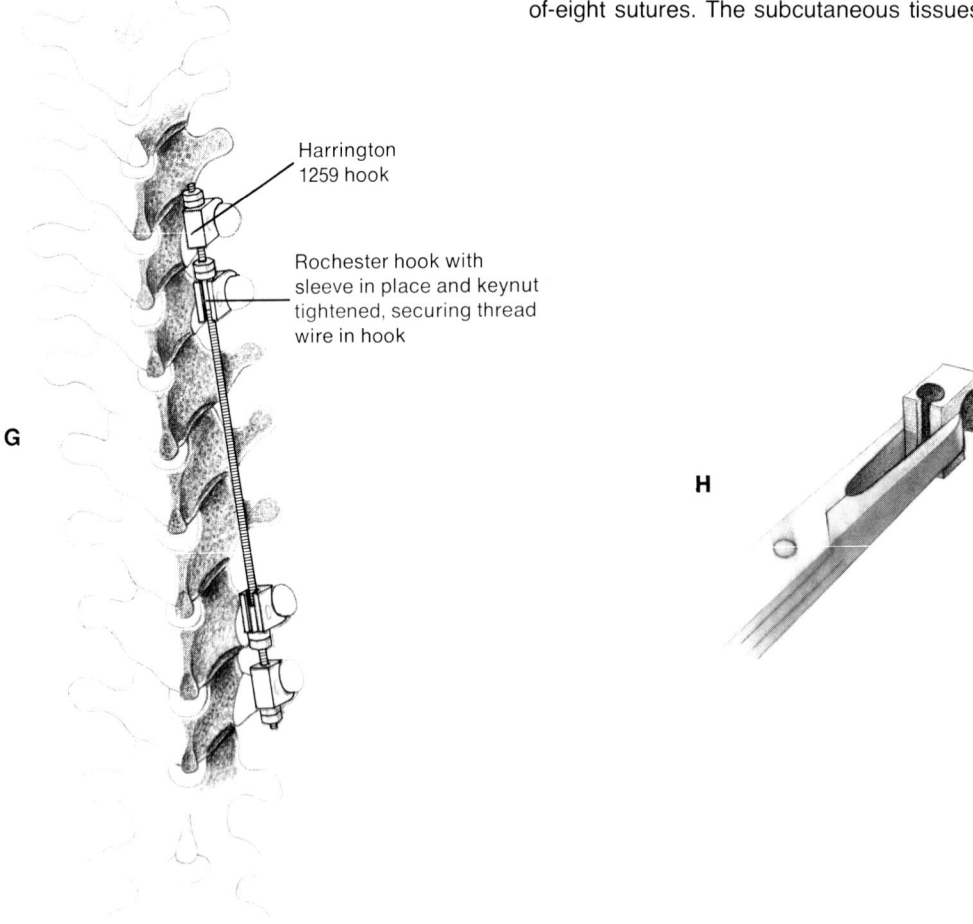

Fig. 30, cont'd

interrupted sutures of fine catgut, eliminating dead space. The skin edges are approximated with a subcuticular wire suture or a continuous monofilament nylon suture. The sacral bar of the plaster cast, if it was removed preoperatively, is replaced and secured with a couple of rolls of plaster. The posterior plaster lid is replaced and fastened in place, and the patient is ready to be turned and returned to bed.

Blood replacement and monitoring. The blood loss is accurately measured during operation. Sponges are weighed. Blood loss is replaced as it occurs. Since the introduction of the use of the MacKay operating frame for the scoliosis fusions, eliminating all pressure on the abdomen, the intraoperative blood loss has been decreased significantly. Prior to the use of the MacKay frame, 5 to 6 units of blood during surgery was usual, 3 units rarely. In occasional patients who bled excessively, particularly if the blood pressure during operation was running in the range of 120 to 130 mm of mercury and if extensive fusion was done, 7 to 10 units of blood might be required for replacement. Now, with the MacKay frame, 2 to 3 units of blood is the usual replacement required. A systolic blood pressure of about 90 mm Hg is desirable and can usually be obtained by using deep halothane anesthesia with controlled hyperventilation or by the use of other hypotensive drugs. When the distraction rod is inserted and distraction force applied, the blood pressure is brought up to 120 to 130 mm Hg.

In all patients direct arterial pressure, central venous pressure, electrocardiogram, arterial blood gases, and rectal or esophageal temperature are monitored.

Postoperative treatment. In the recovery room a nasogastric tube is passed and left in place until the patient recovers from the postoperative ileus and good bowel sounds are heard, usually 48 to 72 hours after surgery. The patient is then started on clear liquids and progresses to full diet slowly as tolerated.

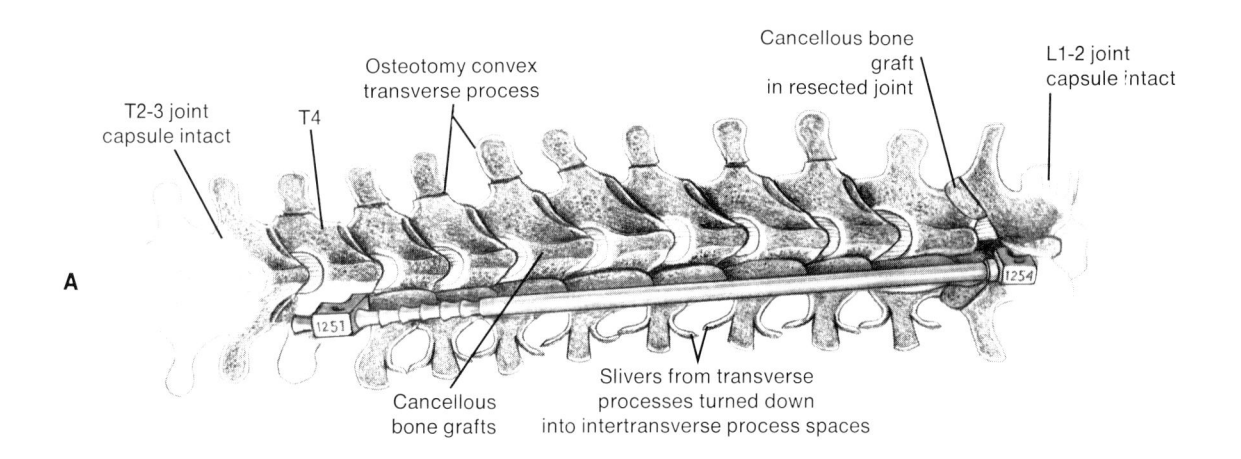

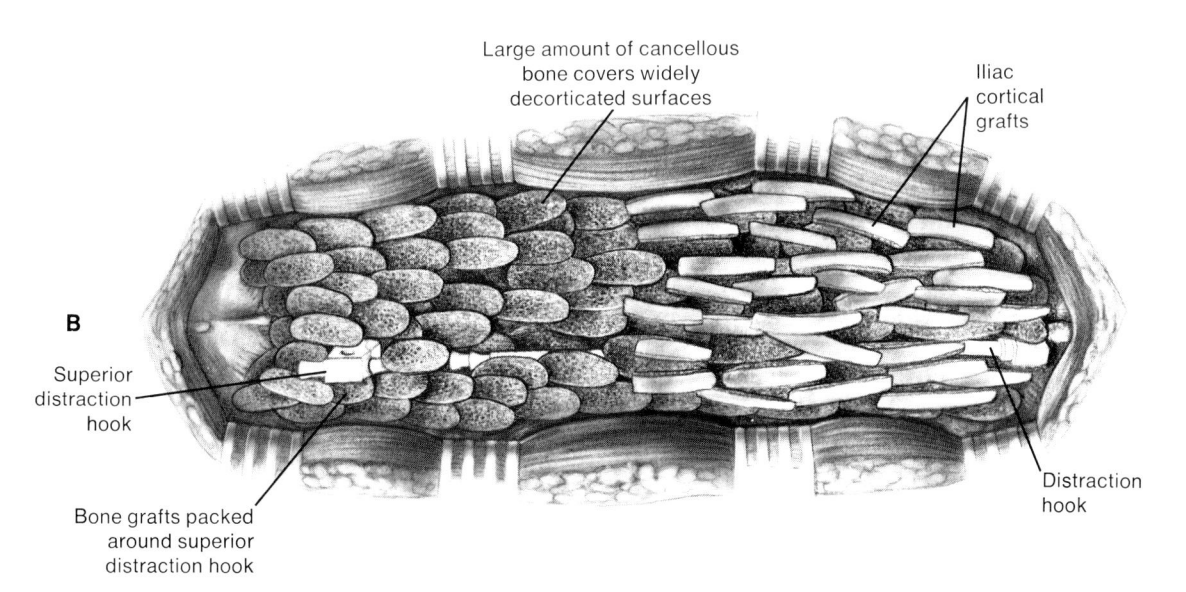

Fig. 31

Prophylactic antibiotics. All scoliosis fusion patients receive a course of prophylactic antibiotics. Methicillin, 1 g, is given intravenously when the skin incision is made. Another gram is given during the course of the surgery. Every 4 hours 1½ g of methicillin are given intravenously (9 grams daily) for 5 days postoperatively.

Comment. A meticulous fusion and the large amount of fresh autogenous iliac bone creates a favorable environment for the prompt formation, organization, and incorporation of a massive bone graft. The effectiveness of a spine fusion to maintain correction depends on a fusion mass of proper length and sufficient strength to withstand the stresses thrust on it when the patient resumes the erect posture without external support. Harrington instrumentation is useful as a major correction modality, a supplemental corrective force, and for *temporary* internal fixation. A low pseudarthrosis rate and maintenance of a high percentage of the preoperatively gained correction is obtained with a meticulous fusion technique, a large amount of fresh autogenous cancellous bone, and adequate external immobilization with instrumentation as a helpful adjunct.

JUVENILE KYPHOSIS (SCHEUERMANN'S DISEASE)

GENERAL DISCUSSION. Treatment depends on skeletal maturity, severity, flexibility of the spine, and structural changes of the vertebral bodies. In addition to the standard erect anteroposterior and lateral roentgenogram of the entire spine, a lateral view of the thoracic spine in maximum extension over a wedge is made to determine the flexibility of the kyphosis.

The flexible kyphosis of less than 70° that corrects 30° or more on maximum extension in patients before skeletal maturity responds favorably to a well-implemented Milwaukee brace and exercise program.

If the kyphosis is rigid with 15° or more of anterior wedging of two to three thoracic vertebrae, one or two antigravitylocalizer casts are applied for preliminary correction before fabrication and fitting of the Milwaukee brace.

In patients with kyphosis of 70° or more that corrects to 45° or less, posterior fusion and compression instrumentation alone can be done. External immobilization with an antigravity cast including the head and neck is used for 10 to 12 months. Failure to support the spine adequately externally may result in loss of correction, pseudarthrosis, and instrument failure. In the immature spine the extended period of immobilization allows the fusion mass to mature and the wedged vertebral bodies to "rectangularize."

Kyphosis over 70° with anterior wedging of vertebral bodies of 15° or more is indication for surgical treatment. The two-stage anterior and posterior procedure is most effective in obtaining and maintaining optimum correction and stabilization of the spine (Fig. 32).

In the mature spine with severe deformity and dis-

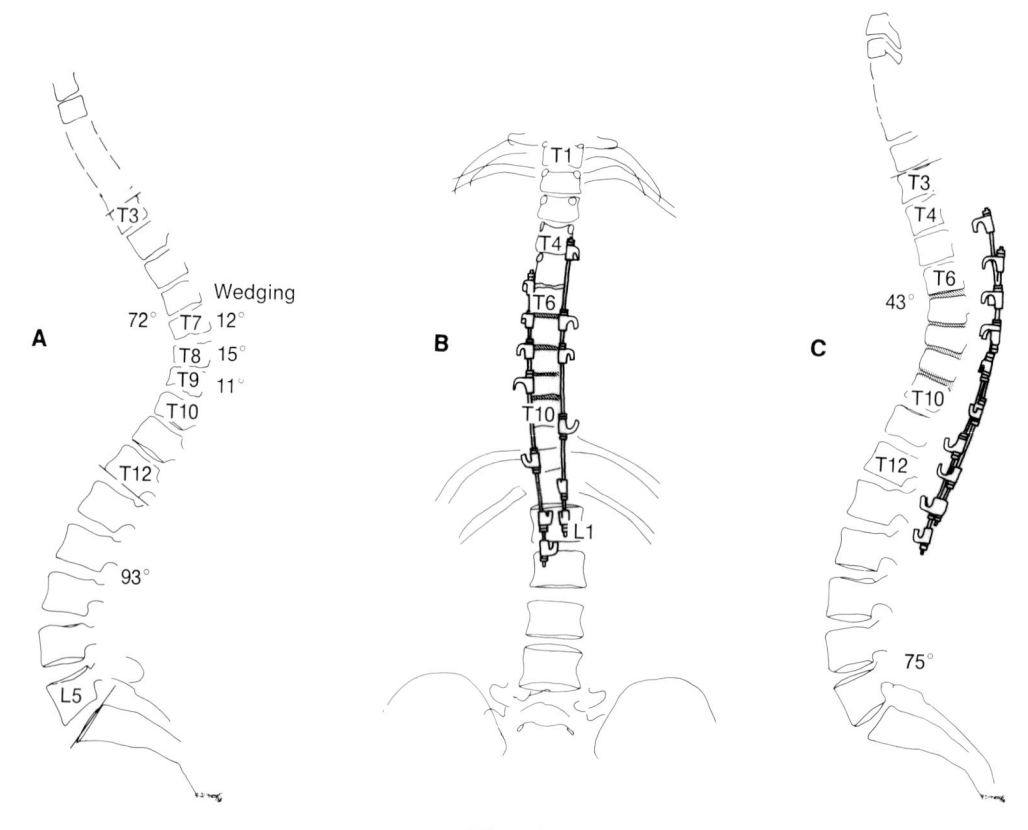

Fig. 32

abling pain, the two-stage anterior and posterior procedure is indicated.

NONOPERATIVE TREATMENT. A hyperkyphosis of less than 70° with vertebral wedging of less than 12° before skeletal maturity will usually respond favorably to a well-implemented Milwaukee brace and exercise treatment program. If the kyphosis corrects less than 20° on hyperextension, preliminary correction is obtained in an antigravity localizer cast. The cast is applied in two stages on the Risser table. First, the lumbar lordosis is eliminated as much as possible with the hips flexed, and a well-molded pelvic girdle is applied. The thoracic spine is then extended over the cross bar of the Risser table after the pelvic girdle has set. Halter traction is applied, and the plaster is extended over the thorax to the chin and occiput. At 6 weeks the cast is removed, a plaster mold is made for fabrication of a Milwaukee brace, and a second antigravity cast is applied that is worn until the Milwaukee brace is fitted. The brace is worn for 23 hours a day, and the patient is instructed in an exercise regime. When the kyphosis is more flexible, treatment with Milwaukee brace can be initiated without preliminary cast correction. Use of the antigravity cast is advantageous when there is a delay of 6 weeks or longer in the fabrication of the Milwaukee brace.

DETAILS OF PROCEDURE IN OPERATIVE TREATMENT. For kyphosis of 70° or more with vertebral wedging over 12° that corrects to 45° or less, posterior spine fusion and compression instrumentation are employed.

With the patient under general anesthesia and in the prone position on the spinal operating frame, the back is prepared and draped. A midline incision is made from T1 to L1. The incision is carried through the subcutaneous and fascia layers. The tips of the spinous processes are incised. Subperiosteal exposure of the spinous processes and the laminae is carried out. Facet capsulectomy and further subperiosteal exposure to the tips of the transverse processes are performed (Fig. 27, A and B). Before instrumentation the inferior articular processes are excised and the superior articular processes decorticated bilaterally, destroying one half to two thirds of the facet joints (Fig. 33, A). Posterior Harrington compression instrumentation is carried out from T3 or T4 to T12 or L1 using three or four hooks proximally and three or four hooks distally. The hooks are placed proximally over the transverse processes and distally under the transverse processes of T10 and T11 and under the lamina of T12 or L1 (Fig. 33, A and B). The spinous processes are removed after they are split. As complete decortication as possible is performed, leaving intact those areas which serve as hook seatings (Fig. 33, C). Fresh autogenous iliac cancellous and cortical bone is used. Bone grafts are placed

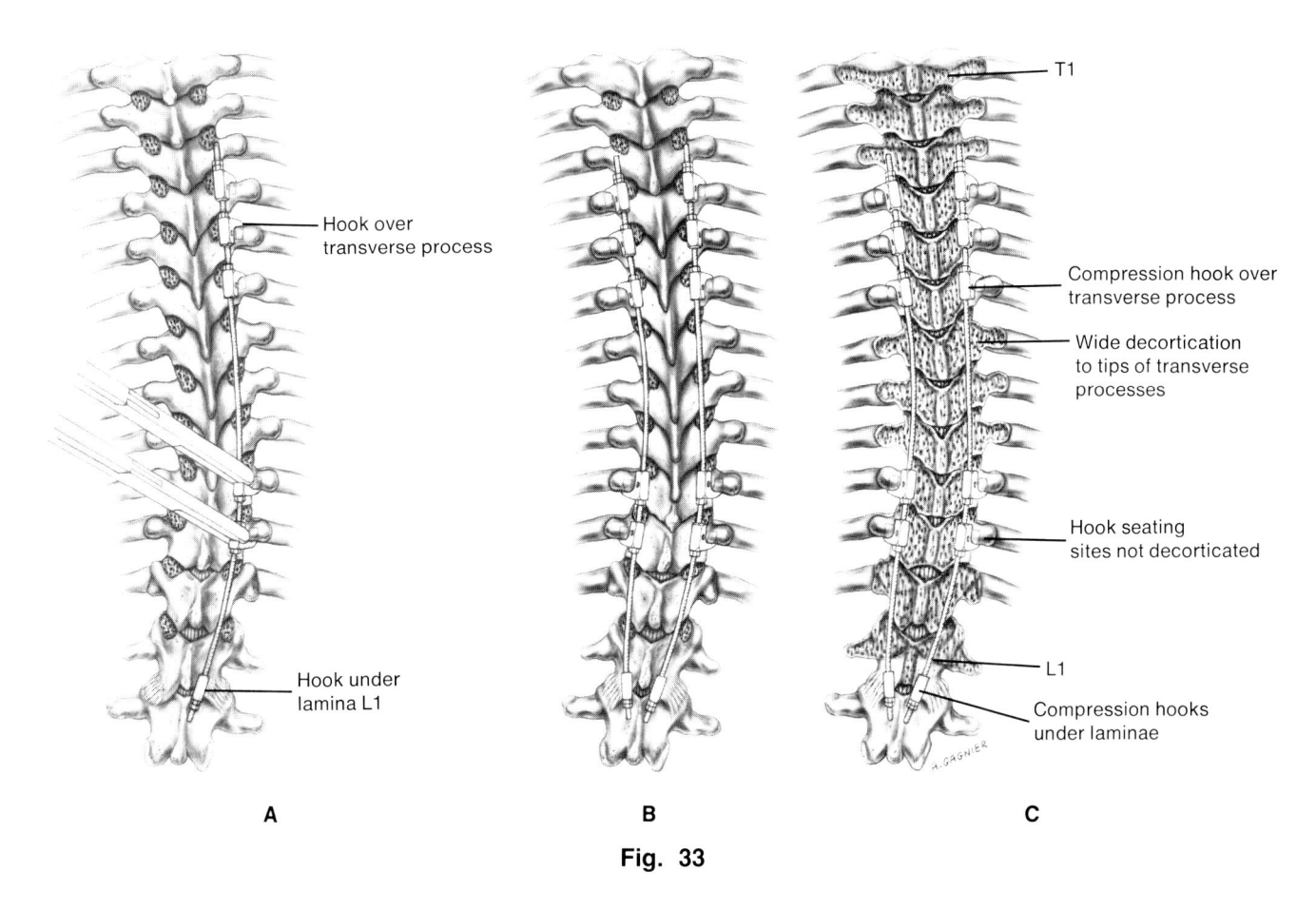

Fig. 33

Fig. 34

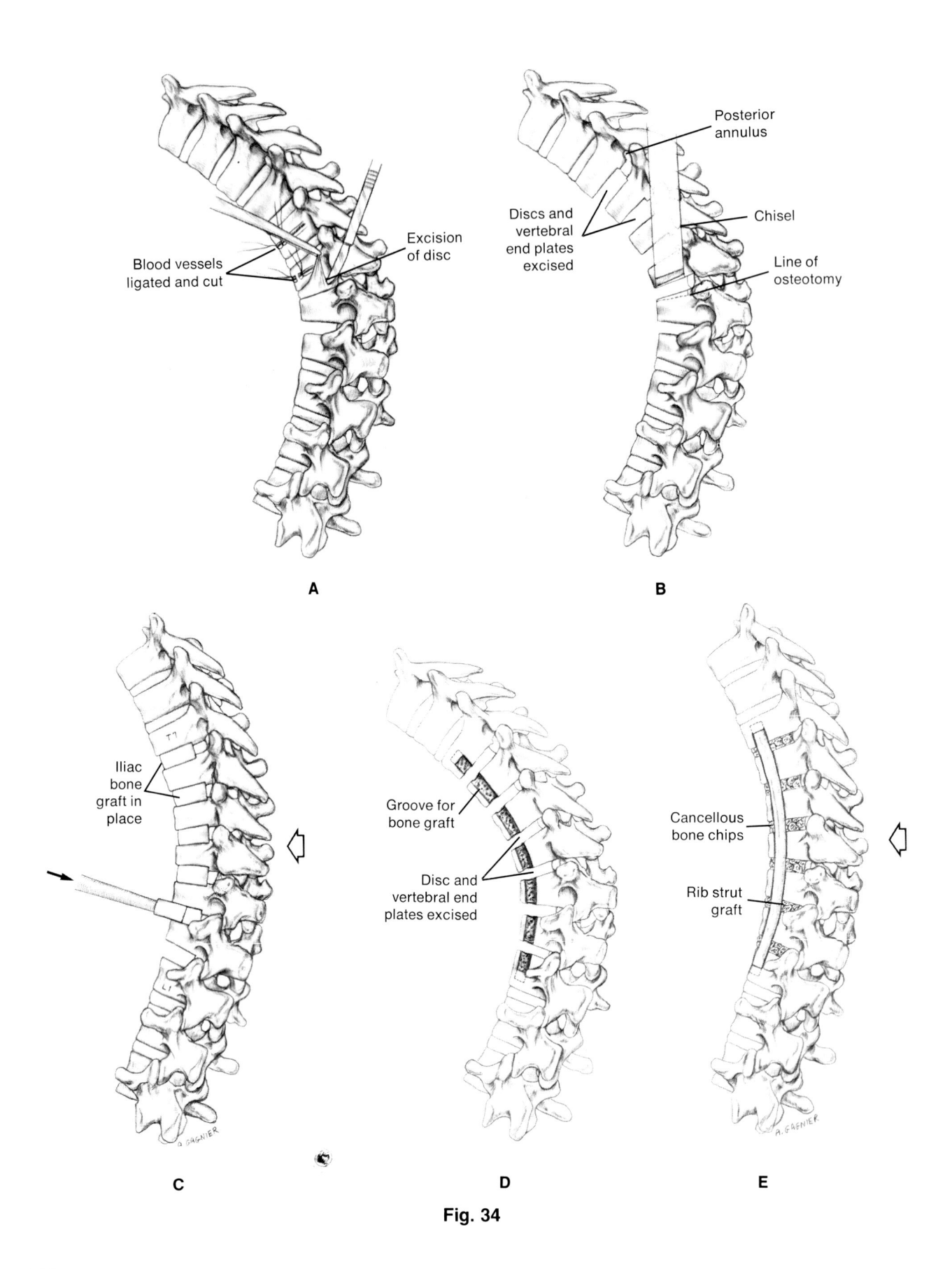

as in posterior fusion for scoliosis (Figs. 28 to 31). The wound is then closed in layers. The patient is nursed on a regular bed. About 10 days postoperatively an antigravity localizer cast is applied, and the patient is allowed to be ambulatory the following day. This cast is worn for 10 to 12 months.

In the patient with the more rigid and severe kyphosis the surgical treatment of choice is a two-stage procedure. The first stage is an anterior release of the contracted, thickened longitudinal ligament with anterior interbody fusion of vertebrae at the apex of the kyphosis. The approach to the thoracic spine is through a standard thoracotomy incision as described in the anterior exposure of the thoracic spine (Plate 8-5).

The intervertebral discs, usually four or five levels, are excised (Fig. 34, A). The end-plates are excised with a thin, sharp chisel (Fig. 34, B). With the application of pressure over the spinous processes and pushing on the kyphosis the excised disc spaces open up (Fig. 34, C). Bicortical iliac bone grafts are placed into the interbody spaces (Fig. 34, C). An alternative method of fusion is illustrated in Fig. 34, D and E. The trough in the vertebral bodies is made to accommodate the rib strut-graft which is countersunk into the end vertebrae. The resected disc spaces are packed with cancellous bone grafts. This allows for further correction of the kyphosis prior to the second-stage posterior instrumentation and fusion. The parietal pleura is closed. A chest drain is inserted, and the thoracotomy wound is closed in layers. A halo is then applied. The patient is nursed in cranial-halo gravity traction in bed and wheelchair. Ten to fourteen days after the first stage an antigravity halo cast is applied. The cast is prepared with large anterior and posterior windows. The second-stage procedure is performed in the cast a few days later. Posterior compression instrumentation is performed (Fig. 33). After 7 to 9 days the posterior window in the halo cast is boxed in, and the patient is allowed to be ambulatory. After 3 months the cranial halo is removed, and a new antigravity underarm body cast is applied. This is worn for another 6 months.

Recent use of the Rochester modification of the Harrington compression hook (Fig. 30, B and C) has facilitated application of compression instrumentation for kyphosis. Adequate postoperative immobilization is essential.

NEUROMUSCULAR SCOLIOSIS

The complete preoperative evaluation of the patient with neuromuscular scoliosis includes detailed cardiorespiratory function studies. There is often an associated pelvic obliquity. If the obliquity is due to contractures distal to the iliac crest, correction of pelvic obliquity is accomplished before treatment of the spine deformity. When the pelvic obliquity is part of the scoliosis due to contractures of trunk musculature, it is treated along with the spine deformity. The spine fusion required is longer than in idiopathic scoliosis, and it must be protected by external support for a longer period of time. The rigid, severe deformities require preliminary halo-femoral traction. The introduction of Harrington instrumentation and, subsequently, of anterior Dwyer instrumentation and anterior fusion has simplified the overall management of these deformities, improved the degree of correction obtained and maintained, and reduced the period of immobilization and recumbency. Early ambulation is often possible. When a fixed pelvic obliquity is part of the spine deformity, fusion must extend to the sacrum. The major objective is a stable spine with a balanced torso over a level pelvis.

The collapsing type of paralytic spine deformity with pelvic obliquity is best treated with the combination of anterior Dwyer instrumentation for correction of a thoracolumbar or lumbar curve and its associated pelvic obliquity followed by a second-stage long posterior fusion extending to the sacrum with Harrington instrumentation (Fig. 35). In the absence of pelvic obliquity, posterior fusion and Harrington instrumentation with adequate postoperative immobilization have successfully managed the noncollapsing paralytic spine deformity.

Fig. 35, A, shows a collapsing type of neuromuscular scoliosis with pelvic obliquity in a patient with cerebral palsy. The patient is wheelchair bound because of severe disability in the lower extremities. The objective of treatment is a stable spine balanced over a level pelvis. There is a long thoracolumbar curve, T5 to L4, measuring 50°, with pelvic obliquity, left side high. Treatment is in two stages. First an anterior Dwyer instrumentation with disc excision and interbody fusion from T11 to L5 is performed. The lumbar portion of the curve, T11 to L4, was reduced to 28° (Fig. 35, B). The pelvic obliquity was almost completely corrected, although the sacrum was not involved in the instrumentation. After 2 to 3 weeks the second-stage procedure is performed. This is posterior Harrington instrumentation and spine fusion. The Harrington rod is bent to accommodate the contours of the spine, and the spine fusion extends from T4 to the sacrum (Fig. 35, C and D). The postoperative radiographs show a stable, well-balanced spine over a level pelvis. Postoperative immobilization is in a pantaloon localizer cast with thigh extensions bivalved to allow passive hop motion daily. The patient remains recumbent for 3 months, after which an ambulatory localizer cast is applied to allow the patient to sit. This is followed at 6 months postoperative with a removable plastic jacket that is worn for 6 months. In general, scoliosis due to neuromuscular disturbance requires longer periods of immobilization than does idiopathic scoliosis. Early upright activity is encouraged in keeping with the general condition of the patient and the degree of disability. A postoperative halo cast may allow ambulation at an earlier date.

CONGENITAL SPINE DEFORMITY

The problem in congenital spine deformity is one of asymmetric growth. These patients do not have normal growth potential in the spine. There is no valid objection to early fusion of the congenital curvature that is progressing. Fusion of the anomalous segment

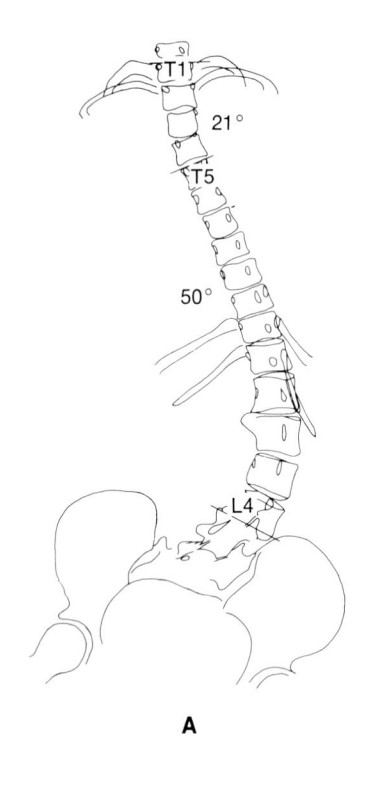

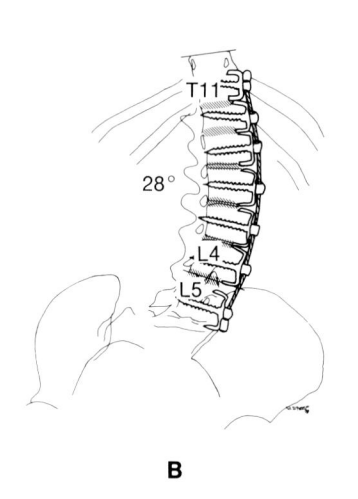

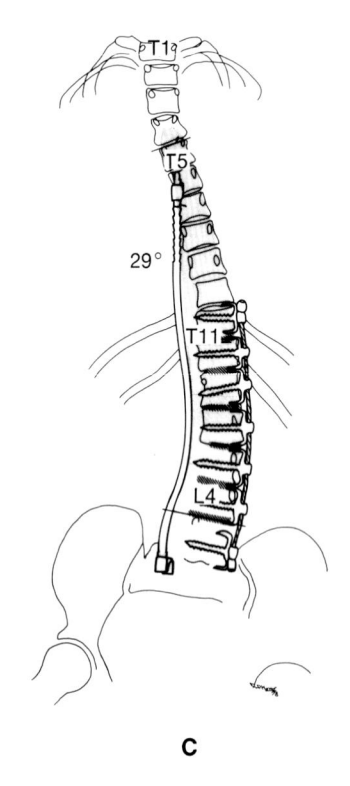

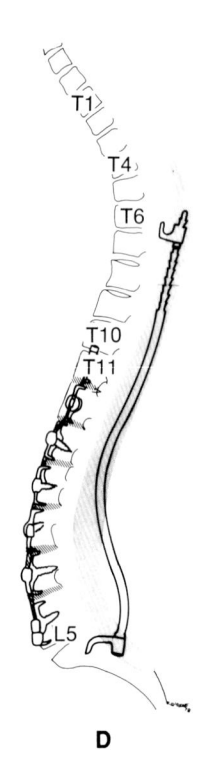

Fig. 35

will prevent progression and result in a short, relatively straight spine rather than a shorter crooked spine in which the curvature was allowed to increase. Documentation of 10° of progression of the congenital curve is sufficient indication for fusion. A study of untreated patients with congenital scoliosis shows that about 75% of congenital curves progress. Radiographic criteria of a bad prognosis in a congenital curve are the following: the presence of an unsegmented bony bar that has no potential growth, significant asymmetric growth potential such as 2 or 3 hemivertebrae on the same side, and the microvertebra associated with kyphosis. Adequate management requires surgical treatment early in the evolution of the curve followed by long-term use of the Milwaukee brace to control the unpredictable behavior of the unfused segments of the spine and prevent bending of the fusion. In general, treatment depends on the severity and location of the curve.

GUIDELINES FOR THE SURGICAL MANAGEMENT OF CERTAIN CONGENITAL SPINE DEFORMITIES

1. With a curve of poor prognosis, the ideal treatment is fusion of the anomalous segment in situ before significant deformity requiring correction has occurred, the long-term use of the Milwaukee brace to control the unfused segments of the spine and prevent the fused segment from bending with growth, as well as the prevention of lengthening of the fused curve by the addition of vertebrae distal to the curve.

2. Osteotomy of the unsegmented bar and fusion of the anomalous segment and usually one normal vertebra proximal and distal is followed by correction of the curve in halo-femoral traction or turnbuckle cast, which in turn is followed by long-term use of the Milwaukee brace.

3. Excision of a hemivertebra, a two-stage procedure, is shown in Fig. 36: excision of vertebral body and a portion of the pedicle through an anterior approach (Fig. 36, B) and excision of the appropriate posterior elements with correction and fusion of the appropriate segment of the spine 2 weeks later (Fig. 36). This method of management may be necessary in the hemivertebra at L4-5 or lumbosacral levels with pelvic obliquity. After consolidation of the fusion, long-term bracing during the growth period is indicated.

4. A clear-cut indication for Dwyer anterior instrumentation (Plate 8-4) is the myelomeningocele patient with progressive scoliosis or lordoscoliosis. The wide defect in the laminae prevents or makes it difficult to perform a satisfactory posterior fusion. The anterior approach (Plate 8-4, N to Y), excision of the discs, and internal fixation with Dwyer's flexible cable system has definite advantages.

All patients with congenital spine deformity should have an intravenous pyelogram early during the period of observation because of the high incidence of genitourinary tract abnormalities. Special preoperative studies include tomograms, which help define the details of the anomalous development and aid in planning the surgical approach. Myelograms are performed on patients with congenital spine deformity before surgery to rule out diastematomyelia and other subarachnoid abnormalities.

When there is a fixed pelvic obliquity associated with a congenital lumbar scoliosis, the pelvic obliquity must be corrected and the fusion must be extended to include the sacrum to maintain correction of the obliquity.

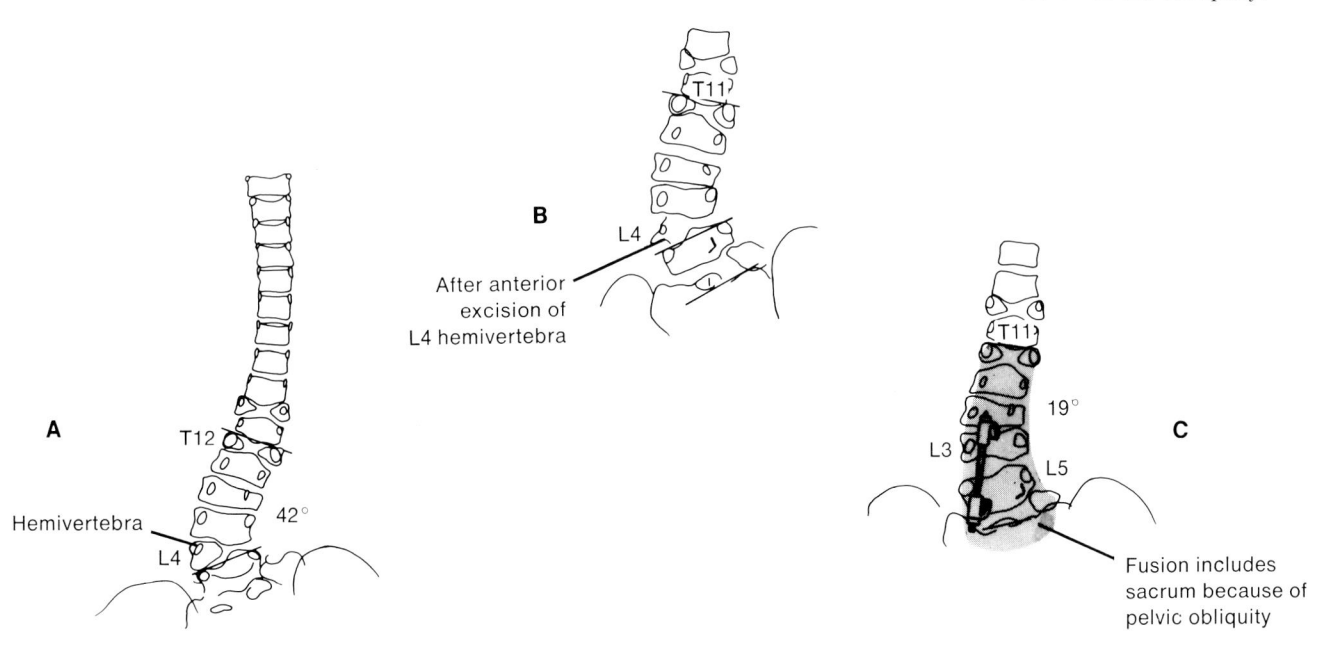

Fig. 36

POSTERIOR LUMBOSACRAL SPINE FUSION (Plate 8-1)

GENERAL DISCUSSION. Spondylolisthesis is most common at the lumbosacral level. It does occur at L4-5 and occasionally at levels above. Spondylolysis is a defect in the pars interarticularis without olisthesis for which surgery is rarely indicated.

Following is a classification of lumbosacral spondylolisthesis (by Wiltse et al., 1976):

Dysplastic: Congenital abnormality of the upper sacrum and/or the arch of L5 allowing forward slip of L5

Isthmic: Defective or elongated pars interarticularis in the lumbosacral spine with olisthesis at one or several levels

Degenerative: Associated with osteoarthritic changes in the lumbosacral spine with olisthesis at one or several levels

Traumatic: Fracture of posterior structures

Pathologic: Generalized or localized bone disease

Defects in the pars interarticularis (isthmic) are the most common cause of spondylolisthesis in the child and young adult. The incidental finding of a spondylolisthesis in a child under 10 years of age warrants spot lateral roentgenograms of the lumbosacral area made in the erect posture at about 6-month intervals to monitor olisthesis. If there is evidence of progressive forward slip, spine fusion is indicated.

Meyerding classified forward slip: grade I, less than 25%; grade II, 25% to 50%; grade III, 50% to 75%; grade IV, greater than 75%. Grade V has been added to designate the fifth lumbar vertebra anterior to the sacrum.

Following are indications for spine fusion in children:
1. Progressive slipping with or without symptoms
2. Slip of 30% to 50% even if patient is asymptomatic
3. Persistent symptoms not relieved by conservative treatment

In adults the indication for surgery is presence of disabling symptoms not relieved by nonoperative treatment. Spondylolisthesis usually occurs before age 20, and olisthesis rarely increases in the adult, except for the degenerative type and instability secondary to surgical intervention.

If there are symptoms of nerve root disturbance with or without objective evidence of neurologic deficit, the loose posterior arch of L5 and the fibrous and cartilaginous tissue in the pars defect are removed followed by spine fusion. In patients with severe degrees of spondylolisthesis, fusion is performed from L4 to the sacrum. Fusion of L5 to the sacrum is adequate for the mild slip. Transverse processes are always included in the fusion. A large amount of fresh autogenous iliac bone is always used. Spine exposure may be through a midline incision exposing the transverse processes of L4 and L5 and the ala of the sacrum (Plate 8-1, *B*). Alternative approaches are through two lateral incisions with the deep approach to the spine by either Watkins' paraspinal approach (Plate 8-2, *A* to *C*) or Wiltse's muscle-splitting exposure (Plate 8-2, *D*).

In a limited experience with the traction and hyperextension cast method of reduction of severe spondylolisthesis described by Scaglietti, a partial reduction of the slip has been obtained (not illustrated). Posterolateral fusion was performed in the corrective bilateral pantaloon cast, followed by 4 months of bed rest in the cast. More time and experience are required to clearly define the indications, safety, and techniques of reduction and stabilization of severe spondylolisthesis.

DETAILS OF PROCEDURE. A longitudinal incision is made over the spinous processes from the third lumbar vertebra to the third sacral segment **(A)**. With pressure applied to either side of the spinous process of L4, the supraspinous ligament and cartilaginous tip of the spinous process (if the patient is a child) are sharply incised down to bone. This allows clean subperiosteal reflection of soft tissues off the spinous process. There is often a spina bifida of the first and second sacral segments, and there may be a defect in the lamina of the fifth lumbar vertebra. This is determined preoperatively from the roentgenographs. If there is a spina bifida, care must be taken in initiating subperiosteal reflection of the soft tissues so the dura mater is not penetrated.

The subperiosteal reflection of soft tissues is carried laterally, exposing the posterior arch of L4, L5, and the first two sacral segments **(B)**. It is helpful to incise the attachment of the joint capsules to the inferior articular process. This will facilitate reflection of the capsule and allow continued reflection of tissues off the lateral aspect of the superior articular process of L5. If the degree of forward slip is severe, the transverse process of L5 may not be visualized. The transverse processes of L4 and the ala of the sacrum are exposed. Care is taken to leave the facet joint capsule between L3 and L4 intact. The distal one third of the spinous process of L3 is exposed, however, to facilitate retraction of reflected tissues. The interspinous ligaments are excised if they have not already been removed with the subperiosteal reflection of tissues.

The lamina of L5 is usually underdeveloped and very mobile. If it is to be decorticated, a rongeur is more effective than a gouge because of the mobility of the lamina **(C)**. The spinous processes of L4 and L5 are excised. The lamina of L4 is deeply decorticated, exposing cancellous bone. The decortication is continued over the lateral aspect of the superior articular process out to the tip of the transverse process. The inferior articular process of the fifth lumbar lamina is excised, exposing the superior articular process of the first sacral segment. This allows removal of the cartilage from these articular processes and decortication of the ala of the sacrum **(C)**. The first and second sacral segments are decorticated with care. Usually, the sacral laminae are very thin and entirely cortical so that very thin slivers have to be reflected to avoid exposure of the dura. As the exposure progresses and decortication of the sacrum is done, blood is aspirated from the wound into a basin. The decorticated bone slivers are placed in the basin and immersed in the aspirated blood until replaced in the wound. The spine wound is packed.

(Plate 8-1) POSTERIOR LUMBOSACRAL SPINE FUSION

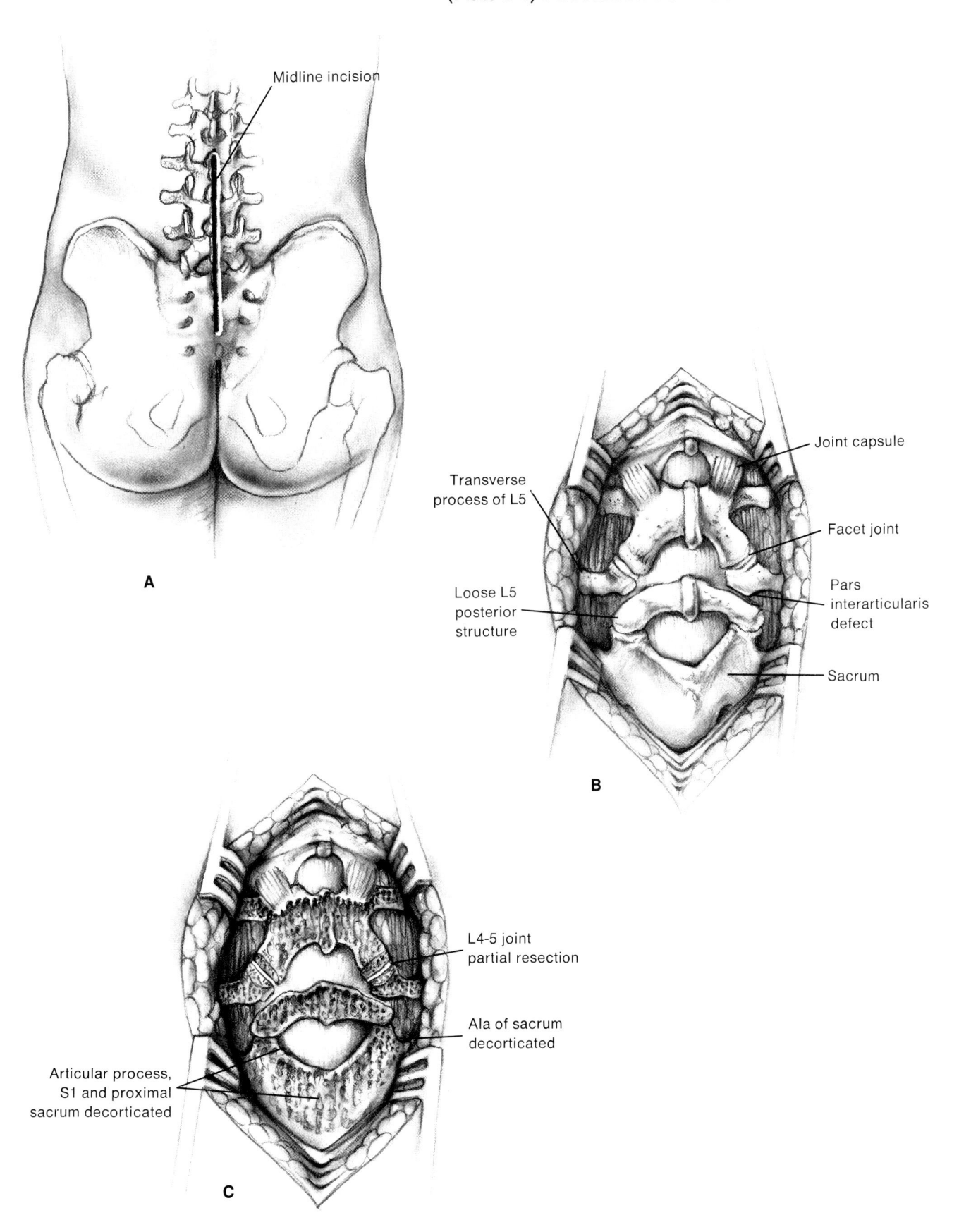

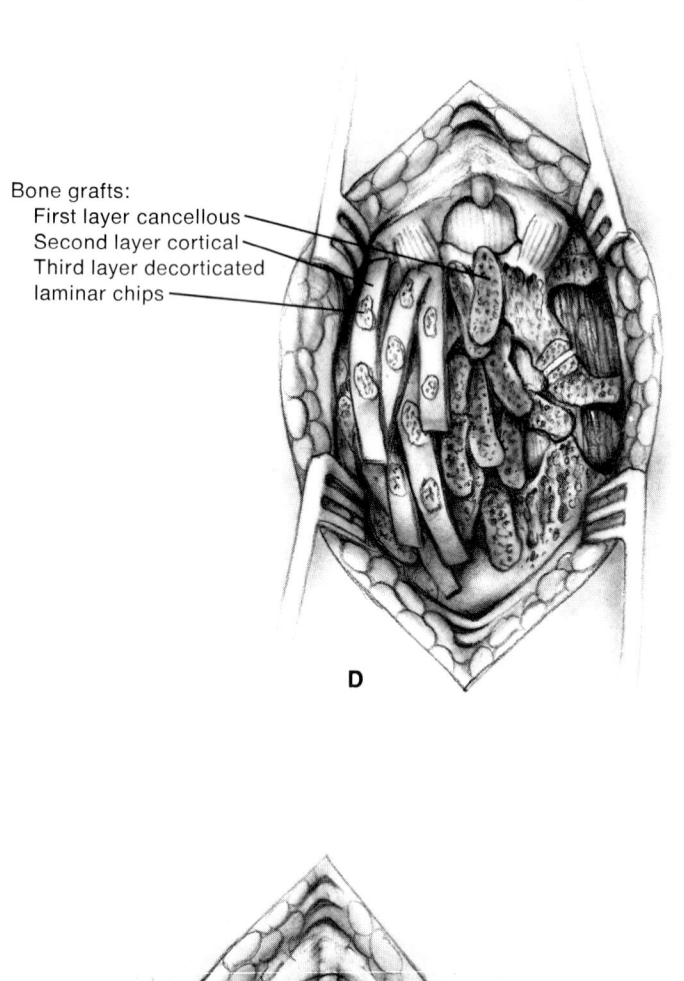

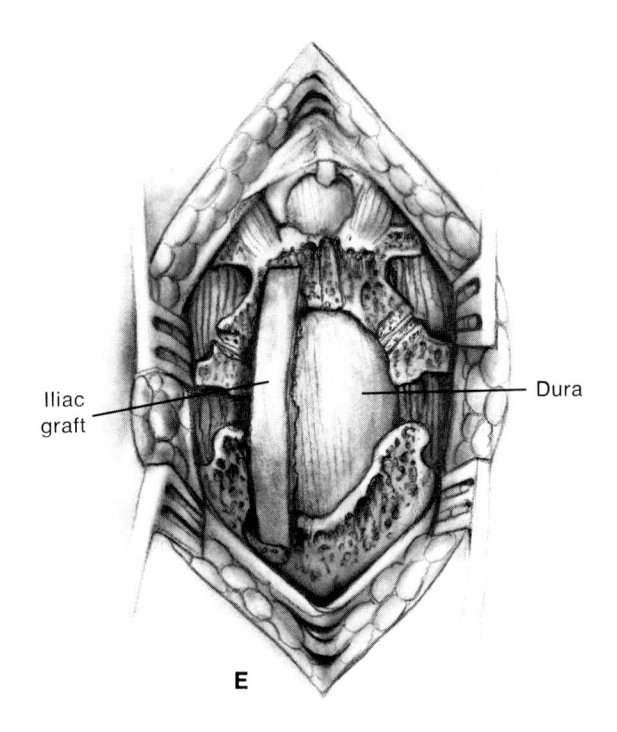

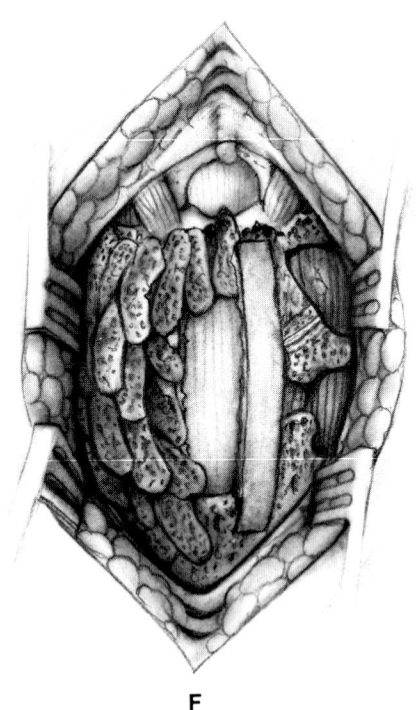

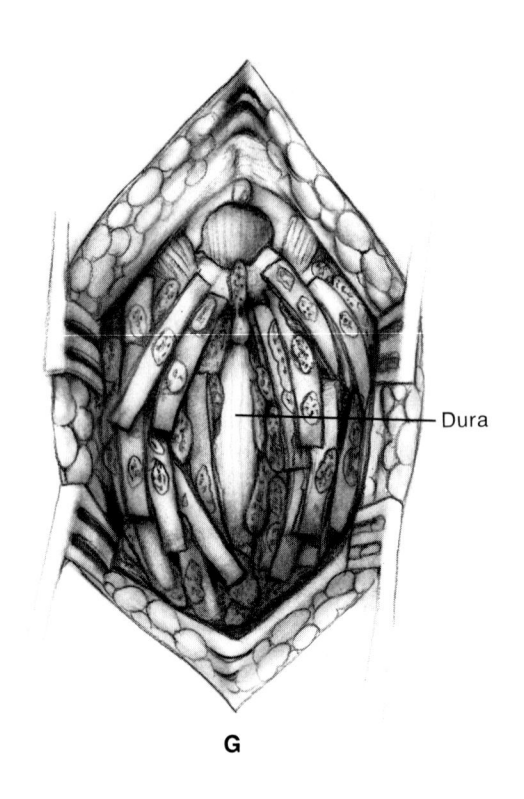

POSTERIOR LUMBOSACRAL SPINE FUSION (Plate 8-1)

Bone grafts:
 First layer cancellous
 Second layer cortical
 Third layer decorticated laminar chips

D

Iliac graft — Dura

E

F

Dura

G

256

(Plate 8-1) POSTERIOR LUMBOSACRAL SPINE FUSION

The outer table of one ilium is then widely exposed (as described on p. 283). A large amount of outer table cortex and cancellous bone is obtained and placed in the basin containing blood from the wounds. The iliac wound is closed. The packing is removed from the spinal wound.

Cancellous iliac bone slivers are laid down in and over the facet joints between L4 and L5, and L5 and the sacrum, as well as in the gutter over the lateral aspect of the superior articular processes and the transverse processes, and out over the ala of the sacrum (**D**). All the cancellous bone is laid down first, followed by slivers of iliac cortical bone, and finally the decorticated lamina bone, which has been cut into small chips. The grafts are gently packed down with a flat retractor. The wound is closed using figure-of-eight heavy absorbable sutures for the deeper structures and finer absorbable sutures for the more superficial tissues.

When the loose L5 lamina is removed, a rather large area of dura is exposed in the defect (**E**). The technique of fusion is the same as with the lamina left in place. The exposed dura is covered with a layer of Gelfoam, and long, wide iliac cortical grafts span the defect on each side (**E** and **F**), overlapping the decorticated L4 lamina and the proximal sacrum and leaving a narrow defect in the midline (**G**). The large amount of iliac cancellous and cortical bone is placed in the gutter on each side over transverse processes, the laminae and proximal sacrum overlapping the two iliac cortical grafts (**G**).

POSTOPERATIVE MANAGEMENT. The child or adolescent is treated postoperatively on a turning frame or a firm bed for 10 to 14 days. The patient is usually more comfortable in bed with knees slightly flexed. If treated in bed, the patient is instructed to logroll when turning. At about 10 days postoperatively, after skin suture removal, a snug bilateral pantaloon hip spica cast is applied incorporating the lower ribs. After 3 to 4 months of recumbency, ambulation is started in a well-molded light plaster jacket, which is worn for 2 to 3 months.

The adult with more than a 25% slip is treated in recumbency for 4 months in a pantaloon plaster cast followed by 2 to 3 months in a light ambulatory, well-molded plaster jacket.

In a child or adult with a mild slip or in the occasional patient with spondylolysis requiring surgical treatment, the fusion may be limited to the L5-sacrum level (**H** and **I**). The same technique is used with a generous amount of iliac cancellous and cortical grafts over the widely decorticated area up to the tips of the transverse processes, over the ala of the sacrum and the proximal sacrum. The child or adolescent is immobilized in a pantaloon spica cast in recumbency for 3 months and then allowed to increase upright activity gradually.

When posterolateral fusion is performed in situ, in a patient with a minimal slip, immobilization is with a single pantaloon body cast, and limited ambulation is allowed.

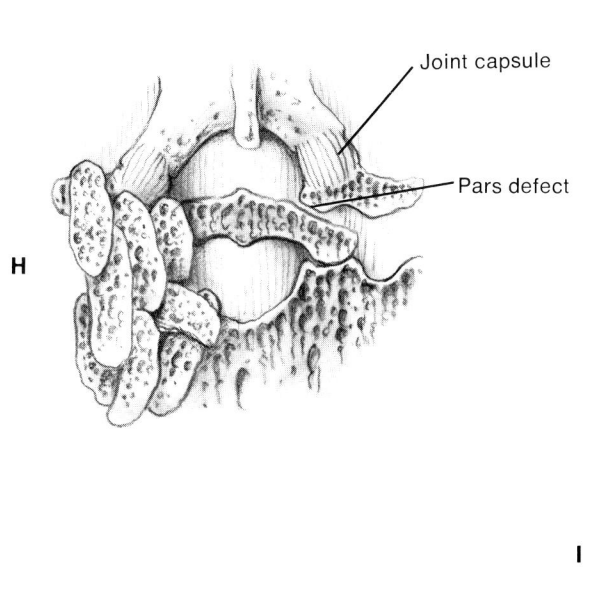

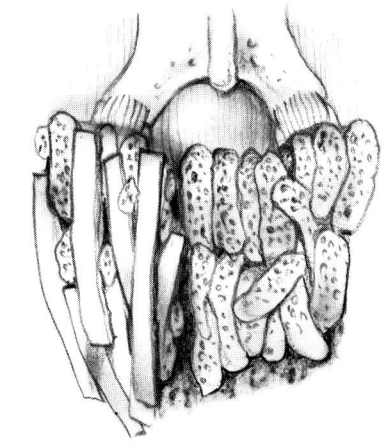

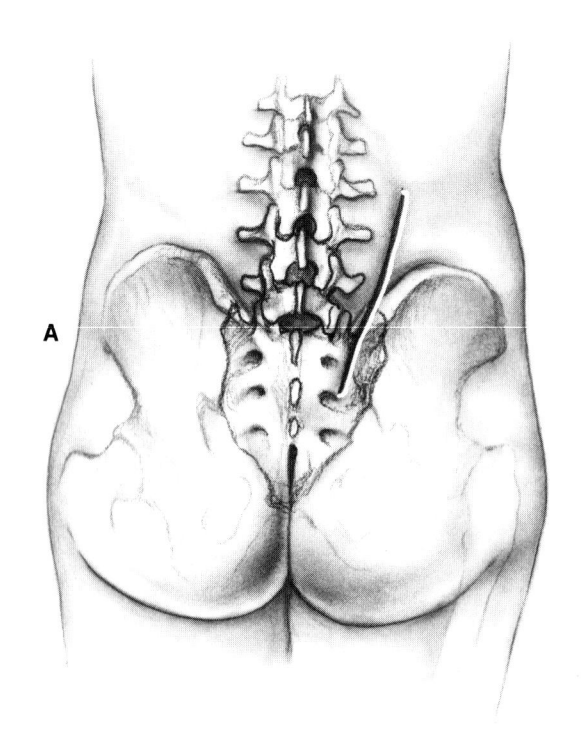

POSTEROLATERAL SPINE FUSION BY BILATERAL, LATERAL APPROACH (Plate 8-2)

GENERAL DISCUSSION. An alternative method of posterolateral spine fusion may be performed through a bilateral, lateral approach as described by Watkins (**A** to **C**) and Wiltse (**D**). This is particularly suitable in patients with extensive midline scarring from previous operations and defects in the posterior elements of the spine.

DETAILS OF PROCEDURE. The patient is positioned completely prone. The surgical approach on either side requires a longitudinal incision along the outer border of the paraspinal muscles that then curves medially at the caudal end as the incision crosses the posterior superior iliac spine **(A)**.

The lumbodorsal fascia is incised **(B)**. The dissection plane is established between the paraspinal muscles medially and the fascia overlying the transversus abdominus muscle laterally. In this plane, one can palpate the tips of the transverse processes in the depth of the wound. Three centimeters of the posterior crest of the ilium, including the posterosuperior spine, are superficially osteotomized **(B)**. Wiltse exposes the spine through a more medial muscle-splitting approach **(D)**.

The osteotomized superficial crest of the ilium is retracted medially along with the reflected sacrospinalis muscle, thus exposing the ala of the sacrum **(C)**. The lateral skin flap is retracted laterally. An incision is made along the posterior third of the iliac crest, and subperiosteal exposure of the posterior portion of the ilium is accomplished **(C)**. The sciatic notch is visualized or palpated. This allows sufficient exposure to subsequently remove enough iliac bone to be used on both sides of the spine. The exposure is then carried medially from the tips of the transverse processes, clearing the tissues off the superior articular process. The joint capsule is excised and the exposure is carried medially, exposing the lamina to the base of the spinous process except in patients with laminar defects. The exposure is continued distally to uncover the first two sacral segments. At the completion of exposure for L4 to sacrum fusion, the transverse process and superior articular process of L4 will be exposed, leaving the capsule of the facet joint between L3 and L4 intact **(C)**. The facet joint between L4 and L5 is clearly visualized along with adjacent laminae. If the patient has a spondylolisthesis at the lumbosacral level, the defect in the pars interarticularis is visualized and the fibrofatty tissue is removed from the defect. The transverse processes of L4 and L5 are decorticated along with the pars interarticularis and the lateral aspect of the superior articular process of L4 and L5. Cartilage is excised from the joint between L4 and L5 **(E)**.

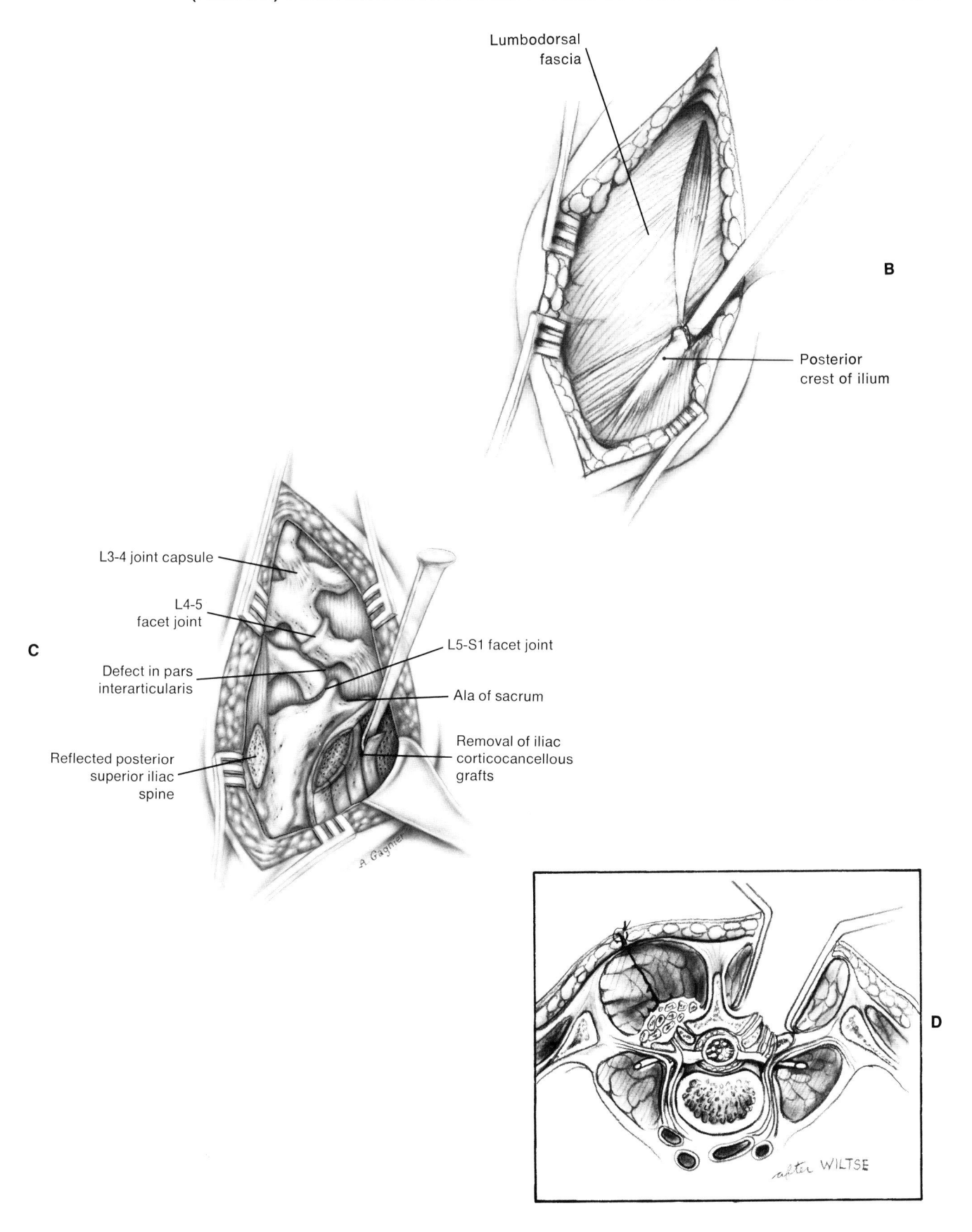

(Plate 8-2) POSTEROLATERAL SPINE FUSION BY BILATERAL, LATERAL APPROACH

Lumbodorsal fascia

Posterior crest of ilium

B

L3-4 joint capsule
L4-5 facet joint
Defect in pars interarticularis
L5-S1 facet joint
Ala of sacrum
Removal of iliac corticocancellous grafts
Reflected posterior superior iliac spine

C

after WILTSE

D

259

POSTEROLATERAL SPINE FUSION BY BILATERAL, LATERAL APPROACH (Plate 8-2)

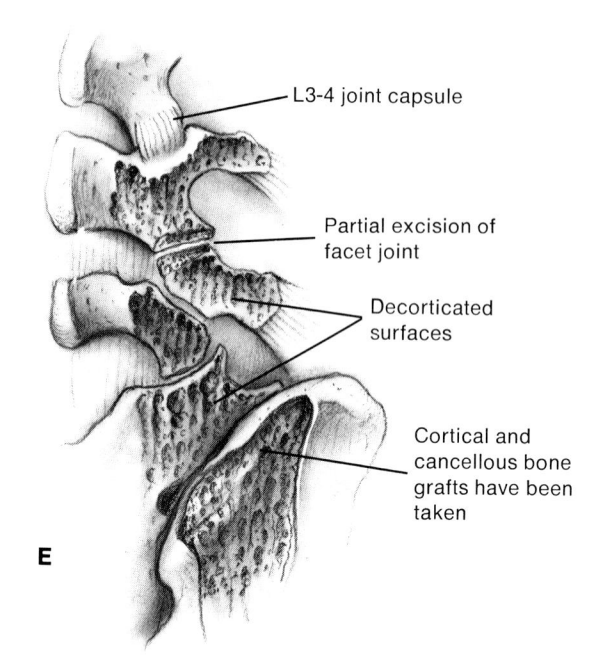

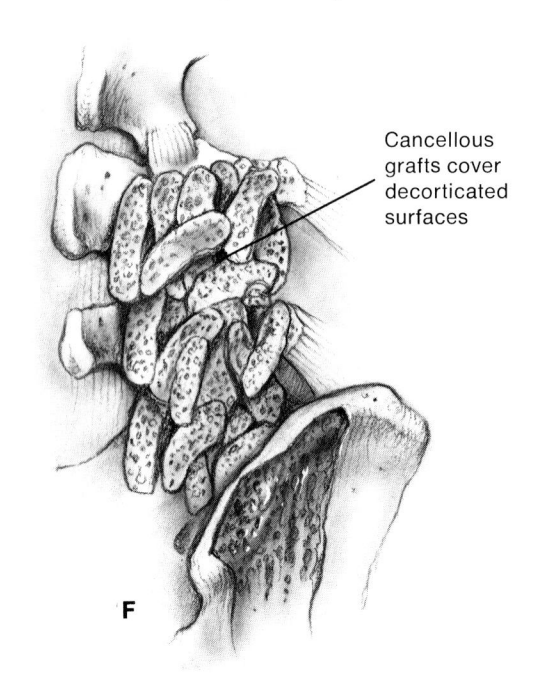

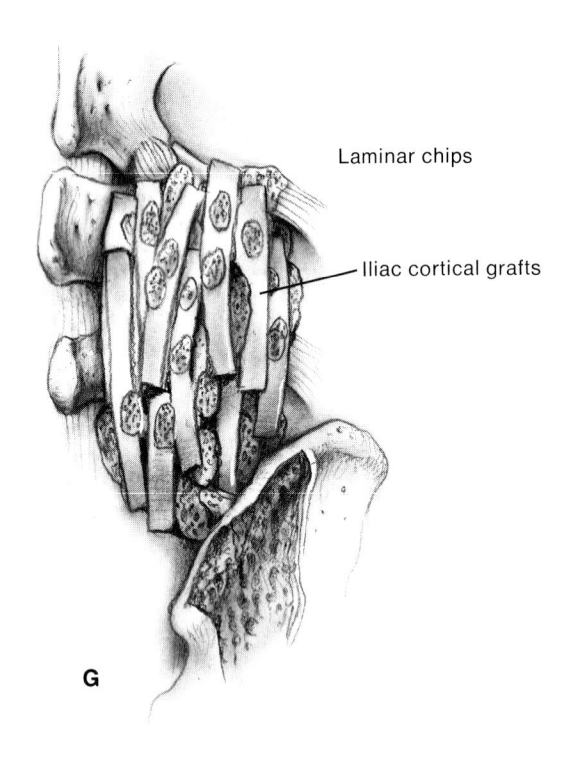

The lateral portion of the lamina of L4 is decorticated. The inferior articular process of L5 is excised, exposing the articular surface of the superior articular process of the first sacral segment. This is decorticated along with the ala of the sacrum and the remainder of the exposed sacral laminae (**E**). The decorticated bone slivers are placed in a basin and submerged in blood aspirated from the wound until they are replaced in the wound. This wound is temporarily packed. The exposed outer table of the ilium is then osteotomized. Cortical grafts are removed, and as much cancellous bone as possible is taken (**C** and **E**).

A cancellous graft is packed into the resected joint between L4 and L5. Half of the graft material removed from the ilium is set aside for use for the fusion on the opposite side of the spine. The cancellous slivers are placed in several overlapping layers over the widely decorticated area, which includes the transverse process, the articular process and laminae to the base of the spinous process, the ala, and the adjacent sacrum (**F**). The iliac cortical strips and laminar bone are then laid down (**G**). The retractors are removed, and the soft tissues are allowed to fall into place. Several holes are made in the intact medial crest of the posterior ilium with a towel clip. The gluteal muscle and fascia are securely approximated with interrupted heavy chromic catgut sutures through the drill holes. The rest of the wound is closed in layers.

Through a similar incision, the opposite side of the spine is exposed and treated in the same manner. The other half of the iliac bone grafts is used. Final wound closure is accomplished by approximation of the fascial structures, subcutaneous tissue, and skin.

POSTOPERATIVE MANAGEMENT. The patient is cared for in the manner outlined earlier for posterior lumbosacral spine fusion.

(Plate 8-3) ANTERIOR SPINE FUSION BY RETROPERITONEAL APPROACH TO THE LUMBAR SPINE

GENERAL DISCUSSION. The anterior aspect of the lumbar spine, including the lumbosacral disc, may be exposed through a retroperitoneal approach. This allows wide exposure of the vertebral bodies and discs. If there is an option, the approach through the left side is technically slightly easier and preferred. The aorta and common iliac artery are more easily protected from injury. Care must be taken to avoid injury to the inferior vena cava and the common iliac vein with retraction. When L1 and L2 are to be exposed, the twelfth rib is resected. For exposure to the lower lumbar spine and the lumbosacral disc, a lower incision is used. Indications for using this approach to perform anterior spine surgery are the following:

1. For diagnosis and treatment of diseases of the lumbar vertebrae or discs (e.g., debridement and grafting for osteomyelitis, biopsy of vertebral bodies, excision of hemivertebra, wedge resection or osteotomy [Fig. 36]).

2. To perform anterior interbody fusion for failed repair of posterior spine fusion in the adult idiopathic scoliosis.

3. An alternative exposure to the lumbosacral joint is a transperitoneal approach, which is useful when there is a high bifurcation of the aorta and vena cava or in patients who have had previous retroperitoneal surgery.

DETAILS OF PROCEDURE. When the approach is through the left side, the patient is placed in the lateral position with the body tilted 30° from the horizontal. This position is preferred because it allows the surgeon to have a more direct anterior view while standing on the left side behind the patient. A "beanbag," which on suction can be firmly contoured, is placed under the patient, thus holding the patient stably in the desired position during the procedure. The "beanbag" is also flexible enough so that the operating table can be "broken" or flexed as desired during the procedure.

A curved flank incision starts from the lateral border of the erector spinae muscles on the left side and extends around the flank toward a point between the umbilicus and the symphysis pubis just lateral to the rectus abdominus muscle **(A)**. The dissection is carried through the subcutaneous tissue; the external oblique and the transversus abdominus are divided along the line of the incision **(B)**. During division of the transversus abdominus muscle, care must be taken not to violate the peritoneum. It is easiest to enter the retroperitoneal space near the posterior aspect, where there is usually a good amount of retroperitoneal fat and loose areolar tissue. When this plane has been entered, the peritoneum is gently swept away from the abdominal wall; the peritoneum, kidney, and ureter are retracted anteriorly and toward the opposite side. The 30° lateral position of the patient allows the viscera to move away

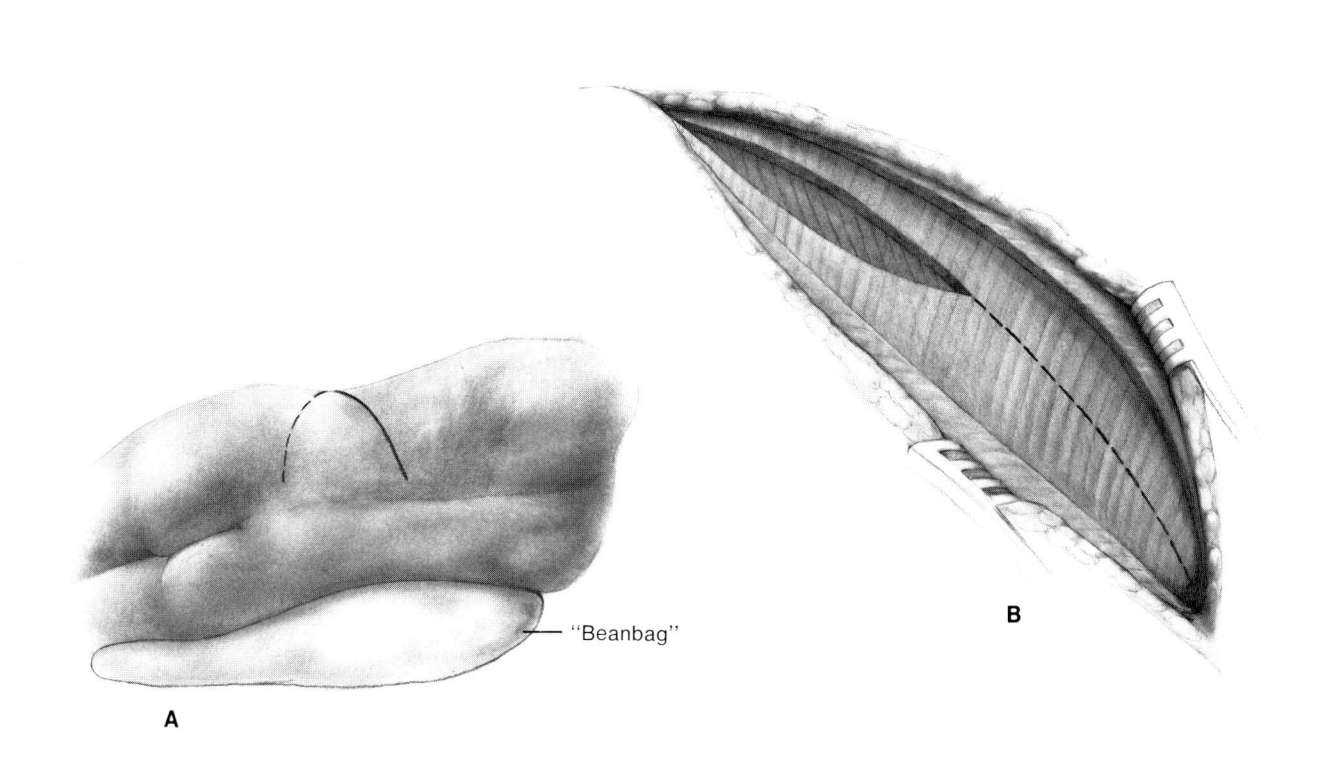

ANTERIOR SPINE FUSION BY RETROPERITONEAL APPROACH TO THE LUMBAR SPINE (Plate 8-3)

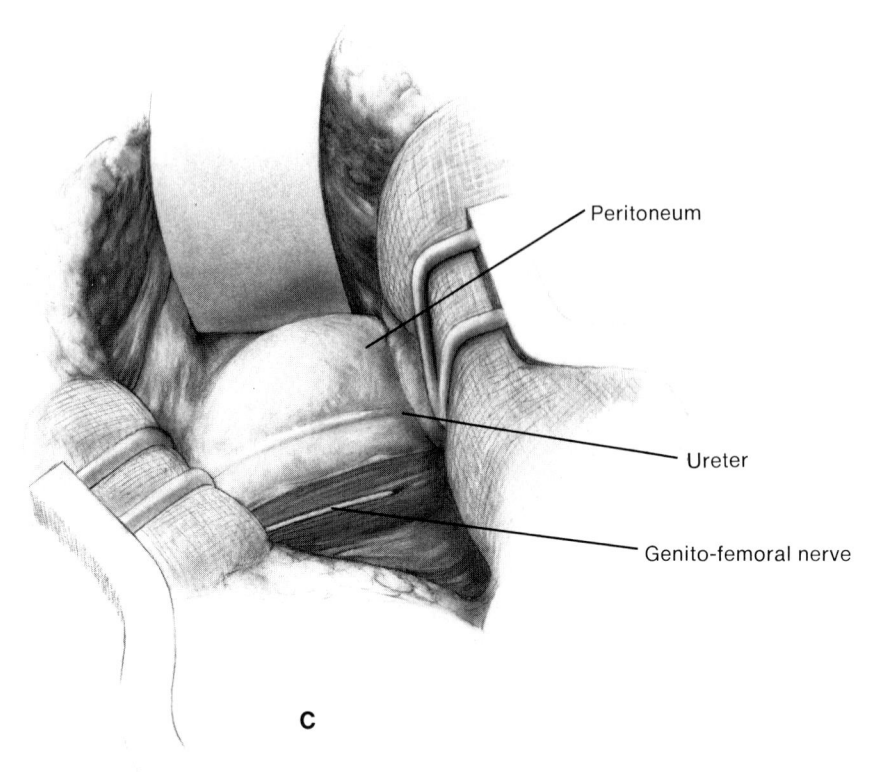

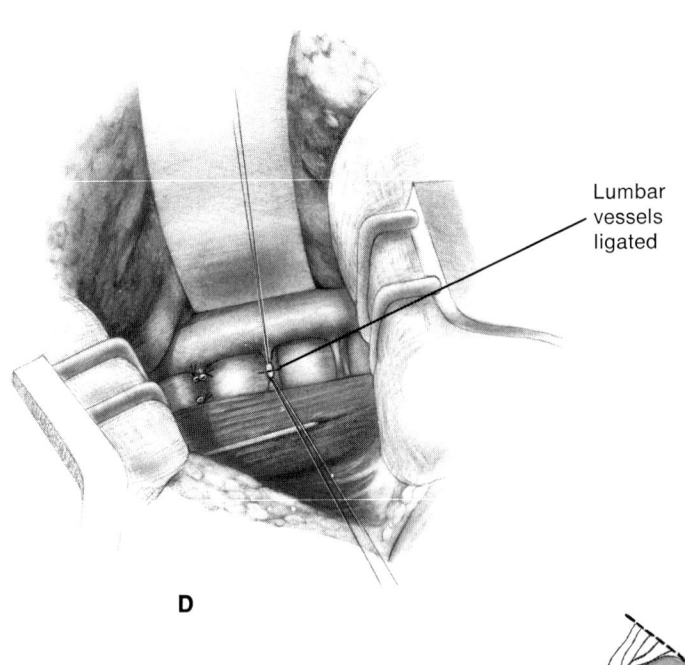

- Peritoneum
- Ureter
- Genito-femoral nerve

C

- Lumbar vessels ligated

D

E

262

(Plate 8-3) ANTERIOR SPINE FUSION BY RETROPERITONEAL APPROACH TO THE LUMBAR SPINE

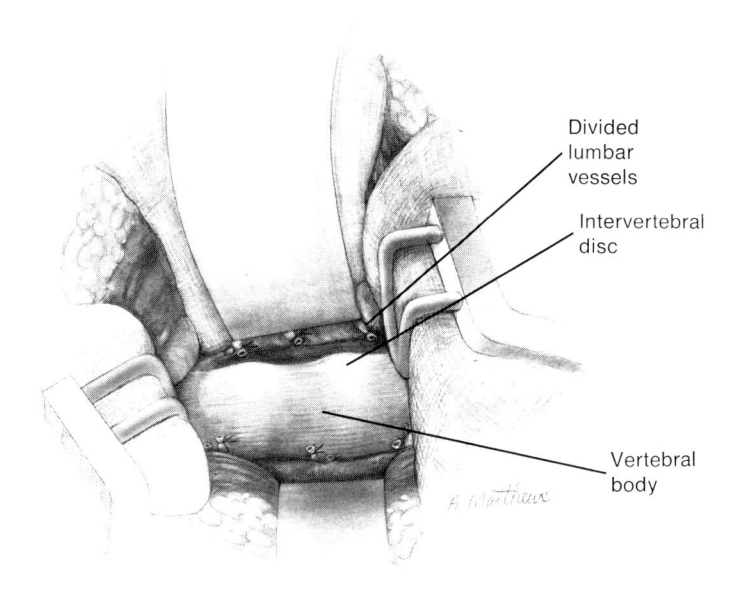

Divided lumbar vessels
Intervertebral disc
Vertebral body

F

with gravity, requiring less retraction. As the peritoneum is reflected forward, the ureter may be seen through the surface of the peritoneum and must be protected from injury. As the reflection of the peritoneum is continued, the psoas muscle and the genitofemoral nerve come into view **(C)**. Further reflection of the peritoneum toward the midline allows visualization of the aorta. Peritoneal reflection in the inferior part of the wound may sometimes be difficult, particularly over the area of the left lower quadrant.

As the dissection progresses, the medial border of the psoas muscle is exposed, providing visualization of the sympathetic chain with lymphatics between the psoas muscle and the aorta. The sympathetics should be protected from injury. The segmental vessels pass across the vertebral bodies in loose areolar and adipose tissue, allowing easy mobilization of the vessels with either a small sponge or a blunt instrument **(D)**. These vessels are divided between ligatures, which allows the aorta and the inferior vena cava to be retracted over the front of the vertebral bodies toward the opposite side **(E)**. The anterior longitudinal ligament is visualized. Occasionally, small vessels entering the vertebral bodies may require cauterization. When exposure of the lumbosacral disc is required, care is taken to ligate and divide between ligatures the iliolumbar vein, which may be duplicated and drains into the common iliac vein. If the iliolumbar vein or the ascending lumbar vein is not ligated, forceful retraction of the inferior vena cava could cause a laceration and troublesome bleeding from the common iliac vein.

The psoas muscle should be stripped with a Cobb elevator in a posterolateral direction to expose the lateral aspect of the vertebral bodies. With patience and careful exposure, it is possible to visualize about three fourths of the anterior circumference of the vertebral bodies **(F)**. With this exposure, definitive procedures on the vertebrae and the discs as listed in the discussion of indications may be carried out satisfactorily.

The vertebral levels are identified. The annulus fibrosus is incised, and with a rongeur the disc material is removed to the posterior longitudinal ligament. Care is taken during dissection in the region of the intervertebral foramina to avoid injury to the nerve roots and important collateral vessels. The vertebral end-plates are removed with ring curets and sharp chisels until cancellous bone is visualized on opposing surfaces. The above steps are as illustrated for anterior interbody fusion (p. 268) (Fig. 34, *A* and *B*). The raw surfaces are packed with Gelfoam while iliac bone graft is obtained from the ipsilateral anterior iliac crest. Corticocancellous iliac strut-grafts of appropriate size are punched gently but firmly into the prepared interbody spaces (Fig. 34, *C*). Closure is performed in layers. The internal oblique and the transversus abdominus are sutured in one layer, followed by closure of the external oblique muscle, the subcutaneous and fascia plane, and finally the skin. Drains are not used even after debridement for infection.

POSTOPERATIVE MANAGEMENT. The patient is kept at bed rest for 10 to 14 days. When the wound is healed, the sutures are removed and a double pantaloon spica cast is applied that extends from the knees to the lower rib cage. At 3 months after surgery the cast is removed and walking is permitted with the protection of an ambulatory plaster jacket, which is worn for an additional 3 months.

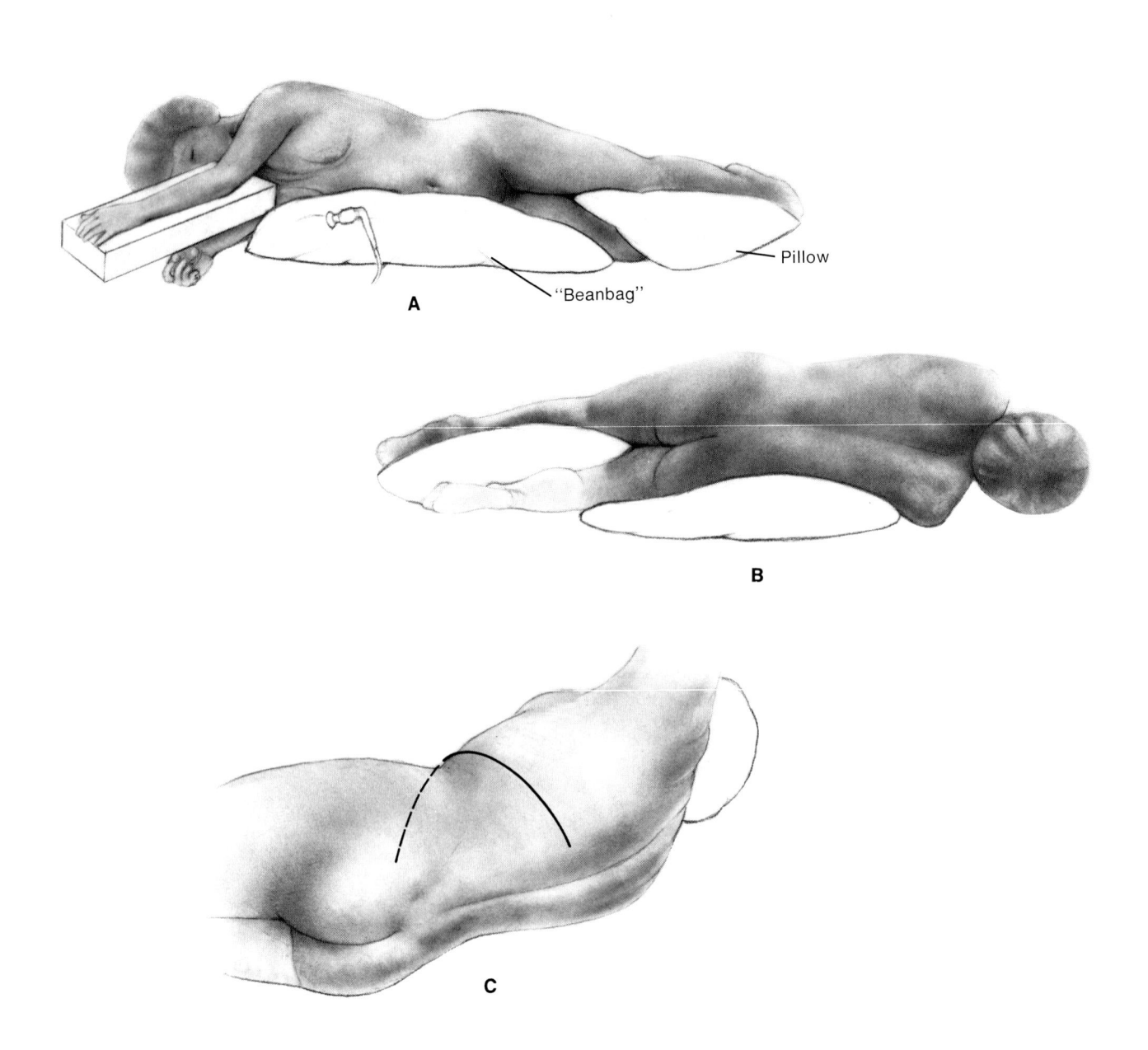

ANTERIOR SPINE FUSION BY THORACOABDOMINAL APPROACH (Plate 8-4)

GENERAL DISCUSSION. Thoracoabdominal approach allows exposure of the lower thoracic and lumbar spine.

DETAILS OF PROCEDURE. The patient is placed on a "beanbag" in the lateral decubitus position with the convex side upward. The bean bag is used to prevent pressure on the neurovascular structures in the axilla of the down side (**A** and **B**). A 60° tilt, or 30° short of the true lateral position, gives the surgeon a better working position. The arm and the shoulder of the "up side" are supported appropriately (**A**). The operative field is then prepared and draped. The prepared area extends from the midline anteriorly and posteriorly from the shoulder down to the midthigh. The draping is applied from just below the anterior superior spine to just below the axilla above and from the midline in the front to the midline posteriorly along the spinous processes.

The incision is along the rib to be excised, which is the one attached to the vertebral body one or two levels above the uppermost vertebra that is to be exposed (**C**). The incision is made along the rib and then forward and downward to a point about midway between the umbilicis and the symphysis pubis (**D** and **E**). The incision is carried down through the subcutaneous and fascia layers. The trapezius posteriorly and the latissimus dorsi are divided along the line of the incision (**F** and **G**).

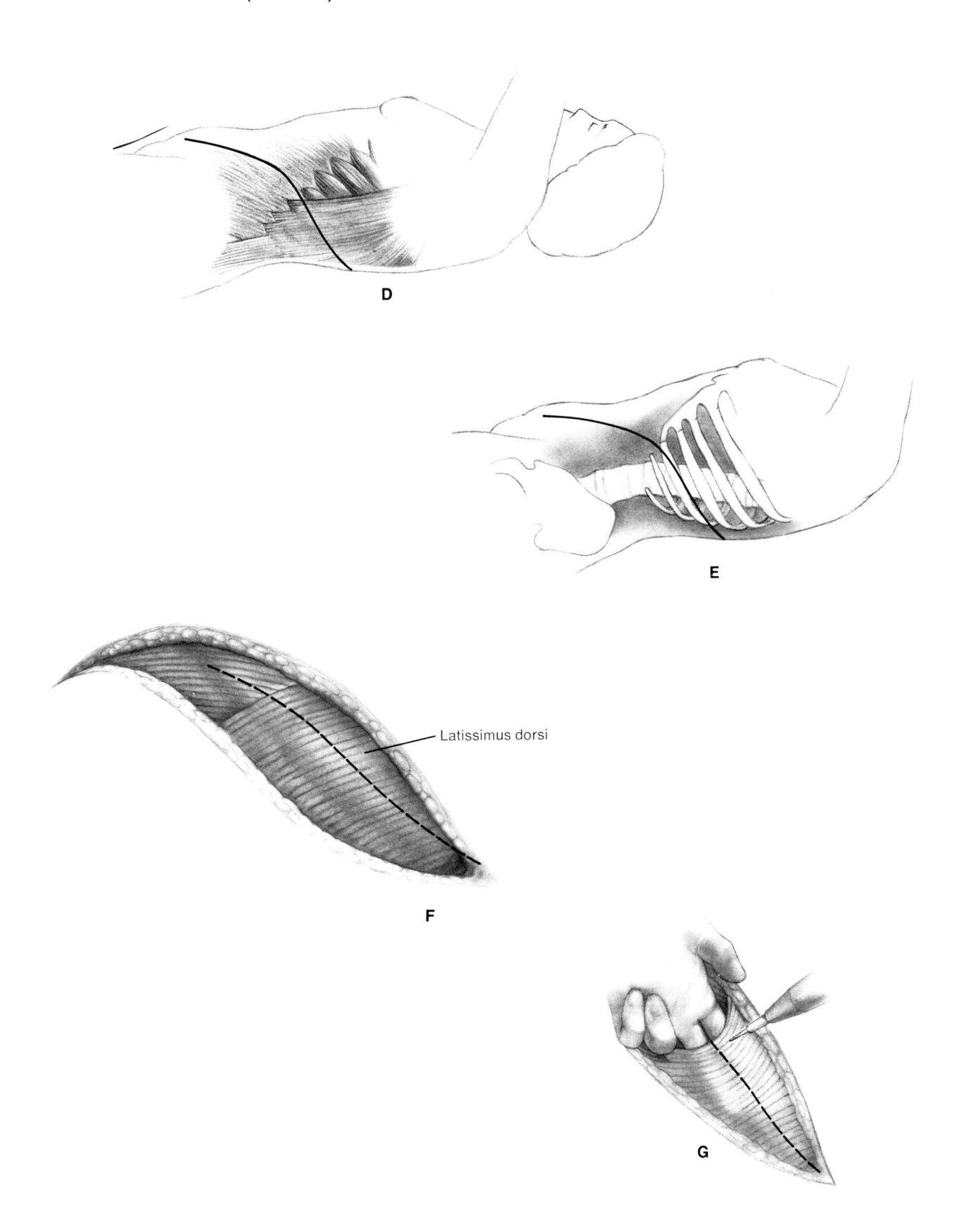

(Plate 8-4) ANTERIOR SPINE FUSION BY THORACOABDOMINAL APPROACH

Latissimus dorsi

D

E

F

G

265

ANTERIOR SPINE FUSION BY THORACOABDOMINAL APPROACH (Plate 8-4)

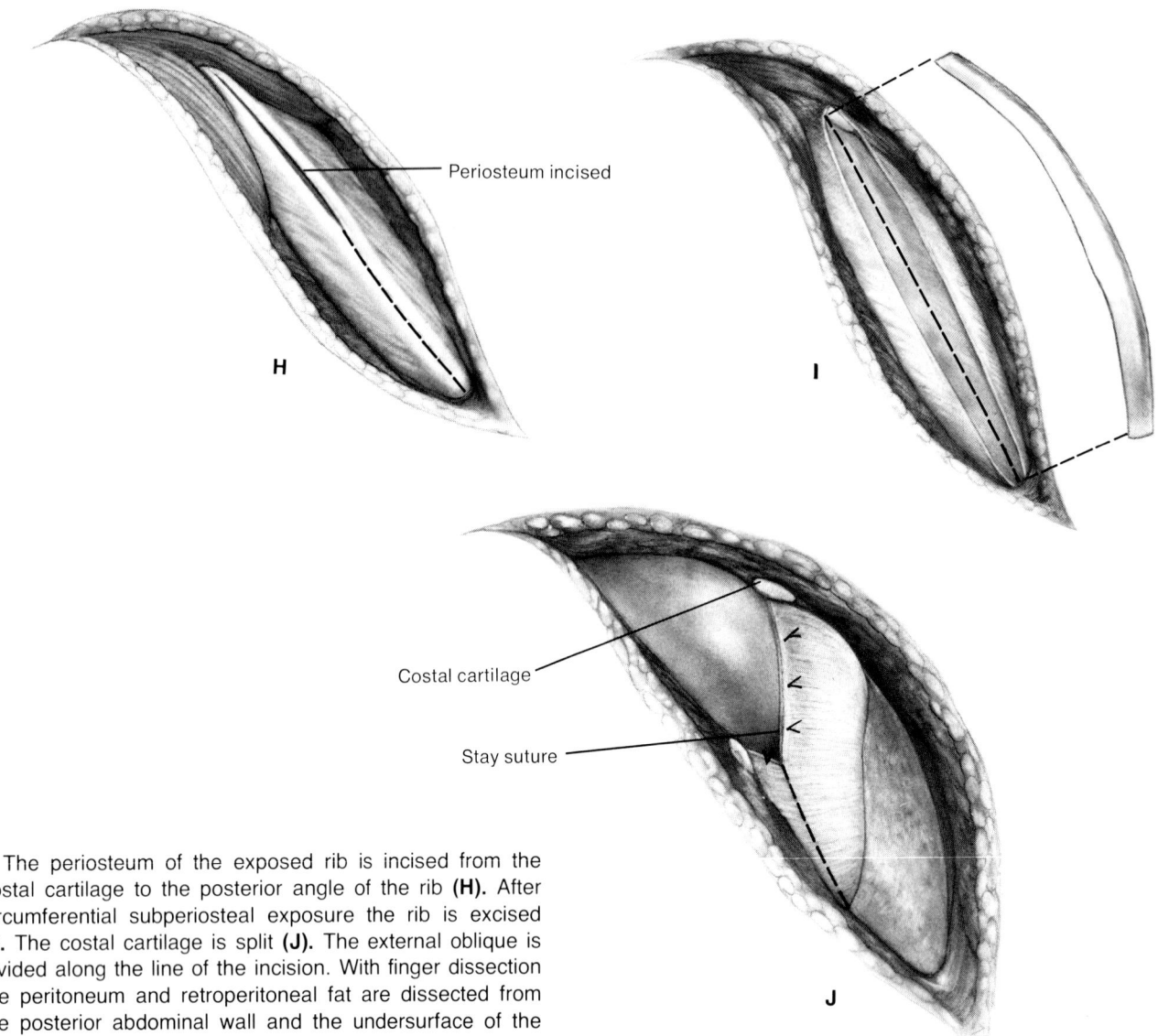

Periosteum incised

H

I

Costal cartilage

Stay suture

J

The periosteum of the exposed rib is incised from the costal cartilage to the posterior angle of the rib (**H**). After circumferential subperiosteal exposure the rib is excised (**I**). The costal cartilage is split (**J**). The external oblique is divided along the line of the incision. With finger dissection the peritoneum and retroperitoneal fat are dissected from the posterior abdominal wall and the undersurface of the diaphragm. Once a plane is developed retroperitoneally, the internal oblique and the transversus abdominus are divided along the line of the incision. Usually the rectus sheath is also divided along this line to facilitate anteromedial retraction of the viscera. The rib bed is incised and the thoracic cavity entered. The lung is retracted. The diaphragm being visualized from below and above is incised, and a 1.5 cm margin of its peripheral attachment is left (**J**). As the diaphragmatic detachment is being performed, stay sutures are placed at 3 or 4 cm intervals as markers, allowing subsequent repair of the diaphragm (**K** and **L**). The crus of the diaphragm is also tagged with stay sutures.

In the retroperitoneal space the peritoneum with the ureter is reflected anteriorly and medially. With gentle retraction using Deavor retractors the vertebral bodies are clearly visualized. The parietal pleura over the anterolateral aspect of the vertebral bodies is incised. The intercostal vessels are divided between ligatures close to its anterior midpoint (**M**). Cautery is never used near the costovertebral junction.

The ligation of the intercostal vessels is done anteriorly to avoid the anastomotic branches close to the intervertebral foramen. The lumbar vessels are also divided between ligatures.

In an approach through the left side, the aorta is gently dissected away from the front of the vertebral bodies and retracted. When the approach is through the right side, the inferior vena cava is mobilized in similar fashion and retracted. This approach allows exposure of the lumbar spine. When the lumbosacral area is exposed, care must be taken to divide the iliolumbar vessels between ligatures to allow reflection of the common iliac vessels medially. Further exposure of the vertebral bodies is obtained by stripping off the attachments of the psoas muscle from the side of the vertebral bodies. Care is taken not to damage the sympathetic chain or genitofemoral nerve.

(Plate 8-4) ANTERIOR SPINE FUSION BY THORACOABDOMINAL APPROACH

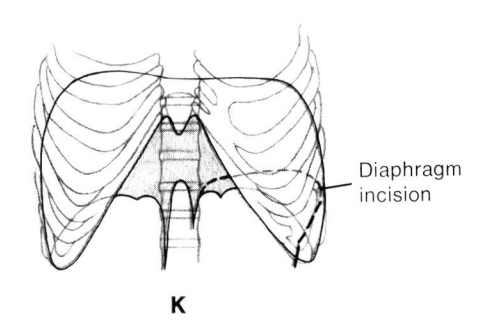

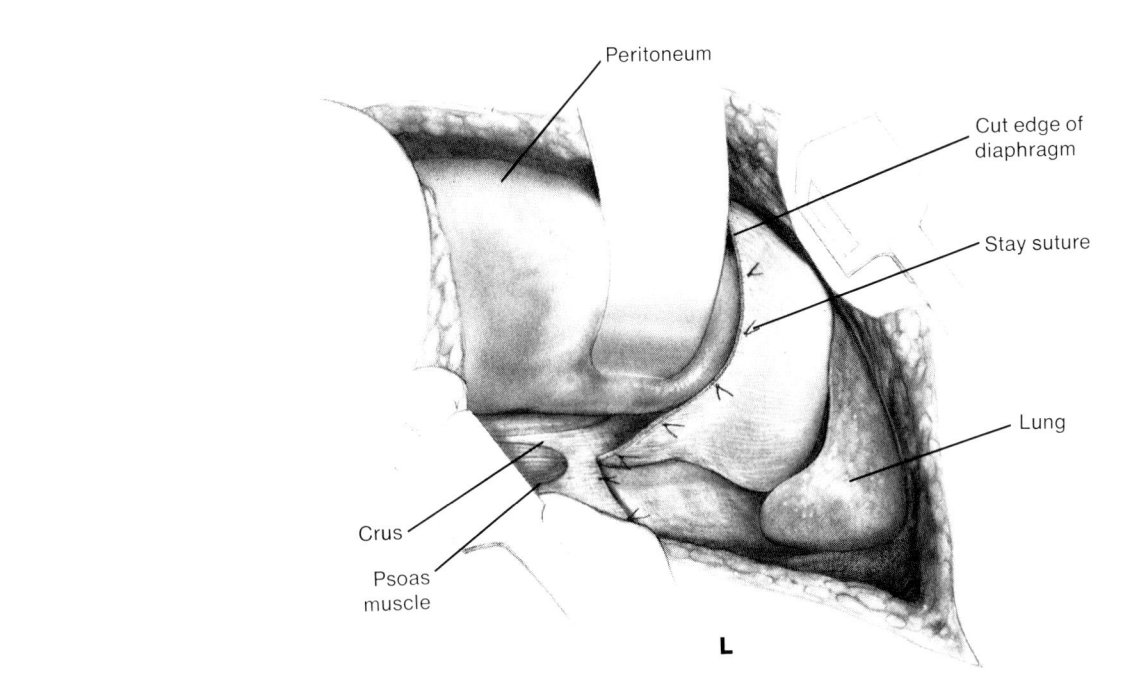

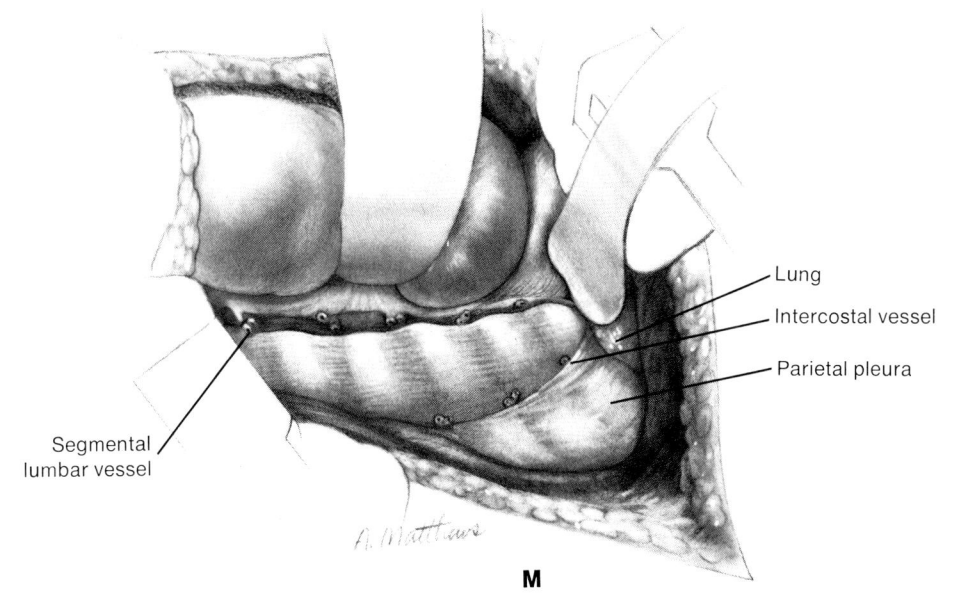

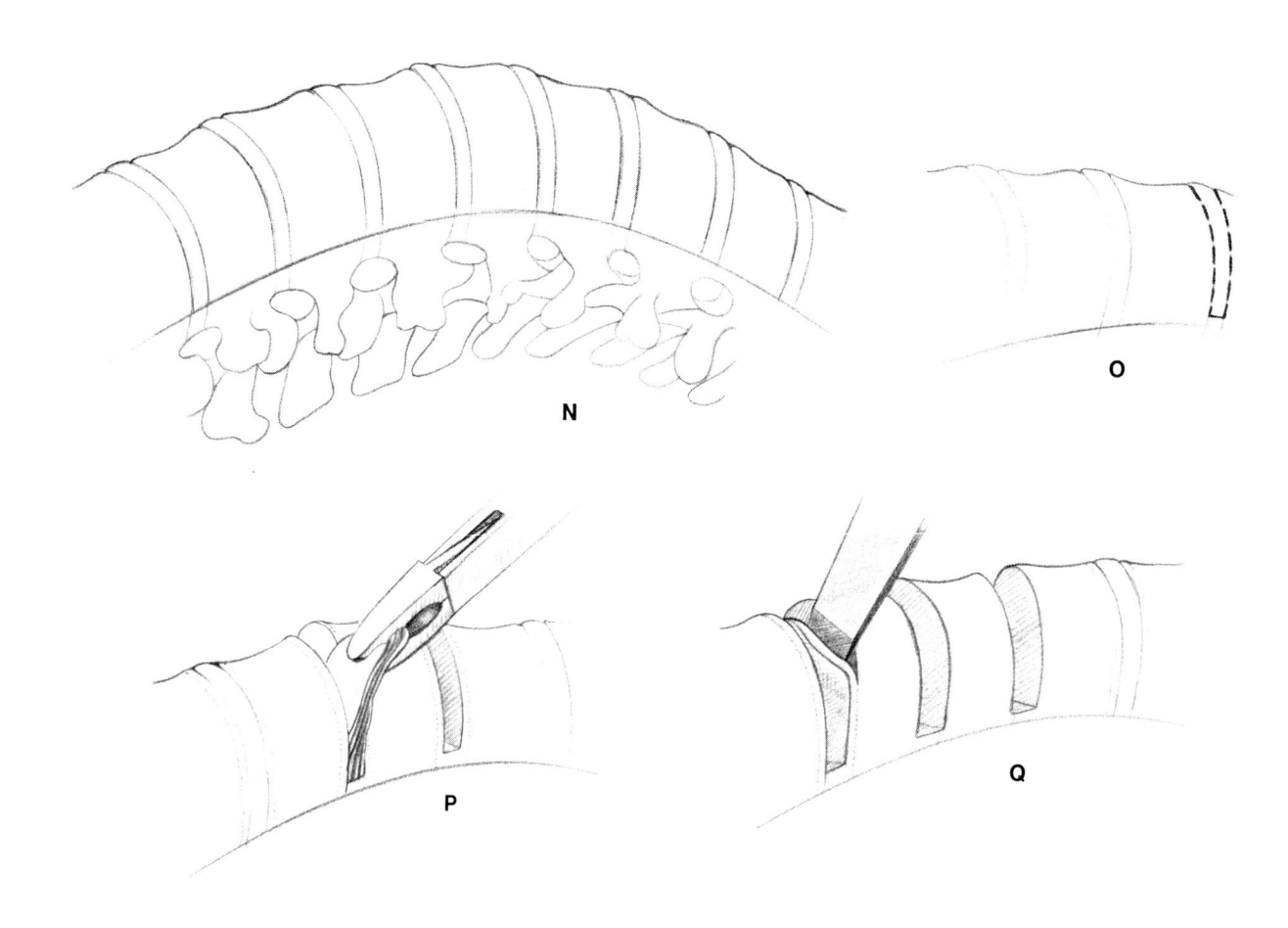

ANTERIOR INTERBODY FUSION WITH DWYER INSTRUMENTATION (Plate 8-4)

GENERAL DISCUSSION. Patients with severe lordoscoliosis who require multiple-level anterior interbody fusion and Dwyer instrumentation usually need a surgical approach to expose the lower thoracic and the lumbar spine. The thoracoabdominal approach is therefore used as described.

DETAILS OF PROCEDURE. The vertebral bodies and discs are exposed over the entire length of the area to be fused and instrumented (N). It is important that the anterior aspect of the spine be stripped so that the palpating finger can be easily placed on the opposite side to feel the opposite transverse processes.

The discs are excised by first incising the annulus fibrosus (O) and then taking out the nucleus pulposus with rongeurs (P). Care is taken not to injure the discs above and below the upper and lower limits of the area to be instrumented. The end-plates are curetted or osteotomized (Q) until cancellous bone is exposed. The posterior longitudinal ligament and posterior annulus fibrosus are not violated.

After preparation of the disc spaces, instrumentation is carried out. The procedure may be performed from above downward or from below upward, as is sometimes necessary. A starter is used to make a slot in the vertebral body of the uppermost vertebra to be instrumented to avoid violating the disc above. A staple of appropriate width is chosen and, with use of the staple holder, tapped into position (R). A screw length–measuring device is used to measure the width of the vertebral body, making the measurement in the interbody space just under the inferior end-plate. The screw is inserted and directed toward the opposite cortex, the screw being aimed at the pulp of the palpating finger placed against the transverse process on the opposite side of the vertebra (S). It is important that the finger on the opposite side of the vertebral body be able to feel the tip of the screw, and preferably one or two threads should emerge from the opposite side for more secure fixation (T). The next staple is then placed on the vertebra below. The staples in patients with small vertebrae are usually placed astride the vertebral body. In the lumbar spine and in vertebral bodies that are larger, the staples may be placed into the bodies themselves as in T. After the second screw is placed, the cable is passed through the upper screw head and into the second screw head.

(Plate 8-4) ANTERIOR INTERBODY FUSION WITH DWYER INSTRUMENTATION

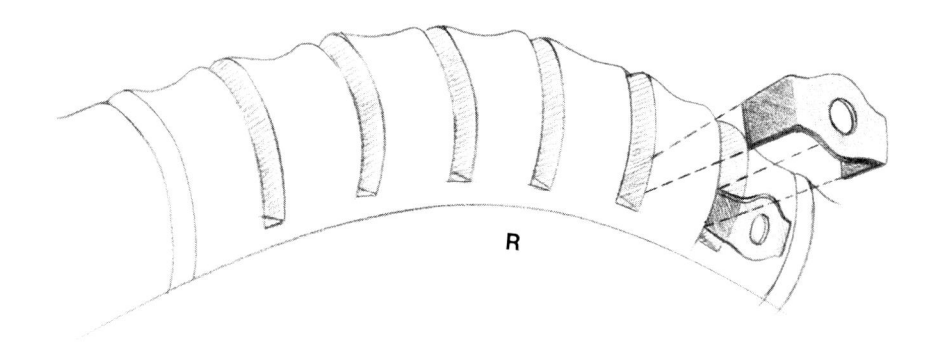

R

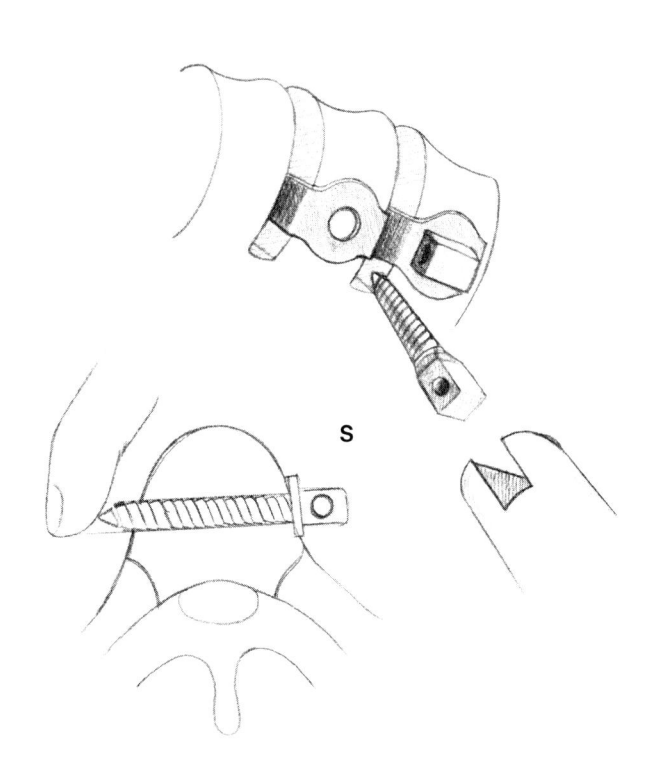

S

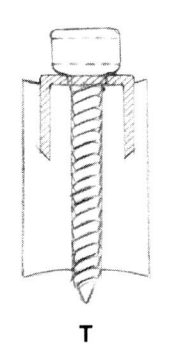

T

269

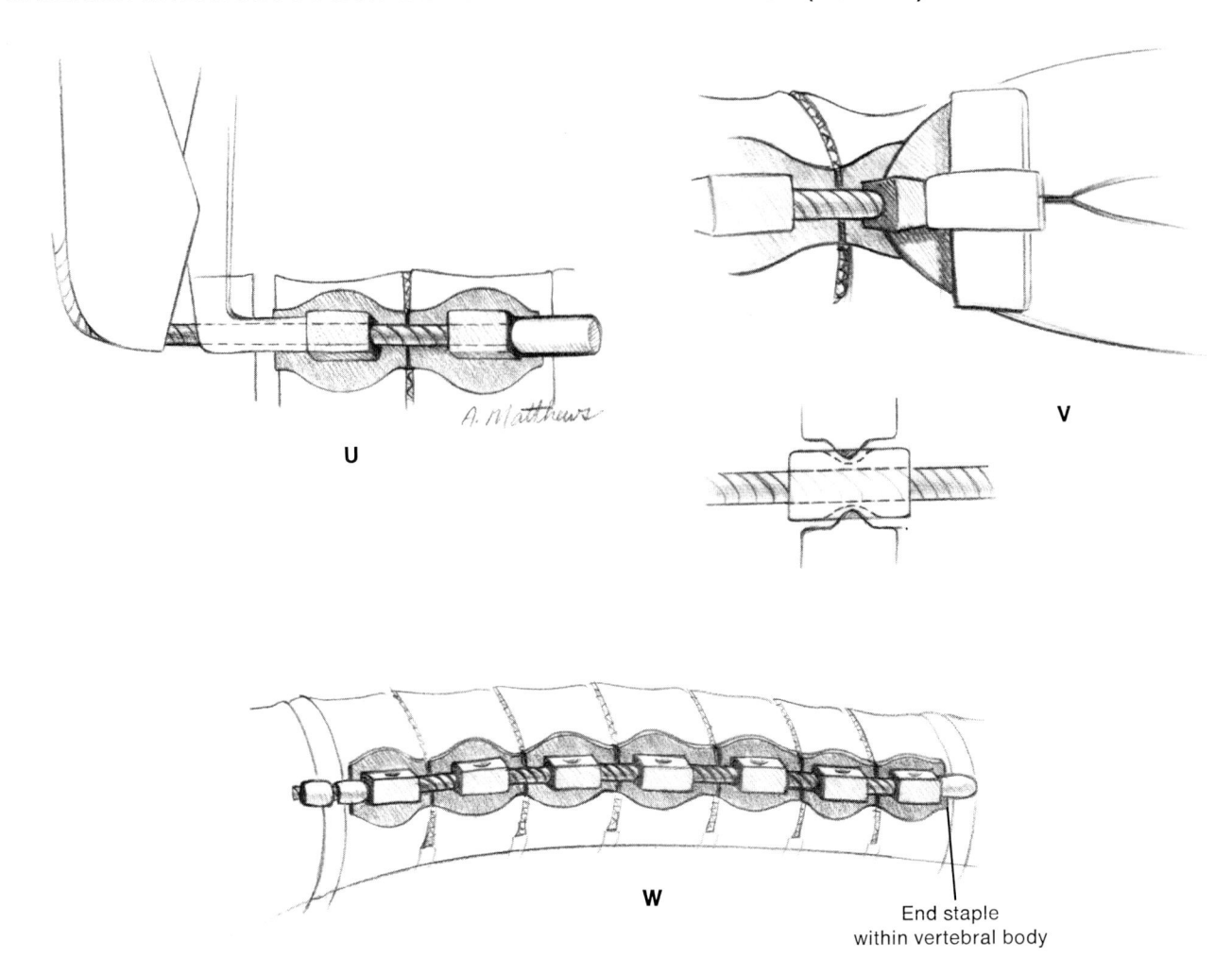

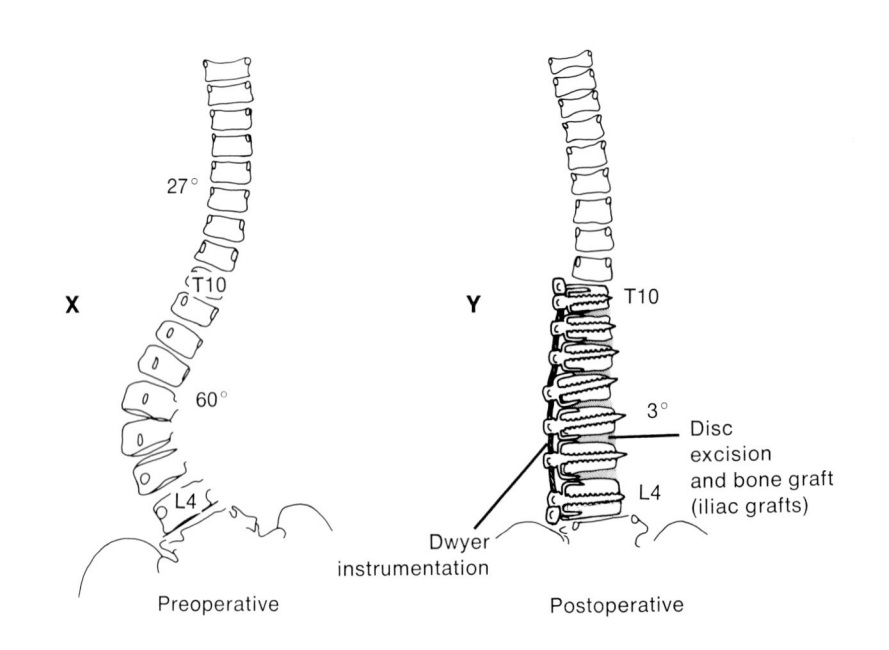

ANTERIOR INTERBODY FUSION WITH DWYER INSTRUMENTATION (Plate 8-4)

U

V

W — End staple within vertebral body

X Preoperative — 27°, T10, 60°, L4

Y Postoperative — T10, 3°, L4, Disc excision and bone graft (iliac grafts), Dwyer instrumentation

270

(Plate 8-4) ANTERIOR INTERBODY FUSION WITH DWYER INSTRUMENTATION

Cancellous bone graft usually obtained through a separate incision is packed into the interbody space and tensioning carried out with the tensioning device until the interbody space is closed (**U**). The screw heads are then crimped with the crimping clamp (**V**). The instrumentation is likewise carried out until the entire selected fusion area has been instrumented (**W**). The lowermost staple is punched into the vertebral body without violating the disc space below the lowest vertebra to be fused (**W** to **Y**).

After the cable has passed through the last screw, a holding button is placed over the cable and against the screw head. Tensioning is carried out as before, and the screw head and the holding end button are both crimped. A second end button is applied against the first and crimped. The cable is cut off with the cable cutter just below the buttons. Care should be taken to cut the cable as close to the button as possible to avoid exposure of frayed ends of the multifilament cable. The psoas muscle is sutured to the anterior longitudinal ligament over the cut end of the cable to avoid erosion of the major vessels.

After the fusion and instrumentation, the parietal pleura is closed over the instruments with absorbable suture. Sometimes the parietal pleura is unable to completely cover the instruments and a piece of Gelfoam is placed under the sutures to cover the instruments. The diaphram is repaired with interrupted sutures starting at the crus. A chest drain is inserted exiting from a separate hole one or two intercostal spaces below the thoracotomy wound. The lung is expanded. Circumferential interrupted 0 chromic catgut sutures are used to approximate the ribs. The intercostal muscle layer is repaired with 2-0 chromic catgut sutures. The serratus anterior and the latissimus dorsi muscles are repaired. The abdominal portion of the thoracoabdominal wound is closed in layers. The internal oblique and transversus abdominus muscles are closed in one layer and the external oblique in a separate layer. The subcutaneous layer and skin are sutured in standard fashion. Dwyer instrumentation is contraindicated in the presence of kyphosis.

Ventral derotation system (Zielke). Zielke's anterior instrumentation, which uses a flexible compression rod, affords remarkable correction of vertebral rotation, corrects kyphosis, and can produce some lordosis. Our early experience with this system as illustrated (**AA** to **CC**) has been encouraging.

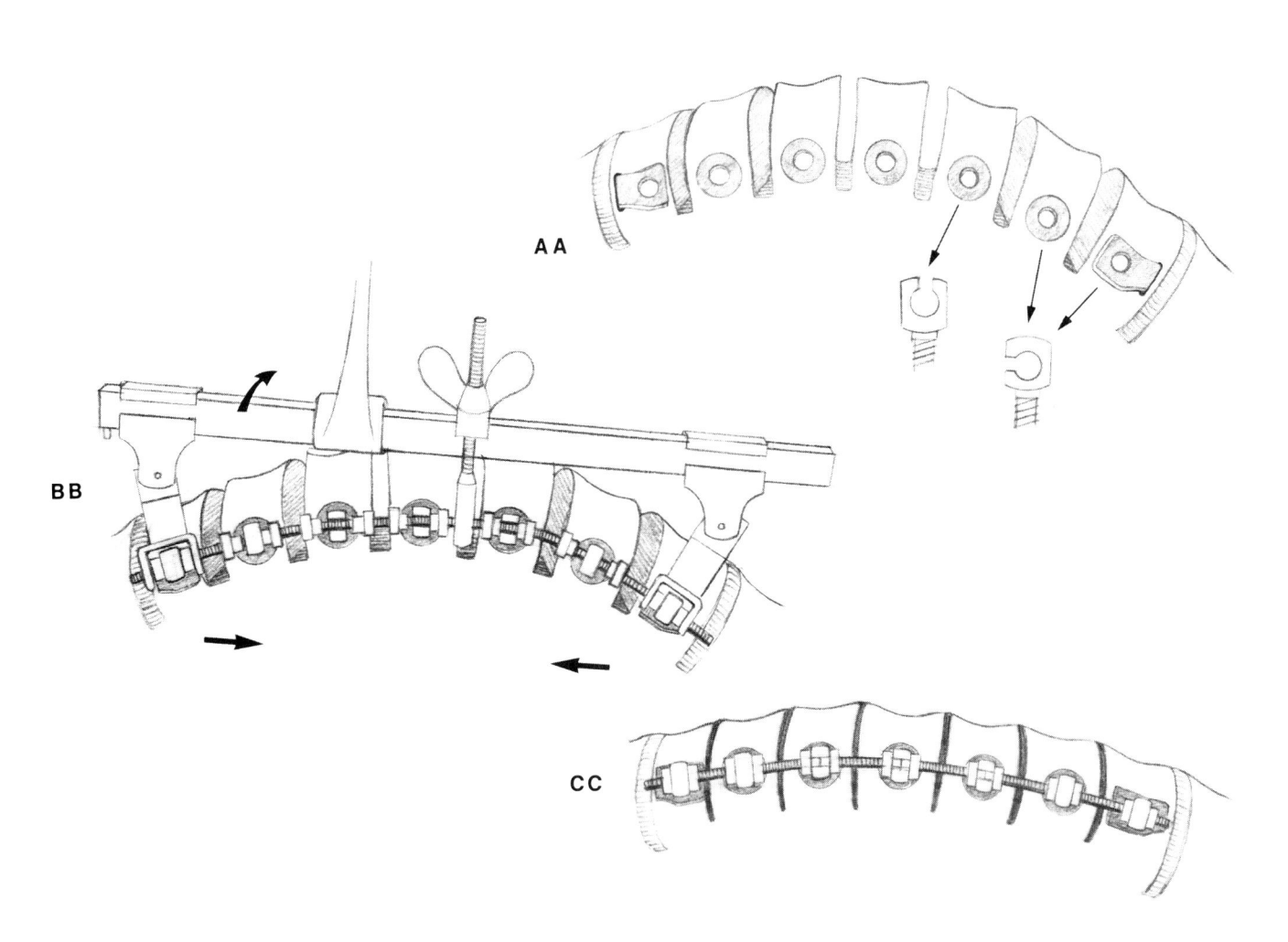

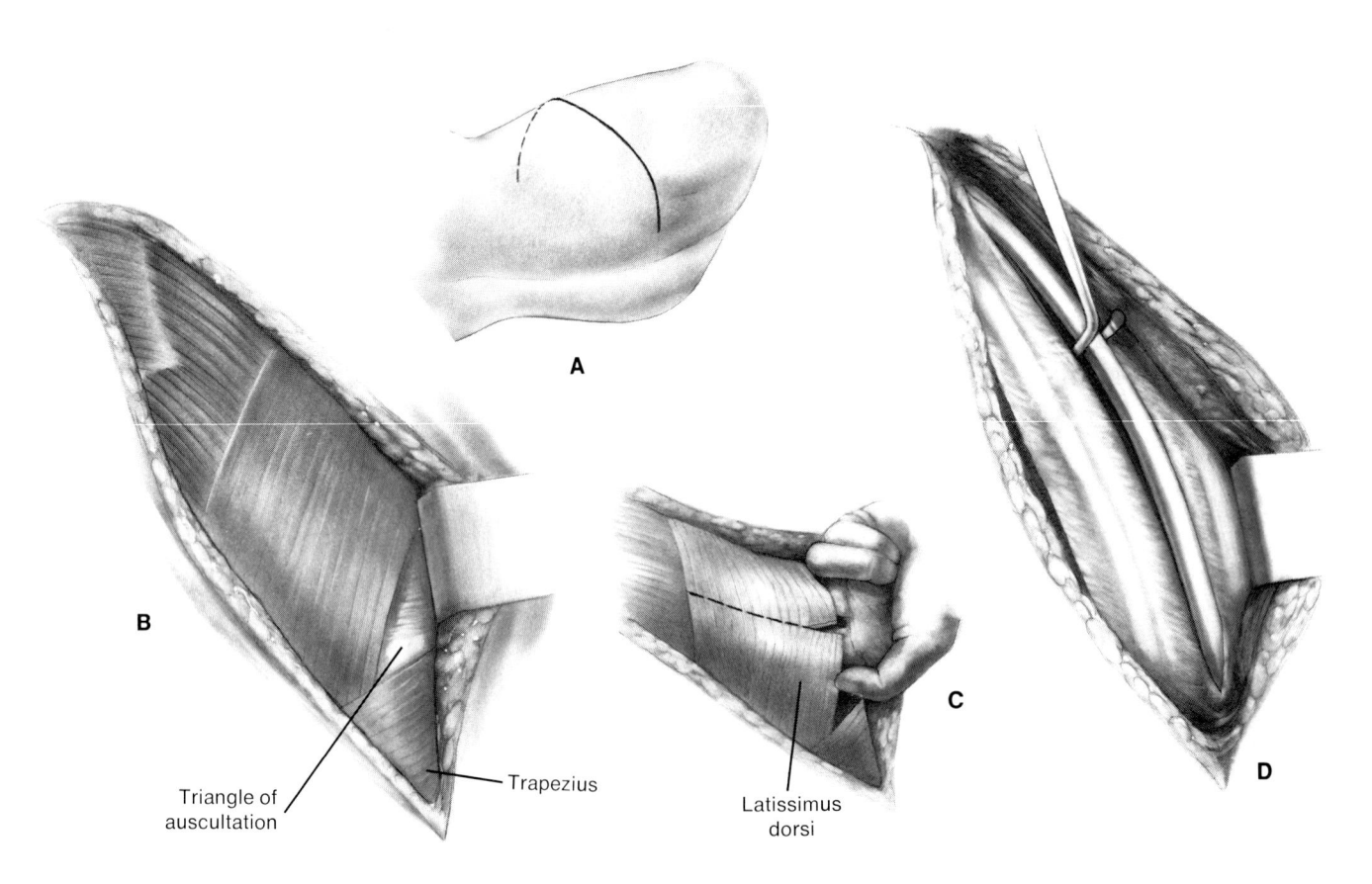

TRANSTHORACIC APPROACH TO THE THORACIC SPINE (Plate 8-5)

GENERAL DISCUSSION. The vertebral bodies and discs of the thoracic spine may be approached through a thoracotomy approach, either from the right or the left side. The left side is preferred because technically it is easier to mobilize the aorta. The selection of the rib through which the chest is entered depends on the levels of vertebrae that need to be approached. Usually the rib chosen is the one attached to the vertebra two levels above the uppermost vertebra that is to be exposed. Sometimes, in certain chest cage configurations, where the ribs are more horizontal than sloping, the chest may be entered through the rib attached to the top vertebra to be exposed. When the upper thoracic vertebral bodies are to be exposed, the third or fourth ribs are excised. In this case the incision is medial to the medial border of the scapula, extending downward toward the angle of the scapula and then curving forward and slightly upward to a submammary point. The muscles along the medial border of the scapula and the serratus anterior and incised, and the scapula is mobilized and moved forward and upward. When the upper thoracic spine is exposed through the left thoracotomy approach, care should be taken not to damage the thoracic duct.

DETAILS OF PROCEDURE. The lateral decubitus position is used with the patient 30° from the true lateral position, and we have used the "beanbag" between the patient and the operating table for this purpose. Care should be taken to relieve the pressure of the neurovascular structures in the axilla by giving adequate support of the thoracic cage just below the shoulder. The upper extremity of the side to be approached has to be supported in the forward flexed position with the arm horizontal (Plate 8-4, *A* and *B*). The sides of the thorax and trunk are prepared from the shoulder down to the upper thigh. This is to allow removal of iliac crest bone graft when necessary.

The incision extends from the lateral border of the erector spinae muscles along the slope of the rib to be resected to a point near the costal cartilage **(A)**. The incision is carried down through the subcutaneous layer and onto the muscles. The triangle of auscultation is a useful landmark for finding the areolar plane between the scapula and the thoracic cage **(B)**. The latissimus dorsi muscle is isolated and lifted from the thoracic cage through this triangle and is divided along the rib from posterior toward the anterior margin **(C)**. Posterior to this triangle, fibers of the trapezius are divided along the line of the incision. The serratus anterior is incised over the rib to be excised. The periosteum over the rib is incised, and the rib is exposed widely subperiosteally **(D)**. The rib is excised from the posterior angle to the articulation with the costal cartilage anteriorly **(E)**. The rib bed is incised and a self-retaining retractor is placed. The lung is retracted anteriorly and medially **(F)**. The parietal pleura covering the vertebral bodies is visualized and incised over the vertebrae that are to be exposed **(G)**. These intercostal vessels are ligated near the anterior aspect of the vertebral bodies and divided

(Plate 8-5) TRANSTHORACIC APPROACH TO THE THORACIC SPINE

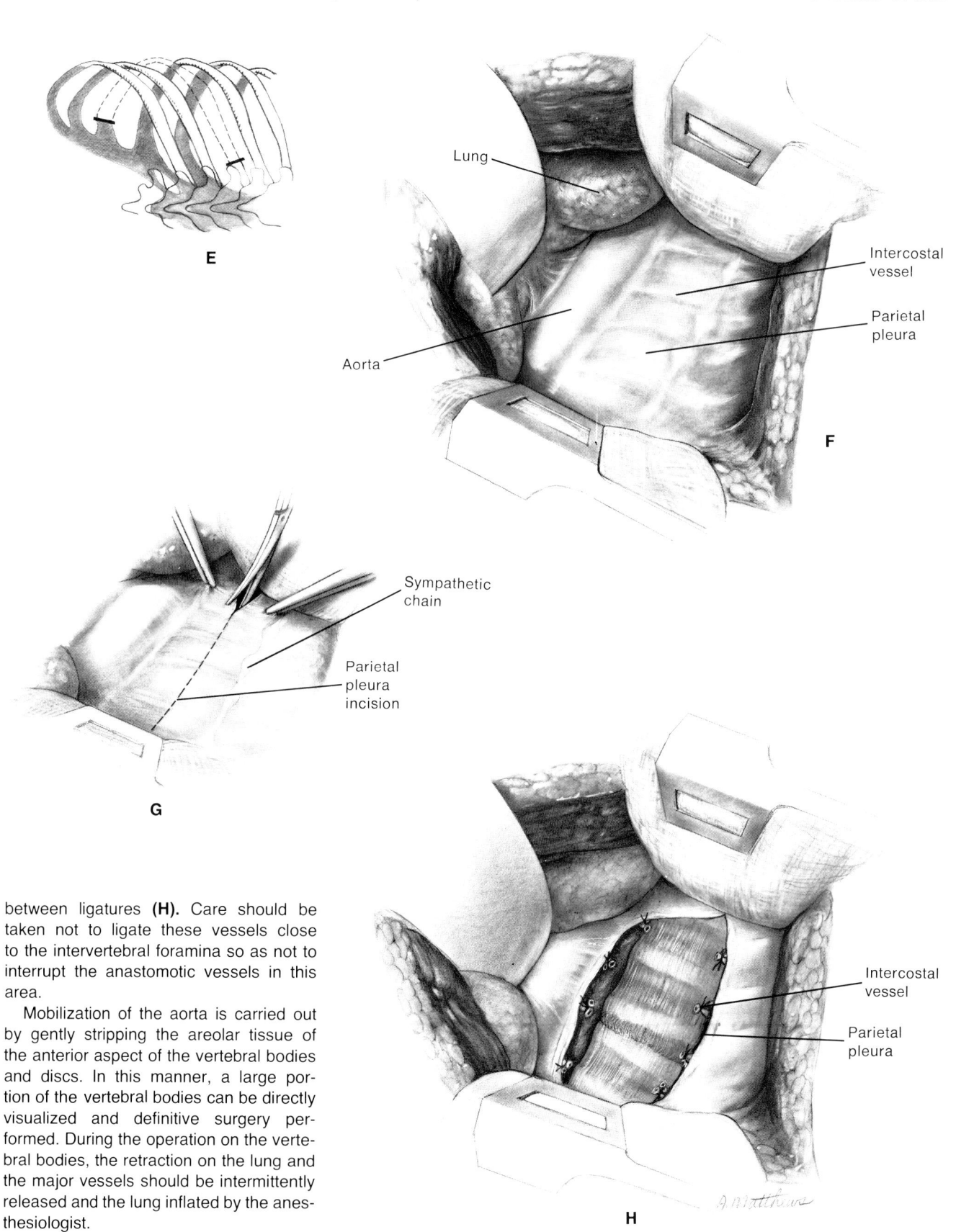

between ligatures **(H)**. Care should be taken not to ligate these vessels close to the intervertebral foramina so as not to interrupt the anastomotic vessels in this area.

Mobilization of the aorta is carried out by gently stripping the areolar tissue of the anterior aspect of the vertebral bodies and discs. In this manner, a large portion of the vertebral bodies can be directly visualized and definitive surgery performed. During the operation on the vertebral bodies, the retraction on the lung and the major vessels should be intermittently released and the lung inflated by the anesthesiologist.

273

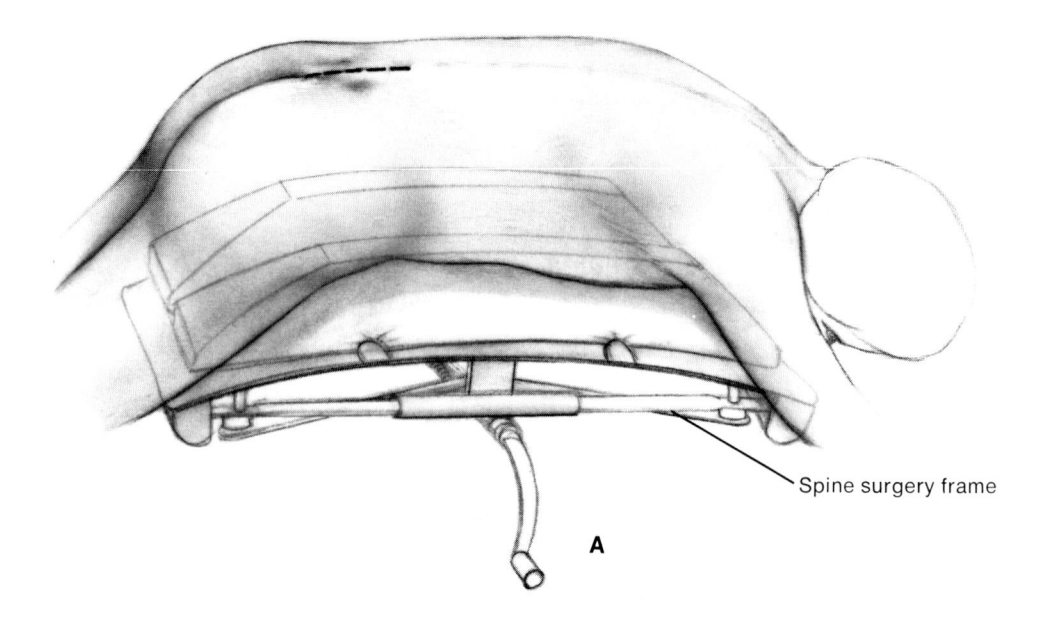

LAMINECTOMY (LUMBAR INTERVERTEBRAL DISC LESION) (Plate 8-6)

GENERAL DISCUSSION. The typical history of the lumbar disc syndrome is that of dull, aching, low back pain, developing after a bending or lifting strain. Pain in the buttock or lower extremity may develop at the same time, but this is unusual. Sciatica generally develops later in the course of the acute episode but sometimes not at all during the initial or early attacks. It is usually unilateral, but even when it is bilateral, one limb is more painful than the other. The distribution of the limb pain is often the same whether the protrusion is at the fourth lumbar or the lumbosacral interspace. The intensity of the pain seems to have no direct relationship to the size of the disc protrusion. In the typical disc syndrome the back pain is static or mechanical in nature. Activity or use of the back aggravates it, and rest relieves it at least partially.

Sensory change in the foot, manifested by paresthesias, is common in the typical syndrome and is much more common than muscle weakness.

Occasionally a patient may have sciatica but no back pain, or foot pain and paresthesias but no back pain and no true sciatica. Some patients with lumbar disc protrusion present after suddenly developing a severe foot drop without preceding pain in either the back or lower extremity. Occasionally patients suddenly and completely lose bowel and bladder function with the onset of back and lower extremity pain. This unfortunate situation is most likely caused by a huge disc protrusion and requires immediate operation.

The essential physical findings result from nerve irritation and muscle spasm caused by the disc protrusion. Although the findings vary considerably from patient to patient, flexion and extension of the spine will be limited to some degree. The normal lumbar lordosis may be absent, or a list may be present. This list is usually away from the side of the disc protrusion, but this is not always so.

The straight-leg raising test is significant if the back or limb discomfort is reproduced during the test, regardless of the angle that the limb makes with the horizontal when the typical pain is experienced. Reproduction of the sciatic symptoms in one leg by contralateral straight-leg raising is almost pathognomonic for lumbar disc protrusion or extrusion.

Although myelography is useful in the preoperative assessment of patients with persistent nerve root irritation, the decision to operate cannot be dependent on myelographic findings alone but should be based on the clinical evaluation of the patient. There are five clinical criteria that are generally regarded as indications for laminectomy: impairment of bladder or bowel function, gross motor weakness, evidence of increasing impairment of nerve root conduction (despite complete bed rest), severe sciatic pain persisting or increasing (despite 1 or more weeks of complete bed rest) and associated with evidence of nerve root irritation on examination, and recurrent incapacitating episodes of sciatic pain with evidence of nerve root irritation.

DETAILS OF PROCEDURE. The patient is placed prone on an adjustable spine-operating frame. The frame is adjusted to flatten the lumbar lordosis to widen the interlamina spaces **(A)**. A midline incision 7 to 10 cm long from the spine of the third lumbar vertebra to the first sacral spine should allow full exploration of the fourth and fifth intervertebral disc spaces. The supraspinatus ligament is incised from the fourth lumbar to the first sacral spinous process. The paravertebral muscles are then reflected subperiosteally from the spines **(B)** and the laminae of these vertebrae on each side of the lesion. A self-retaining retractor is placed to hold these muscles retracted **(C)**. The position of the sacrum is verified by palpation and direct vision to be absolutely certain about identification of the correct interspace intended for explora-

Spine surgery frame

A

(Plate 8-6) LAMINECTOMY (LUMBAR INTERVERTEBRAL DISC LESION)

tion. Hemostasis is obtained using electrocautery, bone wax, and packs (part of the packs should always remain outside of the wound). The ligamentum flavum is then grasped and incised where it fuses with the interspinous ligament. During the dissection of the ligamentum flavum, the point of the scalpel should be kept in view so the dura is not opened. Then the flap of ligamentum flavum should be turned outward and removed by sharp dissection **(C)**.

The lumbosacral interspace may be large enough to permit exposure and removal of a herniated nucleus without removal of any bone. If not, a small part of the inferior margin of the fifth lamina, and sometimes the superior edge of the sacrum, should be removed **(D)**. The interspaces between the fourth and fifth lumbar laminae and between the third and fourth lumbar laminae are never wide enough to permit the exploration of a disc space without removal of some bone.

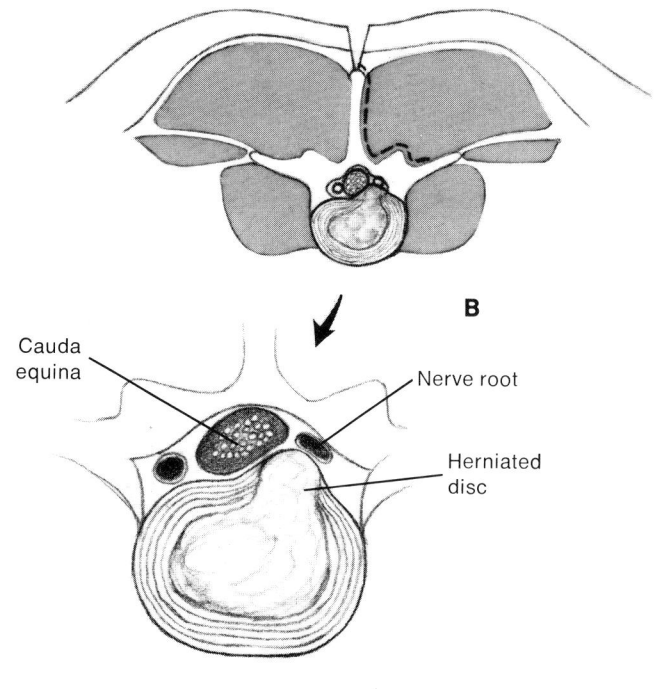

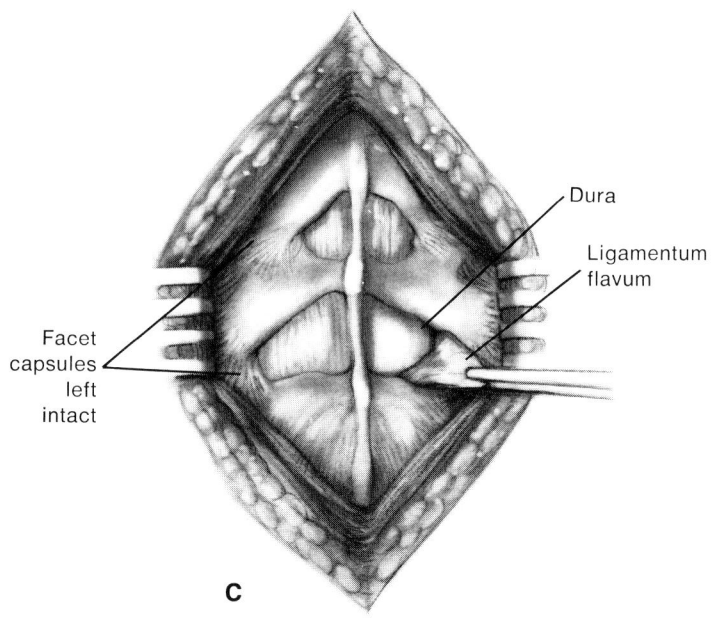

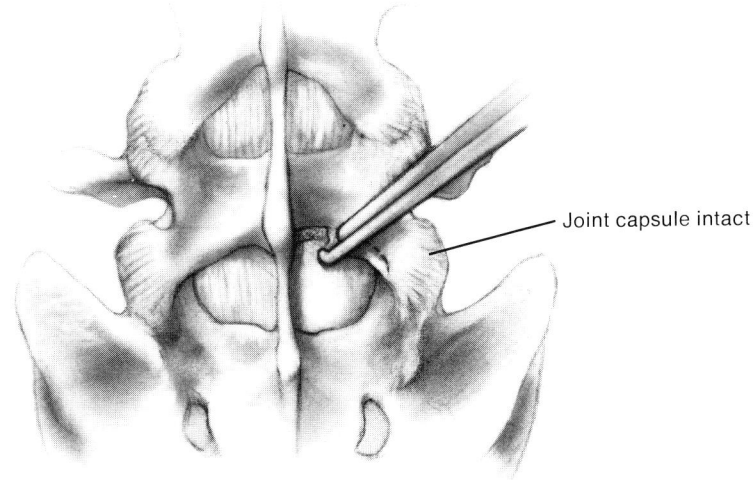

275

LAMINECTOMY (LUMBAR INTERVERTEBRAL DISC LESION) (Plate 8-6)

When adequate exposure has been obtained, the dura is retracted medially **(E)** and the nerve gently palpated with a blunt dissector. If the nerve root is compressed by a herniated disc, it will usually be elevated. The nerve root is retracted medially with a Love root retractor or a blunt dissector to expose the herniated fragment **(F)**. If the herniated fragment is a particularly large one, it is much better to sacrifice the medial edge of the facet so that a more lateral exposure may be obtained than to risk injury to the cauda equina by excessive medial retraction. With adequate exposure, the nerve root can usually be elevated and retracted away from the herniated disc **(F)**. An incision is made over the bulging disc, and the fragments are removed with rongeurs. The disc space is carefully curetted. If the herniation is upward or downward, additional removal of bone from the lamina and facet edges may be required. Bleeding from the epidural veins is controlled by packing pledgets of cotton to which black threads have been attached for identification whenever they are placed within the wound.

One must remember that the anterior part of the annulus fibrosus is adjacent to the aorta, vena cava, and iliac arteries, and that these structures may be injured if the dissection is extended too deeply. Before wound closure, a complete search must be carried out, and any loose fragments of annulus are lifted out by suction or with pituitary rongeurs. The cotton pledgets are removed and any residual bleeding is controlled with pieces of Gelfoam dipped in thrombin. These are removed after the bleeding has stopped. The wound is closed in layers with interrupted sutures.

POSTOPERATIVE MANAGEMENT. Turning in bed is allowed as tolerated from the beginning. If the patient is unable to void, various bladder stimulants are tried before catheterization; if necessary, the patient is helped to stand to try to void rather than resorting to catheterization. The patient is otherwise allowed to be out of bed as soon as wound discomfort subsides, generally on the second or third postoperative day. At the time of discharge from the hospital, the patient is reminded about lifting objects properly with minimum strain on the back and advised against lifting heavy objects. External support for the back is sometimes recommended. Postural and muscle-strengthening exercises are recommended as soon as the soft tissues have healed sufficiently.

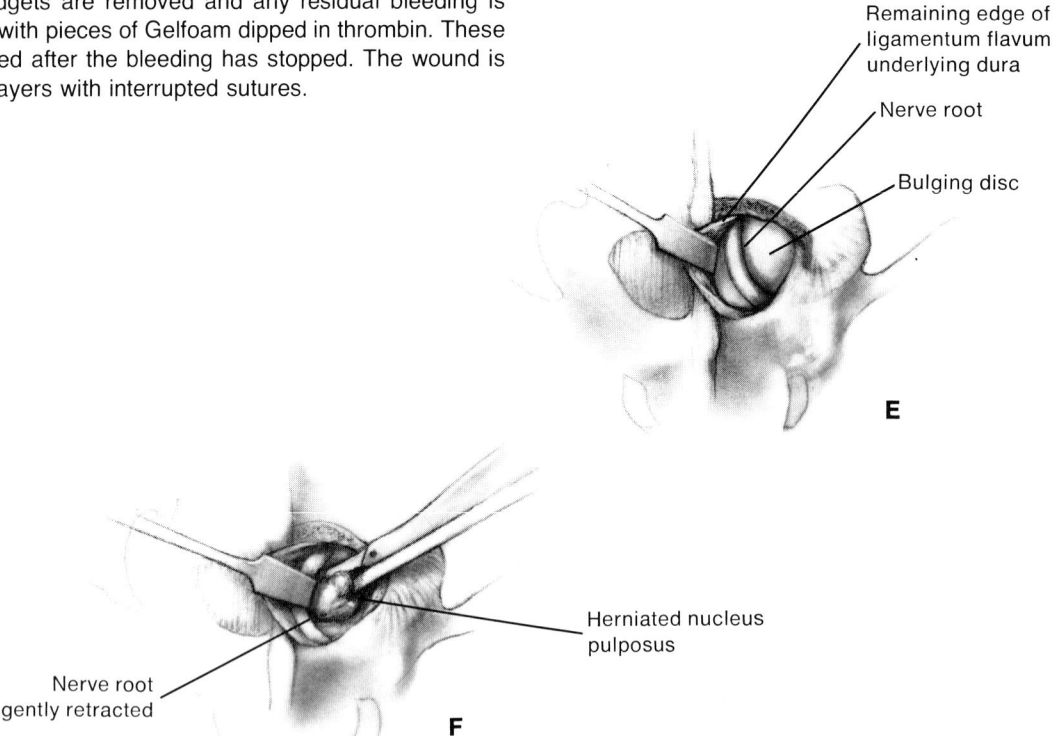

REFERENCES
General

Adson, A. W.: Technique of removal of intervetebral discs and surgical results, American Academy of Orthopaedic Surgeons Instructional Course Lectures, vol. 1, Ann Arbor, Mich., 1943, J. W. Edwards, p. 111.

Akeson, W. H., Woo, S. L-Y., Taylor, T. K. F., Ghosh P., and Bushell, G. R.: Biomechanics and biochemistry of the intervertebral disks: the need for correlation studies, CORR **129:**4, 1977.

Albee, F. H.: Bone-graft surgery, Philadelphia, 1915, W. B. Saunders Co.

Anderson, T. P., Cole, T. M., Gullickson, G., Hudgens, M. S. W., and Roberts, A. H.: Behavior modification of chronic pain: a treatment program by a miltidisciplinary team, CORR **129:**4, 1977.

Andersson, G. B. J., Ortengren, R., and Nachemson, A.: Intradiskal pressure, intra-abdominal pressure and myoelectric back muscle activity related to posture and loading, CORR **129:**4, 1977.

Aronson, H. A., and Dunsmore, R. H.: Herniated upper lumbar discs, J. Bone Joint Surg. **45-A:**311, 1963.

Barr, J. S.: Sciatica caused by intervetebral disc lesions, J. Bone Joint Surg. **19:**323, 1937.

Barr, J. S.: Ruptured intervertebral disc and sciatic pain, J. Bone Joint Surg. **29:**429, 1947.

Barr, J. S.: The operative management of low back pain, American Academy of Orthopaedic Surgeons Instructional Course Lectures, vol. 5, Ann Arbor, Mich., 1948, J. W. Edwards, p. 291.

Barr, J. S.: Lumbar disk lesions in retrospect and prospect, CORR **129:**4, 1977.

Barr, J. S., et al.: Evaluation of end results in treatment of ruptured lumbar intervertebral discs, Surg. Gynecol. Obstet. **125:**250, 1967.

Barr, J. S., Hampton, A. O., and Mister, W. J.: Pain low in the back and "sciatica" due to lesions of the intervertebral discs, J.A.M.A. **109:**1265, 1937.

Batson, O. V.: The vertebral vein system as a mechanism for the spread of metastases, Am. J. Roentgenol. Radium Ther. Nucl. Med. **48:**715, 1942.

Bianco, A. J., Jr.: Low back pain and sciatica: diagnosis and indications for treatment, J. Bone Joint Surg. **41-B:**4, 1969.

Birkeland, I. W., and Taylor, T. K. F.: Major vascular injuries in lumbar disc surgery, J. Bone Joint Surg. **41-B:**4, 1969.

Bosworth, D. M., Wright, H. A., Fielding, J. W., and Goodrich, E. R.: A study in the use of bonak bone for spine fusion in tuberculosis, J. Bone Joint Surg. **35-A:**329, 1953.

Brady, L. P., Parker, L. B., and Vaughen, J.: An evaluation of the electromyogram in the diagnosis of the lumbar-disc lesion, J. Bone Joint Surg. **51-A:**539, 1969.

Calandruccio, R. A., and Benton, B. F.: Anterior lumbar fusion, Clin. Orthop. **35:**63, 1964.

Caldwell, A. B., and Chase, C.: Diagnosis and treatment of personality factors in chronic low back pain, CORR **129:**4, 1977.

Campbell, W. C.: Operative measures in the treatment of affections of the lumbosacral and sacroiliac articulation, Surg. Gynecol. Obstet. **51:**381, 1930.

Coventry, M. B.: Symposium: Low back and sciatic pain. Introduction to symposium, including anatomy, physiology, and epidemiology, J. Bone Joint Surg. **50-A:**167, 1968.

DePalma, A. F., and Ray, R. D.: Surgery of the lumbar spine, Clin. Orthop. **63:**162, 1969.

Flesch, J. R., et al.: Harrington instrumentation and spine fusion for unstable fractures and fracture-dislocations of the thoracic and lumbar spine, J. Bone Join Surg. **59-A:**143, 1977.

Gertzbein, S. D.: Degenerative disk disease of the lumbar spine: immunologic implications, CORR **129:**4, 1977.

Ghormley, R. K.: Results of combined operation, American Academy of Orthopaedic Surgeons Instructional Course Lectures, vol. 1, Ann Arbor, Mich., 1943, J. W. Edwards, p. 120.

Goldthwait, J. E.: Low-back lesions, J. Bone Joint Surg. **19:**810, 1937.

Harris, R. I., and Macnab, I.: Structural changes in the lumbar intervertebral discs. Their relationship to low back pain and sciatica, J. Bone Joint Surg. **38-B:**304, 1954.

Hirsch, C.: Efficiency of surgery in low-back disorders. Pathoanatomical, experimental, and clinical studies, J. Bone Joint Surg. **47-A:**991, 1965.

Holdsworth, F. W.: Fractures, dislocations, and fracture-dislocations of the spine, J. Bone Joint Surg. **46-B:**5, 1963.

Holscher, E. C.: Vascular and visceral injuries during lumbardisc surgery, J. Bone Joint Surg. **50-A:**383, 1968.

Howorth, M. B.: Management of problems of the lumbosacral spine, J. Bone Joint Surg. **45-A:**1487, 1963.

Howorth, B.: Low backache and sciatica: results of surgical treatment. I. Spine fusion only, J. Bone Joint Surg. **46-A:**1485, 1964.

Howorth, B.: Low backache and sciatica: results of surgical treatment. II. Removal of nucleus pulposus and spine fusion, J. Bone Joint Surg. **46-A:**1500, 1964.

Howorth, B.: Low backache and sciatica: results of surgical treatment. III. Surgical treatment of spondylolisthesis, J. Bone Joint Surg. **46-A:**1515, 1964.

Kambin, P., Smith, J. M., and Hoerner, E. F.: Myelography and myography in diagnosis of herniated intervertebral disc, J.A.M.A. **181:**472, 1962.

Key, J. A.: Intervertebral disc lesions and low back and leg pain, American Academy of Orthopaedic Surgeons Instructional Course Lectures, vol. 11, Ann Arbor, Mich., 1954, J. W. Edwards, p. 99.

Keyes, D. C., and Compere, E. L.: The normal and pathological physiology of the nucleus pulposus of the intervertebral disc. An anatomical, clinical, and experimental study, J. Bone Joint Surg. **14:**897, 1932.

Knutsson, B.: Comparative value of electromyographic, myelographic and clinical-neurological examinations in diagnosis of lumbar root compression syndrome, Acta Orthop. Scand. (Suppl.) 49, 1961.

Lindblom, K.: Protrusions of disks and nerve compression in the lumbar region, Acta Radiol **25:**195, 1944.

Macnab, I.: Negative disc exploration. An analysis of the causes of nerve root involvement in sixty-eight patients, J. Bone Joint Surg. **53-A:**891, 1971.

Macnab, I., and Dall, D.: The blood supply of the lumbar spine and its application to the technique of intertransverse lumbar fusion. J. Bone Joint Surg. **53-B:**628, 1971.

Meyerding, H. W.: Low backache and sciatic pain associated with spondylolisthesis and protruded intervertebral disc: incidence, significance and treatment (symposium), J. Bone Joint Surg. **23:**461, 1941.

Mixter, W. J., and Barr, J. S.: Rupture of the intervertebral disc with involvement of the spinal canal, N. Engl. J. Med. **211:**210, 1934.

Murphy, R. W.: Nerve roots and spinal nerves in degenerative disk disease, CORR **129:**4, 1977.

Norton, P. L., and Brown, T.: The immobilizing efficiency of back braces. J. Bone and Joint Surg. **39-A:**111, 1957.

Odell, R. I., and Key, J. A.: Results of the operative treatment of ruptured intervertebral discs, American Academy of Orthopaedic Surgeons Instructional Course Lectures, vol. 6, Ann Arbor, Mich., 1949, J. W. Edwards, p. 43.

Rothman, R. H., and Simeone, F. A.: The spine, Philadelphia, 1975, W. B. Saunders Co.

Schlesinger, P. T.: Low lumbar nerve-root compression and adequate operative exposure, J. Bone Joint Surg. **39-A:**541, 1953.

Smyth, M. J., and Wright, V. J.: Sciatica and the intervertebral disc: An experimental study, CORR **129:**4, 1977.

Stauffer, R. N., and Coventry, M. B.: Anterior interbody lumbar spine fusion. Analysis of Mayo Clinic series, J. Bone Joint Surg. **54-A:**756, 1972.

Sternach, R. A.: Psychological aspects of chronic pain, CORR **129:**4, 1977.

Stinchfield, F. E., and Cruess, R. L.: Indications for spine fusion in conjunction with removal of herniated nucleus pulposus, American Academy of Orthopaedic Surgeons Instructional Course Lectures, vol. 18, St. Louis, 1961, The C. V. Mosby Co., p. 41.

Truchly, G., and Thompson, W. A. L.: Posterolateral fusion of the lumbosacral spine, J. Bone Joint Surg. **44-A:**505, 1962.

Willis, T. A.: Low-back pain. The anatomical structure of the lumbar region, including variations, J. Bone Joint Surg. **19:** 745, 1937.

Wiltse, L. L.: Surgery for intervertebral disk disease of the lumbar spine, CORR **129:**4, 1977.

Young, H. H.: Additional lesions simulating protruded intervertebral disk, Int. Surg. **17:**831, 1952.

Young, H. H., and Love, J. G.: End results of removal without fusion, American Academy of Orthopaedic Surgeons Instructional Course Lectures, vol. 16, Ann Arbor, Mich., 1959, J. W. Edwards, p. 213.

Scoliosis

Adamkiewicz, A.: Die Blutgefasse des Menschilicken Ruckenmarkes, Sitzungsb. d.k. Akad. d. Wissensch. Math.-Naturw. Cl. 3 Abt., Wein **85:**101, 1882.

Adamkiewicz, A.: Die Blutgefasse des Menschlicken Ruckenmarkes, Stizungsb. d.k. Akad. d. Wissensch. Math.-Naturw. Cl. 3 Abt., Wein **85:**101, 1882.

Bergofsky, E. H., Turnio, G. M., and Fishman, A. P.: Cardiorespiratory failure in kyphoscoliosis, Medicine **38:**263, 1959.

Blount, W. P.: Scoliosis and the Milwaukee brace, Bull. Hosp. Joint Dis. **19:**152, 1958.

Blount, W. P.: Congenital scoliosis, Acta Medica Belgica p. 748, 1960.

Blount, W. P.: Congenital scoliosis, Huitième Congrès, Société Internationale de Chirurgie Orthopédique et de Traumatologie, New York, 1960.

Blount, W. P.: The Milwaukee brace in the treatment of the young child with scoliosis, Acta. Orthop. Unfallchir. **56:**363, 1964.

Blount, W. P.: Early recognition and prompt evaluation of spinal deformity, Wis. Med. J. **68:**245, 1969.

Blount, W. P.: Use of the Milwaukee brace, Orthop. Clin. North Am. **3:**3, 1972.

Blount, W. P., and Moe, J. H.: The Milwaukee brace, Baltimore, 1973, The Williams & Wilkins Co.

Cobb, J. R.: Outline for the study of scoliosis, American Academy of Orthopaedic Surgeons Instructional Course Lectures, vol. 5, Ann Arbor, Mich., 1948, J. W. Edwards, p. 261.

Cobb, J. R.: Technique after treatment and results of spine fusion for scoliosis, American Academy of Orthopaedic Surgeons Instructional Course Lectures, vol. 9, Ann Arbor, Mich., 1952, J. W. Edwards, p. 65.

Cotrel, Y., and Morel, G.: La technique de L'E.D.F. dans la correction des scolioses, Rev. Clin. Orthop. **50:**59, 1964.

Dewald, R. L., and Ray, R. D.: Skeletal traction for treatment of severe scoliosis. The University of Illinois halo-hoop apparatus, J. Bone Joint Surg. **52-A:**233, 1970.

Dommisse, G. F.: The arteries and veins of the human spinal cord from birth, Edinburgh, 1975, Churchill Livingstone, Publisher.

Doppman, J. O., Di Chiro, G., Omnaya, A. K.: Selective arteriography of the spinal cord, St. Louis, 1969, Warren H. Green, Inc.

Dwyer, A. F., Newton, N. C., and Sherwood, A. A.: An anterior approach to scoliosis. A preliminary report, Clin. Orthop. **62:** 192, 1969.

Fang, H. S. Y., Ong, G. B., and Hodgson, A. R.: Anterior spinal fusion. The operative approaches, Clin. Orthop. **35:**16, 1964.

Garrett, A. L., Perry, J., and Nickel, V. L.: Stabilization of the collapsing spine, J. Bone Joint Surg. **43-A:**474, 1961.

Gazioglu, K., Goldstein, L. A., Femi-Pearse, D., and Yu, P. N.: Pulmonary function in idiopathic scoliosis. Comparative evaluation before and after orthopaedic correction, J. Bone Joint Surg. **50-A:**1391, 1968.

Ginsburg, H., Goldstein, L. A., Devanny, J. R., Haake, P. W., Chan, D. P. K., and Robinson, S.: An evaluation of the upper thoracic curve in idiopathic scoliosis. Guideline in the selection of the fusion area. Orthop. Trans. **2:**267, 1978.

Ginsburg, H., Goldstein, L. A., Robinson, S., Haake, P. W., Devanny, J. R., Chan D. P. K., and Suk, S.: Back pain in postoperative idiopathic scoliosis. Long-term follow-up. Orthop. Trans. **3:**50, 1979.

Goldstein, L. A.: Results of treatment of scoliosis with turnbuckle plaster cast correction and fusion, J. Bone Joint Surg. **41-A:**321, 1959.

Goldstein, L. A.: The surgical treatment of scoliosis, Springfield, Ill., 1959, Charles C Thomas, Publisher.

Goldstein, L. A.: The surgical management of scoliosis, Clin. Orthop. **35:**95, 1964.

Goldstein, L. A.: Surgical management of scoliosis, J. Bone Joint Surg. **48-A:**167, 1966.

Goldstein, L. A.: Concave rib resection and ligament release for correction of idiopathic thoracic scoliosis. In Symposium on the Spine, American Academy of Orthopaedic Surgeons, St. Louis, 1969, The C. V. Mosby Co., pp. 241, 254.

Goldstein, L. A.: Terminology committee report, presented at the Fourth Annual Meeting of the Scoliosis Research Society, Los Angeles, 1969.

Goldstein, L. A.: Treatment of idiopathic scoliosis by Harrington instrumentation and fusion with fresh autogenous iliac bone grafts. Results in 80 patients, J. Bone Joint Surg. **1-A:**209, 1969.

Goldstein, L. A.: The surgical management of scoliosis, Clin. Orthop. **77:**32, 1971.

Goldstein, L. A.: The surgical treatment of idiopathic scoliosis. Selection of the fusion area, Clin. Orthop. **93:**131, 1973.

Goldstein, L. A.: The surgical treatment of idiopathic scoliosis. II. Indications, technique, results, Clin. Orthop. **93:**137, 1973.

Goldstein, L. A., and Evarts, C. M.: Further experiences with the treatment of scoliosis by cast correction and spine fusion with fresh autogenous iliac bone grafts, J. Bone Joint Surg. **48-A:**962, 1966.

Goldstein, L. A., and Waugh, T. R.: Classification and terminology of scoliosis, Clin. Orthop. **93:**10, 1973.

Harrington, P. R.: Treatment of scoliosis. Correction and internal fixation by spine instrumentation, J. Bone Joint Surg. **44-A:**591, 1962.

Harrington, P. R., and Tullos, H. S.: Reduction of severe spondylolisthesis in children, South. Med. J. **62:**1, 1969.

Hibbs, R. A.: An operation for progressive spinal deformities, N.Y. Med. J. **93:**1013, 1911.

Hibbs, R. A., Risser, J. C., and Ferguson, A. B.: Scoliosis treated by the fusion operation. An end result study of 360 cases, J. Bone Joint Surg. **13:**91, 1931.

Hodgson, A. R.: Correction of fixed spinal curves, J. Bone Joint Surg. **47-A:**1221, 1965.

Hodgson, A. R., and Stock, F. E.: Anterior spinal fusion. In Rob, C., and Smith, R., editors: Operative surgery, vol. 9, London, 1960, Butterworth & Co., Ltd.

Huebert, H. T., and MacKinnon, W. B.: Syringomyelia and scoliosis, J. Bone Joint Surg. **51-B:**2, 1969.

James, C. C. M., and Lassman, L. T.: Spinal dysraphism. An orthopaedic syndrome in children accompanying occult forms, Arch. Dis. Child. **35:**315, 1960.

James, J. I. P.: Idiopathic scoliosis. The prognosis, diagnosis, and operative indications related to curve patterns and the age at onset, J. Bone Joint Surg. **36-B:**36, 1954.

James, J. I. P.: Paralytic scoliosis, Ann. R. Coll. Surg. Engl. **21:**21, 1957.

Keim, H. A., and Hilal, S. K.: Spinal angiography in scoliosis patients, J. Bone Joint Surg. **53-A:**904, 1971.

Leider, L., Moe, J., and Winter, R. B.: Early ambulation after the surgical treatment of idiopathic scoliosis, presented at Annual Meeting, American Orthopaedic Association, Bermuda, June, 1972.

Lloyd-Roberts, G. C., and Pilcher, M. F.: Structural idiopathic scoliosis in infancy: A study of the natural history of 100 patients, J. Bone Joint Surg. **47-B:**520, 1965.

MacKay, I. M.: A new frame for the positioning of patients for surgery on the back, Can. Anaesth. Soc. J. **3:**279, 1956.

Moe, J. H.: The maangement of paralytic scoliosis, South. Med. J. **50:**67, 1957.

Moe, J. H.: Critical analysis of methods of fusion for scoliosis. An evaluation in 266 patients, J. Bone Joint Surg. **40-A:**529, 1958.

Moe, J. H.: Complications of scoliosis treatment, Clin. Orthop. **53:**21, 1967.

Moe, J. H.: Methods and technique of evaluating idiopathic scoliosis. Symposium on the Spine, American Academy of Orthopaedic Surgeons, St. Louis, 1969, The C. V. Mosby Co., p. 196.

Moe, J. H.: The nonoperative treatment of scoliosis and round back with the Milwaukee brace, American Academy of Orthopaedic Surgeons Instructional Course Lecture, personal communication.

Moe, J. H., and Gustilo, R. B.: Treatment of scoliosis. Results in 196 patients treated by cast correction and fusion, J. Bone Joint Surg. **46-A:**293, 1964.

Moe, J. H., Winter, R. B., Bradford, D. S., and Longstein, J. E.: Scoliosis and other spinal deformities, Philadelphia, 1978, W. B. Saunders Co.

Nachemson, A.: A long-term follow-up study of nontreated scoliosis, Acta Orthop. Scand. **39:**446, 1968.

Nickel, V. L., Perry, J., Garrett, A., and Heppenstall, M.: The halo. A spinal skeletal traction fixation device, J. Bone Joint Surg. **50-A:**1400, 1968.

Perry, J.: The halo in spinal abnormalities. Practical factors and avoidance of complications. Orthop. Clin. North Am. **3:**69, 1972.

Perry, J., and Nickel, V. L.: Total cervical-spine fusion for neck paralysis. J. Bone Joint Surg. **41-A:**37, 1959.

Relton, J. E. S., and Hall, J. E.: Reduction of hemorrhage during spinal fusion combined with internal metallic fixation using a new scoliosis operating frame, J. Bone Joint Surg. **49-B:**327, 1967.

Risser, J. C.: Important practical facts in the treatment of scoliosis, American Academy of Orthopaedic Surgeons. Instructional Course Lectures, vol. 5, Ann Arbor, Mich., 1948, J. W. Edwards, p. 248.

Risser, J. C., Lauder, C. H., Narquist, D. H., and Craig, W. A.: Three types of body casts, American Academy of Orthopaedic Surgeons Instructional Course Lectures, vol. 10, Ann Arbor, Mich., 1953, J. W. Edwards, p. 131.

Steindler, A.: Nature and course of scoliosis, American Academy of Orthopaedic Surgeons Instructional Course Lectures, vol. 7, Ann Arbor, Mich., 1950, J. W. Edwards, p. 150.

Taddonio, R. F., and McNeill, T. W.: Lower hook placement and its effect on end vertebra obliquity in idiopathic thoracolumbar and lumbar scoliosis, Orthop. Trans. **2:**267, 1978.

Tambornino, J. M., Armbrust, E. N., and Moe, J. H.: Harrington instrumentation in correction of scoliosis. A comparison with cast correction, J. Bone Joint Surg. **45-A:**313, 1964.

VanGrouw, A., Jr., Nadel, C. I., Weierman, R. J., and Lowell, H. A.: Long term follow up of patients with idiopathic scoliosis treated surgically. A Preliminary Subjective Study, CORR **117:**197, 1976.

Vanzelle, C., Stagnara, P., and Jouvinvoux, P.: Functional monitoring of spinal cord activity during spinal surgery, CORR **93:**173, 1973.

Winter, R. B., Moe, J. H., and Eilers, V. E.: Congenital scoliosis. A study of 234 patients treated and untreated. I. Natural history, J. Bone Joint Surg. **50-A:**1, 1968.

Winter, R. B., Moe, J. H., and Eilers, V. E.: Congenital scoliosis. A study of 234 patients treated and untreated. II. Treatment, J. Bone Joint Surg. **50-A:**15, 1968.

Winter, R. B., Moe, J. H., and Wang, J. F.: Congenital kyphosis, 1971. (Unpublished.)

Winter, R. B., Moe, J. H., and Wang, J. F.: Congenital kyphosis. Its natural history and treatment as observed in a study of one hundred and thirty patients, J. Bone Joint Surg. **55-A:**223, 1973.

Zielke, K., and Pellin, B.: Ergebuisse operativer skoliosen und Kyphoskoleosen behandlung beun adoleszenten uber 18 jahre und beun erwachsgenen, Z. Orthop. **113:**157, 1975.

Zorab, P. A.: Scoliosis and growth. Proceedings of a third symposium held at the Institute of Diseases of the Chest, Brompton Hospital, London, Nov., 1970, Edinburgh, 1971, Churchill Livingstone, Publisher.

Zorab, P. A., editor: Scoliosis. Proceedings of a fifth symposium held at Cardiothoracic Institute, Brompton Hospital, London, New York, 1977, Academic Press, Inc.

Zuege, R. C., Blount, W. P., and Haskell, D. S.: The push-pull treatment of decompensated lumbosacral curves, presented at the Annual Meeting of the Scoliosis Research Society, Sept., 1972.

Spondylolisthesis

Bosworth, D. M., Fielding, J. W., Demarest, L., and Bonaquist, M.: Spondylolisthesis, J. Bone Joint Surg. **37-A:**707, 1955.

Boxall, D., Bradford, D. S., Winter, R. B., Moe, J. H.: Management of severe spondylolisthesis in children and adolescents, J. Bone Joint Surg. **61-A:**479, 1979.

Bradford, D. S.: Neurological complications in Scheuermann's disease, J. Bone Joint Surg. **51-A:**657, 1969.

Bradford, D. S.: Juvenile kyphosis, CORR **128:**45, 1977.

Bradford, D. S.: Spondylolysis and spondylolisthesis. In Chou,

S. N. editor: Spinal deformity and neurologic dysfunction, New York, Raven Press, 1977.

Bradford, D. S.: Treatment of severe spondylolisthesis. A combined approach for reduction and stabilization, Spine **4:**423, 1979.

Bradford, D. S., Moe, J. H., Montalbo, F. J., and Winter, R. B.: Scheuermann's kyphosis and round back deformity: results of Milwaukee brace treatment, J. Bone Joint Surg. **56-A:**749, 1974.

Bradford, D. S., Moe, J. H., Montalbo, F. J., and Winter, R. B.: Scheuermann's kyphosis: results of surgical treatment in 22 patients, J. Bone Joint Surg. **57-A:**439, 1975.

Bradford, D. S., Winter, R. B., Longstein, J. E., and Moe, J. H.: Techniques of anterior spinal surgery for the management of kyphosis. CORR **128:**129, 1977.

Chou, S. N.: The treatment of paralysis associated with kyphosis. Role of anterior decompression, CORR **128:**149, 1977.

Davis, I. S., and Bailey, R. W.: Spondylolisthesis: indications for lumbar nerve root decompression and operative technique, Clin. Orthop. **117:**129, 1976.

Fisk, J., Winter, R. B., and Moe, J. H.: Scoliosis, spondylolysis, and spondylolisthesis: their relationship as reviewed in 539 patients. (In press.)

Goldstein, L. A., Haake, P. W., Devanny, J. R., and Chou, P. K.: Guidelines for the management of lumbosacral spondylolisthesis associated with scoliosis, Clin. Orthop. **117:**135, 1976.

Harrington, P. R., and Dickson, J. H.: Spinal instrumentation in the treatment of severe progressive spondylolisthesis, Clin. Orthop. **117:**157, 1976.

Harrington, P. R., and Tullos, H. S.: Spondylolisthesis in children. Observations and surgical treatment, Clin. Orthop. **79:** 75, 1971.

Harris, R. I.: Spondylolisthesis, Ann. R. Coll. Surg. Engl. **8:**259, 1951.

Hensinger, R. N., Lang, J. R., and MacEwen, G. D.: Surgical management of spondylolisthesis in children and adolescents, Spine **1:**207, 1976.

Hodgson, A. R., and Wong, S. K.: A description of a technic and evaluation of results in anterior spinal fusion for deranged intervertebral disc and spondylolisthesis, Clin. Orthop. **56:**133, 1968.

Jackson, D. W., Wiltse, L. L., and Cirincione, R. J.: Spondylolysis in the female gymnast, Clin. Orthop. **117:**68, 1976.

Jenkins, J. A.: Spondylolisthesis, Br. J. Surg. **24:**80, 1936.

Laurent, L. E., and Osterman, K.: Operative treatment of spondylolisthesis in young patients, Clin. Orthop. **117:**85, 1976.

Lowe, R. W., Hayes, T. D., Kaye, J., Bagg, R. J., and Leukens, C. A.: Standing roentgenograms in spondylolisthesis, Clin. Orthop. **117:**85, 1976.

McPhee, I. B., and O'Brien, J. P.: Reduction of severe spondylolisthesis. A preliminary report, Spine **4:**430, 1979.

Moe, J. H.: Treatment of adolescent kyphosis by non-operative and operative methods, Manitoba Med. Review **45:**41, 1965.

Moe, J. H., Winter, R. B., Bradford, D. S., Longstein, J. E.: Scoliosis and other spinal deformities, Philadelphia, 1978, W. B. Saunders Co., pp. 331-357, 537-554.

Myerding, H. W.: Spondylolisthesis, Surg. Gynecol. Obstet. **54:** 371, 1932.

Nachemson, A.: Repair of the spondylolisthetic defect and intertransverse fusion for young patients, Clin. Orthop. **117:**101, 1976.

Nachemson, A., and Wiltse, L. L.: Editorial comment: spondylolisthesis, Clin. Orthop. **117:**4, 1976.

Neugebauer, F. L.: The classic: a new contribution to the history and etiology of spondylolisthesis, Clin. Orthop. **117:**4, 1976.

Newman, P. H.: A clinical syndrome associated with severe lumbosacral subluxation, J. Bone Joint Surg. **47-B:**472, 1965.

Newman, P. H.: Surgical treatment for spondylolisthesis in the adult, Clin. Orthop. **117:**106, 1976.

Newman, P. H., and Stone, K. H.: The etiology of spondylolisthesis with a special investigation, J. Bone Joint Surg. **45-B:** 39, 1963.

Phalen, G. S., and Dickson, J. A.: Spondylolisthesis and tight hamstrings, J. Bone Joint Surg. **43-A:**505, 1961.

Riseborough, E. J.: The anterior approach to the spine for correction of deformities of the axial skeleton, Clin. Orthop. **93:** 207, 1973.

Risser, J. C., Lauder, C. H., Norquist, D. H., and Craig, W. A.: Three types of body casts, American Academy of Orthopaedic Surgeons Instructional Course Lectures, vol. 10, Ann Arbor, Mich., 1953, J. W. Edwards, pp. 131-142.

Risser, J. C., and Norquist, D. M.: Sciatic scoliosis in growing children, Clin. Orthop. **21:**137, 1961.

Roche, M. B.: Healing of bilateral fracture of the pars interarticularis of a lumbar neural arch, J. Bone Joint Surg. **32-A:** 428, 1950.

Rosenberg, N. J.: Degenerative spondylolisthesis, Clin. Orthop. **117:**112, 1976.

Scaglietti, O., Frontino, G., and Bartolozzi, P.: Technique of anatomical reduction of lumbar spondylolisthesis and its surgical stabilization, Clin. Orthop. **117:**164, 1976.

Scheuermann, H. W.: Kyphosis dorsalis juvenilis, The classic, CORR **128:**5, 1977.

Stagnara, P.: Deviations et deformations sagittales du tachis, Encycl. Med. Chir., Paris, Appareil locomoteur, 4.1.01, 15865 E-10.

Streitz, W., Brown, J. C., and Bonnett, C. A.: Anterior fibular strut grafting in the treatment of kyphosis, CORR **128:**140, 1977.

Taillard, W. F.: Etiology of spondylolisthesis, Clin. Orthop. **117:** 30, 1976.

Taylor, T. C., Wenger, D. R., Stephen, J., Gillespie, R., and Dobechko, W. P.: Surgical management of thoracic kyphosis in adolescents, J. Bone Joint Surg. **61-A:**496, 19 9.

Tojner, H.: Olisthetic scoliosis, Acta Orthop. Scand. **33:**291, 1963.

Turner, R. H., and Bianco, A. J.: Spondylolysis and spondylolisthesis in children and teenagers, J. Bone Joint Surg. **53-A:** 1298, 1971.

White, A. A., III, Panjabi, M. M., and Thomas, C. L.: The clinical biomechanics of kyphotic deformities. CORR **128:**8, 1977.

Wiltse, L. L.: Spondylolisthesis in children, Clin. Orthop. **21:** 156, 1961.

Wiltse, L. L.: The etiology of spondylolisthesis, J. Bone Joint Surg. **44-A:**539, 1962.

Wiltse, L. L., and Hutchinson, R. H.: Surgical treatment of spondylolisthesis, Clin. Orthop. **35:**116, 1964.

Wiltse, L. L., and Jackson, D. W.: Treatment of spondylolisthesis and spondylolysis in children, Clin. Orthop. **117:**92, 1976.

Wiltse, L. L., Newman, P. H., and MacNab, I.: Classification of spondylolysis and spondylolisthesis, Clin. Orthop. **117:**23, 1976.

Wiltse, L. L., Widell, E. H., and Jackson, D. W.: Fatigue fracture: the basic lesion in intrinsic spondylolisthesis, J. Bone Joint Surg. **57-A:**17, 1975.

9
PELVIS

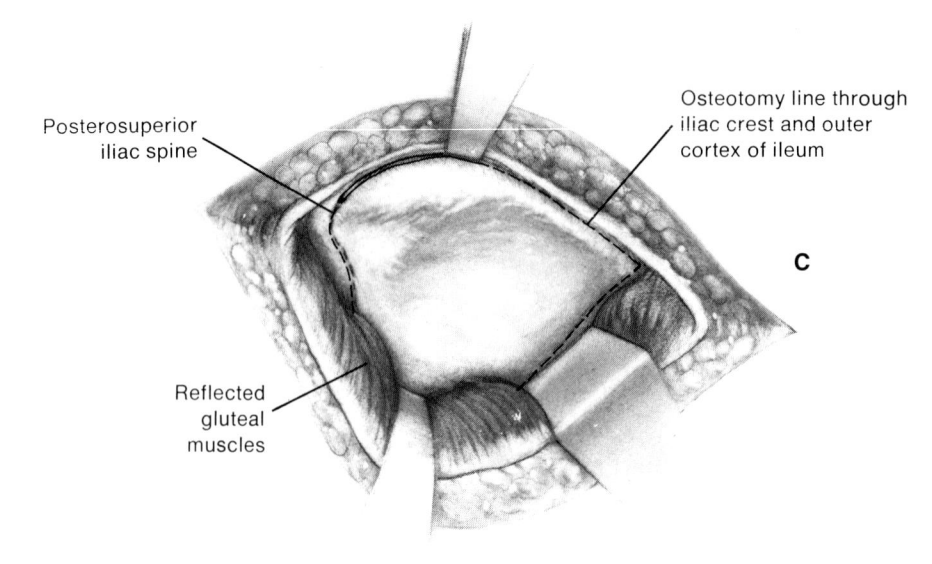

REMOVAL OF DONOR BONE FROM ILIAC WING FOR BONE GRAFT (Plate 9-1)

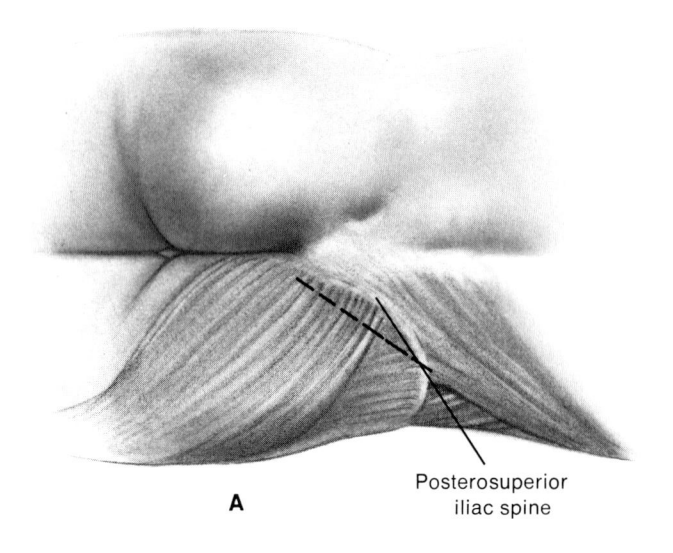

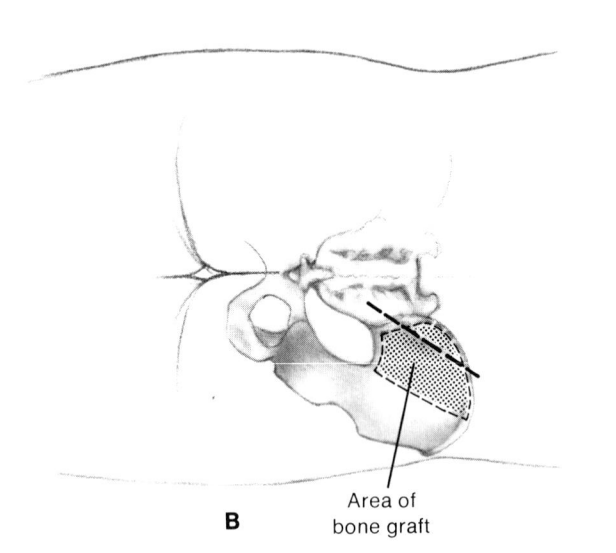

GENERAL DISCUSSION. The ilium is the best source of fresh autogenous cancellous and cortical bone for use in bone grafting for almost any purpose. Depending on the type of bone graft required, the ilium will provide a full-thickness bone graft of cortical and cancellous tissue, purely cancellous bone, or single-thickness cortical grafts. With the proper technique, bone can be removed from the inner or outer table of the anterior ilium or the outer table of the posterior ilium without permanent sequelae with regard to the pelvis or sacroiliac joints. The complication of subluxation of the sacroiliac joint following the removal of bone from the posterior ilium is caused by disturbance of the stabilizing ligaments or violation of the integrity of the joint. In well over 500 spine fusions for which a large amount of iliac bone was removed from the posterior half of the ilium, there have been no sacroiliac joint complications. The most abundant source of cancellous bone is found in the posterior portion of the iliac wing where it is wide and thick, just under the iliac crest from the anterior superior iliac spine to the posterior superior iliac spine, and the very thick portion of the ilium just above the sciatic notch. The least productive area for obtaining cancellous bone from the ilium is in the midportion of the ilium between the anterior and inferior gluteal lines where the inner and outer tables are almost in contact with each other.

When the anterior ilium is the bone graft donor site for cancellous or single-thickness cortical grafts, discomfort to the patient in the early postoperative period is significantly less if the bone is removed from the medial aspect of the ilium. The attachments of the external and internal oblique abdominal muscles and the transversus abdominis muscle are reflected from the anterior iliac crest and the iliacus muscle is reflected subperiosteally to expose the iliac fossa and inner table. Removing bone from the outer table of the anterior ilium requires subperiosteal reflection of the tensor fascia lata

(Plate 9-1) REMOVAL OF DONOR BONE FROM ILIAC WING FOR BONE GRAFT

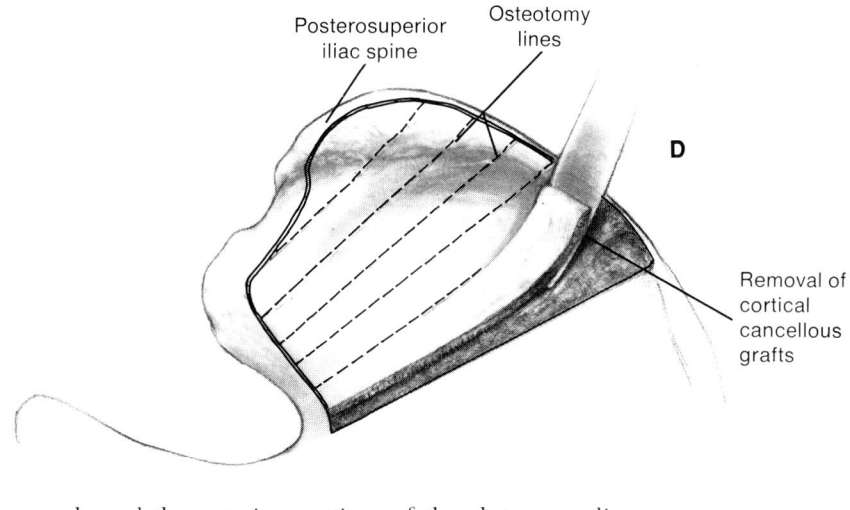

muscle and the anterior portions of the gluteus medius and the gluteus minimus.

Exposure of the outer table of the posterior ilium is illustrated here, but the method of obtaining donor bone from the anterior ilium is basically the same.

DETAILS OF PROCEDURE. An oblique straight incision is made from the highest point of the iliac crest, downward and medially (**A** and **B**). The subcutaneous tissues are divided by sharp dissection, exposing the iliac crest (**C**). The gluteal fascia is incised 2 cm distal to the posterosuperior iliac spine and the gluteal muscles separated in the direction of their fibers (**C**). In a child the white line of the iliac apophysis is easily visualized. The superior cluneal nerve and vessels may be visualized crossing the crest under the deep fascia in the lateral third of the wound. An incision is made through the iliac apophysis down to bone extending the length of the exposed crest and joining the split in the gluteal fascia medially. The lateral half of the iliac apophysis is reflected off the crest and a wide subperiosteal reflection of tissues is made, exposing the posterior one half or two thirds of the ilium (**C**). The 2 cm split in the gluteal muscles facilitates wide exposure of the operative field.

The sciatic notch is identified. An osteotomy cut is made with a sharp chisel around the periphery of the exposed outer table of the ilium leaving a 1.5 cm rim around the sciatic notch. Multiple osteotomy cuts are made through the outer table outlining rectangles of cortical bone, which are removed with a thin layer of cancellous bone, using curved, sharp osteotomes (**D**). As much of the exposed cancellous bone as possible is obtained with assorted bone gouges (**E**). There is a large amount of cancellous bone available just superior to the sciatic notch. If all this bone is taken, there are always one or two vigorous nutrient artery bleeders that will need to be plugged with bone wax. At completion of removal of the bone, the inner table is almost completely bare of cancellous bone. Blood is aspirated from the wound as the bone is removed, and saved in a basin. The removed bone is kept in the blood until ready for use. The cortical rectangles are cut into the desired size. The cancellous grafts are usually used as they were obtained.

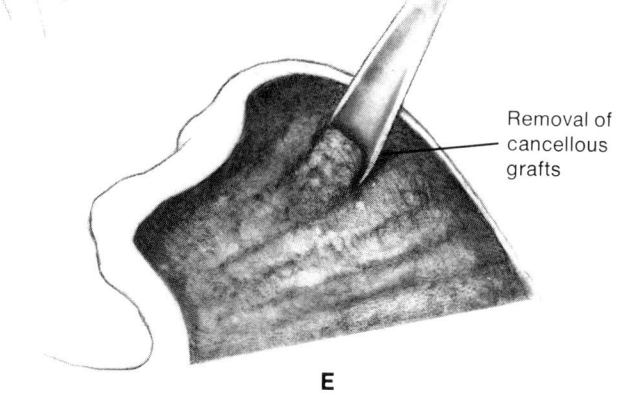

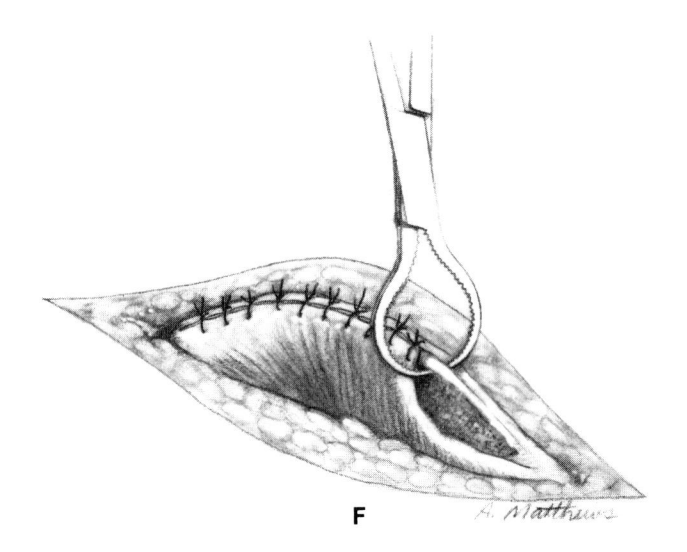

Closure of the wound is important. The gluteal structures must be firmly reattached to the crest of the ilium. In a child the periosteal flap, gluteal fascia, and lateral half of the apophysis can be reattached to the medial half of the apophysis with a heavy cutting-edge needle using figure-of-eight No. 1 chromic catgut sutures. In the adult, an awl or a towel clip (**F**) is used to perforate the medial crest of the ilium, and the gluteal fascia–periosteum layer is resutured securely to bone. The remainder of the wound is closed in routine fashion.

ACETABULOPLASTY (Plate 9-2)

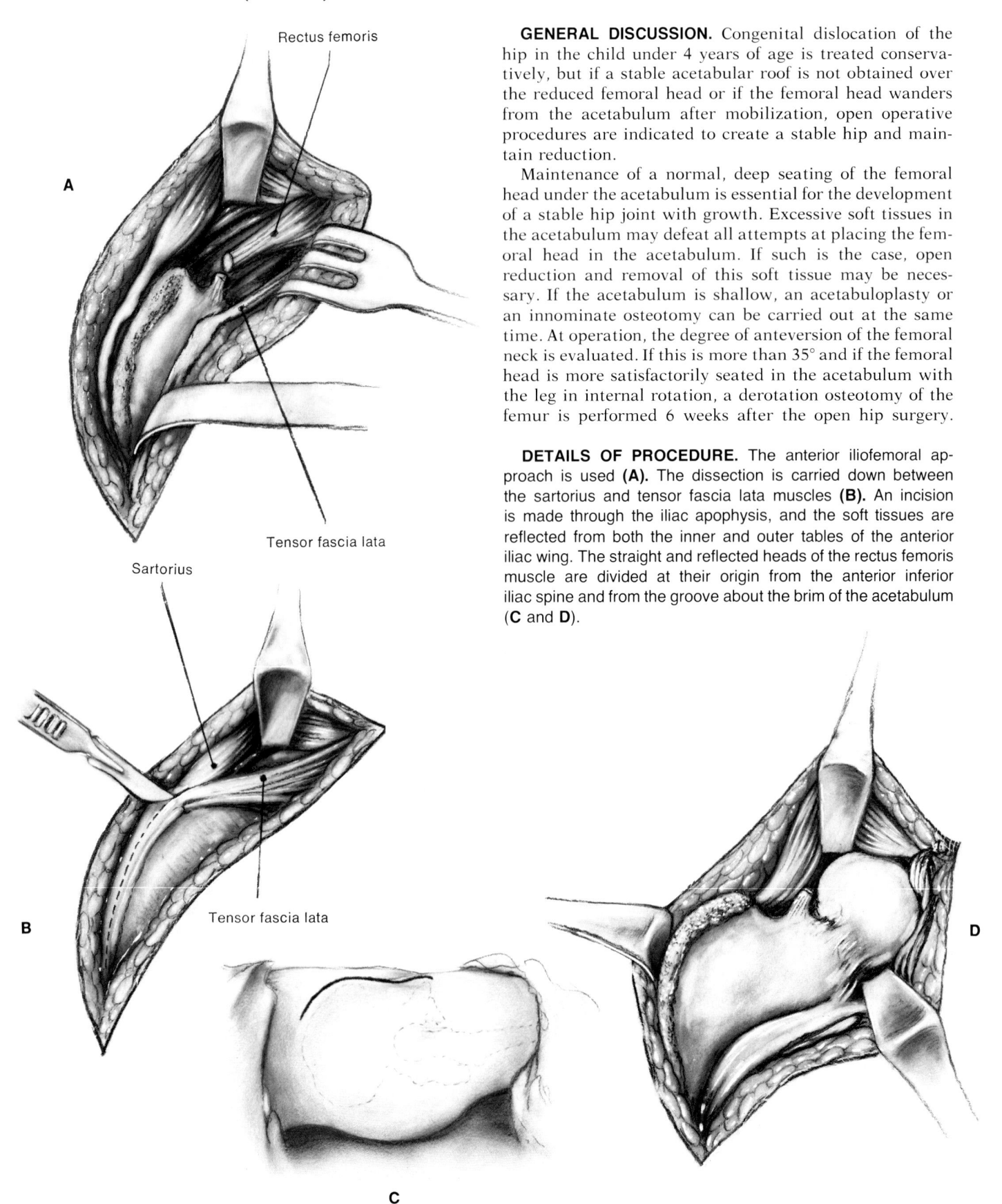

GENERAL DISCUSSION. Congenital dislocation of the hip in the child under 4 years of age is treated conservatively, but if a stable acetabular roof is not obtained over the reduced femoral head or if the femoral head wanders from the acetabulum after mobilization, open operative procedures are indicated to create a stable hip and maintain reduction.

Maintenance of a normal, deep seating of the femoral head under the acetabulum is essential for the development of a stable hip joint with growth. Excessive soft tissues in the acetabulum may defeat all attempts at placing the femoral head in the acetabulum. If such is the case, open reduction and removal of this soft tissue may be necessary. If the acetabulum is shallow, an acetabuloplasty or an innominate osteotomy can be carried out at the same time. At operation, the degree of anteversion of the femoral neck is evaluated. If this is more than 35° and if the femoral head is more satisfactorily seated in the acetabulum with the leg in internal rotation, a derotation osteotomy of the femur is performed 6 weeks after the open hip surgery.

DETAILS OF PROCEDURE. The anterior iliofemoral approach is used **(A)**. The dissection is carried down between the sartorius and tensor fascia lata muscles **(B)**. An incision is made through the iliac apophysis, and the soft tissues are reflected from both the inner and outer tables of the anterior iliac wing. The straight and reflected heads of the rectus femoris muscle are divided at their origin from the anterior inferior iliac spine and from the groove about the brim of the acetabulum **(C and D)**.

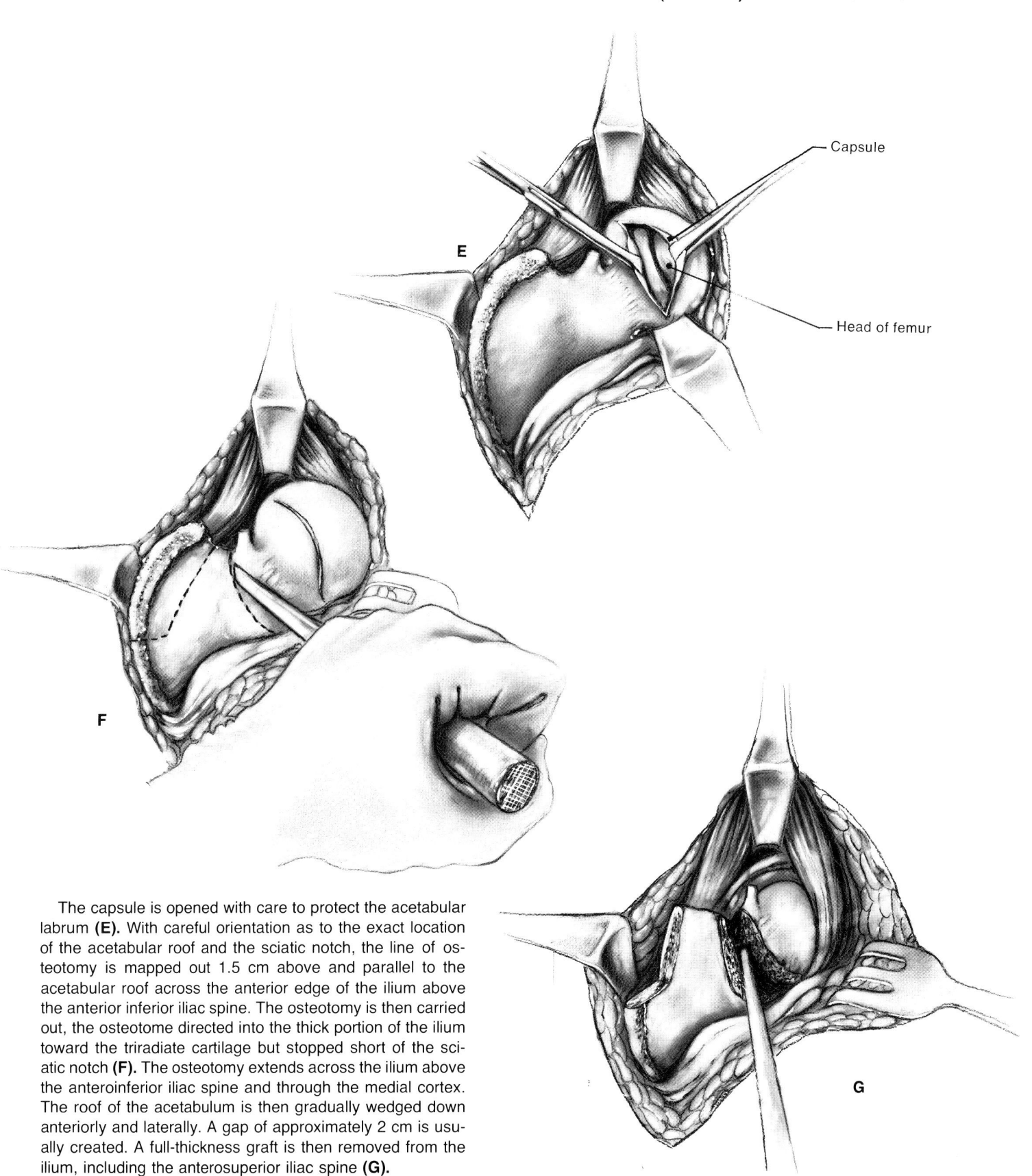

(Plate 9-2) ACETABULOPLASTY

The capsule is opened with care to protect the acetabular labrum **(E)**. With careful orientation as to the exact location of the acetabular roof and the sciatic notch, the line of osteotomy is mapped out 1.5 cm above and parallel to the acetabular roof across the anterior edge of the ilium above the anterior inferior iliac spine. The osteotomy is then carried out, the osteotome directed into the thick portion of the ilium toward the triradiate cartilage but stopped short of the sciatic notch **(F)**. The osteotomy extends across the ilium above the anteroinferior iliac spine and through the medial cortex. The roof of the acetabulum is then gradually wedged down anteriorly and laterally. A gap of approximately 2 cm is usually created. A full-thickness graft is then removed from the ilium, including the anterosuperior iliac spine **(G)**.

ACETABULOPLASTY (Plate 9-2)

Three wedges are cut from the full-thickness iliac graft, and these are placed into the gaping osteotomy (H). The grafts are tapped in lightly and should be firmly anchored under pressure (I). Each area between the wedges is packed with iliac chips (J).

As the osteotomy is wedged down, as assistant maintains the leg in moderate internal rotation under traction or the femoral head is dislocated so that there is no interference with adequate displacement of the acetabular roof.

The head is then reduced after the osteotomy is stabilized with the bone wedges.

The capsule is closed with interrupted sutures after excision of any redundant capsule. The rectus tendon is resutured, and the iliac apophysis is reapproximated. The remainder of the wound is closed in the usual manner. A one and one-half plaster hip spica is applied with the leg in slight flexion, slight abduction, and moderate internal rotation.

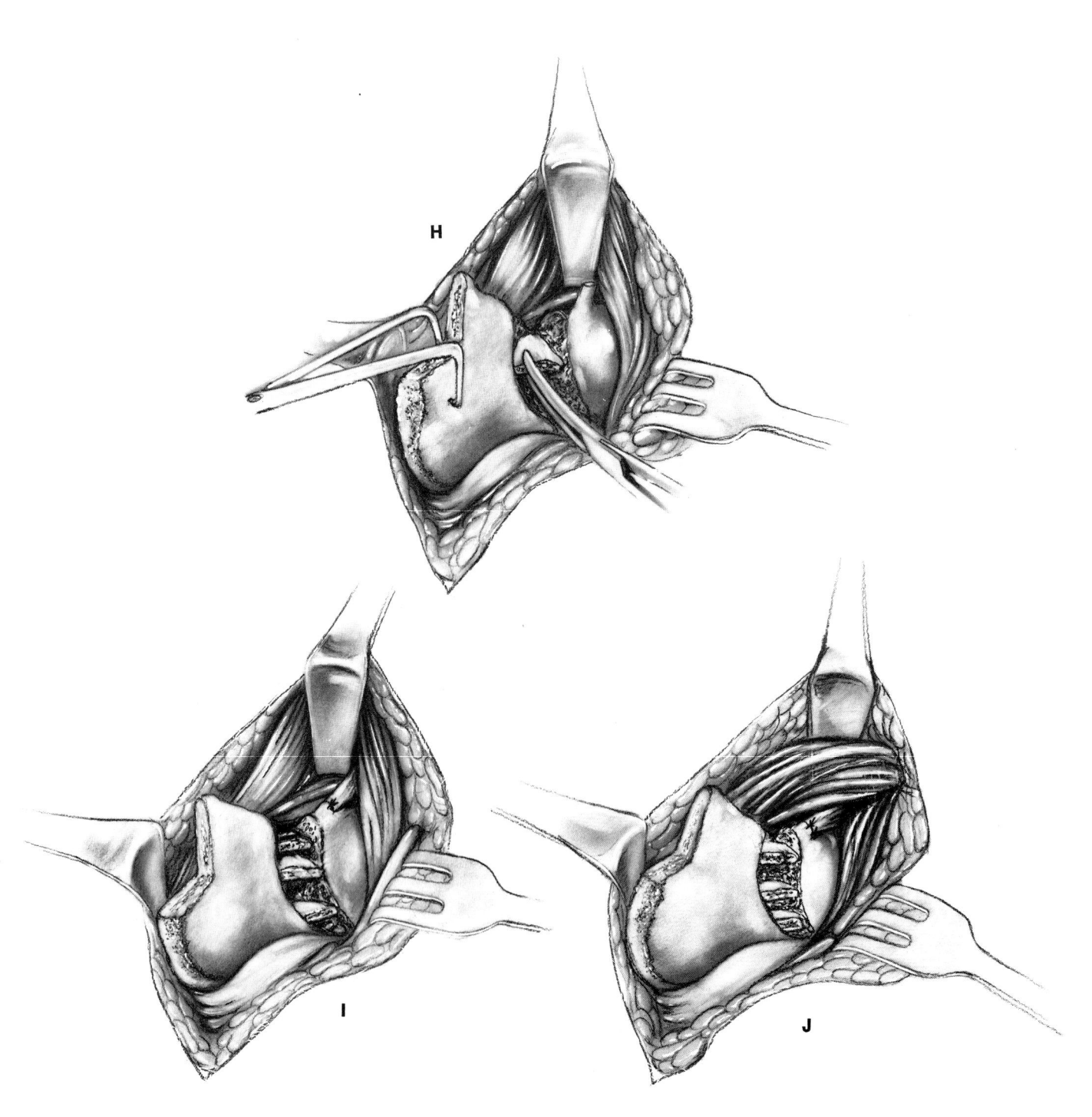

(Plate 9-2) ACETABULOPLASTY

POSTOPERATIVE MANAGEMENT. Immobilization is continued for 8 weeks. If a femoral derotation osteotomy is to be done, the cast is removed 6 weeks after the derotation procedure.

Preoperative (**K** and **L**) and postoperative (**M** and **N**) roentgenograms are shown. Anteroposterior and "frog leg" views are shown but a tube-lateral view is more useful generally than the "frog leg" view for two-dimensional roentgenographic evaluation of the hip joint.

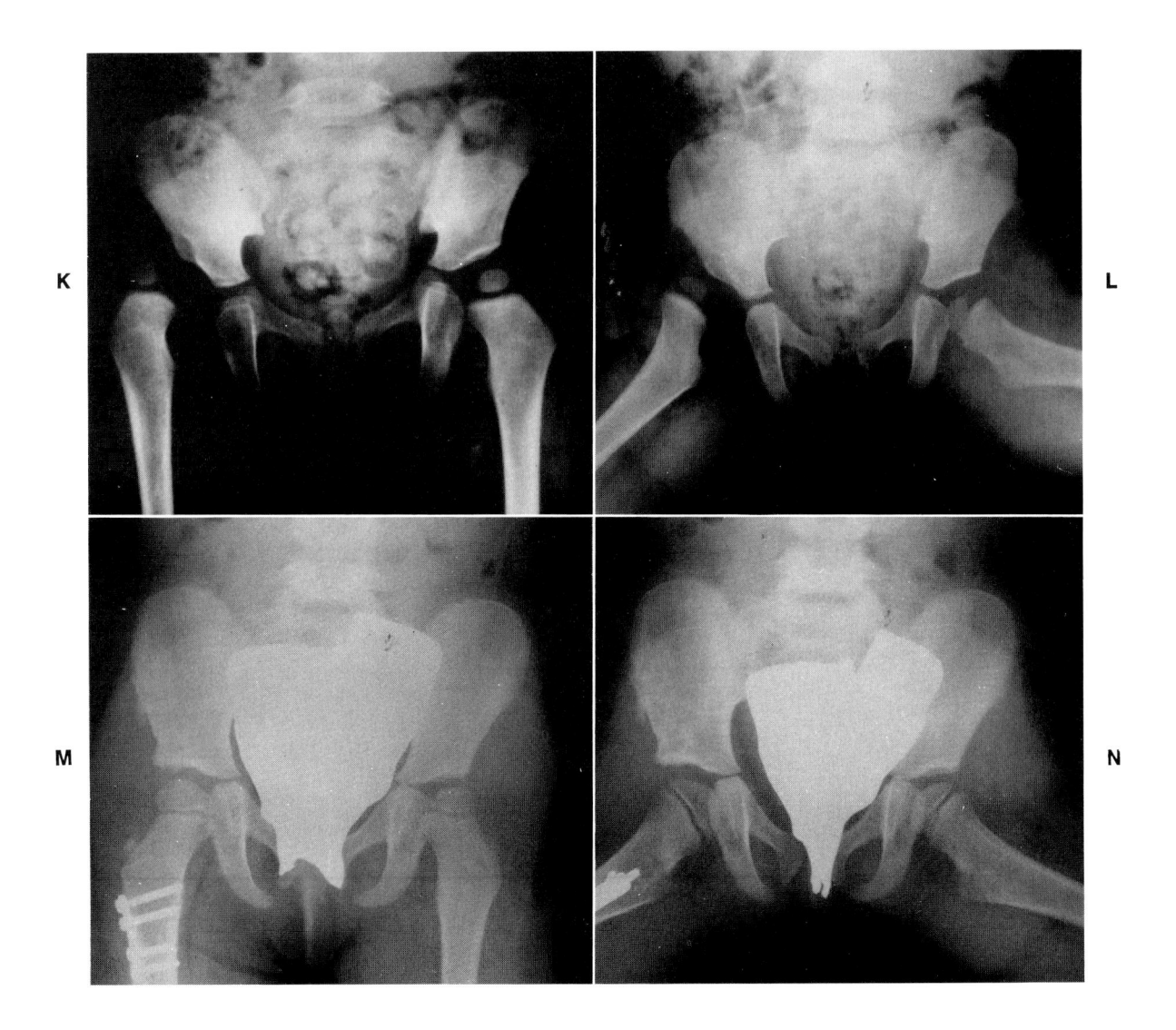

INNOMINATE OSTEOTOMY (Plate 9-3)

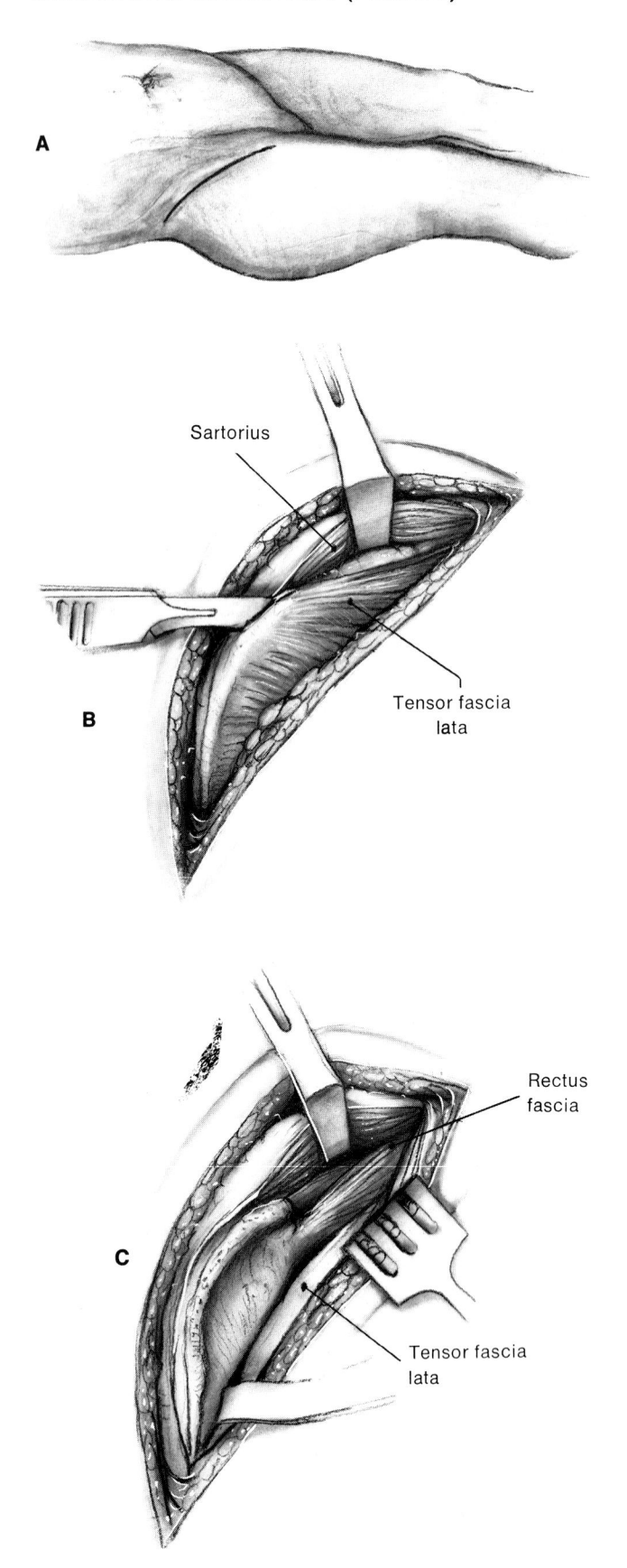

GENERAL DISCUSSION. The principle of innominate osteotomy as described by Salter is applicable to both congenital dislocation and congenital subluxation in the age group of children more than 18 months of age. Complete reduction of the hip is an essential prerequisite for innominate osteotomy. To achieve absolute concentric reduction of a complete dislocation in this age group, it is usually necessary to open the joint at the time of operation. Preliminary traction is essential in a child over the age of 18 months with a complete dislocation, and the traction should be maintained for a period of at least 2 to 3 weeks.

This procedure is indicated in the treatment of the unstable congenital subluxation or dislocation of the hip in children from 18 months to 6 years of age. The procedure has usefulness up to adult life for those children with persisting subluxation of the hip after other methods of treatment. For the older child requiring surgery for an inadequate acetabulum, innominate osteotomy is preferred to acetabuloplasty because it has the advantage of improving the direction of a defective acetabulum while, at the same time, avoiding any alteration in the congruity or capacity of the acetabulum.

If there is any residual tightness of the adductor muscles after the period of skin traction, a subcutaneous adductor tenotomy should be carried out prior to any gentle attempt at closed reduction. If the hip can be completely reduced and is found to be stable after closed reduction, this operation is deferred. If a stable reduction is not obtained with gentle, closed manipulation, innominate osteotomy combined with open reduction of the hip may be required. If the problem is that of persisting subluxation of the hip in spite of closed methods, innominate osteotomy may be carried out without opening of the hip joint.

Salter has defined six prerequisites for innominate osteotomy: (1) ability to bring the head of the femur opposite the acetabulum, (2) release of contractures of adductors and iliopsoas muscle, (3) complete and concentric reduction of the femoral head in the depth of the true acetabulum, (4) reasonable congruity of the hip joint surfaces, (5) a good range of hip joint motion, and (6) correct age of the patient. Innominate osteotomy is recommended as primary treatment for congenital dislocation of the hip between 1½ and 6 years of age as well as for primary treatment for congenital subluxation between 1½ years and adult life or in the same age range after failed treatment for congenital dislocation or subluxation of the hip.

DETAILS OF PROCEDURE. A sandbag is placed under the chest, and the buttock on the affected side and the leg is draped to permit free movement of the entire lower extremity during the operative procedure. If there is any adductor tightness about the hip that has not been corrected previously, a subcutaneous adductor tenotomy is done at this time.

(Plate 9-3) INNOMINATE OSTEOTOMY

An oblique incision is made beginning just below the middle of the iliac crest, extending forward just below the anterosuperior iliac spine **(A)**. The dissection is carried down between the sartorius and tensor fasciae latae muscles **(B)**. The iliac epiphysis is split longitudinally over its anterior half, and the medial and lateral aspects of the ilium are exposed subperiosteally down to the sciatic notch **(C)**. The straight head of the rectus femoris is divided at its attachment to the anteroinferior iliac spine, and any portion of the fibrous capsule that is found adherent to the outer table of the ilium is freed subperiosteally. The iliopsoas muscle is identified, and the tendinous portion that lies on the posterior surface of the muscle is divided **(D)**. Care must be taken at all times to protect the femoral nerve and femoral vessels lying medial to the iliopsoas.

The joint capsule is incised parallel to the acetabular margin, preserving the limbus (**E** and **F**). Fibro-fatty tissue is removed from the acetabulum, and any inferior tight capsular

289

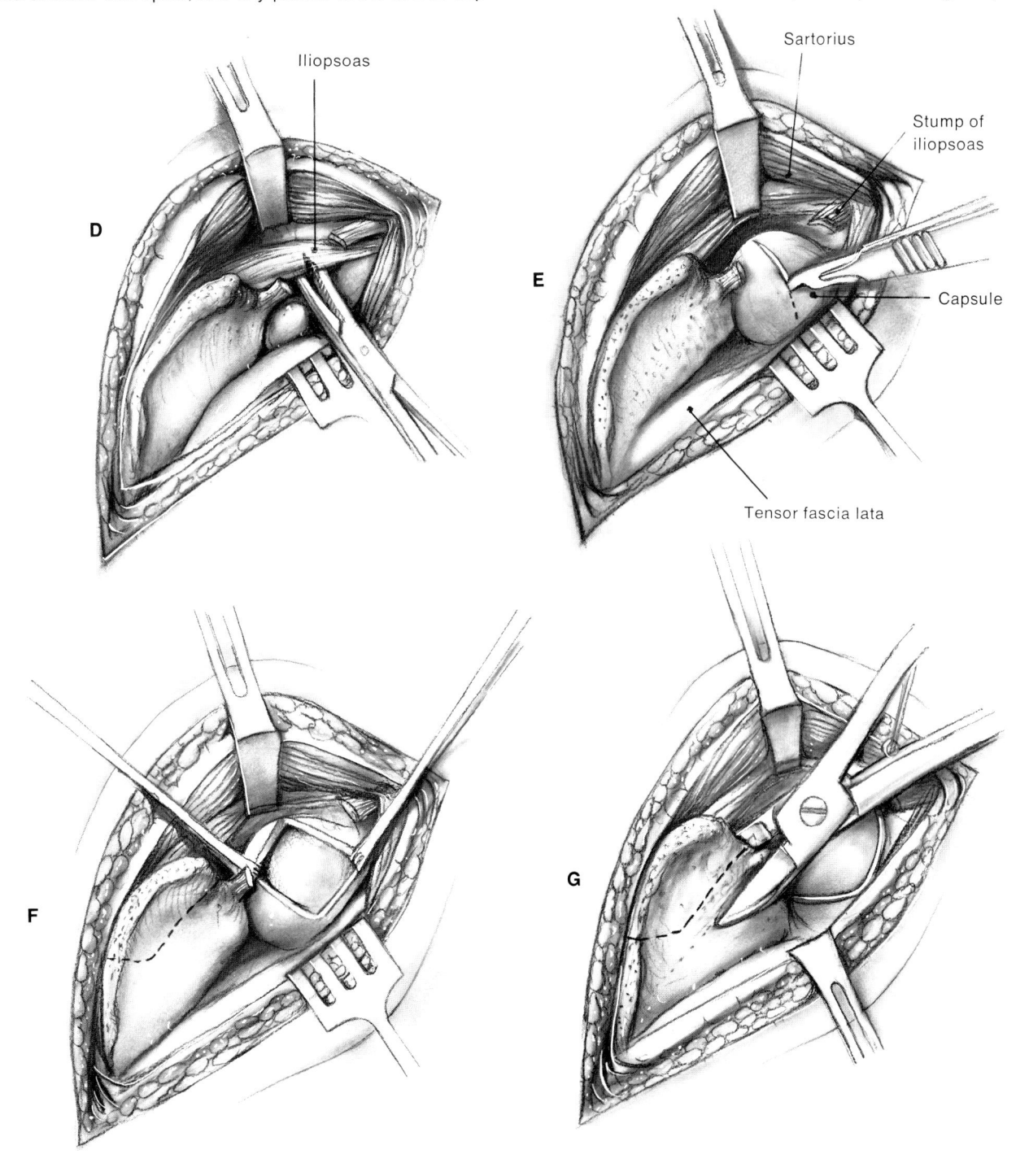

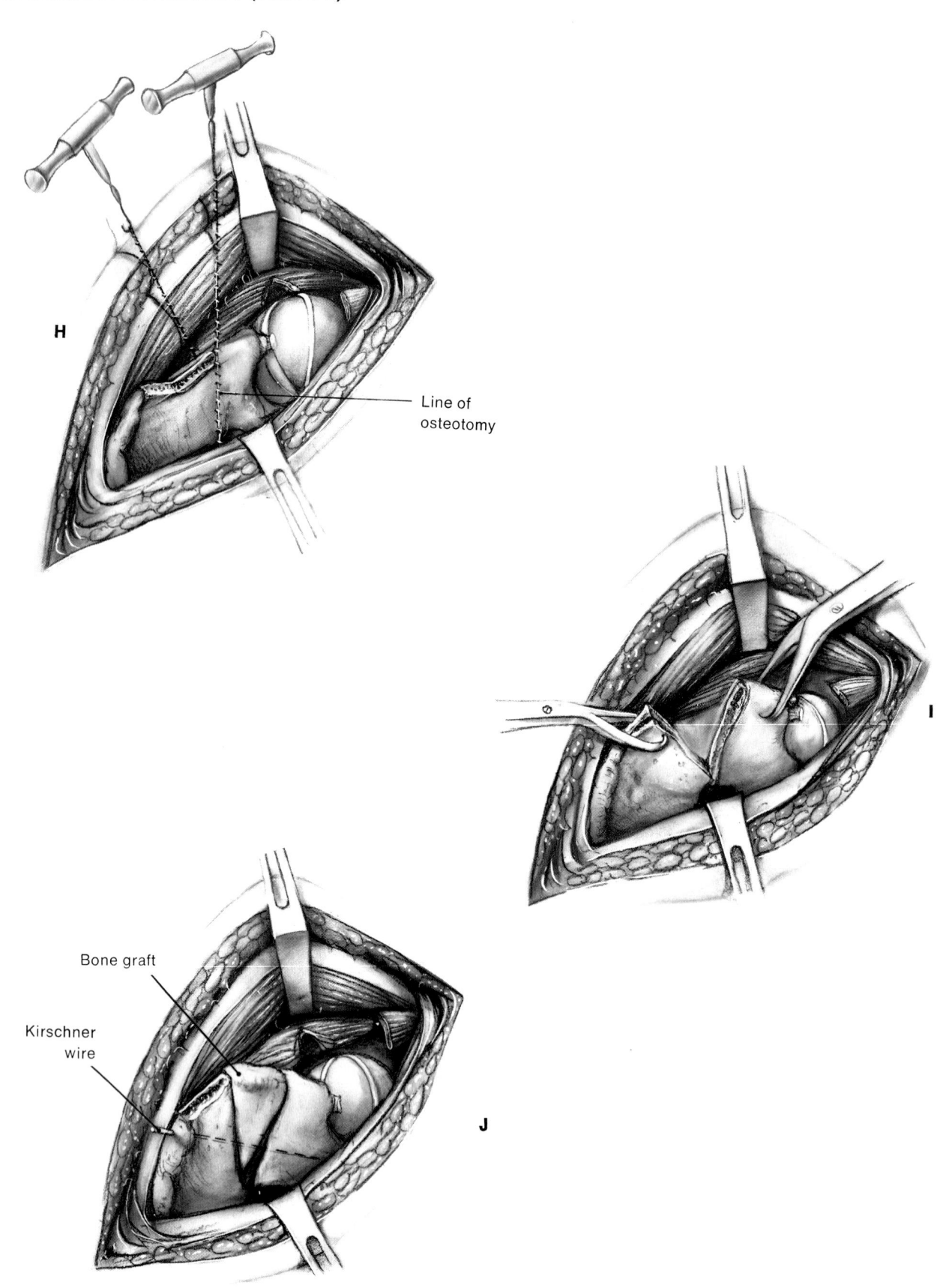

INNOMINATE OSTEOTOMY (Plate 9-3)

H

Line of osteotomy

I

Bone graft

Kirschner wire

J

290

(Plate 9-3) INNOMINATE OSTEOTOMY

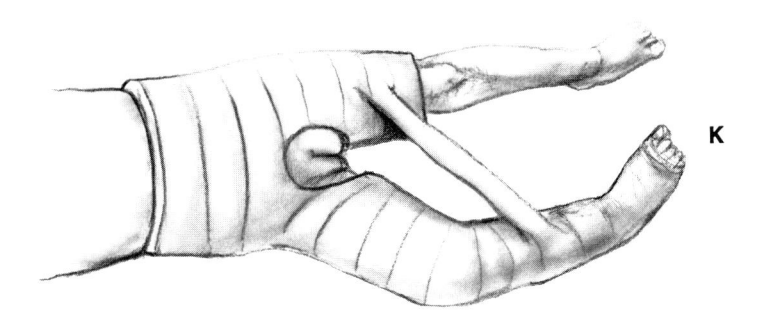

structures are incised. If the ligamentum teres is long and redundant, it may be necessary to resect it to accomplish optimum seating of the femoral head within the acetabulum. Under direct vision, the femoral head is gently reduced. A large, full-thickness graft is taken from the anterior iliac crest and put aside for later use **(G)**.

The margin of the sciatic notch is visualized, and a Gigli saw is drawn through the sciatic notch immediately adjacent to bone in the subperiosteal plane throughout **(H)**. The osteotomy of the ilium is then carried out in a straight line from the sciatic notch to the anteroinferior iliac spine and perpendicular to the vertical plane of the ilium. The hip is redislocated because it is easier to displace the acetabular fragment optimally with the femoral head out of the acetabulum. Both sides of the osteotomy are then grasped with strong towel clips, and the distal fragment is displaced downward, anteriorly and laterally **(I)**. Care must be taken, with the assistance of a periosteal elevator in the region of the sciatic notch if necessary, to prevent any medial displacement of the acetabular fragment.

The full-thickness graft from the anterior iliac crest is then fashioned to be placed in the osteotomy, which should have its base anteriorly and laterally. When the graft is in place, it may be held firmly by the two segments of the innominate bone, but it is further stabilized by the insertion of one or two Kirschner wires from the superior fragment of the pelvis, through the full-thickness graft, and into the inferior portion of the pelvis posterior to the acetabulum **(J)**. The femoral head is again gently reduced into the acetabulum. The leg is held with the hip in slight abduction, slight flexion, and some internal rotation throughout the remainder of the procedure (and until the child is placed securely in a spica cast after wound closure). After reevaluation of the position of the femoral head to ensure that it is in optimum position, any excess capsule is excised, and the capsule is closed. The straight head of the rectus femoris muscle is resutured, and the split iliac apophysis is resutured. The Kirschner wires are divided so their superficial ends will remain in subcutaneous tissue after wound closure.

A one and one-half hip spica is applied with the hip in slight flexion, abduction, and internal rotation **(K)**.

POSTOPERATIVE MANAGEMENT. The child is kept in the hip spica for 8 weeks, at which time the Kirschner wires are removed under local or general anesthesia. Free active motion of the hip is then permitted, and partial weight bearing with crutches is encouraged. In the older child the period of plaster immobilization and partial weight bearing is extended appropriately.

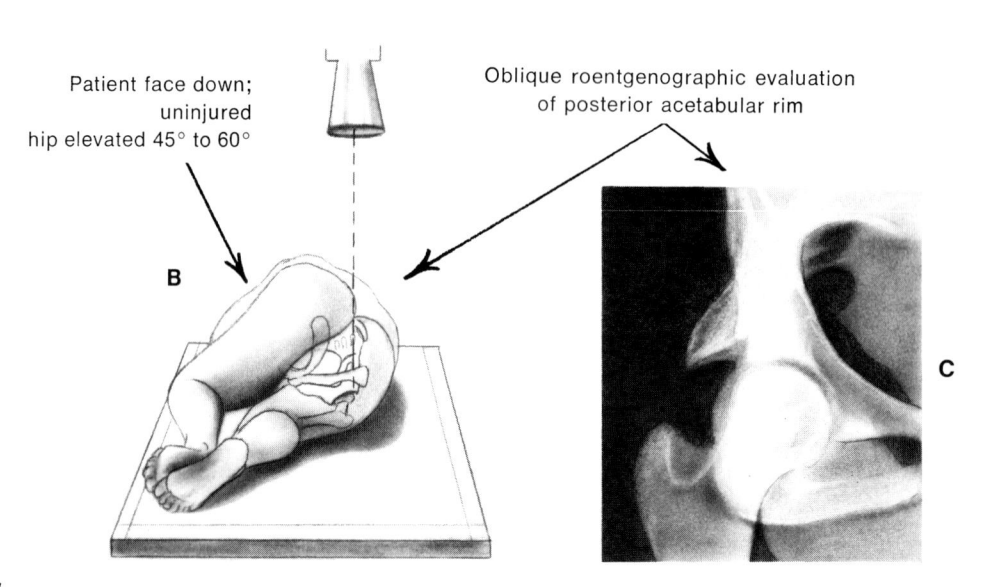

OPEN REDUCTION AND INTERNAL FIXATION FOR DISPLACED ACETABULAR FRACTURE (Plate 9-4)

GENERAL DISCUSSION. The incidence of fractures of the acetabulum appears to be increasing in partial relation to the number of automobiles on our roads and highways. Unsatisfactory results following nonoperative treatment of displaced fractures of the acetabulum are usually not caused by failure to reduce the dislocation of the femoral head but, rather, by the inability to reduce the acetabular fracture. Reduction of the dislocation of the femoral head by traction, closed manipulation, or both may be relatively easy, but exact restoration of the fractured acetabulum is generally impossible by closed means. Surgical treatment cannot be expected to correct any vascular damage to the femoral head caused by the original trauma, but accurate reduction can reduce or eliminate additional mechanical aggravation in the production of posttraumatic arthritis. Open reduction and reconstruction of fragments of the acetabulum are recommended except when there is no displacement or when the displaced acetabular fragment constitutes a negligible portion of the articular surface. Undisplaced fractures are treated with complete bed rest and gentle, passive, range of motion exercises for the first 3 to 6 weeks. The possibility of secondary displacement of these fractures must be kept in mind. Crutch walking without weight bearing on the involved limb is begun subsequently and continued for at least an additional 6 weeks. This is followed by gradually increasing weight bearing.

For roentgenographic examination of the acetabular fracture, oblique views are indispensable. An anteroposterior view of the hip may indicate very little in posterior quadrant fractures of the acetabulum. Oblique views of the acetabulum, taken with the patient face down on the x-ray table, will show clearly the extent of any subluxation of the femoral head. When these views are taken, it is important that the surgeon or an assistant accompany the patient to the x-ray department to maintain control of the extremity. If this is done, little discomfort will be experienced by the patient. In the technique for x-raying the posterior acetabular rim, the patient is placed face down on the x-ray table with the x-ray tube overhead and the uninjured hip is elevated 45° to 60° (**A** to **C**). Displaced fractures of the acetabulum may be treated surgically by either an anterior or a posterolateral approach. The posterolateral approach is required more frequently.

To reach the anterior aspect of the acetabulum, an anterior iliofemoral (Smith-Petersen) approach is used. This approach extends along the anterior half of the crest of the ilium as far as the anterior superior iliac spine and then runs obliquely anteriorly and medially along the lateral aspect of the sartorius muscle for approximately 15 cm. The external aspect of the ilium is not stripped of the gluteal muscles. The medial aspect of the ilium is exposed above the acetabulum by reflecting the iliopsoas. The sartorius muscle is detached from the iliac crest with care to preserve the innervation of the sartorius. Through this approach, the internal iliac fossa of the pelvis can be exposed from the sacroiliac joint to the iliopectineal prominence. Flexing the thigh facilitates release of the lateral edge of the deep surface of the iliopsoas muscle to give access to the horizontal ramus of the pubis. This approach does not endanger the crural nerve provided the thigh is flexed. If the dissection is subperiosteal, the femoral vessels are easily avoided. The only problem is the femoral cutaneous nerve, which is often cut in this incision.

For fractures of the posterior margin of the acetabulum, the posterolateral approach is best.

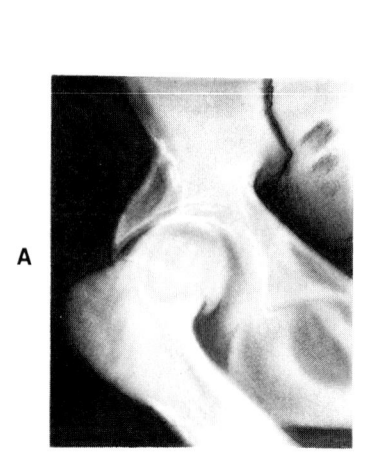

A

Anteroposterior roentgenographic view
(posterior fracture-dislocation)

B

Patient face down;
uninjured
hip elevated 45° to 60°

C

Oblique roentgenographic evaluation
of posterior acetabular rim

(Plate 9-4) OPEN REDUCTION AND INTERNAL FIXATION FOR DISPLACED ACETABULAR FRACTURE

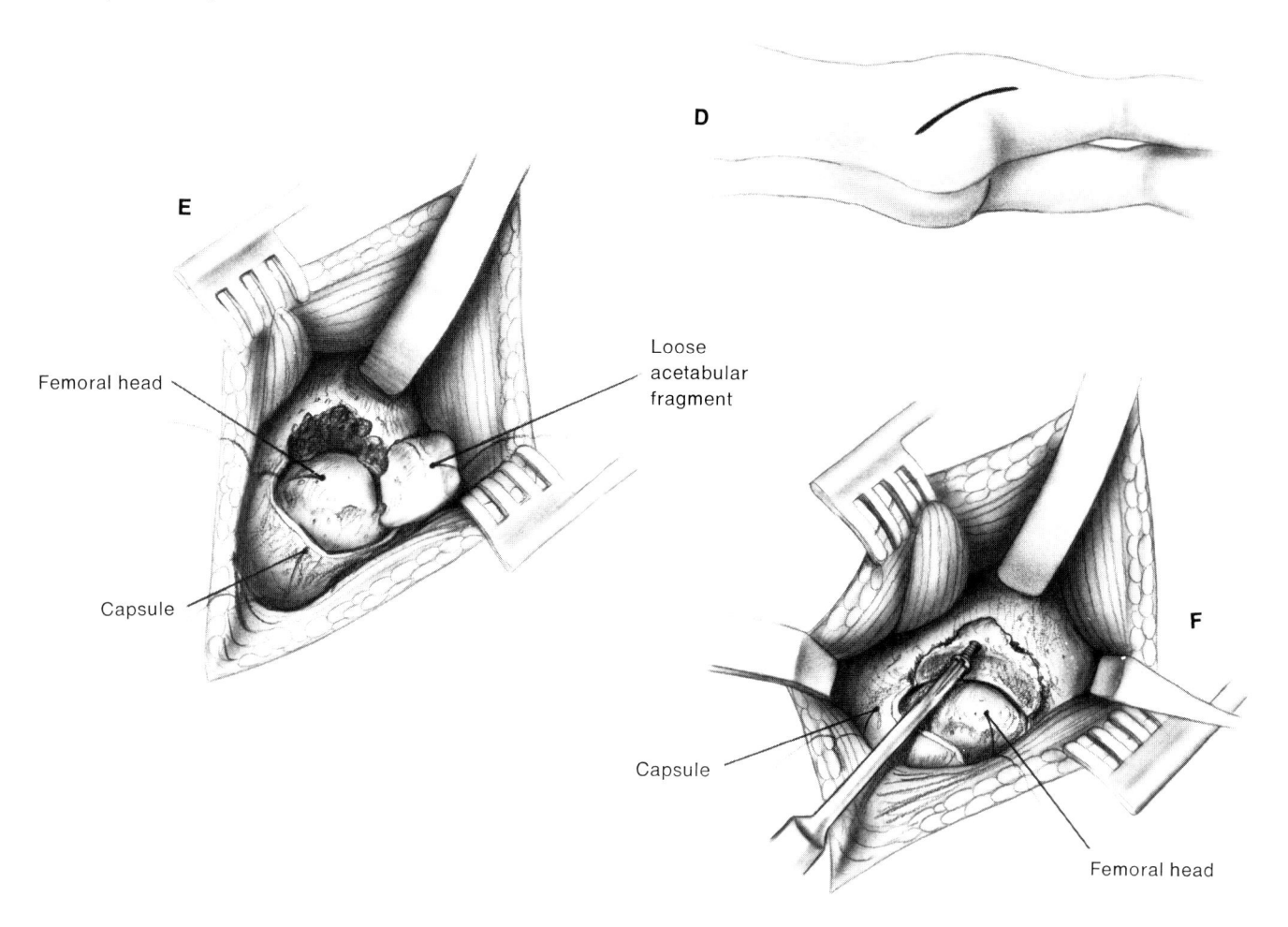

DETAILS OF PROCEDURE. For the posterolateral approach, the patient is placed on the unaffected hip in a lateral position. The center of the incision is over the superior portion of the greater trochanter. The proximal limb is directed toward the posterosuperior iliac spine. The inferior part of the incision descends vertically along the lateral side of the greater trochanter (**D**).

The fascia lata is opened longitudinally, and in the upper portion of the wound the fibers of the gluteus maximus are separated to expose the posterior aspect of the hip joint. The sciatic nerve is identified and protected throughout the procedure. The tendon of the piriformis is cut to gain a better view of the sciatic notch and the emerging sciatic nerve. The short external rotator muscles are also divided. If necessary, the lower portion of the external iliac fossa can be exposed subperiosteally and, with the sciatic nerve isolated, an instrument may be slipped into the greater sciatic notch.

After adequate visualization and reduction of the fracture of the acetabulum, one or more screws or plates may be used for internal fixation depending on the individual circumstances. For posterior rim fractures, one or two screws are generally sufficient for internal fixation (**E** to **G**).

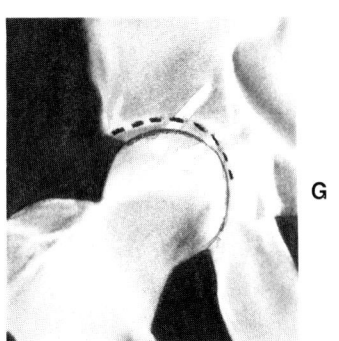

POSTOPERATIVE MANAGEMENT. The management of the patient postoperatively depends on the nature of the injury and the security of fixation of the acetabular fracture. If good internal fixation has been obtained, the patient is generally allowed to be sitting in bed with some gentle, passive mobilization of the hip joint beginning on the second or third postoperative day. The patient is permitted to walk with crutches, but full weight bearing is not permitted on the involved limb until 4 months following the injury.

HEMIPELVECTOMY (Plate 9-5)

GENERAL DISCUSSION. Hemipelvectomy may occasionally be necessary in treatment of malignant tumors of the upper thigh, particularly those of soft tissue and bone in which hip joint disarticulation would give a questionable margin of clearance. The modified hemipelvectomy, retaining a major portion of the ilium and pubic symphysis, may be able to give a reasonable margin of uninvolved and healthy tissue.

According to Duthie and Sherman, the modified hemipelvectomy procedure is much simpler than the standard hemipelvectomy, with less operative shock, blood loss, and morbidity. The adjustment to a prosthesis is better with the leaf of the ilium and pubic rami being left as supporting points for the socket.

DETAILS OF PROCEDURE. The incision is made parallel to and approximately 2 cm above the inguinal ligament. The incision extends laterally and posteriorly just superior to the anterosuperior iliac spine, curving back as a racquet-type incision from this spine toward the posterosuperior iliac spine. The incision is continued posteriorly near the distal crease below the buttocks to meet a second incision carried from the region of the external inguinal ring around the perineum on the medial side of the leg (**A** and **B**). Dissection is carried to the peritoneum, with displacement of the ureter medially and division of the external iliac vessels just distal to the internal iliac branches. Lymph nodes along the common iliac artery may or may not require dissection and removal. The femoral nerve, obturator nerve, and obturator vessels are divided (**C** and **D**). The corpus cavernosum is reflected medially along with the remaining soft tissues to visualize the symphysis pubis, which is then divided with a Gigli saw **(E)**. The psoas and iliac muscles are separated off the ilium extraperiosteally by finger dissection and are divided.

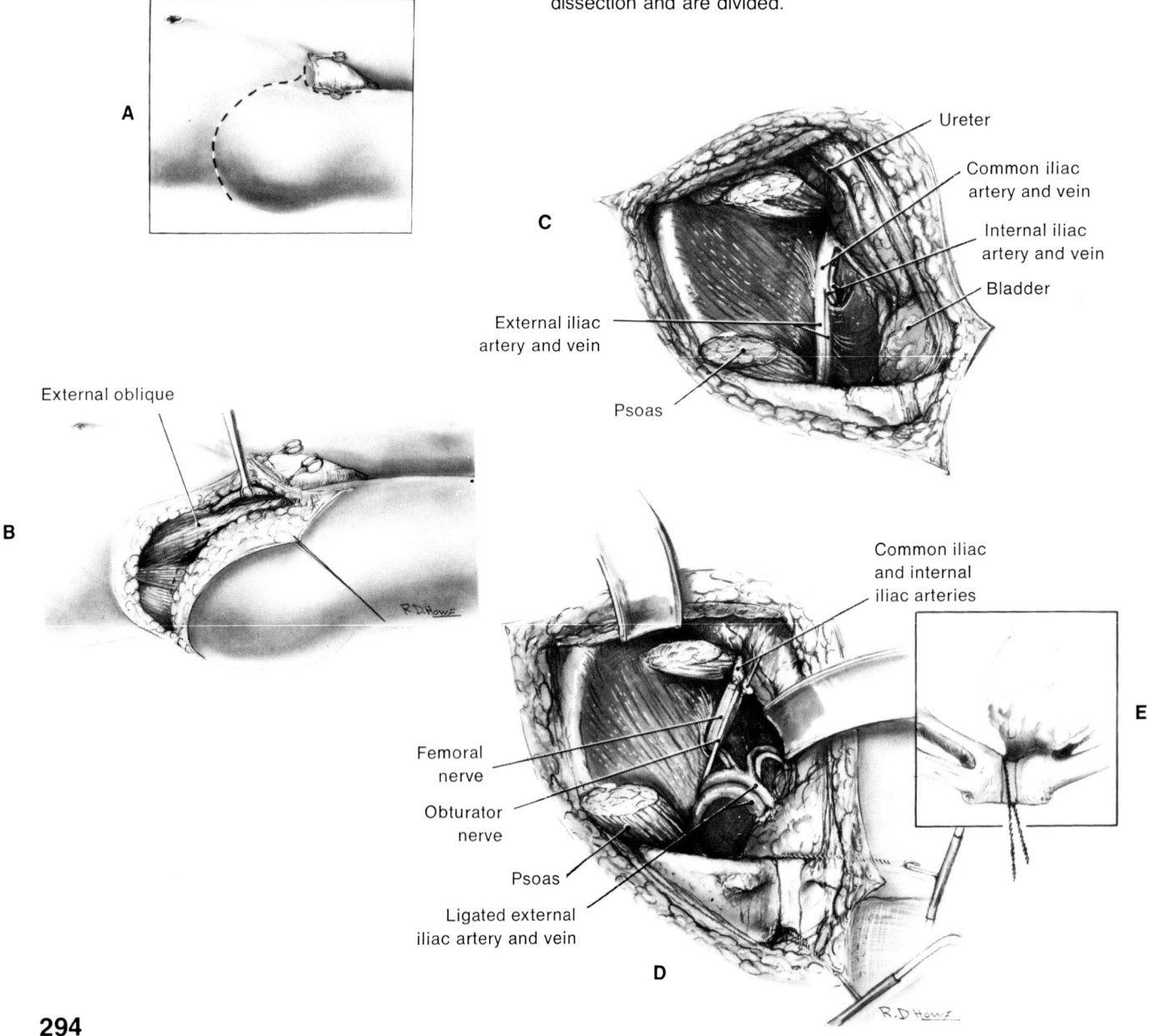

(Plate 9-5) HEMIPELVECTOMY

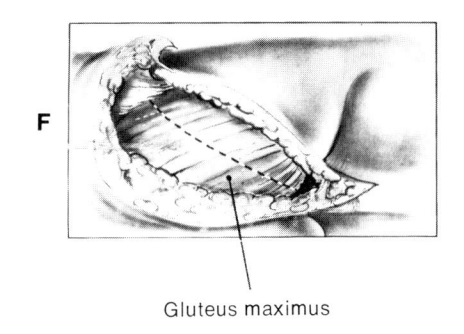

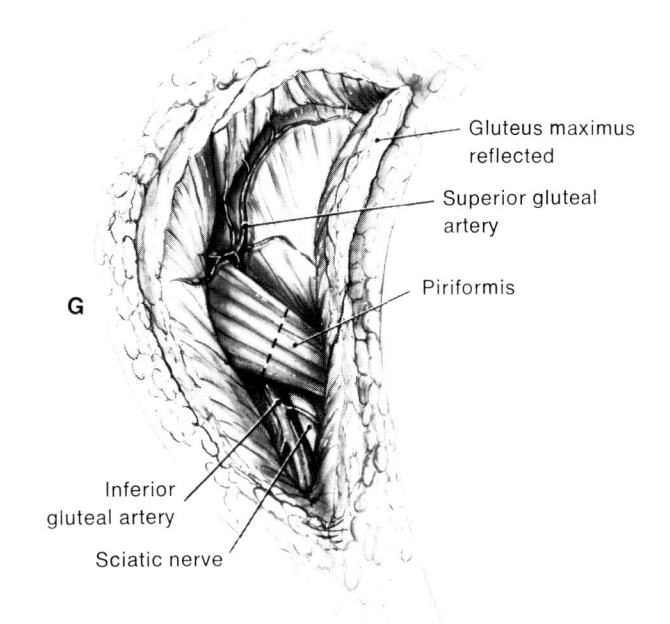

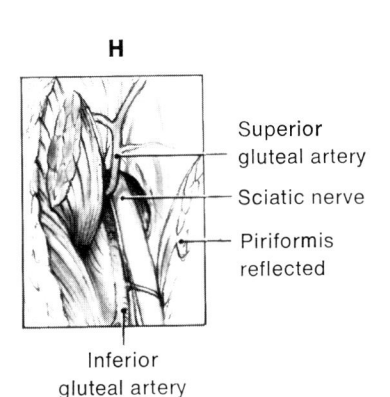

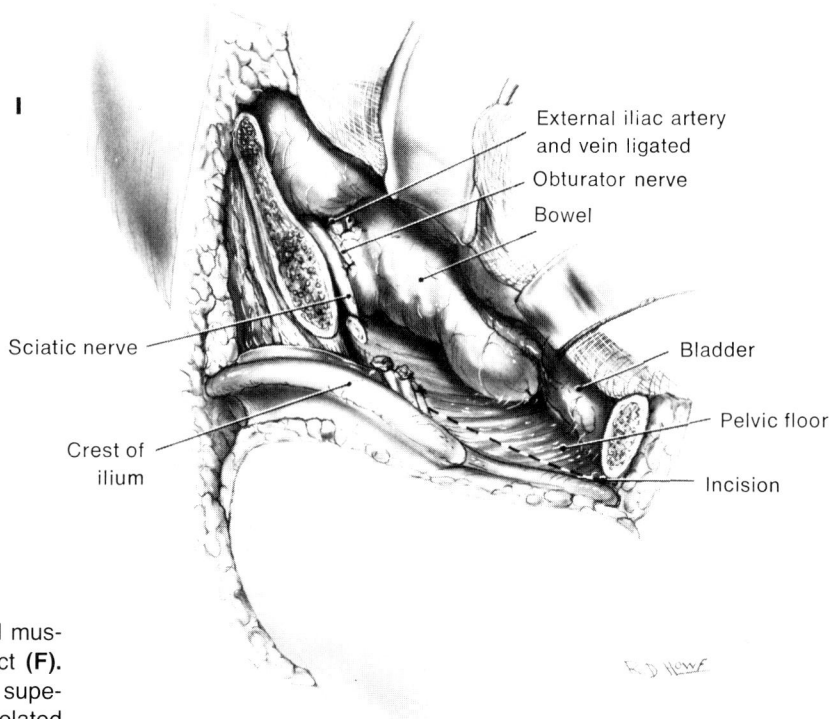

Similar dissection separates the gluteal muscles from the ilium on its posterior aspect (**F**). The piriformis muscle, sciatic nerve, and superior and inferior gluteal arteries are each isolated and divided (**G** and **H**). After the sarcospinalis muscle and iliolumbar ligament are divided, a Gigli saw is used to divide the posterior ilium or the lateral aspect of the sacrum adjacent to the sacroiliac joint (**I**).

295

HEMIPELVECTOMY (Plate 9-5)

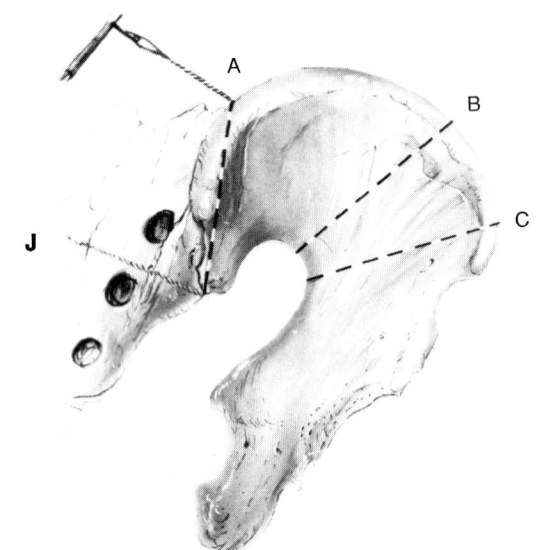

If the individual circumstances permit, a variable amount of the ilium can be left by starting the osteotomy with the Gigli saw in the greater sciatic notch (**J**). The wound is closed by suturing the posterior flap (and any remaining proximal portion of the gluteal muscles) to the anterior soft tissues (**K**).

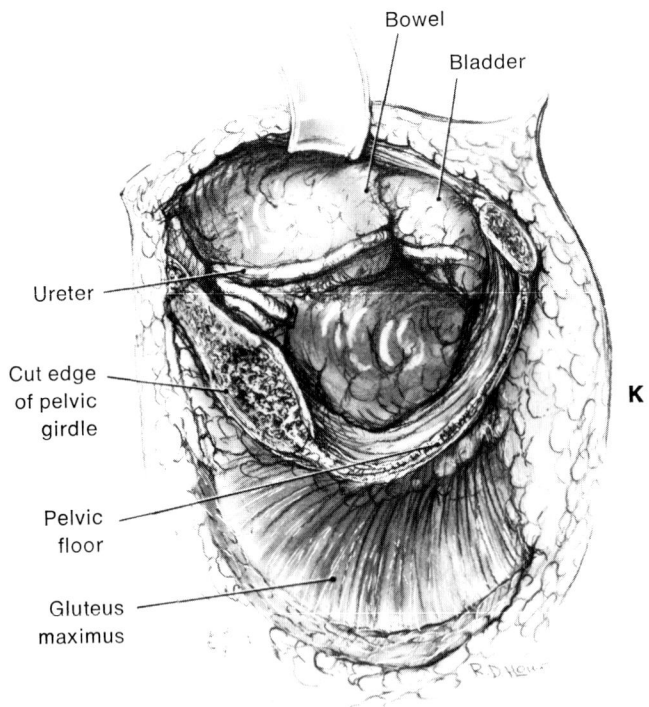

(Plate 9-6) COCCYGECTOMY

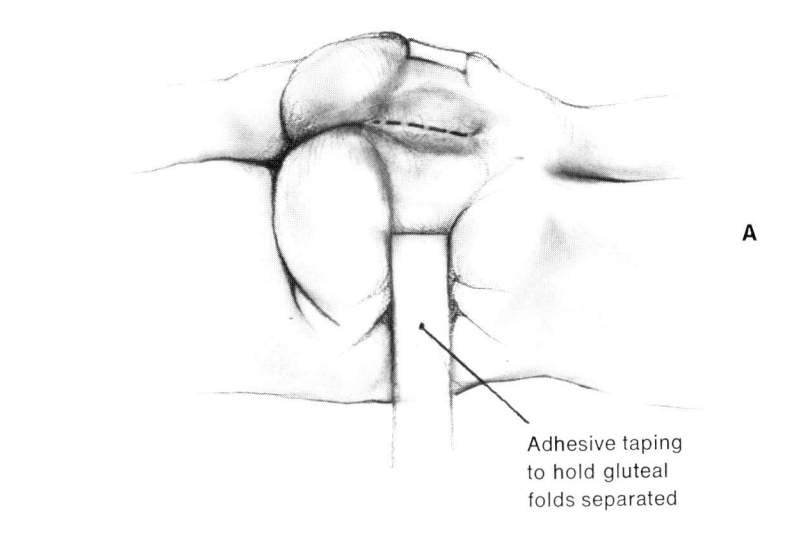

GENERAL DISCUSSION. Surgery is indicated only rarely for coccygodynia (painful coccyx). Surgery is contraindicated when injuries of the sacrococcygeal joint are acute, even when the coccyx is severely angulated anteriorly; these injuries should be treated conservatively for at least 6 months. Along with other conservative measures, the use of local injections of hydrocortisone preparations in the treatment of the painful coccyx can be most satisfying. This treatment will definitely decrease the necessity for coccygectomy, which should be an operation of "last resort."

DETAILS OF PROCEDURE. The patient is positioned prone, and the buttocks are separated and taped in position to provide optimum access to the sacrococcygeal area (**A**). The skin and subcutaneous tissue can be excised longitudinally or transversely over the sacrococcygeal joint. The sacrococcygeal joint is then incised transversely with caution because of the close proximity of the rectum anteriorly (**B**). The proximal end of the coccyx is grasped with a firm forceps or clamp and, by careful dissection close to the bone, the coccyx is carefully dissected free from the remaining soft tissue attachments (**C**). Following wound closure, a collodion dressing is applied.

POSTOPERATIVE MANAGEMENT. Care should be taken to prevent contamination of the wound with feces or urine. In the initial postoperative days, a commode should be used rather than a bedpan. The patient is advised to use a horseshoe-shaped pillow for 2 or 3 months after surgery to avoid pressure on the distal portion of the sacrum.

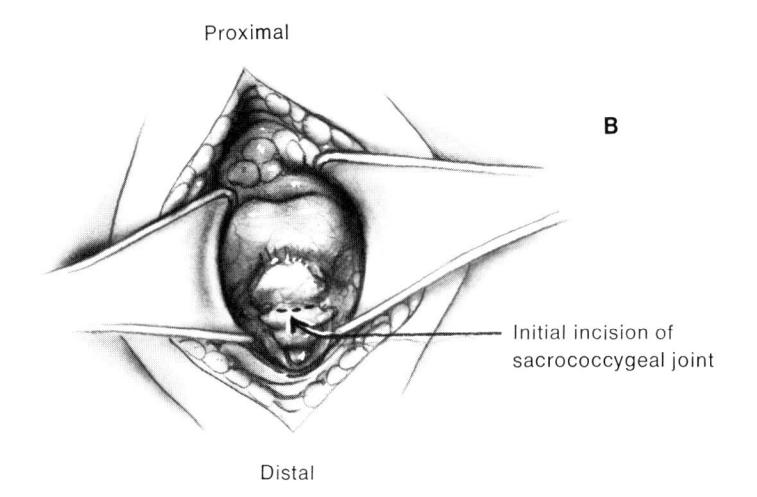

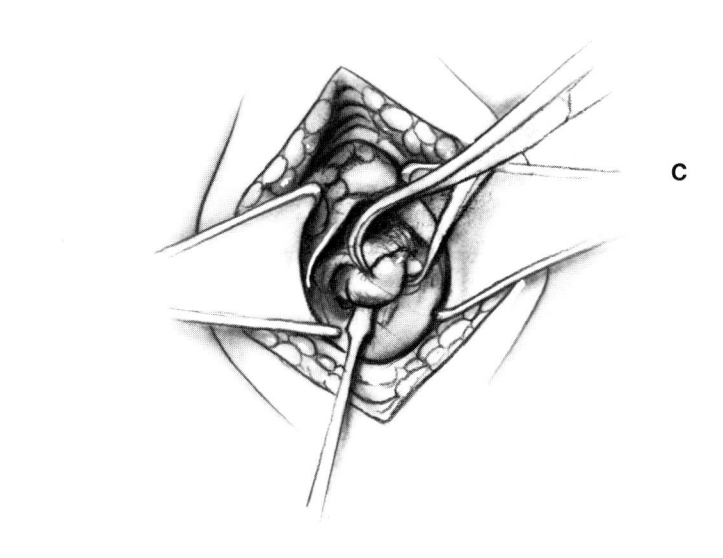

REFERENCES

Abbott, L. C.: The use of iliac bone in the treatment of ununited fractures, American Academy of Orthopaedic Surgeons Instructional Course Lectures, vol. 2, Ann Arbor, Mich., 1944, J. W. Edwards.

Albee, F. H.: The bone graft wedge. Its use in the treatment of relapsing, acquired, and congenital dislocation of the hip, N.Y. State J. Med. **102**:433, 1915.

Braund, R. R., and Pigott, J. D.: Acetabulectomy with preservation of the extremity. Operative technic and report of three cases, Am. Surg. **32**:112, 1966.

Brittain, H. A.: Hindquarter amputation, J. Bone Joint Surg. **31-B**:104, 1949.

Carnesale, P. G., Stewart, M. J., and Barnes, S. N.: Acetabular disruption and central fracture-dislocation of the hip. A long-term study, J. Bone Joint Surg. **57-A**:1054, 1975.

Eyre-Brook, A. L.: Treatment of congenital dislocation or subluxation of the hip in children over the age of three years, J. Bone Joint Surg. **48-B**:682, 1966.

Frey, C., Matthews, L. S., and Benjamin, H., and Fidler, W. J.: New technique for hemipelvectomy, Surg. Gynecol. Obstet. **143**:753, 1976.

Gaenslen, F. J.: Sacro-iliac arthrodesis: indications, author's technic and end results, J.A.M.A. **89**:2031, 1927.

Gill, B.: Plastic construction of an acetabulum in congenital dislocation of the hip—the shelf operation, J. Bone Joint Surg. **17**:48, 1935.

Henderson, M. S.: The massive bone graft in ununited fractures, J.A.M.A. **107**:1104, 1936.

Heyman, C. H.: Long-term results following a bone-shelf operation for congenital and some other dislocations of the hip in children, J. Bone Joint Surg. **45-A**:1113, 1963.

Howorth, M. B.: Shelf stabilization of the hip, J. Bone Joint Surg. **17**:945, 1935.

Howorth, M. B.: Congenital dislocation of the hip. Technique of open reduction, Ann. Surg. **135**:508, 1952.

Howorth, M. B.: The painful coccyx, Clin. Orthop. **14**:145, 1959.

Hunter, G. A.: Posterior dislocation and fracture-dislocation of the hip. A review of fifty-seven patients, J. Bone Joint Surg. **51-B**:38, 1969.

Judet, R., Judet, J., and Letournel, E.: Fractures of the acetabulum: classification and surgical approaches for open reduction. Preliminary report, J. Bone Joint Surg. **46-A**:1615, 1964.

Key, J. A.: Operative treatment of coccygodynia, J. Bone Joint Surg. **19**:759, 1937.

King, D., and Richards, V.: Fracture-dislocations of the hip joint, J. Bone Joint Surg. **23**:533, 1941.

Knight, R. A., and Smith, H.: Central fractures of the acetabulum, J. Bone Joint Surg. **40-A**:1, 1958.

McCarroll, H. R.: Primary anterior congenital dislocation of the hip, J. Bone Joint Surg. **30-A**:416, 1948.

Pack, G. T.: Major exarticulations for malignant neoplasms of the extremities: interscapulothoracic amputation, hip-joint disarticulations, and interilio-abdominal amputation. A report of end results in 228 cases, J. Bone Joint Surg. **38-A**:249, 1956.

Pack, G. T., and Miller, T. R.: Exarticulation of the innominate bone and corresponding lower extremity (hemipelvectomy) for primary and metastatic cancer. A report of 101 cases with analysis of the end results, J. Bone Joint Surg. **46-A**:91, 1964.

Pemberton, P. A.: Rotation of the acetabular roof for treatment of congenital dysplasia of the hip (in Proceedings of Société International de Chirurgie Orthopédique et de Traumatologie), J. Bone Joint Surg. **43-A**:287, 1961.

Pemberton, P. A.: Pericapsular osteotomy of the ilium for treatment of congenital subluxation and dislocation of the hip, J. Bone Joint Surg. **47-A**:65, 1965.

Phemister, D. B.: Splint grafts in the treatment of delayed and non-union of fractures, Surg. Gynecol. Obstet. **52**:376, 1931.

Phemister, D. B.: Treatment of ununited fractures by onlay bone grafts without screw or tie fixation and without breaking down of the fibrous union, J. Bone Joint Surg. **29**:946, 1947.

Rowe, C. R., and Lowell, J. D.: Prognosis of fractures of the acetabulum, J. Bone Joint Surg. **43-A**:30, 1961.

Salter, R. B.: Innominate osteotomy in the treatment of congenital dislocation and subluxation of the hip, J. Bone Joint Surg. **43-B**:518, 1961.

Salter, R. B.: The present state of innominate osteotomy in congenital dislocation of the hip, J. Bone Joint Surg. **48-B**:853, 1966.

Salter, R. B.: Role of innominate osteotomy in the treatment of congenital dislocation and subluxation of the hip in the older child, J. Bone Joint Surg. **48-A**:1413, 1966.

Salter, R. B.: Etiology, pathogenesis and possible prevention of congenital dislocation of the hip, Can. Med. Assoc. J. **98**:933, 1968.

Sherman, C. D., Jr., and Duthie, R. B.: Modified hemipelvectomy, Cancer **13**:51, 1960.

Smith-Petersen, M. N.: A new supra-articular subperiosteal approach to the hip joint, Am. J. Orthop. Surg. **15**:592, 1917.

Somerville, E. W.: Open reduction in congenital dislocation of the hip, J. Bone Joint Surg. **35-B**:363, 1953.

Spence, K. F., Jr.: Coccygectomy, Am. J. Surg. **102**:850, 1961.

Steel, H. H.: Partial or complete resection of the hemipelvis. An alternative to hindquarter amputation for peracetabular chondrosarcoma of the pelvis, J. Bone Joint Surg. **60-A**:719, 1978.

Stewart, M. J., and Milford, L. W.: Fracture-dislocation of the hip. An end-result study, J. Bone Joint Surg. **36-A**:315, 1954.

Thibodeau, A.: The bridging of defects by autogenous grafts and bone chips, American Academy of Orthopaedic Surgeons Instructional Course Lectures, vol. 2, Ann Arbor, Mich., 1944, J. W. Edwards.

Waller, A.: Dorsal acetabular fractures of the hip (dashboard fractures), Acta Chir. Scand (Suppl.) 205, 1955.

Westerborn, A.: Central dislocation of the femoral head treated with mold arthroplasty, J. Bone Joint Surg. **36-A**:307, 1954.

10
HIP

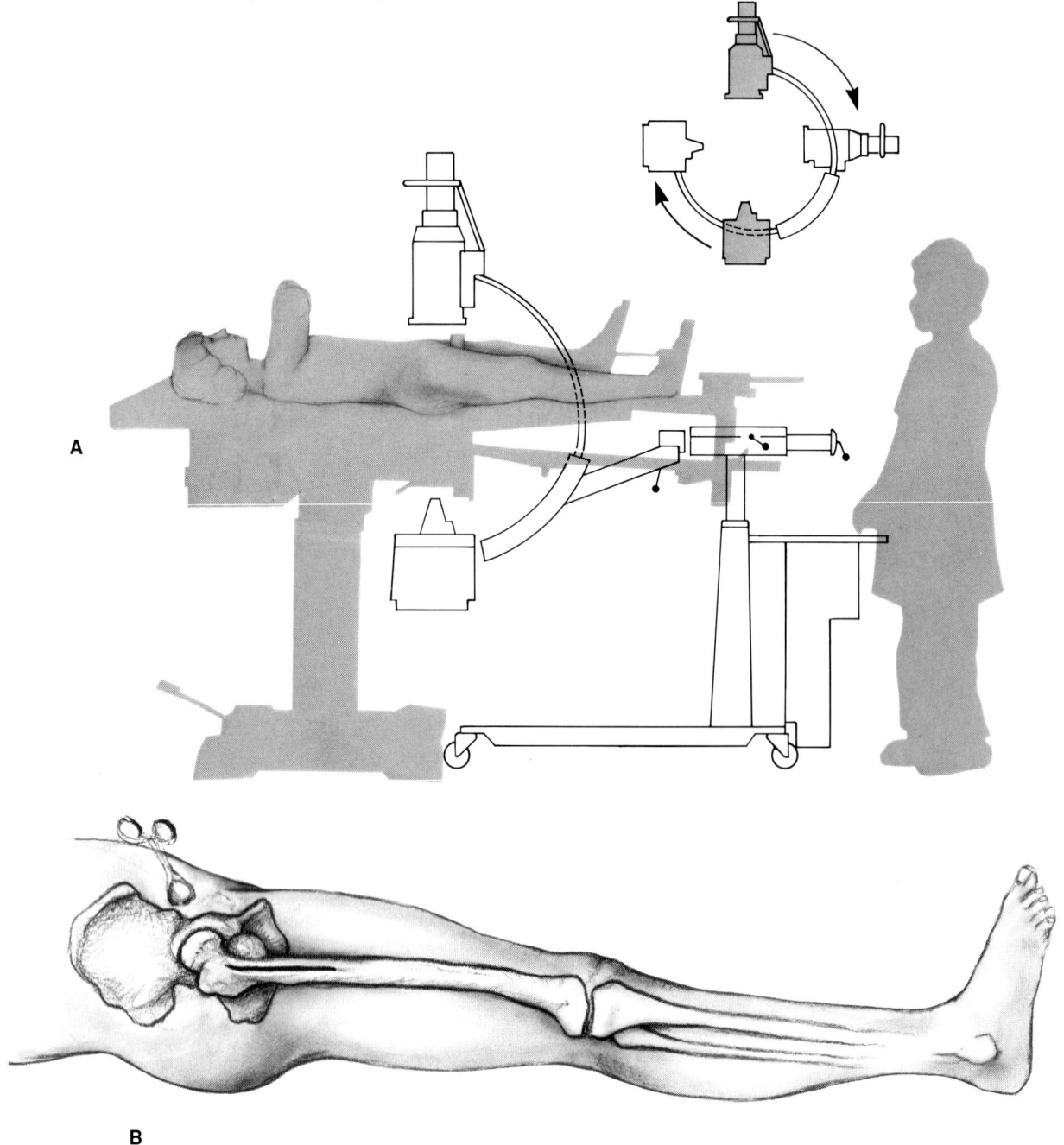

HIP PINNING FOR SUBCAPITAL FRACTURE OF FEMUR (MULTIPLE PIN FIXATION) (Plate 10-1)

GENERAL DISCUSSION. For the subcapital fracture of the femur, the use of multiple Knowles pins is a satisfactory method for internal fixation of the reduced subcapital fracture. Insertion of multiple Knowles pins parallel to each other across the fracture site carries no hazard of distracting the fracture and permits maintained apposition with any absorption of bone.

DETAILS OF PROCEDURE. Of utmost importance is good reduction of any displaced subcapital fracture prior to the insertion of any type of internal fixation. In contrast to intertrochanteric fractures, it may be necessary to hold the involved leg in 45° to 60° internal rotation on the orthopaedic operating table **(A)** to obtain good reduction of a subcapital fracture. Caution must be exercised against distraction of the fracture when traction is applied with the patient on the orthopaedic operating table under anesthesia. A towel clip is placed in the skin midway between the anterosuperior iliac spine and the pubic symphysis for use as a reference guide during the operative procedure. Satisfactory initial roentgenograms in the anteroposterior and tube-lateral projections must be obtained before the skin incision is made. A lateral thigh incision is used **(B)**.

(Plate 10-1) HIP PINNING FOR SUBCAPITAL FRACTURE OF FEMUR (MULTIPLE PIN FIXATION)

The dissection continues through the fascia lata **(C)** in the same line as the skin incision. The vastus lateralis is opened in line with its muscle fibers **(D)**. The previously placed towel clip, which can be palpated through the sterile drapes, in the inguinal area is used as an aid, and a drill hole larger than the diameter of a guide wire is made in preparation for insertion of a guide wire **(E)**.

The wire is inserted into the femoral neck and head at an angle between 130° and 150° to the longitudinal axis of the shaft of the femur **(F)**. With biplane roentgenographic

301

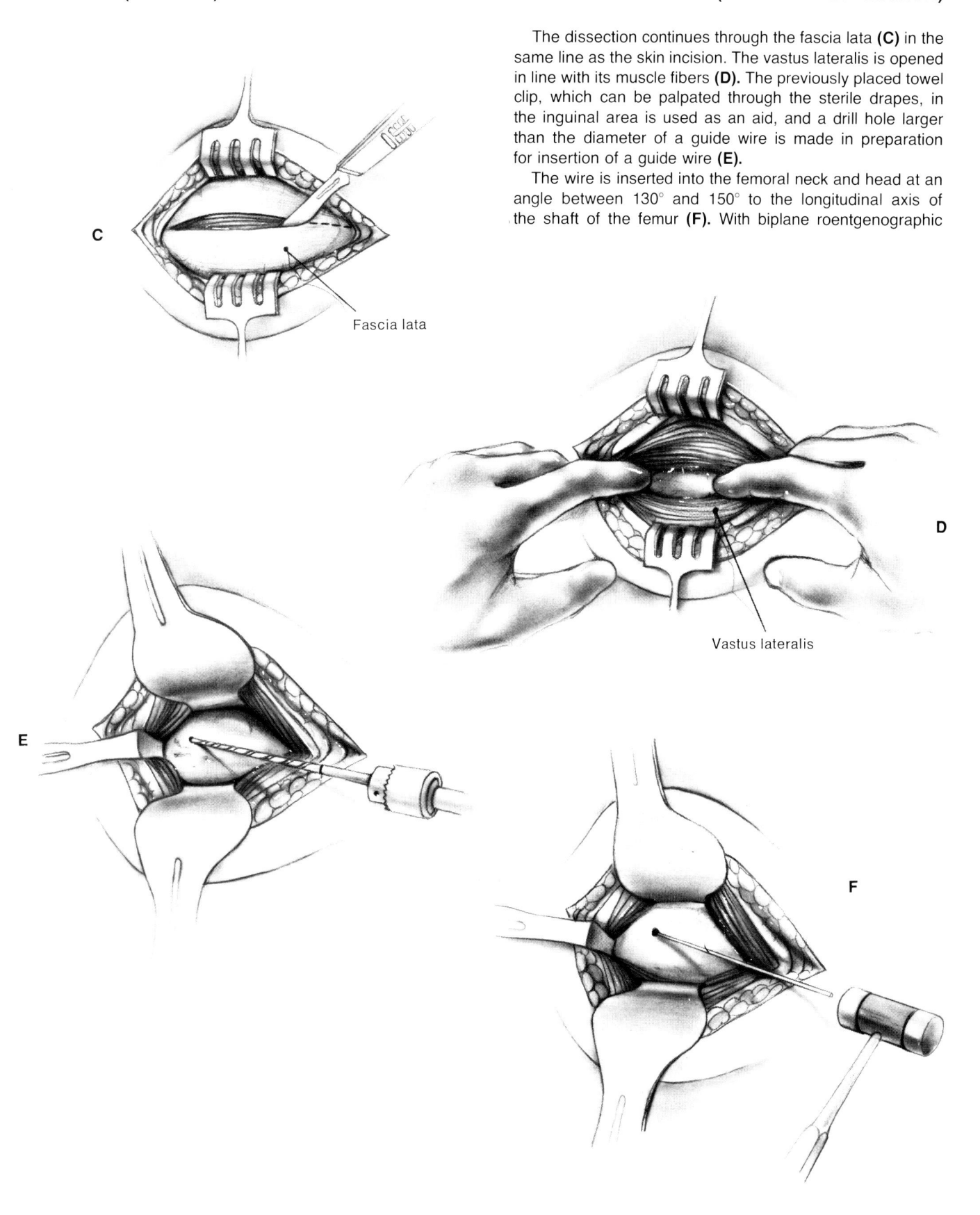

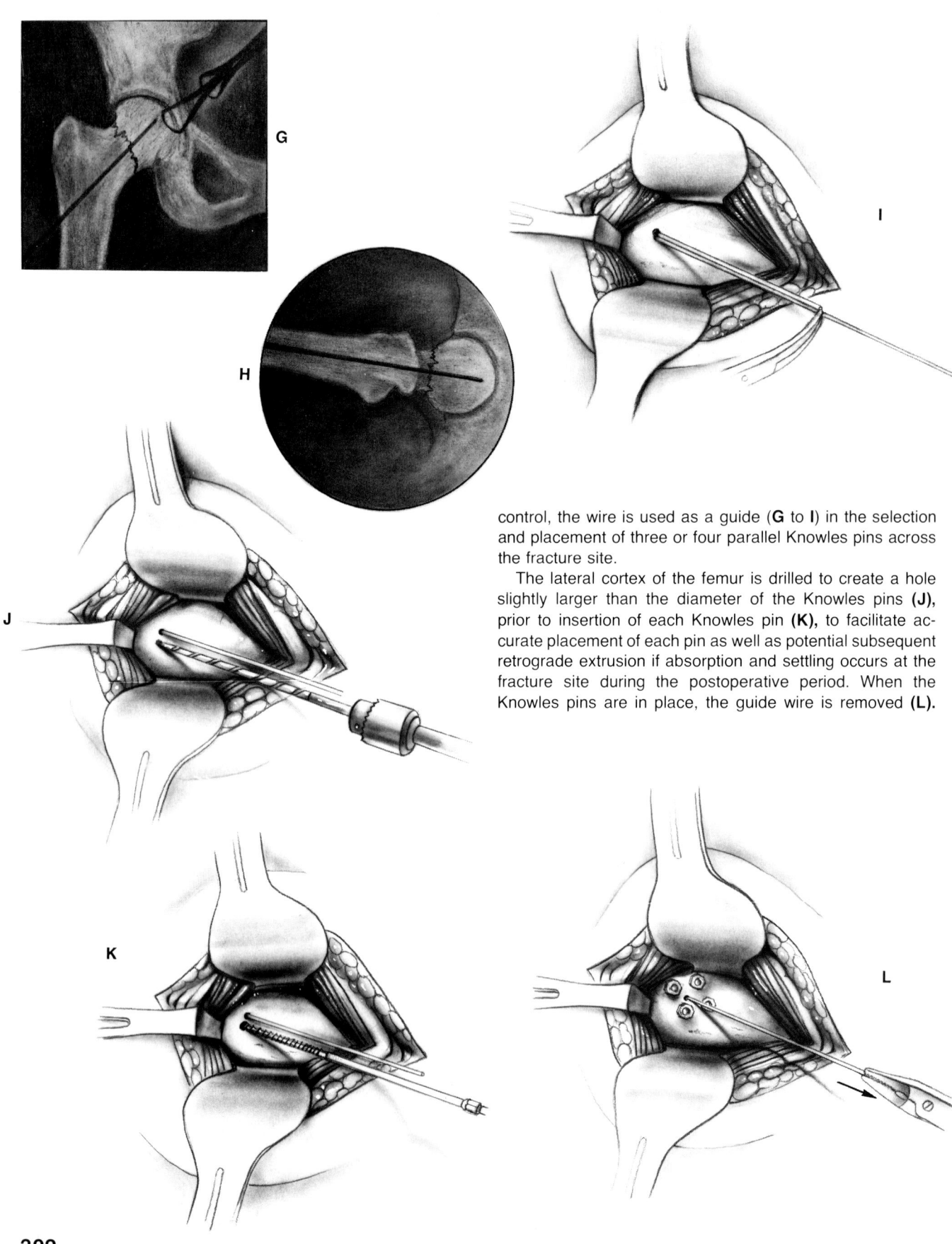

HIP PINNING FOR SUBCAPITAL FRACTURE OF FEMUR (MULTIPLE PIN FIXATION) (Plate 10-1)

control, the wire is used as a guide (**G** to **I**) in the selection and placement of three or four parallel Knowles pins across the fracture site.

The lateral cortex of the femur is drilled to create a hole slightly larger than the diameter of the Knowles pins (**J**), prior to insertion of each Knowles pin (**K**), to facilitate accurate placement of each pin as well as potential subsequent retrograde extrusion if absorption and settling occurs at the fracture site during the postoperative period. When the Knowles pins are in place, the guide wire is removed (**L**).

(Plate 10-1) HIP PINNING FOR SUBCAPITAL FRACTURE OF FEMUR (MULTIPLE PIN FIXATION)

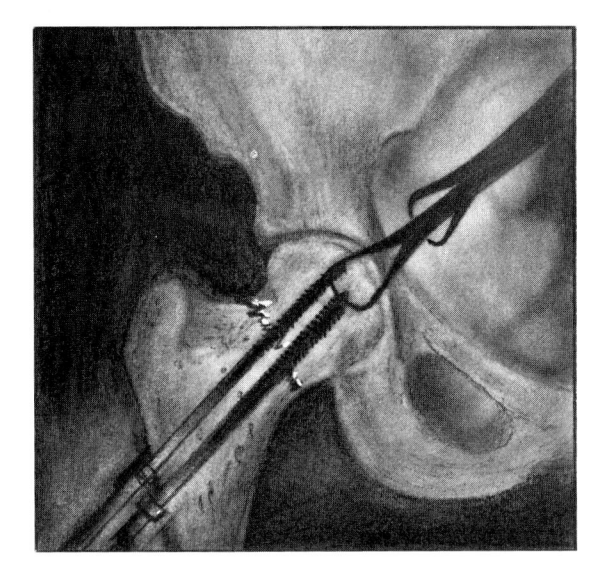

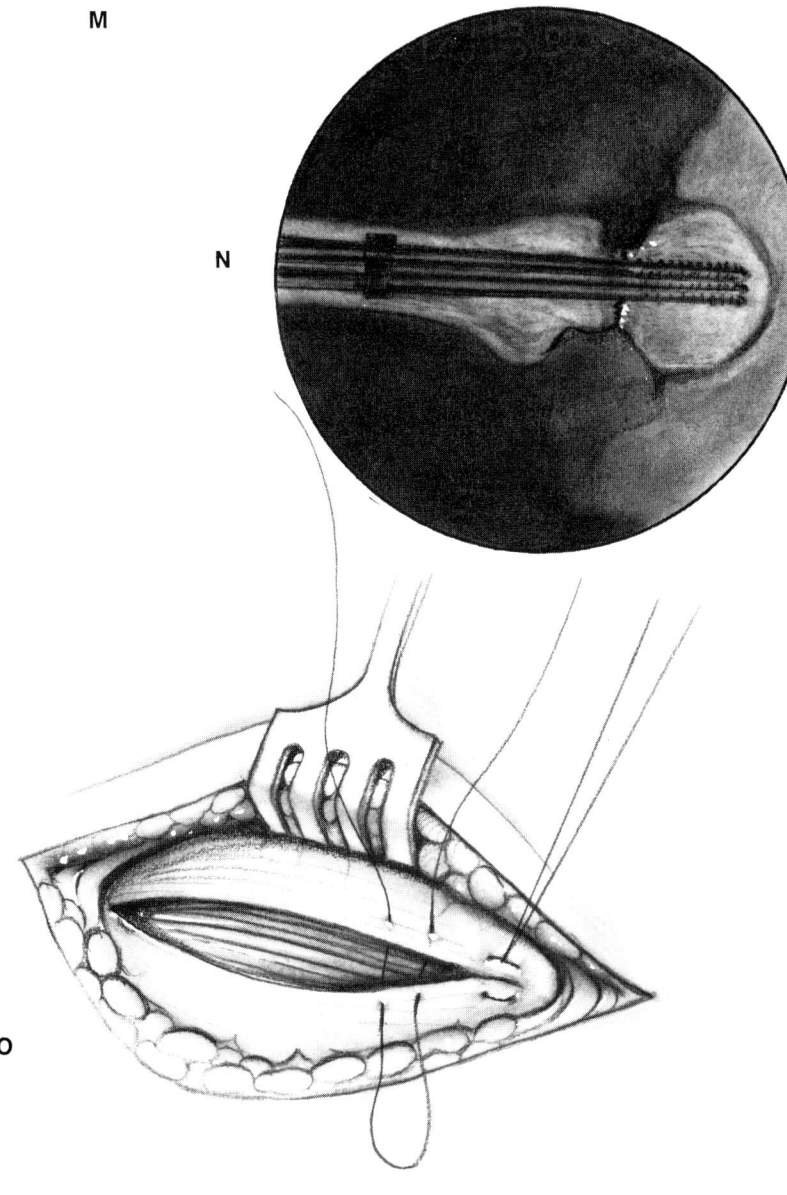

Each Knowles pin should obtain as much purchase in the proximal fragment as possible without entering the articular surface of the femoral head (**M** and **N**). It is best to have the entire threaded portion of each pin on the proximal side of the fracture. The Knowles pins should be evenly distributed in relation to the transverse cross-sectional diameter of the femoral neck and head for optimum fixation of the fracture, and the base of each Knowles pin should abut the lateral cortex of the femur in its final placement position. When good position of each of the pins has been confirmed roentgenographically in two planes at the operating table, the removable lateral portion of each Knowles pin is removed. The wound is closed in layers **(Q)**, including vastus lateralis muscle, fascia lata, subcutaneous tissue, and skin.

POSTOPERATIVE MANAGEMENT. The patient is helped to sit up in a chair on the first postoperative day and is given assistance in walking with crutches or a walkerette in the next few days. No weight bearing is permitted on the involved leg the first 4 weeks after surgery. With good reduction of a subcapital fracture and good internal fixation, healing of a subcapital fracture can usually be anticipated within 6 months, but the development of nonunion and/or avascular necrosis of the femoral head are constant potential complications with any complete fracture (and especially those severely displaced initially) in the subcapital area of the femoral neck. It is possible for nonunion of a fracture of the femoral neck to develop with good viability of the femoral head, and, conversely, avascular necrosis of the femoral head may develop as a delayed complication even several years after solid union of a fractured femoral neck.

Avascular necrosis of the femoral head is more likely to occur with the subcapital fracture that is severely displaced initially, but it can occur after an undisplaced subcapital fracture and is unpredictable as a potential late complication. On the other hand, nonunion of a subcapital fracture is unlikely to develop unless there has been some breakdown in the sequence of good fracture reduction, good operative internal fixation, and controlled aftercare.

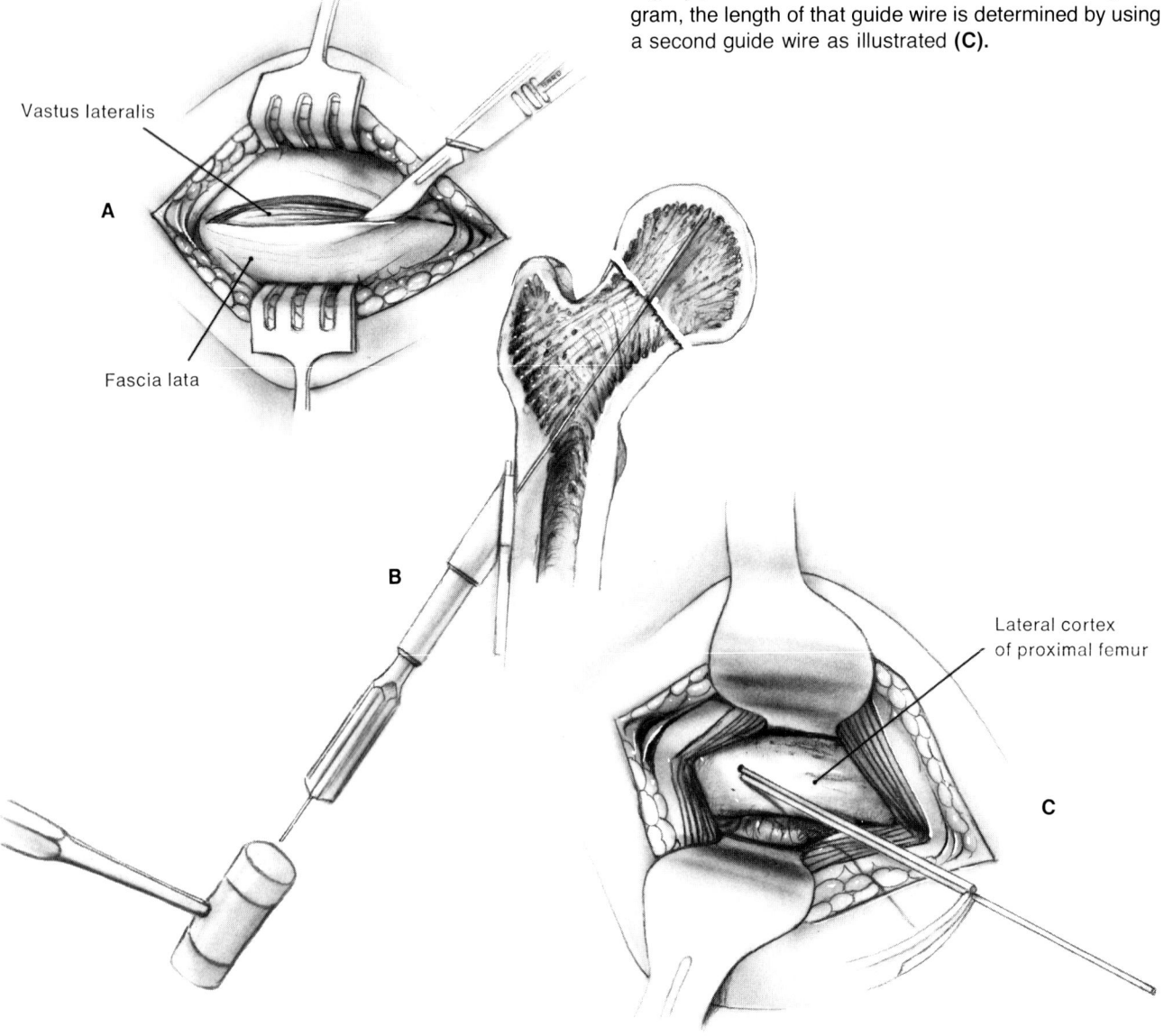

HIP PINNING FOR SUBCAPITAL FRACTURE OF FEMUR (TELESCOPING APPLIANCE) (Plate 10-2)

GENERAL DISCUSSION. A sliding or telescoping nail designed to permit firm impaction of the fracture at operation and to avoid any maintained distraction postoperatively may be used for internal fixation of the subcapital fracture. The quality of reduction of the fracture regardless of the appliance selected for internal fixation is of paramount importance. On the anteroposterior roentgenogram, a slight valgus position at the fracture site is acceptable, but there should be no medial displacement of the proximal fragment. If there is any displacement at the fracture site on the anteroposterior roentgenogram, the distal fragment must be medial to the proximal fragment and preferably not more than the thickness of the femoral calcar. On the lateral roentgenogram the head, neck, and shaft should be in the same plane.

DETAILS OF PROCEDURE. The lateral exposure to the proximal femur is used **(A)**. The incision should not be made until good reduction of the fracture has been obtained and confirmed with anteroposterior and lateral roentgenograms with the patient securely in place on the orthopaedic operating table.

After exposure of the lateral aspect of the proximal femur, the barrel and plate are held in reverse position against the shaft of the femur **(B)** as a ⅛-inch (0.32 cm) guide wire is inserted at the desired 150° angle to the longitudinal axis of the femoral shaft. A second or third hole may be drilled in the same manner at short intervals distally on the shaft. One-eight-inch guide wires are inserted through each of the prepared drill holes and tapped in with a small hammer. When a guide wire has been inserted into a position that is near the femoral calcar on the anteroposterior roentgenogram and in the midline or slightly posterior to the midline on the lateral roentgenogram, the length of that guide wire is determined by using a second guide wire as illustrated **(C)**.

(Plate 10-2) HIP PINNING FOR SUBCAPITAL FRACTURE OF FEMUR (TELESCOPING APPLIANCE)

A ½-inch drill bit is used to ream a hole in the lateral femoral cortex around the selected guide wire **(D)**. The nail-barrel telescoping assembly is fully extended, the entire assembly is driven into the femoral neck over the guide wire **(E)**, and roentgenograms are obtained. With the nail portion of the appliance in place extending to the subchondral region of the femoral head, the lateral plate is placed on the barrel of the assembly. The impactor is fitted to the plate and the barrel-plate assembly is driven inward, telescoping itself over the nail **(F)**. The plate is secured to the shaft of the femur with two transfixion screws. With the appliance in satisfactory position and secured to the shaft of the femur (**G** and **H**), all traction is removed from the affected leg and the impactor is fitted against the plate laterally and used to firmly impact the fracture before closure of the wound is started.

POSTOPERATIVE MANAGEMENT. The patient is helped to sit up in a chair on the first postoperative day and then, beginning on the second and third postoperative days, is helped to walk with a walkerette or crutches. The patient is permitted to "touch down" for balance on the involved leg but is advised against any greater weight on the involved hip until there is evidence of healing at the fracture site. Although these patients may lie directly on the involved side, they are advised against straight-leg hip flexion exercises from the supine position or side-lying abduction exercises of the involved leg until union of the fracture is complete. Massie states that usually by the end of a 6-week period the fracture line is no longer visible roentgenographically and full weight bearing can be permitted.

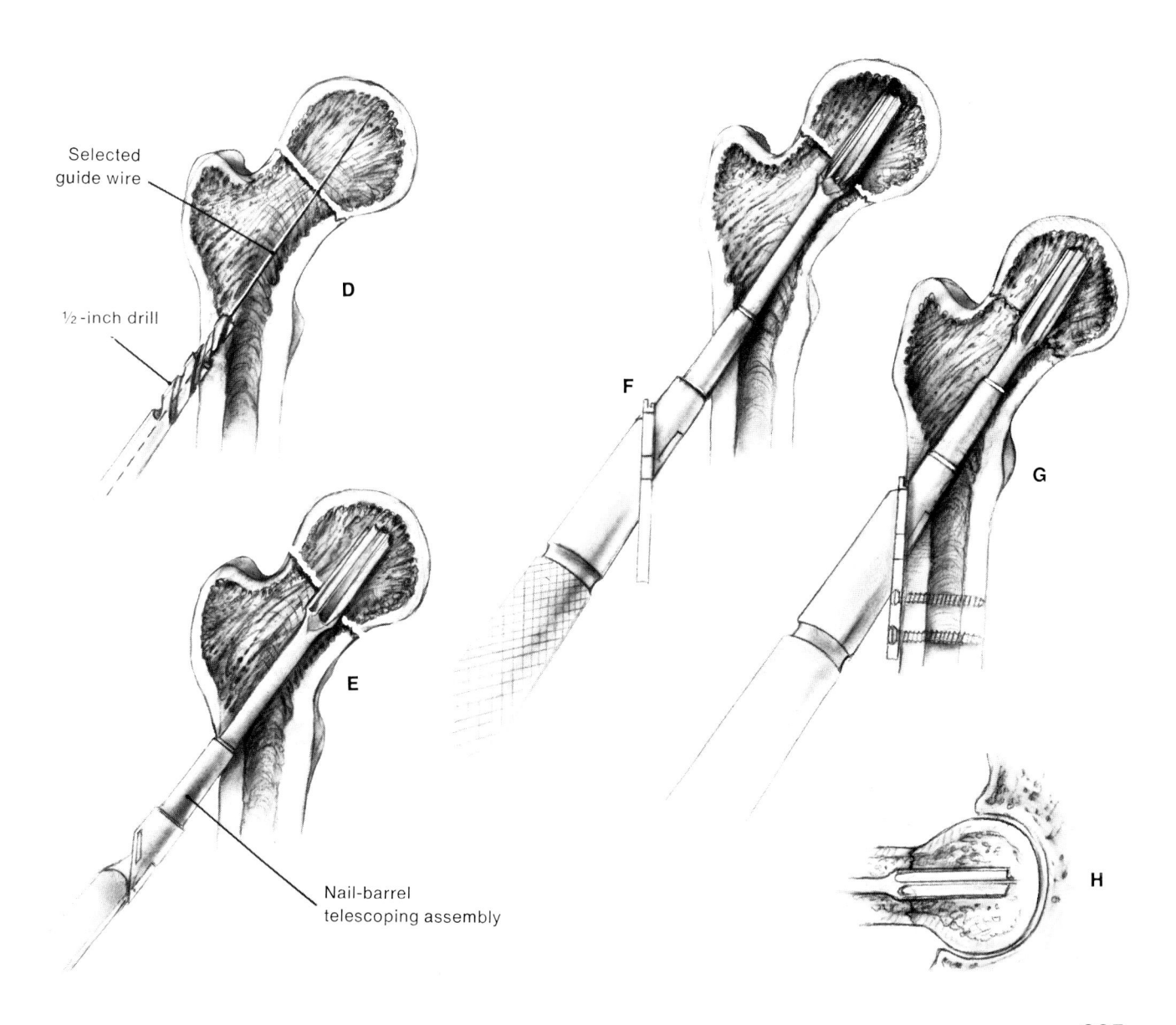

HIP PINNING FOR PERITROCHANTERIC FRACTURE OF FEMUR (COMPRESSION SCREW FIXATION) (Plate 10-3)

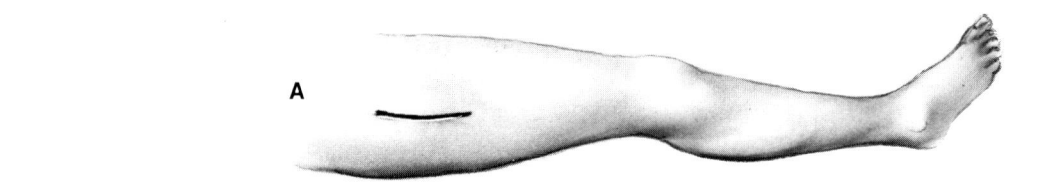

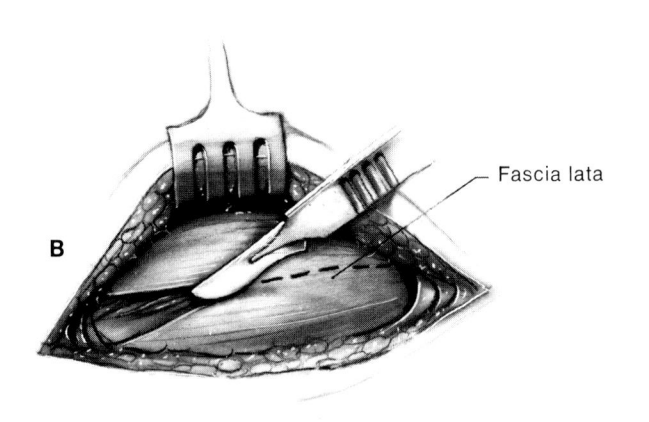

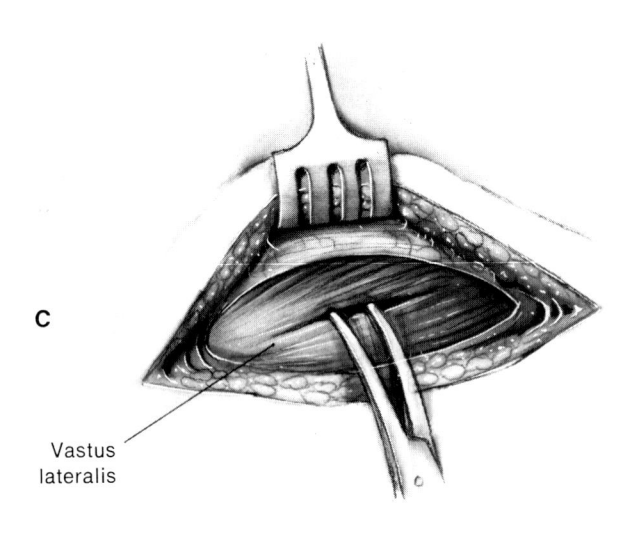

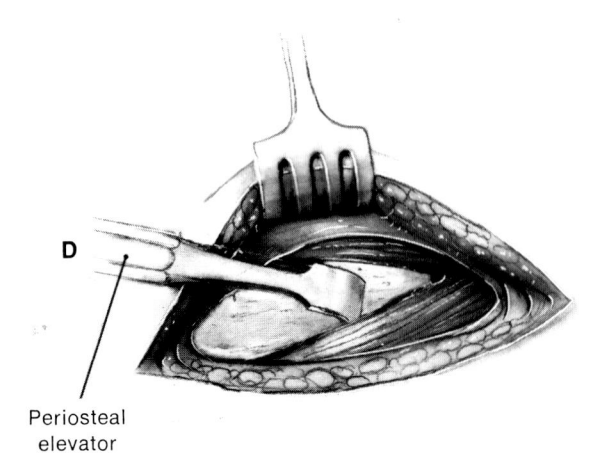

GENERAL DISCUSSION. Fractures in the intertrochanteric area respond well to internal fixation, and these fractures are best treated by reduction and internal fixation as soon after injury as possible. Operative fixation is conservative in the sense of preserving the vitality of the elderly patient who has sustained an intertrochanteric fracture. When these fractures occur in elderly people who are not ideal operative risks, prompt internal fixation of the fracture, if at all possible, may be critical to the survival of these patients. A number of appliances are in common usage, and one of the most satisfactory of these is the compression hip screw.

There are several advantages in using the compression hip screw for peritrochanteric fractures of the femur. It provides optimal fixation in the femoral head. Its integral sliding feature greatly reduces the problem of penetration of the acetabulum, and permits weight bearing forces to be transferred to bone rather than to the device itself. It allows maintenance of good apposition of the fracture surfaces, thus reducing the incidence of delayed union or nonunion. It is also possible to impact the reduction directly on the operating room table in a controlled manner.

DETAILS OF PROCEDURE. The patient is carefully placed on the orthopaedic traction table, and if any reduction of the fracture is required, this is carried out under anesthesia by applying gentle longitudinal traction and placing the hip and leg in approximately 10° abduction and the foot in a position of rotation between neutral and 15° internal rotation.

Biplane roentgenographic control is necessary initially to check the reduction of the fracture and subsequently throughout the procedure. Before the initial roentgenograms, a towel clip is placed in the inguinal area midway between the anterosuperior iliac spine and the pubic symphysis to coincide in the anteroposterior plane with the central portion of the hip joint and to serve as a guide during the subsequent insertion of one or more guide wires. The incision should not be made until a satisfactory reduction has been obtained and the capability of reproducing good quality roentgenograms in both the anteroposterior and tube-lateral projections has been demonstrated by the x-ray technician.

The lateral incision **(A)** is begun approximately 3 cm distal to the lateral prominence of the greater trochanter and is extended distally for a distance of 17 to 20 cm. The dissection is carried down to the fascia lata, which is divided longitudinally throughout the length of the skin incision **(B)**. Some fibers of the tensor fascia lata muscle may be encountered in dividing the upper portion of the fascia lata. The fibers

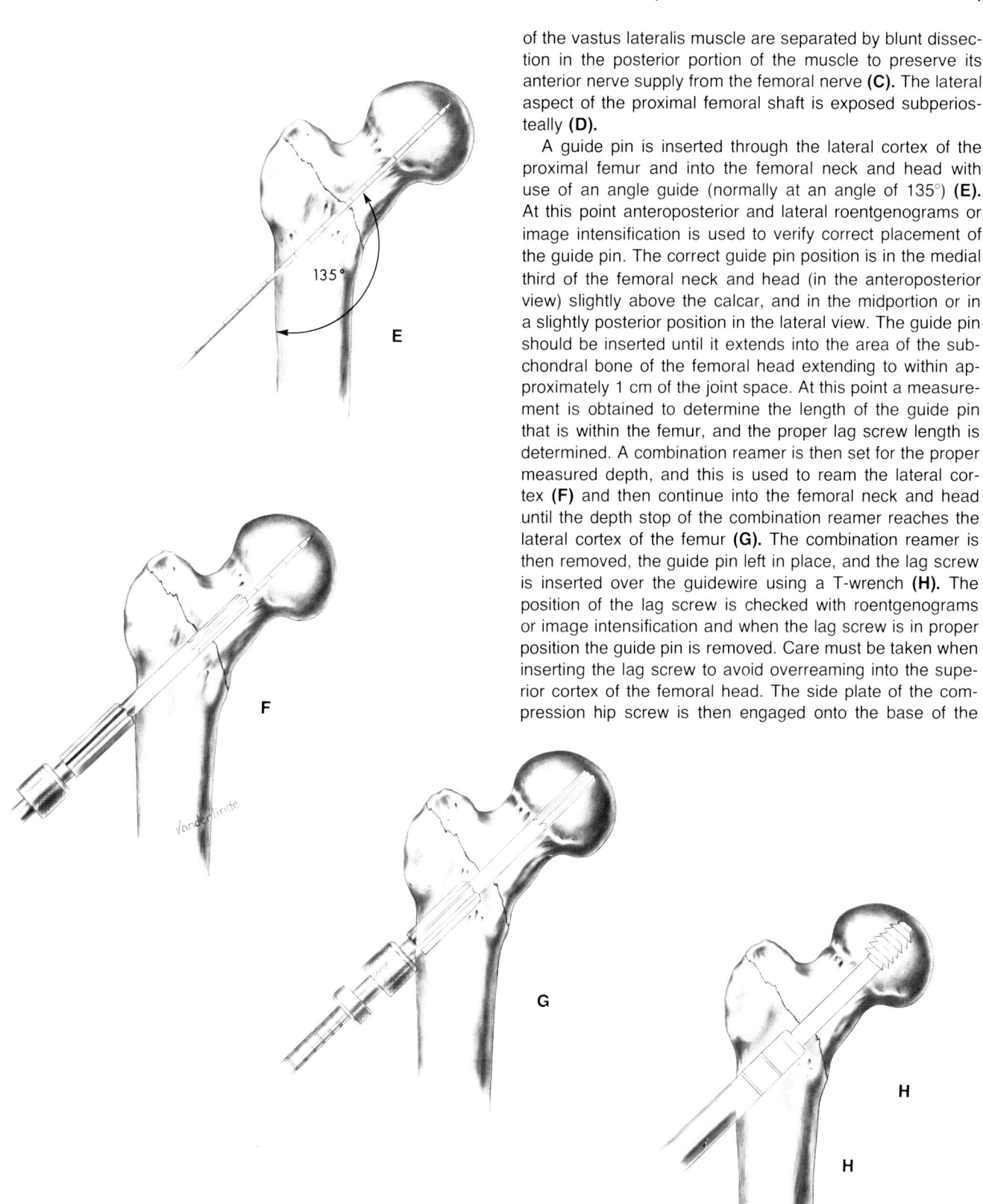

(Plate 10-3) HIP PINNING FOR PERITROCHANTERIC FRACTURE OF FEMUR (COMPRESSION SCREW FIXATION)

of the vastus lateralis muscle are separated by blunt dissection in the posterior portion of the muscle to preserve its anterior nerve supply from the femoral nerve **(C)**. The lateral aspect of the proximal femoral shaft is exposed subperiosteally **(D)**.

A guide pin is inserted through the lateral cortex of the proximal femur and into the femoral neck and head with use of an angle guide (normally at an angle of 135°) **(E)**. At this point anteroposterior and lateral roentgenograms or image intensification is used to verify correct placement of the guide pin. The correct guide pin position is in the medial third of the femoral neck and head (in the anteroposterior view) slightly above the calcar, and in the midportion or in a slightly posterior position in the lateral view. The guide pin should be inserted until it extends into the area of the subchondral bone of the femoral head extending to within approximately 1 cm of the joint space. At this point a measurement is obtained to determine the length of the guide pin that is within the femur, and the proper lag screw length is determined. A combination reamer is then set for the proper measured depth, and this is used to ream the lateral cortex **(F)** and then continue into the femoral neck and head until the depth stop of the combination reamer reaches the lateral cortex of the femur **(G)**. The combination reamer is then removed, the guide pin left in place, and the lag screw is inserted over the guidewire using a T-wrench **(H)**. The position of the lag screw is checked with roentgenograms or image intensification and when the lag screw is in proper position the guide pin is removed. Care must be taken when inserting the lag screw to avoid overreaming into the superior cortex of the femoral head. The side plate of the compression hip screw is then engaged onto the base of the

307

HIP PINNING FOR PERITROCHANTERIC FRACTURE OF FEMUR (COMPRESSION SCREW FIXATION) (Plate 10-3)

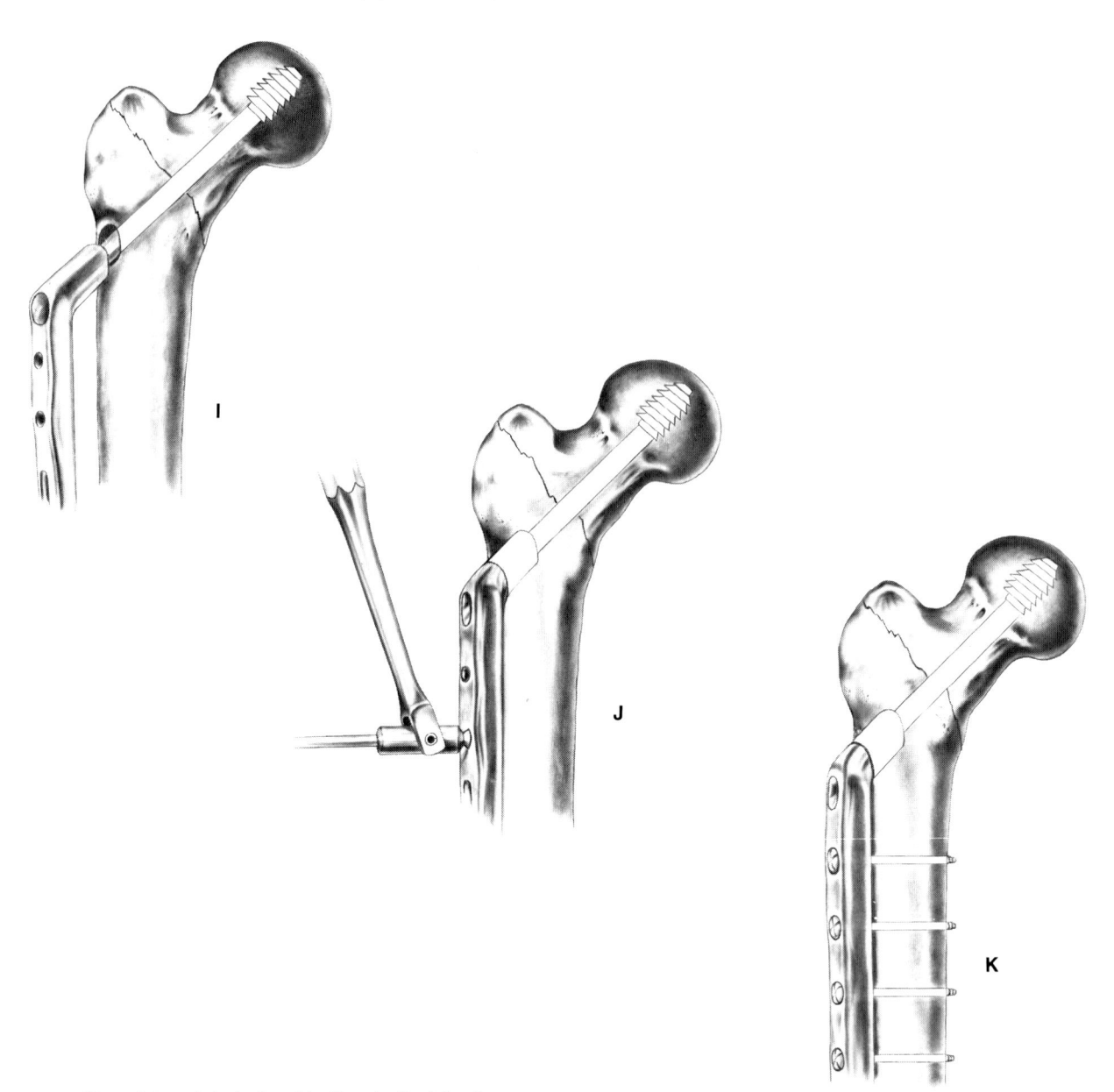

lag screw **(I)** and the plate is fixed to the shaft of the femur with transfixion screws **(J, K)**. When the bone screws are securely in place, any traction on the patient's leg may be released and the fracture may be impacted by screwing the compression screw into the proximal end of the side plate. Final roentgenograms or image intensification should be used prior to closing the wound not only to check the final position of the compression lag screw but also to make certain that the fracture is completely compressed and there is no gap or abnormal angulation at the fracture site.

The wound is irrigated with sterile saline solution and then closed in layers by successively approximating the vastus lateralis muscle, fascia lata, subcutaneous tissue, and skin.

At the end of the procedure the involved leg is carefully protected as the patient is transferred from the operating table to bed.

POSTOPERATIVE MANAGEMENT. The patient is permitted to be out of bed, sitting in a chair on the first-day after surgery. The "extended knee" position while sitting in a chair is avoided. Assistance in walking with crutches or a walkerette is begun on the second or third postoperative day. If the fracture is stable, the patient may be permitted to "touch down" with the foot of the involved leg for balance only, but otherwise no additional weight bearing is allowed until there is roentgenographic evidence of healing at the fracture site. Unprotected full weight bearing is not permitted until evidence of adequate healing is noted, usually a matter of 4 to 5 months.

(Plate 10-4) HIP PINNING FOR PERITROCHANTERIC FRACTURE OF FEMUR (EXTRASTRONG NAIL AND BOLT FIXATION)

GENERAL DISCUSSION. The use of a strong appliance like that designed by Holt to permit early weight bearing for hip fractures in the trochanteric region is a good alternative method for operative fixation of these fractures. The proper use of this appliance permits early walking on the involved leg and earlier return to self-sufficiency for patients with intertrochanteric and base-of-neck fractures of the femur. For patients with fractures of the trochanteric region who will not be capable of handling crutches or walking without weight bearing in the postoperative period (for example, very elderly patients or patients with unrelated disorders such as parkinsonism), the use of a Holt appliance for internal fixation can make the difference between early walking or a bed and chair existence until the fracture is healed. A patient is a mental institution, incapable of comprehending or maintaining a non-weight-bearing status on one hip, would also be a good candidate for the use of this appliance for a base-of-neck or intertrochanteric fracture. There would be no advantage in using this appliance if, for any reason, the patient was incapable of walking before the fracture was sustained.

DETAILS OF PROCEDURE. The procedure is carried out in the same manner as outlined for insertion of a Jewett appliance with a few specific modifications. Accurate reduction of the femoral calcar is essential, because without integrity of the femoral calcar on both the anteroposterior and lateral roentgenograms, weight bearing may cause significant migration of the nail or loss of reduction or both. The necessary accessories include a ½-inch cannulated drill, a $^5/_{32}$-inch drill bit, Barr bolts and nuts, and a special wrench for the hexagonal nuts in addition to a full set of different size Holt nails. The incision should be 3 to 5 cm longer than usual to facilitate application of the hexagonal nuts to the Barr bolts on the medial aspect of the femoral shaft. Use of the Barr bolts and nuts necessitates reflection of the muscles from the medial aspect of the proximal femoral shaft. The wound exposure must permit the muscles to be reflected easily without any additional bleeding. The nail-plate angle is 130°, and an angle guide must be used for insertion of one or more initial guide wires (**A** and **B**).

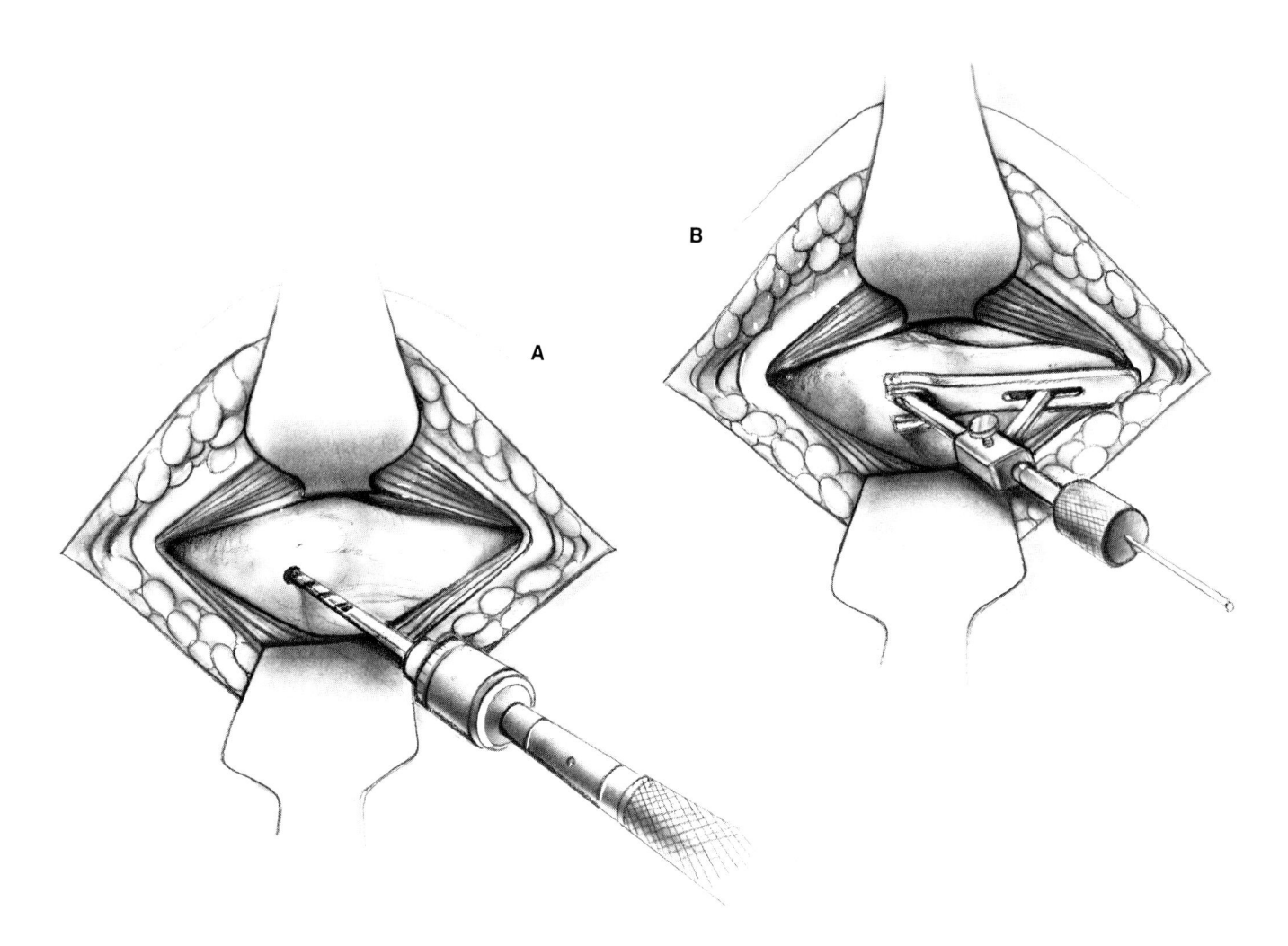

HIP PINNING FOR PERITROCHANTERIC FRACTURE OF FEMUR (EXTRASTRONG NAIL AND BOLT FIXATION) (Plate 10-4)

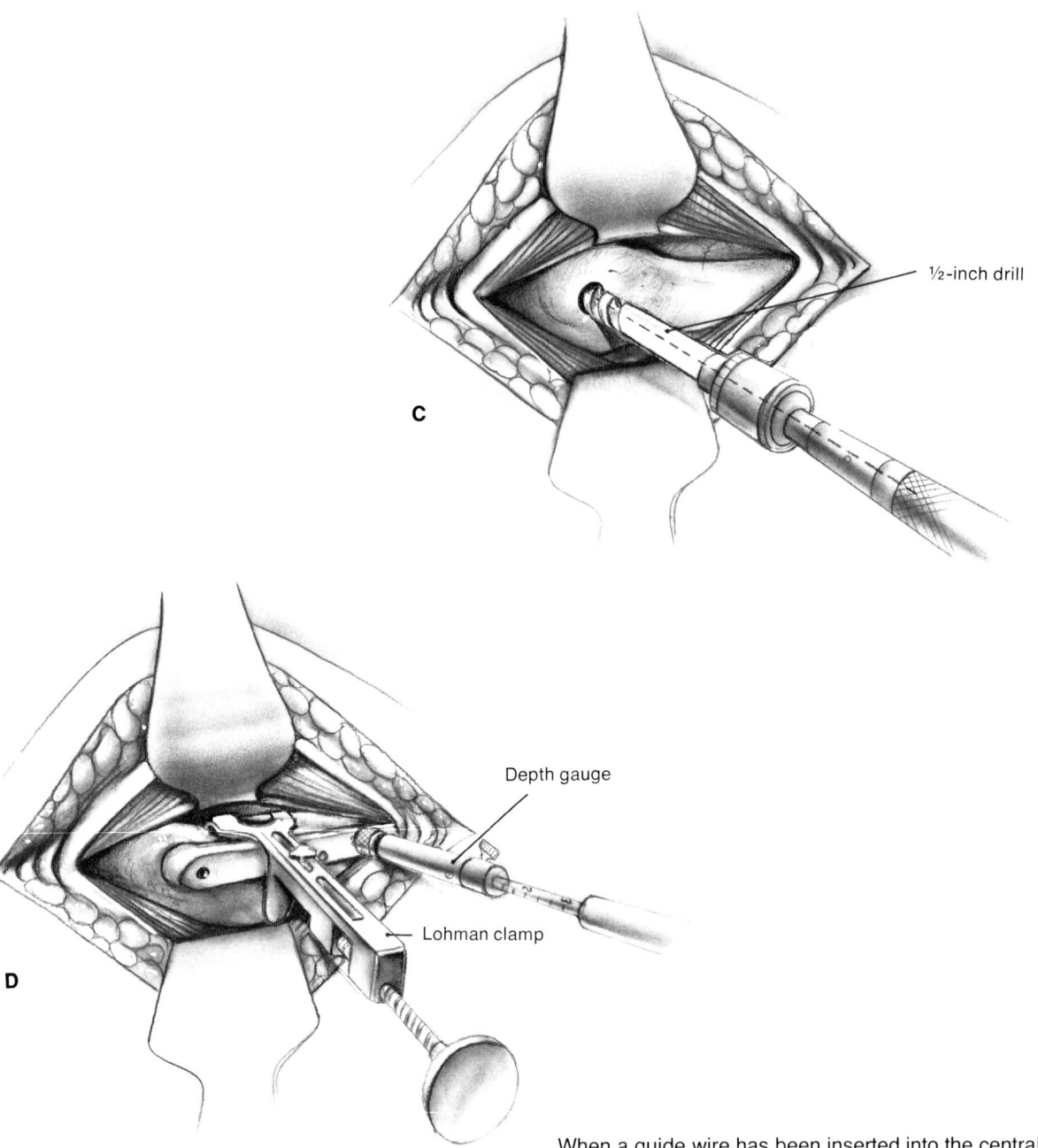

When a guide wire has been inserted into the central portion of the femoral head on both the anteroposterior and lateral projections, a ½-inch cannulated drill is used to bore into the femoral neck and head **(C)**. Caution must be exercised to avoid excessive penetration of the ½-inch-diameter drill to the cartilaginous surface of the femoral head. A Holt appliance is selected that will extend beyond the central portion of the femoral head, but it must remain at least 0.5 cm from the joint and this appliance is placed (not hammered or driven) into the ½-inch hole so that the plate conforms to the shaft of the femur **(D)**. Distraction of the fracture fragments must be avoided. A Lohman clamp holds the appliance in place until roentgenograms have confirmed satisfactory length and position of the nail.

(Plate 10-4) HIP PINNING FOR PERITROCHANTERIC FRACTURE OF FEMUR (EXTRASTRONG NAIL AND BOLT FIXATION)

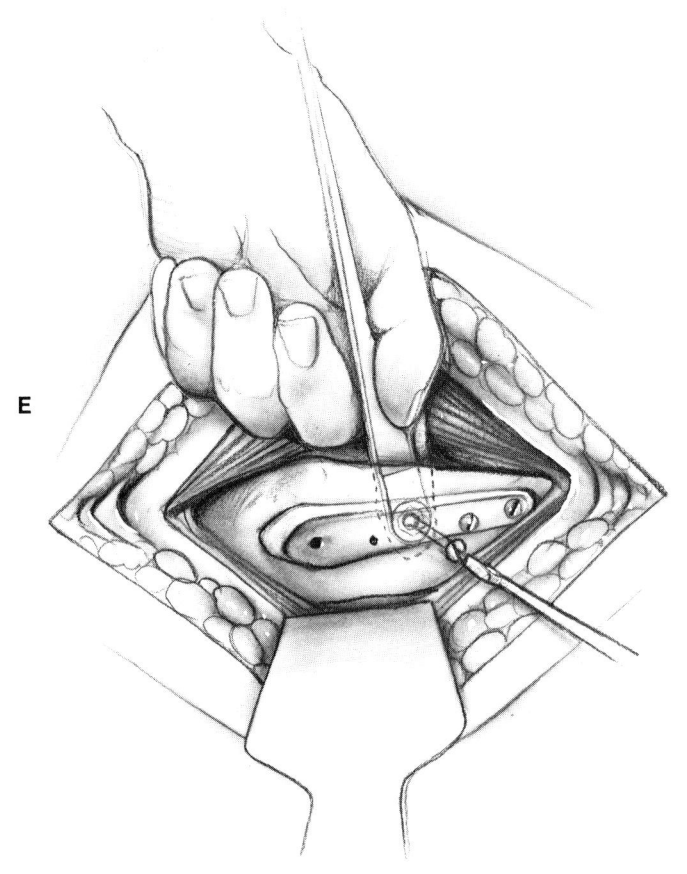

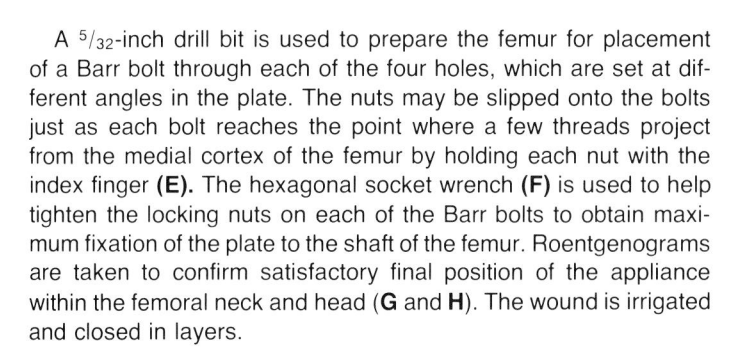

A $^5/_{32}$-inch drill bit is used to prepare the femur for placement of a Barr bolt through each of the four holes, which are set at different angles in the plate. The nuts may be slipped onto the bolts just as each bolt reaches the point where a few threads project from the medial cortex of the femur by holding each nut with the index finger **(E)**. The hexagonal socket wrench **(F)** is used to help tighten the locking nuts on each of the Barr bolts to obtain maximum fixation of the plate to the shaft of the femur. Roentgenograms are taken to confirm satisfactory final position of the appliance within the femoral neck and head **(G** and **H)**. The wound is irrigated and closed in layers.

POSTOPERATIVE MANAGEMENT. The patient is helped to sit up in a chair on the first postoperative day, and as soon as wound discomfort will permit, is helped to walk with a light walkerette. He is permitted to bear full weight as tolerated on the involved limb. As soon as the patient is able to use a cane in the opposite hand, he is encouraged to do so. The cane is discontinued when the patient can walk comfortably and with confidence without it. With a stable trochanteric fracture and proper insertion of the Holt appliance, the patient can be walking with minimal assistance a few weeks after hip pinning, and, as a rule, the fracture will be well healed clinically and roentgenographically within 3 to 4 months.

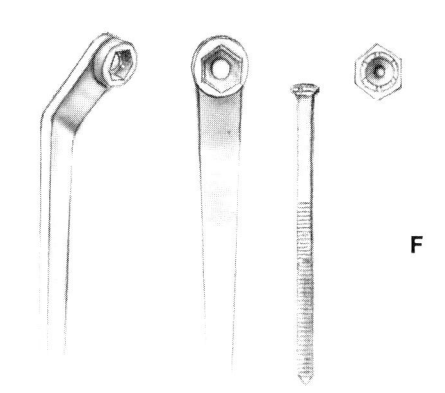

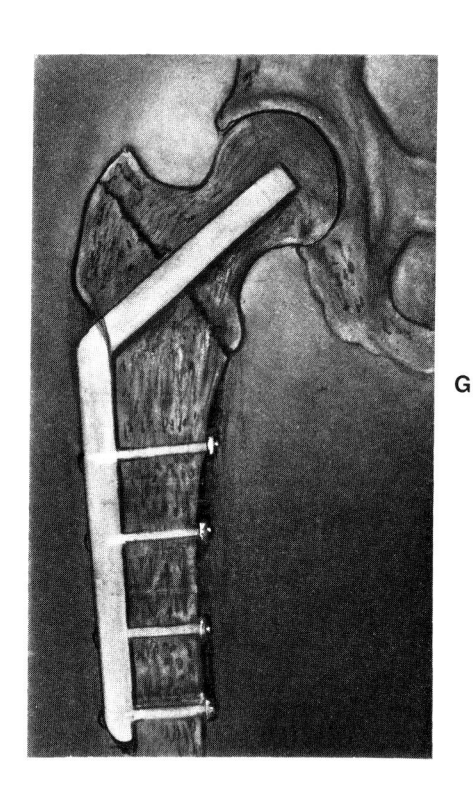

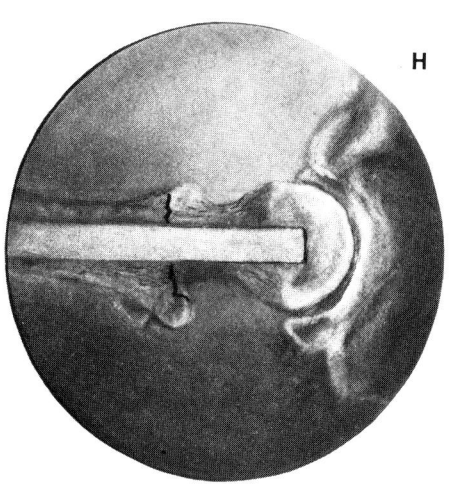

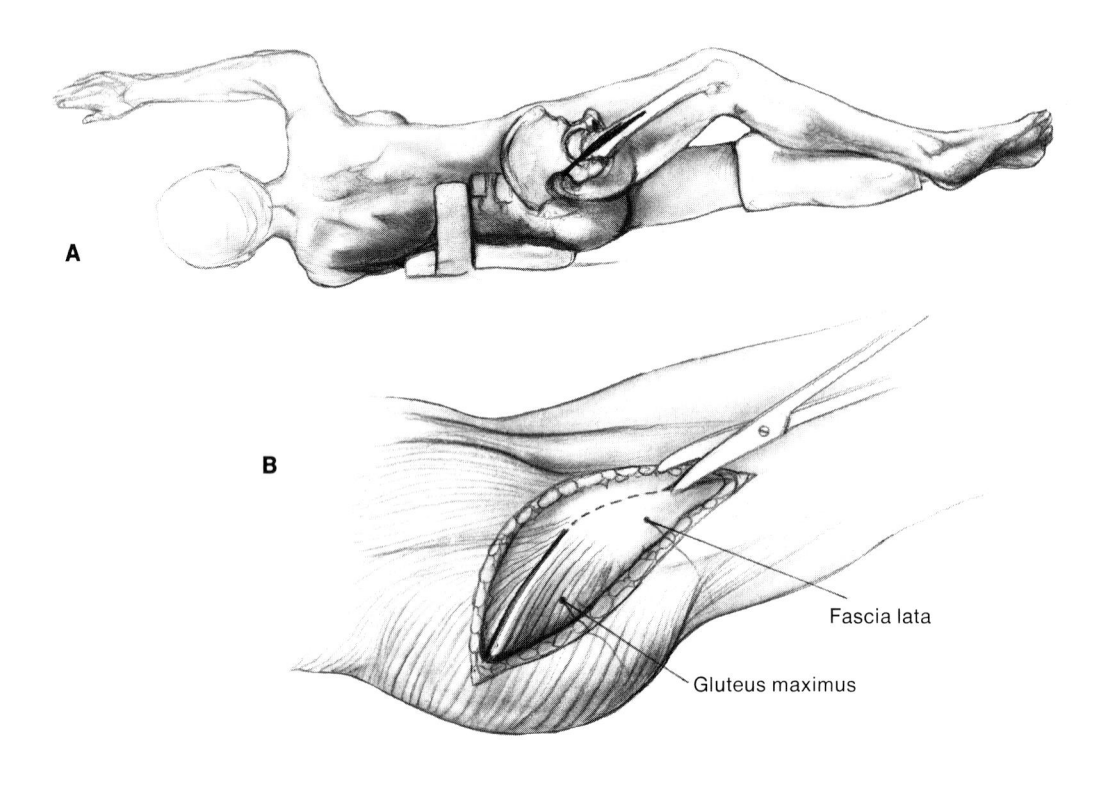

INSERTION OF FEMORAL HEAD PROSTHESIS (Plate 10-5)

GENERAL DISCUSSION. Controversy still exists over the routine use of an endoprosthesis for the treatment of all displaced femoral neck fractures. The decision-making process for the use of an endoprosthesis occurs in three phases: first, the decision must be made whether to use internal fixation or an endoprosthesis; next it is necessary to identify the circumstances that will require the use of methylmethacrylate for added fixation; and finally it is important to determine whether total hip reconstruction should be performed as an initial procedure.

Certain situations warrant the use of an endoprosthesis: a displaced high subcapital comminuted fracture of the femoral neck; an irreducible intracapsular fracture of the femur; nonunion and/or avascular necrosis following pinning of an intracapsular fracture of the femoral neck; a pathologic fracture of the femoral head or neck; and severe osteoporosis of the proximal femur in a patient with mental disease, Parkinsonism, hemiplegia, or blindness. Age alone is not an absolute indication.

The specific indications for the use of a cemented endoprosthesis are irreducible intracapsular fracture of the femur; severe osteoporosis of the proximal femur in which fixation in the cancellous bone by an interference fit would be inappropriate; a pathologic fracture of the femoral head or neck; avascular necrosis of the femoral head in a patient with a shortened life span following chronic kidney disease and renal transplantation, systemic lupus erythematosis, or other diseases; and associated illnesses such as Parkinsonism, mental illness, or blindness.

On occasion total hip reconstruction may be indicated for the treatment of an intracapsular fracture of the femur in a patient with preexisting osteoarthritis of the hip, in a rheumatoid patient with severe hip involvement, or in a patient with acetabular involvement following collapse of an avascular femoral head.

DETAILS OF PROCEDURE. The hip prosthesis may be inserted through an anterior, lateral, or posterior approach. The posterior approach is most commonly used.

The patient is placed in the lateral position on the unaffected side and securely supported in this position with kidney rests anteriorly and posteriorly **(A)**. The entire leg is draped free to permit movement of the extremity throughout the procedure.

The incision extends from a point 5 cm below the postero-inferior iliac spine toward the posterior aspect of the greater trochanter and then distally along the posterior aspect of the proximal femur approximately 7 cm **(A)**. The dissection is continued to expose the fibers of the gluteus maximus muscle and the fascia lata. The leg is abducted, and the fascia lata is opened longitudinally posterior to the shaft of the femur **(B)**. The opening in the fascia lata is extended superiorly until fibers of the gluteus maximus muscle are encountered, and the gluteus maximus is then divided bluntly along the oblique course of its muscle fibers toward the posterior ilium. At this time, the sciatic nerve should be identified just posterior to the piriformis muscle, coursing distally parallel to and 2 to 3 cm posterior to the proximal shaft of the femur **(C)**. The sciatic nerve must be protected throughout the procedure.

(Plate 10-5) INSERTION OF FEMORAL HEAD PROSTHESIS

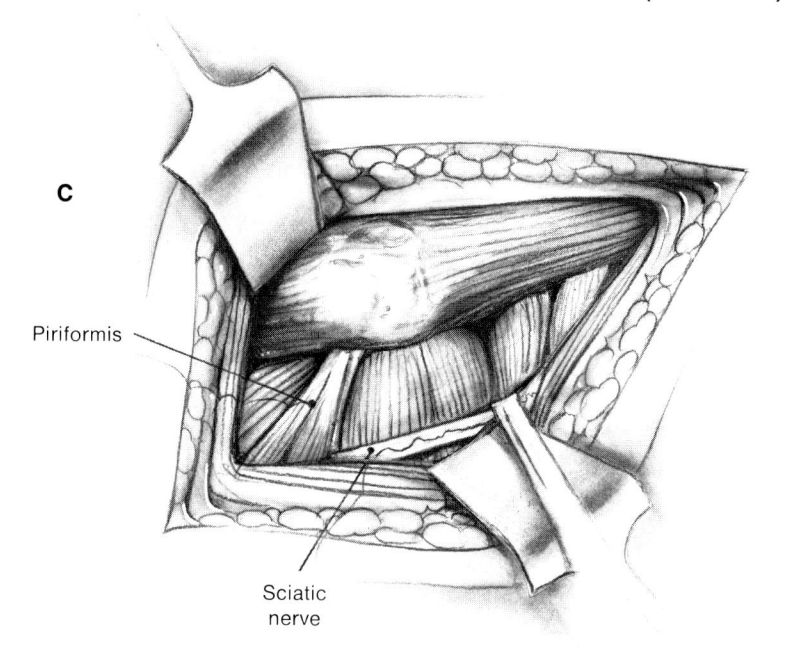

The short external rotators (the gemelli and obturator internus muscles) are divided at their point of insertion into the proximal femur. The tendinous insertion of the piriformis into the tip of the greater trochanter should be divided to improve exposure. A linear incision is made in the posterior aspect of the hip joint capsule parallel to the femoral neck and extending up to, but not into, the acetabular labrum (**D** and **E**). The femoral head is removed. The femoral head fragment is retained for subsequent caliper measurement to determine the proper prosthetic head diameter **(F)**. The lesser trochanter is identified, and the femoral neck is shaped to conform to the base of the prosthesis in a manner that retains an anteversion angle of 15° and 1.5 cm of femoral calcar (one finger's breadth) above the lesser trochanter for seating of the prosthesis.

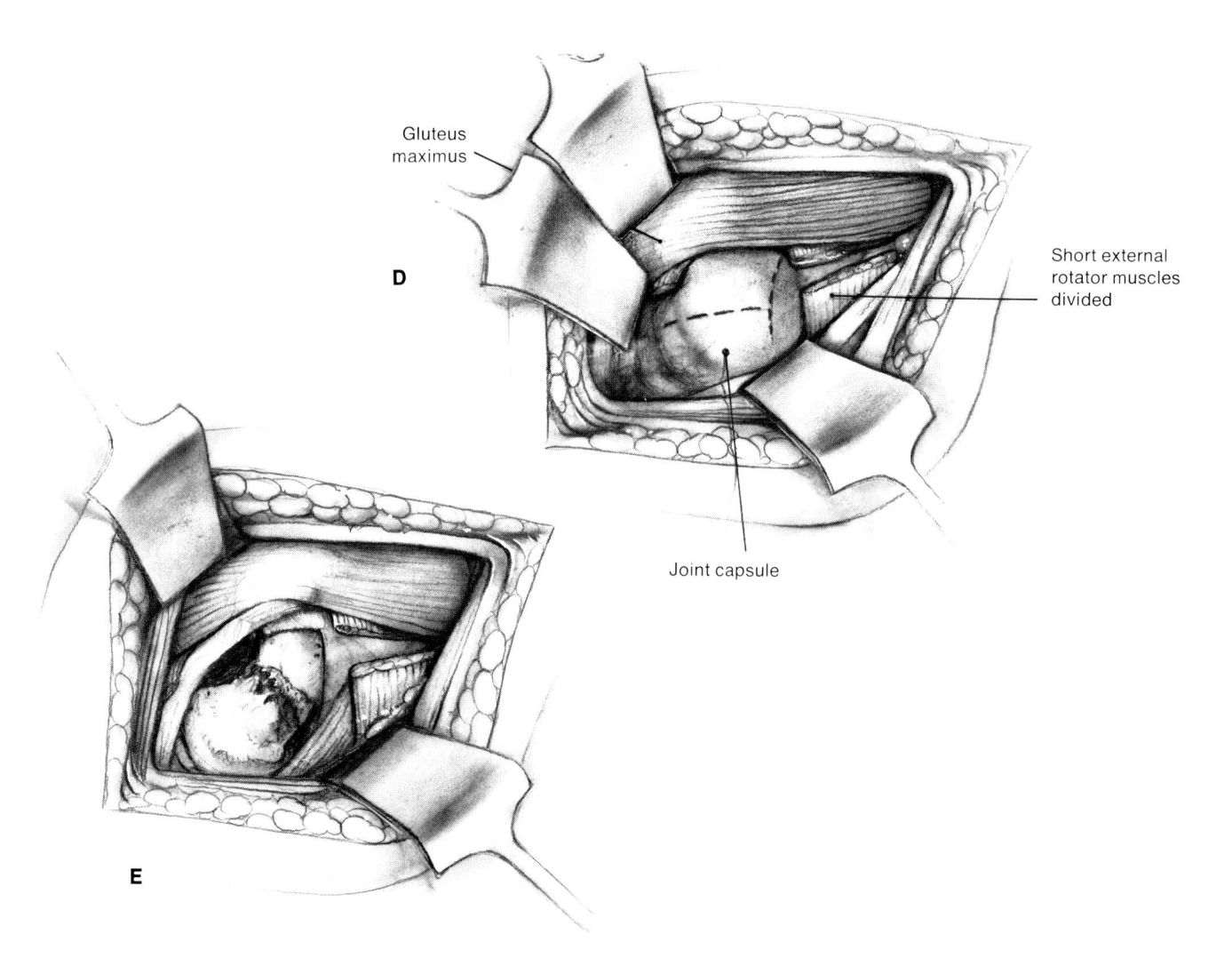

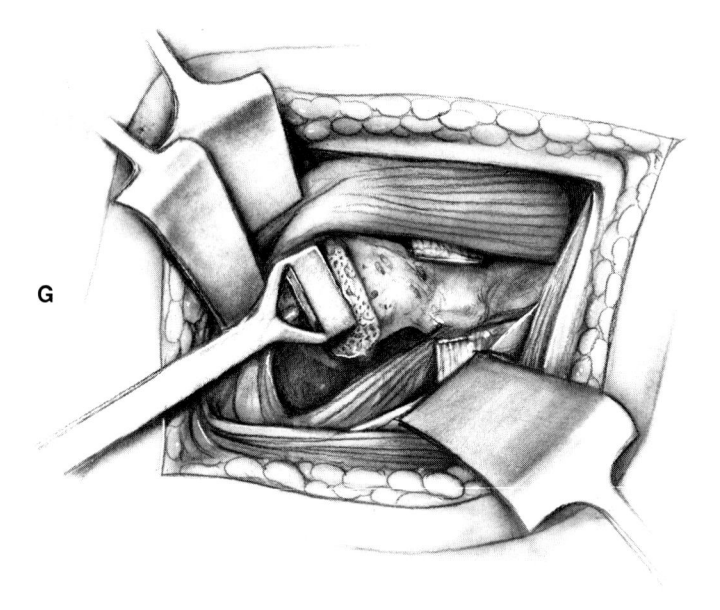

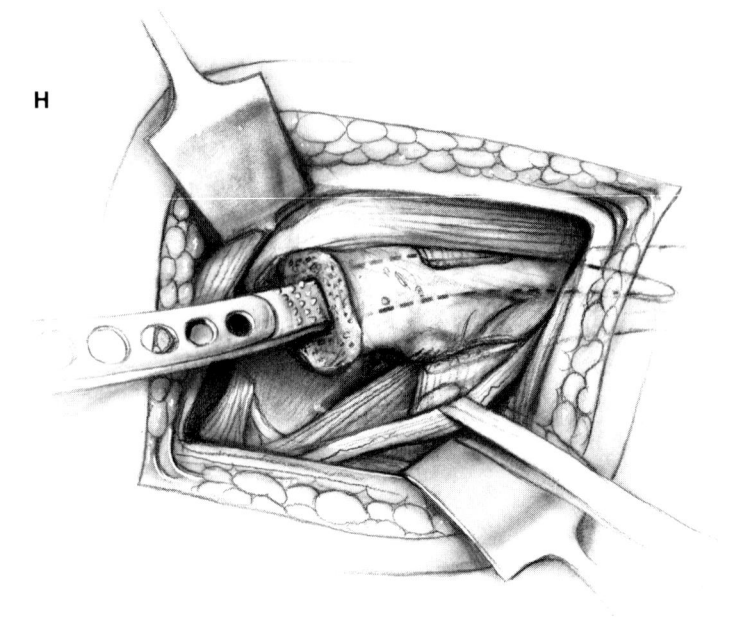

INSERTION OF FEMORAL HEAD PROSTHESIS (Plate 10-5)

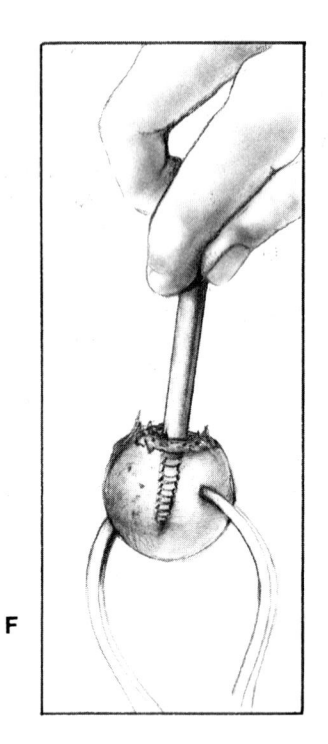

A rectangular punch (**G**) is used to remove bone from the trochanteric region of the femur in preparation for rasping (**H**) and ultimate seating of the prosthetic stem. Caution should be exercised against removing too much bone from the femoral shaft. Periodic testing by placement of the prosthesis in the shaft of the femur is useful in determining the proper amount of bone that should be removed with the rasp while the channel is prepared within the proximal femur so the base of the prosthesis can be easily inserted to within 1 cm of the femoral calcar. The prosthesis is then removed, and the prosthetic fenestrations are filled with cancellous bone (taken from the femoral neck or femoral head).

(Plate 10-5) INSERTION OF FEMORAL HEAD PROSTHESIS

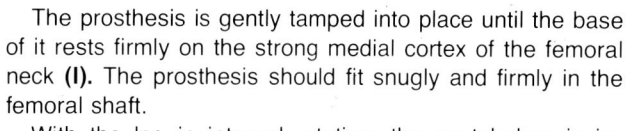

The prosthesis is gently tamped into place until the base of it rests firmly on the strong medial cortex of the femoral neck (I). The prosthesis should fit snugly and firmly in the femoral shaft.

With the leg in internal rotation, the acetabulum is inspected, irrigated thoroughly, and suctioned to be certain that no bone fragments remain within or near the acetabulum. Reaming of acetabular cartilage is avoided unless absolutely necessary. Routine removal of the ligamentum teres serves no useful purpose. Reduction of the prosthesis (K) should be a combination of manual placement of the prosthetic head into the acetabulum with carefully coordinated gentle extension and external rotation of the leg by an assistant. The prosthetic head should not be reduced into the acetabulum by forceful manipulation of the leg alone.

Closure of the joint capsule is facilitated by placing the leg in some degree of external rotation as previously placed sutures in the capsule are tied (J). The short external rotator muscles are resutured. The leg is placed in slight abduction to facilitate reapproximation of the fascia lata, gluteus maximus muscle, and the remainder of the wound. The patient's leg is carefully protected as the patient is moved directly to bed from the operating table.

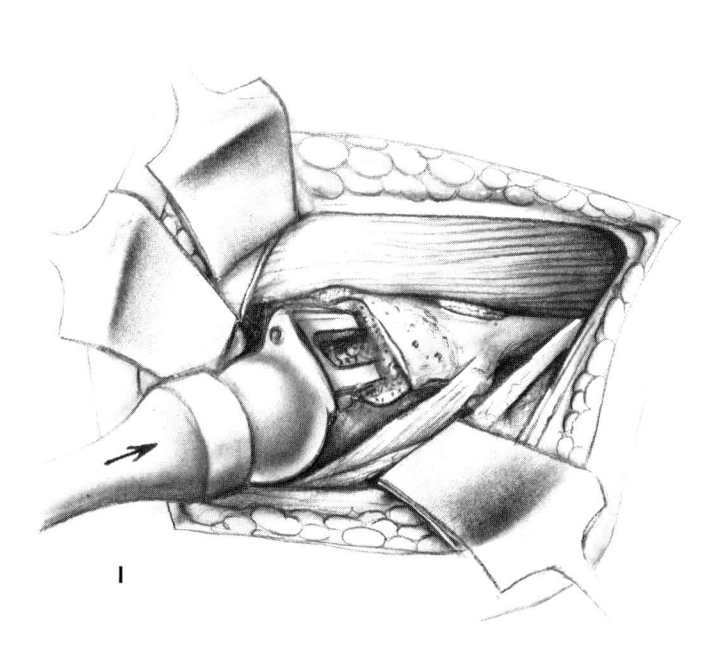

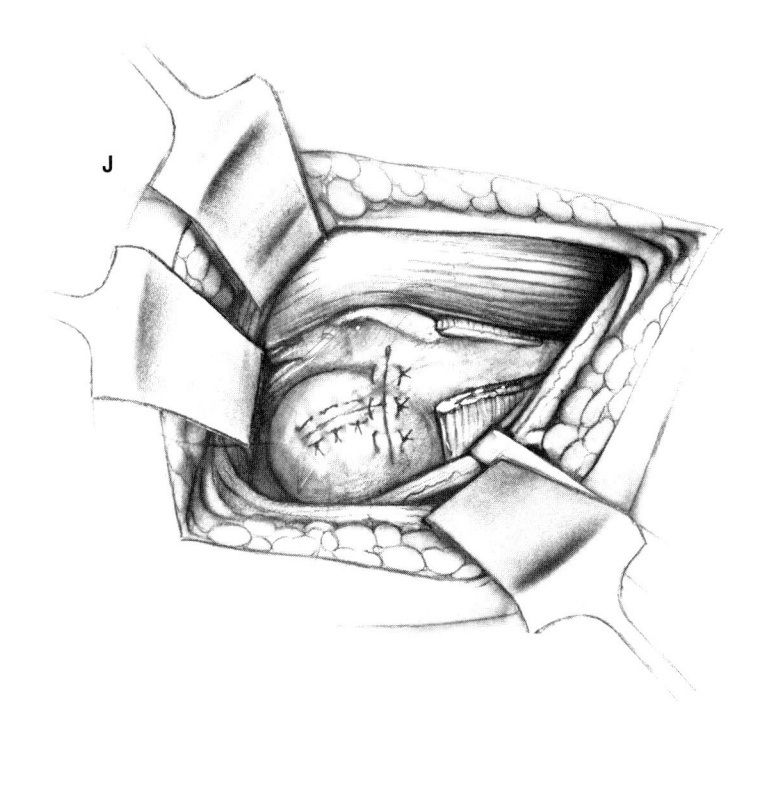

315

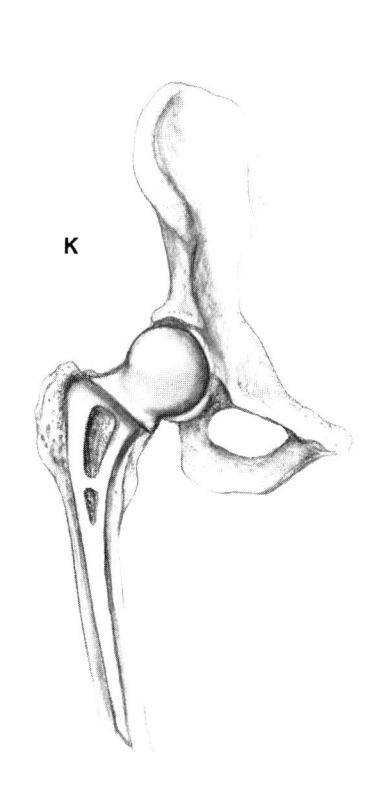

INSERTION OF FEMORAL HEAD PROSTHESIS (ANTEROLATERAL APPROACH) (Plate 10-6)

DETAILS OF PROCEDURE. An anterolateral approach may also be utilized for insertion of a femoral head prosthesis. The patient is placed in a supine position with a support beneath the involved leg and buttocks. The involved leg is draped free to allow full movement of the leg during the operative procedure. A curvilinear incision centered over the greater trochanter is used, as shown. The fascia lata is incised longitudinally, and the interval between the tensor fascia lata and gluteal muscles is identified. The fat overlying the anterior capsule of the femoral head and neck is dissected, and a retractor is placed beneath the femoral neck medially and laterally, increasing the exposure. After incision of the capsule the fracture line is visible and the femoral head can be removed with a corkscrew.

After the femoral shaft has been reamed to accommodate the trial prosthesis, careful attention is paid to preparation of the cancellous bed. If the prosthesis is to be cemented, a bristle brush is used to remove all loose cancellous bone and other debris, and the entire proximal femoral wound is cleansed with a Water Pic jet stream. The prepared cavity is kept dry until the insertion of bone cement.

The stem of the femoral endoprosthesis is slightly oversized in regard to the Charnley-Muller stem of a total hip prosthesis. This allows for removal of the endoprosthesis at a later date and replacement with a total hip prosthesis without removal of the bone cement. The tip of the femoral prosthesis is directed into valgus positioning toward the medial cortex. Care is used to maintain a steady pressure on the prosthesis during insertion, and calcar-collar fit should be accurate.

A prompt closure can be accomplished with interrupted chromic catgut sutures and skin staples.

POSTOPERATIVE MANAGEMENT. The patient is helped to sit up in a chair on the first or second postoperative day. The patient is instructed to avoid any acute flexion, adduction, and internal rotation of the involved hip but is otherwise encouraged to move about in bed or in chair as tolerated. The patient uses crutches or a walkerette with partial weight bearing or "touching down" on the involved leg until pain free. Thereafter, gradually increasing weight bearing on the involved leg is allowed. Finally, a cane in the opposite hand may be used indefinitely.

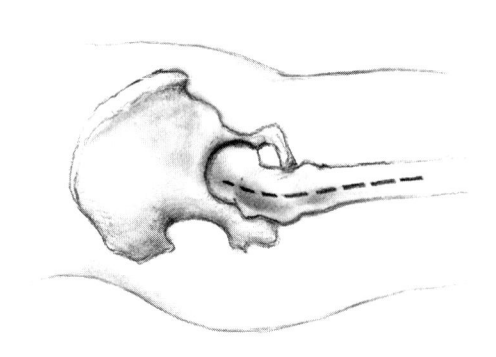

(Plate 10-7) INTERTROCHANTERIC DISPLACEMENT OSTEOTOMY OF FEMUR (COMPRESSION PLATE FIXATION)

GENERAL DISCUSSION. Osteotomy of the hip is helpful in patients with early degenerative arthritis of the hip. This procedure may result in relief of pain, restoration of joint space, and occasionally some improvement in motion of the hip joint as well as apparently spontaneous healing of degenerative cysts.

Osteotomy of the hip is not recommended for patients with rheumatoid arthritis of the hip or advanced avascular necrosis because it is much less likely to bring about relief of pain in these patients and reversal of joint changes cannot be expected in the rheumatoid hip following intertrochanteric osteotomy of the femur.

Osteotomy of the hip is one of the preferable procedures for consideration in the young person for treatment of early symptomatic degenerative arthritis of the hip.

Fair to good motion of the hip, preferably 70° of flexion, should still be present if a good result is to be obtained with intertrochanteric osteotomy. If x-ray films of the hip show an increased joint space and a better weight-bearing surface when the involved hip is adducted, a valgus osteotomy is indicated. If varus osteotomy is to be done, the patient should be able to abduct the involved hip at least 20° preoperatively. When bony spurs are present on both medial and lateral aspects of the hip joint, displacement without any change in angulation may be indicated. A small amount of displacement is likely to provide as much relief to the patient as a large degree. Delay in healing is also less likely when overdisplacement is avoided. Percutaneous adductor tenotomy may be combined with this procedure and may be done before or after the osteotomy.

DETAILS OF PROCEDURE. The procedure is carried out with the patient on the fracture table with the involved leg fastened to the footpost in neutral position. X-ray machines should be positioned for anteroposterior and lateral roentgenograms of the femoral neck and intertrochanteric area. The proximal femur is approached through a lateral incision **(A),** and a Kirschner wire is inserted into the femoral neck as a guide for the position of the blade of the appliance. The site for insertion of the blade of the appliance should be selected so at least 2 cm of bone remains between the blade and the planned osteotomy. The blade should be as close to the calcar as possible. The position of the Kirschner wire is checked by roentgenograms. Several drill holes are placed to outline the location for insertion of the blade of the compression appliance adjacent to the Kirschner wire, and a special chisel **(B)** coinciding with the contour of the blade of a compression appliance is inserted through the lateral cortex of the femur adjacent to the Kirschner wire. The special chisel in the proximal fragment is removed, and the blade of the compression appliance is inserted into the same prepared channel. With a Lohman clamp holding the plate of the appliance to the shaft of the femur, the femur is divided with a Gigli saw **(C)** or with an oscillating saw. A relatively transverse osteotomy is made **(C).** Any fixed deformity is corrected.

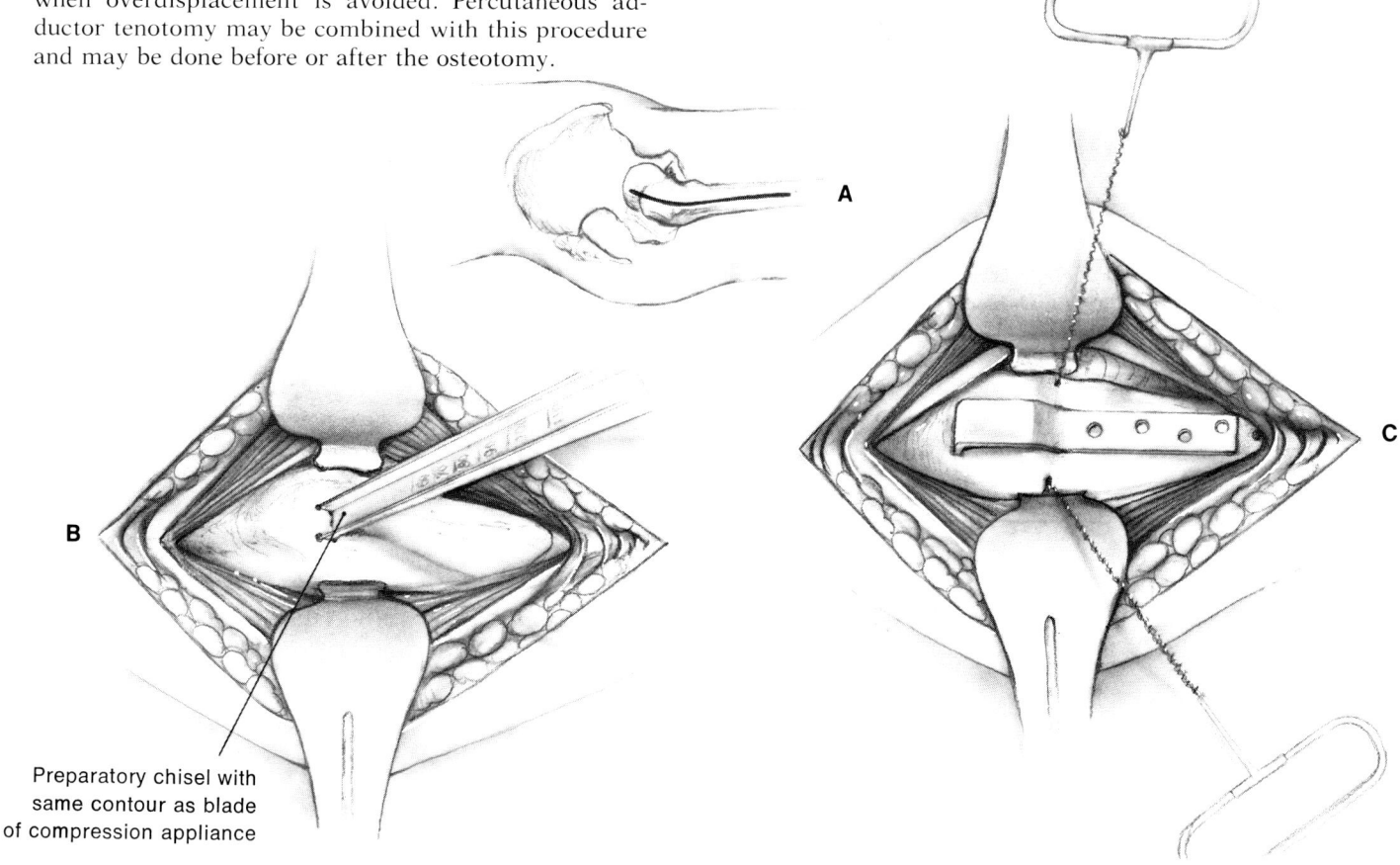

317

INTERTROCHANTERIC DISPLACEMENT OSTEOTOMY OF FEMUR (COMPRESSION PLATE FIXATION) (Plate 10-7)

The distal fragment is displaced medially about 1 cm until the plate of the compression appliance is apposed to and in alignment with the femoral shaft. The separated compression clamp is inserted. Any Lohman type of clamp applied to hold the plate to the femoral shaft is loosened slightly or removed to allow the osteotomy site to be compressed as the compression clamp is tightened **(D).** If there is good cortical bone, strong compression can be applied manually. If the bone is osteoporotic, one should avoid applying excessive compression that might cause the bone to fragment with loss of the rigid fixation. The osteotomy surfaces should be clearly visualized as the compression is applied. As the compression is maintained, three transfixion screws are inserted and a fourth is placed after removal of the compression clamp (**E** and **F**). The wound is closed in routine fashion, and the patient is carefully moved directly to his bed.

POSTOPERATIVE MANAGEMENT. The patient should be able to sit up on the first or second postoperative day if stable compression fixation of the osteotomy site was obtained. Crutch walking without weight bearing on the involved leg is usually started within 3 to 4 days. After 1 week, partial weight bearing is permitted. By 3 to 4 months after surgery radiographs will demonstrate early bony union, and the patient is usually able to discard crutches and begin using a cane in the opposite hand.

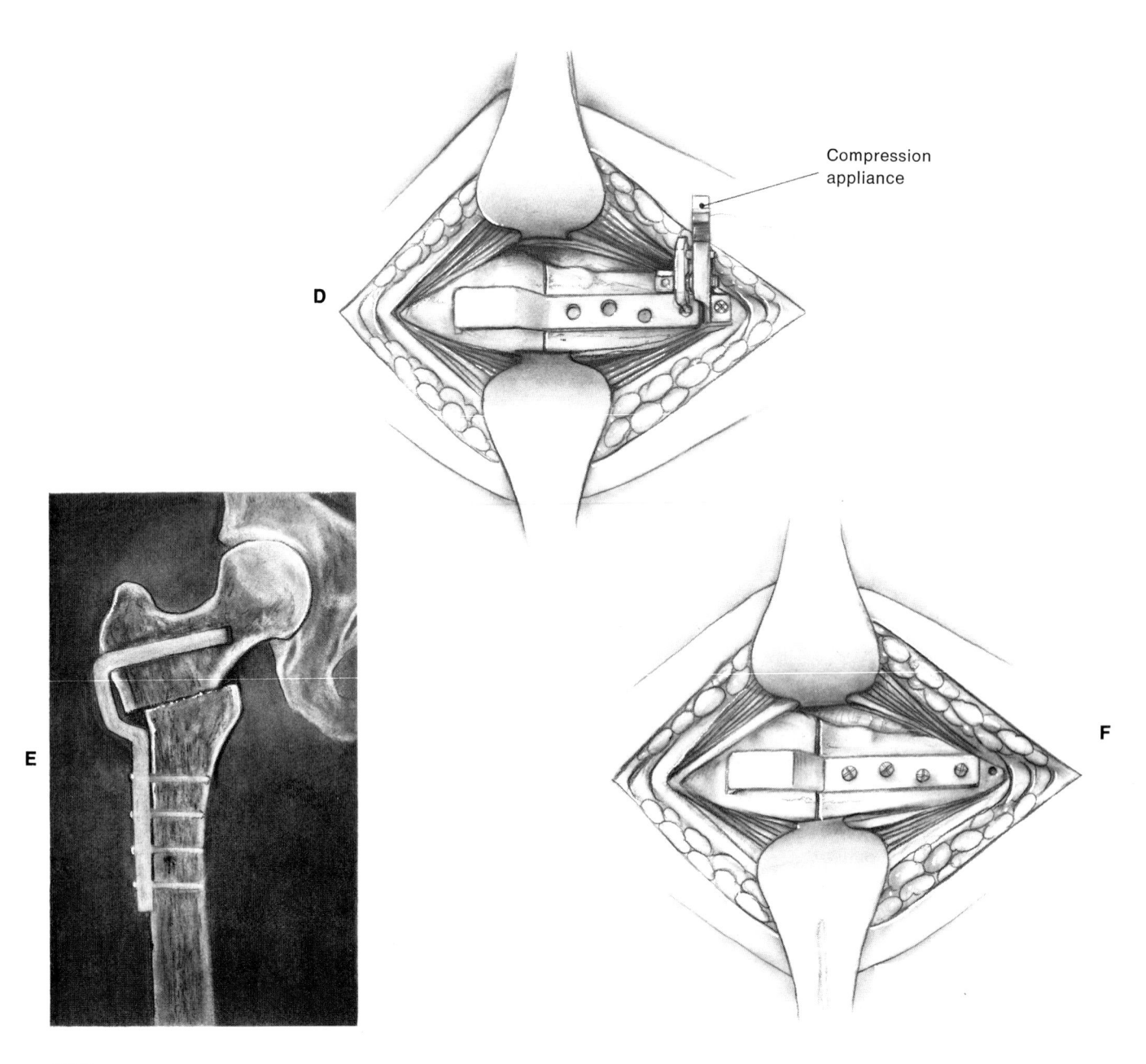

(Plate 10-8) TOTAL HIP RECONSTRUCTION—CHARNLEY-MÜLLER

GENERAL DISCUSSION. The remarkable advances made in total hip reconstruction in the last decade have added new dimensions to the management of patients with musculoskeletal disorders. Indeed, it is the most successful "organ transplant" available for human use. Tens of thousands of patients worldwide have benefitted from this form of reconstructive surgery of the hip.

It is indicated in patients with symptomatic severe degenerative arthritis of the hip or disabling rheumatoid arthritis of the hip. Many other disorders may result in hip destruction, including the childhood hip disorders such as slipped capital femoral epiphysis, congenital hip dysplasia, and Legg-Perthes disease. Hip destruction may follow trauma to the femoral head or acetabulum. Surgery is indicated in patients who have undergone previous reconstructive procedures of the hip joint, including osteotomy, cup arthroplasty, and prosthetic replacement, and who have subsequently become symptomatic.

DETAILS OF PROCEDURE. The patient is placed in the supine position with a small roll measuring 36 × 10 cm beneath the buttocks and lower back. The roll serves to accentuate the hip joint structures anteriorly and is removed at the time of acetabular cup insertion. A Watson-Jones incision is used to expose the hip. The incision is made with the midpoint directly over the greater trochanter and extending 6 cm proximally and distally, curving anteriorly at both ends **(A)**. After the skin and subcutaneous tissues are divided, the fascia lata overlying the vastus lateralis is excised and incised distally.

The next step is to locate the interval between the gluteus medius and tensor fascia lata muscles **(B)**. This may be difficult and can best be accomplished by proceeding proximally from the origin of the vastus lateralis. After this interval has been identified, the gluteus medius and other abductors are retracted by a smooth Hohman retractor placed just behind the neck in front of the greater trochanter. A second sharp Hohman retractor is placed along the medial aspect of the neck, allowing retraction of the tensor fascia lata muscles and exposing the precapsular fat. Precapsular fat is cleared with a periosteal elevator, and the reflected head of the rectus is identified. A third retractor with a sharp point and broad blade is placed over the anteromedial rim of the acetabulum, allowing full exposure of the capsule of the hip **(C)**. The hip capsule is then incised, and hip joint fluid is obtained for culture. The remainder of the capsule visible anteriorly, medially, and laterally is dissected and removed. A cartilage forceps is used to grasp the capsule **(D)**.

Without dislocating the hip, the surgeon then turns attention toward the femoral neck **(E)**. A power saw is used to divide the femoral neck at 45° to the long axis and in neutral version. This cut is approximately 1 cm proximal to the lesser trochanter **(F)**. An osteotome may be introduced into the cut in the neck, and with a slight amount of leverage

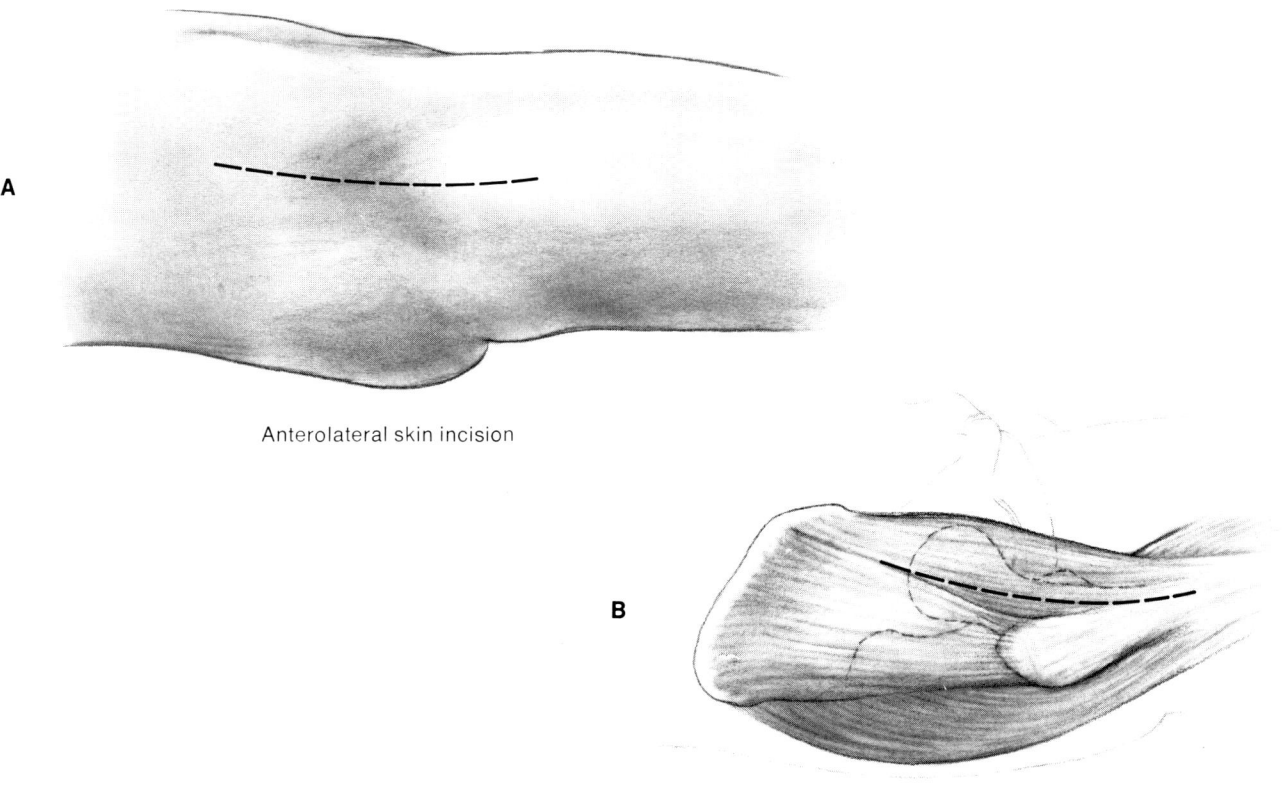

A

Anterolateral skin incision

B

Interval between fascia lata and glutei

319

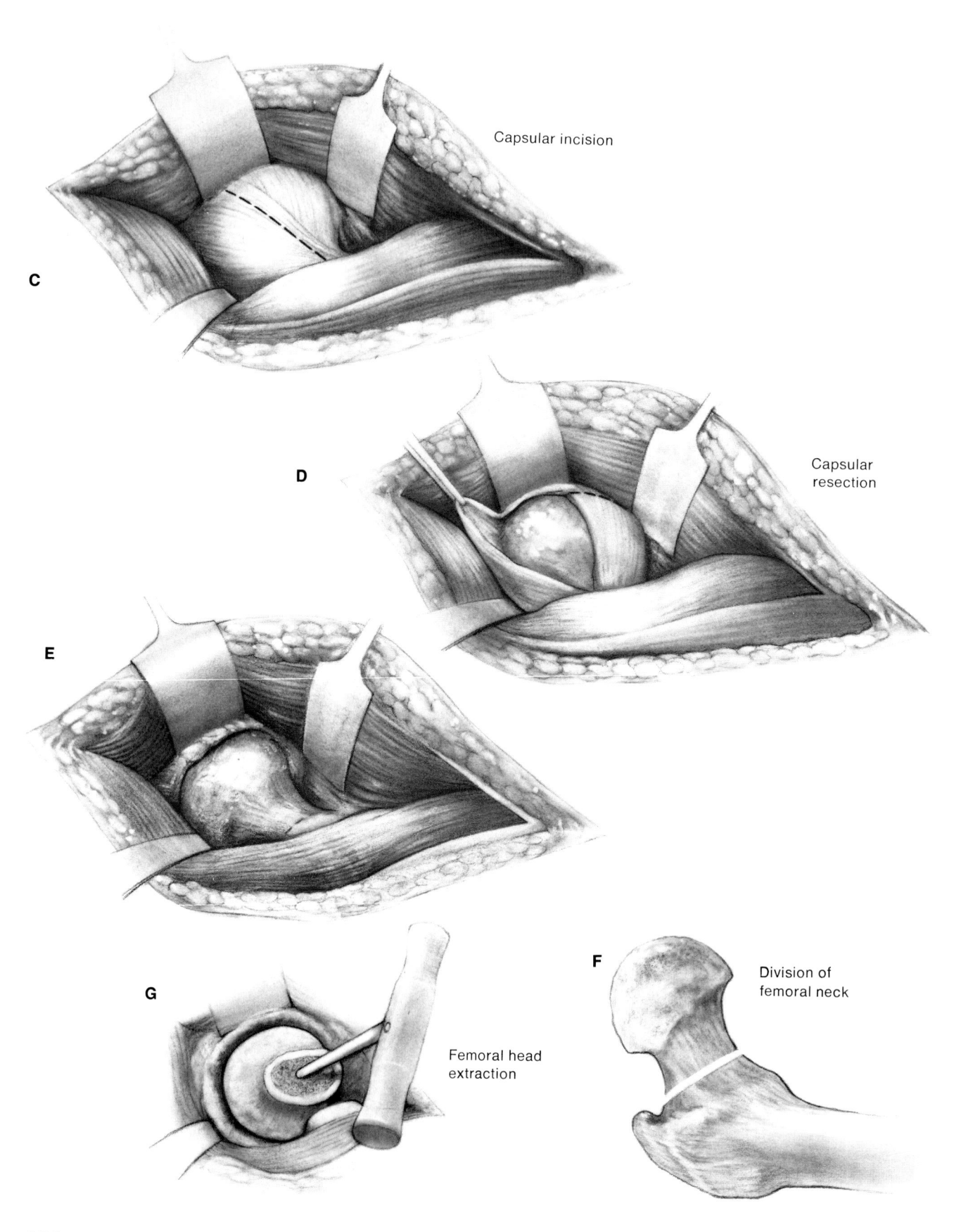

TOTAL HIP RECONSTRUCTION—CHARNLEY-MÜLLER (Plate 10-8)

C

Capsular incision

D

Capsular resection

E

G

Femoral head extraction

F

Division of femoral neck

320

(Plate 10-8) TOTAL HIP RECONSTRUCTION—CHARNLEY-MÜLLER

a corkscrew can be introduced into the cut surface and the femoral head can be removed **(G)**. The anterolateral acetabular lip may be overgrown with osteophytes, which will have to be excised to allow removal of the femoral head.

Care is taken to remove the remainder of the posterior capsule. The curved beaver blade should be used to remove the medial and posterior portions of the hip capsule and synovium **(H)**. Occasionally it is necessary to divide the short external rotators of the hip. This must be done with a right-angle clamp, and care is taken to divide the rotators at the bony origin. A special retractor is then placed beneath the acetabular rim and allows for posterior displacement of the femur, exposing the entire acetabulum and its margins **(I)**.

After complete removal of the soft tissue from the rim of the acetabulum along with other acetabular debris, the acetabulum is ready for deepening.

A Charnley centering ring and drill are directed toward the acetabulum approximately 40° to the long axis of the body and in 10° of anteversion. A centering hole is drilled through the acetabulum into the pelvis **(J)**. The Charnley deepening reamer allows for preparation of the acetabular bed and effects medial displacement of the acetabulum **(K)**.

H Posterior capsular resection

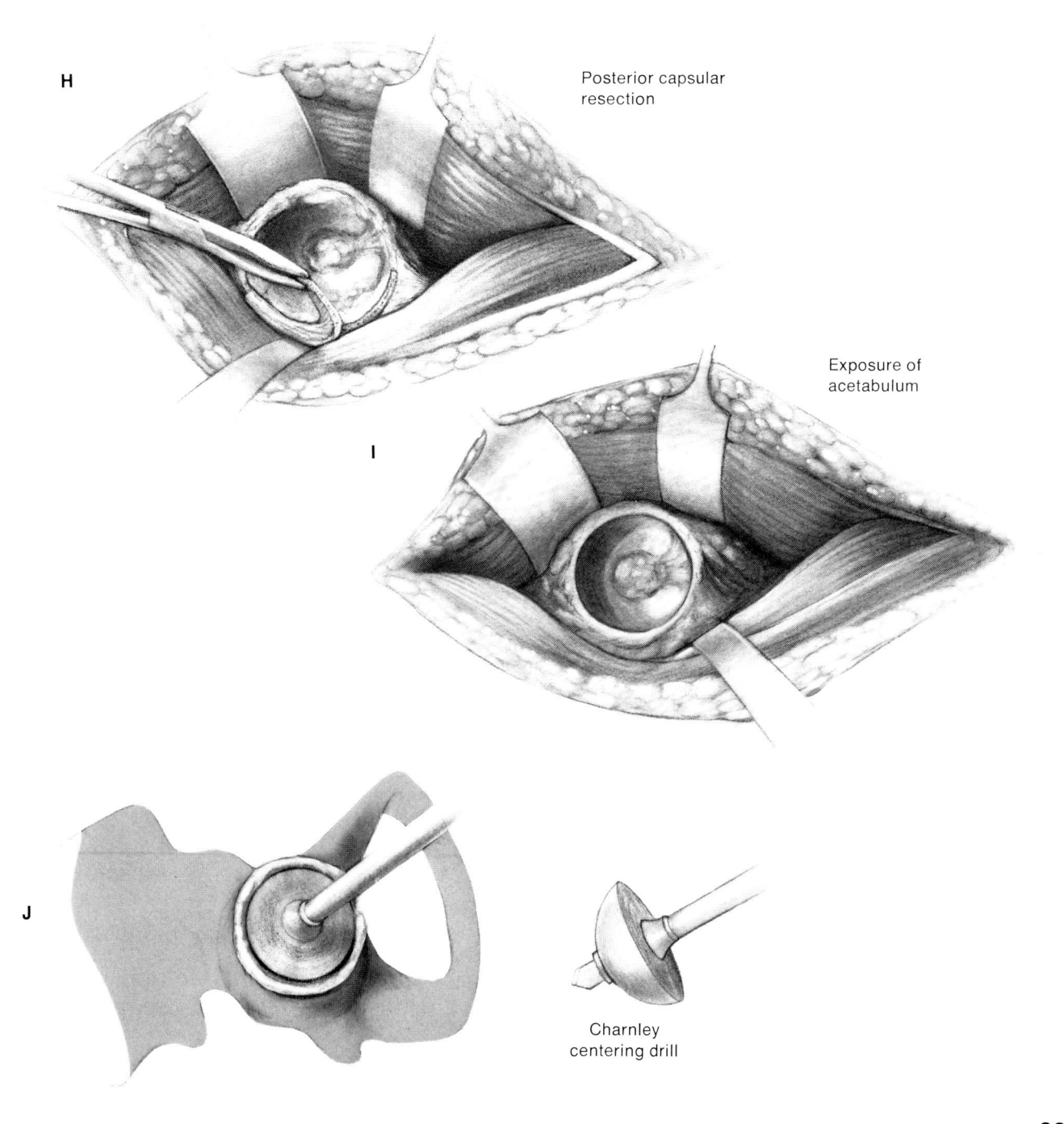

I Exposure of acetabulum

J

Charnley centering drill

321

TOTAL HIP RECONSTRUCTION—CHARNLEY-MÜLLER (Plate 10-8)

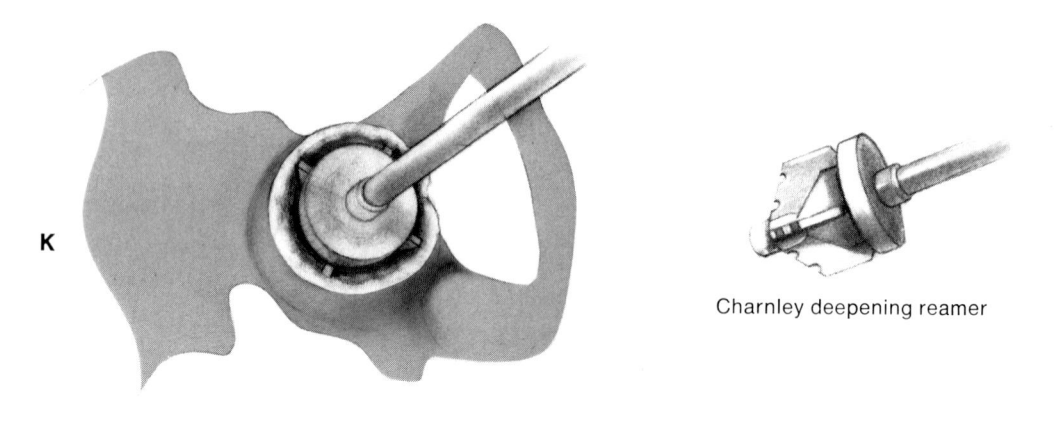

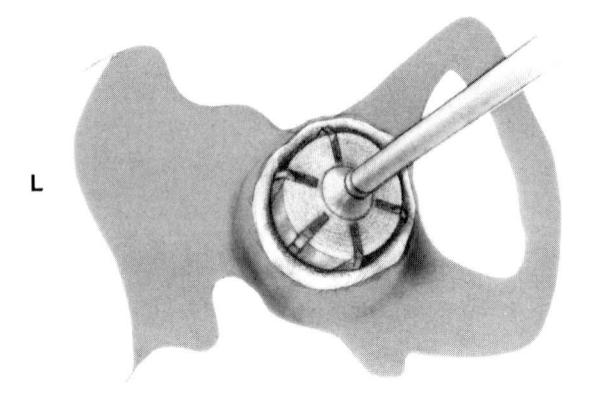

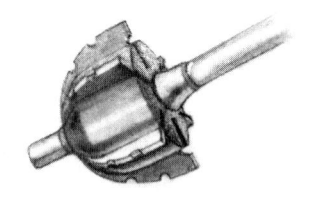

K

Charnley deepening reamer

L

Charnley expandable reamer

M

Acetabular cup

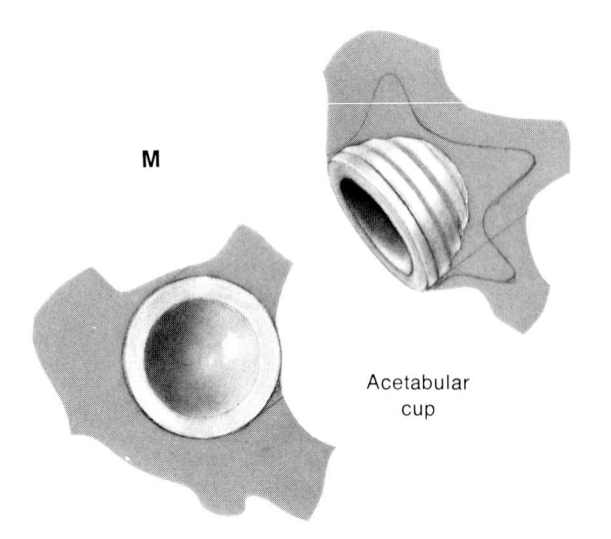

One can determine the depth of bone stock in the acetabulum by measuring the depth of the centering hole. Medial displacement of the acetabular component remains a vital step in true reconstruction of the hip joint.

Care is taken to leave an acetabular thickness of at least 0.5 cm. The Charnley expandable reamer is used to increase the diameter of the acetabulum to its desired size **(L)**. A small patient with a shallow and small acetabulum may require an acetabular cup of 44 mm outside diameter.

Following preparation of the acetabulum a trial acetabular cup is placed in the acetabulum to determine bony coverage. The cup must be covered with bone, especially along the superior, posterior and lateral margins **(M)**.

To prepare the acetabulum for cementing, the centering hole drill is used to create holes in the ilium, ischium, and pubis. The drill should not penetrate the pelvis at any point. The depth of the holes should vary from 0.75 to 1 cm. Each hole is then undercut with a curet, and special attention must be paid to the seating holes in a patient whose acetabulum is eburnated and smooth. Additional smaller seating holes may be required. Surfaces must be roughened. The entire surface of the acetabulum is then cleansed with a Water Pic spray. This will remove the debris and clean out the interstices of the cancellous bone. A cement restrictor is placed in the centering hole that penetrates the pelvis **(N)**.

(Plate 10-8) TOTAL HIP RECONSTRUCTION—CHARNLEY-MÜLLER

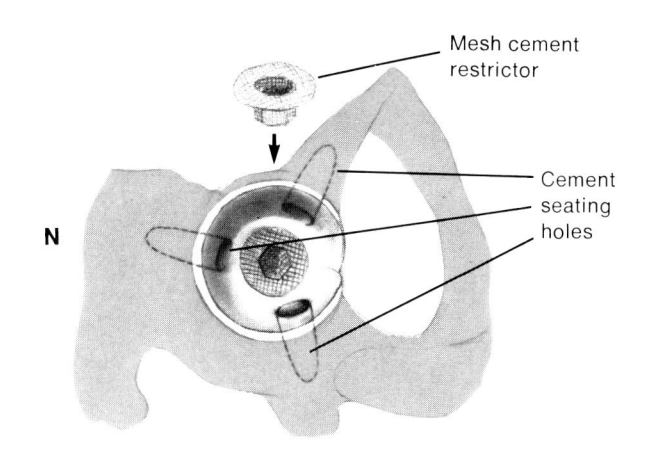

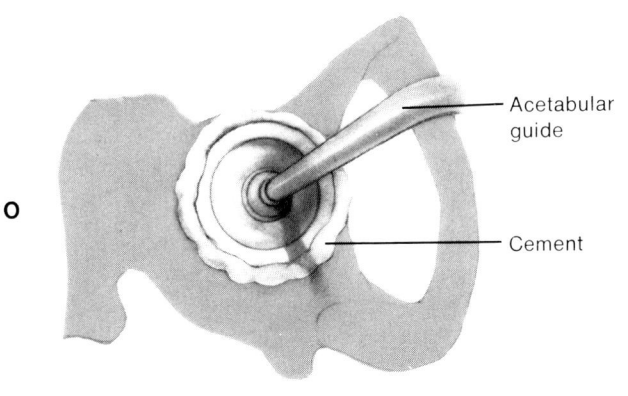

A pillow is removed from beneath the hip, and care is taken to dry completely the acetabulum with an absorbant gauze. Methylmethacrylate is applied firmly into the acetabulum, including the cementing holes and centering hole. The cup is guided into place initially with fingertip pressure and then with the guide (O). The cup should not be forced into the acetabulum, since this will cause the cement to extrude. Gentle pressure is applied with an acetabular guide. The cup must be placed in a 45° angle to the long axis of the body and 10° of anteversion. An acetabular protractor passing across the anterosuperior iliac spines helps to position the acetabular cup accurately (P). Excess cement is removed from the edges of the acetabulum. Firm inward pressure is applied with a hip guide, and care is taken to tamp all the margins to provide firm fixation of the methylmethacrylate. It is important to fill in all the margins around the cup with methylmethacrylate under pressure following tamping.

After the cement cup is placed, the femur is prepared to accept the femoral prosthesis. If trouble is encountered in assuming a figure-of-four positioning of the femur, then further attention should be directed to releasing the posterior capsule and short external rotators. A few fibers of the gluteus medius and minimus at their insertion at the greater trochanter may have to be divided. In short, for obese patients it may be necessary to actually move the opposite leg off the operating table. After the leg is properly positioned, a femoral rasp is placed into the shaft of the femur. Care is taken not to penetrate the femur, and most often the rasp can be directed with hand pressure alone (Q). The final 2 cm of movement can be achieved with mallet pressure.

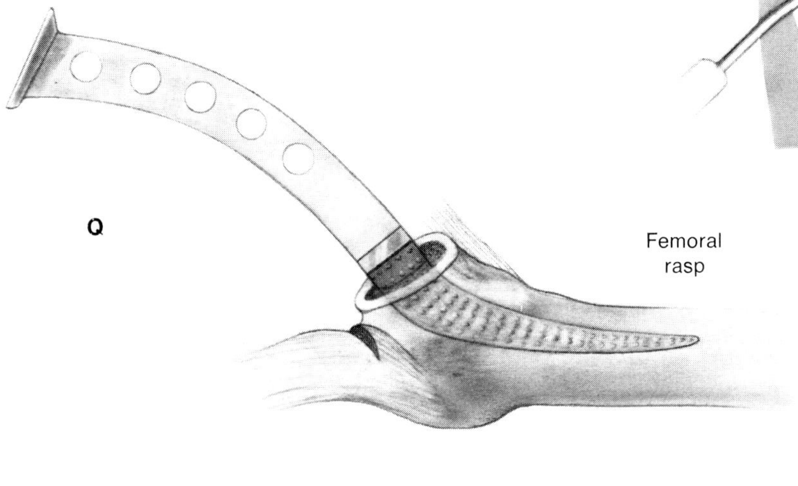

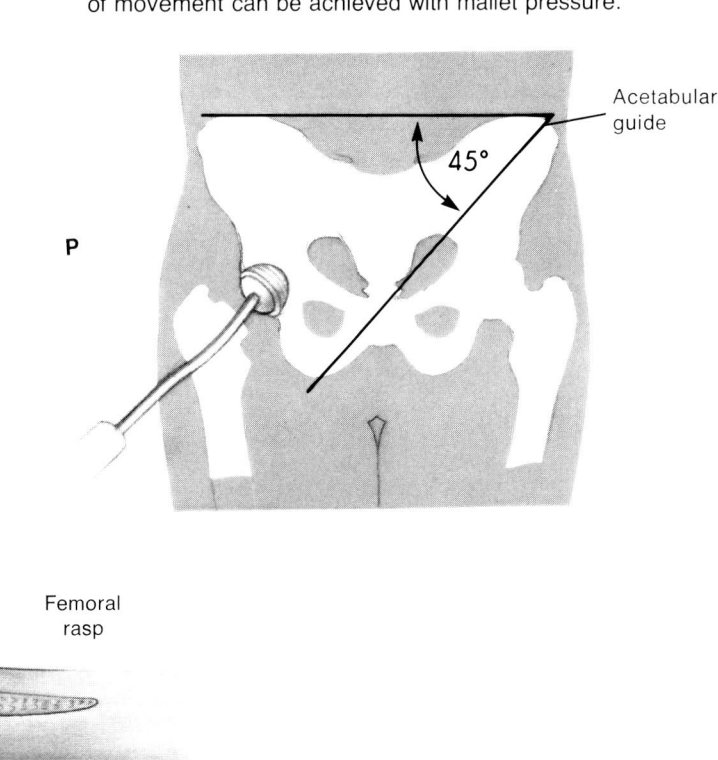

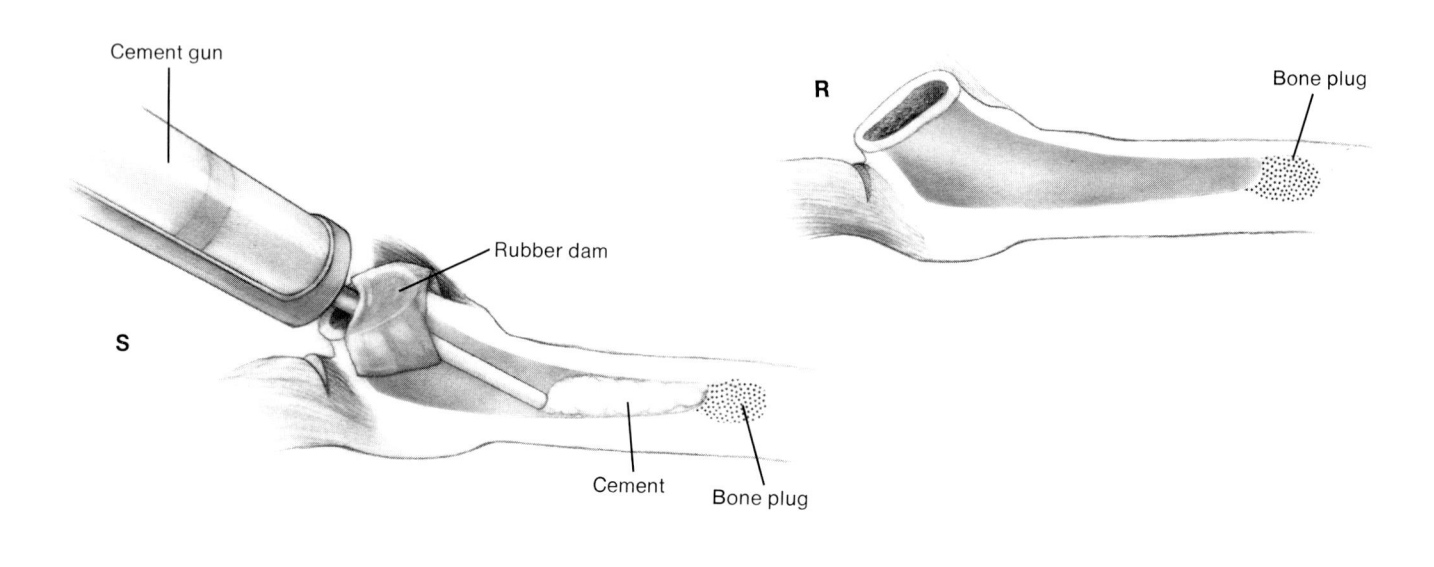

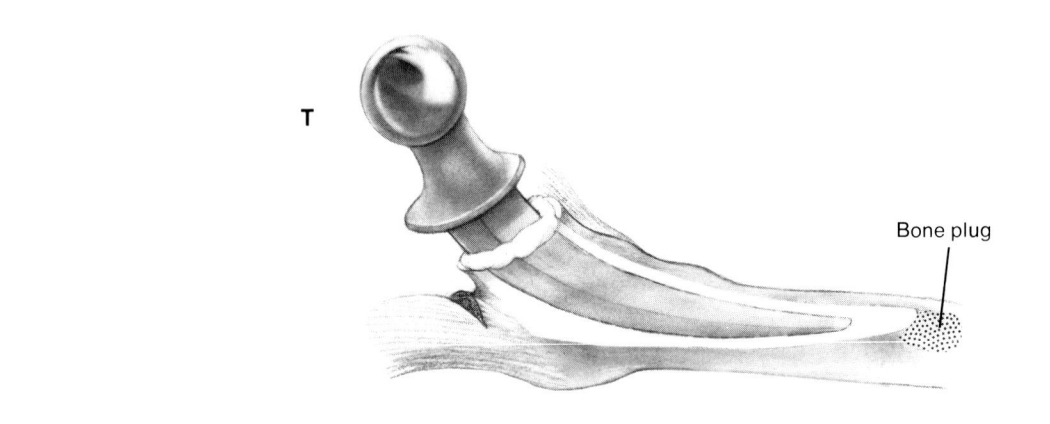

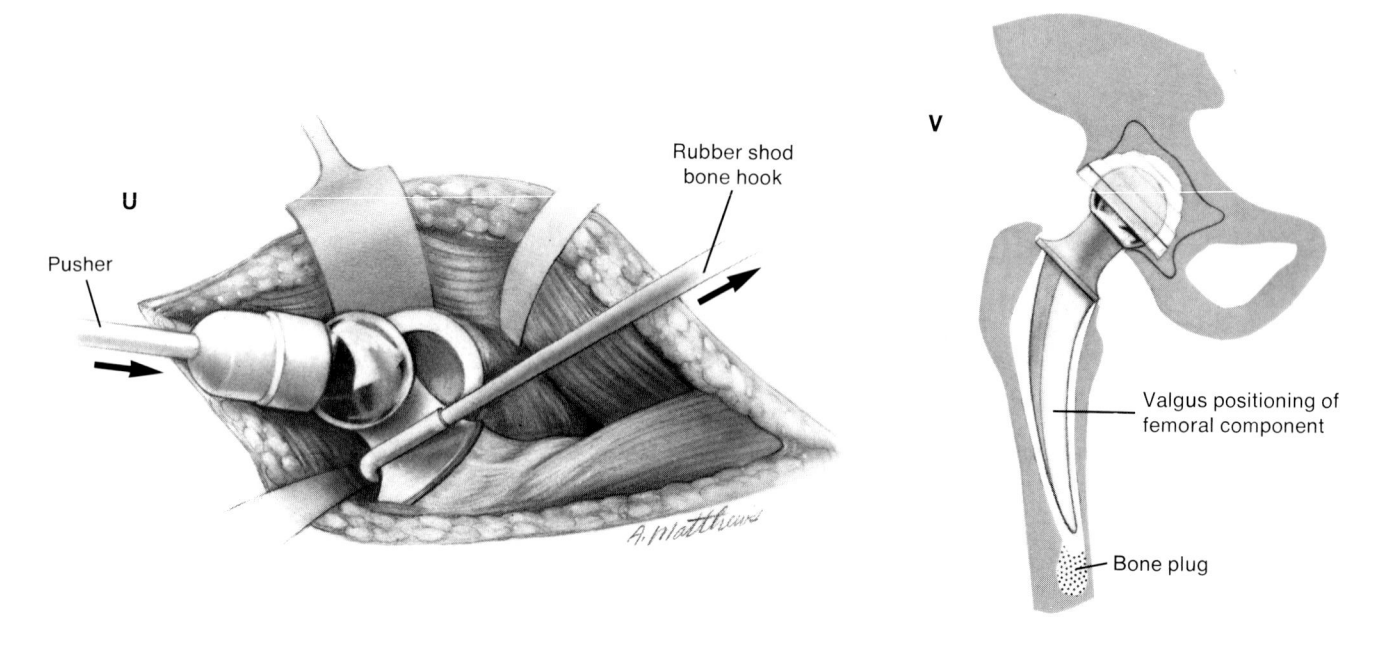

TOTAL HIP RECONSTRUCTION—CHARNLEY-MÜLLER (Plate 10-8)

324

(Plate 10-8) TOTAL HIP RECONSTRUCTION—CHARNLEY-MÜLLER

A reverse curret should be used to remove the cancellous bone at the calcar femoral area, and if trochanteric osteotomy has not been performed, a trough should be created toward the greater trochanter in the proximal femur **(R)**. This will allow for better cement fixation. After preparation of the femoral shaft a trial reduction with a trial prosthesis is performed. The femoral component should be placed at 0° to 5° of anteversion and in a valgus position. It is important to maintain proper abductor tension and neck length because only by maintaining neck length and abductor tension can greater trochanteric osteotomy be avoided. A rubber shod bone hook is used in the reduction of the prosthesis.

After measurement of both legs has been obtained by using positioning of the patella and medial malleoli, the shaft of the femur is cleansed with a bristle brush or plastic brush to remove all the debris and a Water Pic jet stream is directed into the femoral shaft. Methylmethacrylate is placed in a gun and inserted from distal to proximal in the femoral shaft **(S)**. It may be necessary in the osteoporotic patient to place a bone plug in the distal femoral shaft at the level of the tip of the prosthesis, just beneath the tip of the prosthesis. This will allow for firmer fixation. The femoral prosthesis is introduced in the shaft in the femur with great care to obtain the valgus position **(T)**. During the curing period of methylmethacrylate the leg must be held absolutely still, and no motion should be allowed between the prosthesis and methylmetacrylate. After the cement is hardened, the femoral prosthesis is reduced into the acetabular cup and moved through a range of motion (**U** and **V**). A hemovac tube is placed deep in the hip joint, and a second tube may be placed in the subcutaneous area. The fascia is closed with interrupted sutures, and the skin may be closed with staples.

Certain precautions must be taken before undertaking a total hip replacement. An entire supply of femoral prostheses should be available before the procedure is begun. Special sizes can be obtained for use in exceptional circumstances.

POSTOPERATIVE MANAGEMENT. After the wound is closed, the hip is placed in a cotton hip spica. Occasionally Buck's traction and a rotator strap must be applied to the extremity and the extremity held in abduction. The bed is equipped with a flexion assist, and active motion is begun the day following surgery. After 3 to 4 days of bed rest during which quadriceps setting exercises, gluteal setting exercises, and movement via the assisted flexion sling are emphasized, the patient begins active quadriceps and hip exercises. The patient begins crutch walking with partial weight bearing only. This continues for 8 weeks following surgery. Gradual weight bearing is then allowed for the patient when activities are resumed. Occasionally a patient will need to the assistance of a cane in the opposite hand.

TOTAL HIP RECONSTRUCTION—RESURFACING (Plate 10-9)

GENERAL DISCUSSION. Resurfacing of the hip joint is an arthroplastic procedure designed to replace the deformed articular surfaces of the hip joint. It is an extension of an old concept, the cup arthroplasty, and involves cementing a high-density polyethylene acetabular cup into a deepened and enlarged acetabulum and a metal cup onto the femoral head. The major advantage of this form of total hip reconstruction is the transfer of loads across the hip joint to the proximal end of the femur in a physiologic manner. It is a procedure that can be performed in a younger age group of patients in that it preserves bone stock and allows salvage procedures such as conventional hip reconstruction, head and neck resection, or arthrodesis.

Several types of resurfacing prosthesis are available, including those introduced by Gerard in France; Nishio and Furya in Japan; Freeman in England, Trentani in Italy; Eicher, Capello, and Amstutz in the United States; and Wagner in Germany. This discussion will center on the use of the Indiana conservative hip designed by Eicher in 1973 and later modified by Capello.

DETAILS OF PROCEDURE. The patient is placed in the supine position with a roll underneath the involved hip and buttocks (**A**). A lateral incision is made, exposing the greater trochanteric area (**B** and **C**). The greater trochanteric osteotomy is performed in a vertical manner, and care is taken not to invade the attachments of the hip capsule superiorly, laterally, or posteriorly (**D** and **E**). Following greater trochanteric removal the hip is dislocated and the femoral head is prepared for the placement of the metal cup. The femoral head is prepared in a manner that will allow the cup to be placed in a valgus positioning of 145°. The medial osteophytes are removed with a saw (**F** and **G**). Other osteophytes are removed, and a concentric reamer is used to smooth the femoral head (**H**). Great care is taken to preserve the length of the femoral head and neck and to avoid notching of the neck in any manner during the procedure. The cup is placed over the prepared femoral head and observed to lie in a valgus, slightly retroverted position (**I**).

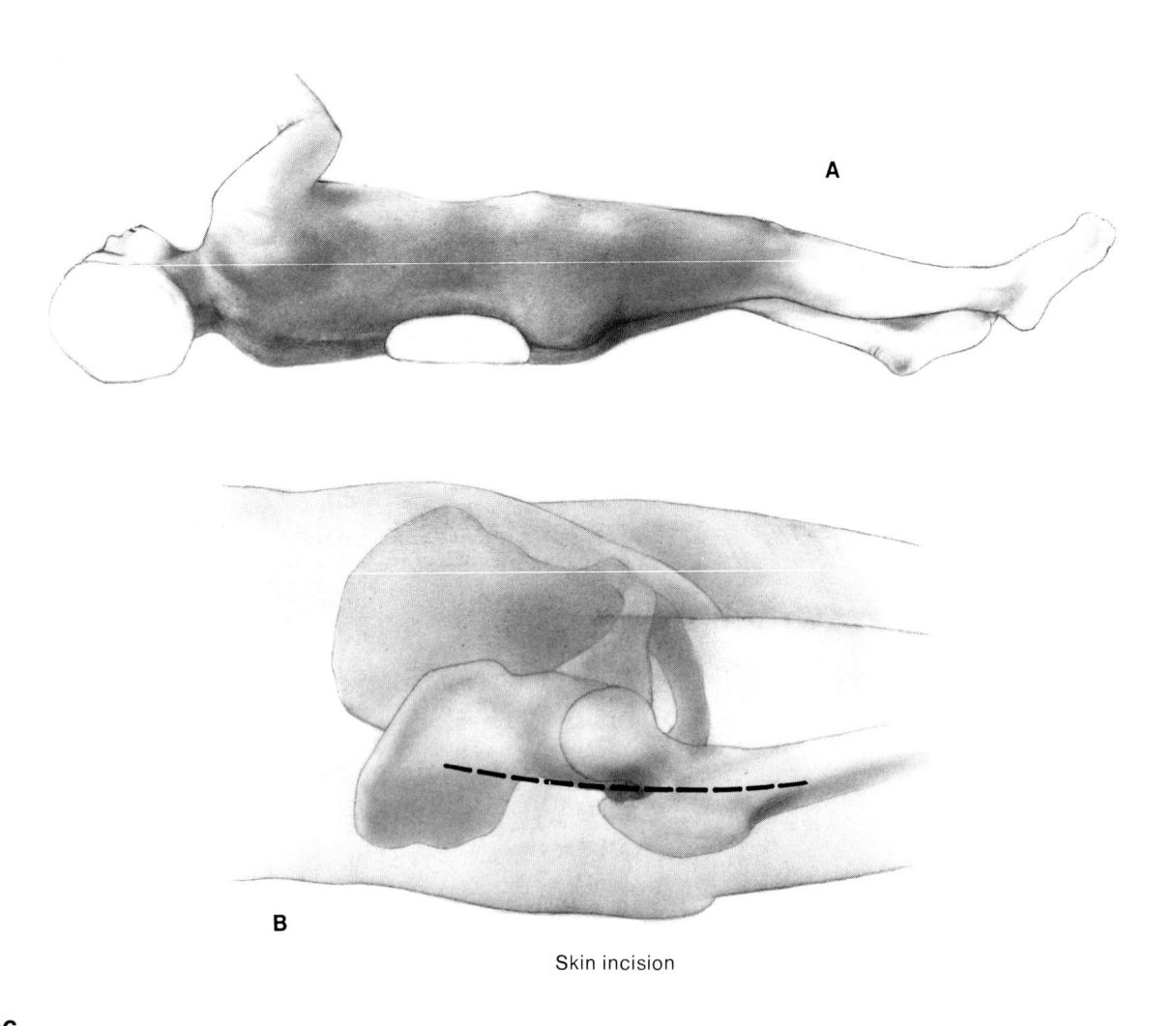

Skin incision

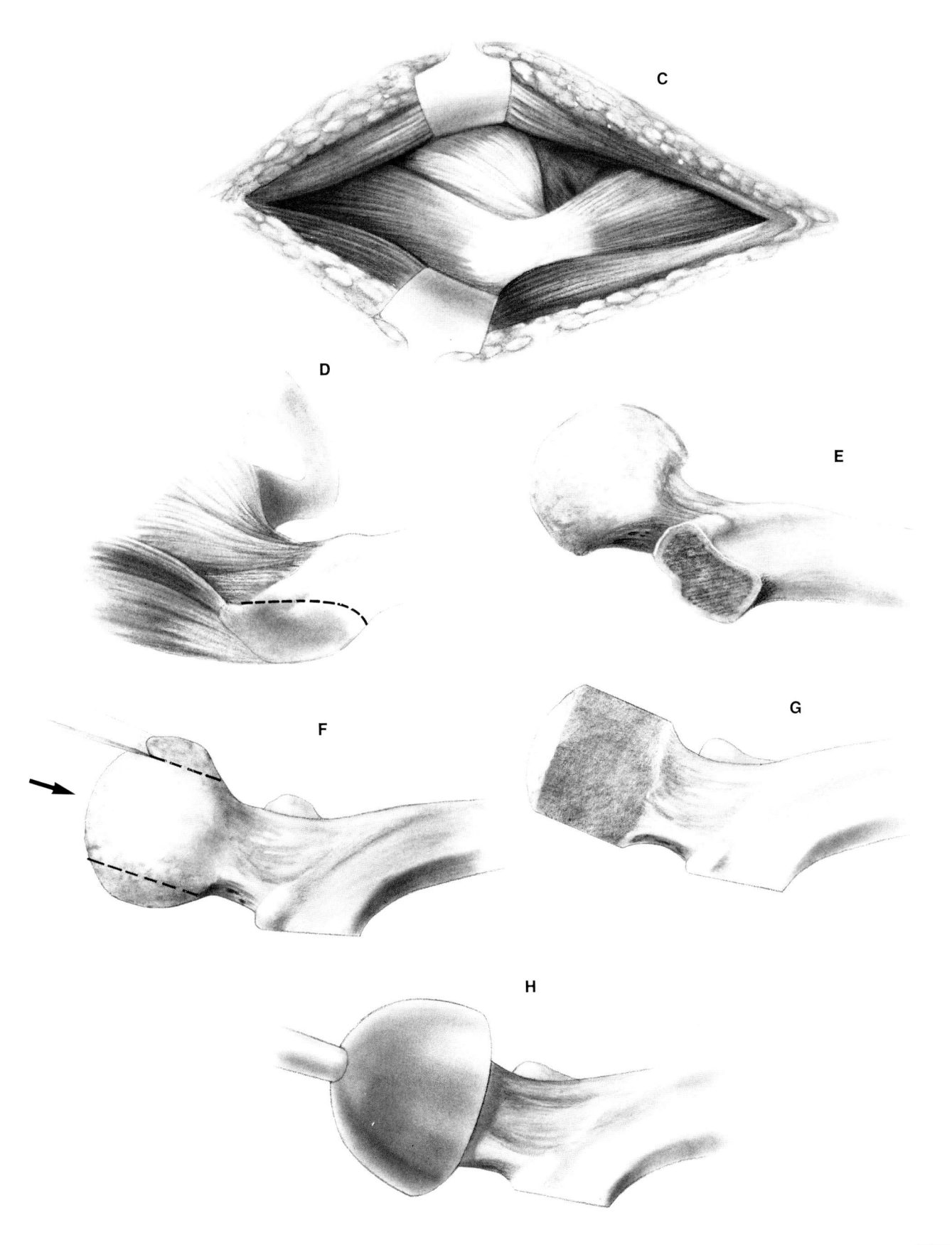

(Plate 10-9) TOTAL HIP RECONSTRUCTION—RESURFACING

C

D

E

F

G

H

327

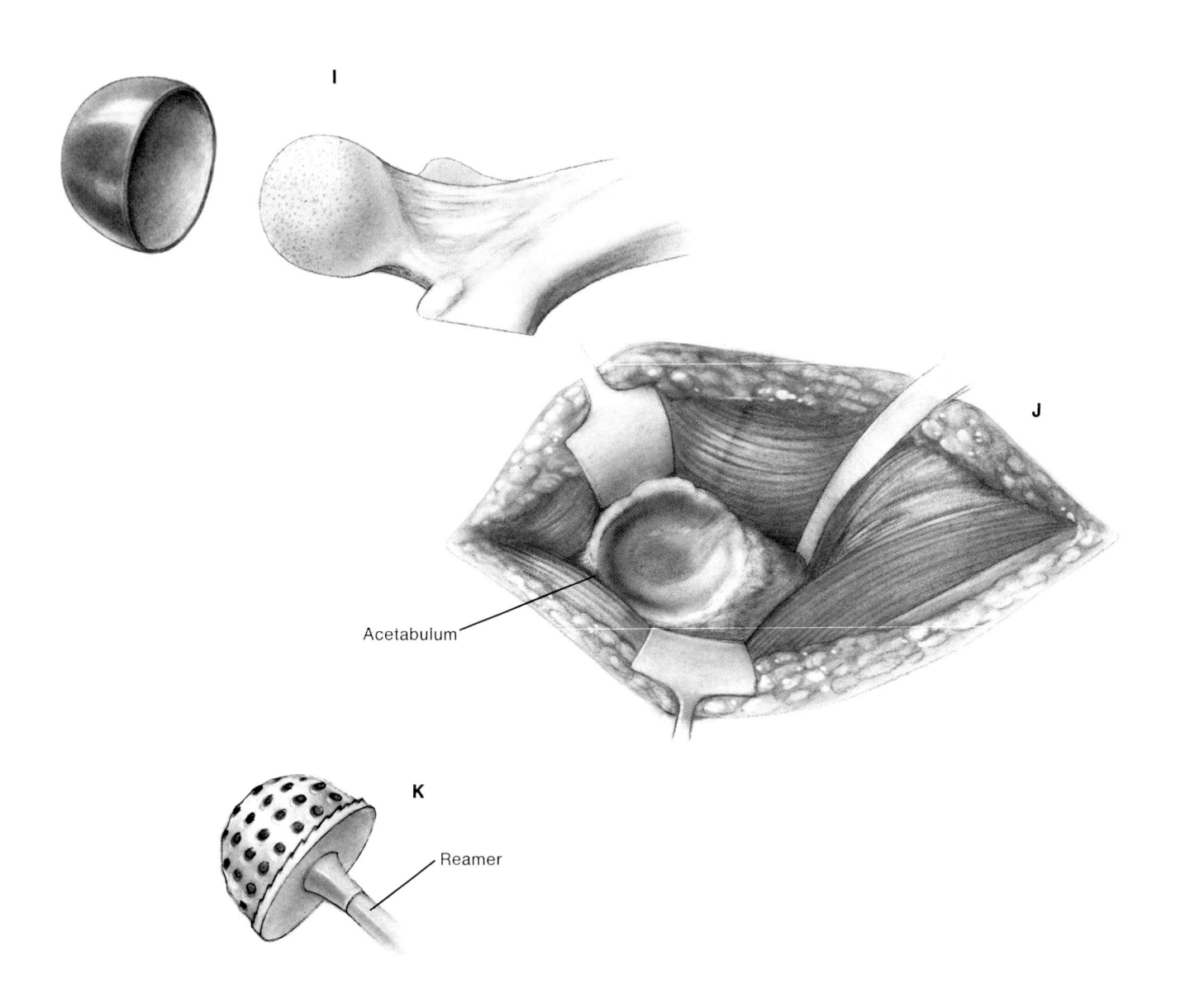

TOTAL HIP RECONSTRUCTION—RESURFACING (Plate 10-9)

The acetabulum is deepened and enlarged to accommodate the thin polyethylene cup, which corresponds to the femoral cup size (**J** and **K**). Seating holes are drilled into the ischium and ilium. The cup is cemented in place following thorough cleansing of the acetabulum with a Water Pic spray (**L**). Following cementing of the acetabular cup a trial femoral cup is placed on the femoral head and a trial reduction is carried out. The hip is moved through a full range of motion without dislocation. The femoral cup is cemented in place.

The greater trochanter is reattached with two screws (**M** and **N**). If advancement of the greater trochanter is deemed necessary to restore abductor tension, it can be performed with screw fixation. Closure of the wound is carried out in layers over suction drainage tubes. The skin is closed with staples.

POSTOPERATIVE MANAGEMENT. A Robert Jones single hip compression dressing is applied and is retained for 5 days. Immediately after surgery, isometric exercises are begun on the operated hip joint. At 10 days postoperatively the patient is allowed out of bed, and partial weight bearing supported by walker or crutches is begun. This weight-bearing mode is maintained for 8 weeks following surgery. Continued efforts are made to achieve a full range of motion of the hip joint.

(Plate 10-9) TOTAL HIP RECONSTRUCTION—RESURFACING

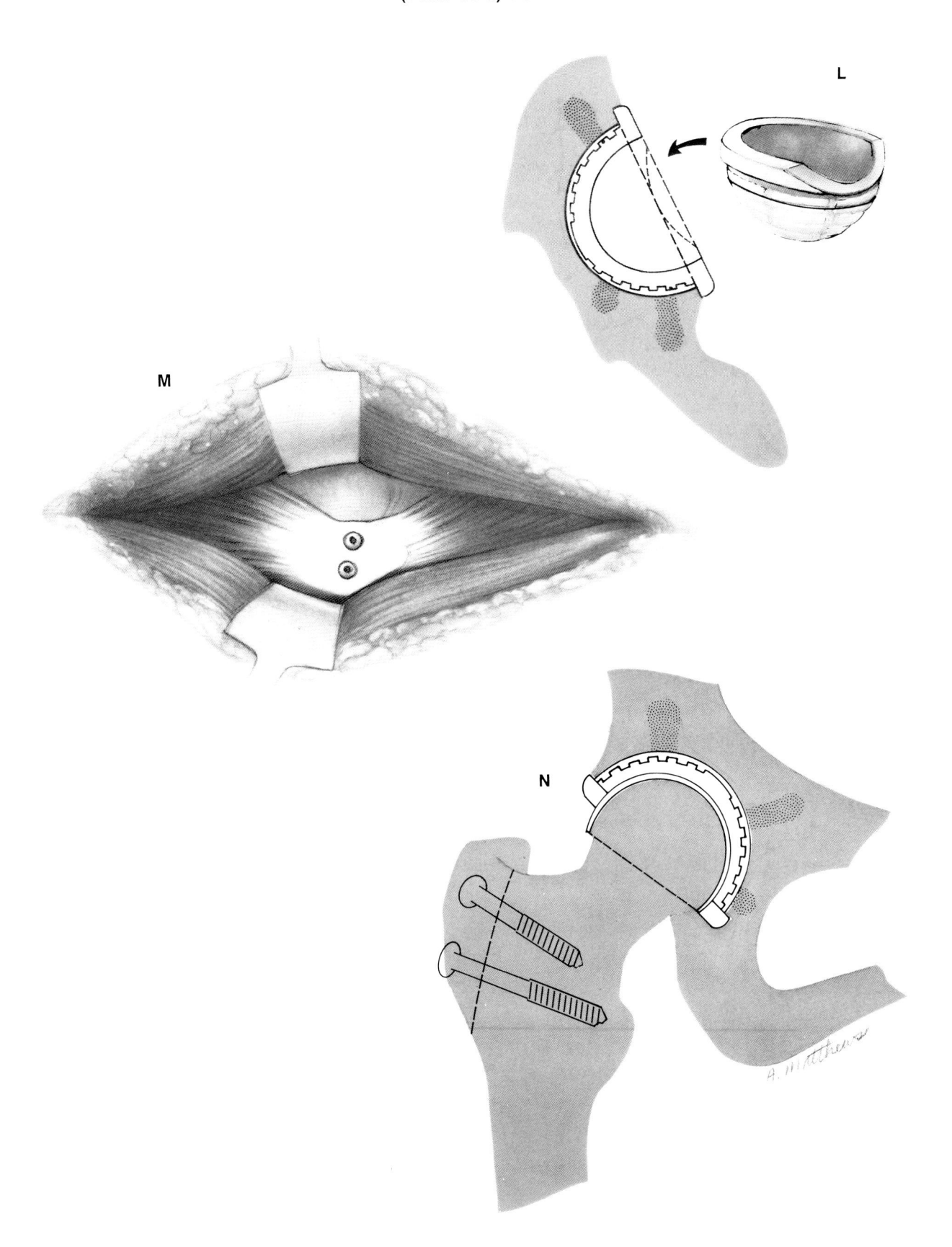

CUP ARTHROPLASTY (Plate 10-10)

GENERAL DISCUSSION. On occasion in the younger patients cup arthroplasty with a Vitallium mold may be used to relieve or decrease hip pain, to restore, maintain or improve function, and to correct deformities.

The lateral approach to the hip for cup arthroplasty provides full visualization of the femoral head and a direct, complete view of the acetabulum. It permits powered tools to be used for shaping the acetabulum and femoral head. Osteotomy of the greater trochanter is an essential component of the procedure. The functional capacity of the abductor muscles is enhanced by transplanting the greater trochanter distally. The lateral approach to the hip is particularly suitable for cup arthroplasty but can also be used for other procedures.

DETAILS OF PROCEDURE. The patient is placed in a semilateral position with the involved side raised 60°. The buttock should hang completely free without compression of the posterior soft tissues to facilitate posterior dislocation of the femoral head during the procedure. A U-shaped incision is made **(A)** with the base of the U at the level of the greater trochanter, as recommended by W. H. Harris, or a longer straight incision may also be used. The fascia lata is opened in the distal portion of the wound parallel to the skin incision. With an index finger deep to the fascia lata as it is incised in a proximal direction, it is possible to palpate the femoral insertion of the gluteus maximus on the gluteal tuberosity and to guide the incision in the fascia lata as far posteriorly as possible without cutting into the femoral insertion of the gluteus maximum **(B)**. The fascia is incised proximally overlying the gluteus medius, between the gluteus maximus and the tensor fascia lata. Keeping the incision in the fascia lata along the posterior border of the greater trochanter will allow the best exposure subsequently, but if the incision is placed too far behind the posterior border of the greater trochanter, the gluteus maximus may be damaged.

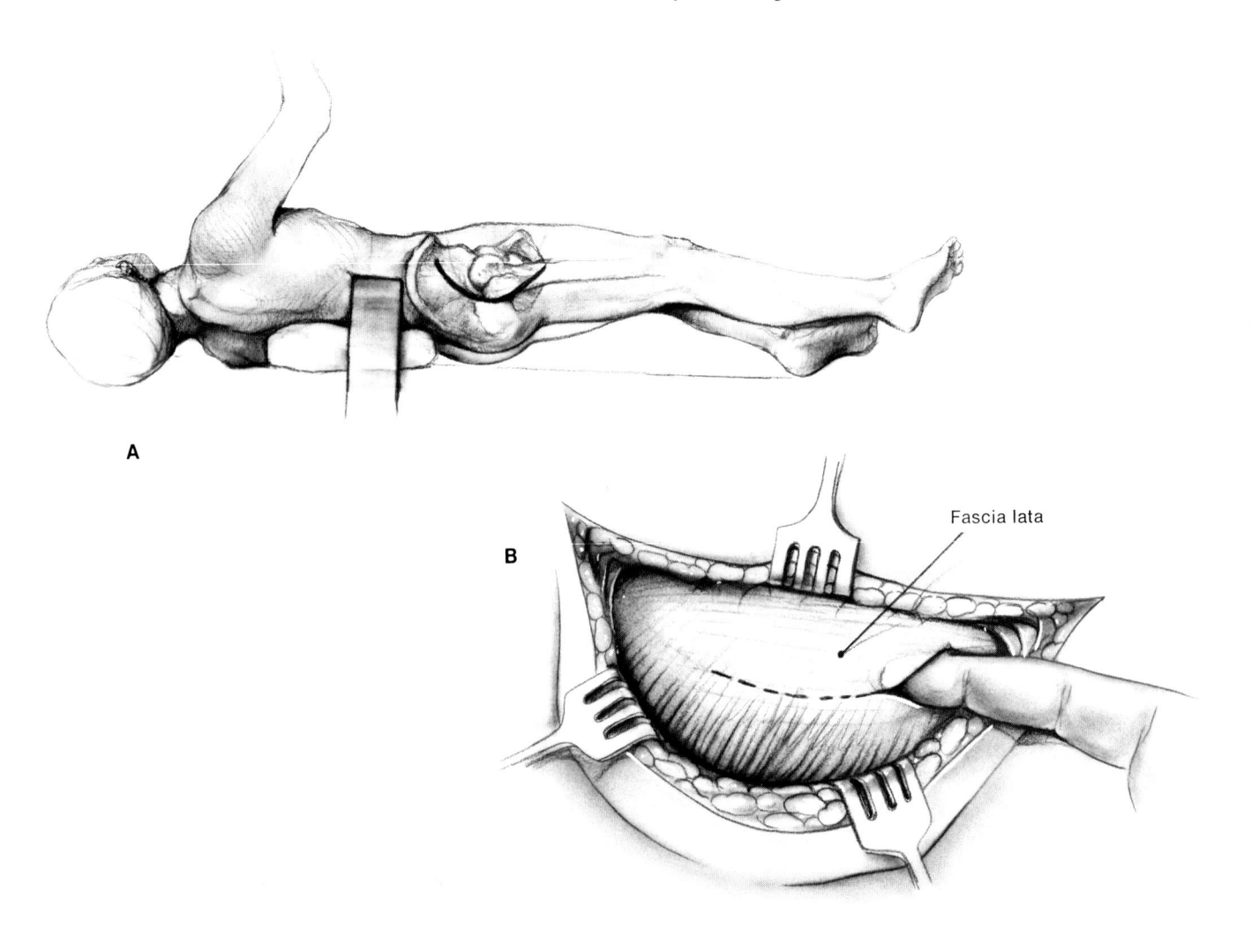

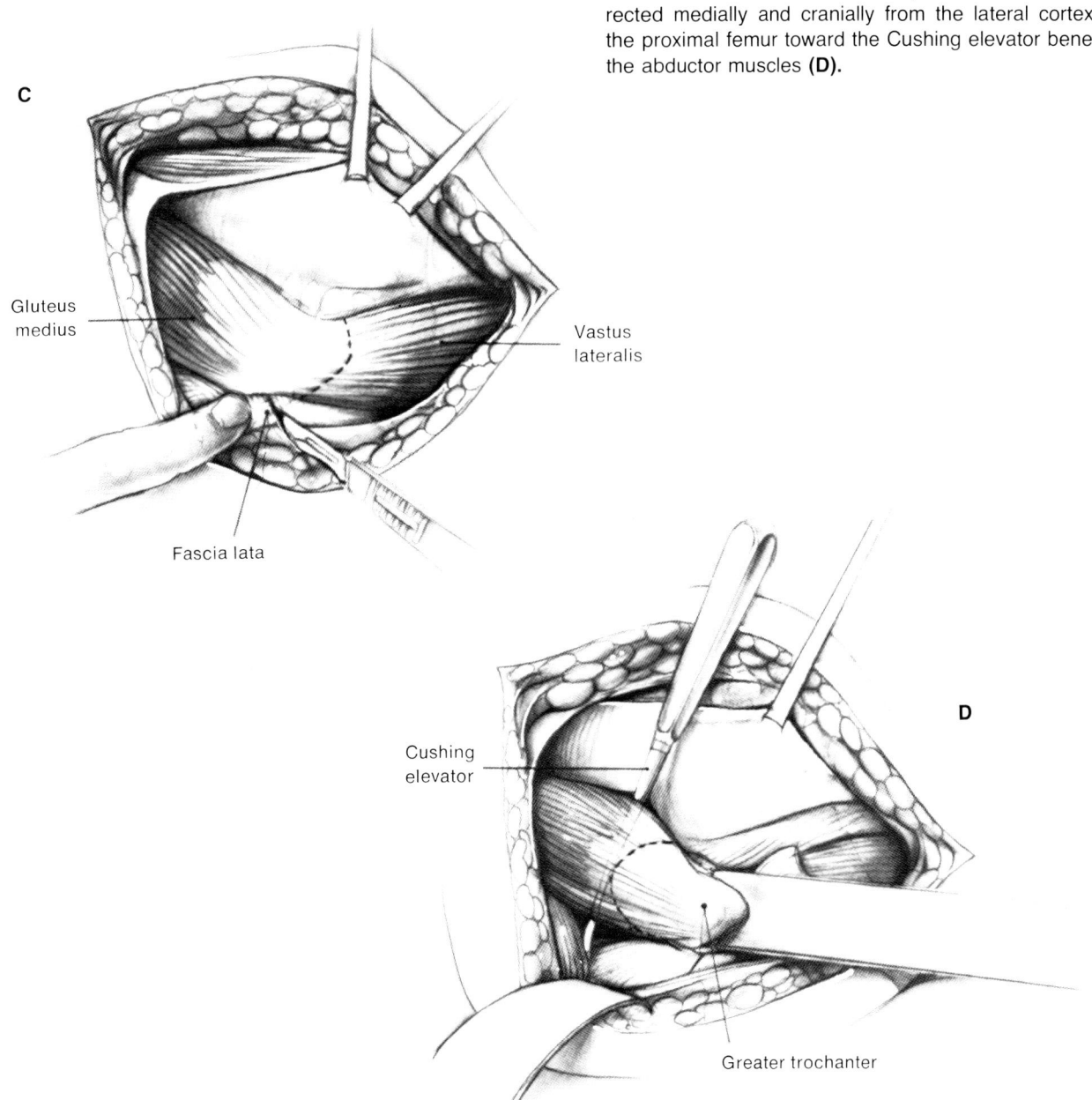

(Plate 10-10) CUP ARTHROPLASTY

A short oblique incision is made in the deep surface of the posteriorly reflected fascia lata, extending into the substance of the gluteus maximus **(C)** to obtain wide exposure of the posterior aspect of the joint capsule and to provide a space into which the femoral head can subsequently be dislocated posteriorly for a complete view of the acetabulum. This incision in the posterior fibers of the fascia lata begins at the level of the superior tip of the greater trochanter and extends posteriorly and proximally into the gluteus maximus for 3.5 cm, keeping parallel to the muscle fibers. The tensor fascia lata along with the anterior portion of the iliotibial band is retracted anteriorly, a periosteal elevator being used along the anterior capsule of the femoral neck to the border of the acetabulum. A Cushing elevator is passed from anterior to posterior along the superior surface of the capsule at the base of the medial surface of the greater trochanter beneath the fibers of the gluteus minimus and gluteus medius to direct the plane for osteotomy of the greater trochanter. Before the greater trochanter is osteotomized, the proximal portion of the vastus lateralis is reflected distally to expose the proximal femur below the greater trochanter to allow a wide, sharp osteotome to be directed medially and cranially from the lateral cortex of the proximal femur toward the Cushing elevator beneath the abductor muscles **(D)**.

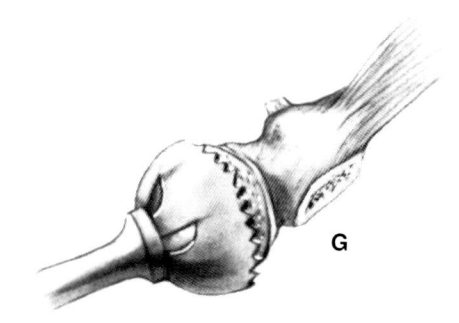

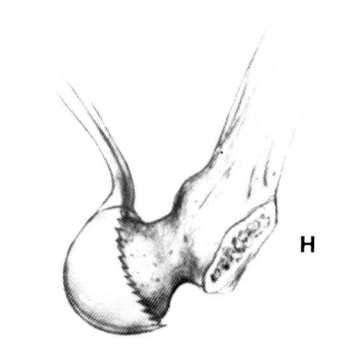

CUP ARTHROPLASTY (Plate 10-10)

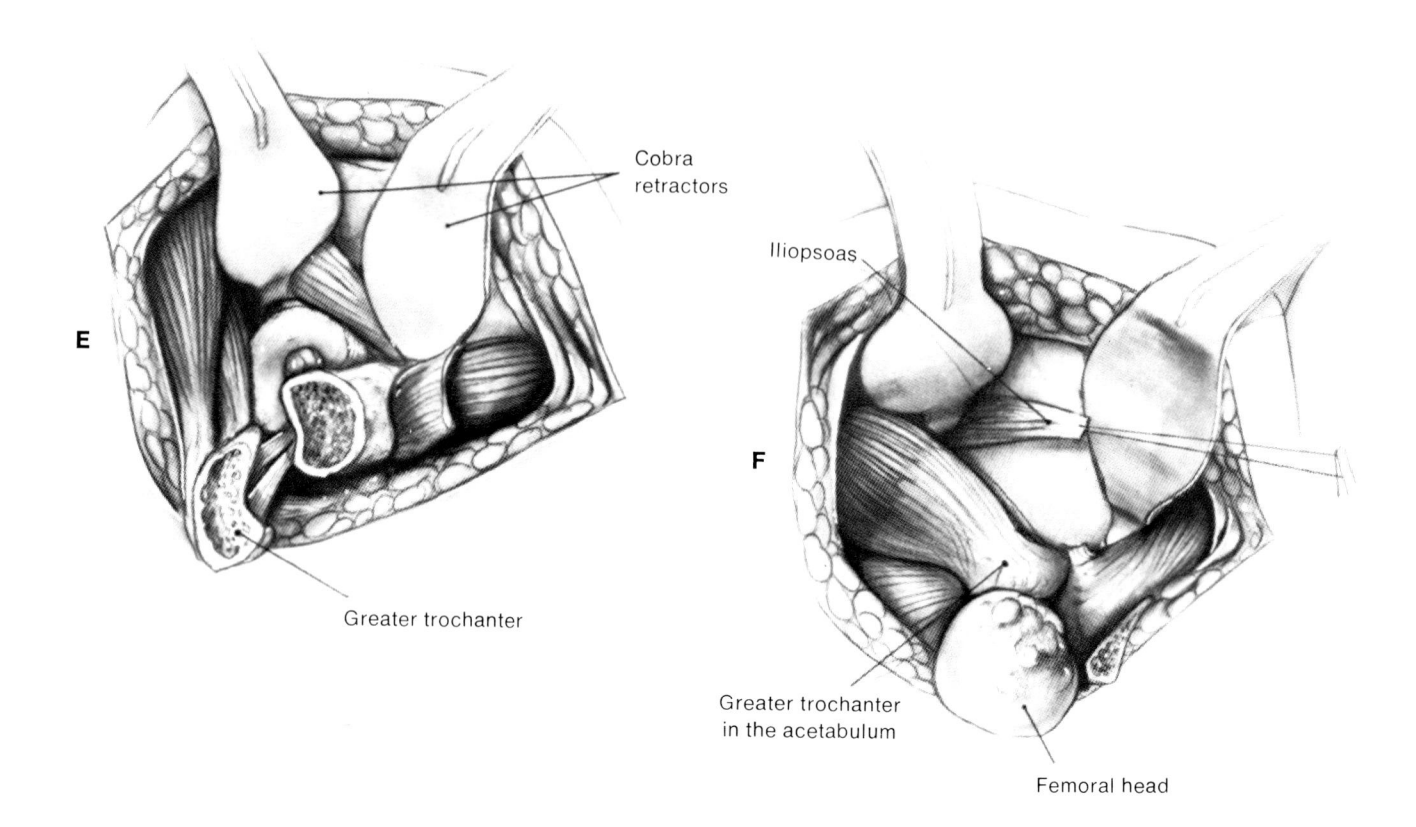

When the greater trochanter and its attached muscles are reflected proximally, the superior portion of the capsule will be visualized (E). The piriformis, obturator internus, and obturator externus are cut from the detached greater trochanter. The superior portion of the capsule is incised in line with the neck of the femur from the rim of the acetabulum to the osteotomy of the greater trochanter. Internal rotation of the femur then allows visualization of the posterior aspect of the capsule, which is excised under direct vision. The sciatic nerve is specifically protected during this procedure.

Attention is now directed to the anterior aspect of the hip. A cobra-type-retractor with a small blunt tip is inserted deep to the straight head of the rectus femoris over the anterior inferior iliac spine. This should provide exposure of the superior and anterior aspect of the capsule. Another cobra retractor is placed between the capsule and the iliopsoas to provide exposure of the anterior and inferior aspect of the capsule. The remainder of the capsule is then excised, the surgeon working from both the anterior and posterior aspects of the hip and leaving only the stump of the insertion of the anterior capsule, which is saved for subsequent reattachment of the iliopsoas tendon.

The femoral head is now dislocated anteriorly by extension, adduction, and external rotation of the hip as traction is applied in a lateral direction with a bone hook around the femoral neck. This will bring the iliopsoas and lesser trochanter into view. The iliopsoas tendon is divided at its insertion under direct vision (F). The greater trochanter with its muscle attachments is placed into the acetabulum, and the leg is externally rotated to bring the femoral head anteriorly into the wound. This allows the entire circumference of the femoral head to be visualized where it can be shaped appropriately with gouges and reamers (G and H).

332

(Plate 10-10) CUP ARTHROPLASTY

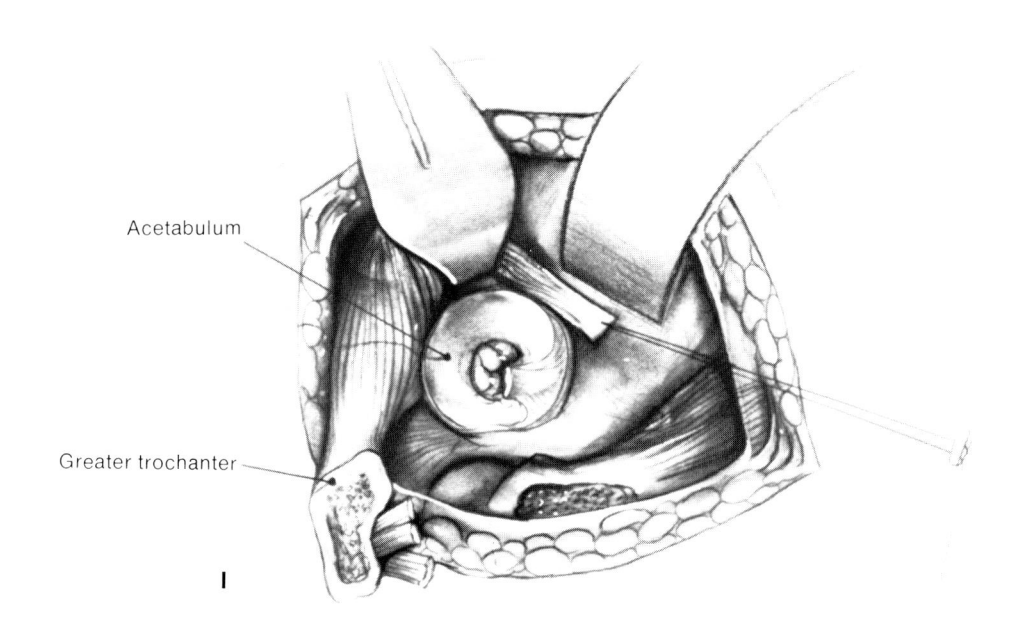

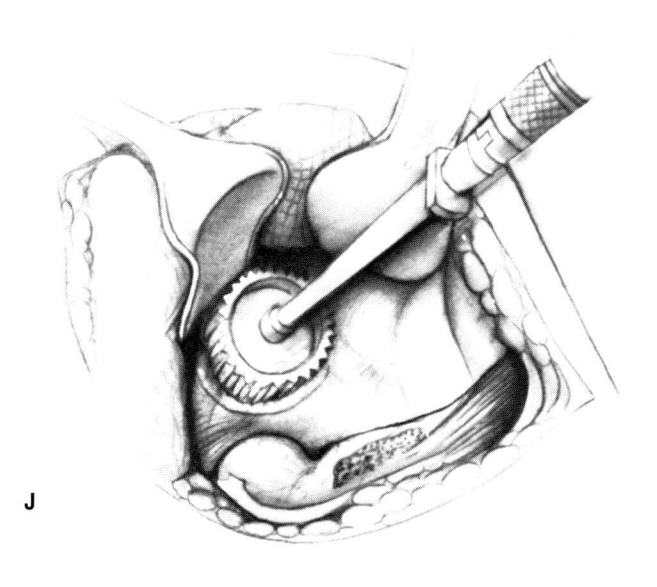

Acetabulum

Greater trochanter

I

J

For exposure of the acetabulum, the greater trochanter is again retracted proximally and the femoral head is moved into a position posterior to the acetabulum (I). This is accomplished by adduction, flexion, and internal rotation of the hip (together with flexion of the knee). Flexing the knee reduces the tension on the hamstrings and sciatic nerve when the femoral head is moved into a position posterior to the acetabulum. A cobra retractor is placed behind the posterior rim of the acetabulum to retract the femur and posterior soft tissues to provide an unobstructed view of the entire acetabulum. The acetabulum is prepared with gauges and acetabular reamers (J).

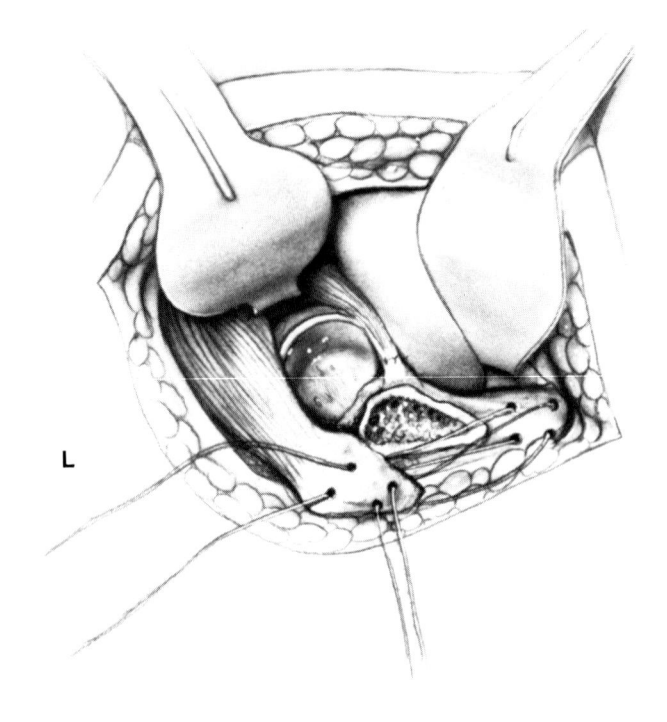

CUP ARTHROPLASTY (Plate 10-10)

The wound is debrided thoroughly, and the mold is inserted when the acetabulum has been completely prepared. The prepared femoral head is reduced into the concavity of the mold. The behavior of the mold is visualized as the hip is moved through a range of motion. If the cup mold moves properly, the iliopsoas tendon is then transplanted anteriorly and laterally to the distal stump of the remaining portion of the capsule (**K**).

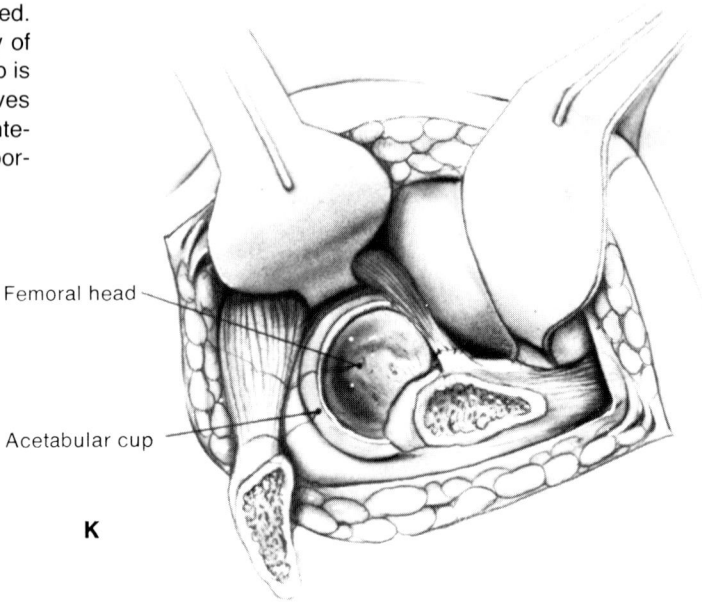

The greater trochanter is transplanted distally and wired directly to the lateral side of the femoral shaft with the leg in a position just short of maximum abduction and in approximately 10° of external rotation. The greater trochanter is secured to the proximal shaft of the femur by placing four drill holes in the lateral cortex of the femoral shaft and comparable holes in the greater trochanter for the placement of two 18-gauge wires that are used to tighted and secure the greater trochanter in the desired position (**L**).

(Plate 10-10) CUP ARTHROPLASTY

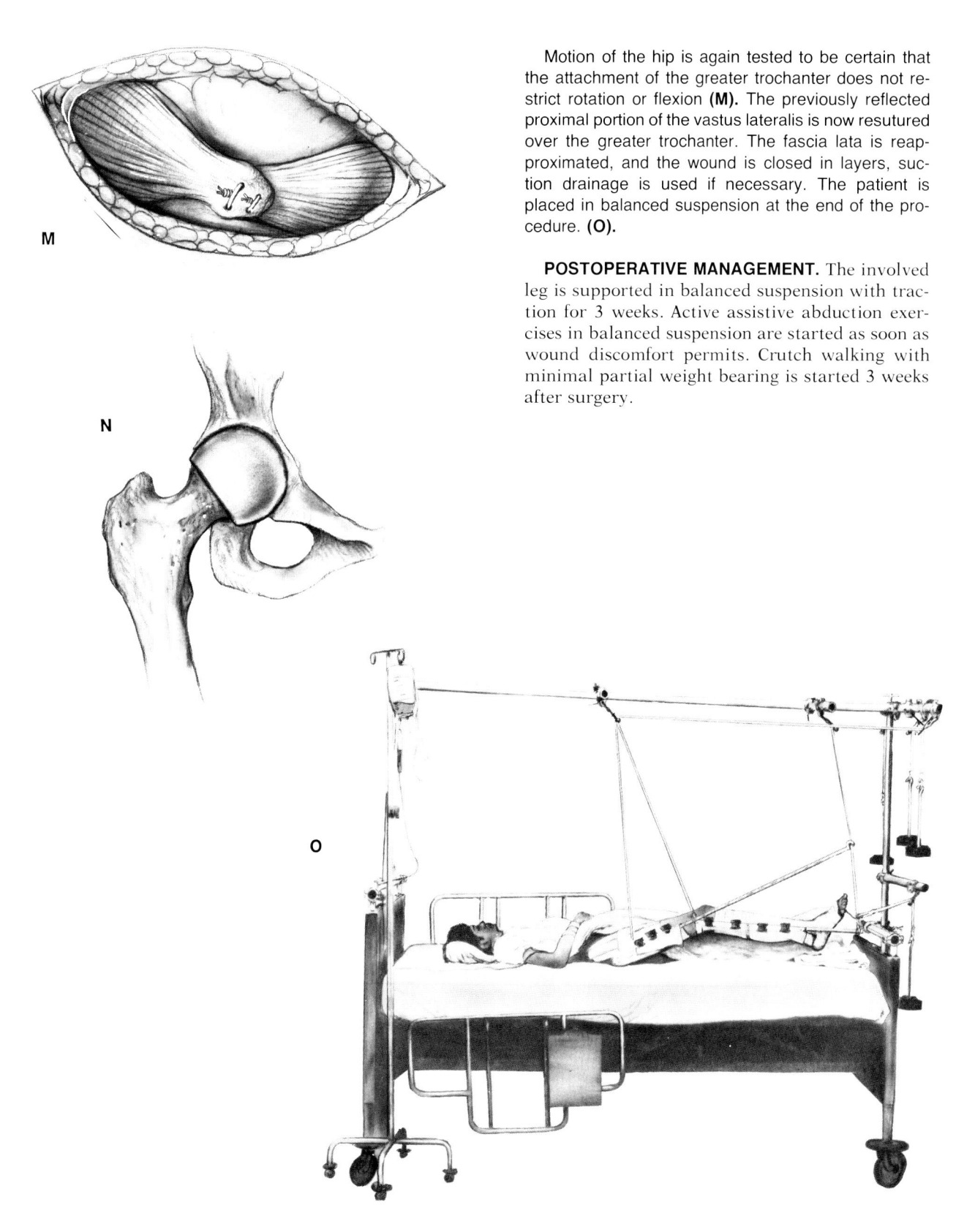

M

Motion of the hip is again tested to be certain that the attachment of the greater trochanter does not restrict rotation or flexion **(M)**. The previously reflected proximal portion of the vastus lateralis is now resutured over the greater trochanter. The fascia lata is reapproximated, and the wound is closed in layers, suction drainage is used if necessary. The patient is placed in balanced suspension at the end of the procedure. **(O)**.

POSTOPERATIVE MANAGEMENT. The involved leg is supported in balanced suspension with traction for 3 weeks. Active assistive abduction exercises in balanced suspension are started as soon as wound discomfort permits. Crutch walking with minimal partial weight bearing is started 3 weeks after surgery.

N

O

ADDUCTOR TENOTOMY (Plate 10-11)

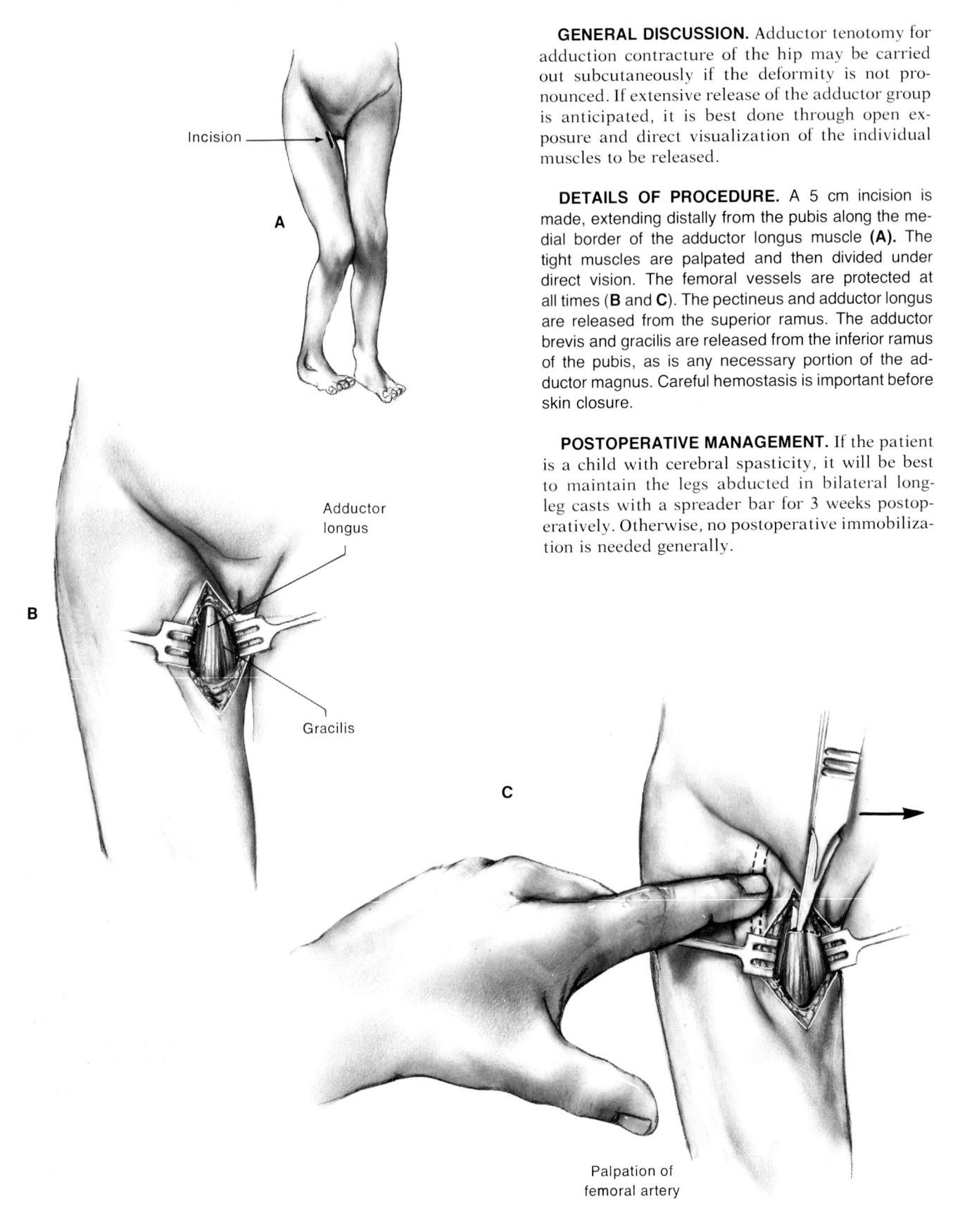

GENERAL DISCUSSION. Adductor tenotomy for adduction contracture of the hip may be carried out subcutaneously if the deformity is not pronounced. If extensive release of the adductor group is anticipated, it is best done through open exposure and direct visualization of the individual muscles to be released.

DETAILS OF PROCEDURE. A 5 cm incision is made, extending distally from the pubis along the medial border of the adductor longus muscle (**A**). The tight muscles are palpated and then divided under direct vision. The femoral vessels are protected at all times (**B** and **C**). The pectineus and adductor longus are released from the superior ramus. The adductor brevis and gracilis are released from the inferior ramus of the pubis, as is any necessary portion of the adductor magnus. Careful hemostasis is important before skin closure.

POSTOPERATIVE MANAGEMENT. If the patient is a child with cerebral spasticity, it will be best to maintain the legs abducted in bilateral long-leg casts with a spreader bar for 3 weeks postoperatively. Otherwise, no postoperative immobilization is needed generally.

(Plate 10-12) RELEASE OF HIP FLEXION CONTRACTURE

GENERAL DISCUSSION. For flexion and abduction contracture of the hip, conservative measures may not be successful and surgical release may be necessary to correct the deformity. Tightness of the iliotibial band may be associated with several deformities: flexion and abduction contracture of the hip, flexion contracture of the knee, and genu valgus. If the flexion and abduction contracture of the hip are recent and mild, division of the iliotibial band and fascia lata proximal to the lateral femoral condyle (as described by Yount) may correct the contracture. For the severe flexion and abduction contracture of the hip, more extensive release of muscle attachments at their proximal origin will be necessary.

DETAILS OF PROCEDURE. The skin is incised as for an anterior iliofemoral approach **(A)**. Skin and subcutaneous tissue are retracted, and the entire thickness of the fascia is divided from the anterosuperior iliac spine to the greater trochanter. The sartorius is released from the anterosuperior iliac spine. An incision is made along the lateral aspect of the iliac crest to permit reflection of muscles from the outer cortex of the ilium **(B)**.

Muscles are reflected subperiosteally from the outer cortex of the anterior portion of the ilium **(C)**. Since there is often an associated knee flexion contracture, release of the origin of the rectus femoris from the anteroinferior iliac spine **(D)** should be omitted unless release of the other muscles does not correct the hip flexion contracture. The hip is now hyperextended, which allows each of these muscles to retract distally. Skin and subcutaneous tissues are closed in layers.

POSTOPERATIVE MANAGEMENT. The patient is placed in a hip spica postoperatively, maintaining the hip in that degree of extension which could be obtained at the time of operation. The hip spica is removed 3 to 4 weeks after surgery. If correction is incomplete, further correction may be obtained with wedging of the cast.

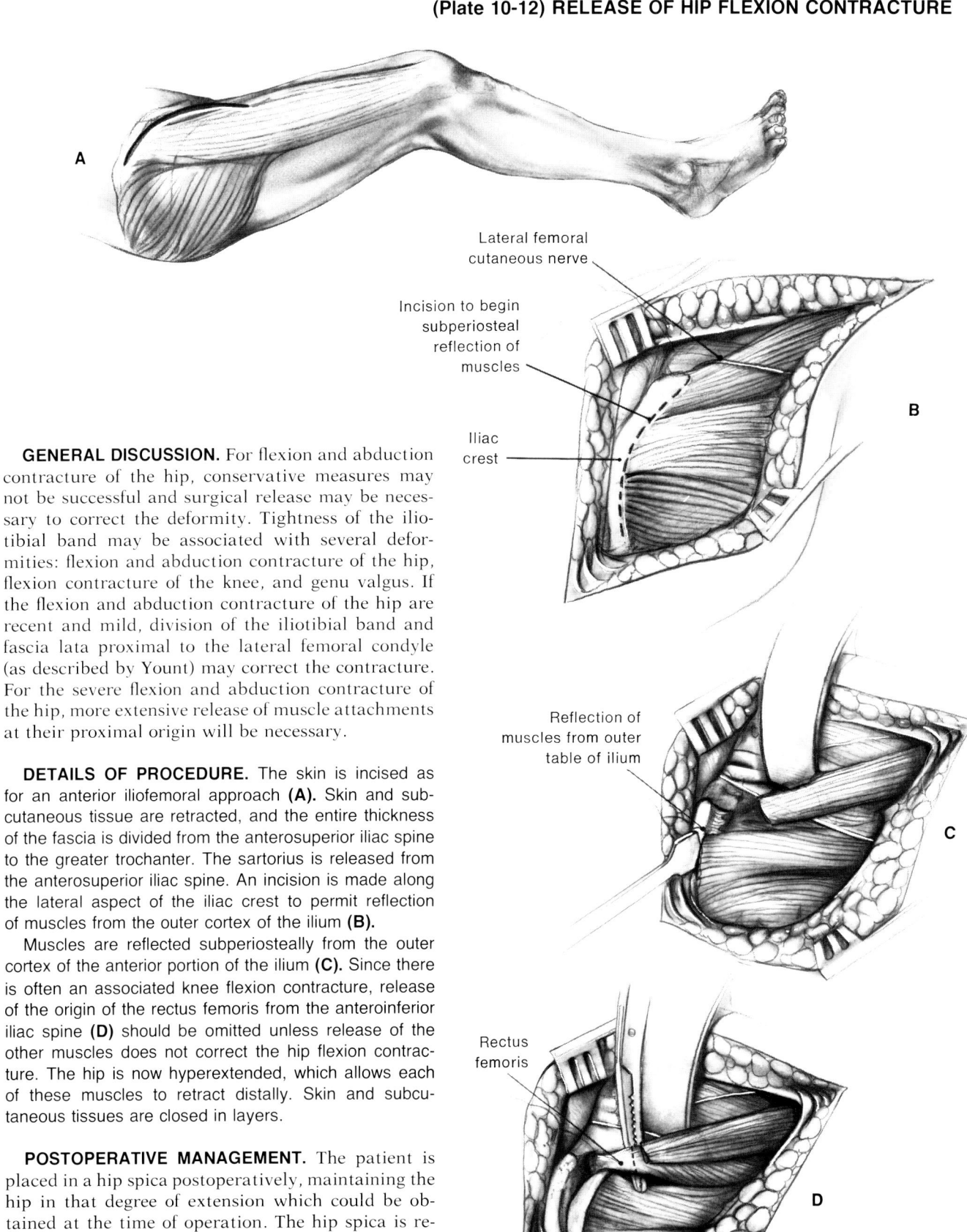

OBTURATOR NEURECTOMY (Plate 10-13)

GENERAL DISCUSSION. A total obturator neurectomy performed through an intrapelvic approach will give a dramatic release of the spastic adduction deformity of the hip, but it is also possible to produce an uncontrolled abduction deformity. It is more conservative in most cases to combine an extrapelvic neurectomy of the anterior branch of the obturator nerve with an adductor tenotomy (through the same incision) before sacrificing the entire obturator nerve, which can be done at a subsequent date if it should prove to be necessary.

DETAILS OF PROCEDURE. In the *extrapelvic* procedure a 5 cm incision is made beginning at the symphysis pubis and extending parallel to the adductor longus muscle **(A)**. The adductor longus muscle is retracted laterally to expose the underlying adductor brevis muscle around which the anterior and posterior divisions of the obturator nerve normally separate (**B** and **C**). The anterior division is identified on the anterior surface of the adductor brevis muscle and a portion of the anterior division of the obturator nerve is resected **(D)**, thereby removing innervation to the gracilis, adductor longus, and adductor brevis muscle (plus sensory branches to the hip joint and medial aspect of the upper thigh). The posterior division of the obturator nerve **(E)** is located between the adductor brevis and the adductor magnus, and this portion of the obturator nerve may or may not be transected, depending on the degree of adductor deformity and the individual circumstances. If there is any element of fixed adduction contracture, the tendinous origins of the adductor muscles are easily divided along the pubis through the same exposure.

In the *intrapelvic* procedure a transverse incision is made across the lower portion of the rectus abdominis muscle 2.5 cm above the pubis. The anterior rectus fascia is divided longitudinally in the midportion of the muscle. The lateral border of the rectus abdominis muscle is outlined and retracted medially. The index finger is used as a blunt dissector to follow the posterior surface of the superior pubic ramus. It should be possible to palpate the obturator nerve as it enters the superior aspect of the obturator foramen. Flat retractors are placed to allow direct visualization and separation of the obturator nerve from the accompanying vessels before resection of a portion of the nerve is carried out between proximal and distal nerve ligatures. This sacrifices all innervation to the adductor musculature except the femoral nerve supply to the pectineus and the sciatic nerve supply to the portion of the adductor magnus that arises from the ischial tuberosity.

(Plate 10-13) OBTURATOR NEURECTOMY

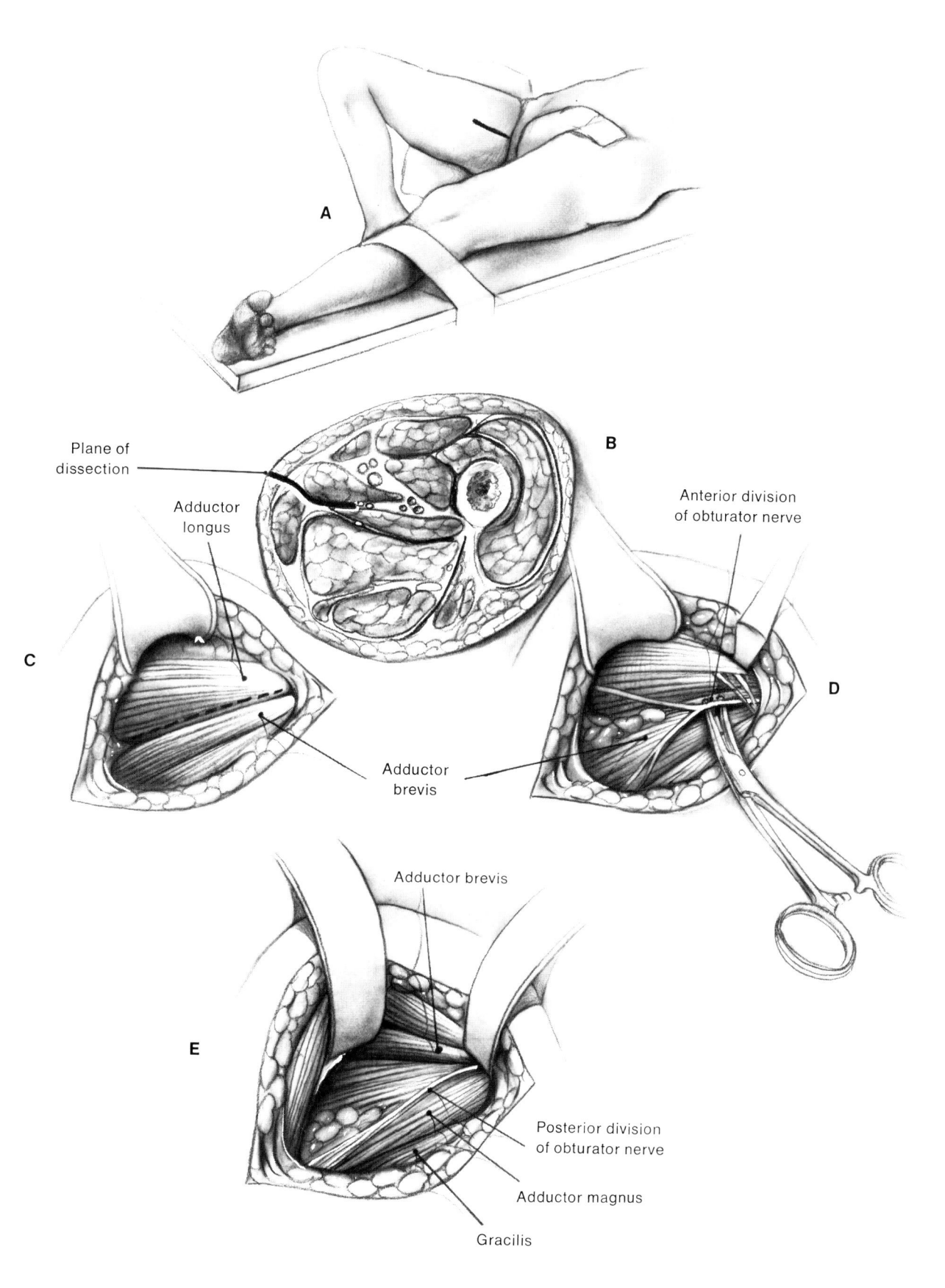

Plane of dissection

Adductor longus

Adductor brevis

Anterior division of obturator nerve

Adductor brevis

Posterior division of obturator nerve

Adductor magnus

Gracilis

339

RELEASE OF ILIOPSOAS (Plate 10-14)

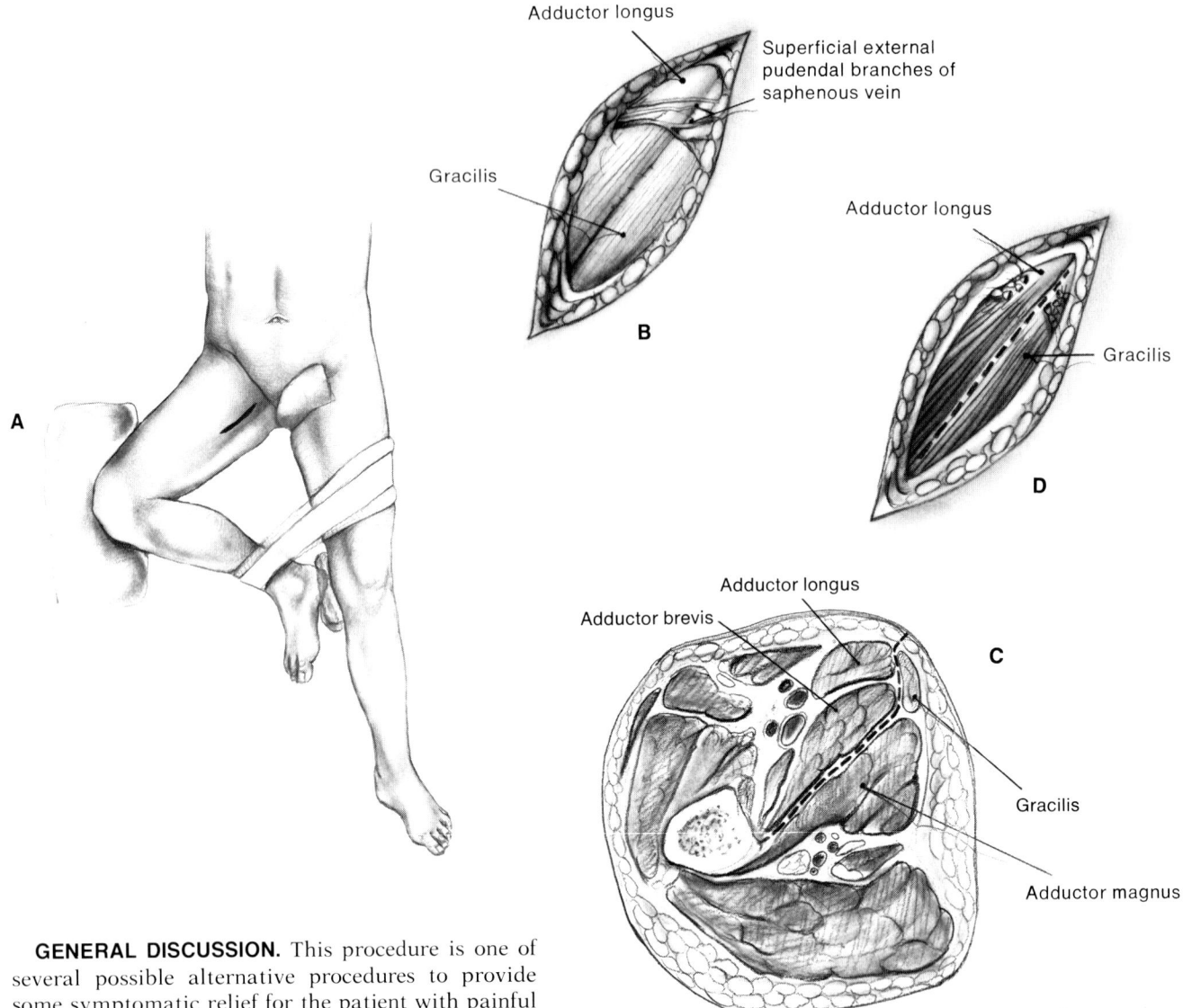

GENERAL DISCUSSION. This procedure is one of several possible alternative procedures to provide some symptomatic relief for the patient with painful degenerative arthritis of the hip. An advantage of this soft tissue procedure is the minimal convalescence compared with alternative procedures involving surgical alterations of the femur or hip joint. However, the extent and duration of symptomatic relief resulting from this procedure is difficult to predict. It is probably most likely to be helpful when the painful hip has been associated with a flexion adduction position and some degree of spasm of the adductor musculature. Depending in part on the extent of the degenerative change existing with the hip joint and the duration of any maintained flexion adduction contracture, some improvement in terms of abduction and extension can be anticipated. However, although this and the diminished muscle tension across the hip joint may provide some clinical improvement, the patient should understand that this procedure will not alter the prexisting changes or basic underlying disease process of the hip joint.

DETAILS OF PROCEDURE. If the patient's knees can be separated by at least 46 cm by any combination of movements with both hips, the medial approach described by Ludloff permits good exposure by dissection between normal muscle planes without any necessary detachment or transection of muscles. With the hip in slight flexion and maximum abduction and external rotation, the contour of the adductor longus muscle can be easily identified. A longitudinal incision is made along its posterior border beginning 2.5 cm distal to the pubic tubercle and extending 15 cm distally **(A)**. The plane is developed between the adductor longus muscle anteriorly and the gracilis muscle posteriorly (**B** to **D**). It is usually necessary to ligate the superficial external pudendal branches of the saphenous vein in the proximal portion of the wound **(D)**.

(Plate 10-14) RELEASE OF ILIOPSOAS

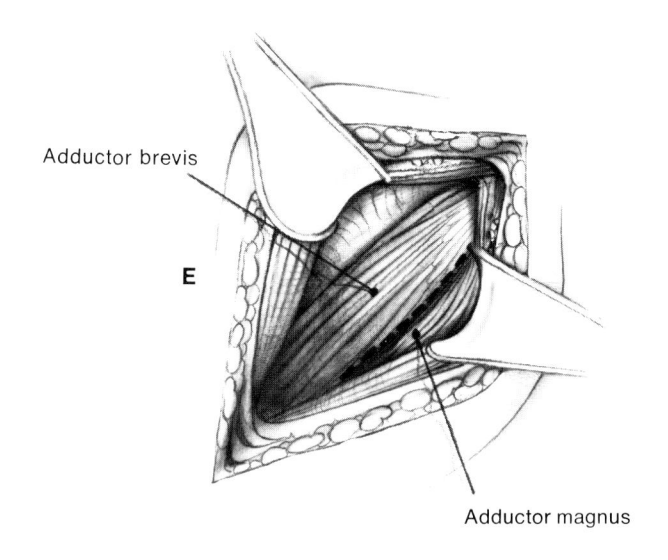

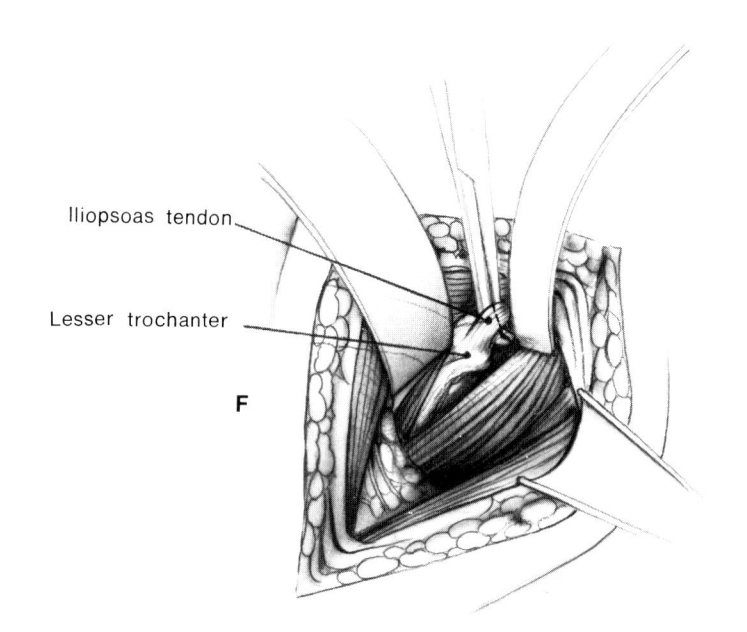

Next the plane is developed between the adductor brevis muscle anteriorly and the adductor magnus muscle posteriorly **(E)** while the neurovascular bundle to the gracilis muscle and the posterior branch of the obturator nerve (innervating the adductor magnus), which emerge together in the distal portion of the wound between the adductor brevis and adductor magnus muscles, are protected.

By retracting the gracilis and adductor magnus muscles posteriorly, the medial aspect of the proximal femoral shaft and the iliopsoas tendon inserting into the lesser trochanter can be visualized. A deep right-angle clamp is placed around the iliopsoas tendon at its insertion into the lesser trochanter, and the iliopsoas tendon is completely sectioned **(F)**. If an adductor tenotomy is also indicated, this may be carried out under direct vision in the upper portion of the wound either just prior to wound closure or earlier, if desired, to facilitate exposure of the lesser trochanter and iliopsoas tendon through this medial approach.

341

RELEASE OF ILIOPSOAS (Plate 10-14)

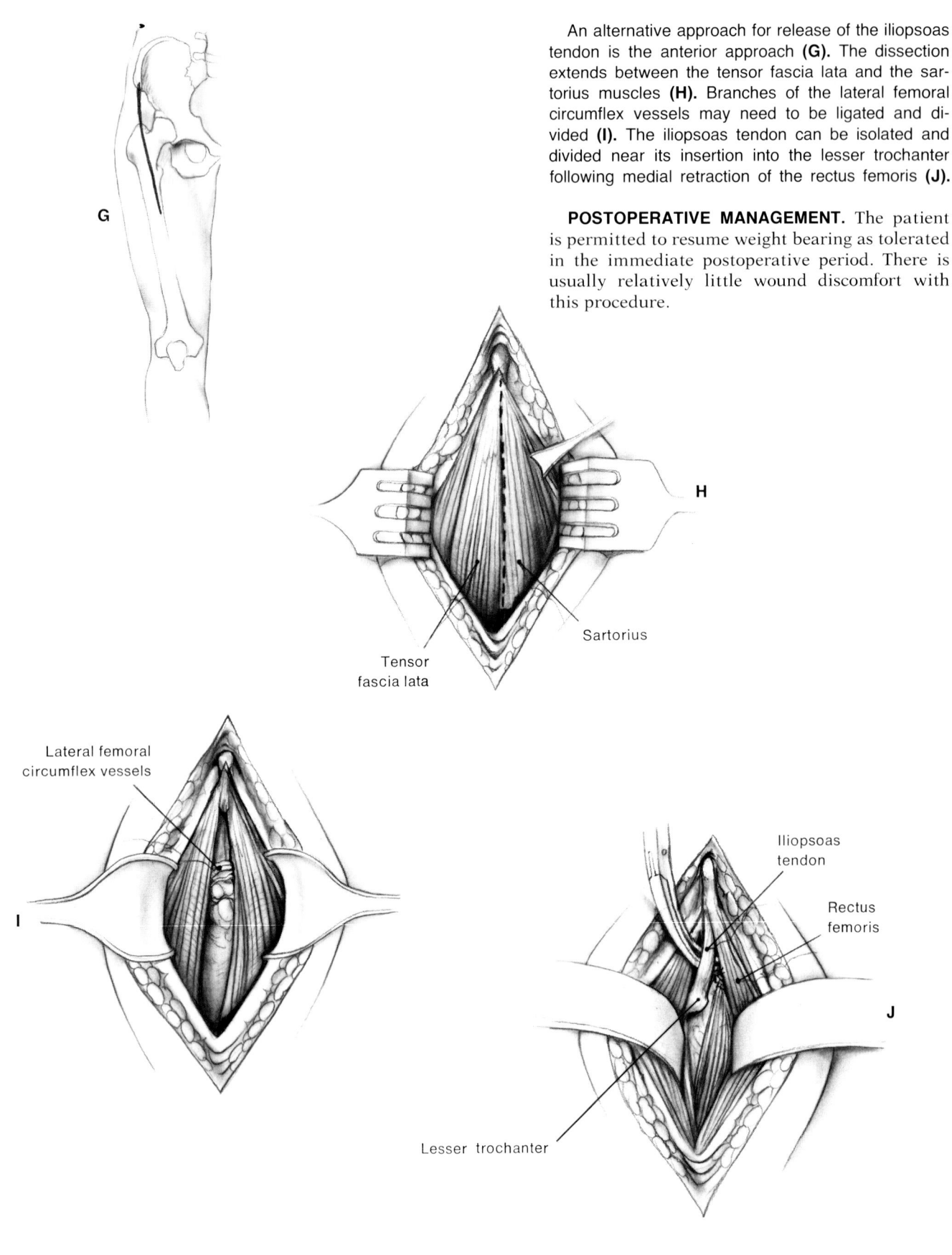

An alternative approach for release of the iliopsoas tendon is the anterior approach **(G)**. The dissection extends between the tensor fascia lata and the sartorius muscles **(H)**. Branches of the lateral femoral circumflex vessels may need to be ligated and divided **(I)**. The iliopsoas tendon can be isolated and divided near its insertion into the lesser trochanter following medial retraction of the rectus femoris **(J)**.

POSTOPERATIVE MANAGEMENT. The patient is permitted to resume weight bearing as tolerated in the immediate postoperative period. There is usually relatively little wound discomfort with this procedure.

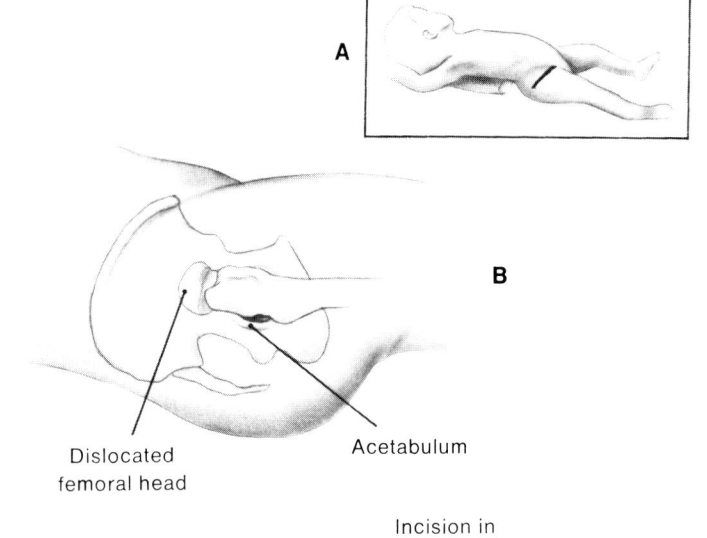

(Plate 10-15) OPEN REDUCTION FOR CONGENITAL DISLOCATION OF HIP

GENERAL DISCUSSION. If the diagnosis of congenital dislocation of the hip is made and treatment is started within the first year of life, open reduction of the hip is rarely necessary.

Open reduction for congenital dislocation of the hip may be indicated occasionally in patients under 5 or 6 years of age if it has been impossible to obtain concentric seating of the femoral head within the acetabulum by closed treatment methods. Open reduction is indicated when it becomes evident during the course of closed treatment that unyielding soft tissue structures are obstructing a satisfactory reduction of the femoral head into the acetabulum.

Open reduction for congenital dislocation of the hip is unlikely to be sufficient treatment by itself after 4 years of age because by that age the acetabular roof may be too oblique and an operation on the pelvis to provide a more satisfactory acetabular roof is often also indicated. In patients under 4 years of age, if open reduction is performed, the acetabular roof should be examined, and if it is too oblique, innominate osteotomy may be indicated.

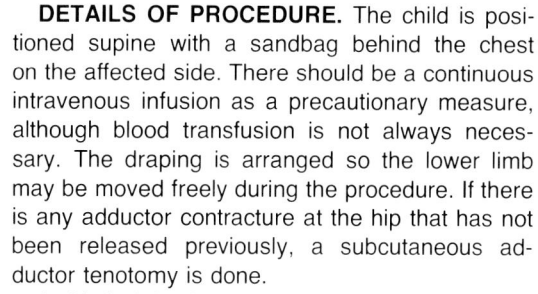

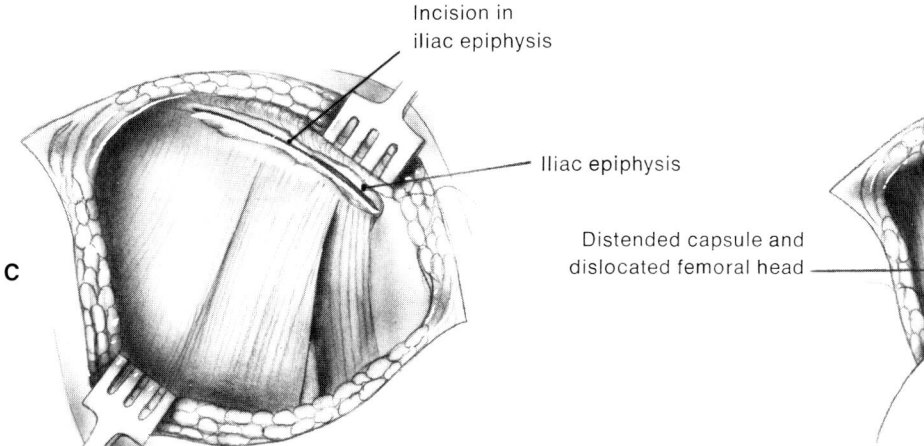

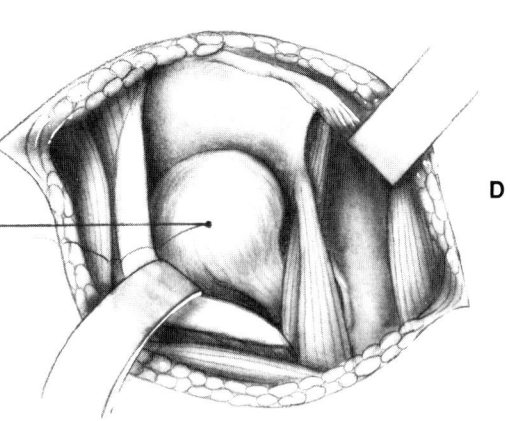

DETAILS OF PROCEDURE. The child is positioned supine with a sandbag behind the chest on the affected side. There should be a continuous intravenous infusion as a precautionary measure, although blood transfusion is not always necessary. The draping is arranged so the lower limb may be moved freely during the procedure. If there is any adductor contracture at the hip that has not been released previously, a subcutaneous adductor tenotomy is done.

A skin incision is made beginning below the middle of the iliac crest and passing obliquely forward distal to the anterosuperior iliac spine almost to the midpoint of the inguinal ligament (**A** and **B**). The plane is developed between the tensor fascia lata laterally and the sartorius and rectus femoris medially, and this interval is then packed. An incision is made in the iliac epiphysis down to bone along the iliac crest (**C**) from its midpoint to the anterosuperior iliac spine and then distally to the anteroinferior iliac spine. The lateral portion of the epiphysis with the periosteum on the external surface of the ilium is then reflected in a continuous sheet inferiorly to the lateral edge of the acetabulum and posteriorly to the greater sciatic notch (**D**). This area is also packed. The fibrous capsule of the hip may have become adherent to the lateral aspect of the ilium above the acetabulum as a result of being stretched upward by the intracapsular dislocation; if this is the situation, it should be freed from the outer table of the ilium with a periosteal elevator. The anterior and lateral portions of the hip capsule are exposed by blunt dissection in the interval between the fibrous capsule and the abductor muscles.

OPEN REDUCTION FOR CONGENITAL DISLOCATION OF HIP (Plate 10-15)

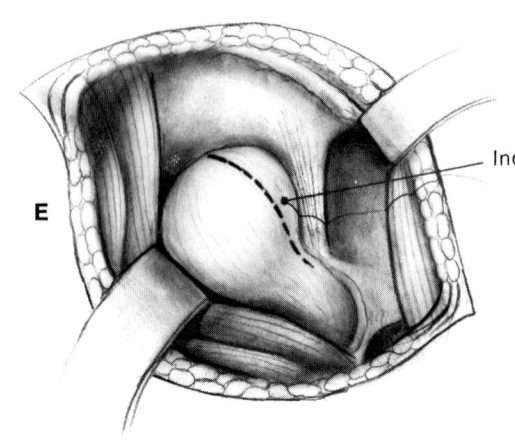

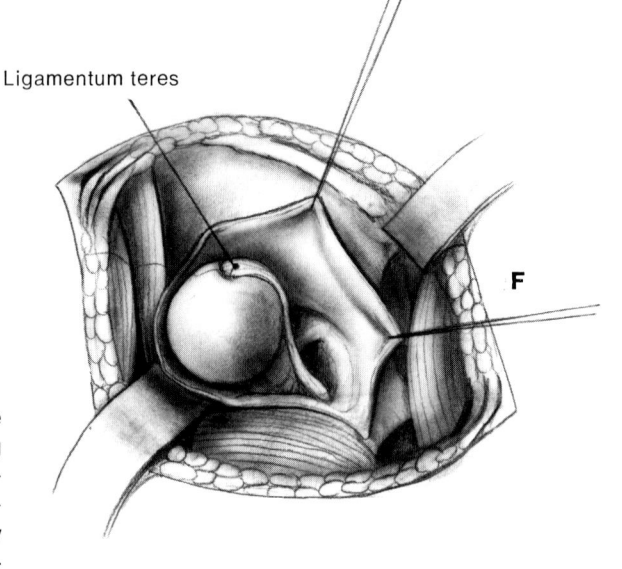

The capsule of the hip joint is opened widely close to the superior and anterior margin of the acetabulum **(E)**. Identifying the ligamentum teres and tracing it into the depth of the acetabulum is useful in determining the location of the true acetabulum **(F)**. The ligamentum teres is left intact unless it is grossly hypertrophied. Any excessive fibrofatty tissue in the acetabulum is removed gently. If the capsule has been opened widely, the limbus usually presents no obstacle to reduction and should be preserved. The femoral head should be gently reduced under direct vision. The tightness of the iliopsoas should be noted specifically. If the iliopsoas is tight, making reduction difficult and preventing abduction and medial rotation when the hip is reduced, the tendinous portion of the iliopsoas should be divided. The stability of the reduction should be assessed carefully. The reduction is generally stable with the hip in abduction, flexion, and variable degrees of internal rotation. Redislocation may occur laterally when the hip is adducted and anteriorly when the hip is either extended or externally rotated. If the hip has been gently reduced but remains unstable because of inadequacy of the acetabular roof, an innominate osteotomy (as described by Salter) should be carried out.

The affected limb is held in the stable position as any redundant capsule is excised and as the capsule and the remainder of the wound are closed **(G)**, and until the child has been immobilized in a one and one-half hip spica **(H)** retaining the leg in the desired position of abduction, flexion, and some internal rotation.

POSTOPERATIVE MANAGEMENT. Plaster immobilization in a one and one-half hip spica is continued for 3 to 4 months after surgery depending on the age of the child and the degree of stability of the reduction. Active motion of the hip is then permitted. Any subsequent splinting that holds the hip in external rotation is specifically avoided. The position, stability, and development of the hip are followed clinically and roentgenographically at intervals until it is apparent that the hip is remaining stable under conditions of full weight bearing and unrestricted activity.

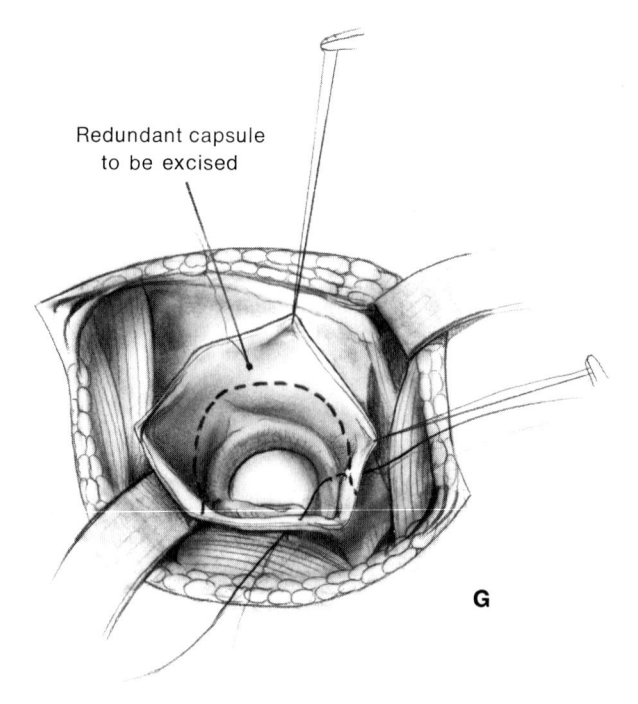

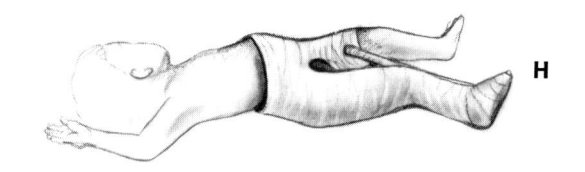

(Plate 10-16) MEDIAL APPROACH TO THE HIP JOINT

GENERAL DISCUSSION. In 1908 Ludloff described the medial approach to the hip. It is a useful alternative exposure in the young child with congenital dislocation of the hip. It is also helpful to gain exposure to the lesser trochanteric region for tumor resection.

DETAILS OF PROCEDURE. The leg is placed in the flexed abducted, externally rotated position. A longitudinal incision is made over the interval between the gracilis and adductor longus muscles (**A** and **B**). The plane between the adductor brevis and magnus is developed and separated (**C**). Once the magnus and brevis are reflected, the lesser trochanter, iliopsoas tendon, and hip capsule are immediately adjacent in the wound (**D** and **E**). The iliopsoas tendon is divided. The neurovascular bundle of the gracilis muscle will be distal in the wound. One must be careful to protect the posterior branch of the abductor nerve.

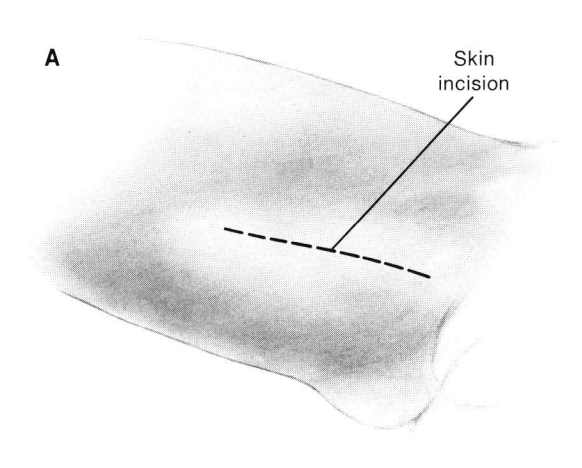

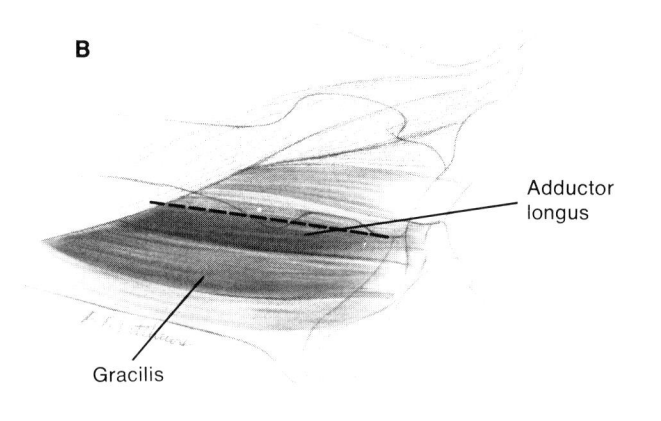

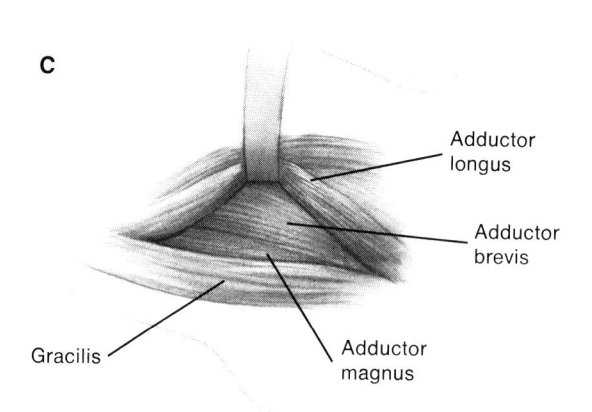

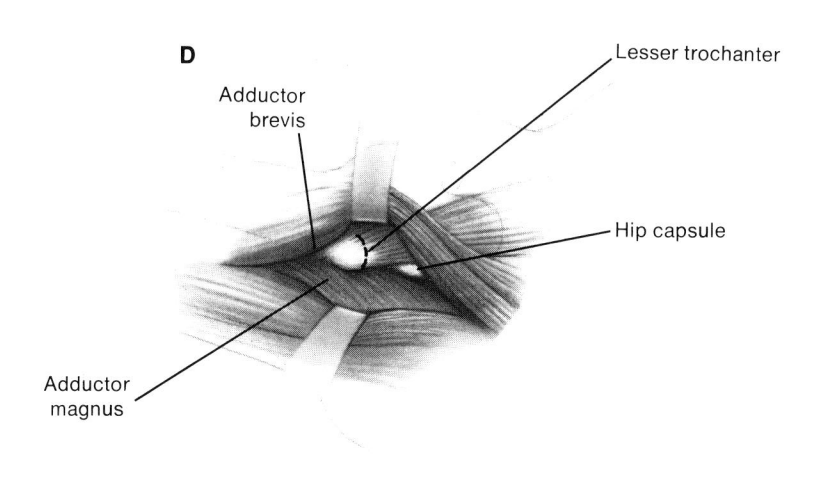

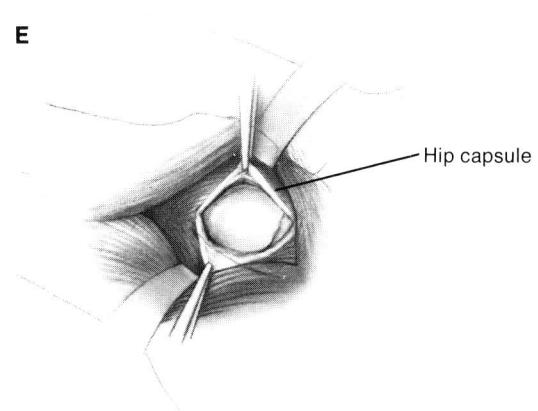

SUBTROCHANTERIC DEROTATION OSTEOTOMY (Plate 10-17)

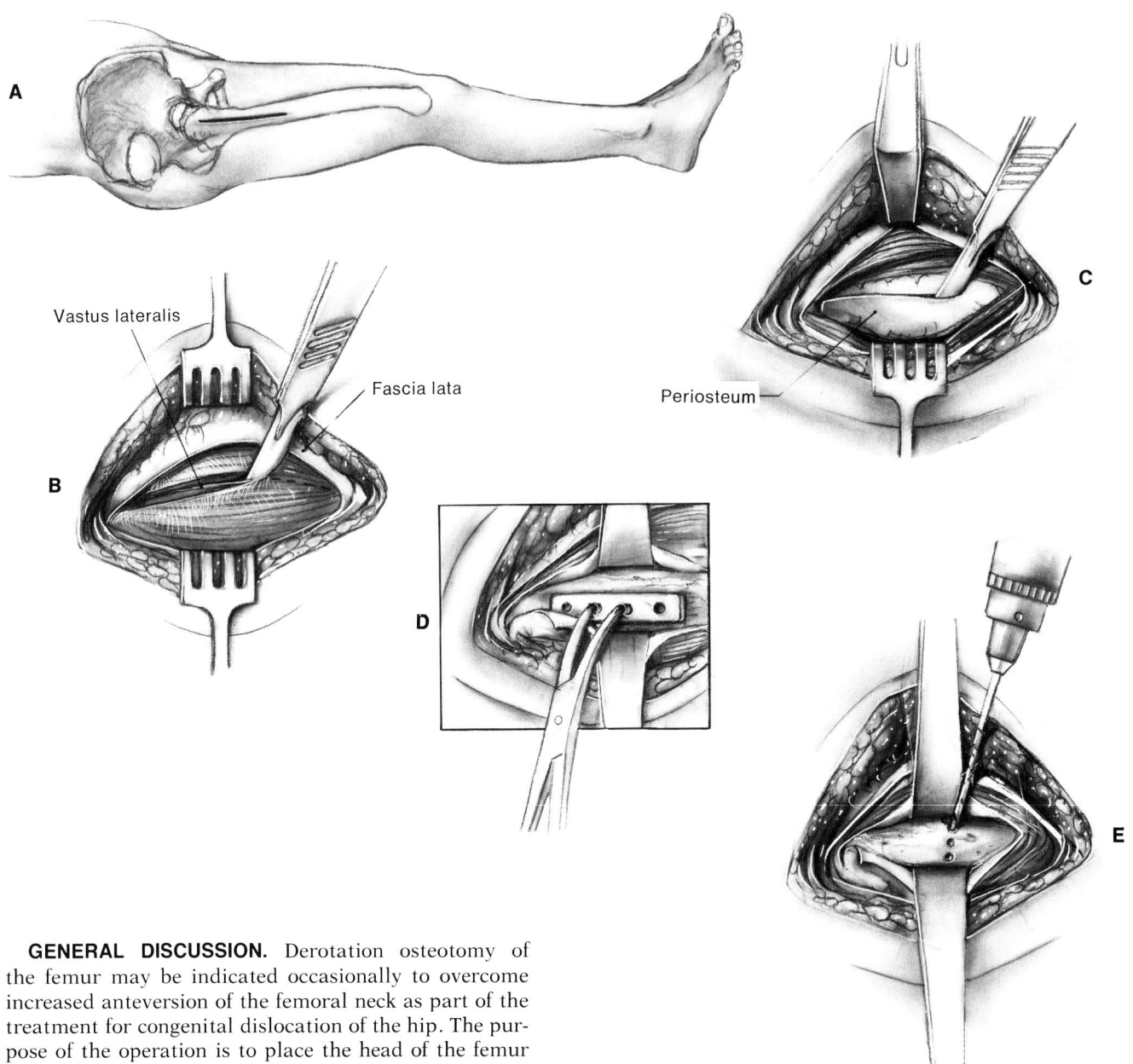

GENERAL DISCUSSION. Derotation osteotomy of the femur may be indicated occasionally to overcome increased anteversion of the femoral neck as part of the treatment for congenital dislocation of the hip. The purpose of the operation is to place the head of the femur in an optimal position in the acetabulum for molding a deep acetabulum.

The derotation osteotomy may be performed in the subtrochanteric or supracondylar region (see Chapter 11) of the femur. With derotation osteotomy in the subtrochanteric area, any excessive valgus of the femoral neck may be overcome at the same time. If the derotation osteotomy is carried out as a second-stage procedure after open reduction and/or acetabuloplasty, 6 weeks should be allowed to elapse between procedures.

DETAILS OF PROCEDURE. At the operating table the child is draped to permit subsequent movement of the entire limb. With the hip held in the optimum position of internal rotation, a lateral, longitudinal incision is made **(A)**. The dissection is carried down through the fascia lata **(B)**. The fibers of the vastus lateralis muscle are split in the direction of their fibers to expose the lateral aspect of the proximal shaft of the femur from the tip of the greater trochanter to approximately 5 cm below the lesser trochanter, and the periosteum is incised **(C)**. The leg is held in full internal rotation, and a small Steinmann pin is inserted through the greater trochanter into the femoral neck. An assistant then holds the pin and the hip in this internally rotated position. A four-hole Lane plate is placed along the lateral aspect of the femur distal to the prominence of the greater trochanter **(D)**. The femur is marked at the midportion of the plate position, and drill holes are made to facilitate the osteotomy **(E)**.

(Plate 10-17) SUBTROCHANTERIC DEROTATION OSTEOTOMY

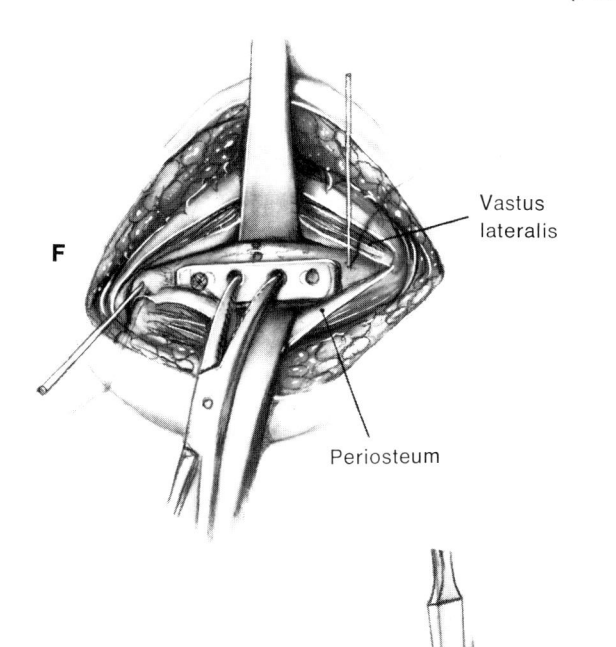

A second Steinmann pin is drilled through the femoral shaft in an anteroposterior direction through both cortices distal to the ultimate plate position (F). The osteotomy is then partially carried out with a thin osteotome to divide the lateral cortex of the femur (G). The Lane plate is secured to the proximal fragment with two screws, and the osteotomy is completed. The distal leg is then externally rotated (often 45° to 60°) while the pin in the proximal fragment is maintained so that the proximal fragment remains internally rotated. The movement of the distal femoral pin indicates the degree of derotation of the femur at the osteotomy site (H). The plate is fixed to the distal fragment with two screws while both sections of the femur are held in firm apposition (I and J). The curved contour of the lateral cortex of the proximal fragment may fix the osteotomy and femoral neck in a somewhat varus position if a straight plate is used. The two Steinmann pins are removed. The wound is closed in layers, and a one and one-half plaster spica is applied with the hip in slight flexion and the foot in neutral rotation.

POSTOPERATIVE MANAGEMENT. Plaster immobilization in the hip spica is continued for 6 weeks in the young child and up to 10 weeks in the older child. The child is then allowed to use the limb actively without any further external splinting.

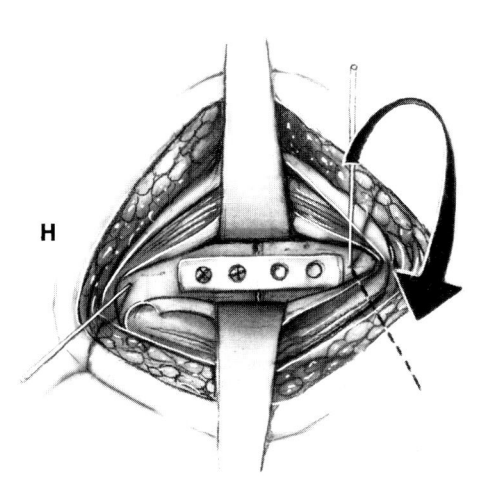

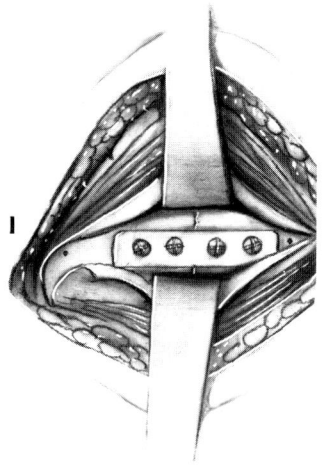

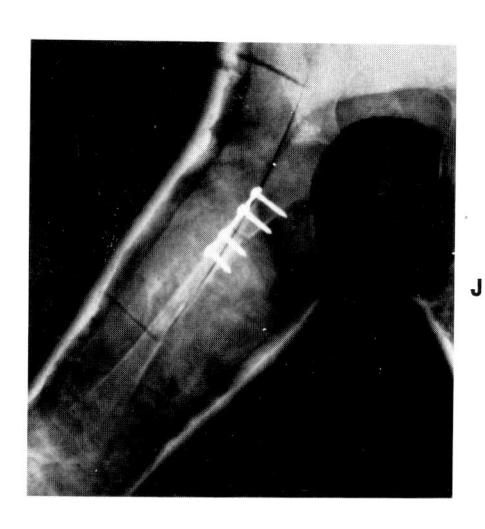

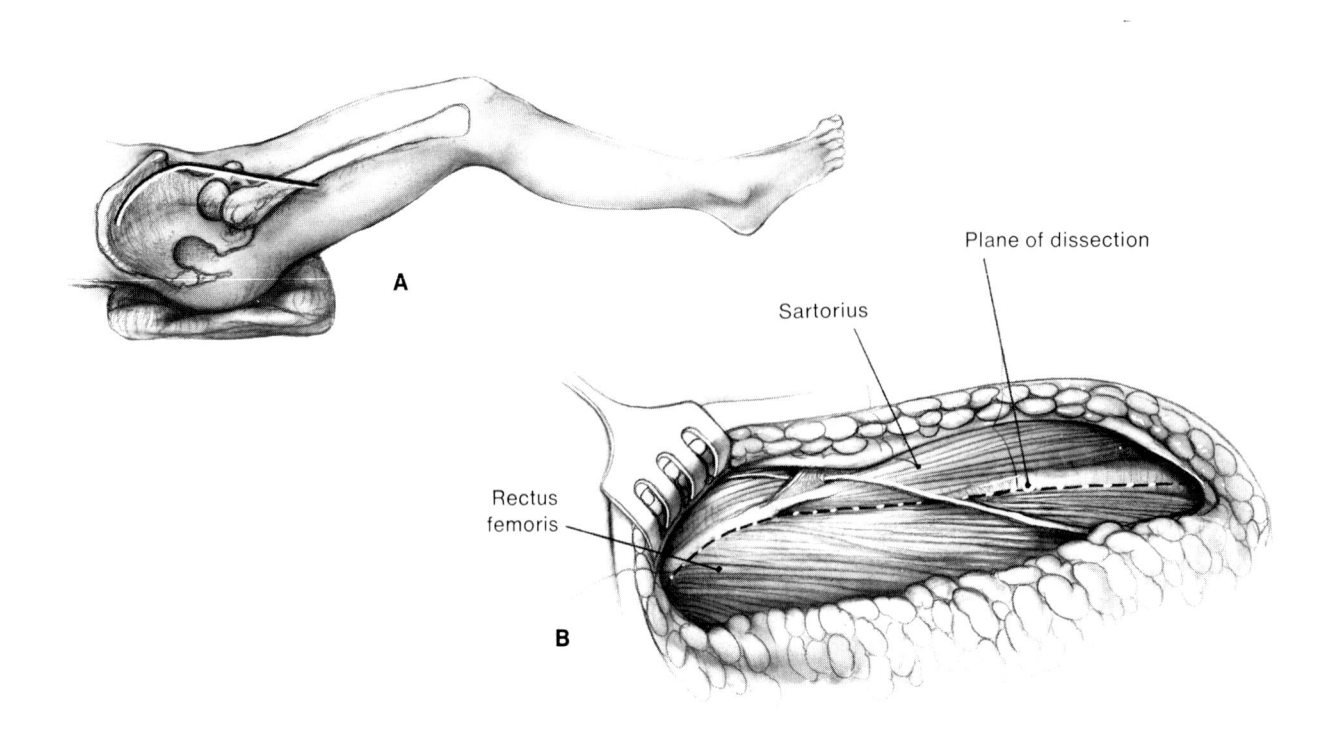

TRANSFER OF ILIOPSOAS TENDON FOR PARALYSIS OF HIP ABDUCTORS (MUSTARD) (Plate 10-18)

GENERAL DISCUSSION. The object of this operation is to improve the stability of the hip and to decrease limp associated with paralysis of the hip abductor muscles. The iliopsoas should have normal or near-normal power preoperatively if it is to function effectively following transfer of its insertion. The iliopsoas tendon may be transferred to the area of the greater trochanter of the femur through a trough in the anterior portion of the ilium (Mustard), as illustrated here, or through a large oval foramen in the wing of the ilium (Sharrard). Although the ideal patient for this procedure would be one with isolated paralysis of the gluteus medius muscle, it is uncommon to encounter such a purely isolated muscle weakness. However, gratifying results can be obtained when there is weakness or paralysis of other abductor or extensor muscles about the hip if a strong functioning iliopsoas is available and is transferred to the region of the great trochanter. In patients over 3 years of age with neuromuscular disorders such as poliomyelitis or myelomeningocele who have an intact iliopsoas mechanism (which is best tested between 90° hip flexion and full hip flexion) and inadequate hip abductors, the age of the patient does not appear to critically affect the functional end result of this procedure.

If the patient has an intact adductor muscle compartment and associated weakness of hip extensors, it may be useful to consider combining (1) lateral transfer of the iliopsoas tendon and (2) posterior transfer of the origins of the adductor longus and brevis muscles to the ischial tuberosity as a two-stage procedure to synergistically improve hip abduction and extension.

DETAILS OF PROCEDURE. The patient is positioned supine with a small sandbag under the pelvis of the affected side and with the leg draped free to permit internal and external rotation during the procedure. The incision is made beginning along the crest of the ilium 7 cm posterior to the anterosuperior iliac spine. After it is extended forward along the anterior iliac crest and slightly medial to the anterosuperior iliac spine, the incision is continued in a curvilinear fashion distally and posteriorly to end by crossing the lateral aspect of the thigh at a level approximately two fifths of the distance from the greater trochanter to the knee **(A)**. This will provide the broad exposure necessary to isolate and detach the lesser trochanter and the insertion of the iliacus fibers, and will allow adequate exposure for reattachment for the iliopsoas tendon on the lateral aspect of the femoral shaft just below the greater trochanter.

The plane between the sartorius muscle and the tensor fascia lata muscle is identified in the distal portion of the wound after reflection of skin and subcutaneous tissue **(B)**. The lateral femoral cutaneous nerve is encountered superficially just below the anterosuperior iliac spine crossing the sartorius muscle. The tensor fascia lata muscle and the remnants of the gluteal muscles are reflected subperiosteally to expose the anterior portion of the iliac crest laterally. The abdominal muscles are reflected from the iliac crest to identify the iliacus muscle in the iliac fossa. By subperiosteal dissection on the lateral side of the iliacus muscle, the anterosuperior iliac spine with the origin of the sartorius muscle is caused to stand out in relief.

(Plate 10-18) TRANSFER OF ILIOPSOAS TENDON FOR PARALYSIS OF HIP ABDUCTORS (MUSTARD)

The anterosuperior iliac spine with the origin of the sartorius muscle is resected. The sartorius muscle is reflected medially by dissecting along its lateral side and then carefully on its medial border to identify and protect the motor branch of the femoral nerve to the sartorius muscle that enters the muscle from the medial side **(C)**.

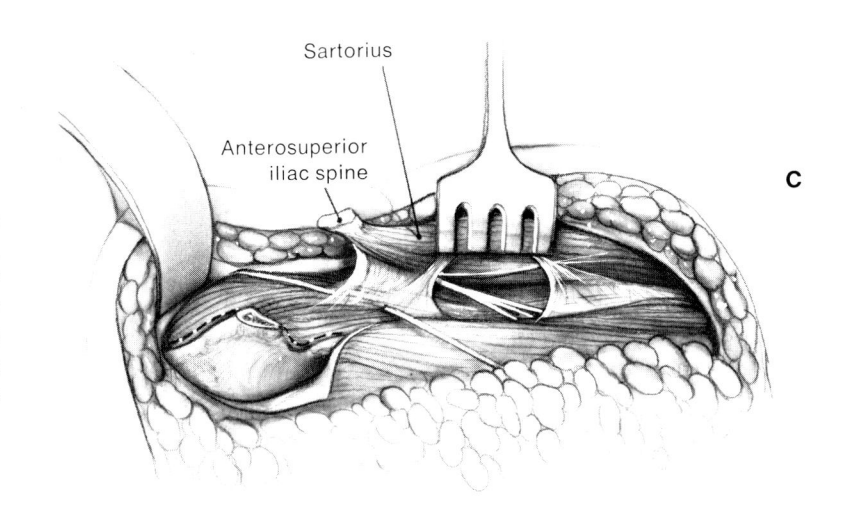

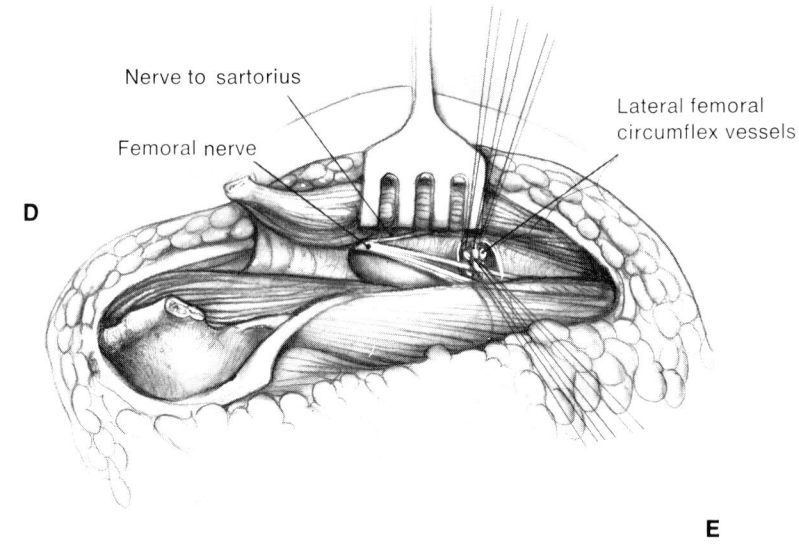

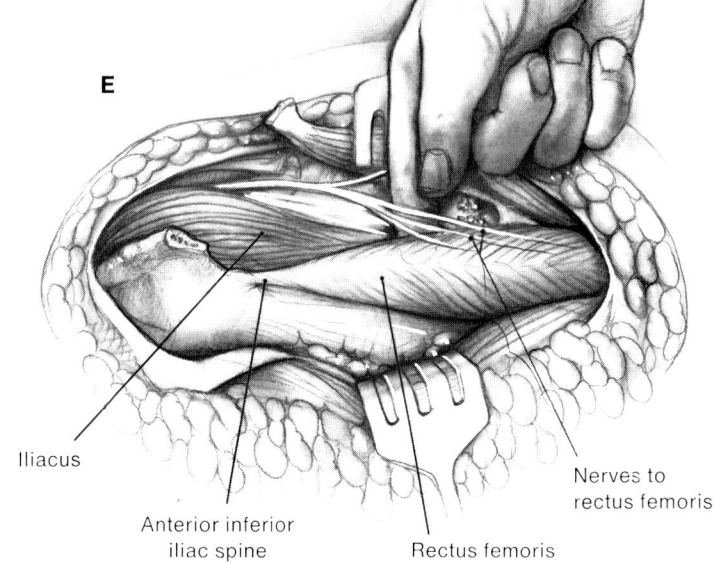

When the motor nerve to the sartorius muscle has been identified **(D)**, this is traced retrograde to the femoral nerve. The dissection is then carried distally along the femoral nerve until the nerve to the rectus femoris is visualized. There may be several nerves leaving the main femoral nerve "fanning out" to the rectus femoris **(E)**. Next, while these motor nerves are protected, the lateral femoral circumflex artery and veins are isolated at a level just proximal to the lesser trochanter. If the nerve to the rectus femoris originates more proximally than these vessels, it will be necessary to dissect between the nerve to the rectus femoris and the femoral nerve itself to isolate, ligate, and divide the lateral femoral circumflex vessels **(D)**. The sartorius muscle and the femoral nerve, artery, and vein are now retracted medially with careful protection of the motor nerve supply to the rectus femoris muscle.

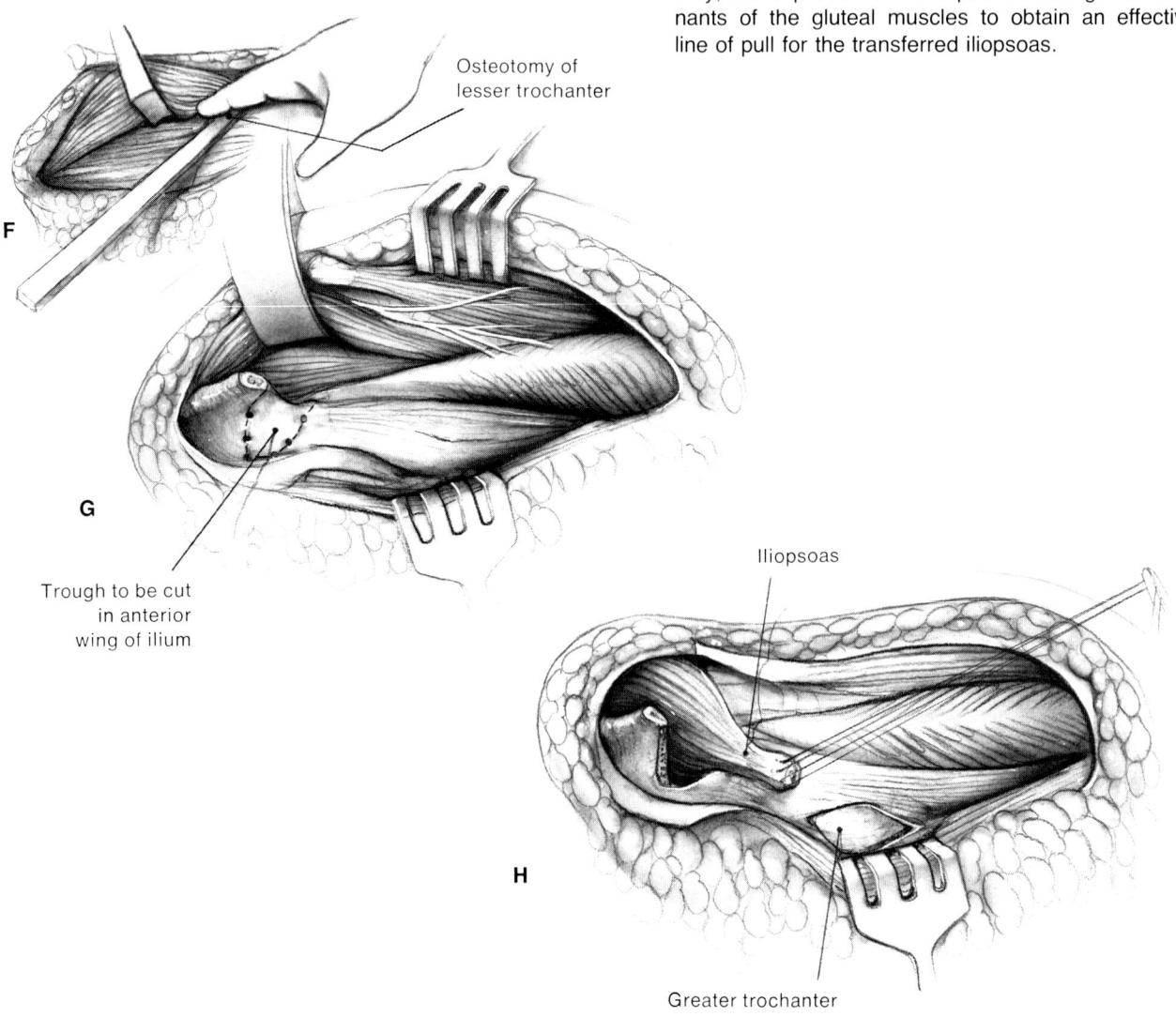

TRANSFER OF ILIOPSOAS TENDON FOR PARALYSIS OF HIP ABDUCTORS (MUSTARD) (Plate 10-18)

At this point it should be possible to trace the fibers of the iliacus muscle from the iliac fossa to the lesser trochanter. The leg is flexed slightly and externally rotated, and the finger is used to clear a space proximal to the lesser trochanter (between femur and iliopsoas insertion) as well as distal to the lesser trochanter (between the iliopsoas and the pectineus muscle). If necessary for exposure, the straight head of the rectus femoris may be released from the anteroinferior iliac spine. A plane is developed deep to the muscle belly of the iliacus in the iliac fossa, and dissection along this plane is continued distally until the lateral aspect of the iliacus is free down to the level of the lesser trochanter.

With a finger on the anterior and medial aspect of the lesser trochanter to guide an osteotome to the deep superior edge **(F)**, the lesser trochanter is carefully osteotomized and the adjacent fibers of the iliacus muscle inserting into the linea aspera are released. After release of the lesser trochanter and the iliacus muscle fibers inserting into the femur, the iliopsoas tendon is drawn proximally under the nerve to rectus femoris for delivery into the wound. A trough is cut into the anterior aspect of the ilium. It is cut as far proximally and posteriorly as possible to accommodate the transferred iliopsoas and to permit as straight a path as possible toward its planned insertion into the femur below the greater trochanter **(G)**.

The hip is internally rotated and the fascia lata and vastus lateralis are divided laterally to expose the greater trochanter and the proximal aspect of the femoral shaft laterally. With the leg abducted and in slight internal rotation, the iliopsoas is pulled down with strong tension to determine the proper site for its insertion into the lateral aspect of the femoral shaft. As this is done, the proper area to cut a trough in the anterior wing of the ilium is mapped out **(H)**. If necessary, the iliopsoas tendon is passed through the remnants of the gluteal muscles to obtain an effective line of pull for the transferred iliopsoas.

(Plate 10-18) TRANSFER OF ILIOPSOAS TENDON FOR PARALYSIS OF HIP ABDUCTORS (MUSTARD)

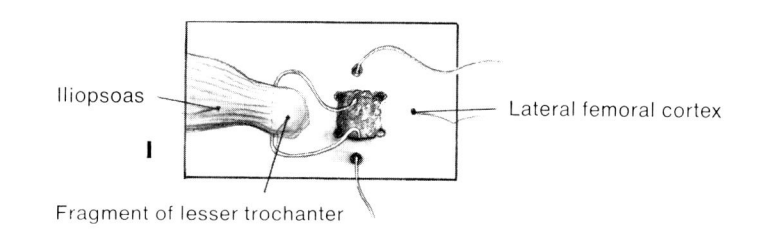

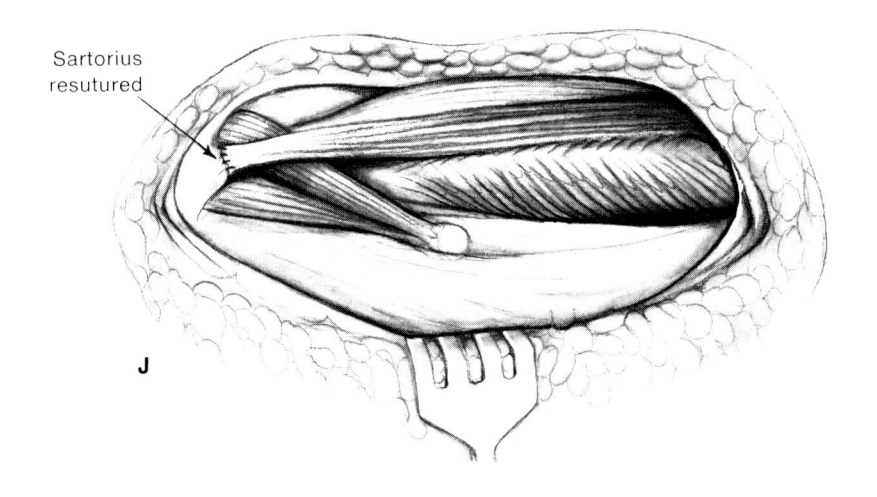

A small window is cut in the cortex of the femur, and the iliopsoas tendon and fragment of the lesser trochanter are anchored through this opening into the lateral aspect of the femur with heavy wire (**I** and **K**). The combined psoas and iliacus muscles pass through the prepared trough in the ilium as illustrated while the leg is held in abduction and slight internal rotation.

The vastus lateralis muscle and the fascia lata are closed. If previously released, the straight head of the rectus femoris muscle is reattached to the anteroinferior iliac spine. The sartorius is resutured to the anterosuperior iliac spine (**J**). The tensor fascia lata is resutured to the abdominal muscles over the iliac crest. The leg is held carefully in abduction, slight internal rotation, and slight flexion during wound closure and until a one and one-half hip spica has been applied with the hip in this position (**L**).

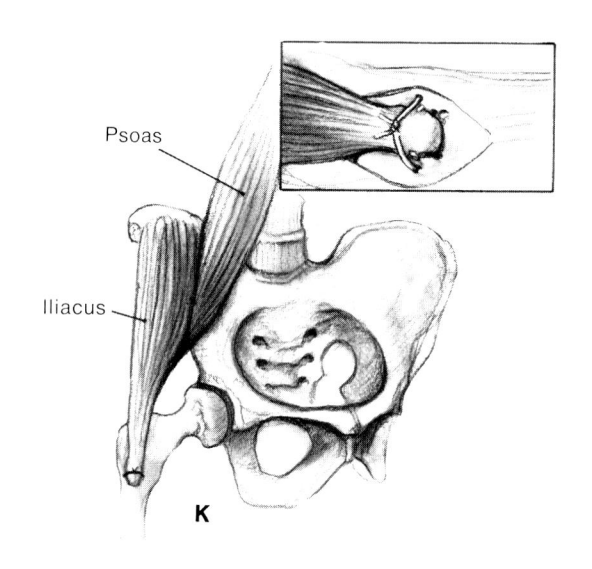

POSTOPERATIVE MANAGEMENT. Immobilization in the hip spica is continued for 6 weeks postoperatively. At this time the patient is readmitted for cast removal and physiotherapy, including active assistive and underwater exercises in a Hubbard tank. The patient continues with crutches and only token weight bearing on the involved leg until at least 10 weeks postoperatively, at which time full weight bearing is allowed.

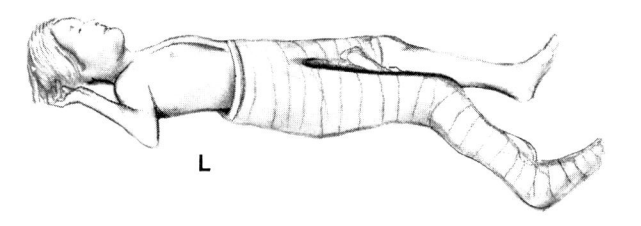

POSTERIOR TRANSFER OF ILIOPSOAS TENDON FOR PARALYSIS OF HIP ABDUCTORS (SHARRARD) (Plate 10-19)

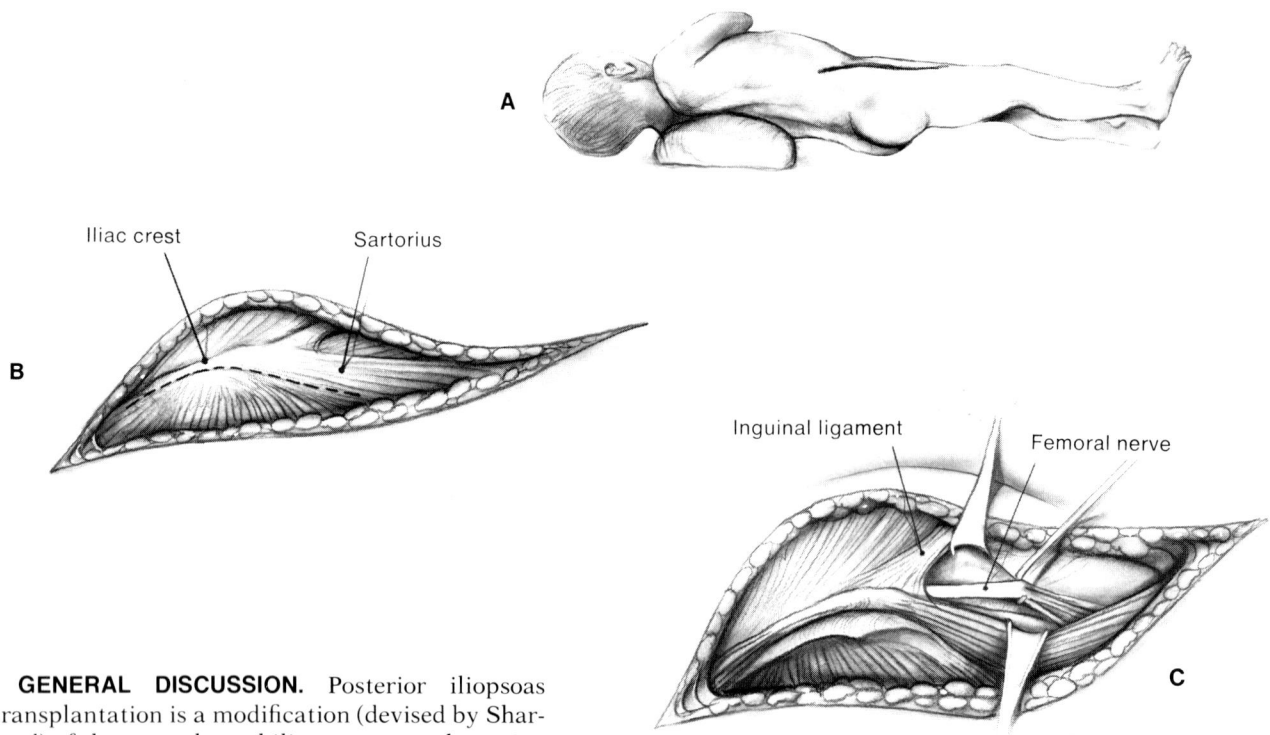

GENERAL DISCUSSION. Posterior iliopsoas transplantation is a modification (devised by Sharrard) of the anterolateral iliopsoas transplantation (recommended by Mustard). Posterior transfer of the iliopsoas involves release of both ends of the iliopsoas muscle and is a more extensive procedure than anterolateral iliopsoas transplantation.

For paralytic dislocation of the hip, four operations offer potential benefit: adductor tenotomy, varus osteotomy of the proximal femur, anterolateral iliopsoas transplantation, and posterior iliopsoas transplantation. The choice of operation or a combination of procedures depends on the degree of paralysis and deformity at the hip.

Although predominance of an adductor contracture may be a primary factor causing paralytic dislocation of the hip, iliopsoas action is a significant secondary deforming force. The iliopsoas becomes a strong lateral rotator of the hip when there is valgus deformity of the femoral neck or when the hip is dislocated. Posterior iliopsoas transplantation leaves the sartorius, rectus femoris, and pectineus as adequate flexors of the hip. When the iliopsoas is transferred posterior and lateral to the hip joint, it can become capable of extending as well as abducting the hip, thus balancing the activity of the remaining flexors and adductors. According to Sharrard, when the posterior iliopsoas transplantation is carried out before the age of 4 years, the muscle can abduct and extend the hip when the leg is off the ground and can partake in the normal rhythm of muscle action and walking.

DETAILS OF PROCEDURE. The child is positioned supine with the involved hip elevated slightly by placement of a small sandbag behind the same side of the chest and the upper lumbar area. The incision is made along the anterior two thirds of the iliac crest and extended distally along the medial border of the sartorius muscle to the midportion of the thigh **(A)**. The deep fascia is opened, and dissection is continued to define the iliac crest in the proximal portion of the incision **(B)**. The atrophic gluteus medius and minimus muscles are divided, and the outer surface of the ilium is exposed subperiosteally. The sartorius muscle in its proximal portion is exposed but not released (unless there is a severe flexion contracture of the hip). Next, the rectus femoris origin is identified but not released (again unless there is a flexion contracture of the hip related to tightness of the rectus femoris). The inferior border of the inguinal ligament is defined. The femoral nerve must be identified as it emerges from the pelvis and then mobilized in a distal and lateral direction **(C)**.

(Plate 10-19) POSTERIOR TRANSFER OF ILIOPSOAS TENDON FOR PARALYSIS OF HIP ABDUCTORS (SHARRARD)

Muscles are reflected from the inner table of the ilium (**D**) by detaching the abdominal muscles from the anterior two thirds of the iliac crest; in a young child, this is done by incising the iliac epiphysis superiorly and gently prying it from the ilium posteriorly. At this time, the hip should be flexed and externally rotated to bring the lesser trochanter anteriorly. The lesser trochanter is identified and detached from the femur along with that portion of the iliopsoas tendon which inserts into it. During this dissection, care must be taken to preserve the lateral femoral circumflex vessels. The origin of the iliacus muscle is reflected from the inner table of the ilium with care to identify and preserve the branches of the femoral nerve that enter the iliacus muscle from a location between the psoas muscle and the iliacus itself; there are usually two, one being given off soon after the nerve enters the pelvis and the other about halfway along the course of the nerve within the pelvis. While the hip is flexed to relax the femoral nerve, the iliopsoas tendon and the attached lesser trochanter are passed beneath the nerve to its lateral side. The more distal portion of the iliopsoas should then be mobilized until the entire iliopsoas is freed proximally into the pelvis, the bursa deep to the psoas indicating the plane of separation.

An oval opening is made through the iliac wing just lateral to the sacroiliac joint with its long axis longitudinal; its anteroposterior width slightly more than one third that of the iliac wing and its longitudinal length one and one-half times its width (**E** and **F**).

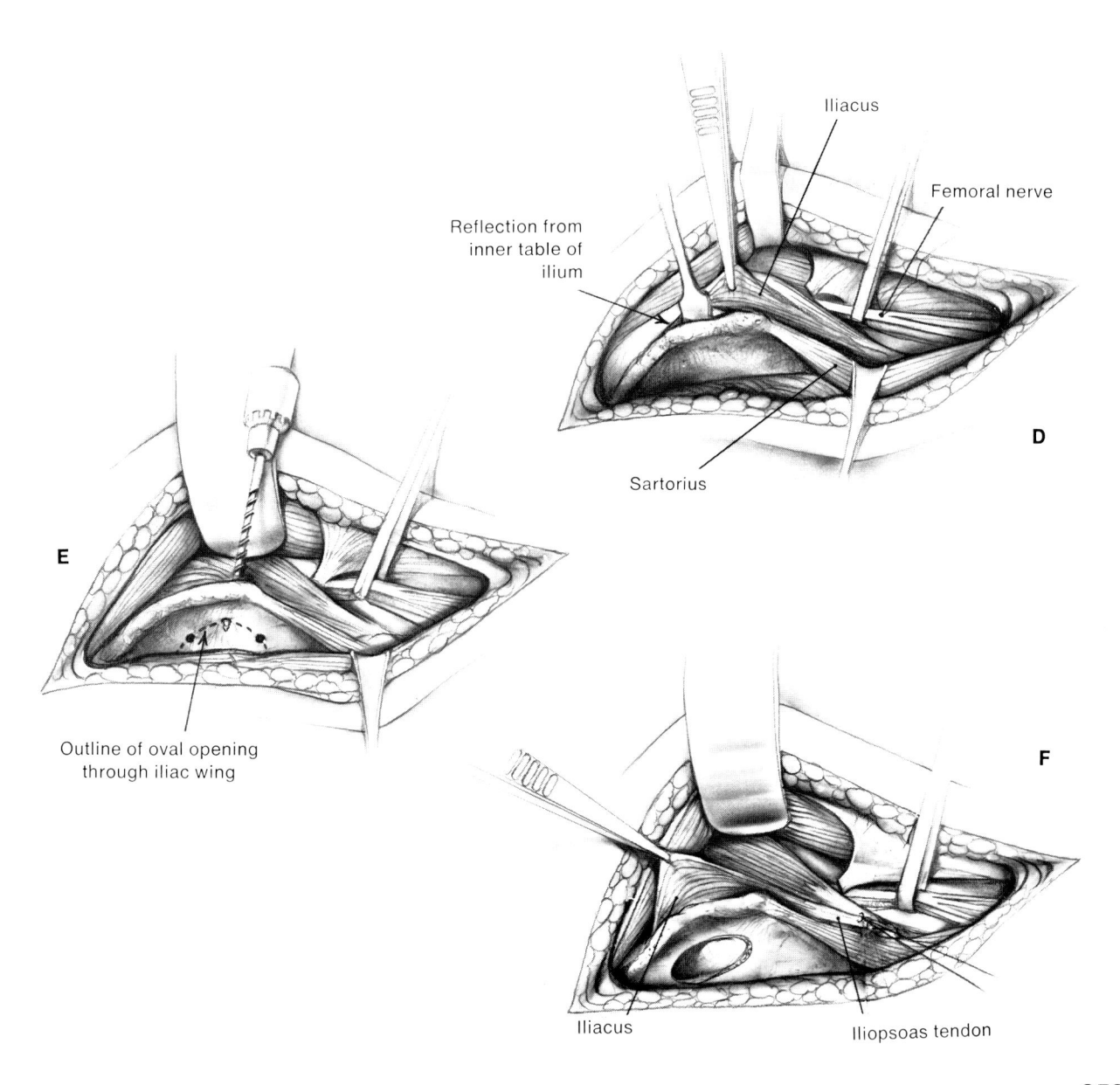

353

POSTERIOR TRANSFER OF ILIOPSOAS TENDON FOR PARALYSIS OF HIP ABDUCTORS (SHARRARD) (Plate 10-19)

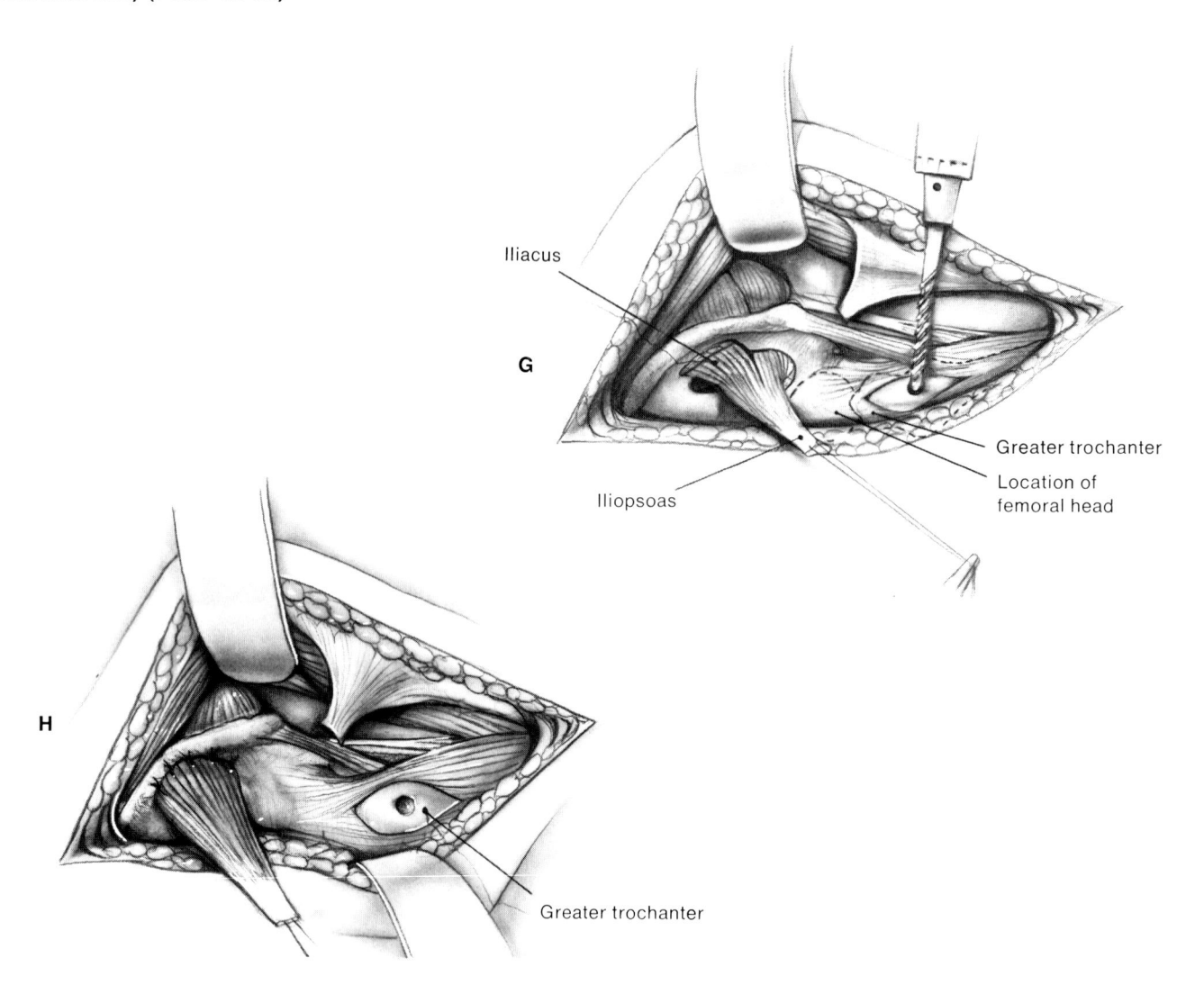

The iliopsoas tendon and the entire iliacus muscle are then passed through this hole (if the origin of the iliacus is passed through the hole first, the iliopsoas tendon will follow easily) **(G)**.

With a finger one should bluntly dissect distally and posteriorly into the bursa deep to the gluteus maximus tendon to identify the posterolateral aspect of the greater trochanter where the iliopsoas transfer should be anchored. Referring to this same point, the corresponding anterior aspect of the greater trochanter is exposed by dissecting through the fascia and the fatty and fibrous tissue over the trochanter. A hole is made from anterior to posterior through the greater trochanter until it is big enough to receive the iliopsoas tendon. The origin of the iliacus muscle is sutured to the ilium just inferior to the iliac crest in the position corresponding to the origin of the gluteus medius **(H)**.

(Plate 10-19) POSTERIOR TRANSFER OF ILIOPSOAS TENDON FOR PARALYSIS OF HIP ABDUCTORS (SHARRARD)

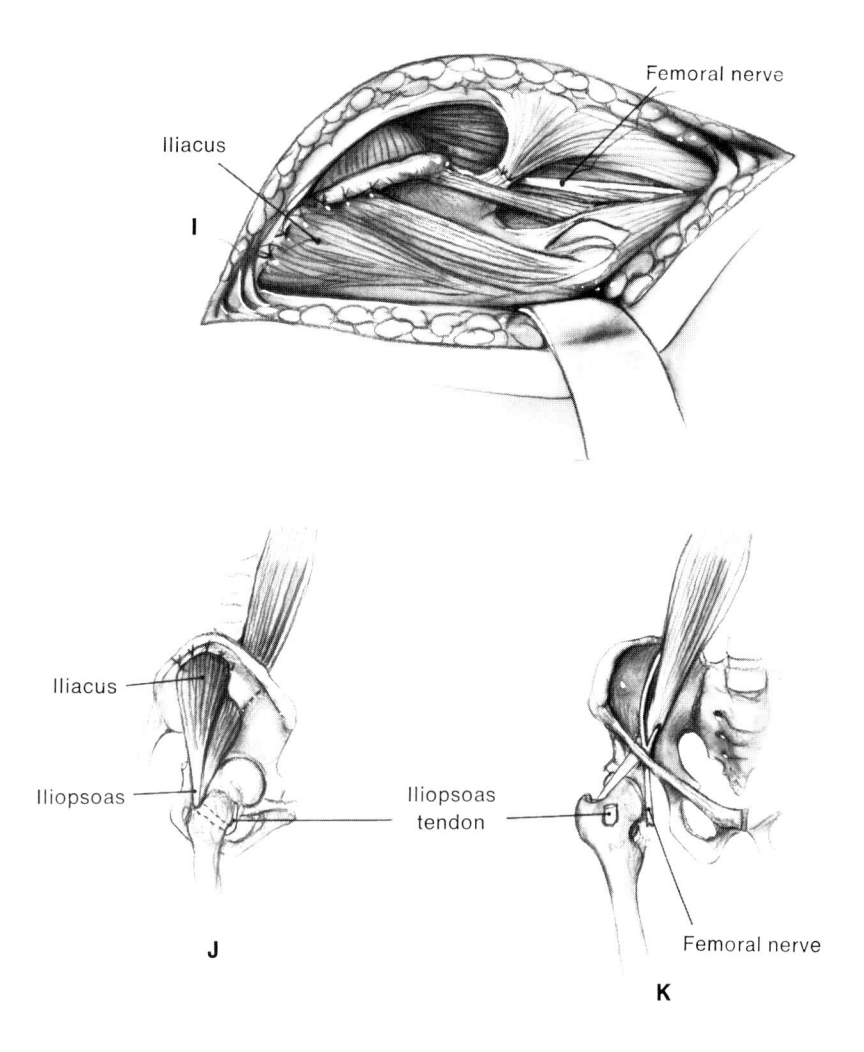

If the lateral end of the inguinal ligament was previously released to improve exposure, it is now resutured (I). With the hip held in abduction, extension, and neutral rotation, the end of the iliopsoas is passed through the buttock and from posterior to anterior through the tunnel in the greater trochanter (J and K). Several strong sutures are used to anchor the tendon securely under tension to the anterior surface of the trochanter. The abdominal muscles and gluteal fascia are sutured to the iliac crest, and the space is closed between the inguinal ligament and the pubic bone by suturing the ligament to the iliopectineal line. The deep fascia and skin are sutured.

With the hip in full abduction, extension, and neutral rotation, a hip spica cast is applied that extends distally to the toes on the involved side. In children with bladder paralysis, which includes almost all of those with myelomeningocele, an area above the pubic area must be left to permit bladder emptying by expression. Also, the feet in almost all patients with myelomeningocele have a sensory deficit as well as almost complete motor paralysis, and it is advisable to cover the entire foot on the operated side with generous padding to avoid pressure on the foot or heel.

The principal technical difficulties in this procedure are exposing the lesser trochanter between the femoral nerve and vessels, separating the origin of the iliacus muscle from the most posterior and medial aspects of the inner table of the ilium, and passing the iliopsoas from posterior to anterior through the greater trochanter (the tendon tends to be caught at the entrance of the tunnel in the bone, resulting in inadequate tension on the transfer).

POSTOPERATIVE MANAGEMENT. The hip spica is discontinued at 3 weeks in children up to 3 years of age, at 4 weeks in children up to 6 years of age, and at 5 weeks in children up to 10 years. If the same procedure is carried out on the opposite side, it may be done 1 week or more postoperatively depending on the child's condition.

TRANSFER OF EXTERNAL OBLIQUE MUSCLE FOR PARALYSIS OF HIP ABDUCTORS (Plate 10-20)

GENERAL DISCUSSION. The external oblique muscle is a good potential substitute when there is paralysis of the hip abductors. Its nerve supply is from a different spinal segment than that of the gluteus medius and minimus, and it is relatively unlikely to be paralyzed when the gluteal muscles are involved.

The aponeurosis of the external oblique muscle is long and broad. Anatomically, this muscle arises by eight digitations, one from each of the lower eight ribs at their anterior angles. From this muscular origin, the muscle fans out to a wide insertion, much of which is aponeurotic. Beginning posteriorly at the twelfth rib, the external oblique muscle can be traced to its insertion as muscle fibers attached into the anterior one half of the outer portion of the iliac crest. Aponeurotic fibers, directed obliquely downward and forward, are attached to the pubic crest and interdigitate with each other above the symphysis pubis across the front of the rectus abdominis to the whole length of the linea alba up to the xiphisternum. The free upper border of the aponeurosis, extending from the fifth rib to the xiphisternum, runs horizontally. The free lower border, lying between the anterosuperior iliac spine and the pubic tubercle, forms the inguinal ligament.

If the external oblique muscle should be transferred, the other abdominal muscles are almost always strong enough to maintain the integrity of the abdominal wall.

DETAILS OF PROCEDURE. The initial skin incision is made as illustrated beginning at the posterior axillary line and at the costal margin extending over and around the crest of the ilium to end at the pubic tubercle **(A)**. Skin and subcutaneous tissue are reflected to expose the external oblique muscle. Two incisions are made in the aponeurosis of the external oblique muscle 2 cm apart, parallel with each other and with the inguinal ligament. The two incisions in the aponeurosis are joined at a point 1 cm proximal to the pubis. The dissection is carried along the superior incision in a proximal direction to outline the medial border of the external oblique muscle to the rib cage to free the muscle from the remainder of its aponeurosis. The inferior incision in the aponeurosis is extended proximally and laterally to the anterosuperior iliac spine. A blunt dissector beneath the muscle fibers of the external oblique muscle is inserted as an aid prior to incision of the insertion of this muscle into the ilium. The remainder of the muscle and its distal aponeurosis is freed from the underlying tissues by blunt dissection **(B)**.

The distal portion of the external oblique aponeurosis is folded into a tube and sutured to form a cone-shaped structure. The remaining free edge of the residual aponeurosis of the external oblique muscle is sutured to the underlying internal oblique muscle **(C)**.

A second skin incision is made longitudinally over the most prominent portion of the greater trochanter approximately 6 cm in length. The greater trochanter is exposed, and two separate drill holes are made, each approximately 1 cm in diameter, in the greater trochanter.

A subcutaneous tunnel extending proximally from the greater trochanter toward the origin of the external oblique muscle is prepared. This tunnel must be wide over the iliac crest, for the transferred muscle will form a mass 5 to 6 cm in diameter at this level. The cone-shaped strip of external oblique muscle is passed distally through this subcutaneous tunnel. The hip is placed in wide abduction. The aponeurotic tube of the distal portion of the external oblique is passed through the holes in the greater trochanter and sutured securely to itself as illustrated **(C)**. Both wounds are closed, and a hip spica is applied holding the hip in wide abduction and some extension.

POSTOPERATIVE MANAGEMENT. The spica cast is removed 4 weeks postoperatively. Hydrotherapy (Hubbard tank) exercises are started at that time and continued on a daily basis until satisfactory muscle reeducation has been obtained. Full weight bearing is allowed beginning 8 weeks after surgery.

(Plate 10-20) TRANSFER OF EXTERNAL OBLIQUE MUSCLE FOR PARALYSIS OF HIP ABDUCTORS

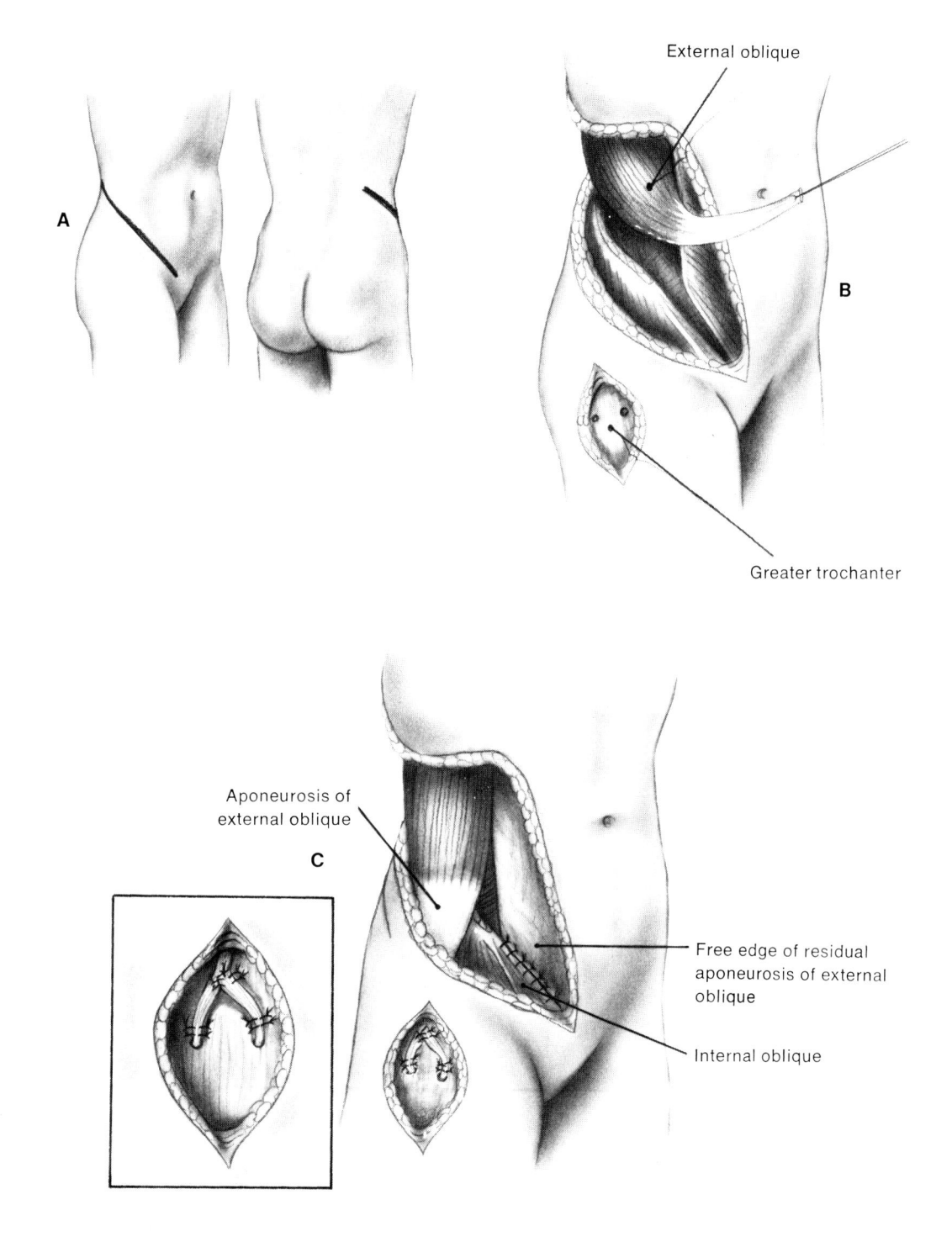

A

External oblique

B

Greater trochanter

Aponeurosis of external oblique

C

Free edge of residual aponeurosis of external oblique

Internal oblique

357

TRANSFER OF ORIGIN OF ADDUCTOR LONGUS AND BREVIS TO ISCHIAL TUBEROSITY (Plate 10-21)

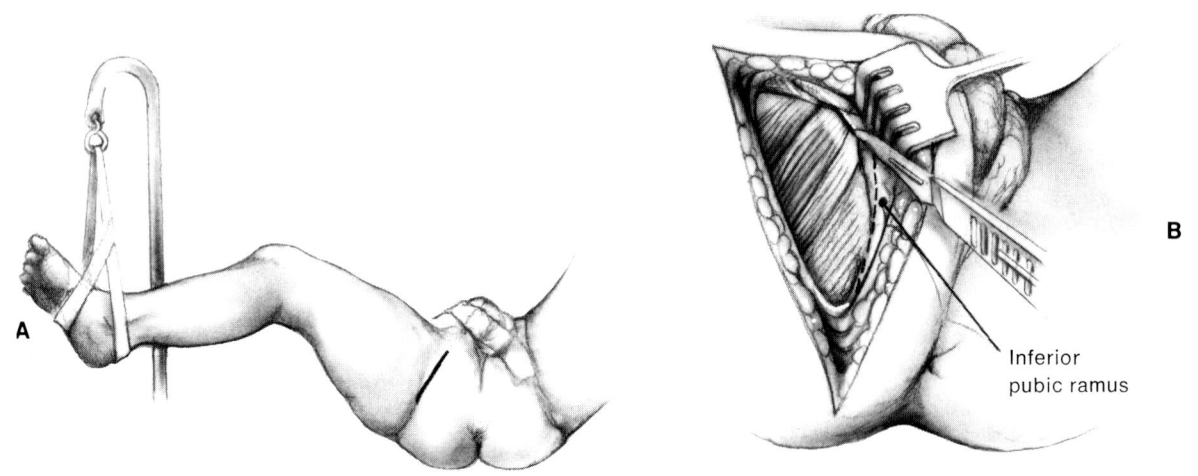

GENERAL DISCUSSION. When there is weakness or paralysis of the hip extensors but normal power in the adductor compartment of the thigh, transfer of the origin of the adductor longus and adductor brevis to the ischial tuberosity can be helpful.

DETAILS OF PROCEDURE. The patient is placed in the lithotomy position. The ischial tuberosity is palpated, and the incision is made along the inferior ramus of the pubis as illustrated **(A)**. The gracilis is identified where it attaches to the pubis superficial to the adductor longus, and the gracilis is retracted anteriorly. The adductor longus and the adductor brevis are detached from their origin near the symphysis pubis and from the anterior portion of the inferior ramus of the pubis **(B)**. These muscles are freed distally for a short distance and then resutured posteriorly to the periosteum of the inferior pubic ramus near the ischial tuberosity (**C** and **D**). Subcutaneous tissue and skin are closed and a soft dressing is applied.

POSTOPERATIVE MANAGEMENT. Sutures are removed 10 days postoperatively. Unlimited activity is permitted as the wound discomfort subsides.

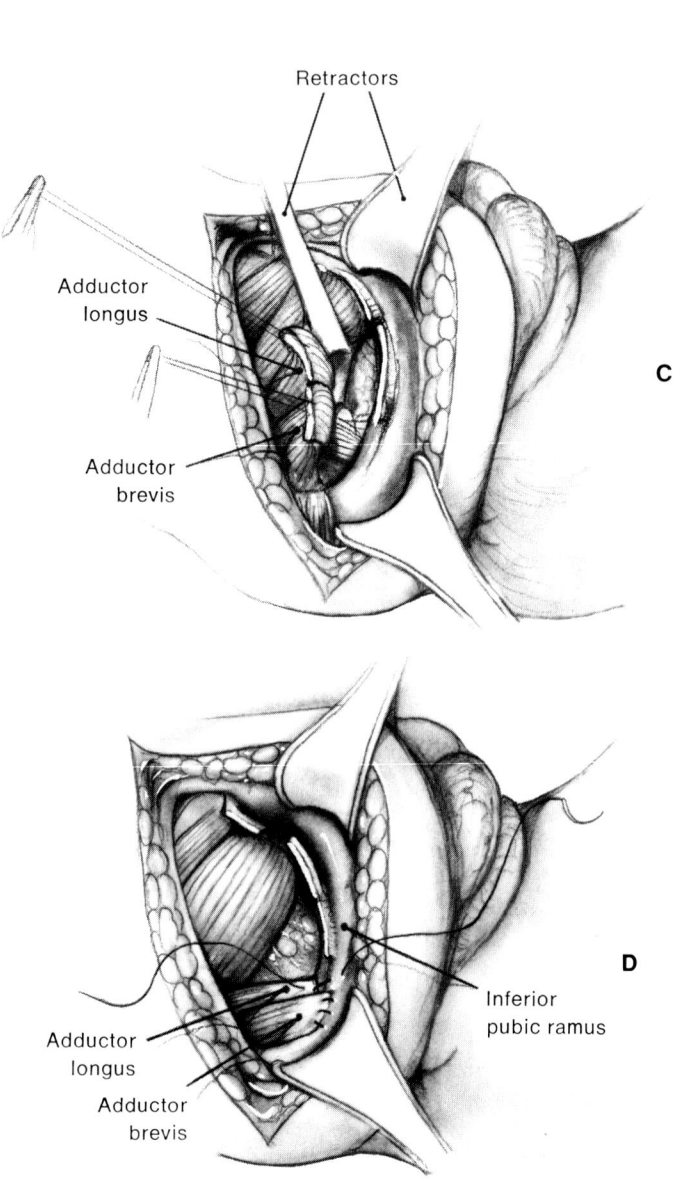

(Plate 10-22) DRAINAGE OF HIP JOINT

GENERAL DISCUSSION. A septic process involving the hip joint can be treated nonoperatively if treatment is prompt and intensive.

There are two basic indications for open drainage of an infected joint (including the hip joint). The first is that material obtained on diagnostic aspiration from the joint is flocculent and grossly purulent with the initial aspiration. The second is failure of the joint to improve under an adequate medical regimen that includes rest of the involved joint and intensive, appropriate antibiotic coverage.

When a septic joint is being treated with intensive antibiotics and rest, the total evaluation of the situation must include changes noted on clinical examination of the involved joint and the following frequent observations during the acute period: temperature recordings, blood counts, and the relative gross appearance and cell count of fluid aspirated from the joint on successive taps after treatment has been instituted.

In general, if there is doubt as to whether a septic joint should be drained or not, it is best to drain the joint promptly. Drainage of the hip joint may be carried out through either an anterior or a posterior approach, but postoperative drainage and general management of the patient are facilitated if the drainage can be accomplished through a posterior approach. Consequently, in the absence of altering factors, preference should be given to drainage through a posterior exposure.

DETAILS OF PROCEDURE. For *anterior drainage* a longitudinal incision approximately 7 cm is made, extending distally from the anterosuperior iliac spine **(A)**. Care is taken to protect the lateral femoral cutaneous nerve, which passes over the sartorius muscle just below the anterosuperior iliac spine. The dissection is carried down between the sartorius muscle medially and the tensor fascia lata muscle laterally **(B)**. The interval between these muscles can usually be identified more easily in the distal portion of the longitudinal wound. The straight head of the rectus femoris muscle is retracted medially, whereupon the bulging joint capsule will become evident **(C)**. A cruciate incision is made in the joint capsule and synovium **(D)**. Cultures are taken of the joint fluid. The incision in the capsule should avoid any damage to the acetabular labrum.

If indicated, a biopsy of the joint capsule and synovium is obtained at this point, and then a rubber tissue drain is sutured to the joint capsule with chromic catgut to maintain effective postoperative drainage from the hip joint **(E)**. The muscles are allowed to fall together over a loose Vaseline gauze pack. One or two sutures approximate the proximal and distal ends of the incision **(F)**. A bulky dressing is applied.

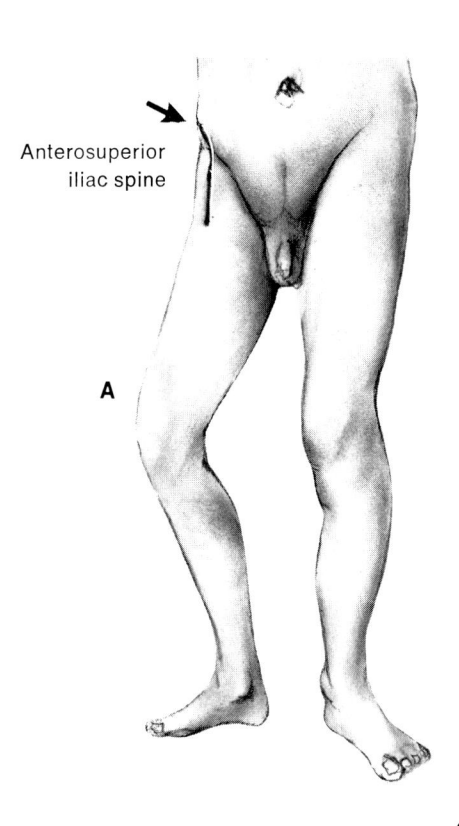

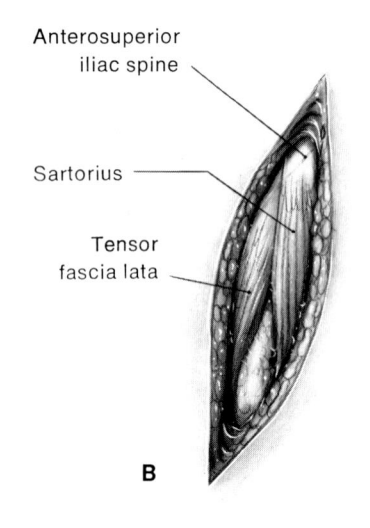

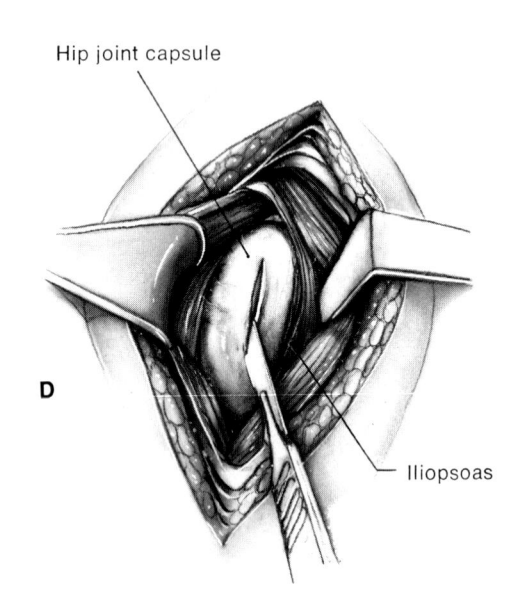

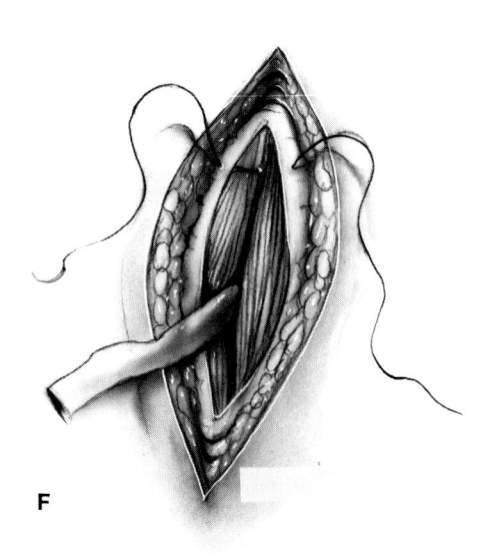

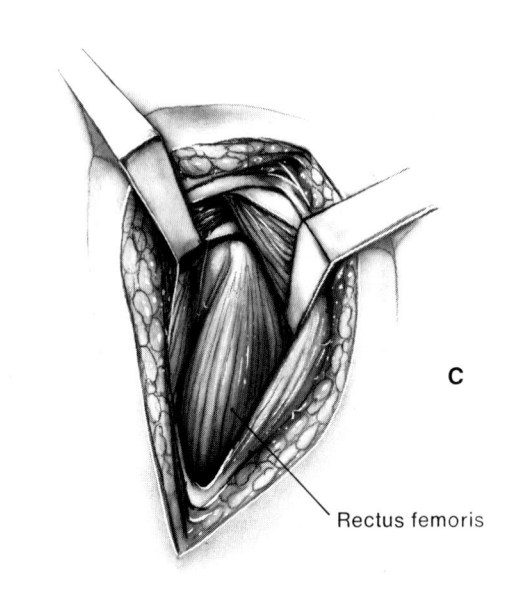

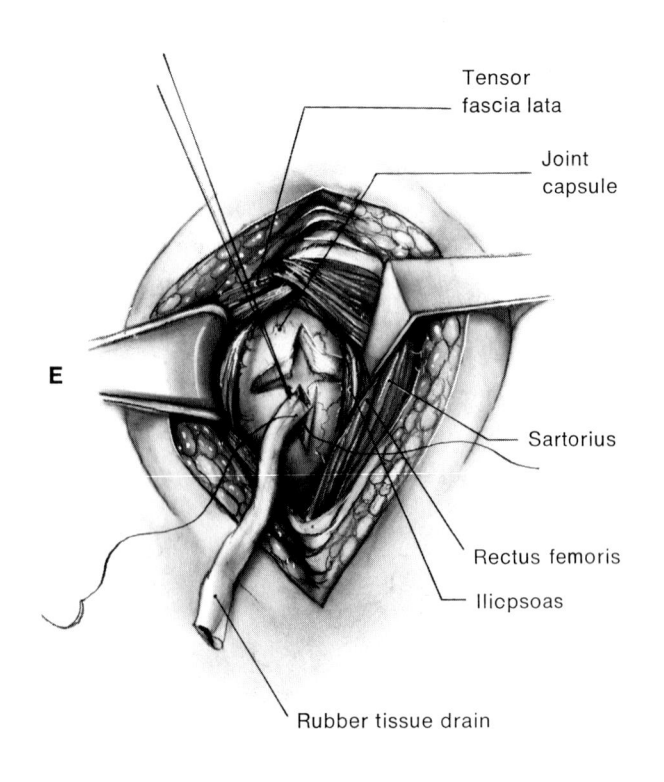

DRAINAGE OF HIP JOINT (Plate 10-22)

- Anterosuperior iliac spine
- Sartorius
- Tensor fascia lata

B

- Rectus femoris

C

- Hip joint capsule
- Iliopsoas

D

- Tensor fascia lata
- Joint capsule
- Sartorius
- Rectus femoris
- Iliopsoas
- Rubber tissue drain

E

F

360

(Plate 10-22) DRAINAGE OF HIP JOINT

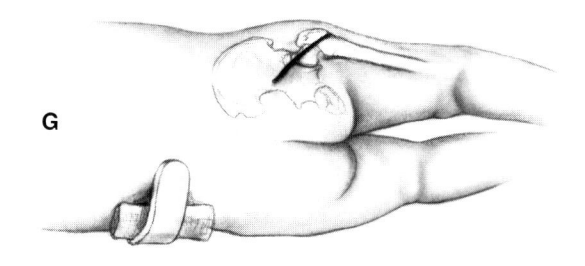

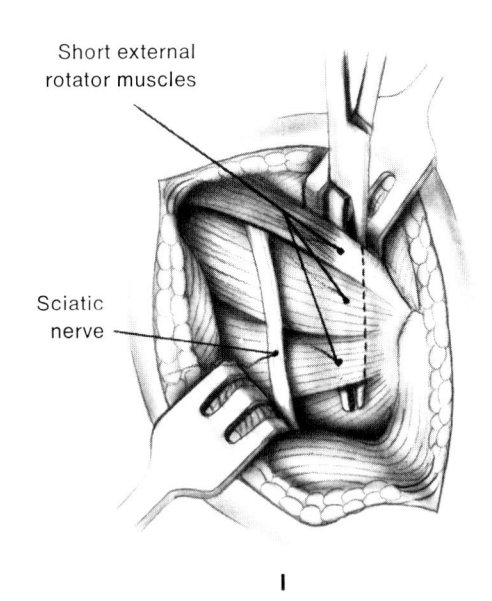

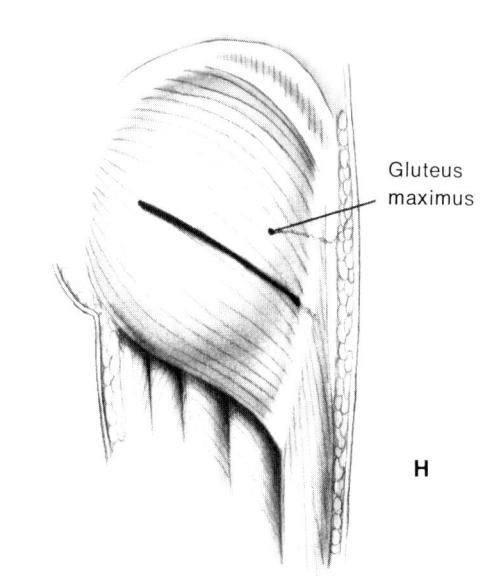

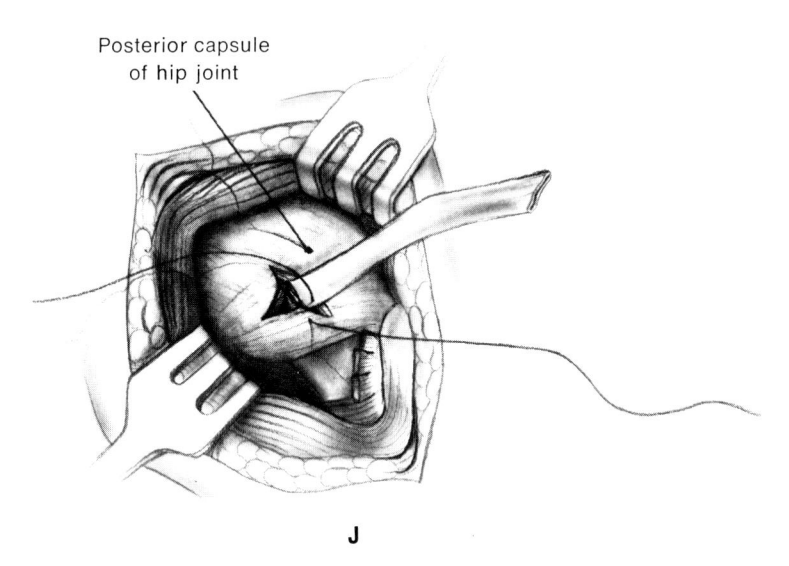

For *posterior drainage*, with the patient in a lateral position on the uninvolved hip, a linear incision is made extending from the posterosuperior aspect of the greater trochanter to within 2.5 cm of the posterosuperior iliac spine (**G** and **H**). The gluteus maximum muscle is separated in the direction of its fibers. Several branches of the superior gluteal artery invariably require ligation. The sciatic nerve is identified in the medial aspect of the wound as it emerges from under the piriformis muscle and is carefully retracted. The insertions of the short external rotator muscles are partially divided **(I)**. The capsule of the hip joint (which is easily seen if distended) is divided parallel to the femoral neck to expose the acetabular rim and femoral head. If necessary, a cruciate opening is made in the capsule to facilitate drainage. One or two Penrose drains are sutured with chromic catgut to the edge of the opened capsule **(J)**. The drains are also sutured to the skin.

POSTOPERATIVE MANAGEMENT. After the procedure for anterior drainage, Buck's traction is usually applied. The patient is turned to the prone position frequently to facilitate gravity drainage.

After the procedure for posterior drainage, Buck's traction is usually applied postoperatively. The patient is kept in the supine position as much as possible as long as any drainage continues from the wound.

361

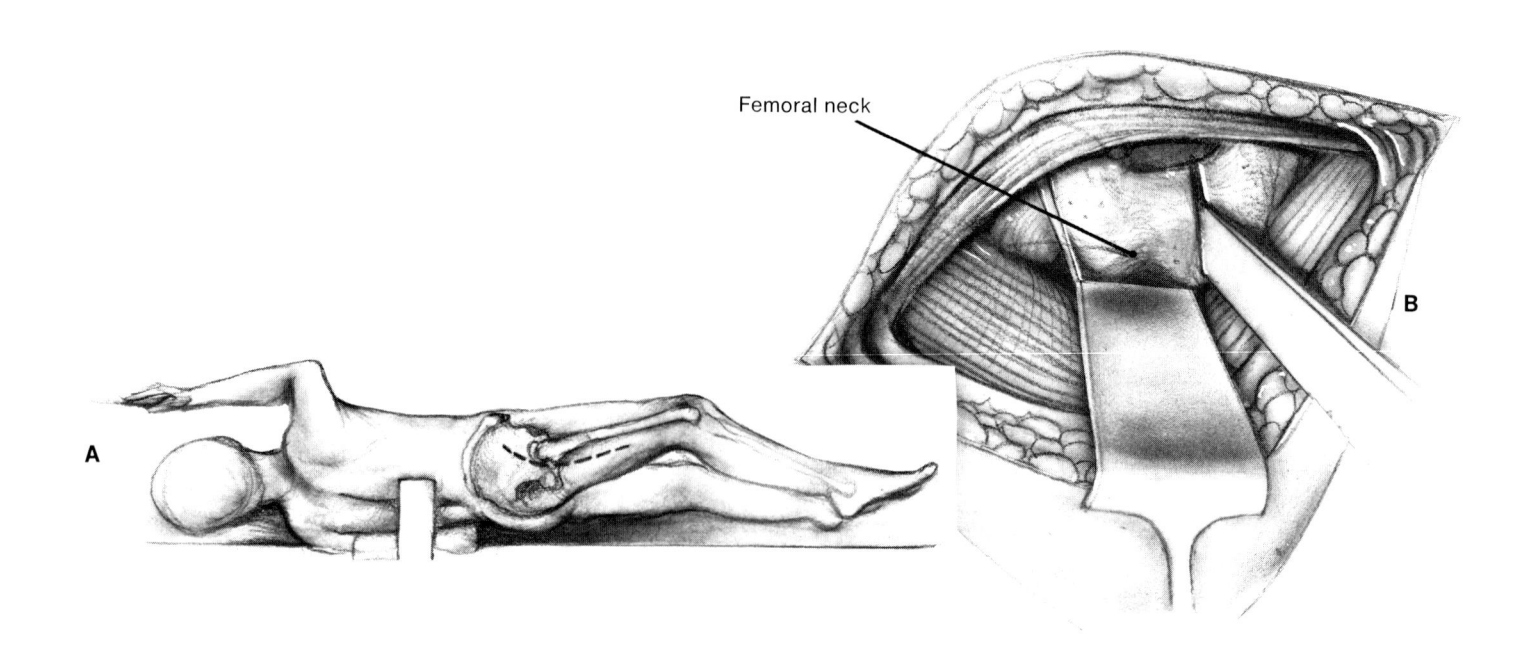

RESECTION OF HIP (GIRDLESTONE) (Plate 10-23)

GENERAL DISCUSSION. Girdlestone described this procedure for treatment of tuberculosis of the hip in 1928, and later, in 1943, modified the technique slightly for debridement of a septic hip. Batchelor and Milch used the Girdlestone procedure combined with angulation osteotomy of the femur as treatment for degenerative arthritis of the hip. With more recent reconstructive procedures, such as cup arthroplasty, prosthetic femoral head replacement, and total hip replacement, resection of the femoral head and neck has come to be a salvage procedure, used only when other procedures have failed. The Girdlestone procedure is seldom indicated as a primary form of treatment except occasionally for joints with chronic sepsis. It is most commonly employed as a salvage proceedure following failed hip arthroplasty.

This procedure can be a satisfactory method for relieving pain, and it restores movement of the hip. The disadvantages of the procedure are instability of the hip and shortening of the limb. Any patient undergoing the procedure should understand that some form of external support may be required postoperatively.

DETAILS OF PROCEDURE. The patient is placed in the lateral position with the affected leg uppermost for a posterior approach to the hip. An incision is made from the area of the posterosuperior iliac spine toward the greater trochanter, then extending distally in line with the femur to a point approximately 10 cm below the tip of the greater trochanter **(A)**. The deep fascia is incised in line with the skin incision to expose the trochanteric bursa. The conjoined tendon of the gluteus maximus muscle is divided near the gluteal tuberosity of the femur, and this muscle is separated proximally along the direction of its fibers to expose the external rotators of the hip joint. The sciatic nerve is identified and protected. The thigh is brought into a position of maximum internal rotation, and the tensed insertions of the external rotators are divided sharply near their insertion into the femur. If possible, only the tendons of the piriformis, gemellus superior, obturator internus, and gemellus inferior are sectioned.

The hip joint is opened with a longitudinal incision directly over the posterior aspect of the femoral neck, and the posterior capsule is excised. It may be possible to easily dislocate the femoral head from the acetabulum with a blunt elevator while the thigh is brought into maximum flexion, adduction, and internal rotation. If difficulty is encountered, the femoral neck should be osteotomized with use of multiple drill holes and osteotomes **(B)** or a reciprocating saw to avoid injury to the femoral shaft or unnecessary stress on the patient's knee while the femoral head is removed from the acetabulum **(C)**.

(Plate 10-23) RESECTION OF HIP (GIRDLESTONE)

With the thigh maintained in a position of flexion, adduction, and internal rotation, the entire intertrochanteric line will lie directly in the wound, permitting full visualization of both the greater and lesser trochanters and the base of the femoral neck. The lateral margin of the acetabulum should be removed with an osteotome (**D** and **E**). Any free bony and soft tissue fragments within the acetabular cavity are removed.

If an osteotomy is to be carried out in the subtrochanteric area in conjunction with resection of the femoral head and neck (Milch), this is accomplished through the same wound, by exposing the lateral aspect of the proximal femur by separating the vastus lateralis muscle in the plane of its muscle fibers.

Following wound closure, the patient's leg is placed in balanced suspension.

POSTOPERATIVE MANAGEMENT. The patient's leg is maintained in balanced suspension for 2 weeks after surgery. During this time the patient is encouraged to actively move the involved leg as the wound discomfort subsides. Crutch walking is started 2 weeks postoperatively. Progressive weight bearing is encouraged. Full weight bearing, without any support, is occasionally possible by 8 to 12 weeks following operation. An ischial weight-bearing brace may be prescribed if the patient is unable to bear full weight on the involved limb by 3 months postoperatively. A gradual increase in range of motion can be anticipated during the following year.

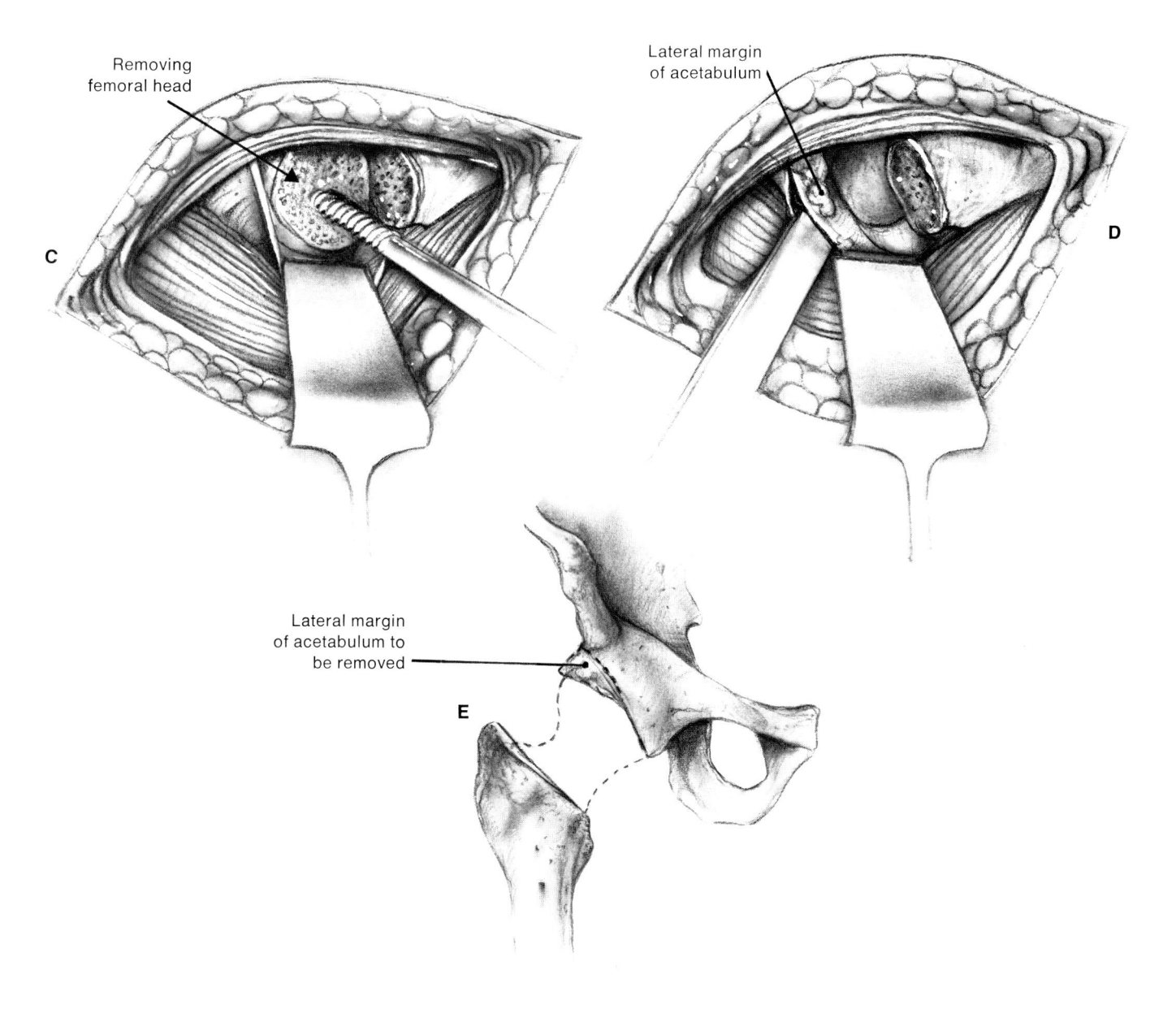

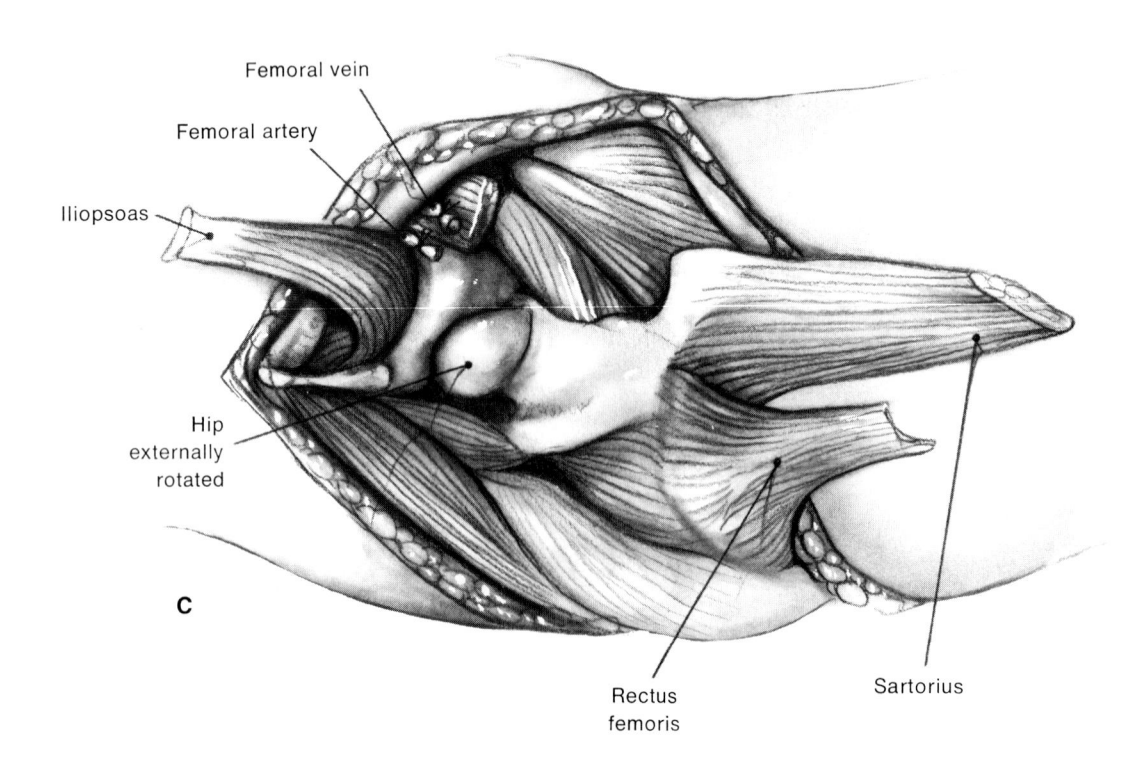

DISARTICULATION OF HIP (Plate 10-24)

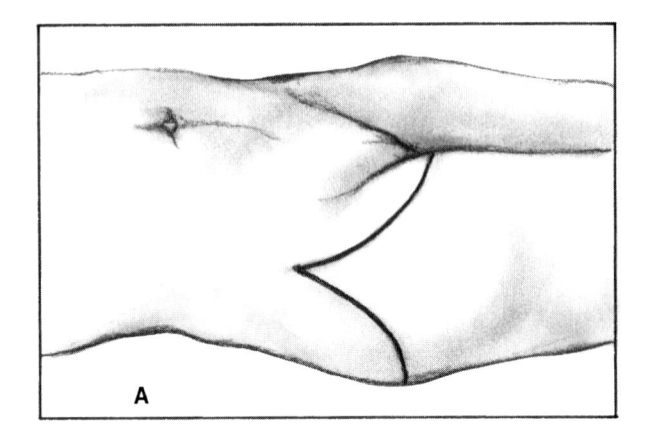

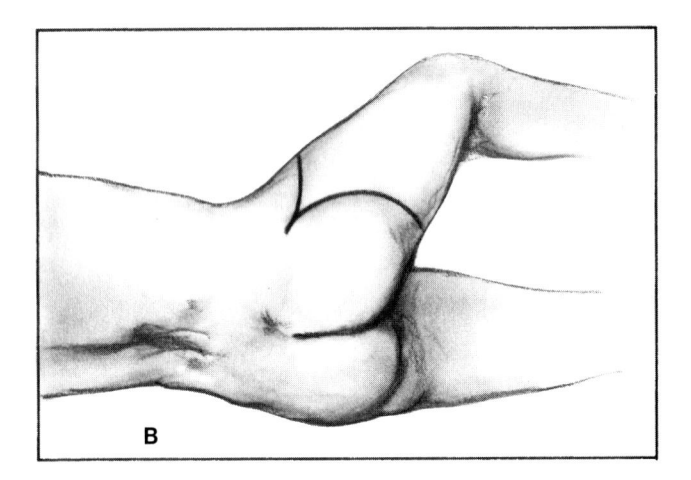

GENERAL DISCUSSION. Disarticulation of the hip may occasionally be indicated for a diseased or severely injured lower extremity.

DETAILS OF PROCEDURE. An incision is made as illustrated similar to an inverted V with apex proximally over the lateral aspect of the hip (**A** and **B**). The two ends of this incision are connected posteriorly to allow an adequate skin flap for ultimate closure of the stump. After the wound edges are developed, the femoral artery and vein should be isolated, ligated, and divided. The femoral nerve is divided. The sartorius muscle is detached from the anterosuperior iliac spine and the rectus femoris from the anteroinferior iliac spine, both muscles being reflected distally (**C**). The pectineus muscle is divided approximately 1 cm from the pubis. The thigh is externally rotated to bring the lesser trochanter and the iliopsoas tendon into view. The iliopsoas tendon is divided at the lesser trochanter and reflected proximally.

The gracilis and adductor muscles are detached from the pubis, including that portion of the adductor magnus muscle that arises from the ischium.

The branches of the obturator artery are exposed by developing the plane between the pectineus and obturator externus, and the short external rotator muscles. These branches of the obturator artery are ligated and divided. The obturator externus muscle is to be divided later at its attachment on the femur rather than at its origin on the pelvis to minimize the likelihood of injury to any branch of the obturator artery that might retract into the pelvis, which could lead to hemorrhage that could be difficult to control.

(Plate 10-24) DISARTICULATION OF HIP

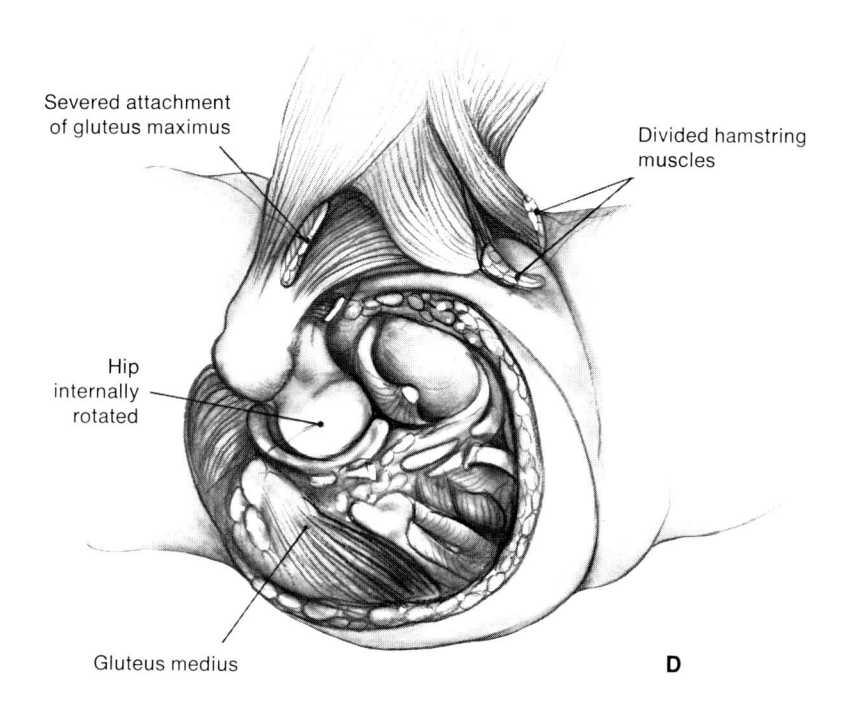

Next, the thigh should be rotated internally. The gluteus medius and minimus muscles are detached from their insertions on the greater trochanter. The fascia lata and the most distal fibers of the gluteus maximus are divided distal to the insertion of the tensor fascia lata muscle. The tendon of the gluteus maximus is severed from its insertion on the linea aspera. The gluteus maximus is then retracted proximally. The sciatic nerve is ligated and divided distal to the ligature. The short external rotators of the hip (piriformis, gemelli, obturator internus, obturator externus, and quadratus femoris) are divided at their insertions into the femur. The attachments of the biceps femoris, semimembranosus, and semitendinosus are divided at their attachment to the ischial tuberosity **(D)**.

The hip joint capsule is incised. The ligamentum teres is divided, and the limb is removed. For wound closure, the gluteal flap is brought anteriorly and the gluteal muscles are sutured to the origin of the pectineus and adductor muscles. A drain is placed in the interior portion of the incision, and the skin edges are approximated with interrupted nonabsorbable sutures **(E)**.

POSTOPERATIVE MANAGEMENT. The patient is helped to be out of bed and to use crutches as soon as possible. Prosthetic fitting is possible as soon as the wound is completely healed.

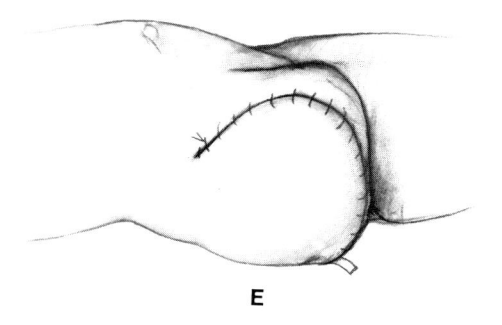

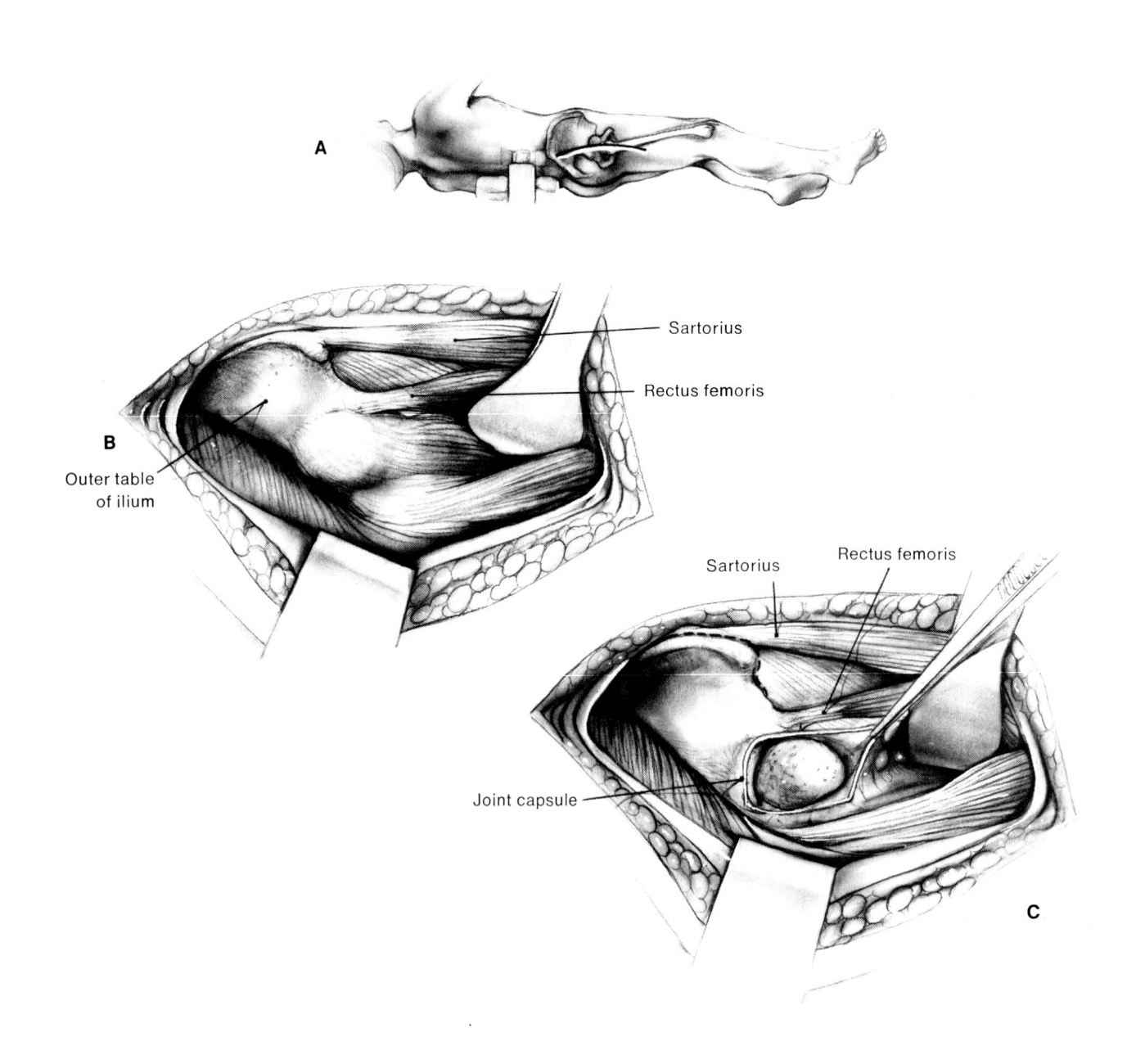

ARTHRODESIS OF HIP (Plate 10-25)

GENERAL DISCUSSION. Arthrodesis of the hip can provide an immobile but symptom-free hip joint. The hip may be arthrodesed by either intra-articular, extra-articular, or combined intra-arcitular and extra-articular methods. No one operative technique is suitable for every patient in whom arthrodesis of the hip is indicated. A combined intra-articular and extra-articular arthrodesis, supplemented in adults by internal fixation of the hip joint and proximal femoral osteotomy (without internal fixation for the proximal femoral osteotomy), is usually the procedure of choice. In tuberculosis, the focus of the disease within the joint should be excised in conjunction with extra-articular arthrodesis.

Subtrochanteric or intertrochanteric osteotomy is a valuable adjunct to arthrodesis of the hip, the fusion being enhanced by the removal of the long lever arm. In adults, fixation of the hip at approximately 20° flexion in either neutral rotation or approximately 5° external rotation is generally best. In children, the hip should be placed in complete extension and neutral rotation. The degree of abduction will depend on the amount of shortening of the affected extremity.

(Plate 10-25) ARTHRODESIS OF HIP

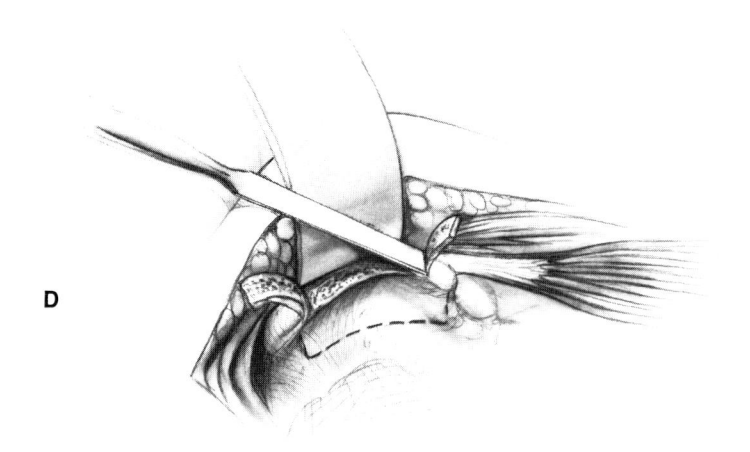

DETAILS OF PROCEDURE. The incision begins over the midportion of the iliac crest and extends distally posterior to the greater trochanter and is then directed anteriorly to end at a level approximately 12 cm distal to the anterosuperior iliac spine (**A**). Skin, subcutaneous tissue, and fascia are retracted anteriorly. Muscular attachments to the outer table of the ilium are reflected subperiosteally (including tensor fascia lata, gluteus medius, and gluteus minimus muscles) (**B**). The capsule of the hip joint is incised on its superior aspect from the acetabulum to the greater trochanter (**C**).

A bone graft, consisting of both tables of the crest of the ilium and the anterosuperior iliac spine, approximately 9 cm in length is removed from the ilium (**D** and **E**). With the hip in the desired position for fusion, a groove is cut from the superior rim of the acetabulum across the superior surface of the head and neck of the femur and into the trochanter to receive the iliac bone graft bridging the hip joint (**F**).

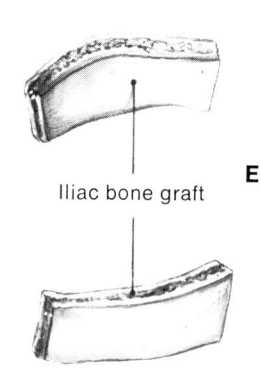

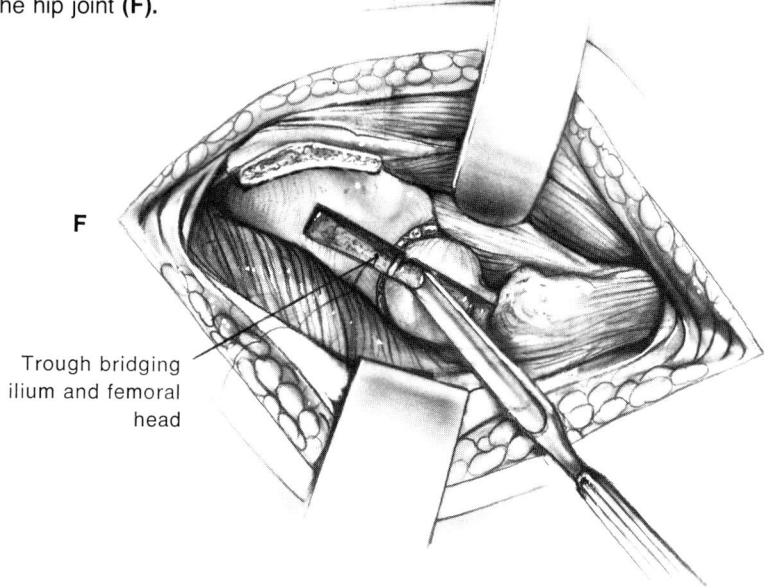

ARTHRODESIS OF HIP (Plate 10-25)

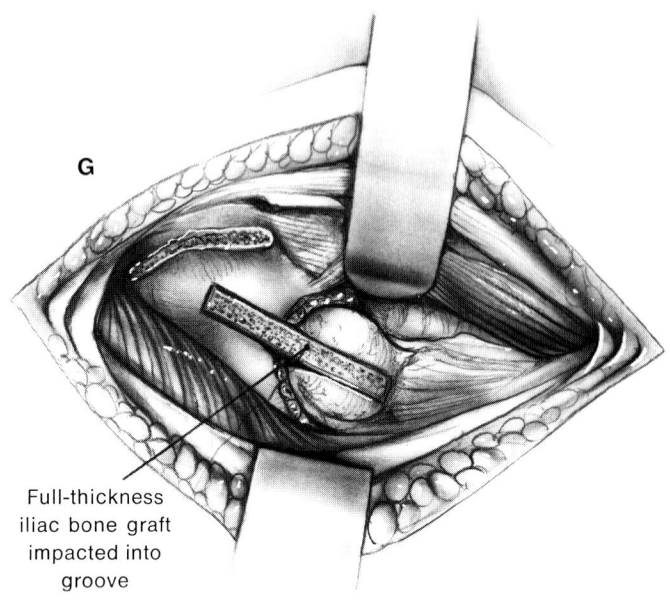

Full-thickness iliac bone graft impacted into groove

The graft is beveled and impacted firmly into this groove **(G)**. Cancellous bone chips are packed into adjacent denuded areas of the hip joint **(H)**.

A subtrochanteric osteotomy should be carried out. The subtrochanteric osteotomy should not be stabilized with internal fixation. Following wound closure, the patient's leg is placed in balanced suspension.

POSTOPERATIVE MANAGEMENT. The skin sutures are removed 10 to 14 days postoperatively, and simultaneously a well-molded one and one-half hip spica is applied with care to position the leg carefully in the desired position. An alternative is to continue traction for 3 to 5 weeks (depending on the patient's age), allowing soft callus to form at the osteotomy site but still permitting position adjustment of the distal fragment when the plaster spica is applied. External plaster immobilization is continued until there is clinical and roentgenographic evidence that both hip joint arthrodesis and the proximal femoral osteotomy are united. Progressive weight bearing with or without external support is permitted thereafter.

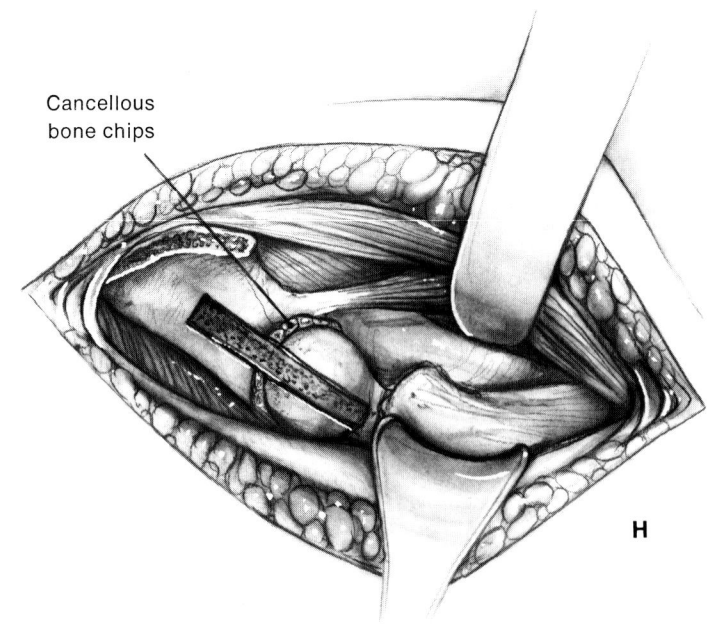

Cancellous bone chips

REFERENCES

Aadalen, R. J., Weiner, D. S., Hoyt, W., and Herndon, C. H.: Acute slipped capital femoral epiphysis, J. Bone Joint Surg. **56-A:**1473, 1974.

Abbott, J. C., and Fischer, F. J.: Arthrodesis of hip: with special reference to a method of securing ankylosis in massive destruction of the joint, Surg. Gynecol. Obstet. **52:**863, 1931.

Abbott, L. C., and Lucas, D. B.: Arthrodesis of the hip. A two-stage method for difficult cases, Surg. Clin. North Am. **36:**1035, 1956.

Adams, J. C.: A reconstruction of cup arthroplasty of the hip, J. Bone Joint Surg. **35-B:**199, 1953.

Ahlbäck, S. O., and Lindahl, O.: Hip arthrodesis. The connection between function and position, Acta Orthop. Scand. **37:**77, 1966.

Albee, F. H.: Extra-articular arthrodesis of the hip for tuberculosis: With a report of 31 cases, Ann. Surg. **89:**404, 1929.

Albee, F. H.: The principles of arthroplasty, J.A.M.A. **96:**245, 1931.

Alexander, J. P., and Barron, D. W.: Biochemical disturbances associated with total hip replacement, J. Bone Joint Surg. **61-B:**101, 1979.

Amstutz, H. C.: Polymers as bearing materials for total hip joint prosthesis. A friction and wear analysis, J. Biomed. Mater. Res. **3:**547, 1969.

Amstutz, H. C.: Complications of total hip replacement, Clin. Orthop. **72:**123, 1970.

Amstutz, H. C., Clarke, I. C., Christie, J., and Graff-Randford, A.: Total hip articular replacement by internal eccentric shells, Clin. Orthop. **128:**261, 1977.

Amstutz, H. C., Graff-Radford, A., Gruen, T. A., and Clarke, I. C.: Thaires surface replacements: a review of the first 100 cases, Clin. Orthop. **134:**87, 1978.

Anderson, L. D., Hamsa, W. R., Jr., and Waring, T. L.: Femoral-head prostheses. A review of three hundred and fifty-six operations and their results, J. Bone Joint Surg. **46-A:**1049, 1964.

Apley, A. G., Millner, W. F., and Porter, D. S.: A follow-up study of Moore's arthroplasty in the treatment of osteoarthritis of the hip, J. Bone Joint Surg. **51-B:** 638, 1969.

Arden, G. P., Taylor, A. R., and Ansell, B. M.: Total hip replacement using the McKee-Farrar prosthesis, Ann. Rheum. Dis. **29:**1, 1970.

d'Aubigne, R. M., and Postel, M.: The treatment of complications in fractures of the femoral neck (Traitement des accidents de la consolidation des fractures cervicales du femur), Rev. Chir. Orthop. **71:**265, 1952.

d'Aubigne, R. M., and Postel, M.: Functional results of hip arthroplasty with acrylic prosthesis, J. Bone Joint Surg. **36-A:** 451, 1954.

d'Aubigne, R. M., et al.: Idiopathic necrosis of the femoral head in adults, J. Bone Joint Surg. **47-B:**612, 1965.

Aufranc, O. E.: Constructive hip surgery with mold arthroplasty, American Academy of Orthopaedic Surgeons Instructional Course Lectures, vol. 11, Ann Arbor, Mich., 1954, J. W. Edwards.

Aufranc, O. E.: Constructive surgery of the hip, St. Louis, 1962, The C. V. Mosby Co.

Aufranc, O. E.: The adaptability of Vitallium mold arthroplasty to difficult hip problems, Clin. Orthop. **66:**31, 1969.

Aufranc, O. E., Jones, W. N., and Harris, W. H.: Severely comminuted intertrochanteric hip fractures, J.A.M.A. **199:**994, 1967.

Aufranc, O. E., and Sweet, E. D.: Study of patients with hip arthroplasty at Massachusetts General Hospital, J.A.M.A. **170:** 507, 1959.

Badgley, C. E., et al.: Study of the end results in one hundred thirteen cases of septic hips, J. Bone Joint Surg. **18:**1047, 1936.

Baitch, A.: Recent observations of acute suppurative arthritis, Clin. Orthop. **22:**157, 1962.

Banks, H. H.: Factors influencing the result in fractures of the femoral neck, J. Bone Joint Surg. **44-A:**931, 1962.

Banks, H. H., and Green, W. T.: Adductor myotomy and obturator neurectomy for the correction of adduction contracture of the hip in cerebral palsy, J. Bone Joint Surg. **42-A:** 111, 1960.

Barlow, T. G.: Early diagnosis and treatment of congenital dislocation of the hip, J. Bone Joint Surg. **44-B:**292, 1962.

Barnes, R.: Fracture of the neck of the femur, Alexander Gibson Memorial Lecture, J. Bone Joint Surg. **49-B:**607, 1967.

Barr, J. S., et al.: A symposium on hip joint prosthesis, American Academy of Orthopaedic Surgeons Instructional Course Lectures, vol. 15, Ann Arbor, Mich., 1958, J. W. Edwards, p. 1.

Barr, J. S., Donovan, J. F., and Florence, D. W.: Arthroplasty of the hip. Theoretical and practical considerations with a follow-up study of prosthetic replacement of the femoral head at the Massachusetts General Hospital, J. Bone Joint Surg. **46-A:**249, 1964.

Batchelor, J. S.: Excision of the femoral head and neck in cases of ankylosis and osteoarthritis of the hips, Proc. R. Soc. Med. **38:**689, 1945.

Batchelor, J. S.: Excision of the femoral head and neck for ankylosis and arthritis of the hip, Postgrad. Med. J. **24:**241, 1948.

Batchelor, J. S.: Pseudarthrosis for ankylosis and arthritis of the hip, J. Bone Joint Surg. **31-B:**135, 1949.

Bechtol, C. O., Ferguson, A. B., and Laing, P. G.: Metals and engineering in bone and joint surgery, London, 1959, Bailliere, Tindall & Cox, Ltd.

Beckenbaugh, R. D., and Ilstrup, D. M.: Total hip arthroplasty. A review of three hundred and thirty-three cases with long follow-up, J. Bone Joint Surg. **60-A:**306, 1978.

Beckenbaugh, R. D., Tressler, H. A., and Johnson, E. W.: Results after hemiarthroplasty of the hip using cemented femoral prosthesis: review of 109 cases with average follow-up of 36 months, Mayo Clin. Proc. **52:**349, 1977.

Bianco, A. J.: Treatment of mild slipping of the capital femoral epiphysis, J. Bone Joint Surg. **47-A:**387, 1965.

Bickel, W. H., and Bryan, R. S.: Results of cup arthroplasty of the hip in patients with rheumatoid arthritis and rheumatoid spondylitis, Surg. Gynecol. Obstet. **123:**243, 1966.

Bleck, E. E.: Postural and gait abnormalities caused by hip-flexion deformity in spastic cerebral palsy. Treatment by iliopsoas recession, J. Bone Joint Surg. **53-A:**1468, 1971.

Blount, W. P.: Blade-plate internal fixation for high femoral osteotomies, J. Bone Joint Surg. **25:**319, 1943.

Blount, W. P.: Proximal osteotomies of the femur, American Academy of Orthopaedic Surgeons Instructional Course Lectures, vol. 9, Ann Arbor, Mich., 1952, J. W. Edwards, p. 1.

Blount, W. P.: Don't throw away the cane, J. Bone Joint Surg. **38-A:**695, 1956.

Blount, W. P.: Osteotomy in the treatment of osteoarthritis of the hip, J. Bone Joint Surg. **46-A:**1297, 1964.

Bonfiglio, M., and Bardenstein, M. B.: Treatment by bone grafting of aseptic necrosis of the femoral head and non-union of the femoral neck (Phemister technique), J. Bone Joint Surg. **50-A**:48, 1968.

Borden, J., Spencer, G. E., Jr., and Herndon, C. H.: Treatment of coxa vara in children by means of a modified osteotomy, J. Bone Joint Surg. **48-A**:1106, 1966.

Bost, F. C., Schottstaedt, E. R., and Larsen, L. J.: Surgical approaches to the hip joint, American Academy of Orthopaedic Surgeons Instructional Course Lectures, vol. 11, Ann Arbor, Mich., 1954, J. W. Edwards.

Boyd, H. B.: Anatomic disarticularion of the hip, Surg. Gynecol. Obstet. **84**:346, 1947.

Boyd, H. B., and Anderson, L. D.: Management of unstable trochanteric fractures, Surg. Gynecol. Obstet. **112**:633, 1961.

Boyd, H. B., and George, I. L.: Complications of fractures of the neck of the femur, J. Bone Joint Surg. **29**:13, 1947.

Boyd, H. B., and Lipinski, S. W.: Nonunion of trochanteric and subtrochanteric fractures, Surg. Gynecol. Obstet. **104**:463, 1957.

Boyd, H. B., and Salvatore, J. E.: Acute fracture of the femoral neck: Internal fixation or prosthesis? J. Bone Joint Surg. **46-A**:1066, 1964.

Boyd, R. J., Burke, J. R., and Colton, T.: A double-blind clinical trial of prophylactic antibiotics in hip fractures, J. Bone Joint Surg. **55-A**:1251, 1973.

Brewster, R. C., Coventry, M. B., and Johnson, E. W., Jr.: Conversion of the arthrodesed hip to a total hip replacement, J. Bone Joint Surg. **57-A**:27, 1975.

Brittain, H. A.: Ischiofemoral arthrodesis, Br. J. Surg. **29**:93, 1941.

Brittain, H. A.: Ischiofemoral arthrodesis, J. Bone Joint Surg. **30-B**:642, 1948.

Brown, J. T., and Abrami, G.: Transcervical femoral fracture: a review of 195 patients treated by sliding nail-plate fixation, J. Bone Joint Surg. **46-B**:648, 1964.

Bulmer, J. H.: Septic arthritis of the hip in adults, J. Bone Joint Surg. **43-B**:289, 1966.

Cabaud, H. E., Westin, G. W., and Connelly, S.: Tendon transfers in the paralytic hip, J. Bone Joint Surg. **61-A**:1035, 1979.

Campbell, R. D., Jr., et al.: The use of intramedullary prosthetic replacement in fractures of the femoral neck, Am. J. Surg. **99**:745, 1960.

Campbell, W. C.: Posterior dislocation of the hip joint with fracture of the acetabulum, J. Bone Joint Surg. **18**:842, 1936.

Canale, S. T., and Bourland, W. L.: Fracture of the neck and intertrochanteric region of the femur in children, J. Bone Joint Surg. **59-A**:431, 1977.

Capello, W. N., Ireland, P. H., Trammel, T. R., and Eicher, P.: Conservative total hip arthroplasty: a procedure to conserve bone stock, Clin. Orthop. **134**:59, 1978.

Carlsson, A. S.: Erythrocyte sedimentation rate in infected and non-infected total hip arthroplasties, Acta Orthop. Scand. **49**:287, 1978.

Carroll, N. C., and Sharrard, W. J. W.: Long-term follow-up of posterior iliopsoas transplantation for paralytic dislocation of the hip, J. Bone Joint Surg. **54-A**:551, 1972.

Cave, E. F.: Fractures of the femoral neck, American Academy of Orthopaedic Surgeons Instructional Course Lectures. vol. 17, St. Louis, 1960, The C. V. Mosby Co., p. 79.

Chacha, P. B.: Suppurative arthritis of the hip joint in infancy, A persistent diagnostic problem and possible complication of femoral venipuncture, J. Bone Joint Surg. **53-A**:538, 1971.

Chan, K. P., and Shin, J. S.: Brittain ischiofemoral arthrodesis for tuberculosis of the hip. An analysis of 76 cases, J. Bone Joint Surg. **50-A**:1341, 1968.

Chandler, F. A.: Hip-fusion operation, J. Bone Joint Surg. **15**:947, 1933.

Chapchal, G., and Muller, W.: Total hip replacement with the McKee prosthesis. A study of 121 follow-up cases using neutral cement, Clin. Orthop. **72**:115, 1970.

Charnley, J.: Compression arthrodesis, including central dislocation as a principle in hip surgery, Edinburgh, 1953, E. & S. Livingstone Ltd.

Charnley, J.: Arthroplasty of the hip. A new operation, Lancet **1**:1129, 1961.

Charnley, J.: The bonding of prostheses to bone by cement, J. Bone Joint Surg. **46-B**:518, 1964.

Charnley, J.: A biomechanical analysis of the use of cement to anchor the femoral head prosthesis, J. Bone Joint Surg. **47-B**:354, 1965.

Charnley, J.: The reaction of bone to self-curing acrylic cement. A long-term histological study in man, J. Bone Joint Surg. **52-B**:340, 1970.

Charnley, J.: Total hip replacement by low-friction arthroplasty, Clin. Orthop. **72**:7, 1970.

Charnley, J., and Crawford, W. J.: Histology of bone in contact with self-curing acrylic cement, J. Bone Joint Surg. **50-B**:228, 1968.

Charnley, J., Kamanger, A., and Longfield, M.D.: The optimum size of prosthetic heads in relation to the wear of the plastic sockets in total hip replacement, Med. Biol. Eng. **7**:31, 1969.

Charnley, J., and Kettlewell, J.: The elimination of slip between prosthesis and femur, J. Bone Joint Surg. **47-B**:56, 1965.

Chen, H.-T., and Lee, T.-S.: Arthrodesis of the tuberculous hip, Int. Surg. **46**:125, 1966.

Christensen, I.: Anteversion deformity and derotation osteotomy in congenital dislocation of the hip, Acta Orthop. Scand. **40**:62, 1969.

Chuinard, E. G.: Early weight-bearing and correction of anteversion in the treatment of congenital dislocation of the hip, J. Bone Joint Surg. **37-A**:229, 1955.

Chuinard, E. G., and Logan, N. D.: Varus-producing and derotational subtrochanteric osteotomy in the treatment of congenital dislocation of the hip, J. Bone Joint Surg. **45-A**:1397, 1963.

Clawson, D. K.: Intertrochanteric fractures of the hip, Am. J. Surg. **93**:580, 1957.

Clawson, D. K., and Seddon, H. J.: Late consequences of sciatic nerve injury, J. Bone Joint Surg. **42-B**:213, 1960.

Cleveland, M.: Traction versus rest in the treatment of hip disease, J. Bone Joint Surg. **39-A**:661, 1957.

Cleveland, M., Bosworth, D. M., and Della Pietra, A.: Subtrochanteric osteotomy and spline fixation for certain disabilities of the hip joint, J. Bone Joint Surg. **33-A**:351, 1951.

Cleveland, M., Bosworth, D. M., and Thompson, F. R.: Infertrochanteric fractures of the femur. A survey of treatment in traction and by internal fixation, J. Bone Joint Surg. **29**:109, 1947.

Clouse, M. E., Aufranc, O. E., and Weber, A. L.: Roentgenologic and clinical evaluation of Vitallium mold arthroplasty of the hip, Surg. Gynecol. Obstet. **127**:1042, 1968.

Cohen, J.: Tissue reactions to metals—the influence of surface finish, J. Bone Joint Surg. **43-A**:687, 1961.

Coleman, S. S.: Treatment of congenital dislocation of the hip in the infant, J. Bone Joint Surg. **47-A**:590, 1965.

Collis, D. K.: Femoral stem failure in total hip replacement, J. Bone Joint Surg. **59-A**:1033, 1977.

Colonna, P. C.: Congenital dislocation of the hip in older subjects, J. Bone Joint Surg. **14**:277, 1932.

Colonna, P. C.: An arthroplastic operation for congenital dislocation of the hip. A two-stage procedure, Surg. Gynecol. Obstet. **63**:777, 1936.

Colonna, P. C.: Capsular arthroplasty for congenital dislocation of the hip: indications and technique. Some long-term results, J. Bone Joint Surg. **47-A**:437, 1965.

Coventry, M. B.: Fresh fracture of the hip treated with prosthesis, American Academy of Orthopaedic Surgeons Instructional Course Lectures, vol. 16, St. Louis, 1959, The C. V. Mosby Co., p. 292.

Coventry, M. B.: Salvage of the painful hip prosthesis, J. Bone Joint Surg. **46-A**:200, 1964.

Coventry, M. B.: Osteotomy of the hip for degenerative arthritis, Mayo Clin. Proc. **44**:505, 1969.

Coventry, M. B., Beckenbaugh, R. D., Nolan, D. R., and Ilstrup, D. M.: 2,012 total hip arthroplasties: a study of postoperative course and early complications, J. Bone Joint Surg. **56-A**:273, 1974.

Cram, R. H.: The unstable intertrochanteric fracture, Surg. Gynecol. Obstet. **101**:15, 1955.

Crawford, H. B.: Conservative treatment of impacted fractures of the femoral neck, J. Bone Joint Surg. **42-A**:371, 1960.

Crawford, H. B.: Experience with the nonoperative treatment of impacted fractures of the neck of the femur, J. Bone Joint Surg. **47-A**:830, 1965.

Crawford, H. B.: Impacted femoral neck fractures, Clin. Orthop. **66**:90, 1969.

Crawford, H. B., Merrill, E. F., and Bridgman, C. F.: Radiography of the hip joint. III. Radiographic procedures during hip-joint operations, Med. Radiogr. Photogr. **26**:106, 1950.

Crego, C. H., Jr., and Schwartzmann, J. R.: Follow-up study of the early treatment of congenital dislocation of the hip, J. Bone Joint Surg. **30-A**:428, 1948.

Crenshaw, A. H.: Muscle pedicle bone graft in arthrodesis of the hip, South. Med. J. **50**:169, 1957.

Crowe, J. F., Mani, V. S., and Ranawat, C. S.: Total hip replacement in congenital dislocation and dysplasia of the hip, J. Bone Joint Surg. **61-A**:15, 1979.

Cruess, R. L.: The pathology of acute necrosis of cartilage in slipping of the capital femoral epiphysis. A report of two cases with pathological sections, J. Bone Joint Surg. **45-A**:1013, 1963.

Cubbins, W. R., Callahan, J. J., and Scuderi, C. S.: Fractures of the neck of the femur, Surg. Gynecol. Obstet. **68**:87, 1939.

Cunha, B. A., et al.: The penetration characteristics of Cefazolin, Cephalothin and Cephradine into bone in patients undergoing total hip replacement, J. Bone Joint Surg. **59-A**:856, 1977.

Curtiss, P. H., and Klein, L.: Destruction of articular cartilage in septic arthritis, J. Bone Joint Surg. **45-A**:797, 1963.

Curtiss, P. H., and Klein, L.: Destruction of articular cartilage in septic arthritis. II. In vivo studies, J. Bone Joint Surg. **47-A**:1595, 1965.

Davis, J. R.: The muscle-pedicle bone graft in hip fusion, J. Bone Joint Surg. **36-A**:790, 1954.

Davis, P. H., and Frymoyer, J. W.: The lateral position in the surgical management of intertrochanteric and subtrochanteric fractures of the femur, J. Bone Joint Surg. **51-A**:1128, 1969.

DeHaven, K. E., Evarts, C. M., Wilde, A. H., Collins, H. R., Nelson, C. L., Jr., and Razzano, C. D.: Early results of Charnley-Muller total hip reconstruction, Orthop. Clin. North Am. **4**:465-472, 1973.

DePalma, A. F., Rothman, R. H., and Klemek, J. S.: Osteotomy of the proximal femur in degenerative arthritis, Clin. Orthop. **73**:109, 1970.

Deyerle, W. M.: Absolute fixation with contact compression in hip fractures, Clin. Orthop. **13**:279, 1959.

Deyerle, W. M.: Multiple-pin peripheral fixation in fractures of the neck of the femur: immediate weight-bearing, Clin. Orthop. **39**:135, 1965.

Dickerson, R. C.: Congenital subluxation of the hip, Pediatrics **41**:977, 1968.

Dickson, F. D.: Davis method for closed reduction of congenital dislocation of the hip, J. Bone Joint Surg. **17**:43, 1935.

Dickson, J. A., et al.: Symposium on Management of Fresh Fractures of the Neck of the Femur, American Academy of Orthopaedic Surgeons Instructional Course Lectures, vol. 17, St. Louis, 1960, The C. V. Mosby Co.

Dickson, J. A., and Willien, L. J.: Arthrodesis of the hip joint in degenerative arthritis: a modified procedure with internal fixation, J. Bone Joint Surg. **29**:687, 1947.

Dimon, J. H., III, and Hughston, J. C.: Unstable intertrochanteric fractures of the hip, J. Bone Joint Surg. **49-A**:440, 1967.

Drutz, D. J., et al.: The penetration of penicillin and other antimicrobiols into joint fluid, J. Bone Joint Surg. **49-A**:1415, 1967.

Dunn, D. M.: Anteversion of the neck of the femur, J. Bone Joint Surg. **34-B**:181, 1952.

Duthie, R. B., and Harris, C. M.: A radiographic and clinical survey of the hip joint in sero-positive rheumatoid arthritis, Acta Orthop. Scand. **40**:346, 1969.

Duthie, R. B., and Howe, W., Jr.: Displacement osteotomy for arthritis of the hip, Clin. Orthop. **31**:65, 1963.

Ecker, M. L., Joyce, J. J., III, and Kohl, E. J.: The treatment of trochanteric hip fractures using a compression screw, J. Bone Joint Surg. **57-A**:23, 1975.

Eggers, G. W. N., and Evans, E. B.: Surgery in cerebral palsy, J. Bone Joint Surg. **45-A**:1275, 1963.

Enneking, W. F.: Local resection of malignant lesions of the hip and pelvis, J. Bone Joint Surg. **48-A**:991, 1966.

Epstein, H. C.: Posterior fracture-dislocations of the hip. Long-term follow-up, J. Bone Joint Surg. **56-A**:1103, 1974.

Evans, E. M.: The treatment of trochanteric fractures of the femur, J. Bone Joint Surg. **31-B**:190, 1949.

Evans, E. M.: Trochanteric fractures, J. Bone Joint Surg. **33-B**:192, 1951.

Evarts, C. M.: Total hip-joint arthroplasty, N.Y. State J. Med. **71**:2082, 1971.

Evarts, C. M.: Advantages of total hip replacement, Geriatrics **12**:52, 1972.

Evarts, C. M.: Acetabular cup alignment in total hip reconstruction, Clin. Orthop. **103**:22-23, 1974.

Evarts, C. M.: Hip surgery: successes and sorrows. Clinics in Rheum. Dis. **4**:375, 1978.

Evarts, C. M., DeHaven, K. E., Nelson, C. L., Jr., Collins, H. R., and Wilde, A. M.: Interim results of Charnley-Muller total hip arthroplasty, Clin. Orthop. **95**:193-200, 1973.

Evarts, C. M., and Feil, E. J.: Prevention of thromboembolic disease after elective surgery of the hip, J. Bone Joint Surg. **53-A**:1271, 1971.

Evarts, C. M., Nelson, C. L., Jr., Collins, H. R., and Wilde, A. H.: The surgical technique of total hip joint arthroplasty: the Charnley-Muller prosthesis, Orthop. Clin. North Am. **4**:449-463, 1973.

Evarts, C. M., Wilde, A. H., DeHaven, K. E., Nelson, C. L., Jr., and Collins, H. R.: Total hip-joint arthroplasties, J. Bone Joint Surg. **52-A:**1562, 1972.

Eyre-Brook, A. L.: Septic arthritis of the hip and osteomyelitis of the upper end of the femur in infants, J. Bone Joint Surg. **42-B:**11, 1960.

Fahey, J. J., and O'Brien, E. T.: Acute slipped capital femoral epiphysis, J. Bone Joint Surg. **47-A:**1105, 1965.

Ferciot, C. F.: Primary prosthetic replacement in fractures of the femoral neck, American Academy of Orthopaedic Surgeons Instructional Course Lectures, vol. 16, St. Louis, 1959, The C. V. Mosby Co.

Ferguson, A. B., Jr.: High intertrochanteric osteotomy for osteoarthritis of the hip. A procedure to streamline the defective joint, J. Bone Joint Surg. **46-A:**1159, 1964.

Ferguson, A. B., Jr.: The pathological changes in degenerative arthritis of the hip and treatment by rotational osteotomy, J. Bone Joint Surg. **46-A:**1337, 1964.

Ferguson, A. B., Jr.: The pathology of degenerative arthritis of the hip and the use of osteotomy in its treatment, Clin. Orthop. **77:**84, 1971.

Ferguson, A. B., Jr.: Primary open reduction of congenital dislocation of the hip using a median adductor approach, J. Bone Joint Surg. **55-A:**671, 1973.

Fielding, J. W., and Magliato, H. J.: Subtrochanteric fractures, Surg. Gynecol. Obstet. **122:**555, 1966.

Fisher, R. H.: Guide for insertion of the F. R. Thompson prosthesis, J. Bone Joint Surg. **45-A:**583, 1963.

Fitzgerald, R. H., et al.: Deep wound sepsis following total hip arthroplasty, J. Bone Joint Surg. **59-A:**847, 1977.

Follacci, F. M., and Charnley, J.: A comparison of the results of femoral head prosthesis with and without cement, Clin. Orthop. **62:**156, 1969.

Forrester-Brown, M.: Slipping of the upper femoral epiphysis. End result after conservative treatment, J. Bone Joint Surg. **23:**256, 1941.

Foster, Y. C.: Trochanteric fractures of the femur treated by the Vitallium McLaughlin nail and plate, J. Bone Joint Surg. **40-B:**684, 1958.

Francis, K. C., et al.: The treatment of pathological fractures of the femoral neck by resection, J. Trauma **2:**465, 1962.

Frangakis, E. K.: Intracapsular fractures of the neck of the femur. Factors influencing nonunion and ischaemic necrosis, J. Bone Joint Surg. **48-B:**17, 1966.

Freeman, M. A. R., Cameron, H. V., and Brown, G. C.: Cemented double cup arthroplasty of the hip: a 5-year experience with the ICLH prosthesis, Clin. Orthop. **134:**45, 1978.

Freiberg, J. A.: Experiences with the Brittain ischiofemoral arthrodesis, J. Bone Joint Surg. **28:**501, 1946.

Friedenberg, Z. B.: Protrusio acetabuli, Am. J. Surg. **85:**764, 1953.

Frejka, B.: Prävention der angeborenen Hüft gelenksluxation durch das Abduktionspolster, Wien Med. Wochenschr. **91:**523, 1941.

Froimson, A. I.: Treatment of comminuted subtrochanteric fractures of the femur, Surg. Gynecol. Obstet. **131:**465, 1970.

Gaenslen, F. J.: The Schanz subtrochanteric osteotomy for irreducible dislocation of the hip, J. Bone Joint Surg. **17:**76, 1935.

Galante, R., et al.: Sintered fiber metal composites as a basis for attachment of implants to bone, J. Bone Joint Surg. **53-A:**101, 1971.

Garrett, J. C., et al.: Treatment of unreduced traumatic posterior dislocations of the hip, J. Bone Joint Surg. **61-A:**2, 1979.

Ghormley, R. K.: Use of the anterior superior spine and crest of ilium in surgery of the hip joint, J. Bone Joint Surg. **13:**784, 1931.

Ghormley, R. K., and Fairchild, R. D.: Diagnosis and treatment of slipped epiphysis, J.A.M.A. **114:**229, 1940.

Gibson, A.: Posterior exposure of the hip joint, J. Bone Joint Surg. **32-B:**183, 1950.

Gill, A. B.: Arthrodesis of the hip for ununited fractures, J. Bone Joint Surg. **29:**305, 1947.

Girdlestone, G. R.: Arthrodesis and other operations for tuberculosis of the hip. In the Robert Jones Birthday volume, London, 1928, Oxford University Press.

Girdlestone, G. R.: Acute pyogenic arthritis of the hip. An operative giving free access and effective drainage, Lancet **1:**419, 1943.

Goodman, A. H., and Sherman, M. S.: Post irradiation fractures of the femoral neck, J. Bone Joint Surg. **45-A:**723, 1963.

Green, W. T.: Slipping of the upper femoral epiphysis: diagnostic and therapeutic considerations, Arch. Surg. **50:**19, 1945.

Groves, E. W. H.: Arthroplasty, Br. J. Surg. **11:**234, 1923.

Groves, E. W. H.: Some contributions to the reconstructive surgery of the hip, Br. J. Surg. **14:**486, 1927.

Haggart, G. E.: Degenerative disease of the hip joint treated by arthrodesis, American Academy of Orthopaedic Surgeons Instructional Course Lectures, vol. 3, Ann Arbor, Mich., 1946, J. W. Edwards, p. 223.

Hahn, D.: Ischio-femoral arthrodesis for tuberculosis of the hip, J. Bone Joint Surg. **45-B:**477, 1963.

Hall, J. E.: The results of treatment of slipped femoral epiphysis, J. Bone Joint Surg. **39-B:**659, 1957.

Harrington, K. D., and Johnston, J. O.: The management of comminuted unstable intertrochanteric fractures, J. Bone Joint Surg. **55-A:**1367, 1973.

Harris, N. H.: A technique for internal fixation of a high femoral osteotomy using the Muller compression device, Proc. Soc. R. Med. **59:**831, 1966.

Harris, N. H., and Kirwan, E.: The results of osteotomy for early primary osteoarthritis of the hip, J. Bone Joint Surg. **46-B:**477, 1964.

Harris, W. H.: A new lateral approach to the hip joint, J. Bone Joint Surg. **49-A:**891, 1967.

Harris, W. H.: Surgical approach and technique of cup arthroplasty, Surg. Clin. North Am. **49:**763, 1969.

Harris, W. H.: Traumatic arthritis of the hip after dislocation and acetabular fractures: treatment by mold arthroplasty. An end-result study using a new method of result evaluation, J. Bone Joint Surg. **51-A:**737, 1969.

Harris, W. H.: Power instrumentation for cup arthroplasty, Clin. Orthop. **72:**219, 1970.

Harris, W. H., and Aufranc, O. E.: Mold arthroplasty in the treatment of hip fractures complicated by sepsis. A report of nine cases, J. Bone Joint Surg. **47-A:**31, 1965.

Harris, W. H., and Crothers, O. D.: Reattachment of the greater trochanter in total hip replacement arthroplasty. A new technique, J. Bone Joint Surg. **60-A:**211, 1978.

Harris, W. H., et al.: Comparison of Warfarin, low-molecular-weight, Dextran, Aspirin, and subcutaneous Heparin in prevention of thromboembolism following total hip replacement, J. Bone Joint Surg. **56-A:**1552, 1974.

Harris, W. H., et al.: Aspirin prophylaxis of venous thromboembolism after total hip replacement, New Engl. J. Med. **297:**1246, 1977.

Harris, W. H., Salzman, E. W., and Desanctis, R. W.: The prevention of thromboembolic disease by prophylactic anticoagulation. A controlled study in elective hip surgery, J. Bone Joint Surg. **49-A:**81, 1967.

Harrison, M. H. M., Schajowicz, F., and Trueta, J.: Osteoarthritis of the hip: A study of the nature and evolution of the disease, J. Bone Joint Surg. **35-B:**598, 1953.

Hartz, M., and Joyce, J. J.: Surgical approaches to the hip and femur, J. Bone Joint Surg. **45-A:**175, 1963.

Hayes, J. T., Gross, H. P., and Dow, S.: Surgery for paralytic defects secondary to myelomeningocele and myelodysplasia, J. Bone Joint Surg. **46-A:**1577, 1964.

Heberling, J. A.: A review of two hundred and one cases of suppurative arthritis, J. Bone Joint Surg. **23:**917, 1941.

Henderson, M. S.: Combined intra-articular and extra-articular arthrodesis for tuberculosis of the hip joint, J. Bone Joint Surg. **15:**51, 1933.

Henderson, M. S.: Treatment of ununited fractures of the hip, Surg. Clin. North Am. **24:**751, 1944.

Henrikson, B.: The incidence of slipped capital femoral epiphysis, Acta Orthop. Scand. **40:**365, 1969.

Herndon, C. H., Heyman, C. H., and Bell, D. M.: Treatment of slipped capital femoral epiphysis by epiphyseodesis and osteoplasty of the femoral neck. A report of further experiences, J. Bone Joint Surg. **45-A:**999, 1963.

Heyman, C. H.: The treatment of slipping of the upper femoral epiphysis, American Academy of Orthopaedic Surgeons Instructional Course Lectures, vol. 13, Ann Arbor, Mich., 1956, J. W. Edwards, p. 45.

Heyman, C. H., Herndon, C. H., and Strong, J. M.: Slipped femoral epiphysis with severe displacement. A conservative operative treatment, J. Bone Joint Surg. **39-A:**293, 1957.

Hibbs, R. A.: A preliminary report of twenty cases of hip joint tuberculosis treated by an operation devised to eliminate motion by fusing the joint, J. Bone Joint Surg. **8:**522, 1926.

Hiertonn, T., and James, U.: Congenital dislocation of the hip. Experiences of early diagnosis and treatment, J. Bone Joint Surg. **50-B:**542, 1968.

Hilgenreiner, H.: 10 Jahre Abduktionsschiene und Fruhbehandlung der angeborenen Hüftverrenkung, Z. Orthop. Chir. **63:**344, 1935.

Hinchey, J. J.: An evaluation of prosthetic replacement in management of fresh fractures of the neck of the femur, American Academy of Orthopaedic Surgeons Instructional Course Lectures, vol. 17, St. Louis, 1960, The C. V. Mosby Co.

Hinchey, J. J., and Day, P. L.: Primary prosthetic replacement in fresh femoral-neck fractures. A review of 294 consecutive cases, J. Bone Joint Surg. **46-A:**223, 1964.

Hirsch, C., and Goldie, I.: Osteotomy in osteoarthritis of the hip joint. A follow-up study, Acta Orthop. Scand. **39:**182, 1968.

Hirsch, C., and Goldie, I.: Walk-way studies after intertrochanteric osteotomy for osteoarthritis of the hip, Acta Orthop. Scand. **40:**334, 1969.

Hirsch, C., and Scheller, S.: Result of treatment from birth of unstable hips. A clinical and radiographic 5-year follow-up, Clin. Orthop. **62:**162, 1969.

Hoaglund, F. T., Yau, A. C. M. C., and Wong, W. L.: Osteoarthritis of the hip and other joints in southern Chinese in Hong Kong. Incidence and related factors, J. Bone Joint Surg. **55-A:**545, 1973.

Hogshead, H. P., and Ponseti, I. V.: Fascia lata transfer to the erector spinae for the treatment of flexion-abduction contractures of the hip in patients with poliomyelitis and meningomyelocele. Evaluation of results, J. Bone Joint Surg. **46-A:**1389, 1964.

Holt, E. P.: Hip fractures in the trochanteric region: treatment with a strong nail and early weight-bearing. A report of one hundred cases, J. Bone Joint Surg. **45-A:**687, 1963.

Howorth, M. B.: Slipping of the upper femoral epiphysis, American Academy of Orthopaedic Surgeons Instructional Course Lectures, vol. 8, Ann Arbor, Mich., 1951, J. W. Edwards, p. 306.

Howorth, M. B.: Congenital dislocation of the hip. Technic of open reduction, Ann. Surg. **135:**508, 1952.

Hughston, J. C.: Unstable intertrochanteric fractures of the hip, J. Bone Joint Surg. **46-A:**1145, 1964.

Hunt, D. D., and Larson, C. B.: Treatment of the residua of hip infections by mold arthroplasty. An end-result study of 33 hips, J. Bone Joint Surg. **48-A:**111, 1966.

Hunter, G. A.: A comparison of the use of internal fixation and prosthetic replacement for fresh fractures of the neck of the femur, Br. J. Surg. **56:**229, 1969.

Hunter, G. A.: Further comparison of use of internal fixation and prosthetic replacement for fresh fractures of the neck of the femur, Br. J. Surg. **61:**382, 1974.

Inge, G. A. L., and Liebolt, F. L.: The treatment of acute suppurative arthritis, Surg. Gynecol. Obstet. **60:**86, 1935.

Ivins, J. C., et al.: Arthroplasty of the hip for idiopathic degenerative joint disease, Surg. Gynecol. Obstet. **125:**1281, 1967.

Jensen, J. S., and Holstein, P.: Long-term follow-up of Moore arthroplasty in femoral neck fractures, Acta Orthop. Scand. **46:**764, 1975.

Jewett, E. L.: One-piece angle nail for trochanteric fractures, J. Bone Joint Surg. **23:**803, 1941.

Jewett, E. L.: Rigid internal fixation of intracapsular femoral neck fractures, Am. J. Surg. **91:**621, 1956.

Johnson, E. W., Jr.: Contractures of the iliotibial band, Surg. Gynecol. Obstet. **96:**599, 1953.

Johnson, L. L., Lottes, J. O., and Arnot, J. P.: The utilization of the Holt nail for proximal femoral fractures, J. Bone Joint Surg. **50-A:**67, 1968.

Johnston, R. C., and Larson, C. B.: Biomechanics of cup arthroplasty, Clin. Orthop. **66:**56, 1969.

Johnston, R. C., and Larson, C. B.: Results of treatment of hip disorders with cup arthroplasty, J. Bone Joint Surg. **51-A:**1461, 1969.

Jones, J. M.: Revisional total hip replacement for failed ring arthroplasty, J. Bone Joint Surg. **61-A:**1029, 1979.

Judet, J., and Judet, R.: The use of an artificial femoral head for arthroplasty of the hip joint, J. Bone Joint Surg. **32-B:**166, 1950.

Judet, J., Judet, R., Lagrange, J., and Dunoyer, J.: Resection-reconstruction of the hip; arthroplasty with acrylic prosthesis. Nissen, K. I., editor, London, 1954, E. & S. Livingstone, Ltd. (Translated from the French publication by L'Expansion Scientifique Française, Paris, 1952).

Judet, R., and Judet, J.: Technique and results with the acrylic femoral head prosthesis, J. Bone Joint Surg. **34-B:**173, 1952.

Kaufer, H., Matthews, L. S., and Sonstegard, D.: Stable fixation of intertrochanteric fractures. A biomechanical evaluation, J. Bone Joint Surg. **56-A:**899, 1974.

Keats, S., and Morgese, A. N.: A simple anteromedial approach to the lesser trochanter of the femur for the release of the iliopsoas tendon, J. Bone Joint Surg. **49-A:**632, 1967.

Keats, S., and Morgese, A. N.: Excessive lumbar lordosis in

ambulatory spactic children. Iliopsoas tenotomy, Clin. Orthop. **65:**130, 1969.

Kelly, P. J., and Lipscomb, P. R.: Primary vitallium-mold arthroplasty for posterior dislocation of the hip with fracture of the femoral head, J. Bone Joint Surg. **40-A:**675, 1958.

Kelly, P. J., Martin, W. J., and Coventry, M. B.: Bacterial arthritis of the hip in the adult, J. Bone Joint Surg. **47-A:**1005, 1965.

Kelsey, J. L., Keggi, K. J., and Southwick, W. O.: The incidence and distribution of slipped capital femoral epiphysis in Connecticut and Southwestern United States, J. Bone Joint Surg. **52-A:**1203, 1970.

Key, J. A., and Reynolds, F. C.: Intrapelvic obturator neurectomy for relief of chronic arthritis of the hip, Surgery **24:**959, 1948.

Kidner, F. C.: Open reduction of congenital dislocation of the hip, J. Bone Joint Surg. **13:**799, 1931.

Kilburn, P.: Psoas release operation in osteoarthritis of the hip, J. R. Coll. Surg. Edinb. **12:**27, 1966.

King, D., Leaf, E., and Terwilliger, C. K.: The importance of accurate roentgenography and interpretation in femoral neck fractures treated by internal fixation, J. Bone Joint Surg. **22:**168, 1940.

Knight, R. A., and Bluhm, M. M.: Brittain ischiofemoral arthrodesis, J. Bone Joint Surg. **27:**578, 1945.

Knodt, H.: Osteoarthritis of the hip joint. Etiology and treatment by osteotomy, J. Bone Joint Surg. **46-A:**1326, 1964.

Knowles, F. L.: Fractures of the neck of femur, Wis. Med. J. **35:**106, 1936.

Korn, M. W., and States, J. D.: Slipping capital femoral epiphysis: A long-term follow-up and review of cases in Rochester, New York, Clin. Orthop. **48:**119, 1966.

Kuderna, H., Bohler, N., and Collon, D. J.: Treatment of intertrochanteric and subtrochanteric fractures of the hip by the Ender method, J. Bone Joint Surg. **58-A:**604, 1976.

Kyle, R. F., and Gustilo, R. B.: Analysis of six hundred and twenty-two intertrochanteric hip fractures. A retrospective and prospective study, J. Bone Joint Surg. **61-A:**216, 1979.

Landmark, J. J., Muldoon, S. M., Nolan, N. G., and Coventry, M. B.: Sequential blood volume changes in patients undergoing total hip arthroplasty, Anesth. Analg. (Cleve.) **54:**391, 1975.

Lang, A. G., and Klassen, R. A.: Cup arthroplasties in teenagers and children, J. Bone Joint Surg. **59-A:**444, 1977.

Langenskiöld, A.: Technical aspects of the operative reduction of congenital dislocation of the hip, Acta Orthop. Scand. **20:**8, 1950.

Langenskiöld, A., and Sarpio, O.: Pathologin vid Kongenital höftledsluxation: Finska läk.-sällsk. handl. **100,** 1957.

Larson, C. B.: The treatment of acute fractures of the neck of the femur, American Academy of Orthopaedic Surgeons Instructional Course Lectures, vol. 11, Ann Arbor, Mich., 1954, J. W. Edwards, p. 72.

Lasda, N. A., Levinsohn, E. M., Yuan, H. A., and Bunnell, W. P.: Computerized tomography in disorders of the hip, J. Bone Joint Surg. **60-A:**1099, 1978.

Law, W. A.: Late results in Vitallium-mold arthroplasty of the hip, J. Bone Joint Surg. **44-A:**1497, 1962.

Lazansky, M. G.: Complications in total hip replacement with the Charnley technic, Clin. Orthop. **72:**40, 1970.

Leadbetter, G. W.: A treatment for fractures of the neck of the femur, J. Bone Joint Surg. **15:**931, 1933.

Leadbetter, G. W.: Cervical-axial osteotomy of the femur. A preliminary report, J. Bone Joint Surg. **26:**713, 1944.

Lewis, R. C., Jr., and Ghormley, R. K.: Colonna reconstruction of the hip: results in 57 cases, Mayo Clin. Proc. **29:**605, 1954.

Liebolt, F. L., Beal, J. M., and Speer, D. S.: Obturator neurectomy for painful hip, Am. J. Surg. **79:**427, 1950.

Lindholm, R. V., Puranen, J., and Kinnunen, P.: Moore vitallium femoral head prosthesis in fractures of the femoral neck, Acta Orthop. Scand. **47:**70, 1976.

Linton, P.: On different types of intracapsular fractures of the femoral neck: surgical investigation of origin, treatment, prognosis and complications in 365 cases, Acta Chir. Scand. (Suppl.) 86, 1944.

Linton, P.: Types of displacement in fractures of the femoral neck and observations on impaction of fractures, J. Bone Joint Surg. **31-B:**184, 1949.

Lippmann, R. K.: Transfixion hip prosthesis. Sequential clinical and roentgenographic observations of 64 patients followed for five to fifteen years, J. Bone Joint Surg. **47-A:**876, 1967.

Lipscomb, P. R: Reconstructive surgery for bilateral hip-joint disease in the adult, J. Bone Joint Surg. **47-A:**1, 1965.

Lipscomb, P. R.: Salvage of the poor result of slipped capital femoral epiphysis, Clin. Orthop. **48:**153, 1966.

Lipscomb, P. R., and Barber, J. R.: A comparison of the Gibson posterolateral and Smith-Peterson iliofemoral approaches to the hip for Vitallium mold arthroplasty, Am. J. Surg. **87:**4, 1954.

Lipscomb, P. R., and McCaslin, F. E., Jr.: Arthrodesis of the hip. Review of 371 cases, J. Bone Joint Surg. **43-A:**923, 1961.

Lloyd-Roberts, G. C.: Suppurative arthritis of infancy. Some observations upon prognosis and management, J. Bone Joint Surg. **42-B:**706, 1960.

Lloyd-Roberts, G. C., and Swan, M.: Pitfalls in the management of congenital dislocation of the hip, J. Bone Joint Surg. **48-B:**666, 1966.

Lorenz, A.: Ueber die Behandlung der irreponiblen angegorenen Hüftluxation und der Schenkelhalspseudarthrosen mittels Gabelung (Bifurkation des oberen Femurendes), Wien, Klin. Wochenschr. **32:**997, 1919.

Lorenz, A.: Die sogennannte angeborene Hüftverrenkung, Stuttgart, 1920, Verlag F. Enke.

Lowell, J. D., and Aufranc, O. E.: The anterior approach to the hip joint, Clin. Orthop. **61:**193, 1968.

Luck, J. V.: A transverse anterior approach to the hip, J. Bone Joint Surg. **37-A:**534, 1955.

Ludloff, K.: Zur blutigen Einrenkung der Angeborenen Huptluxation, Z. Orthop. Chir. **22:**272, 1908.

Lunceford, E. M., Jr.: Use of the Moore self-locking Vitallium prosthesis in acute fractures of the femoral neck, J. Bone Joint Surg. **47-A:**832, 1965.

MacEwen, G. D., and Shands, A. R., Jr.: Oblique trochanteric osteotomy, J. Bone Joint Surg. **49-A:**345, 1967.

MacKenzie, I. G., Seddon, H. J., and Trevor, D.: Congenital dislocation of the hip, J. Bone Joint Surg. **42-B:**689, 1960.

Massie, W. K.: Functional fixation of femoral neck fractures; telescoping nail technique, Clin. Orthop. **12:**230, 1959.

Massie, W. K.: Extra-capsular fractures of the hip treated by impaction using a sliding nail-plate fixation, Clin. Orthop. **22:**180, 1962.

Massie, W. K.: Fractures of the hip, J. Bone Joint Surg. **46-A:** 658, 1964.

Matchett, F.: A new long-stem intramedulary Vitallium hip prosthesis. Preliminary report, J. Bone Joint Surg. **47-A:**43, 1965.

Mayer, L.: The importance of early diagnosis in the treatment of slipping femoral epiphysis, J. Bone Joint Surg. **19:**1046, 1937.

Mayer, L.: Critique of Brittain operation for fusion of the hip, Bull. Hosp. Joint Dis. **9:**4, 1948.

McCarroll, H. R.: Primary anterior congenital dislocation of the hip, J. Bone Joint Surg. **30-A:**416, 1948.

McCarroll, H. R., and Crego, C. H., Jr.: Primary anterior congenital dislocation of the hip, J. Bone Joint Surg. **21:**648, 1939.

McDonough, J. M., Brandfass, W. T., and Stinchfield, F. E.: Idiopathic osteoarthritis of the hip. Comparison of the results of treatment by Austin Moore prosthesis and mold arthroplasty, J. Bone Joint Surg. **49-A:**625, 1967.

McElvenny, R. T.: The immediate treatment of intracapsular hip fracture, Clin. Orthop. **10:**289, 1957.

McFarland, B., and Osborne, G.: Approach to the hip. A suggested improvement of Kocher's method, J. Bone Joint Surg. **36-B:**364, 1954.

McKee, G. K.: Development in total hip replacement. In Proceedings of Institute of Mechanical Engineers, London, 1967, Institute of Mechanical Engineers.

McKee, G. K.: Development of total prosthetic replacement of the hip, Clin. Orthop. **72:**85, 1970.

McKee, G. K., and Watson-Farrar, J.: Replacement of arthritic hips by the McKee-Farrar prosthesis, J. Bone Joint Surg. **48-B:**245, 1966.

McMurray, T. P.: Osteoarthritis of the hip joint, Br. J. Surg. **22:**716, 1935.

McMurray, T. P.: Fracture of the neck of the femur treated by oblique osteotomy, Br. Med. J. **1:**330, 1938.

McMurray, T. P.: Osteoarthritis of the hip joint, J. Bone Joint Surg. **21:**1, 1939.

Medgyesi, S.: Healing of muscle-pedicle bone grafts. An experimental study, Acta Orthop. Scand. **35:**294, 1965.

Menelaus, M. B.: Dislocation and deformity of the hip in children with spina bifida cystica, J. Bone Joint Surg. **51-B:**238, 1969.

Mensor, M. C., and Scheck, M.: Review of six years experience with the hanging-hip operation, J. Bone Joint Surg. **50-A:**1250, 1968.

Metz, C. W., Jr., et al.: The displaced intracapsular fracture of the neck of the femur. Experience with the Deyerle Method of fixation in 63 cases, J. Bone Joint Surg. **52-A:**113, 1970.

Meyer, T. L., and Slager, R. F.: False aneurysm following subtrochanteric osteotomy, J. Bone Joint Surg. **46-A:**581, 1964.

Meyers, M. H., Telfer, N., and Moore, T. M.: Determination of the vascularity of the femoral head with Technetium 99m-sulphur-colloid. Diagnostic and prognostic significance, J. Bone Joint Surg. **59-A:**658, 1977.

Michele, A. A.: Iliopsoas, Springfield, Ill., 1962, Charles C Thomas, Publisher.

Milch, H.: The resection-angulation operation for hip joint disabilities, J. Bone Joint Surg. **37-A:**699, 1955.

Milch, H.: Surgical treatment of the stiff painful hip—the resection-angulation operation, Clin. Orthop. **31:**48, 1963.

Miller, J. A., Jr.: Joint paracentesis from an anatomic point of view. II. Hip, knee, ankle, and foot, Surgery **41:**999, 1957.

Moore, A. T.: Blade-plate internal fixation for intertrochanteric fractures, J. Bone Joint Surg. **16:**52, 1944.

Moore, A. T.: Hip joint fracture (a mechanical problem), American Academy of Orthopaedic Surgeons Instructional Course Lectures, vol. 10, Ann Arbor, Mich., 1953, J. W. Edwards, p. 35.

Moore, A. T.: The self-locking metal hip prosthesis, J. Bone Joint Surg. **39-A:**811, 1957.

Moore, A. T.: The Moore self-locking Vitallium prosthesis in fresh femoral neck fractures. A new low posterior approach (the southern exposure), American Academy of Orthopaedic Surgeons Instructional Course Lectures, vol. 16, St. Louis, 1959, The C. V. Mosby Co., p. 309.

Moore, A. T., and Lunceford, E. M.: The self-locking hip prosthesis in osteoarthritis of the hip and other conditions, Orthopedics **2:**155, 1960.

Moore, R. D.: Aseptic necrosis of the capital femoral epiphysis following adolescent epiphyseolysis, Surg. Gynecol. Obstet. **80:**199, 1945.

Morley, T. R., Short, M. D., and Dowsett, D. J.: Femoral head activity in Perthes' disease: clinical evaluation of a quantitative technique for estimating tracer uptake, J. Nucl. Med. **19:**884, 1978.

Mozan, L., and Thompson, R. G.: Treatment of the minimally slipped capital femoral epiphysis, J.A.M.A. **204:**674, 1968.

Mueller, K. H.: Osteotomies of the hip. Some technical considerations, Clin. Orthop. **77:**117, 1971.

Muller, M. E.: Total hip prostheses, Clin. Orthop. **72:**46, 1970.

Mulroy, R. D.: The iliopsoas muscle complex: iliacus muscle, psoas tendon release, Clin. Orthop. **38:**81, 1965.

Murray, W. R., Lucas, D. B., and Inman, V. T.: Femoral head and neck resection, J. Bone Joint Surg. **46-A:**1184, 1964.

Mustard, W. T.: Iliopsoas transfer for weakness of the hip abductors; preliminary report, J. Bone Joint Surg. **34-A:**647, 1952.

Mustard, W. T.: A follow-up study of iliopsoas transfer for hip instability, J. Bone Joint Surg. **41-B:**289, 1959.

Naiman, P. T., Schein, A. J., and Siffert, R. S.: Medical displacement fixation for severely comminuted intertrochanteric fractures, Clin. Orthop. **62:**151, 1969.

Neufeld, A. J., Janzen, J., and Taylor, G. M.: Internal fixation for intertrochanteric fractures, J. Bone Joint Surg. **26:**707, 1944.

Newman, P. H.: The surgical treatment of slipping of the upper femoral epiphysis, J. Bone Joint Surg. **42-B:**280, 1960.

Nicoll, E. A., and Holden, N.: Displacement osteotomy in treatment of osteoarthritis of the hip, J. Bone Joint Surg. **43-B:**50, 1961.

Nissen, K. I.: The arrest of primary osteoarthritis of the hip, J. Bone Joint Surg. **42-B:**423, 1960.

Nissen, K. I.: The rationale of early osteotomy for idiopathic coxarthrosis (epichondro-osteoarthrosis of the hip), Clin. Orthop. **77:**98, 1971.

Ober, F. R.: Posterior arthrotomy of the hip joint. Report of five cases, J.A.M.A. **83:**1500, 1924.

Ober, F. R.: An operation for relief of paralysis of the gluteus maximus muscle, J.A.M.A. **88:**1063, 1927.

Obletz, B. E.: Acute suppurative arthritis of the hip in the neonatal period, J. Bone Joint Surg. **42-A:**23, 1960.

Obletz, B. E.: Suppurative arthritis of the hip joint in infants, Clin. Orthop. **22:**27, 1962.

Obletz, B. E., Lockie, L. M., Milch, E., and Hyman, I.: Early effects of partial sensory denervation of the hip for relief of pain in chronic arthritis, J. Bone Joint Surg. **31-A:**805, 1949.

Oh, I., Calson, C. E., Tomford, W. W., and Harris, W. H.: Improved fixation of the femoral component after total hip replacement using a methacrylate intramedullary plug, J. Bone Joint Surg. **60-A:**608, 1978.

Olsson, S. S., Goldie, I. F., and Irstam, L. K. H.: Intertrochanteric osteotomy for osteoarthritis of the hip, J. Bone Joint Surg. **57-B:**466, 1975.

Ortolani, M.: La Lussazione congenita dell'anca, Bologna, 1948, Cappelli.

Ortolani, M.: Frühdiagnose und Frühbehandlung der angeborenen Hüftgelenksverrenkung, Kinderaerztl. Prax. **19:**404, 1951.

Ottolenghi, C. E., and Frigerio, E.: Intertrochanteric osteotomies in osteo-arthritis of the hip. Fundamentals, indications, techniques, and results, J. Bone Joint Surg. **44-A:**855, 1962.

Pack, G. T.: Major exarticulations for malignant neoplasms of the extremities: interscapulothoracic amputation, hip-joint disarticulation, and interilio-abdominal amputation. A report of end results in 228 cases, J. Bone Joint Surg. **38-A:**249, 1956.

Pack, G. T., and Ehrlich, H. E.: Exarticulation of the lower extremities for malignant tumors: hip-joint disarticulation (with and without deep iliac dissection) and sacroiliac disarticulation (hemipelvectomy), Ann. Surg. **123:**965, 1946.

Parr, P. L., Croft, C., and Enneking, W. F.: Resection of the head and neck of the femur with and without angulation osteotomy. A follow-up study of thirty-eight patients, J. Bone Joint Surg. **53-A:**935, 1971.

Parrish, T. F., and Jones, J. R.: Fracture of the femur following prosthetic arthroplasty of the hip. Report of nine cases, J. Bone Joint Surg. **46-A:**241, 1964.

Paterson, D. C.: Acute suppurative arthritis in infancy and childhood, J. Bone Joint Surg. **52-B:**474, 1970.

Patterson, R. J., Bickel, W. H., and Dahlin, D. C.: Idiopathic avascular necrosis of the head of the femur. A study of fifty-two cases, J. Bone Joint Surg. **46-A:**267, 1964.

Pauwels, F.: Grundsätzliches uber indikation und technik der "umlagerung" bei schenkelhalspseudarthrosen (Indications and technic of displacement osteotomy in pseudarthrosis of the neck of the femur), Langenbecks Arch. Klin. Chir. **262:**404, 1949.

Pauwels, F.: Des affections de la hanche d'origine mecanique et de leur traitement par l'osteotomie d'adduction (Mechanical disabilities of the hip and their treatment by adduction osteotomy), Rev. Chir. Orthop. **37:**22, 1951.

Pauwels, F.: Neue Richtlinien für die operative Behandlung der Koxarthrose, Verh. Dtsch. Orthop. Ges. **94:**332, 1961.

Pellicci, P. M., Salvati, E. A., and Robinson, H. J.: Mechanical failures in total hip replacement requiring reoperation, J. Bone Joint Surg. **61-A:**28, 1979.

Pemberton, P. A.: Pericapsular osteotomy of the ilium for treatment of congenital subluxation and dislocation of the hip, J. Bone Joint Surg. **47-A:**65, 1965.

Peterson, C. D., Miles, J. S., Solomons, C., Predecki, P. K., and Stephens, J. S.: Union between bone and implants of open pore ceramic and stainless steel. A histologic study (in proceedings of the Orthopaedic Research Society), J. Bone Joint Surg. **51-A:**805, 1969.

Peterson, L. T.: Tenotomy in the treatment of spastic paralysis with special reference to tenotomy of the iliopsoas, J. Bone Joint Surg. **32-A:**375, 1950.

Phelps, W. M.: Long-term results of orthopaedic surgery in cerebral palsy, J. Bone Joint Surg. **39-A:**53, 1957.

Platou, E.: Subtrochanteric osteotomy in relatively old congenital luxation of the hip, arthritis deformans and coxa vara, Acta Orthop. Scand. **9:**132, 1938.

Platou, E.: Open operation for congenital dislocation of the hip; results in 44 cases (50 hip joints), J. Bone Joint Surg. **32-B:**193, 1950.

Platou, E.: Rotation osteotomy in the treatment of congenital dislocation of the hip, J. Bone Joint Surg. **35-A:**48, 1953.

Poigenfurst, J., Marcove, R. C., and Miller, T. R.: Surgical treatment of fractures through metastases in the proximal femur, J. Bone Joint Surg. **50-B:**743, 1968.

Pomeranz, M. M.: Intrapelvic protrusion of the acetabulum (otto pelvis), J. Bone Joint Surg. **14:**663, 1932.

Ponseti, I. V.: Growth and development of the acetabulum in the normal child. Anatomical, histological and roentgenographic studies, J. Bone Joint Surg. **60-A:**575, 1978.

Ponseti, I. V.: Morphology of the acetabulum in congenital dislocation of the hip. Gross, histological, and roentgenographic studies, J. Bone Joint Surg. **60-A:**586, 1978.

Pugh, W. L.: A self-adjusting nail-plate for fractures about the hip joint, J. Bone Joint Surg. **37-A:**1085, 1955.

Putti, V.: Early treatment of congenital dislocation of the hip, J. Bone Joint Surg. **15:**16, 1933.

Ranawat, C. S., Jordan, L. R., and Wilson, P. D.: A technique of muscle-pedicle bone graft in hip arthrodesis. A report of its use in ten cases, J. Bone Joint Surg. **53-A:**925, 1971.

Rapp, G. F., Griffith, R. S., and Hebble, W. M.: The permeability of traumatically inflamed synovial membrane to commonly used antibiotics, J. Bone Joint Surg. **48-A:**1534, 1966.

Reich, R. S.: The selection of patients with hip fractures for prosthetic or other types of hip reconstruction (high osteotomy or bone graft or both), J. Bone Joint Surg. **48-A:**203, 1966.

Ring, P. A.: Treatment of trochanteric fractures of the femur, Br. Med. J. **5331:**654, 1963.

Ring, P. A.: Complete replacement arthroplasty of the hip by the Ring prosthesis, J. Bone Joint Surg. **50-B:**720, 1968.

Ring, P. A.: Total replacement of the hip, Clin. Orthop. **70:**161, 1970.

Ritter, M. A., and Vaughan, B. A.: Ectopic ossification after total hip arthroplasty. Predisposing factors, frequency, and effect on results, J. Bone Joint Surg. **59-A:**345, 1977.

Ritter, M. A., and Wilson, P. D., Jr.: Colonna capsular arthroplasty. A long-term follow-up of 40 hips, J. Bone Joint Surg. **50-A:**1305, 1968.

Roosth, H. P.: Flexion deformity of the hip and knee in spastic cerebral palsy: treatment by early release of spastic hip-flexor muscles. Technique and results in thirty-seven cases, J. Bone Joint Surg. **53-A:**1489, 1971.

Rosen, S. von: Early diagnosis and treatment of congenital dislocation of the hip joint, Acta Orthop. Scand. **26:**136, 1956.

Rosen, S. von: Diagnosis and treatment of congenital dislocation of the hip in the new-born, J. Bone Joint Surg. **44-B:**284, 1962.

Rosen, S. von: Further experience with congenital dislocation of the hip in the newborn, J. Bone Joint Surg. **50-B:**538, 1968.

Rubin, R., Salvati, E. A., and Lewis, R.: Infected total hip replacement after dental procedures, Oral Surg. **41:**18, 1976.

Russe, O. A.: Acute and chronic slipped femoral epiphysis, Clin. Orthop. **77:**144, 1971.

Ryder, C. T.: Congenital dislocation of the hip in the older child: surgical treatment, J. Bone Joint Surg. **48-A:**1404, 1966.

Salenius, P. A.: A new compression plate for the McMurray displacement hip osteotomy, J. Bone Joint Surg. **52-A:**382, 1970.

Salter, R. B.: Innominate osteotomy in the treatment of congenital dislocation and subluxation of the hip, J. Bone Joint Surg. **43-B:**518, 1961.

Salter, R. B.: Role of innominate osteotomy in the treatment of congenital dislocation and subluxation of the hip in the older child, J. Bone Joint Surg. **48-A:**1413, 1966.

Salter, R. B.: Textbook of disorders and injuries of the musculoskeletal system, Baltimore, 1970, The Williams & Wilkins Co.

Salvati, E. A., and Wilson, P. D., Jr.: Long-term results of femoral-head replacement, J. Bone Joint Surg. **55-A:**516, 1973.

Samilson, R. L., Bersani, F. A., and Watkins, M. B.: Acute suppurative arthritis in infants and children, J. Bone Joint Surg. **40-A:**978, 1958.

Samilson, R. L., Bersani, F. A., and Watkins, M. B.: Acute suppurative arthritis in infants and children. The importance of early diganosis and surgical drainage, Pediatrics **21:**798, 1958.

Sarmiento, A.: Intertrochanteric fractures of the femur. 150-degree-angle nail-plate fixation and early rehabilitation: a preliminary report of 100 cases, J. Bone Joint Surg. **45-A:**706, 1963.

Sarmiento, A., and Williams, E. M.: The unstable intertrochanteric fracture: treatment with a valgus osteotomy and I-beam nail-plate. A preliminary report of one hundred cases, J. Bone Joint Surg. **52-A:**1309, 1970.

Scaglietti, O., and Calandriello, B.: Open reduction of congenital dislocation of hip, J. Bone Joint Surg. **44-B:**257, 1962.

Schantz, A.: Ueber die nach schenkelhalsbrüchen zurückbleibenden Gehstörungen, Dtsch. Med. Wochenschr. **51:**730, 1925.

Scheck, M.: Management of fractures of the femoral neck, J. Bone Joint Surg. **47-A:**819, 1965.

Schwartzmann, J. R.: Reconstruction of the hip in rheumatoid arthritis, J. Bone Joint Surg. **49-A:**398, 1967.

Scott, P. J.: Non-union of oblique displacement intertrochanteric osteotomy for osteoarthritis of the hip, J. Bone Joint Surg. **49-B:**475, 1967.

Seinsheimer, F., III.: Subtrochanteric fractures of the femur, J. Bone Joint Surg. **60-A:**300, 1978.

Sharp, N., Guhl, J. F., Sorenson, R. I., and Voshell, A. F.: Hip fusion in poliomyelitis in children. A preliminary report, J. Bone Joint Surg. **46-A:**121, 1964.

Sharrard, W. J. W.: Congenital paralytic dislocation of the hip in children with myelo-meningocele, J. Bone Joint Surg. **41-B:**622, 1959.

Sharrard, W. J. W.: The mechanism of paralytic deformity in spina bifida, Dev. Med. Child Neurol. **4:**310, 1962.

Sharrard, W. J. W.: Posterior iliopsoas transplantation in the treatment of paralytic dislocation of the hip, J. Bone Joint Surg. **46-B:**426, 1964.

Sharrard, W. J. W.: Paralytic deformity in the lower limb, J. Bone Joint Surg. **49-B:**731, 1967.

Simon, W. H., and Wyman, E. T., Jr.: Femoral neck fractures. A study of the adequacy of reduction, Clin. Orthop. **70:**152, 1970.

Smith, D. M., Oliver, C. H., Ryder, C. T., and Stinchfield, F. E.: Complications of Austin Moore arthroplasty. Their incidence and relationship to potential predisposing factors, J. Bone Joint Surg. **57-A:**31, 1975.

Smith, F. G.: Effects of rotatory and valgus malpositions on blood supply to the femoral neck, J. Bone Joint Surg. **41-A:**800, 1959.

Smith, W. S.: Congenital dislocation of the hip in the older child: introduction, J. Bone Joint Surg. **48-A:**1390, 1966.

Smith, W. S., Coleman, C. R., Olix, M. L., and Slager, R. F.: Etiology of congenital dislocation of the hip, J. Bone Joint Surg. **45-A:**491, 1963.

Smith-Peterson, M. N.: A new supra-articular subperiosteal approach to the hip joint, Am. J. Orthop. Surg. **15:**592, 1917.

Smith-Petersen, M. N.: Arthroplasty of the hip. A new method, J. Bone Joint Surg. **21:**269, 1939.

Smith-Petersen, M. N.: Evolution of mould arthroplasty of the hip joint, J. Bone Joint Surg. **30-B:**59, 1948.

Smith-Petersen, M. N.: Approach to and exposure of the hip joint for mold arthroplasty, J. Bone Joint Surg. **31-A:**40, 1949.

Smith-Petersen, M. N., Cave, E. F., and Van Gorder, G. W.: Intracapsular fractures of the neck of the femur. Treatment by internal fixation, Arch. Surg. **23:**707, 1931.

Smith-Petersen, M. N., Larson, C. B., Aufranc, O. E., and Law, W. A.: Complications of old fractures of the neck of the femur: results of treatment by Vitallium-mold arthroplasty, J. Bone Joint Surg. **29:**41, 1947.

Somerville, E. W.: Flexion contractures of the knee, J. Bone Joint Surg. **42-B:**730, 1960.

Somerville, E. W., and Scott, J. C.: The direct approach to congenital dislocation of the hip, J. Bone Joint Surg. **39-B:**623, 1957.

Soto-Hall, R., Johnson, L. H., and Johnson, R. A.: Variations in the intra-articular pressure of the hip joint in injury and disease—a probable factor in avascular necrosis, J. Bone Joint Surg. **46-A:**509, 1964.

Soutter, R.: A new operation for hip contractures in poliomyelitis, Boston Med. Surg. J. **170:**380, 1914.

Speed, K.: Hip joint fusion, Surgery, **1:**740, 1937.

Stewart, M. J., and Coker, T. P., Jr.: Arthrodesis of the hip. A review of 109 patients, Clin. Orthop. **62:**136, 1969.

Stewart, M. J., and Milford, L. W.: Fracture dislocation of the hip: an end-result study, J. Bone Joint Surg. **36-A:**315, 1954.

Stinchfield, F. E.: Low-friction total hip replacement. Advantages and pitfalls, Clin. Orthop. **72:**36, 1970.

Stinchfield, F. E., and Carroll, R. E.: Vitallium-cup arthroplasty of the hip joint, J. Bone Joint Surg. **31-A:**628, 1949.

Stinchfield, F. E., and Cavallaro, W. U.: Arthrodesis of the hip joint. A follow-up study, J. Bone Joint Surg. **32-A:**48, 1950.

Stinchfield, F. E., and Chamberlin, A. C.: Arthroplasty of the hip, J. Bone Joint Surg. **48-A:**564, 1966.

Stinchfield, F. E., Cooperman, B., and Shea, C. E., Jr.: Replacement of the femoral head by Judet or Austin Moore prosthesis, J. Bone Joint Surg. **39-A:**1043, 1957.

Tachdjian, M. O., and Grana, L.: Response of the hip joint to increased intra-articular hydrostatic pressure, Clin. Orthop. **61:**199, 1968.

Taylor, G. M., Neufeld, A. J., and Janzen, J.: Internal fixation for intertrochanteric fractures, J. Bone Joint Surg. **26:**707, 1944.

Taylor, G. M., Neufeld, A. J., and Nickel, V. L.: Complications and failures in the operative treatment of intertrochanteric fractures of the femur, J. Bone Joint Surg. **37-A:**306, 1955.

Taylor, R. G.: Pseudarthrosis of the hip joint, J. Bone Joint Surg. **32-B:**174, 1950.

Thompson, F. R.: Vitallium intermedullary hip prosthesis: preliminary report, N. Y. J. Med. **52:**3011, 1952.

Thompson, F. R.: Two and a half years' experience with a vitallium intramedullary hip prosthesis, J. Bone Joint Surg. **36-A:**489, 1954.

Thompson, F. R.: Combined hip fusion and subtrochanteric osteotomy allowing early ambulation, J. Bone Joint Surg. **38-A:**13, 1956.

Thompson, F. R.: Prosthesis indications in fresh fractures and basic considerations affecting choice of a prosthesis. American Academy of Orthopaedic Surgeons Instructional Course Lectures, vol. 16, St. Louis, 1959, The C. V. Mosby Co.

Tobin, W. J.: The internal architecture of the femur and its clinical significance. The upper end, J. Bone Joint Surg. **37-A:** 57, 1955.

Trueta, J., and Harrison, M. H. M.: The normal vascular anatomy of the femoral head in adult man, J. Bone Joint Surg. **35-B:**442, 1953.

Trumble, H. C.: Fixation of the hip joint by means of an extra-articular bone graft. Late results, Br. J. Surg. **24:**728, 1937.

Urist, M. L.: The principles of hip-socket arthroplasty, J. Bone Joint Surg. **39-A:**786, 1957.

Van Gorder, G. W.: The Trumble operation for fusion of the hip, J. Bone Joint Surg. **31-A:**717, 1949.

Veleanu, C., Rosianu, I., and Ionescu, L.: An improved approach for obturator neurectomy for cerebral spastic paralysis, J. Bone Joint Surg. **52-A:**1693, 1970.

Venable, C. S., Stuck, W. G., and Beach, A.: Effects on bone of presence of metals; based upon electrolysis experimental study, Ann. Surg. **105:**917, 1937.

Vesely, D. G.: Ischiofemoral arthrodesis. An end-result study of forty-four cases, J. Bone Joint Surg. **43-A:**363, 1961.

Voss, C.: Koxarthrose—die "temorare Hängehüfte": Ein neues Verfahren zur operativen Behandlung der schmerzhaften Altershüfte und anderer chronischer deformierender Huftgelenkserkrankungen, Münch. Med. Wochenschr. **98:**954, 1956.

Voss, C.: "Die temorare Hangehufte." Ein neues Verfahren zur operativen Behandlung der Koxarthrose und anderer deformierender Huftgelenkserkrankungen, Verh. Dtsch. Orthop. Ges. **23:**351, 1965.

Wagner, H.: Surface replacement arthroplasty of the hip, Clin. Orthop. **134:**102, 1978.

Watson-Jones, R.: Fractures of the neck of the femur, Br. J. Surg. **23:**787, 1935-1936.

Watson-Jones, R.: Arthrodesis of the osteoarthritic hip, J.A.M.A. **110:**278, 1938.

Watson-Jones, R., and Robinson, W. C.: Arthrodesis of the osteoarthritic hip joint, J. Bone Joint Surg. **38-B:**353, 1956.

Weber, B. G.: Total hip replacement with rotation-endoprosthesis (trunnion-bearing prosthesis), Clin. Orthop. **72:**79, 1970.

Weissman, S. L., and Salama, R.: Trochanteric fractures of the femur. Treatment with a strong nail and early weight-bearing, Clin. Orthop. **67:**143, 1969.

Welsh, R. P., Pilliar, R. M., and Macnab, I.: Surgical implants. The role of surface porosity in fixation to bone and acrylic, J. Bone Joint Surg. **53-A:**963, 1971.

Whitman, R.: Reconstruction operation for ununited fracture of the neck of the femur, Surg. Gynecol. Obstet. **32:**479, 1921.

Whitman, R.: The abduction treatment of fracture of the neck of the femur: An account of the evaluation of a method adequate to apply surgical principles and therefore the exponent of radical reform of conventional teaching and practice, Ann. Surg. **81:**374, 1925.

Whittaker, R. P., Sotos, L. N., and Ralston, E. L.: Fractures of the femur about femoral endoprosthesis, J. Trauma **14:** 675, 1974.

Wiberg, G.: Studies on dysplastic acetabula and congenital subluxation of the hip joint, Acta Chir. Scand. (Suppl.) **83:** 58, 1939.

Wiberg, G.: Shelf operation in congenital dysplasia of the acetabulum and in subluxation and dislocation of the hip, J. Bone Joint Surg. **35-A:**65, 1953.

Wiesman, H. J., Jr., et al.: Total hip replacement with and without osteotomy of the greater trochanter. Clinical and biomedical comparisons in the same patient, J. Bone Joint Surg. **60-A:**203, 1978.

Wiles, P.: The surgery of the osteo-arthritic hip, Br. J. Surg. **45:**488, 1958.

Wilson, P. D.: Trochanteric arthroplasty for fractures of the femur, J. Bone Joint Surg. **29:**313, 1947.

Wilson, P. D., Jacobs, B., and Schecter, L.: Slipped capital femoral epiphysis. An end-result study, J. Bone Joint Surg. **47-A:** 1128, 1965.

Wilson, P. D., and Osgood, R. B.: Reconstructive surgery in chronic arthritis, N. Engl. J. Med. **209:**117, 1933.

Yount, C. C.: The role of the tensor fasciae femoris in certain deformities of the lower extremities, J. Bone Joint Surg. **8:** 171, 1926.

Zickel, R. E.: An intramedullary fixation device for the proximal part of the femur. Nine years experience, J. Bone Joint Surg. **58-A:**866, 1976.

Zickel, R. E., and Mouradian, W. H.: Intramedullary fixation of pathological fractures and lesions of the subtrochanteric region of the femur, J. Bone Joint Surg. **58-A:**1061, 1976.

11
THIGH

OPEN REDUCTION AND INTERNAL FIXATION FOR FEMORAL SHAFT FRACTURE (Plate 11-1)

GENERAL DISCUSSION. Intramedullary fixation for fractures of the femoral shaft in adult patients can offer great advantages under the right conditions. It is possible for internal fixation to be strong and rigid and sufficient to eliminate the need for external plaster immobilization, splints, or braces. Early weight bearing and early mobilization of adjacent joints can shorten hospitalization and convalescence and decrease the amount of total disability. Early mobilization is perhaps the greatest advantage, although this is true only for selected fractures that are properly stabilized.

However, intramedullary fixation is by no means suitable for all fractures of the shaft of the femur. The fracture should be at least 5 cm distal to the lesser trochanter and at least 17 cm proximal to the adductor tubercle. A fracture involving the proximal portion of the middle third of the femur through the isthmus of the medullary canal is the most suitable location. Intramedullary fixation should not be used for fractures of the femoral shaft in children or adolescents who can be managed well with closed treatment methods.

Segmental or multiple fractures of the femoral shaft, if within the acceptable location, can be adequately secured by use of an intramedullary nail. Intramedullary nailing can be a satisfactory procedure in the treatment of malunion, nonunion, and for many pathologic fractures of the femur. The best candidate for the procedure is a young adult patient with a recent (within 2 weeks) transverse fracture through or near the isthmus of the medullary canal, only mild or moderate soft tissue damage, otherwise normal bone, and no other significant injuries.

There is a choice between the cloverleaf design (Küntscher) and the diamond-shaped nail (Hansen-Street). Both of these femoral intramedullary nails can provide secure internal fixation. The cloverleaf nail is slightly compressible and can be doubly stacked if necessary. The proper length of the nail should be determined preoperatively by roentgenograms. A nail of known length is strapped or taped to the lateral side of the normal thigh. An anteroposterior roentgenogram is obtained to determine the relationship of the nail to the knee and the hip. The intramedullary nail that is used should be long enough to extend from a level 1 to 2 cm proximal to the superior aspect of the femoral neck to the level of the adductor tubercle of the femur.

Intramedullary fixation of the femur should not be undertaken lightly. If the femur is exposed for intramedullary nailing (or for any other method of internal fixation), complications, including surgical shock, pulmonary and fat embolism, and infection, are an ever present possibility. Open reduction of a fracture of the femoral shaft is not advisable as an emergency procedure unless necessary in association with emergency repair of a major artery. If intramedullary fixation of a femoral shaft fracture must be postponed for a week or more, the femoral shaft fracture shoud be treated initially with traction to maintain length and alignment (preferably without skeletal traction).

Preparation and draping for intramedullary nailing of a femoral shaft fracture must be done with extreme care, and the procedure should be carried out expeditiously with careful preoperative planning, since the average rate of infection after open reductions of femoral shaft fractures exceeds that for open reductions of other long bones. Blood for transfusion must be available at the time of surgery. Inserting an intramedullary nail blindly into the femur without exposing the fracture is dangerous unless an image intensifier is used.

DETAILS OF PROCEDURE. The fracture of the femoral shaft should be exposed through a lateral or posterolateral incision **(A)**. If a posterolateral incision, which minimizes damage to the quadriceps, is used, the intermuscular septum is followed to the bone and the vastus lateralis and vastus intermedius muscles are retracted anteriorly. After the fracture is exposed, the fracture fragments are mobilized and the fracture is reduced with specific attention to anatomic rotational alignment.

The distal fragment of the femur should be checked in regard to the size of the medullary canal to be sure it will receive the selected nail. The medullary canal of the distal quarter of the femoral shaft is large; so there is no need to have the intramedullary reamer go past the point of definite resistance. The same procedure should be followed in the proximal fragment.

At this time the guide pin should be introduced into the medullary canal of the proximal fragment and drilled through the bone until it is in a subcutaneous position. As this is done, the hip should be adducted and slightly flexed so the guide pin will emerge in the lateral and distal region of the buttock **(B)**.

A small incision is made over the protruding point of the guide pin. The soft tissues are separated to permit introduction of the cannulated trochanteric reamer over the guide pin, and the drill is turned slowly untl the reamer is well seated with one or more of its cutting edges entering the intramedullary space of the proximal femur. After this hole is drilled, the medullary nail that has been selected is introduced over the guide pin with the eye of the Küntscher (or cloverleaf) nail facing posteromedially. The nail is driven into the trochanteric region and proximal portion of the femur **(C and D)**. The guide pin is then withdrawn from the medullary space of the femur **(D)**. The cloverleaf type of nail is compressible, and if the intramedullary space is narrow, the nail potentially can clamp down on the guide pin and make the removal of either a difficult task.

(Plate 11-1) OPEN REDUCTION AND INTERNAL FIXATION FOR FEMORAL SHAFT FRACTURE

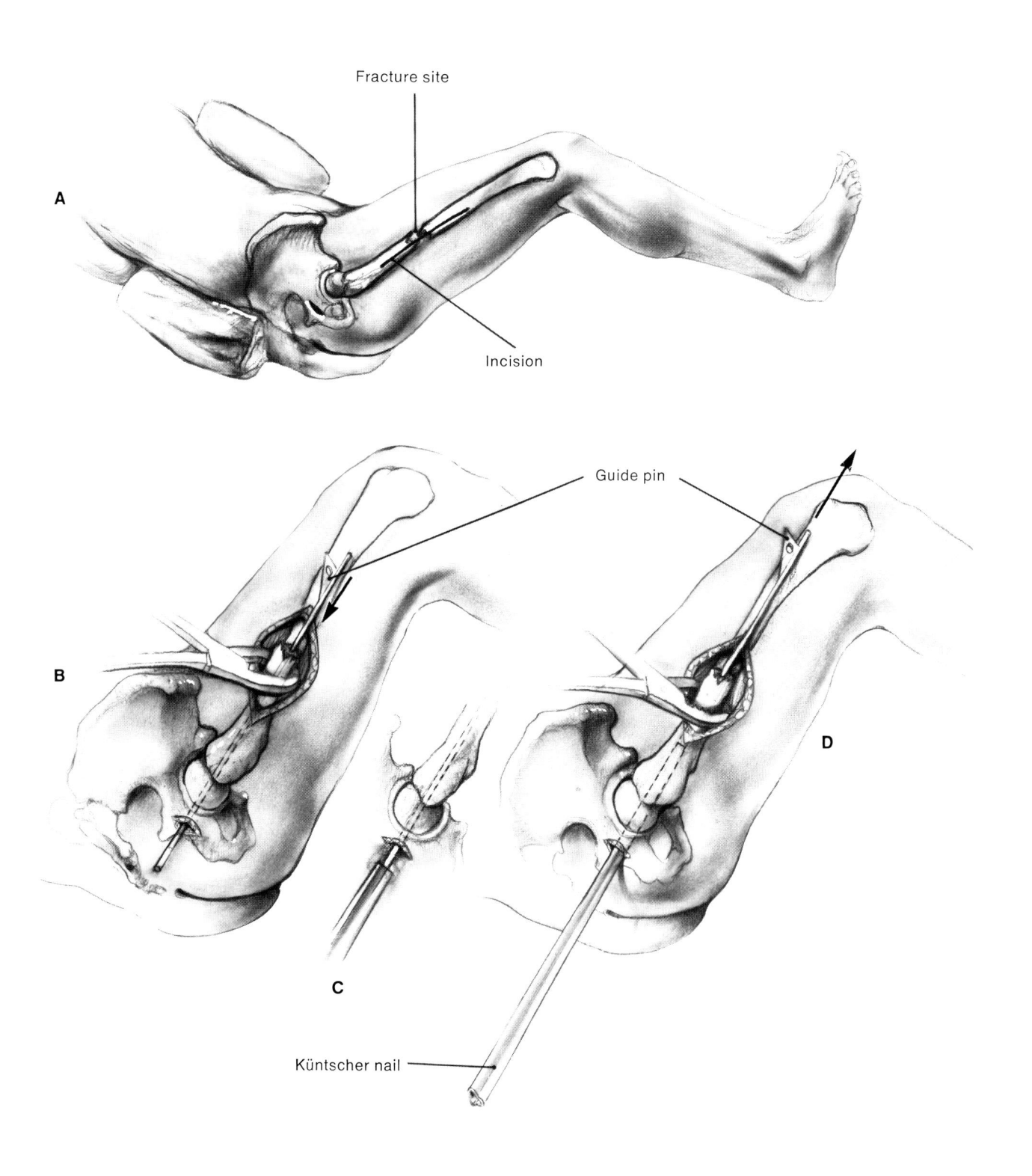

A

Fracture site

Incision

B

Guide pin

C

D

Küntscher nail

381

OPEN REDUCTION AND INTERNAL FIXATION FOR FEMORAL SHAFT FRACTURE (Plate 11-1)

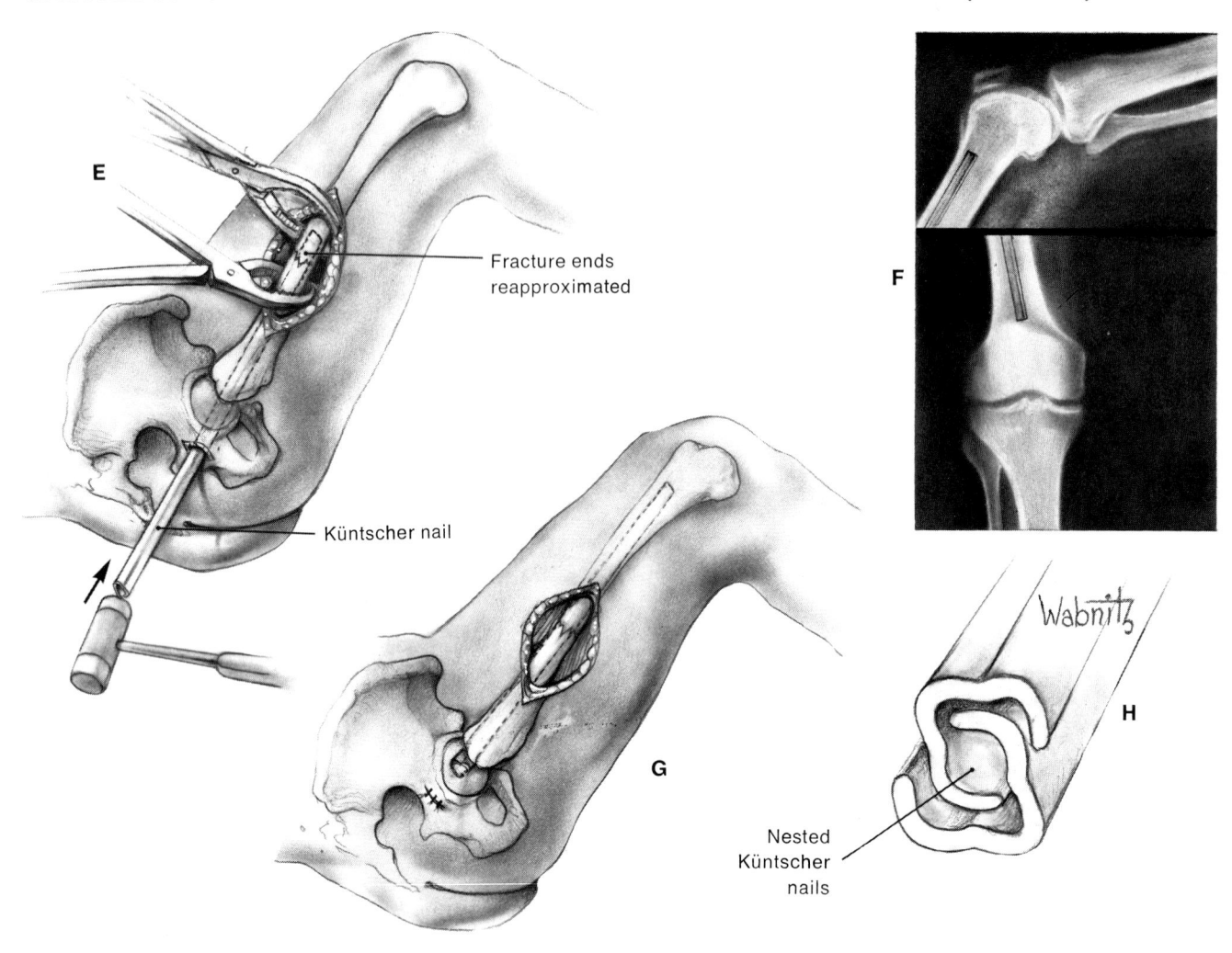

After the cloverleaf nail is driven farther into the proximal fragment to emerge at the fracture site, the fracture is reduced anatomically under direct vision. The distal fragment must be in proper alignment or the intramedullary nail may splinter the distal portion of the femur, impinge on the cortex, distract the fracture, or cut through the cortex when the nail is driven into the distal fragment. The reduction of the fracture should be maintained carefully while an assistant drives the nail across the fracture site into the distal fragment (**E**). Since the femur tends to bow anterolaterally, manual pressure should be exerted to avoid exaggeration of this as the nail is driven into the distal fragment. If undue resistance is encountered while driving the nail into the distal fragment, the situation should be checked immediately before it becomes complicated. If reamers have been used properly in both proximal and distal portions of the femoral shaft, the possibility of incarceration of the cloverleaf nail is unlikely in the young individual. However, in some pathologic conditions and in elderly patients, the normal anterolateral curve is sometimes considerably increased, and the orthopaedic surgeon may be faced with the problem of inserting a straight intramedullary nail down a curved canal. In these instances the distal end of the nail, when seated as far distally as possible, will lie close to the anterolateral cortex of the femur and should not be driven farther to the point where it might perforate the bone and enter the suprapatellar pouch (a complication that should be avoided).

When the cloverleaf nail is properly seated, the open portion faces posteromedially and its end does not protrude more than 2 cm proximal to the greater trochanter (**F** and **G**). The distal end of the nail should extend to the level of the adductor tubercle of the femur. The position of the fracture and the intramedullary nail should be checked roentgenographically with anteroposterior and lateral roentgenograms before final closure of the wounds. Also, the stability of the fracture should be evaluated in the open wound. If the stability of the fracture is unsatisfactory and the length of the nail is correct, the alternatives include replacement of the nail by a larger one, insertion of an additional nail (that is, stacking of two nails) to fill the intramedullary canal (**H**).

(Plate 11-1) OPEN REDUCTION AND INTERNAL FIXATION FOR FEMORAL SHAFT FRACTURE

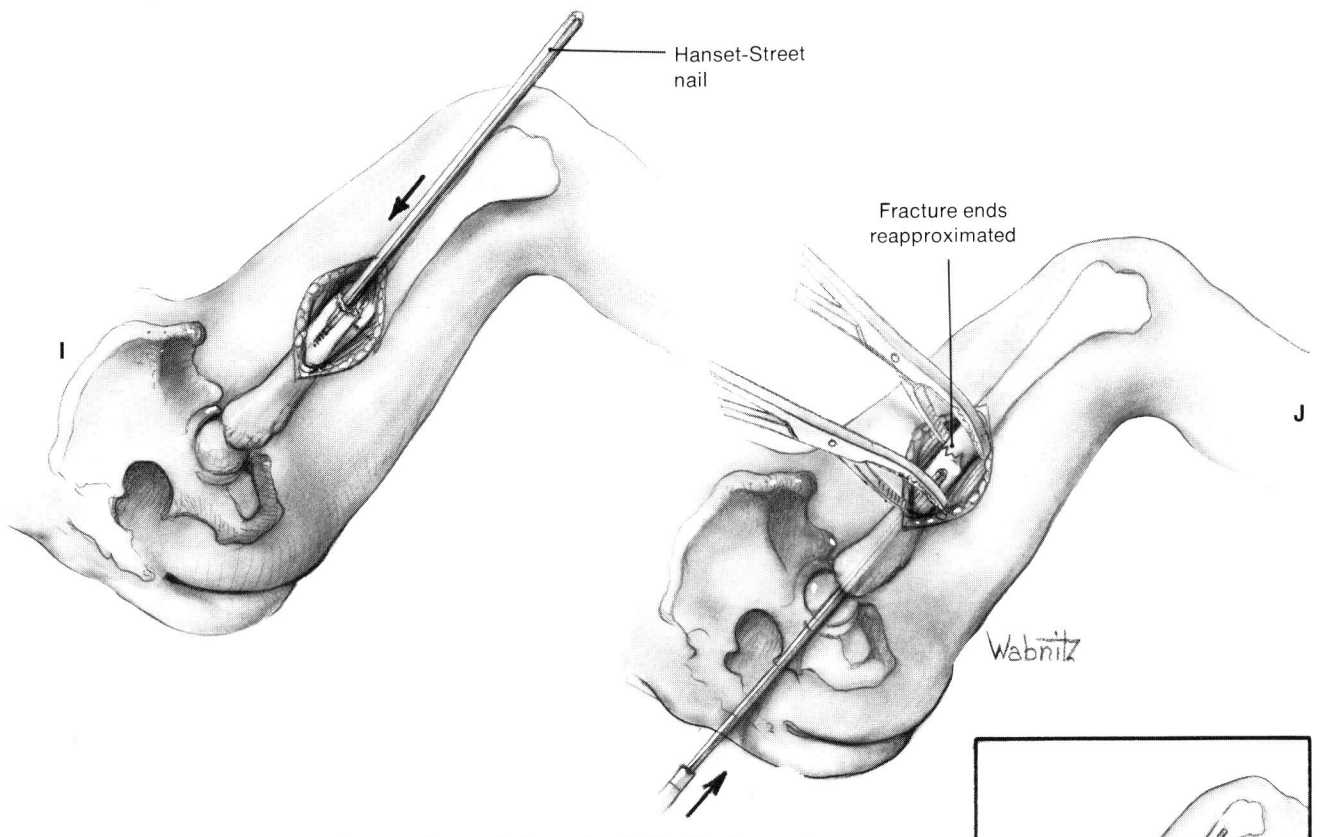

An alternative technique employs a diamond-shaped nail. Positioning and exposure of the fracture are the same as with the cloverleaf nail. The end of the nail with the threaded pointed stud is driven retrograde (**I**) through the proximal femoral fragment until it can be presented through the skin above the greater trochanter. An extractor-driver is screwed on the threaded stud. The fracture is reduced (**J**), and the nail is driven distally until it is seated (**K** and **L**).

POSTOPERATIVE MANAGEMENT. The patient's leg is supported in balanced suspension for 7 to 10 days postoperatively. Quadriceps- and hamstring-setting exercises should be practiced regularly as soon as wound discomfort subsides. These muscle exercises maintain muscle tone and strength, compress the fracture fragments while preventing distraction, and help to stimulate fracture callus and ultimate fracture union.

If the internal fixation has been secure, the patient should be ambulatory 3 to 4 weeks postoperatively. At first, the patient should walk with crutches keeping the knee in extension. Partial and increasing weight bearing may be necessary over a period of several months. During this time, treatment should be directed toward regaining muscle strength, improved hip and knee motion, and improved gait while walking with crutches. Even in younger patients with a stable fracture at an optimum level, full weight bearing without crutches is seldom possible before the third month postoperatively.

In some patients, following intramedullary internal fixation for femoral shaft fractures, there may be a massive and unusual appearance of callus formation roentgenographically. One should not be misled by this and assume that union of the fracture is secure at, for example, 4 or 6 weeks postoperatively. It is only the bridging fracture callus in the area between the fracture fragments that enters into stable union of the fragments, and the exuberant peripheral callus will usually disappear subsequently. The intramedullary nail should not be removed until the area between the fracture fragments is completely obliterated with good fracture callus; otherwise, refracture from minimal trauma is distinctly possible. The intramedullary nail should not be removed less than 1 year postoperatively.

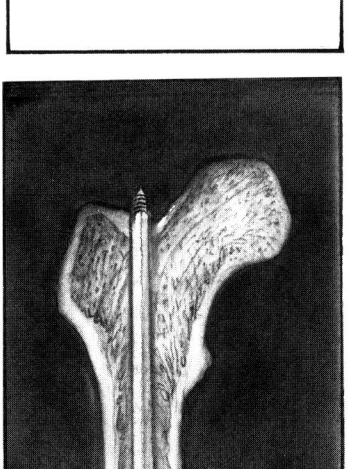

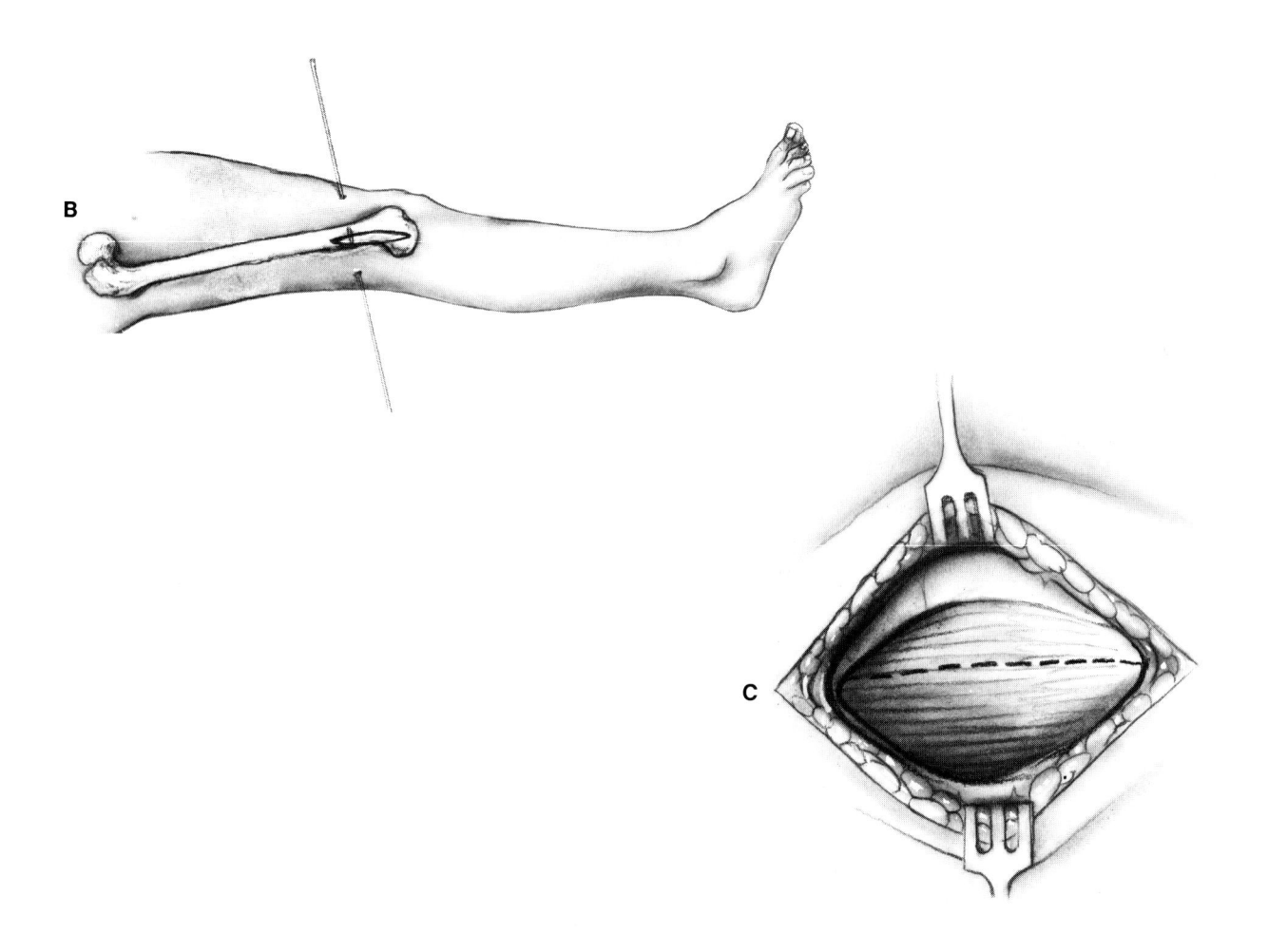

SUPRACONDYLAR DEROTATION OSTEOTOMY (McCARROLL) (Plate 11-2)

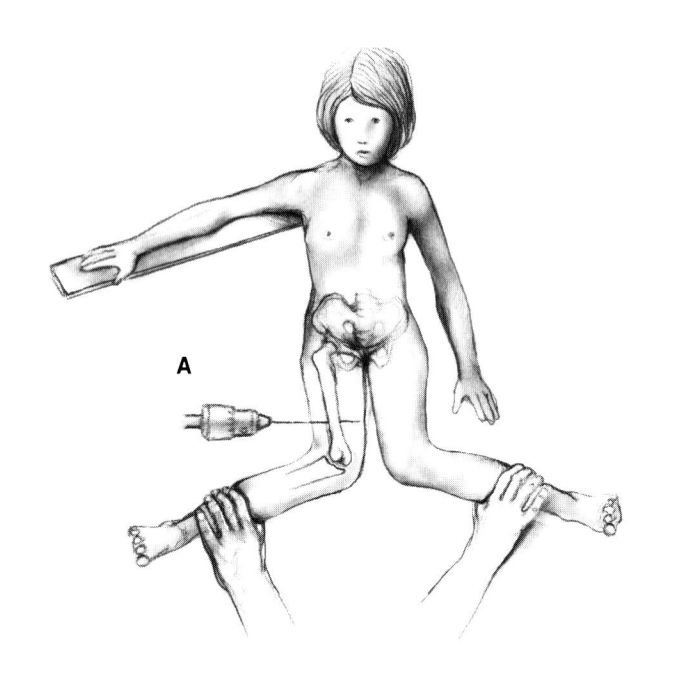

GENERAL DISCUSSION. Derotation osteotomy of the femur is performed to overcome increased anteversion of the femoral neck and may be indicated as part of the treatment for congenital dislocation of the hip. The derotation osteotomy may be carried out in the subtrochanteric region of the femur or in the supracondylar area of the femur, as recommended by McCarroll.

DETAILS OF PROCEDURE. If the child is in a plaster hip spica holding the involved leg in internal rotation to maintain reduction of a congenitally dislocated hip, the child is anesthetized and the cast is removed. An assistant holds the affected leg in internal rotation continually while the child is prepared and draped for surgery. With the leg in internal rotation at the hip, a heavy Kirschner wire is drilled transversely through the distal femur 7 to 8 cm proximal to the distal femoral epiphysis and parallel with the floor (A). A lateral longitudinal incision is then made over the femur just distal to Kirschner wire (B). The fibers of the vastus lateralis muscle are separated (C).

(Plate 11-2) SUPRACONDYLAR DEROTATION OSTEOTOMY (McCARROLL)

The femur is exposed subperiosteally, and a transverse supracondylar osteotomy is carried out by making multiple drill holes and dividing the femur with an osteotome **(D)**. While the proximal fragment is retained in internal rotation with the Kirschner wire parallel to the floor, the distal fragment is rotated externally until the knee, ankle, and foot are positioned normally in alignment with the anterosuperior iliac spine. The wound is closed **(E)** and a spica cast is applied **(F)**, incorporating the Kirschner wire and proximal femur in the same position and with the distal femur and leg externally rotated so the knee, lower leg, and foot are in normal position in relation to the child's body.

POSTOPERATIVE MANAGEMENT. The Kirschner wire is removed through windows in the cast 4 to 5 weeks postoperatively. The spica cast is removed 2 months after surgery and the child is allowed to use the limb without any further external splinting. There should be full active motion of the hip and knee within a few weeks following removal of the cast.

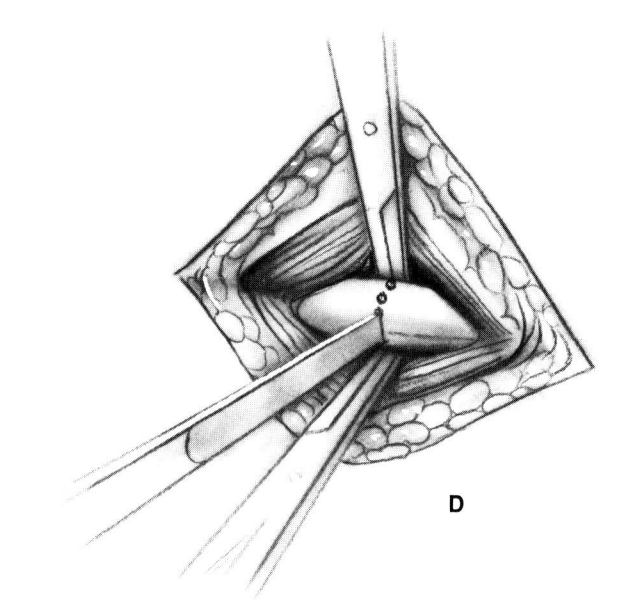

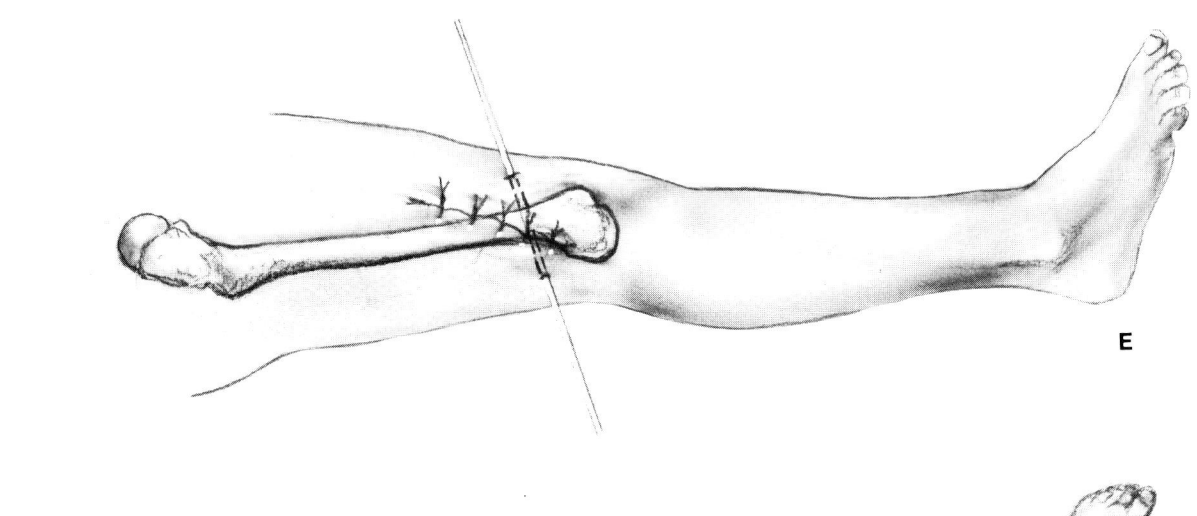

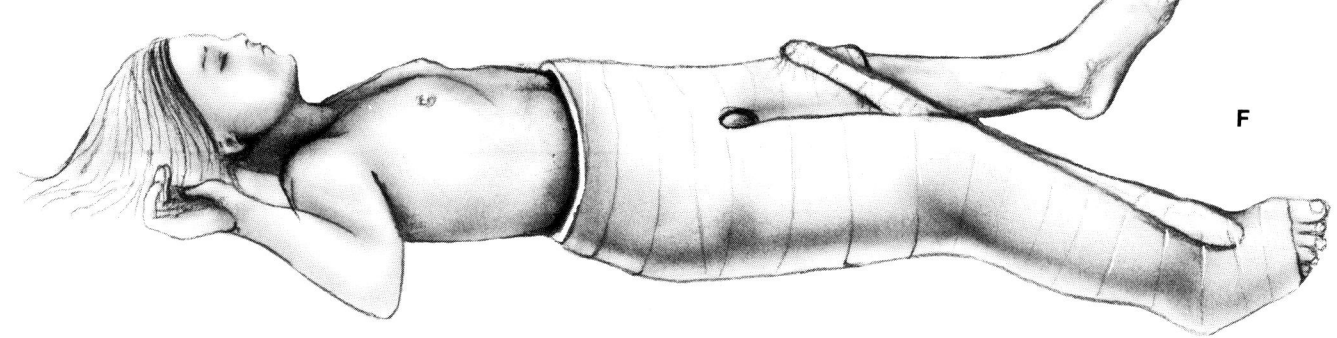

385

QUADRICEPSPLASTY (Plate 11-3)

GENERAL DISCUSSION. Quadricepsplasty can be a useful procedure to correct an extra-articular ankylosis of the knee in extension **(A)** following fractures of the femur. It can also be useful after extensive soft tissue wounds of the anterior aspect of the thigh when the underlying cause of the limited knee flexion is adherence of the vastus intermedius to the femur in the area of the suprapatellar pouch and proximally.

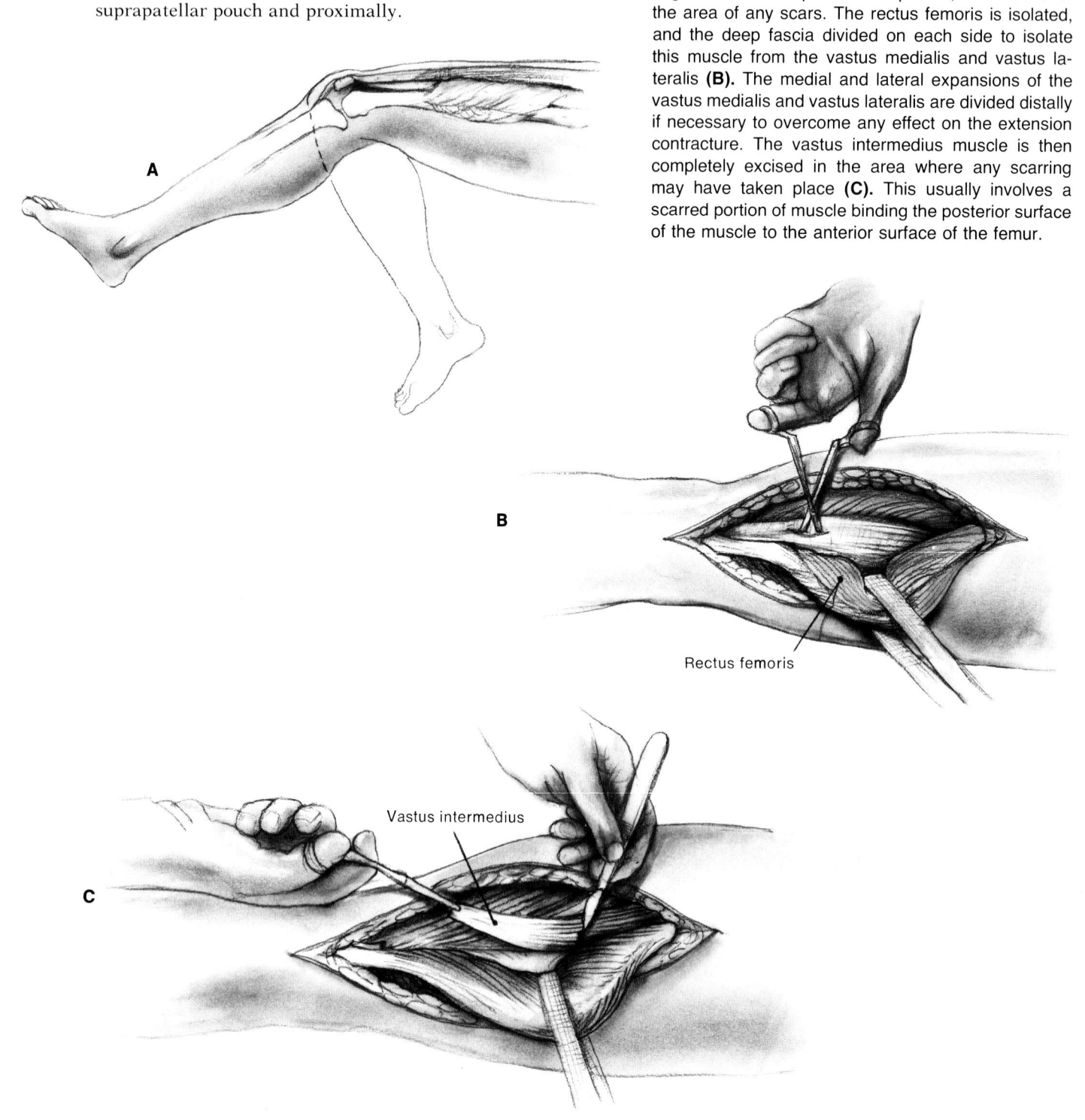

DETAILS OF PROCEDURE. Hemostasis is specifically important in this procedure, and electrocautery or a "vein eraser" should be used throughout the procedure. An S-shaped anterior longitudinal incision is made through the skin, subcutaneous tissue, and the superficial fascia from the proximal third of the thigh to the distal pole of the patella, centered over the area of any scars. The rectus femoris is isolated, and the deep fascia divided on each side to isolate this muscle from the vastus medialis and vastus lateralis **(B)**. The medial and lateral expansions of the vastus medialis and vastus lateralis are divided distally if necessary to overcome any effect on the extension contracture. The vastus intermedius muscle is then completely excised in the area where any scarring may have taken place **(C)**. This usually involves a scarred portion of muscle binding the posterior surface of the muscle to the anterior surface of the femur.

386

(Plate 11-3) QUADRICEPSPLASTY

At this point, the knees should be flexed slowly to at least 110° flexion to release any intra-articular adhesions **(D)**. Subcutaneous fat and/or superficial fascia is interposed between the femur and rectus femoris as much as possible. If a pneumatic trouniquet has been used, this should be removed at this time to obtain complete hemostasis before completion of wound closure **(E)**. The leg is placed in balanced suspension following wound closure.

POSTOPERATIVE MANAGEMENT. Balanced suspension is continued for 3 weeks postoperatively. Active and passive exercises of the knee are instituted in the first few days following surgery and are encouraged regularly and progressively thereafter until a satisfactory range of active motion against resistance has been obtained.

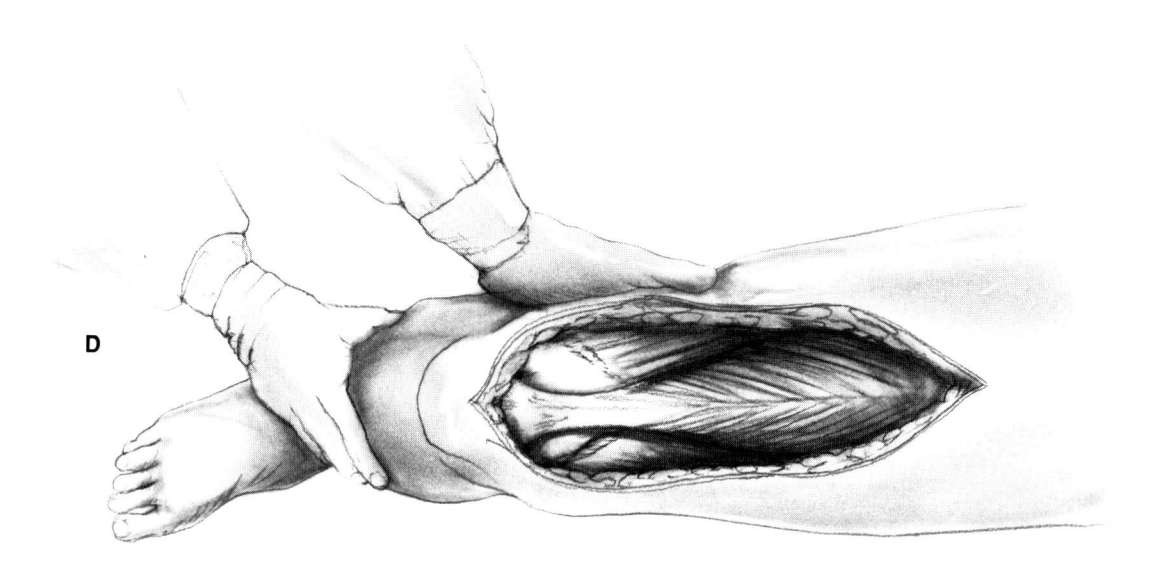

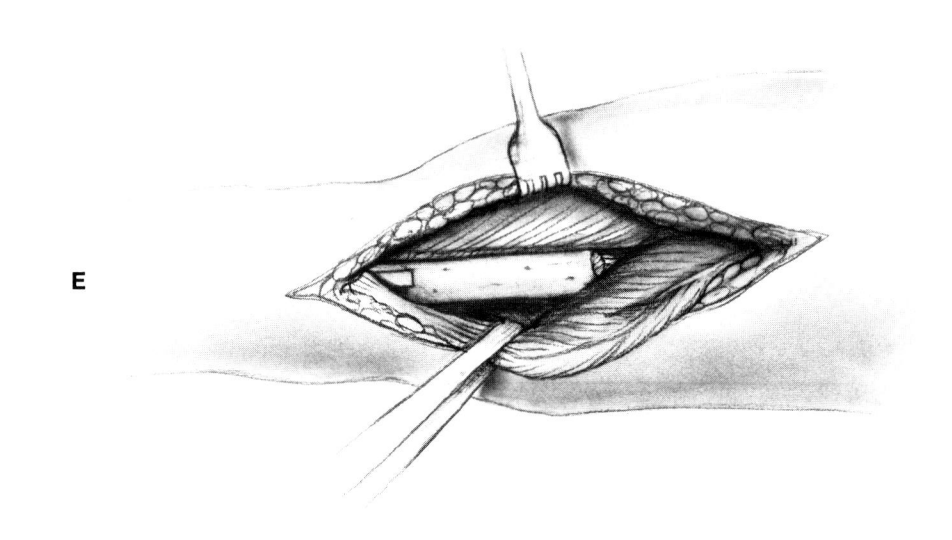

QUADRICEPS LENGTHENING (Plate 11-4)

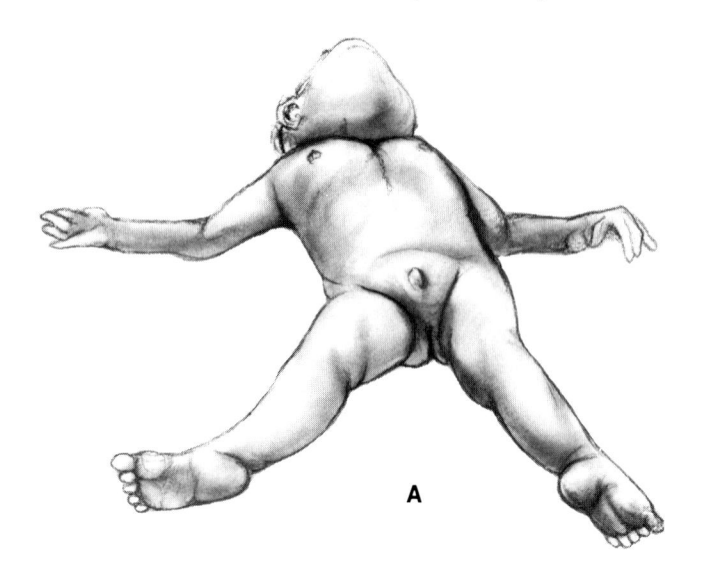

GENERAL DISCUSSION. Quadriceps lengthening may be indicated whenever there is a significant contracture of the quadriceps muscles that does not respond to conservative measures. Such resistant contractures may be encountered in children with myoplasia congenita or congenital hyperextension of the knee **(A)**.

Among children with congenital hyperextension of the knee, there is likely to be fibrous replacement of the quadriceps and lateral placement of the patella. Among these children, anterior capsulotomy and mobilization of the collateral ligaments may be necessary in addition to quadriceps lengthening to correct the fixed extension knee deformity.

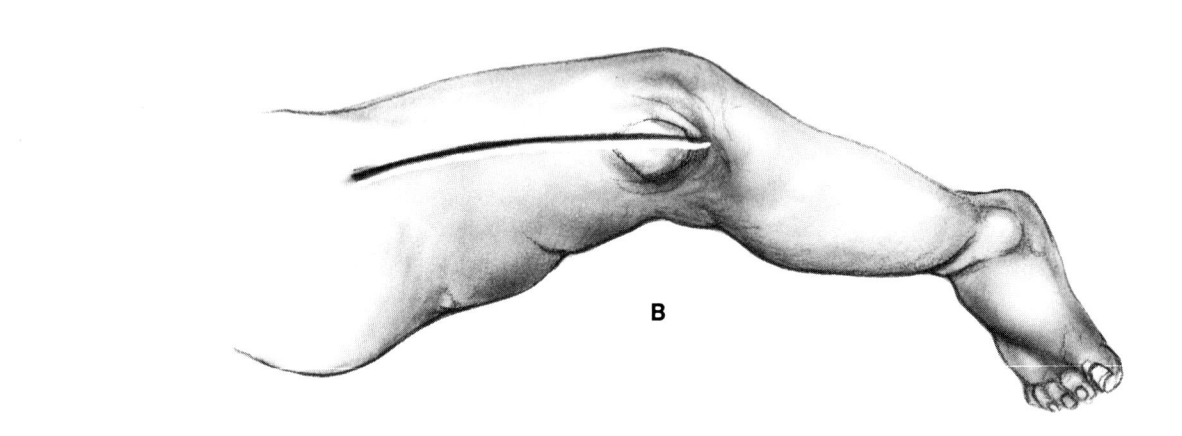

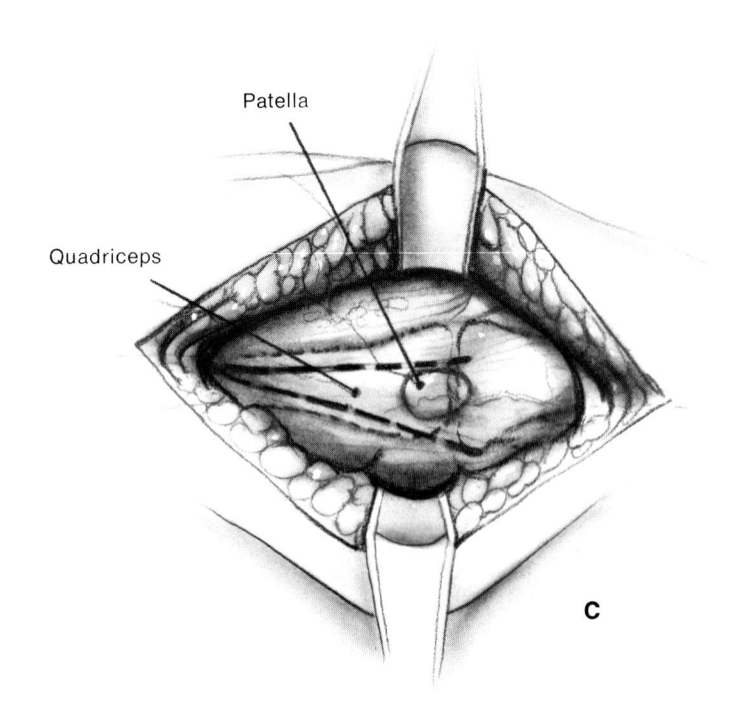

DETAILS OF PROCEDURE. A long anterior incision is made beginning over the medial aspect of the proximal thigh and extending toward the lateral aspect of the distal thigh and knee **(B)**. The incision may need to extend from the level of the lesser trochanter to the tibial tuberosity to obtain sufficient exposure for mobilization and lengthening of the quadriceps. Following exposure of the anterior thigh muscles, the quadriceps mechanism is divided by making an inverted-V incision superior to the patella **(C)**.

(Plate 11-4) QUADRICEPS LENGTHENING

This provides a tongue of tissue superior to the patella that can be attached to any suitable proximal muscle tissue after lengthening the quadriceps **(D)**. The anterior capsule of the knee joint is divided transversely as far posteriorly as the medial and lateral collateral ligaments. Each collateral ligament is then mobilized so each can be displaced posteriorly as the knee is flexed. At this point, the knee is passively flexed **(E)** and, if necessary (an it usually is not), any restricting tightness of the iliotibial band or either collateral ligament is released. It should be possible to flex the knee beyond 90°. The inverted-V tongue of distal quadriceps is sutured to the remaining portion of the quadriceps mechanism on the anteromedial aspect of the thigh **(F)** with the knee in 90° flexion. Following wound closure, the leg is immobilized in a long leg cast holding the knee in normal anteroposterior alignment and 30° flexion.

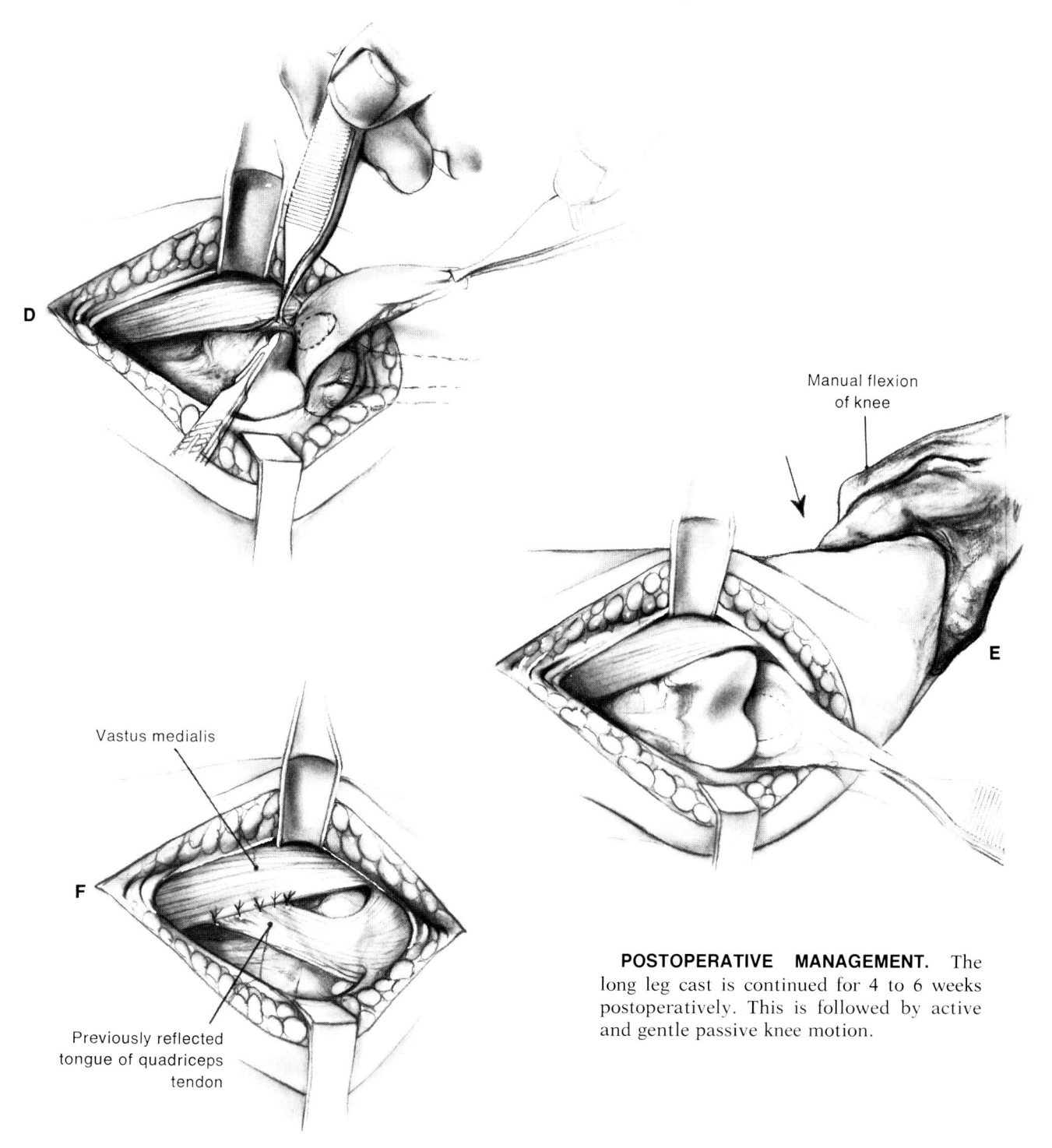

POSTOPERATIVE MANAGEMENT. The long leg cast is continued for 4 to 6 weeks postoperatively. This is followed by active and gentle passive knee motion.

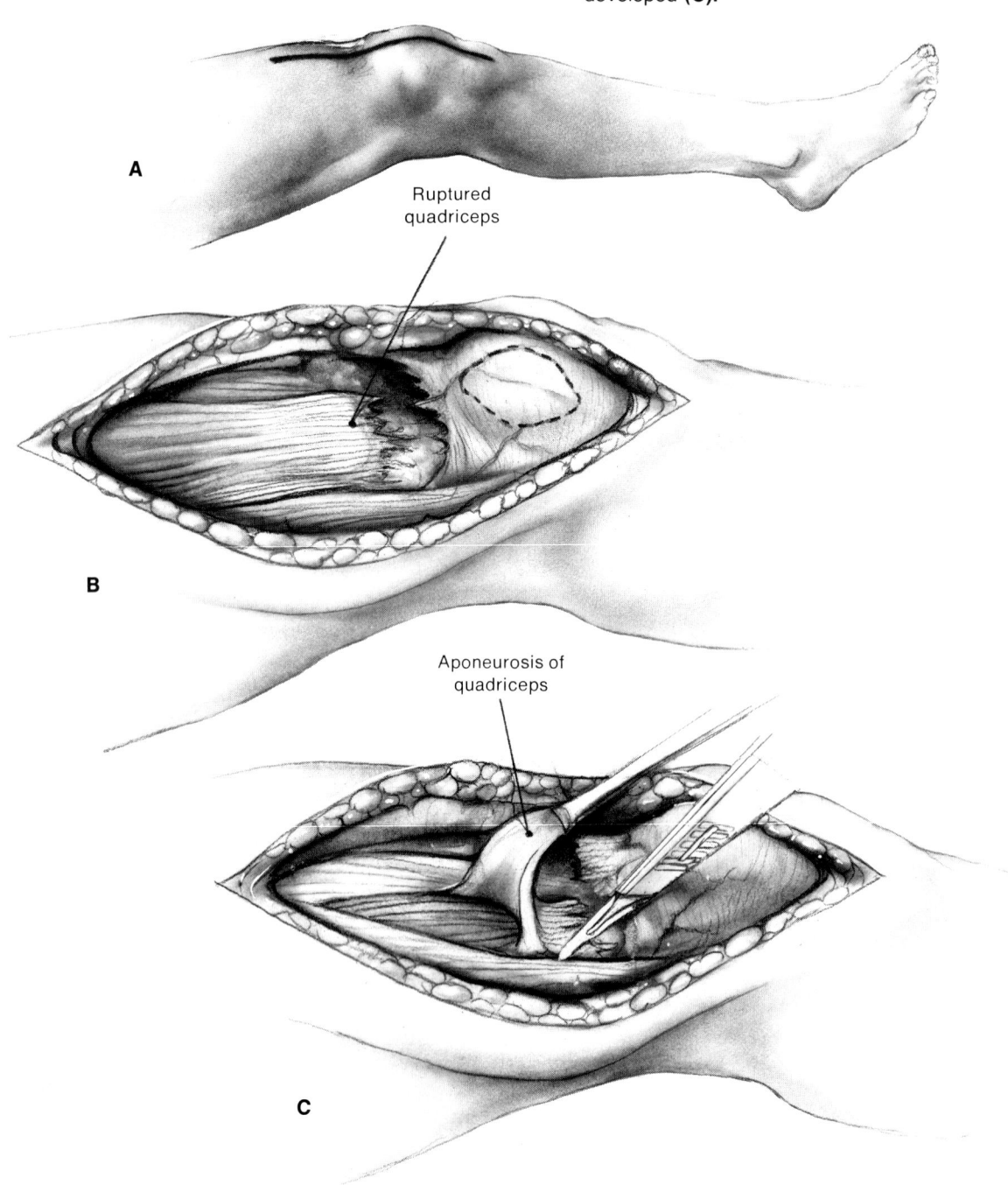

REPAIR OF RUPTURE OF QUADRICEPS TENDON (Plate 11-5)

GENERAL DISCUSSION. When rupture of the tendon of the quadriceps is encountered, this usually occurs transversely at a level just proximal to the patella. The best results will follow operative repair that is carried out within the first few days following injury. Since the rupture frequently occurs through an area of degeneration, some means of reinforcement for the direct end-to-end suture is desirable, for example, turning down a triangular flap of aponeurosis from the proximal portion of the tendon as recommended by Scuderi.

DETAILS OF PROCEDURE. An incision approximately 20 cm in length is made over the anterior aspect of the distal thigh to expose the rupture of the quadriceps femoris (**A** and **B**). The hematoma is evacuated and, with the knee in extension, the ruptured ends of the quadriceps tendon are approximated by moving the proximal portion of the quadriceps mechanism distally. From the anterior aspect of the proximal portion of the quadriceps, a triangular flap of quadriceps aponeurosis, 2 to 3 mm in thickness, approximately 5 cm wide at its base, and 7 to 8 cm long on each side is developed **(C)**.

(Plate 11-5) REPAIR OF RUPTURE OF QUADRICEPS TENDON

Any necrotic or frayed ends of the quadriceps tissue are debrided and the ends are sutured directly with figure-of-eight or mattress sutures **(D)**. The base of the triangular flap of aponeurosis is left attached distally, and the apex is turned down and sutured in place across the first layer of repair for the rupture of the quadriceps **(E)**. A Bunnell-type pull-out wire suture may be placed on the proximal side of the repair in both the medial and lateral aspects of the quadriceps muscle. These sutures are passed distally through the skin and subsequently through the long-leg cast to be tied or twisted together over the plaster to retain a distal pull on the proximal portion os the quadriceps mechanism during the early postoperative period.

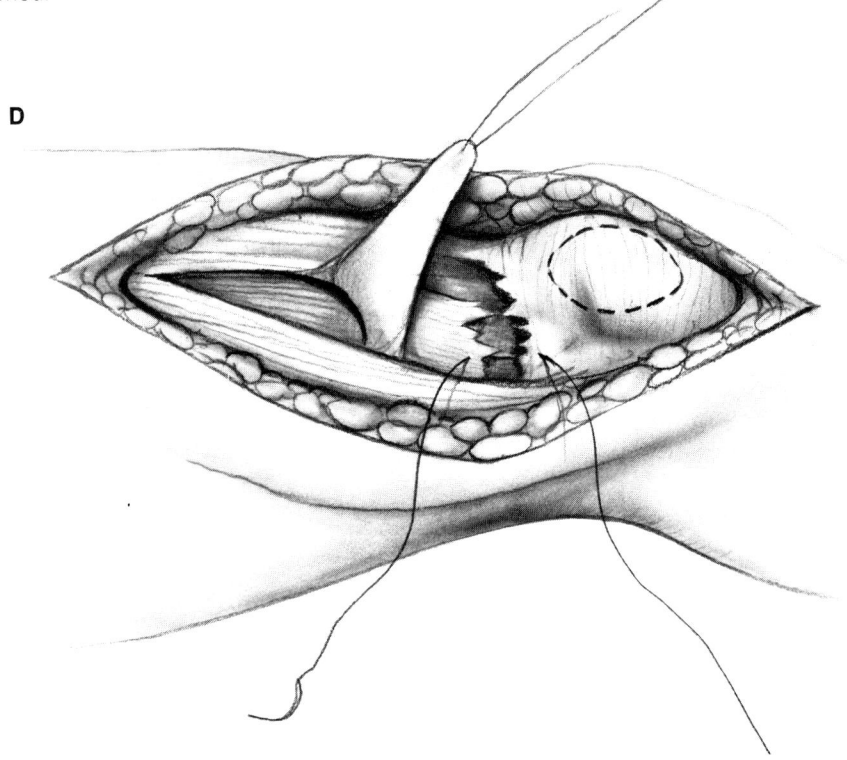

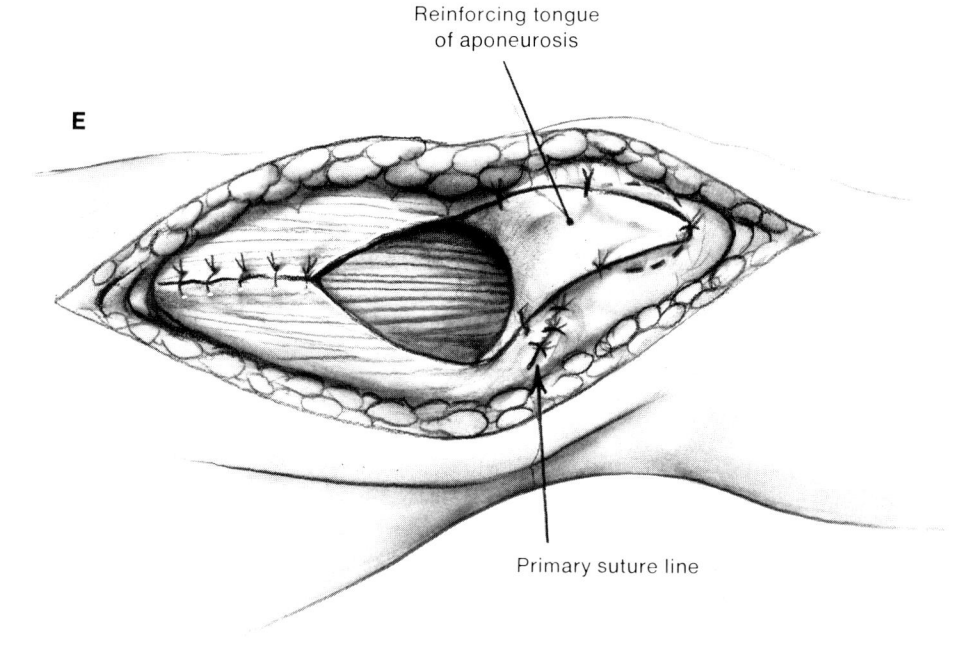

POSTOPERATIVE MANAGEMENT. The long-leg cast is changed 3 weeks postoperatively. The pull-out wires and skin sutures are removed at this time. A new cylinder cast is applied with the knee in extension for an additional 3 weeks. After that, active knee exercise is allowed and encouraged progressively. By 8 weeks postoperatively, complete extension of the knee and flexion to at least 50° should be possible. Three months postoperatively, flexion of the knee to 90° should be possible. After 6 months, additional flexion of the knee should not be anticipated.

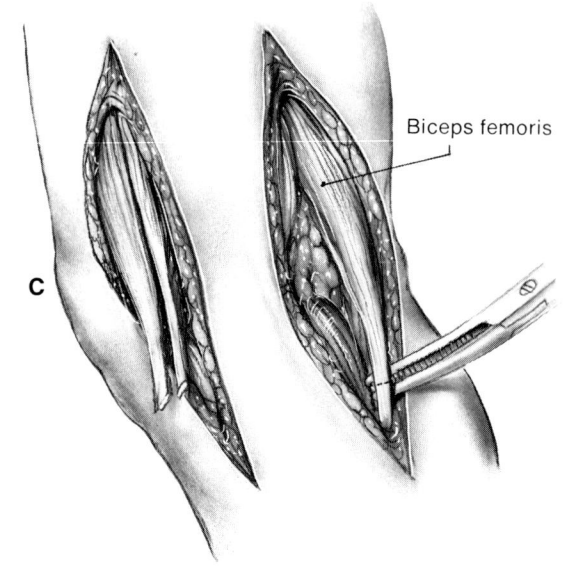

TRANSPLANTATION OF HAMSTRINGS TO FEMORAL CONDYLES (EGGERS) (Plate 11-6)

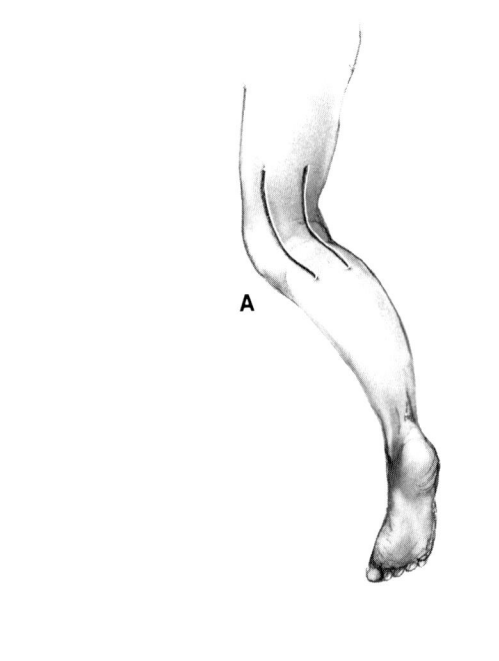

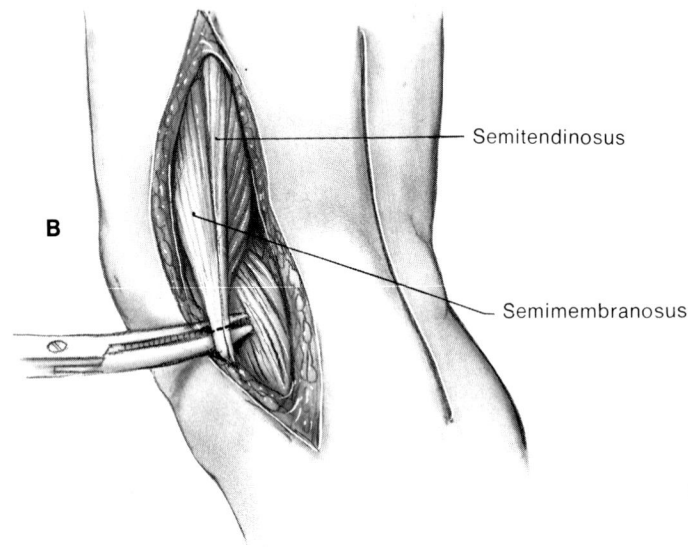

GENERAL DISCUSSION. The choice of the proper procedure for correction of a knee-flexion deformity depends on the specific etiology of the individual deformity.

Knee-flexion deformity without flexed contracture may be secondary to hamstring spasm or to ineffective quadriceps for terminal knee extension. Knee-flexion deformity may also be the result of a fixed posterior contracture.

Transfer of the hamstring tendons to the femoral condyles (Eggers procedure) is the procedure of choice for the spastic knee-flexion deformity. If the problem is basically an ineffective quadriceps, advancement of the patellar tendon is the proper corrective procedure. Posterior capsulotomy is reserved for the fixed knee-flexion contracture.

DETAILS OF PROCEDURE. The patient is positioned prone. A longitudinal curvilinear incision is made over the medial hamstring muscles; the incision is approximately 7 cm in length, ending at the level of the proximal tibia **(A)**. The semitendinosus and semimembranosus tendons are identified and both are sectioned just proximal to their insertion (**B** and **C**). Both tendons are secured together under a periosteal bridge on the posteromedial aspect of the medial femoral condyle **(D)**.

(Plate 11-6) TRANSPLANTATION OF HAMSTRINGS TO FEMORAL CONDYLES (EGGERS)

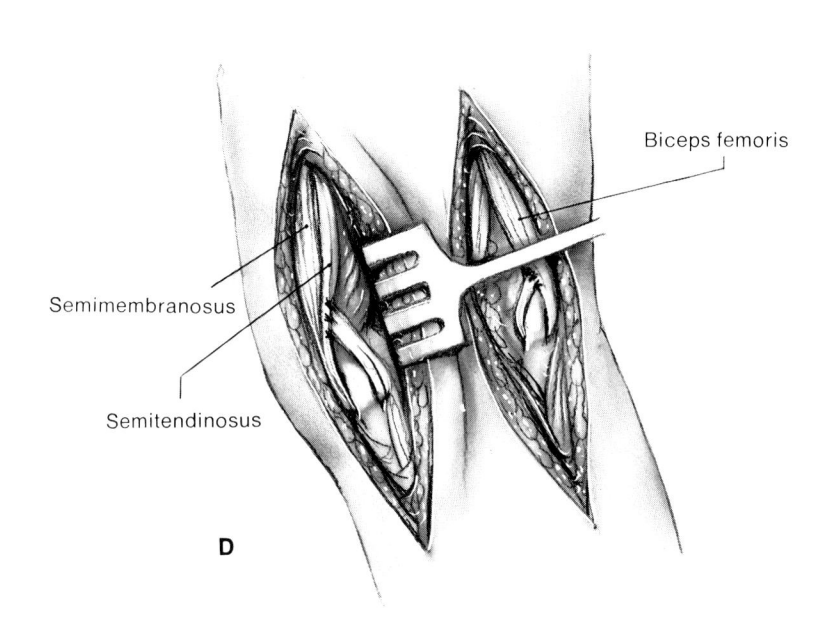

A second longitudinal incision is made in similar fashion laterally **(B)**. Dissection is carried down to expose the common peroneal nerve, which is retracted medially. The biceps femoris tendon is sectioned at its insertion and then secured under a bridge of periosteum on the posterolateral aspect of the lateral femoral condyle as illustrated **(D)**.

POSTOPERATIVE MANAGEMENT. The knee is held in extension in a long-leg cast for 3 weeks postoperatively **(E)**.

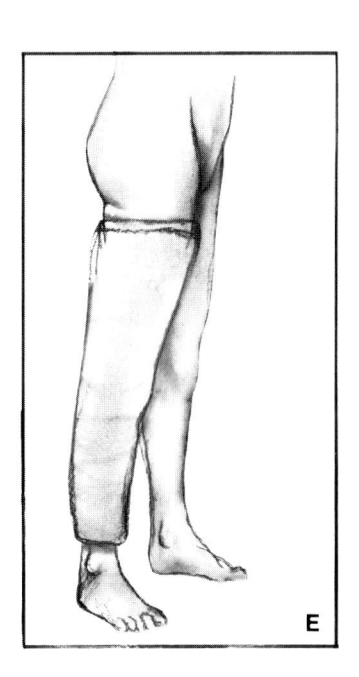

FORWARD TRANSFER OF HAMSTRINGS TO REINFORCE KNEE EXTENSION (Plate 11-7)

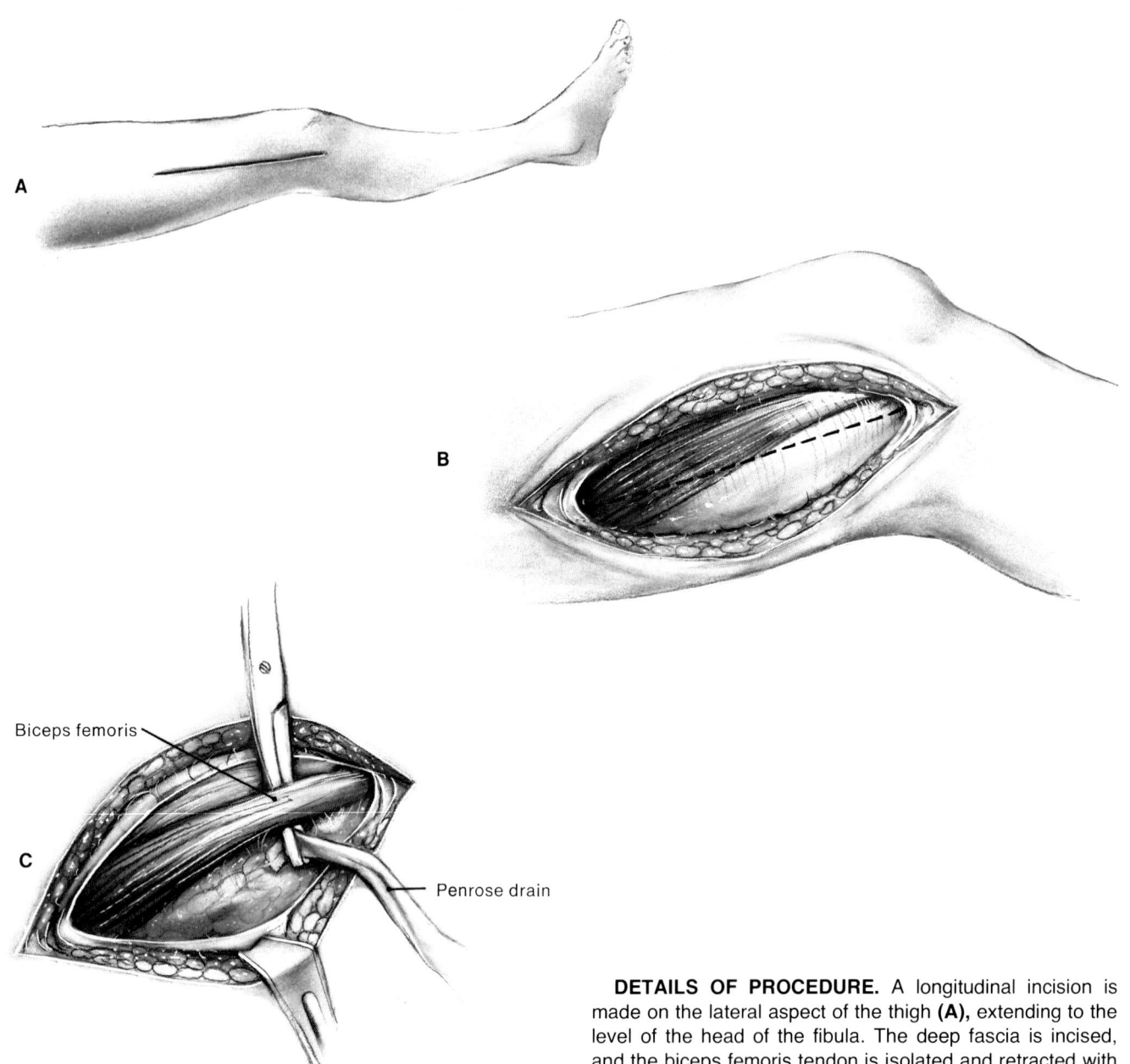

GENERAL DISCUSSION. Forward transfer of hamstrings is effective in restoring active knee extension where there is a weak or paralyzed quadriceps. Both biceps femoris and semitendinosus must have good power preoperatively. The biceps femoris should not be transferred alone (lateral deviation and possible dislocation of the patella may result). Also, activity of the hip flexors should be at least fair or the patient may have difficulty in clearing the extremity from the floor postoperatively. Active knee flexion postoperatively will depend primarily on the gastrocnemius and semimembranosus. Any knee-flexion contracture must be corrected before this procedure is carried out.

DETAILS OF PROCEDURE. A longitudinal incision is made on the lateral aspect of the thigh **(A)**, extending to the level of the head of the fibula. The deep fascia is incised, and the biceps femoris tendon is isolated and retracted with a rubber tape **(B** and **C)**. The common peroneal nerve, which lies medial and posterior to the biceps femoris tendon, is also identified and gently retracted with a rubber tape **(D)**.

The biceps femoris tendon is divided at its insertion into the lateral side of the head of the fibula, care being taken to protect the fibular attachment of the lateral collateral ligament. There is a small slip of insertion of the biceps femoris into the lateral condyle of the tibia, which is also divided. The biceps femoris muscle is dissected free in a proximal direction as far as possible while the nerve and blood supply to both long and short heads of the muscle are carefully preserved **(E)**. The lateral intermuscular septum is incised to bone. A very wide subcutaneous tunnel is prepared for redirection of the biceps femoris to the patella and patellar tendon **(F)**.

(Plate 11-7) FORWARD TRANSFER OF HAMSTRINGS TO REINFORCE KNEE EXTENSION

Biceps femoris

Common peroneal nerve

D

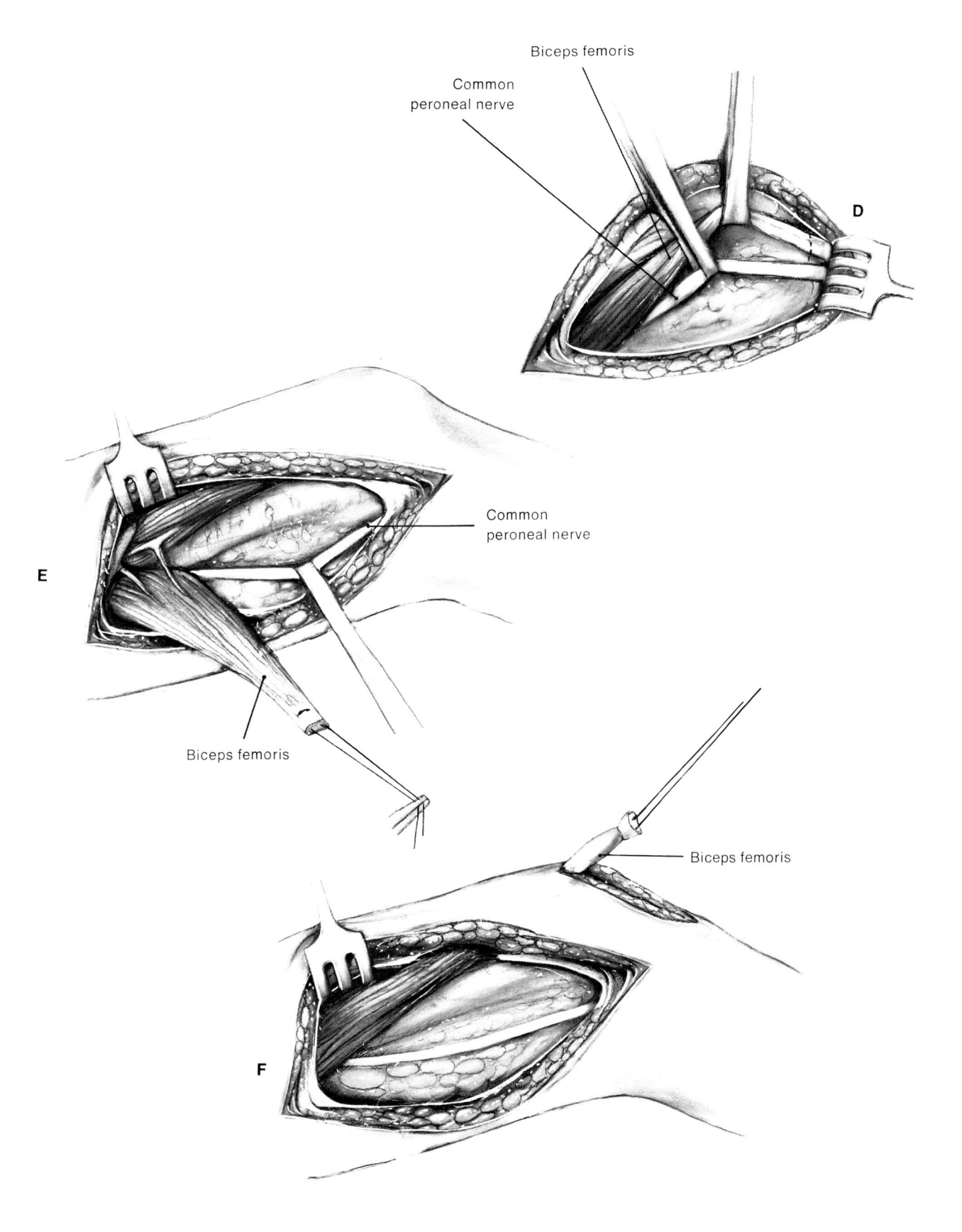

Common peroneal nerve

E

Biceps femoris

Biceps femoris

F

395

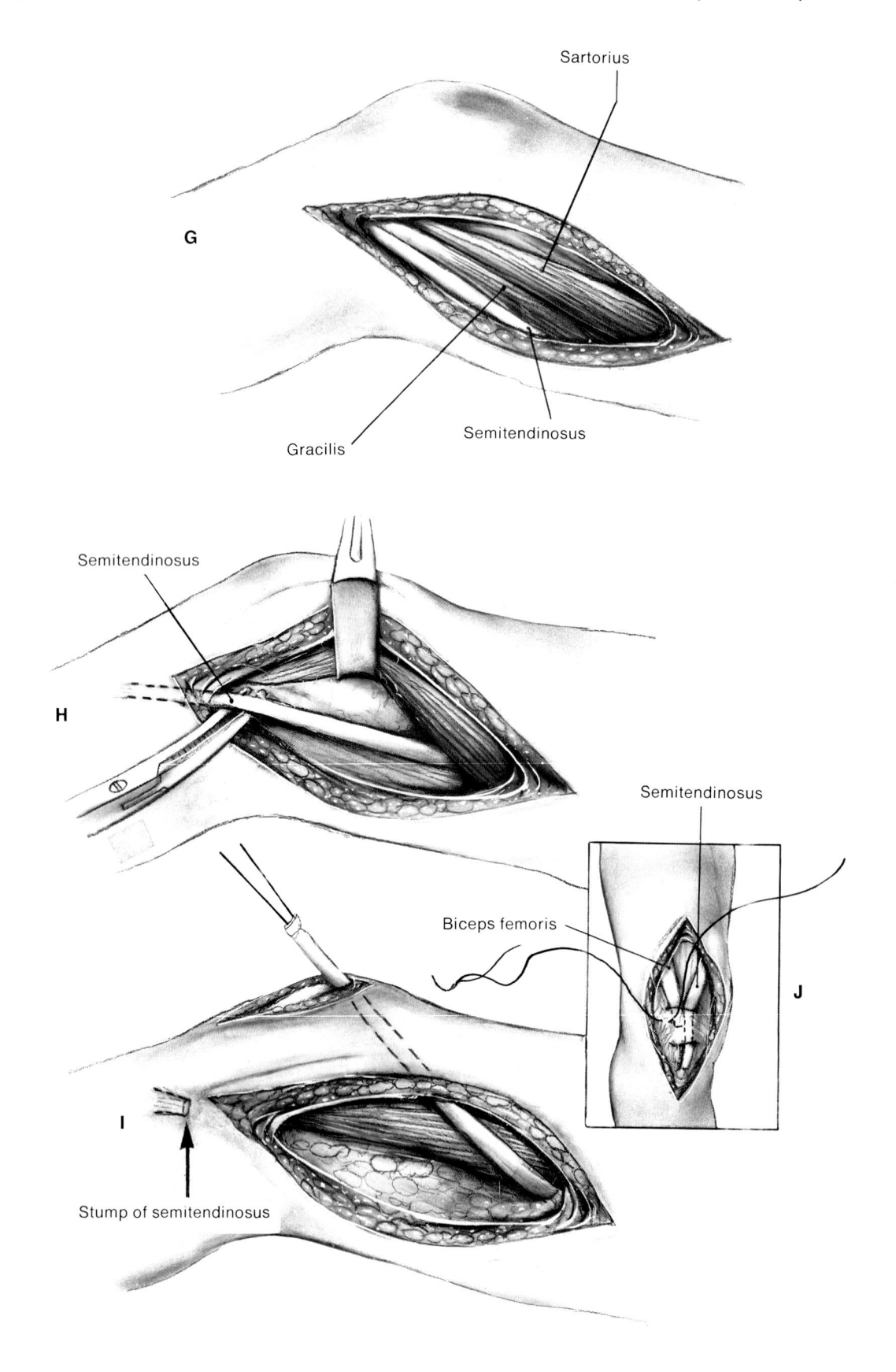

FORWARD TRANSFER OF HAMSTRINGS TO REINFORCE KNEE EXTENSION (Plate 11-7)

(Plate 11-7) FORWARD TRANSFER OF HAMSTRINGS TO REINFORCE KNEE EXTENSION

A medial thigh incision is then made, extending distally to the medial tibial plateau. The dissection is carried down to isolate the semitendinosus tendon, which is divided near its insertion into the tibia (**G** and **H**). The fascia is widely incised proximally, and the mobile, slender semitendinosus muscle belly is readily freed with the surgeon's finger from its surrounding loose areolar tissue. A subcutaneous tunnel is then made from the proximal end of this incision to a third incision anteriorly over the patella. The semitendinosus tendon is passed underneath the sartorius and gracilis muscles and then through a wide subcutaneous tunnel to reach the anterior surface of the patella in as straight a line as possible (**I**). Any restricting fascial edges are incised to avoid any angulation or pressure against the transferred tendon. The biceps femoris tendon is passed through a subcutaneous tunnel to the anterior incision similarly.

A subperiosteal tunnel is fashioned under the tough covering over the anterior patellar surface. The biceps femoris tendon and the semitendinosus tendon are each pulled through the tunnel on the anterior patellar surface, sutured to it, and the ends of each are sutured to the pattellar tendon (**J**).

After closure of the wound, a long-leg cast is applied that holds the knee in 10° flexion. Immobilization with the knee in hyperextension should be avoided.

POSTOPERATIVE MANAGEMENT. Immobilization in the long-leg cast is continued for 3 weeks. Physical therapy is started immediately following cast removal with active knee exercises and reeducation of the transferred hamstring muscles. Protective splinting is continued between exercise periods for an additional 3 weeks.

ABOVE-KNEE AMPUTATION (Plate 11-8)

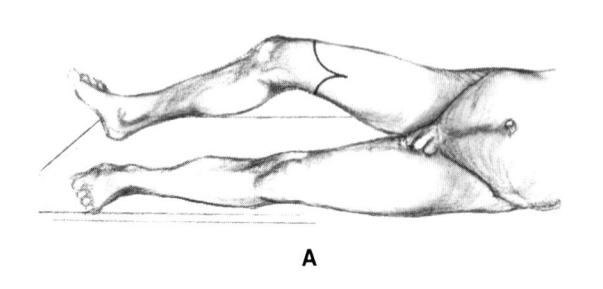

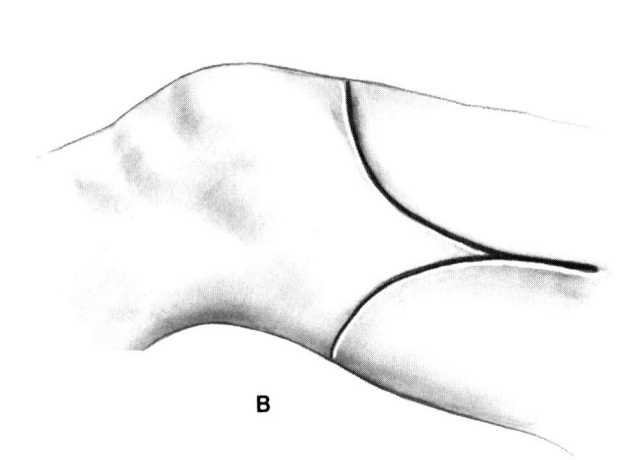

GENERAL DISCUSSION. Above-knee amputation may occasionally by indicated for serious peripheral-vascular disease or other disease or injury involving the lower extremity. The level of amputation is determined by the individual circumstances in each case.

If the amputation level must be above the knee, adequate room should be allowed for the knee mechanism of an artificial limb. Beyond this, the major consideration should be to leave as much length to the above-knee stump as possible with the individual circumstance. For a person of average height, amputation at a level of 25 to 30 cm below the greater trochanter will leave an adequate lever for the prosthesis and will allow room for the mechanism of an artificial knee joint.

DETAILS OF PROCEDURE. Anterior and posterior skin flaps are carefully mapped out to have an anterior flap 2 to 3 cm longer than the posterior flap. The proximal end of the incision on the medial and lateral aspects of the thigh should end 2 to 3 cm above the intended level for division of the femur (**A** and **B**).

Flaps of skin and subcutaneous tissue are reflected proximally (**C**). An anterior myofascial flap is formed by an incision through the fascia and the quadriceps muscles anteriorly and reflected proximally toward the level of planned bone division to create a flap no greater than 2.5 cm in thickness for later suture to the posterior fascia and muscles. All cutaneous nerves are severed and allowed to retract. After division of the quadriceps muscles and creation of the anterior myofascial flap, the femoral vessels are located in the subsartorial canal and are doubly ligated and divided (**D**).

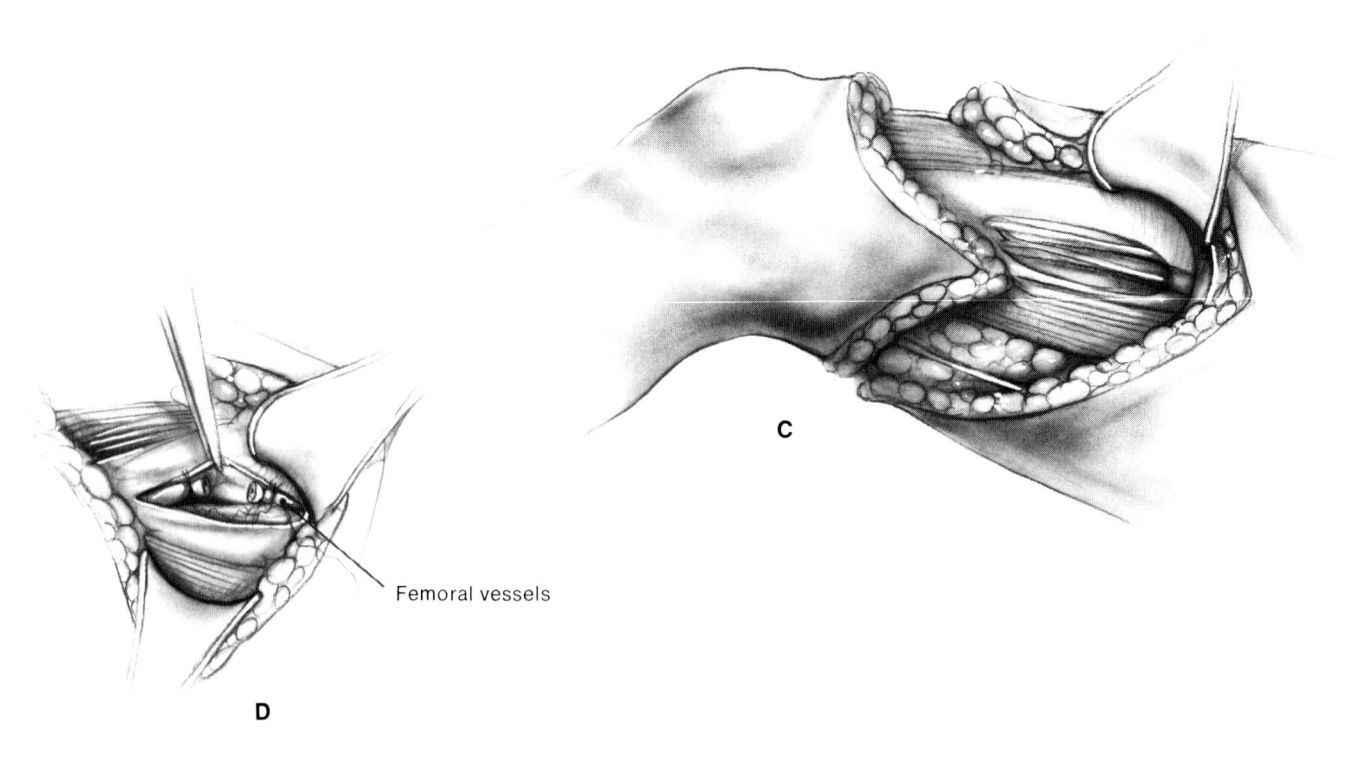

(Plate 11-8) ABOVE-KNEE AMPUTATION

The periosteum of the femur is incised circumferentially and the bone is divided transversely with a saw **(E)**. The sciatic nerve is found in the midline posteriorly deep to the medial hamstrings and between the short head of the biceps femoris muscle and the adductor magnus muscle. The sciatic nerve is ligated and divided **(F)**. The profunda femoris artery will be found close to bone in the midline posteriorly between the bulk of the vastus lateralis muscle and the adductor magnus muscle and must be ligated. The posterior fascia and hamstring muscles are divided transversely so they will retract to the level of the transection of the femur.

399

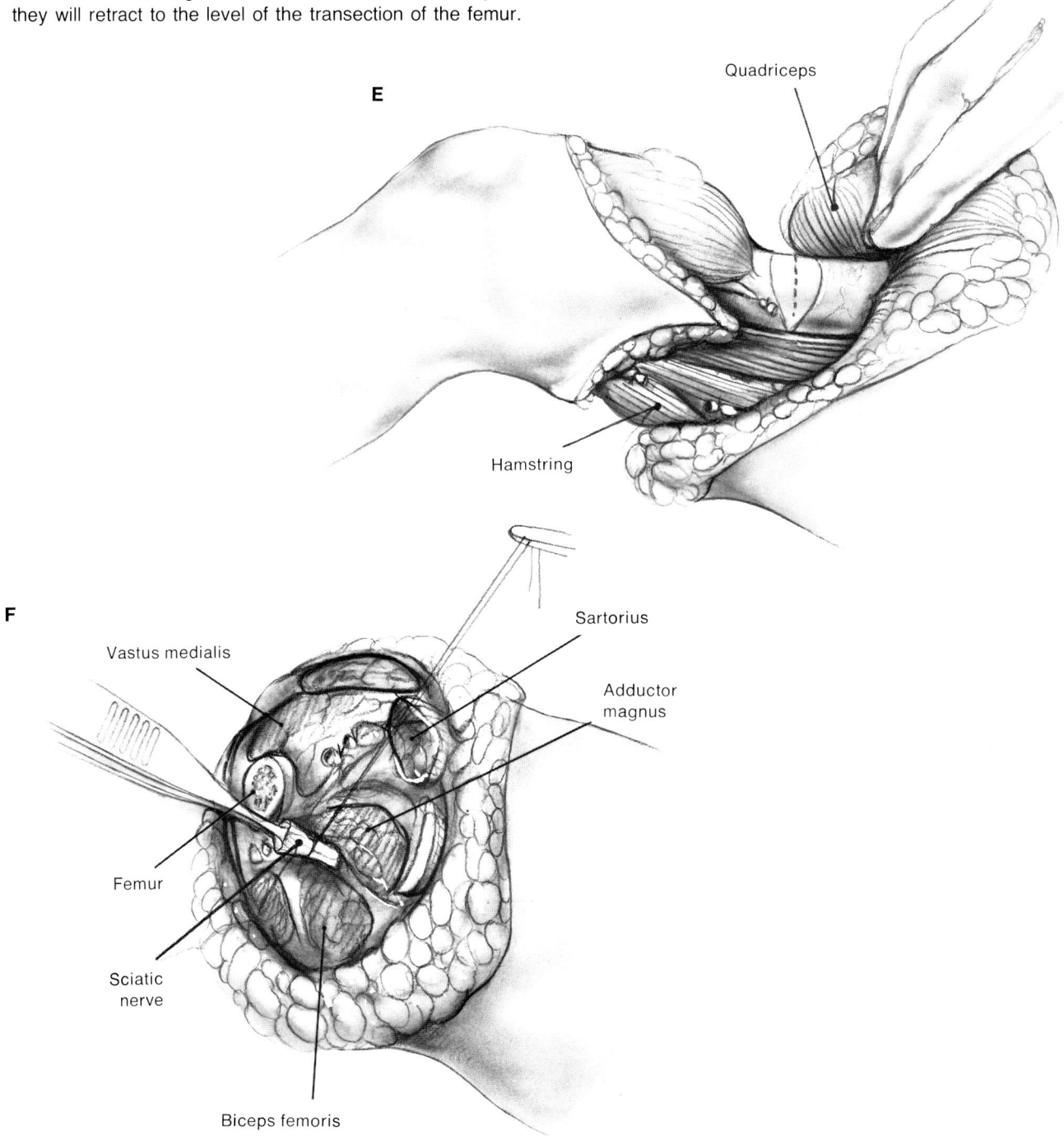

ABOVE-KNEE AMPUTATION (Plate 11-8)

The edges of the bone and the prominence of the linea aspera are smoothed with a file. The wound is irrigated to remove any bone fragments or dust (G). After the wound is carefully checked for hemostasis, the anterior myofascial flap is drawn over the end of the divided femur and sutured to the posterior fascia and hamstring muscles. Skin and subcutaneous tissues are closed with interrupted sutures, and a drain is left at the medial and lateral edges of the wound (H). A bulky compression bandage is applied (I).

POSTOPERATIVE MANAGEMENT. The patient is encouraged to lie in the prone position for part of each day, particularly on teh first postoperative day, to minimize any difficulty with hip flexion contracture. The drains are removed from the wound at 24 to 48 hours postoperatively and the sutures can usually be removed at 14 days. Active exercise of the remaining stump is encouraged. Elastic bandaging of the stump is continued until the initial prosthetic fitting (J).

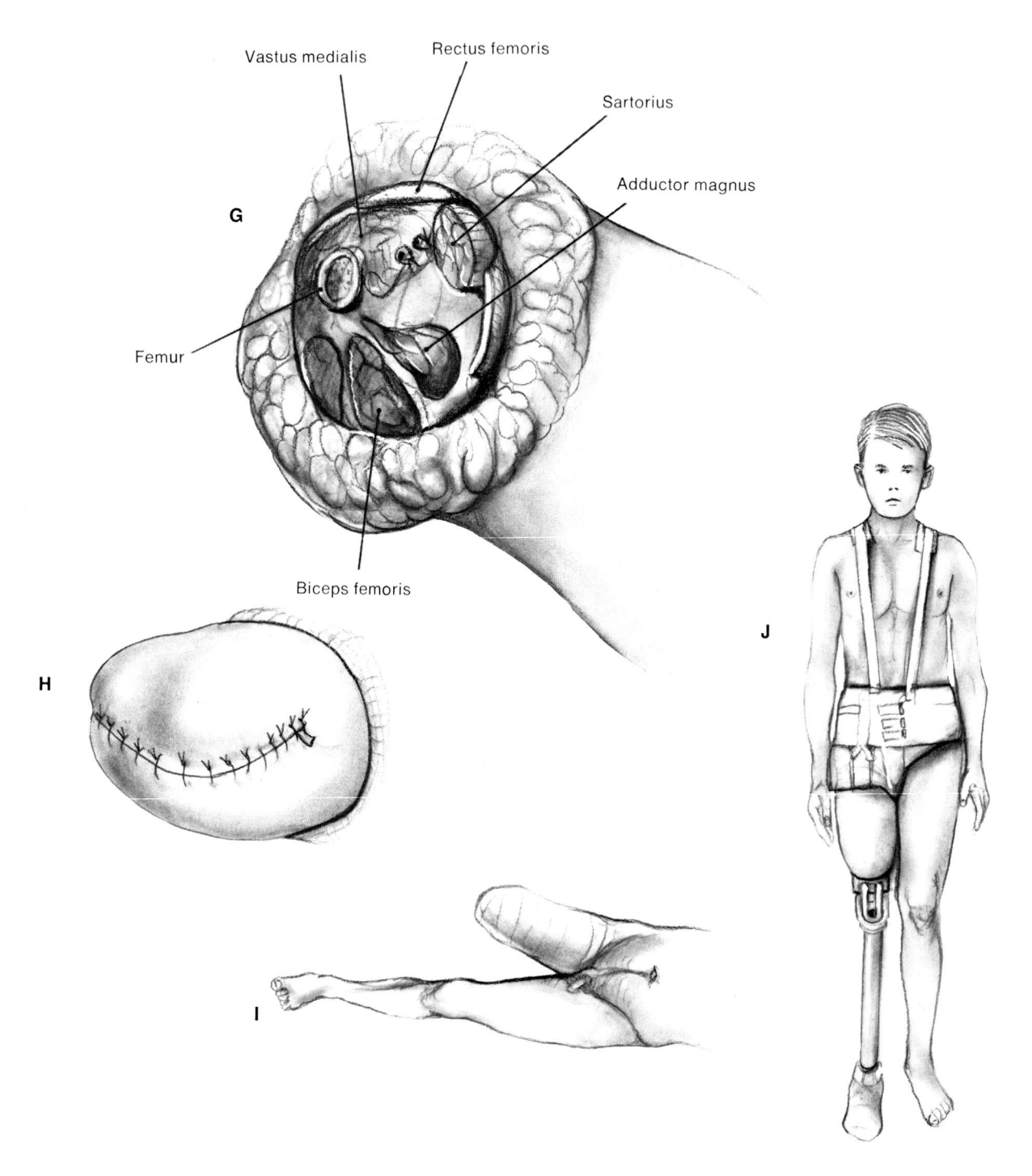

REFERENCES

Alexakis, P. G., and McIvor, R. R.: A practical method of insertion of the Rush rod in the femur, J. Bone Joint Surg. **45-A:**1057, 1963.

Allen, W. C., Piotrowski, G., Burstein, A. H., and Frankel, V. H.: Biomechanical principles of intramedullary fixation, Clin. Orthop. **60:**13, 1968.

Amstutz, H. C., and Wilson, P. D., Jr.: Dysgenesis of the proximal femur (coxa vara) and its surgical management, J. Bone Joint Surg. **44-A:**1, 1962.

d'Aubigne, R. M.: Surgical treatment of non-union of long bones, J. Bone Joint Surg. **31-A:**256, 1949.

Aufranc, O. E., Jones, W. N., and Harris, W. H.: Comminuted intercondylar and supracondylar femoral fracture, J.A.M.A. **187:**293, 1964.

Beals, R. K.: Spastic paraplegia and diplegia. An evaluation of non-surgical and surgical factors influencing the prognosis for ambulation, J. Bone Joint Surg. **48-A:**827, 1966.

Blumenfeld, I.: Pseudarthrosis of the long bones, J. Bone Joint Surg. **29:**97, 1947.

Böhler, J.: Results in medullary nailing of ninety-five fresh fractures of the femur, J. Bone Joint Surg. **33-A:**670, 1951.

Böhler, J.: Closed intramedullary nailing of the femur, Clin. Orthop. **60:**51, 1968.

Böhler, L.: The treatment of fractures, ed. 4, Baltimore, 1935 William Wood & Co.

Böhler, L., and Böhler, J.: Küntscher's medullary nailing, J. Bone Joint Surg. **31-A:**295, 1949.

Bonney, G.: Thrombosis of the femoral artery complicating fracture of the femur. Treatment by endarterectomy, J. Bone Joint Surg. **45-B:**344, 1963.

Boyd, H. B., Lipinski, S. W., and Wiley, J. H.: Observations on non-union of the shafts of the long bones: with a statistical analysis of 842 patients, J. Bone Joint Surg. **43-A:**159, 1961.

Brav, E. A.: The use of intramedullary nailing for nonunion of the femur, Clin. Orthop. **60:**69, 1968.

Brav, E. A., and Jeffress, V. H.: Fractures of the femoral shaft: a clinical comparison of treatment by traction suspension and intramedullary nailing, Am. J. Surg. **84:**16, 1952.

Brav, E. A., and Jeffress, V. H.: Modified intramedullary nailing in recent gunshot fractures of the femoral shaft, J. Bone Joint Surg. **35-A:**141, 1953.

Burgess, E. M., and Romano, R. L.: The management of lower extremity amputees using immediate postsurgical prostheses, Clin. Orthop. 57:137, 1968.

Burgess, E. M., Romano, R. L., and Traub, J. E.: Immediate post-surgical prosthetic fitting. Prosthetic research study report, Bull. Prosthet. Res. **10-4:**42, 1965.

Burgess, E. M., Romano, R. L., and Zettl, J. H.: The management of lower extremity amputations, TR 10-6, Washington, D.C., 1969, Veterans Administration.

Burgess, E. M., Traub, J. E., and Wilson, A. B., Jr.: Immediate postsurgical prosthetics in the management of lower extremity amputees, TR 10-5, Washington, D.C., 1967, Veterans Administration.

Callander, C. L.: Tendinoplastic amputation through femur at knee; further studies, J.A.M.A. **110:**113, 1938.

Carr, C. C., and Turnipseed, D.: Experiences with intramedullary fixation of compound femoral fractures in war wounds, J. Bone Joint Surg. **35-A:**153, 1953.

Carr, C. R., and Wingo, C. H.: Fractures of the femoral diaphysis. A retrospective study of the results and costs of treatment by intramedullary nailing and by traction and a spica cast, J. Bone Joint Surg. **55-A:**690, 1973.

Casey, M. J., and Chapman, M. W.: Ipsilateral concomitant fractures of the hip and femoral shaft, J. Bone Joint Surg. **61-A:**503, 1979.

Cave, E. F.: Medullary nails in pathological conditions of the femur, American Academy of Orthopaedic Surgeons Instructional Course Lectures, vol. 8, Ann Arbor, Mich., 1951, J. W. Edwards.

Cave, E. F.: Femoral-shaft fractures treated by medullary nailing, N. Engl. J. Med. **246:**284, 1952.

Cave, E. F.: Complications of medullary fixation of fractures of long bones, American Academy of Orthopaedic Surgeons Instructional Course Lectures, vol. 15, Ann Arbor, Mich., 1958, J. W. Edwards, p. 86.

Clawson, D. K., Smith, R. F., and Hansen, S. T.: Closed intramedullary nailing of the femur, J. Bone Joint Surg. **53-A:**681, 1971.

Conway, F. M.: Rupture of the quadriceps tendon, Am. J. Surg. **50:**3, 1940.

Crego, C. H., Jr., and Fischer, F. J.: Transplantation of the biceps femoris for the relief of quadriceps femoris paralysis in residual poliomyelitis, J. Bone Joint Surg. **13:**515, 1931.

Curtis, B. H., and Fisher, R. L.: Congenital hyperextension with anterior subluxation of the knee. Surgical treatment and long-term observations, J. Bone Joint Surg. **51-A:**255, 1969.

DeBelder, K. R. J.: Distal migration of the femoral intramedullary nail. Report of seven cases, J. Bone Joint Surg. **50-B:**324, 1968.

Dehne, E., and Immerman, E. W.: Dislocation of the hip combined with fracture of the shaft of the femur on the same side, J. Bone Joint Surg. **33-A:**731, 1951.

Delorme, T. L., West, F. E., and Shriber, W. J.: Influence of progressive-resistance exercises on knee function following femoral fractures, J. Bone Joint Surg. **32-A:**910, 1950.

Eggers, G. W. N.: Surgical division of the patellar retinacula to improve extension of the knee joint in cerebral spastic paralysis, J. Bone Joint Surg. **32-A:**80, 1950.

Eggers, G. W. N.: Transplantation of hamstring tendons to femoral condyles in order to improve hip extension and to decrease knee flexion in cerebral spastic paralysis, J. Bone Joint Surg. **34-A:**827, 1952.

Eggers, G. W. N.: Selective surgery for the cerebral palsy patient, American Academy of Orthopaedic Surgeons Instructional Course Lectures, vol. 12, Ann Arbor, Mich., 1955, J. W. Edwards, p. 221.

Eggers, G. W. N., and Evans, E. B.: Surgery in cerebral palsy, J. Bone Joint Surg. **45-A:**1275, 1963.

Fairbank, T. J., and Barrett, A. M.: Vastus intermedius contracture in early childhood, J. Bone Joint Surg. **43-B:**326, 1961.

Francis, K. C.: Prophylactic internal fixation of metastatic osseous lesions, Cancer **13:**75, 1960.

Funk, F. J., Wells, R. E., and Street, D. M.: Supplementary fixation of femoral fractures, Clin. Orthop. **60:**41, 1968

Gleave, J. A. E.: A plastic socket and stump casting technique for above-knee prostheses, J. Bone Joint Surg. **47-B:**100, 1965.

Golbranson, F. L., et al.: Immediate post surgical fitting and early ambulation, Clin. Orthop. **56:**119, 1968.

Gunn, D. R.: Contracture of the quadriceps muscle. A discussion on the etiology and relationship to recurrent dislocation of the patella, J. Bone Joint Surg. **46-B:**492, 1964.

Herndon, C. H.: Tendon transplantation at the knee and foot, American Academy of Orthopaedic Surgeons Instructional Course Lectures, vol. 18, St. Louis, 1961, The C. V. Mosby Co.

Hesketh, K. T.: Experiences with the Thompson quadricepsplasty, J. Bone Joint Surg. **45-B:**491, 1963.

Holden, W. D.: Technique of low thigh amputation, Surg. Gynecol. Obstet. **87:**739, 1948.

Key, J. A., and Reynolds, F. C.: The treatment of infection after medullary nailing, Surgery **35:**749, 1954.

Kirkup, J. R.: Major arterial injury complicating fracture of the femoral shaft, J. Bone Joint Surg. **45-B:**337, 1963.

Kirkup, J. R.: Traumatic femoral bone loss, J. Bone Joint Surg. **47-B:**106, 1965.

Knutsson, B., and Stahl, F.: Immediate postoperative fitting of prosthesis for lower limbs, Acta Orthop. Scand. **36:**459, 1965-1966.

Küntscher, G.: Die Marknagelung von Knochenbrüchen, Arch. Klin. Chir. **200:**443, 1940.

Küntscher, G.: The Küntscher method of intramedullary fixation, J. Bone Joint Surg. **40-A:**17, 1958.

Küntscher, G.: Intramedullary surgical technique and its place in orthopaedic surgery. My present concept, J. Bone Joint Surg. **47-A:**809, 1965.

Küntscher, G.: Practice of intramedullary nailing, Springfield, Ill., 1967, Chrales C Thomas, Publisher.

Küntscher, G.: The classic; the intramedullary nailing of fractures, Clin. Orthop. **60:**5, 1968.

Levy, M., Seelenfreund, M., Maor, P., Fried, A., and Lurie, M.: Bilateral spontaneous and simultaneous rupture of the quadriceps tendons in gout, J. Bone Joint Surg. **53-A:**510, 1971.

Liao, S. J., and Schnell, A.: A functional above-the-knee prosthesis for geriatric patients, J. Bone Joint Surg. **46-A:**1292, 1964.

Lottes, J. O., and Key, J. A.: Complications and errors in technic in medullary nailing for fractures of the femur, Clin. Orthop. **2:**38, 1953.

MacAusland, W. R., Jr.: Treatment of sepsis after intramedullary nailing of fractures of femur, Clin. Orthop. **60:**87, 1968.

MacAusland, W. R., Jr., and Eaton, R. G.: The management of sepsis following intramedullary fixation for fractures of the femur, J. Bone Joint Surg. **45-A:**1643, 1963.

Marmor, L., and Sollars, R.: Lower extremity amputations and their appropriate prosthesis, J. Trauma **4:**435, 1964.

Martinek, H., and Schmid, L.: Fractures of the distal femur and their treatment with the condylar place, Chirurg. **49:**382, 1978.

McCarroll, H. R.: Early management of congenital dislocation of the hip, American Academy of Orthopaedic Surgeons Instructional Course Lectures, vol. 4, Ann Arbor, Mich., 1948, J. W. Edwards, p. 125.

McCarroll, H. R.: Congenital dislocation of the hip after the age of infancy, American Academy of Orthopaedic Surgeons Instructional Course Lectures, vol. 12, Ann Arbor, Mich., 1955, J. W. Edwards, p. 69.

McCarroll, H. R., and Schwartzmann, J. R.: Spastic paralysis and allied disorders, J. Bone Joint Surg. **25:**745, 1943.

McLaughlin, H. L.: Intramedullary fixation of pathological fractures, Clin. Orthop. **2:**108, 1953.

McLaughlin, H. L., and Francis, K. C.: Operative repair of injuries to the quadriceps extensor mechanism, Am. J. Surg. **91:**651, 1956.

Milgram, J. E.: The reconstruction of some extensor mechanisms in the extremities, American Academy of Orthopaedic Surgeons Instructional Course Lectures, vol. 13, Ann Arbor, Mich., 1956, J. W. Edwards, p. 121.

Murray, W. R., Lucas, D. B., and Inman, V. T.: Treatment of non-union of fractures of the long bones by the two-plate method, J. Bone Joint Surg. **46-A:**1027, 1964.

Neer, C. S., II, Grantham, S. A., and Shelton, M. L.: Supracondylar fracture of the adult femur. A study of 110 cases, J. Bone Joint Surg. **49-A:**591, 1967.

Nicoll, E. A.: Quadricepsplasty, J. Bone Joint Surg. **45-B:**483, 1963.

Nimberg, G. A., and Rosenfeld, H.: Method for removing an incarcerated Küntscher nail, Clin. Orthop. **71:**205, 1970.

Olerud, S., and Danckwardt-Lilliestrom, G.: Fracture healing in compression osteosynthesis in the dog, J. Bone Joint Surg. **50-B:**844, 1968.

Pollock, G. A., and English, T. A.: Transplantation of the hamstring muscles in cerebral palsy, J. Bone Joint Surg. **49-B:**80, 1967.

Ramsey, R. H., and Muller, G. E.: Quadriceps tendon rupture: a diagnostic trap, Clin. Orthop. **70:**161, 1970.

Rokkanen, P., Slatis, P., and Vankka, E.: Closed or open intramedullary nailing of femoral shaft fractures? A comparison with conservatively treated cases, J. Bone Joint Surg. **51-B:**313, 1969.

Rosenthal, J. J., Gaspar, M. B., Gjerdrum, T. C., and Newman, J.: Vascular injuries associated with fractures of the femur, Arch. Surg. **110:**494, 1975.

Rush, L. V., and Rush, H. L.: A technique for longitudinal pin fixation of certain fractures of the ulna and of the femur, J. Bone Joint Surg. **21:**619, 1939.

Rutherford, R. E., and Bell, J. P.: Delayed open reduction of isolated fractures of the femoral shaft, South. Med. J. **68:**1243, 1975.

Sage, F. P.: The second decade of experience with the Küntscher medullary nail in the femur, Clin. Orthop. **60:**77, 1968.

Sarmiento, A.: Recent trends in lower extremity amputations. Surgery and rehabilitation, Nurs. Clin., North Am. **2:**399, 1967.

Sarmiento, A., May, B. J., Sinclair, W. F., McCollough, N. C., III, and Williams, E. M.: Lower-extremity amputation. The impact of immediate postsurgical prosthetic fitting, Clin. Orthop. **68:**22, 1970.

Schneider, H. W.: Use of the four-flanged self-cutting intramedullary nail for fixation of femoral fractures, Clin. Orthop. **60:**29, 1968.

Schwartzmann, J. R., and Crego, C. H., Jr.: Hamstring tendon transplantation for the relief of quadriceps femoris paralysis in residual poliomyelitis, J. Bone Joint Surg. **30-A:**541, 1948.

Scuderi, C.: Ruptures of the quadriceps tendon. Study of twenty tendon ruptures, Am. J. Surg. **95:**626, 1958.

Scuderi, C., and Schrey, E. L.: Ruptures of the quadriceps tendon, Arch. Surg. **61:**42, 1950.

Smith, H., et al.: Symposium on medullary fixation of the femur, American Academy of Orthopaedic Surgeons Instructional Course Lectures, vol. 8, Ann Arbor, Mich., 1951, J. W. Edwards, p. 1.

Smith, J. E. M.: The results of early and delayed internal fixation of fractures of the shaft of the femur, J. Bone Joint Surg. **46-B:**28, 1964.

Sofield, H. A., and Millar, E. A.: Fragmentation, realignment, and intramedullary rod fixation of deformities of the long bones in children, J. Bone Joint Surg. **41-A:**1371, 1959.

Soto-Hall, R., and McCloy, N. P.: Cause and treatment of angulation of femoral intramedullary nails, Clin. Orthop. **2:**66, 1953.

Stewart, M. J., McReynolds, I. S., Lottes, J. O., Street, D. M., and Cave, E. F.: A symposium on intramedullary nailing. American Academy of Orthopaedic Surgeons Instructional Course Lectures, vol. 15, Ann Arbor, Mich., 1958, J. W. Edwards, p. 49.

Stewart, M. J., Sisk, T. D., and Wallace, S. L. Jr.: Fractures of the distal third of the femur: a comparison of methods of treatment, J. Bone Joint Surg. **48-A**:784, 1966.

Street, D. M.: 100 fractures of the femur treated by means of a diamond-shaped medullary nail, J. Bone Joint Surg. **33-A**:659, 1951.

Street, D. M.: Complications in medullary nailing of the femur, Clin. Orthop. **2**:93, 1953.

Street, D. M.: Medullary nailing of the femur, American Academy of Orthopaedic Surgeons Instructional Course Lectures, vol. 10, Ann Arbor, Mich., 1953, J. W. Edwards, p. 27.

Street, D. M.: Intramedullary nailing of the femur, American Academy of Orthopaedic Surgeons Instructional Course Lectures, vol. 15, Ann Arbor, Mich., 1958, J. W. Edwards, p. 78.

Swanson, A. B., Hotchkiss, B., and Meadows, V.: Improving end-bearing characteristics of lower extremity amputation stumps, Inter-Clin. Inform. Bull. **7**:11, 1967.

Taylor, L. W.: Principles of treatment of fractures and nonunion of the shaft of the femur, J. Bone Joint Surg. **45-A**:191, 1963.

Thompson, M. S.: Infections following intramedullary fixation, Clin. Orthop. **2**:60, 1953.

Thompson, R. G., Hanger, H. B., Fryer, C. M., and Wilson, A. B.: Above-the-knee amputations and prosthetics, J. Bone Joint Surg. **47-A**:619, 1965.

Thompson, T. C.: Quadricepsplasty to improve knee function, J. Bone Joint Surg. **26**:366, 1944.

Thorndike, A., and Eberhart, H. D.: Suction socket prosthesis for above-knee amputations, Am. J. Surg. **80**:727, 1950.

Trueta, J., and Cavadias, A. X.: Vascular changes caused by the Küntscher type of nailing. An experimental study in the rabbit, J. Bone Joint Surg. **37-B**:492, 1955.

Vesely, D. G.: Technic for use of the single and the double split diamond nail for fractures of the femur, Clin. Orthop. **60**:95, 1968.

Waters, R. L., Perry, J., Antonelli, E. E., and Hislop, H.: Energy cost of walking of amputees: the influence of level of amputation, J. Bone Joint Surg. **58-A**:42, 1976.

Waters, R. L., Perry, J., McDaniels, J. M., and House, K.: The relative strength of the hamstrings during hip extension, J. Bone Joint Surg. **56-A**:1592, 1974.

Watson-Jones, R., et al.: Medullary nailing of fractures after fifty years, with a review of the difficulties and complications of the operation, J. Bone Joint Surg. **32-B**:694, 1950.

Westin, G. W.: Femoral lengthening using a periosteal sleeve. Report of twenty-six cases, J. Bone Joint Surg. **49-A**:836, 1967.

Wetzler, S. H., and Merkow, W.: Bilateral, simultaneous and spontaneous rupture of the quadriceps tendon, J.A.M.A. **144**:615, 1950.

Wickstrom, J.: Symposium: Surgical mechanics of the internal fixation of fractures. Introduction, J. Bone Joint Surg. **46-A**:397, 1964.

Wickstrom, J., and Corban, M. S.: Intramedullary fixation for fractures of the femoral shaft. A study of complications in 298 operations, J. Trauma **7**:551, 1967.

Wickstrom, J., Corban, M. S., and Vise, G. T., Jr.: Complications following intramedullary fixation of 324 fractured femurs, Clin. Orthop. **60**:103, 1968.

Wilber, M. C., and Evans, E. D.: Fractures of the femoral shaft treated surgically. Comparative results of early and delayed operative stabilization, J. Bone Joint Surg. **60-A**:489, 1978.

Williams, P. F.: Fragmentation and rodding in osteogenesis imperfecta, J. Bone Joint Surg. **47-B**:23, 1965.

Williams, P. F.: Quadriceps contracture, J. Bone Joint Surg. **50-B**:278, 1968.

Yount, C. C.: The role of the tensor fasciae femoris in certain deformities of the lower extremity, J. Bone Joint Surg. **8**:171, 1926.

12

KNEE

ARTHROSCOPY (Plate 12-1)

GENERAL DISCUSSION. Arthroscopy of the knee is proving to be a useful adjunct for the orthopaedic surgeon. The reliability of arthroscopy for accurate diagnosis of internal derangements of the knee is high, and increasingly there are also therapeutic applications (arthroscopic surgery). Arthroscopy should not be used as a substitute for a careful history and physical examination. Although the technique is somewhat demanding and some experience is required before the procedure can be done satisfactorily, it is a safe procedure and through it, patients can often be spared unnecessary knee surgery. When there is pathology of surgical significance, precise diagnosis based on the arthroscopic diagnosis can be of great benefit in selecting the best treatment for each patient. There is the added advantage of being able to examine the synovium and articular surfaces of the joint. In addition, arthroscopy provides a means for morphologic follow-up of patients who have had prior surgery.

DETAILS OF PROCEDURE. Arthroscopy is carried out in an operating room setting under sterile conditions. General, spinal, or local anesthesia can be used depending on the preference of the surgeon. A pneumatic tourniquet is used, but is not inflated unless bleeding obscures vision.

The knee is distended with saline solution via a suprapatellar cannula that later serves as the outflow for irrigation. The arthroscope is inserted anterolaterally, just lateral to the patellar tendon and just above the joint line. The knee joint should always be examined in a routine and complete fashion. Beginning in the suprapatellar pouch the synovium and the patellofemoral joint are visualized. The medial compartment is then examined, including the medial meniscus and articular surfaces; then the intercondylar notch, especially the anterior cruciate ligament; and finally the lateral compartment, including the lateral meniscus. The arthroscope should be maneuvered accurately and gently to avoid inadvertent damage to the articular cartilage.

To increase diagnostic accuracy, the use of a probe inserted percutaneously through the anteromedial portal **(A)** allows palpation of the menisci and other structures under direct vision and greatly enhances the amount of information obtained at arthroscopy. Also, posterior approaches as developed by Johnson, in particular the posteromedial approach **(B)**, can detect posterior peripheral lesions of the menisci and posterior compartment loose bodies that are not visible from anterior approaches.

When a torn meniscus is obvious [e.g., a large tear of the lateral meniscus **(C)**], it is not necessary to probe the lesion to make a diagnosis. However, probing may help define the extent of the tear **(D)** to help in determining whether this lesion can be treated with partial meniscectomy rather than traditional total meniscectomy or, indeed, whether definitive treatment is necessary at all.

When examination from the anterior approaches, including probing, fails to demonstrate any lesion in the medial meniscus, it is recommended that a posteromedial puncture be made, which gives a direct view of the posterior surface of the medial femoral condyle and the rim of the medial meniscus. In the depth of the triangle between those two structures, the posterior cruciate ligament can also be visualized. The normal appearance of the posteromedial compartment as visualized through the posteromedial approach is shown **(E)**, as well as the typical appearance of a posterior peripheral tear of the medial meniscus **(F).**

At the end of the procedure, the knee joint is thoroughly irrigated, and the small arthroscopy wounds closed with subcuticular closure. If arthrotomy and definitive surgical

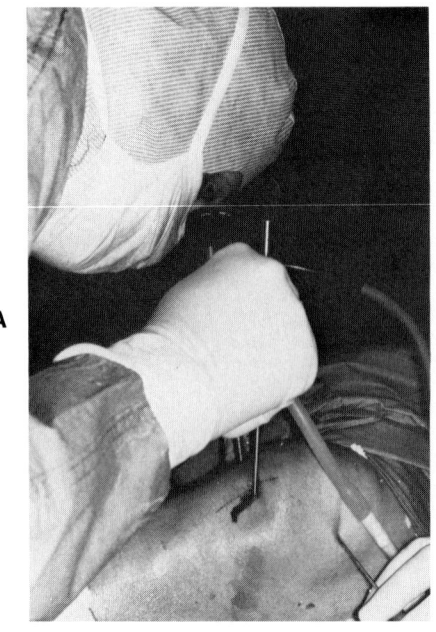

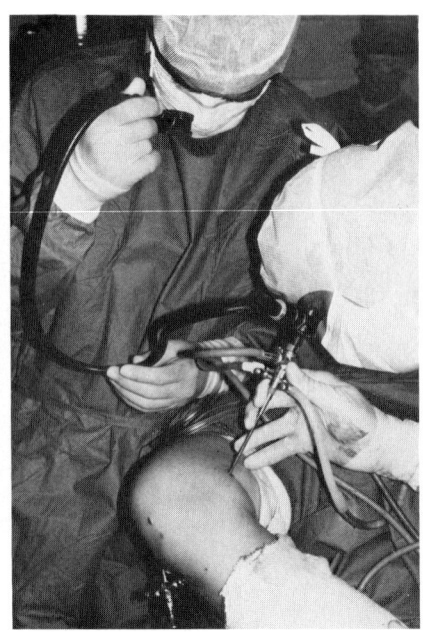

(Plate 12-1) ARTHROSCOPY

intervention are undertaken, it is recommended that the leg be reprepared and redraped before the arthrotomy procedure is started, since it is almost certain that minor breaks in sterile technique have occurred during the arthroscopic examination.

POSTOPERATIVE MANAGEMENT. When arthroscopy has been performed as an independent procedure, a light compression dressing is applied, and the patient is encouraged to begin quadriceps setting and straight leg raising immediately. Since there is almost no quadriceps inhibition following arthroscopy, the patients can be allowed to ambulate, with weight bearing as tolerated, as soon as they have recovered from the anesthesia. Progressive resistance exercises are usually delayed until 10 to 14 days following the procedure. If an operative arthroscopic procedure has been performed, there is usually no reason to alter this postoperative course. If a definitive open operative procedure has been performed, then the postoperative management is dictated by whatever procedure has been performed rather than the arthroscopic portion of the procedure.

C — Torn lateral meniscus

D — Torn lateral meniscus with probe

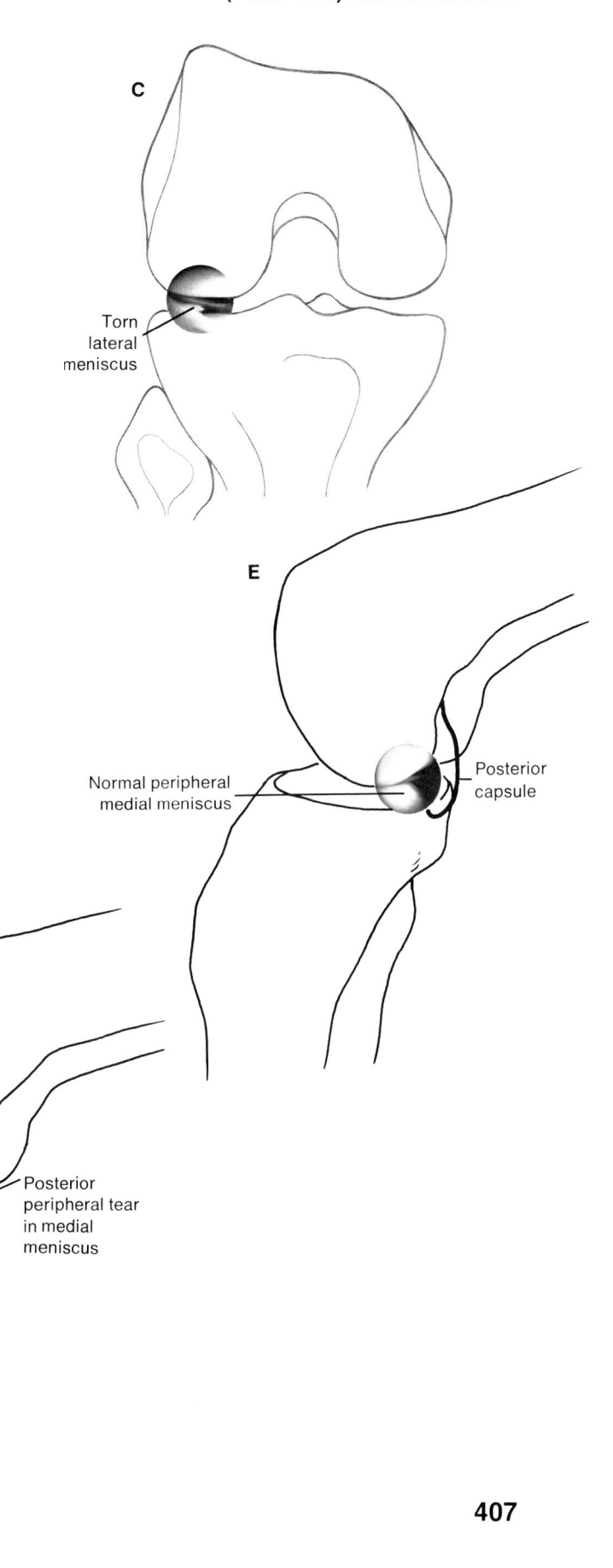

E — Normal peripheral medial meniscus; Posterior capsule

F — Posterior peripheral tear in medial meniscus

KNEE EXPOSURES (Plate 12-2)

GENERAL DISCUSSION. A wide variety of exposures to the medial and lateral aspects of the knee have been described, most of which have advantages and disadvantages depending on the specific procedure to be undertaken. Although there may be alternative skin incisions and exposures that are entirely suitable for a specific procedure, some are more difficult than others to extend to provide a wider exposure when it is necessary to enlarge the scope of the planned procedure. If additional surgical procedures are subsequently necessary, the initial skin incision may be difficult to incorporate into the desired incision to provide adequate exposure without the creation of large subcutaneous flaps with several corners, which may lead to skin necrosis and wound-healing complications.

The system of skin incisions to be described is based on the standard vertical parapatellar incision, which can either be combined with an additional posteromedial or posterolateral incision or extended proximally and distally to provide wider exposure through utility incisions.

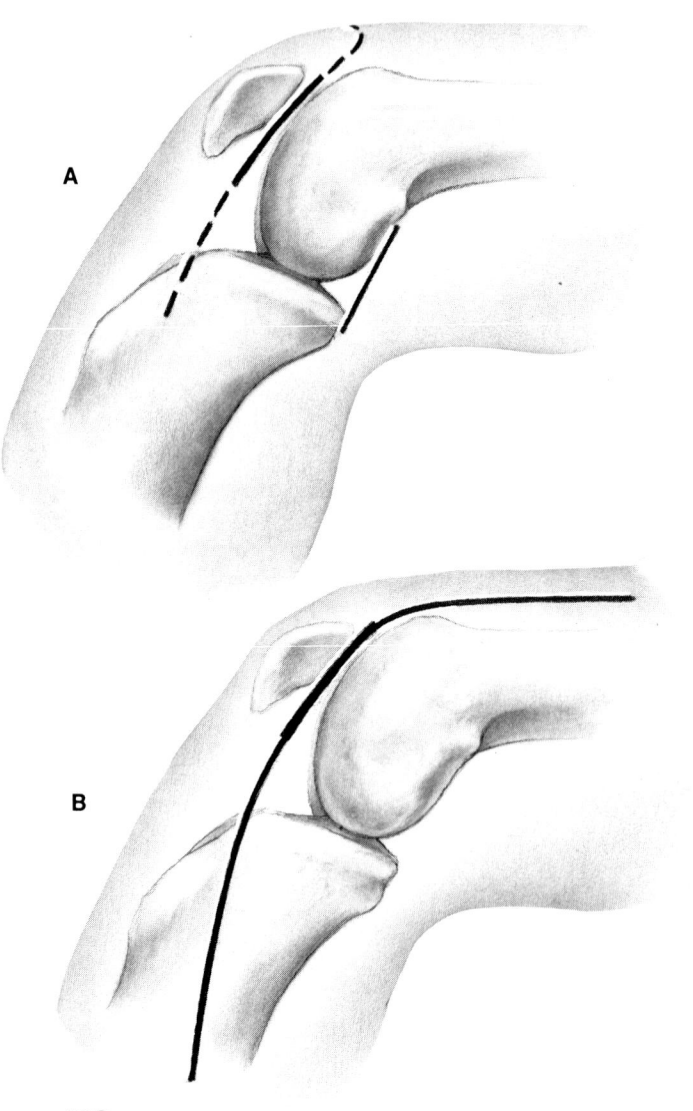

DETAILS OF PROCEDURE. Following are procedures used in *medial approaches.* The basic anteromedial parapatellar incision **(A)** is shown as the solid line, with the incision being located just above the joint line in an effort to avoid sacrificing the infrapatellar branch of the saphenous nerve. This nerve can be protected by retraction, and the capsular incision can then be extended down through the joint line if necessary. The basic parapatellar incision can then be extended proximally, curving around the superomedial pole of the patella and anteriorly over the quadriceps tendon, and extended distally as indicated by the dotted lines **(A)** to facilitate exposure of the anterior and medial aspects of the extensor mechanism. The capsular incision can be extended proximally and medially across the tendon of the vastus medialis and then curved proximally in line with the quadriceps tendon. The capsular incision is then similarly extended distally along the medial border of the patella tendon, so that the patella can be everted for chondroplasty or dislocated laterally to provide exposure of the intracondylar notch to facilitate cruciate ligament repair or reconstruction.

The incision for posteromedial exposure is also shown **(A)**. It is routinely combined with the anteromedial parapatellar approach for medial meniscectomy. It can also be used for exposure for peripheral reattachment of the medial meniscus, for removal of posterior compartment loose bodies, and occasionally for repair of the posterior cruciate ligament. The landmarks are the posterior aspect of the medial femoral epicondyle and adductor tubercle proximally, and the posteromedial joint line distally. This posteromedial incision is parallel with the anteromedial incision, but located slightly inferiorly to reduce the chance of injury of the saphenous nerve. The deep fascia is then incised in line with the skin incision, and the capsular incision is made through the "soft spot" just posterior to the trailing edge of the medial collateral ligament and parallel with that structure.

The standard medial parapatellar incision **(B)** can also be extended proximally and distally in the overall shape of a gentle curve, to make the medial utility approach as described by Slocum and Larson. The skin and subcutaneous tissues are dissected as a single flap, exposing the underlying deep fascia, which can then be incised to provide wide exposure to the medial aspect of the knee from the extensor mechanism anteriorly to the posteromedial corner of the knee posteriorly. Anterior and posterior capsular incisions can be made as appropriate for the particular procedure being performed.

(Plate 12-2) KNEE EXPOSURES

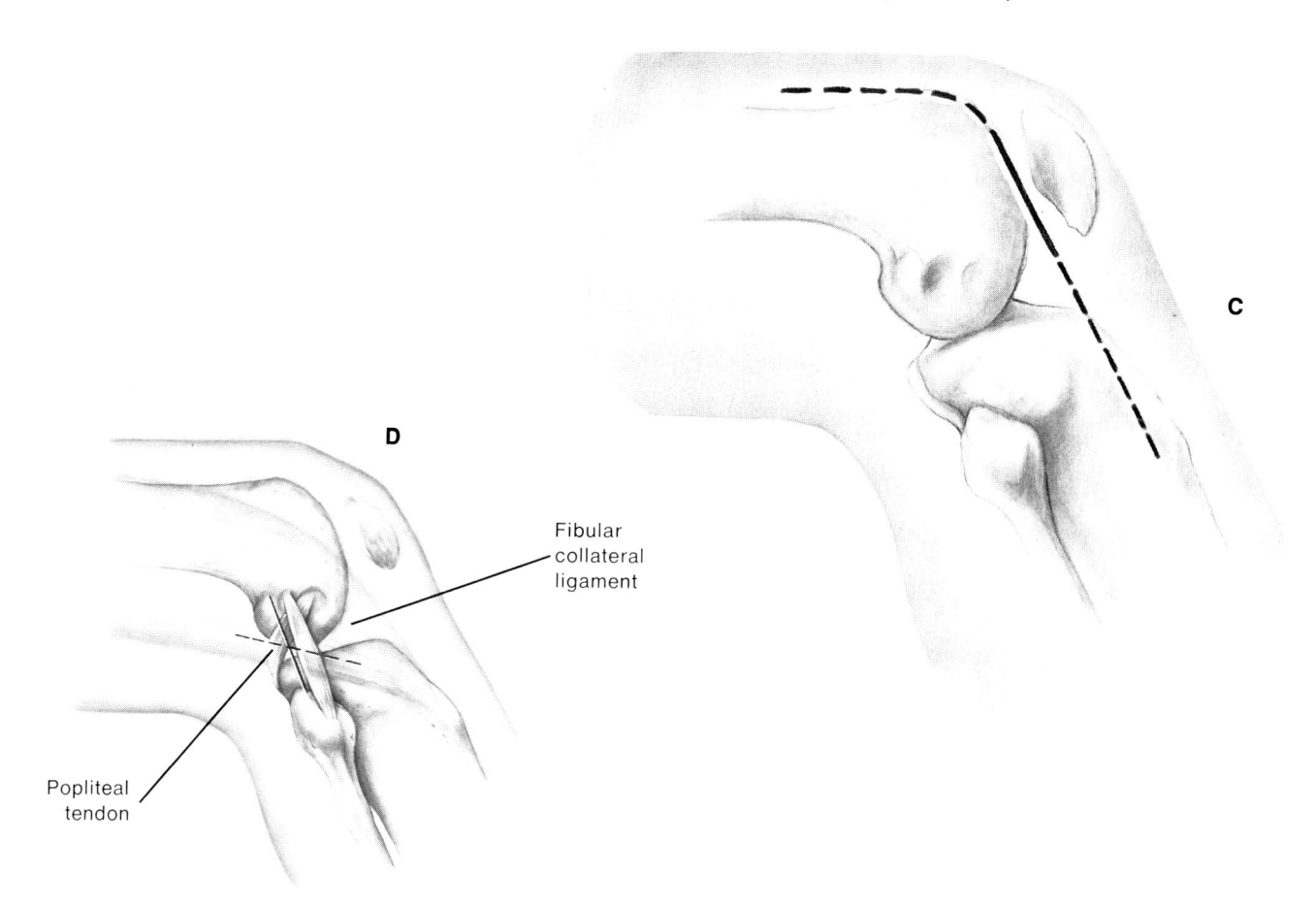

The following are procedures used in *lateral exposures.* The lateral parapatellar incision is similar to the medial and is shown as the solid line **(C)**, which is the basic approach routinely employed for lateral meniscectomy. This incision can be extended proximally and distally into the gentle curve to become the lateral utility incision similar to the medial. The skin and subcutaneous tissue can then be reflected as a single flap, exposing the underlying iliotibial tract and deep fascia.

The posterolateral approach is made through a skin incision running from the posterior aspect of the lateral femoral epicondyle to the fibular head, paralleling the posterior border of the fibular collateral ligament, as shown by the solid line **(D)**. The underlying iliotibial tract is split in line with its fibers along the joint line level, as shown by the dashed line **(D)**, and the iliotibial band is retracted proximally and distally to expose the underlying posterior capsule. The posterolateral capsule is incised vertically behind the posterior border of the fibular collateral ligament with care to protect the popliteus tendon **(D)**.

The completed posterolateral approach is shown **(E)**, illustrating the oblique course of the popliteus tendon and the posterolateral periphery of the lateral meniscus. This approach has been used for reattachment of the lateral meniscus posteriorly and removal of large posterolateral compartment loose bodies.

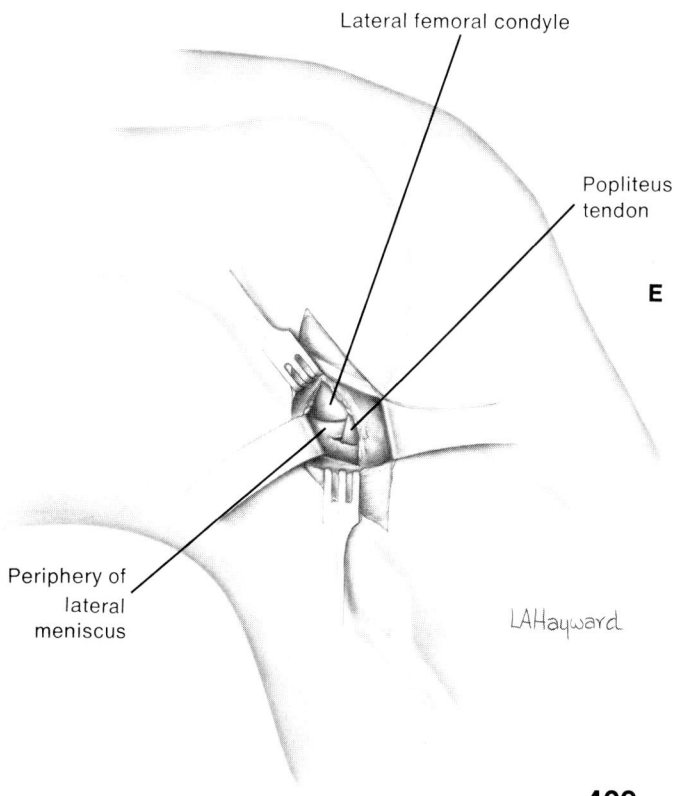

409

MEDIAL MENISCECTOMY (Plate 12-3)

GENERAL DISCUSSION. Arthrotomy of the knee for exploration and possible excision of the medial meniscus may be indicated following either an acute injury with blocking of knee motion (which is unrelieved by conservative measures) or following repetitive episodes of transient blocking and/or knee instability when signs and symptoms point to a tear of the medial meniscus as the probable diagnosis. The extent and manner of excision of the medial meniscus may vary with the nature of the derangement encountered. The most common type of tear causing significant disability is the "bucket handle" tear in which a longitudinal tear of the medial meniscus may be followed by displacement of the inner portion or concave border of the meniscus into the intercondylar notch. When this type of tear is encountered and when the remaining peripheral rim of the medial meniscus remains intact, a partial meniscectomy may be carried out by detaching and removing that portion of the meniscus which has become displaced into the intercondylar notch.

Partial meniscectomy either by open or arthroscopic techniques may be possible for other types of medial meniscus tears such as parrot beak or flap tears. For most extensive lesions, however, the traditional total or subtotal meniscectomy is required.

The diagnostic adjuncts of arthrography and arthroscopy of the knee can be helpful in demonstrating whether a meniscus lesion is present. If a lesion is present, they can facilitate precise determination of the exact type, location, and extent of the lesion so that appropriate treatment can be selected. A meniscus should not be removed unless it can be demonstrated conclusively that a lesion is present. If no pathology can be proved from the anterior incision, the posteromedial incision should be made to directly visualize suspected posterior pathology before the decision is made to proceed with definitive treatment.

DETAILS OF PROCEDURE. The basic steps in the procedure are shown schematically (**A** and **B**). Anteromedial and posteromedial approaches are utilized (**C**) (previously described under medial approaches), with the incisions placed so as to protect the infrapatellar branch of the saphenous nerve. With the posteromedial incision, the plane of dissection is established on the meniscus side of the meniscosynovial junction (**D**), and then the small meniscus knife is used to detach the posterior periphery of the meniscus around to the posterior horn attachment area (**E**).

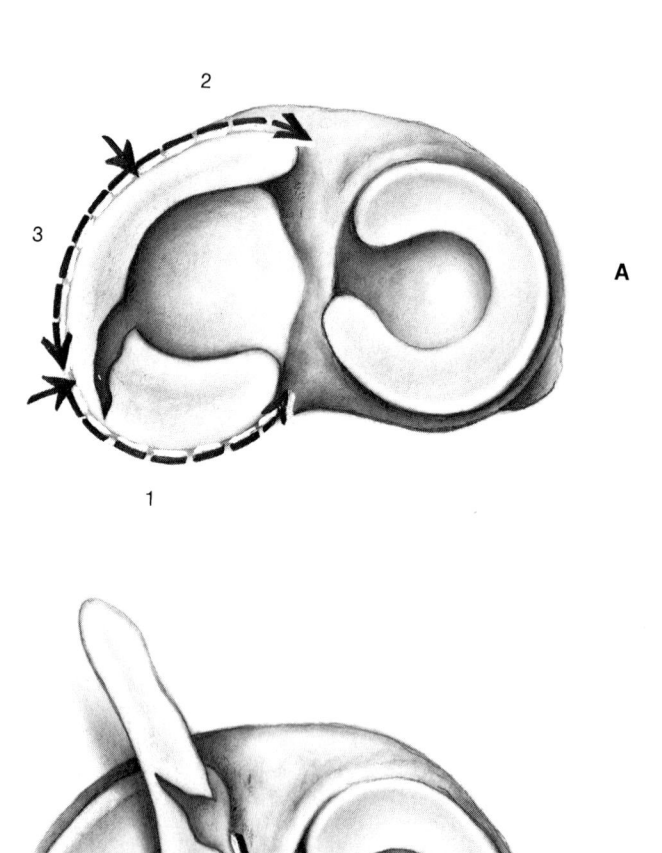

(Plate 12-3) MEDIAL MENISCECTOMY

C — Infrapatellar branch of saphenous nerve

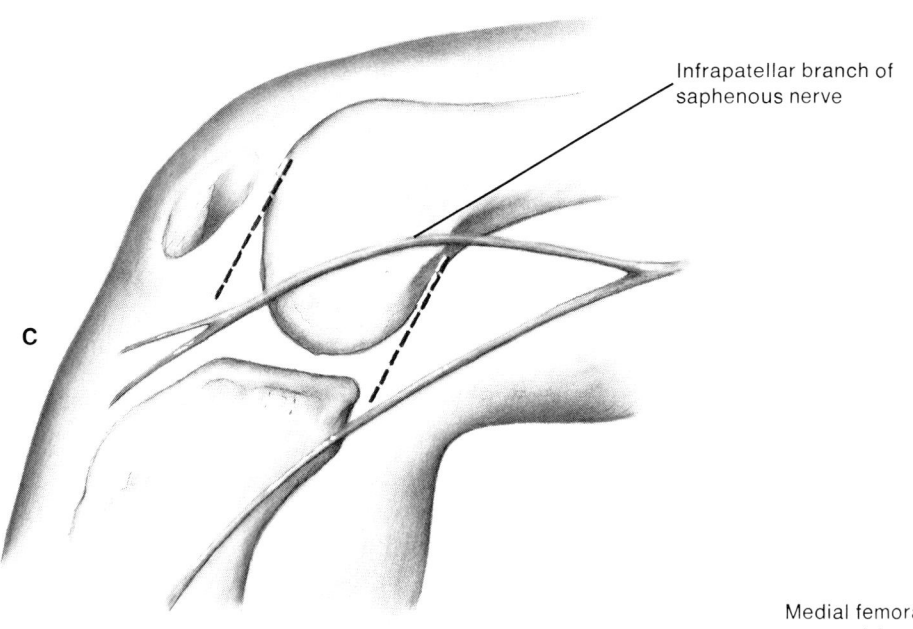

D — Medial femoral condyle; Meniscosynovial junction

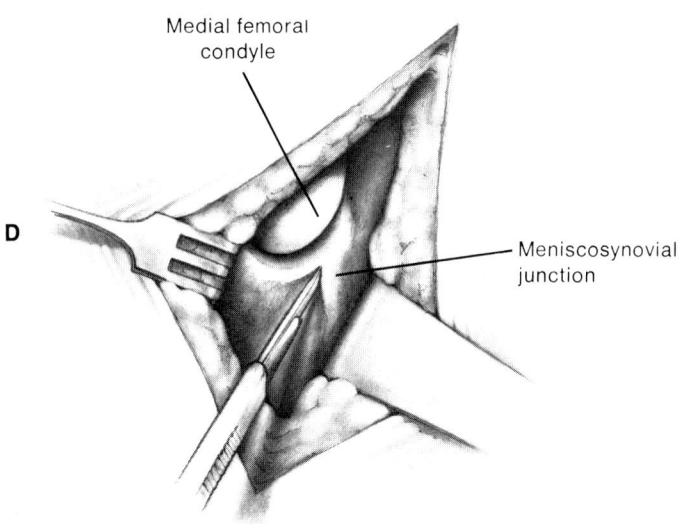

E — Small meniscus knife

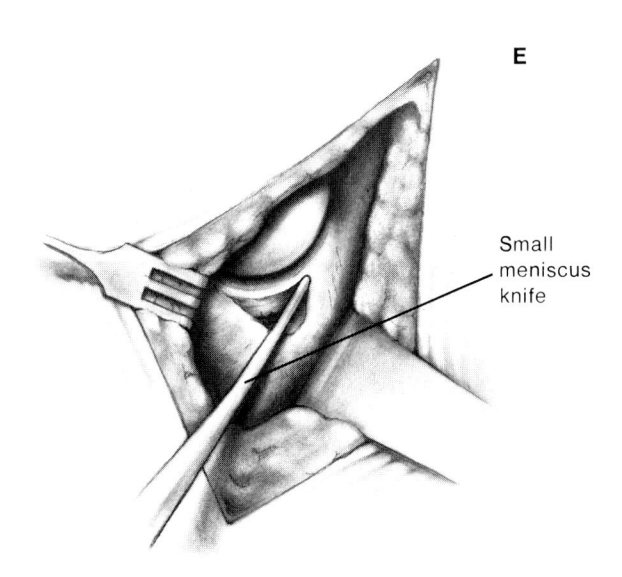

411

MEDIAL MENISCECTOMY (Plate 12-3)

Attention is then turned to the anterior incision (**F**) and the anterior periphery, and the anterior horn attachment of the medial meniscus is similarly released just inside the meniscosynovial junction. The same plane of resection is then developed for the middle third of the meniscus (**G**) and completed by using the small meniscus knife (**H**) to extend the peripheral release back to the posteromedial corner where the posterior peripheral release has previously been completed. This permits the meniscus to be displaced easily and completely into the intercondylar notch. Traction is then placed on the meniscus by means of the meniscus clamp. The small meniscus knife is passed posteriorly in the intercondylar notch along the free margin of the meniscus with care to orient the meniscus knife in the same plane as the femoral condyle and tibial spine so as to not impinge on the articular surfaces. Care is also taken to gradually move the cutting tip of the meniscus knife medially as it is carried more posteriorly in the intercondylar notch to avoid the possibility of injury to the posterior cruciate ligament. The remaining posterior horn attachment is then released by pulling the meniscus anteriorly against the cutting edge of the meniscus knife (**I**) rather than by pushing the meniscus knife posteriorly, thus minimizing the risk of inadvertent posterior penetration of the capsule with possible resultant neurovascular injury.

In younger patients the posteromedial capsular incision is closed with plicating sutures to advance and overlap the posterior capsule over the trailing edge of the medial collateral ligament, to help minimize the instability effect from the meniscectomy. In the older patient in whom return of motion is of more concern than stability, simple side-to-side closure is performed. The anterior incision is closed in layers; first the synovium and then the capsular layer. The remainder of the wounds are closed routinely, and with the knee extended, a bulky compression dressing is applied from the toes to the groin.

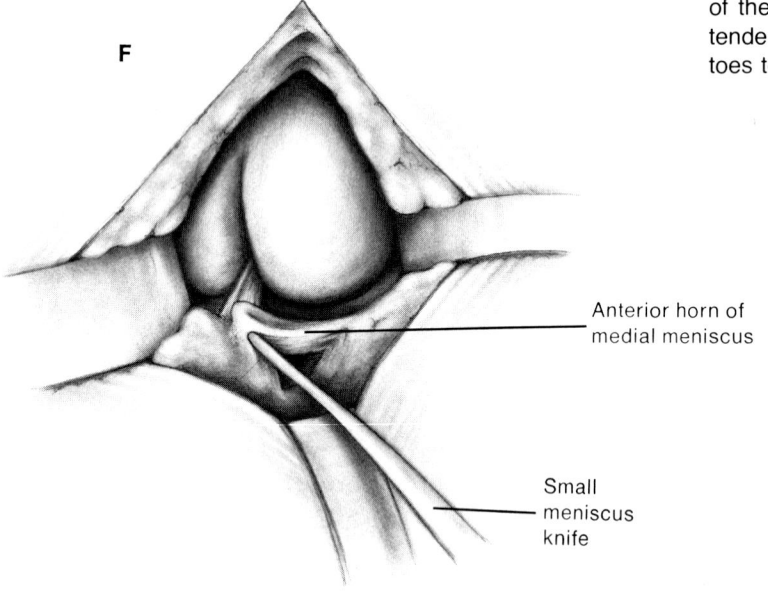

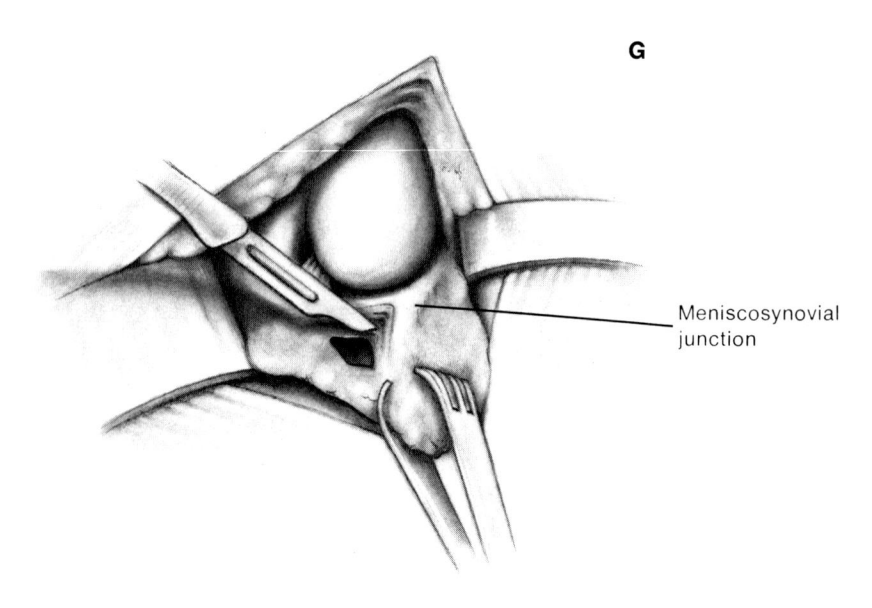

(Plate 12-3) MEDIAL MENISCECTOMY

POSTOPERATIVE MANAGEMENT. The patient is encouraged to begin quadriceps setting exercises and straight leg–raising exercises immediately after recovery from anesthesia, and is permitted out of bed on crutches with touch-down weight bearing as soon as adequate control of the leg has been achieved. Nurses are instructed to help the patient maintain the knee in as much extension as possible and to avoid placement of pillows in the popliteal area, which promotes the insidious development of increasing flexion of the knee. Some degree of intra-articular swelling almost invariably develops postoperatively, but the knee is not aspirated unless required for relief of pain that cannot be managed otherwise. At 72 hours postoperatively the bulky compression dressing is removed and a smaller dressing applied with an elastic stocking below. Active knee flexion and extension exercises are added to the quadriceps-setting and straight leg–raising exercises, and the patient is then discharged from the hospital. The same routine is continued until 2 weeks postoperatively, when the sutures are removed, progressive resistance exercises are instituted, and the remainder of the rehabilitation program is carried out.

PERIPHERAL REATTACHMENT OF MEDIAL MENISCUS (Plate 12-4)

GENERAL DISCUSSION. Peripheral reattachment of the medial meniscus may be considered when there is a vertical tear at or near the periphery, the body of the meniscus is intact, and the extent of the lesion is reasonably limited (usually one half to one third of the total circumference) and is surgically accessible without compromise of ligamentous stability. The amount of time following injury during which successful reattachment may still be accomplished is not known with certainty, but when the technique to be described is used, if the above criteria can be met, there may be no time limit.

Precise knowledge of the exact location and extent of the lesion is critical when reattachment is considered, and the diagnostic adjuncts of arthrography and arthroscopy are of great assistance in making these determinations. On the arthrogram, a vertical peripheral tear with no staining of the body of the meniscus identifies a lesion that can potentially be reattached. It must be emphasized that in the arthroscopic evaluation it is important to evaluate the meniscus with a probe under direct vision (Plate 12-1) to help locate the lesion, define its extent, and evaluate the body of the meniscus. Also, in some cases the posterior peripheral tear in the medial meniscus cannot be visualized adequately from the anterior approach even with probing, and the posteromedial approach is necessary to demonstrate the pathology (Plate 12-1).

DETAILS OF PROCEDURE. When the lesion has been shown to be a posterior peripheral tear of the medial meniscus, this region is exposed by the standard posteromedial approach described in Plate 12-2. This provides exposure of the region with the capsular bed being torn away from the remaining rim of the meniscus. The capsular bed is freshened, including excision of any portion of the meniscus rim that is still attached to the capsule, to ensure a vascular capsular bed to be reattached to the meniscus rim. The remaining peripheral rim of the medial meniscus is also trimmed to remove any tags or partial tears. Direct probing of the remaining meniscus rim is necessary to exclude horizontal cleavage lesions in the body of the meniscus.

The reattachment is accomplished by placing vertically oriented sutures first down through the capsular bed, and then up through the rim of the meniscus with fine absorbable suture material **(A)**. The first suture is placed as far posteriorly toward the posterior horn as possible, and then additional sutures are placed in the same fashion at approximately 5 mm intervals as necessary to provide reapproximation of the prepared capsular bed to the remaining rim of the meniscus **(B)**. The sutures are tagged with hemostats, and tied down at the same time after the required number of sutures have been placed. The posteromedial capsular incision is then closed in a plicating fashion, this is followed by routine skin closure. A bulky compression dressing is applied, with medial and lateral plaster splints to maintain the knee in a position of 45° flexion.

POSTOPERATIVE MANAGEMENT. The leg is immobilized with the knee at 45° flexion for a total of 4 weeks (the splint is changed when the sutures are removed 2 weeks postoperatively). This is followed by 2 additional weeks of protected motion with the patient continuing on crutches. Then a standard knee rehabilitation program is initiated beginning 6 weeks postoperatively.

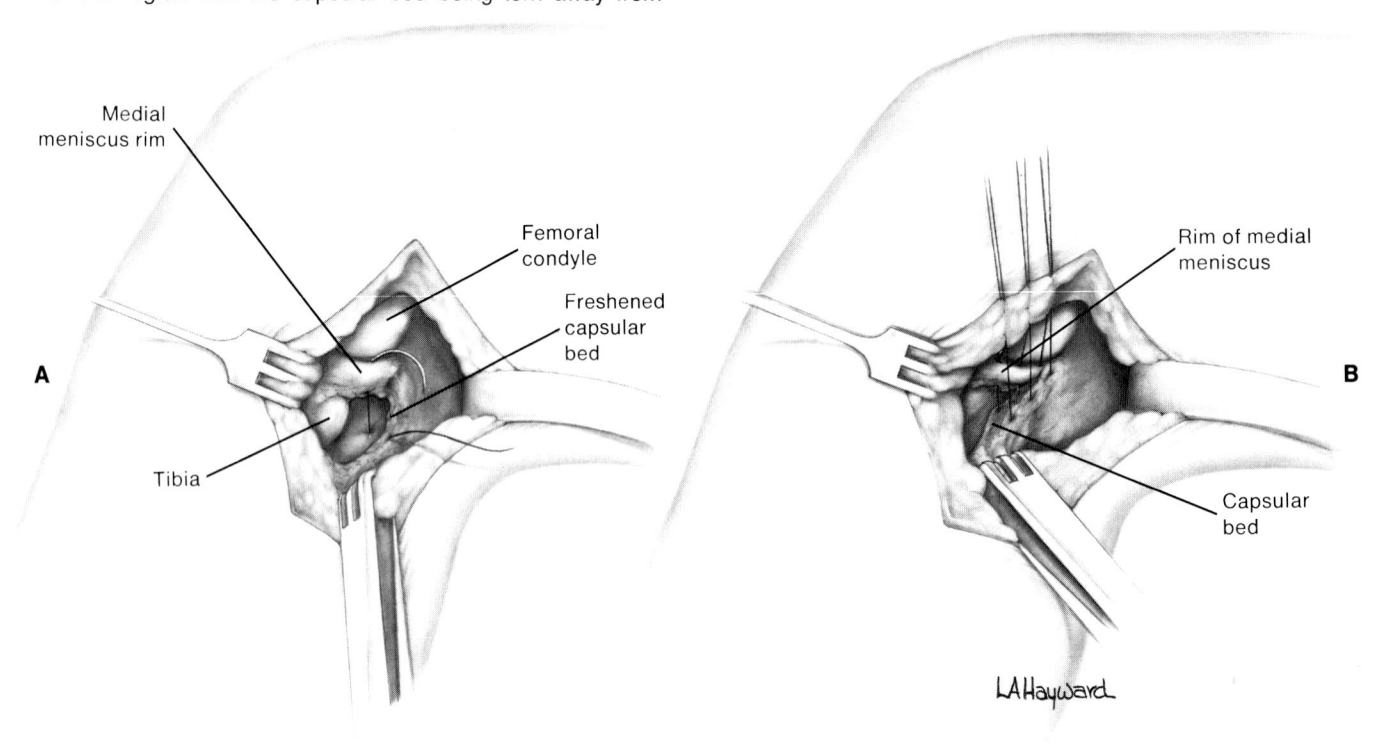

(Plate 12-5) LATERAL MENISCECTOMY

GENERAL DISCUSSION. When localization of the clinical signs and symptoms following knee injury indicates derangement of the lateral meniscus, arthrotomy and lateral meniscectomy may be indicated. Preoperative confirmation of the diagnosis by arthrography and/or arthroscopy can be helpful since tears in the posterior horn of the lateral meniscus may be difficult to visualize at arthrotomy.

Although the lateral meniscus can be excised more easily through a single incision than is possible for the medial meniscus, the popliteus tendon and lateral ligaments must be specifically considered and protected during complete excision of the lateral meniscus.

DETAILS OF PROCEDURE. The basic steps in the procedure are shown schematically (**A** and **B**). An anterolateral parapatellar approach is used, as shown in Plate 12-2, C. The capsular incision follows the skin incision, running from the superolateral pole of the patella to and just below the joint line. The synovium is carefully opened at a level above the joint line to ensure that the lateral meniscus is not inadvertently damaged. The knee joint is then explored as thoroughly as possible to confirm the presence of a lateral meniscus lesion and to identify any associated pathology. The fibularcollateral ligament and the popliteus tendon are protected by the retractor placed at the lateral joint line level.

The desired plane of resection just on the meniscus side of the meniscosynovial junction is created with a scalpel with the No. 15 blade, and this plane is then extended to the anterior horn attachment using the small meniscus knife, which helps to avoid damage to the articular surface of the tibial plateau (**C**). The same plane of resection is then established in a posterior direction (**D**), and once established, the point of resection is then carried posteriorly to and beyond the popliteus hiatus with the small meniscus knife (**E**).

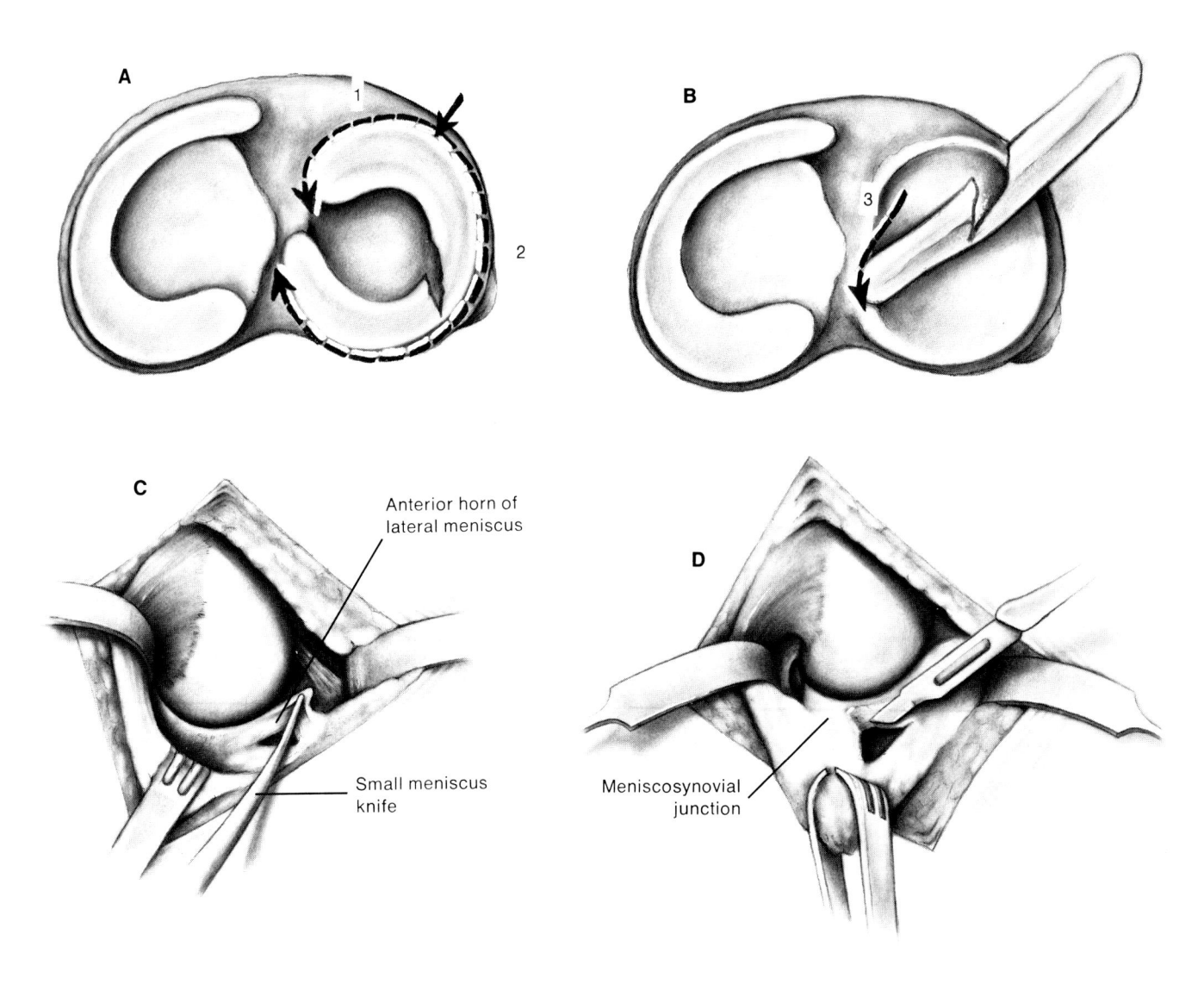

LATERAL MENISCECTOMY (Plate 12-5)

E

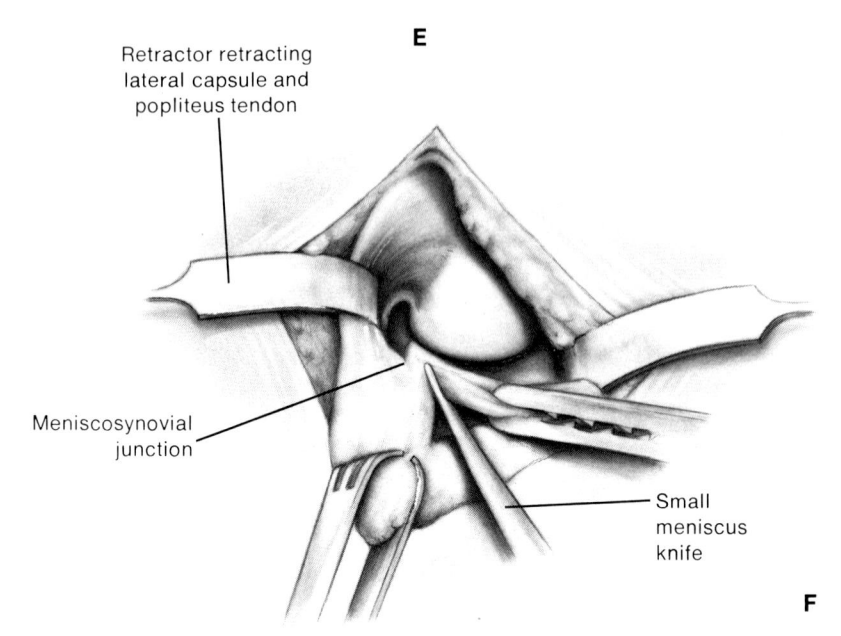

Retractor retracting lateral capsule and popliteus tendon

Meniscosynovial junction

Small meniscus knife

F

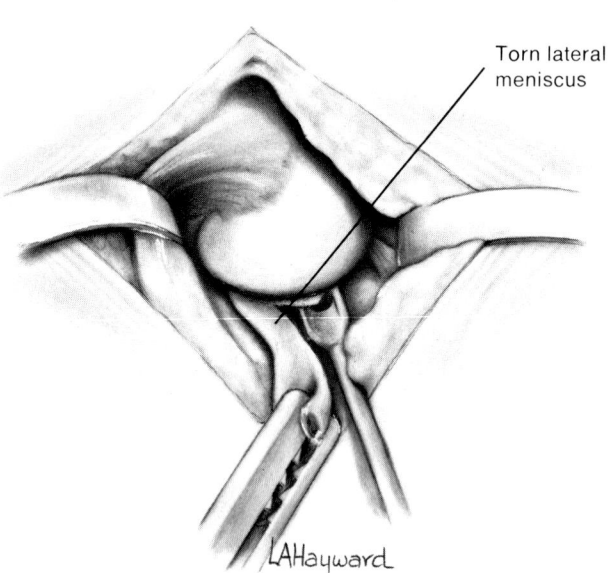

Torn lateral meniscus

When sufficient posterior peripheral release has been achieved, the meniscus can be dislocated into the intercondylar notch. The final posterior horn attachments are then released by passing the meniscus knife back through the lateral side of the intercondylar notch, along the free margin of the lateral meniscus, which is placed under traction using the meniscus clamp **(F)**. The meniscus knife is oriented in the plane of the lateral femoral condyle and the tibial spine to avoid articular damage. The cutting tip of the meniscus knife is gradually moved laterally as it is carried more posteriorly in the intercondylar notch to avoid injury to the posterior cruciate ligament. The remaining posterior horn attachment is then released by pulling the meniscus anteriorly against the cutting edge of the meniscus knife rather than by pushing the meniscus knife posteriorly, which minimizes the risk of inadvertent posterior penetration of the capsule with possible resultant neurovascular injury. The lateral compartment is reexamined, and if any small tags of the meniscus remain, they can be removed with a pituitary rongeur.

(Plate 12-6) PERIPHERAL REATTACHMENT OF LATERAL MENISCUS

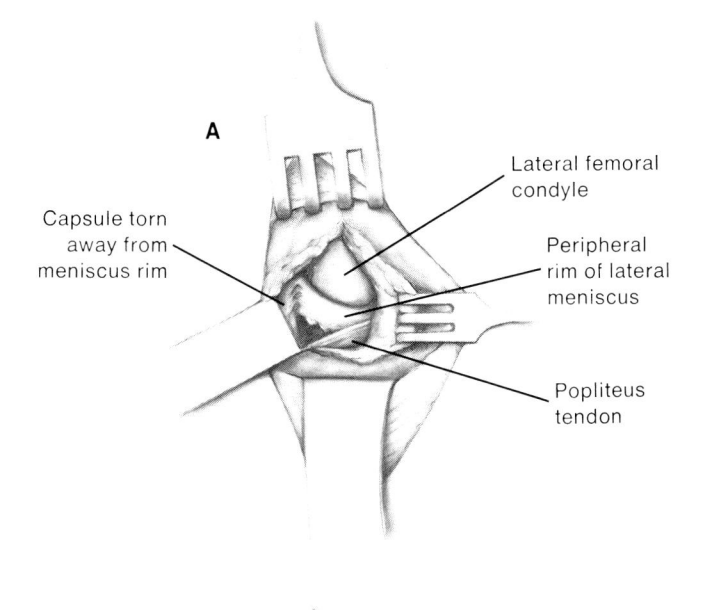

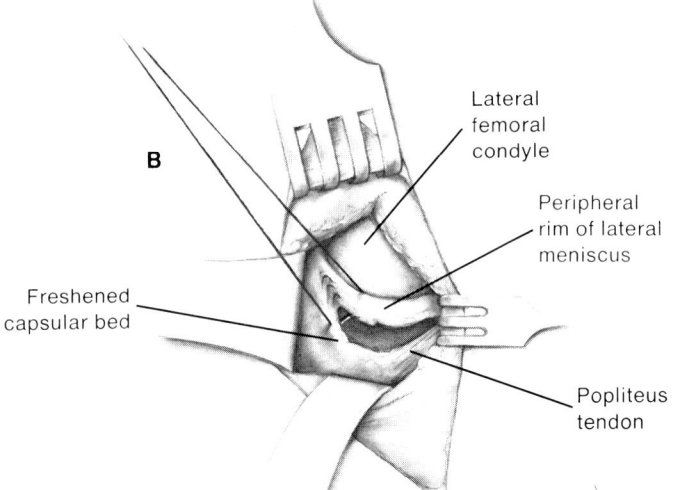

GENERAL DISCUSSION. Selected patients with posterior peripheral tears of the lateral meniscus may be considered for peripheral reattachment. The same criteria described in the discussion of reattachment of the medial meniscus (p. 414) are used.

DETAILS OF PROCEDURE. The posterolateral compartment is exposed by the posterolateral approach, as described in Plate 12-2, D and E. Normally, the capsular structures are attached to the upper half of the periphery of the lateral meniscus from the posterior border of the popliteus hiatus around to the posterior horn, as shown in Plate 12-2, E. A typical posterior peripheral tear is shown **(A)** with no capsular attachment to the meniscus from the popliteus tendon on toward the posterior horn attachment. The rim of the meniscus is probed to be certain there are no major tears into the body, and any small tags are excised. The capsular bed is then freshened back to vascular tissue, including excision of any portion of the meniscus rim still attached to the capsule. The prepared capsular bed is reattached to the rim of the meniscus by placing vertically oriented sutures of fine absorbable suture material down through the meniscus rim and then up through the corresponding area of the capsular bed **(B)**. Additional sutures are placed as necessary to provide adequate reapproximation of the capsular bed to the rim of the meniscus around to the normal location of the popliteus hiatus **(C)**. Care is taken not to suture the meniscus to the portion of the popliteus tendon that normally passes through the popliteus hiatus and normally has no attachment to the rim of the lateral meniscus. The sutures are held until all have been placed and then are tied down. The posterolateral capsule is closed in a plicating fashion.

POSTOPERATIVE MANAGEMENT. Treatment postoperatively is the same as that following peripheral reattachment of the medial meniscus (p. 414).

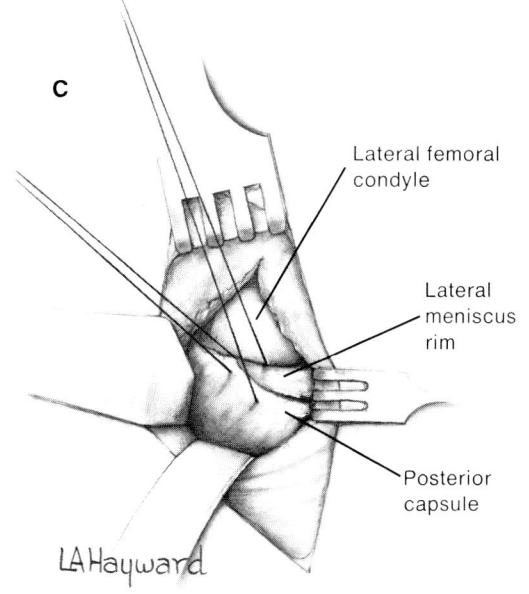

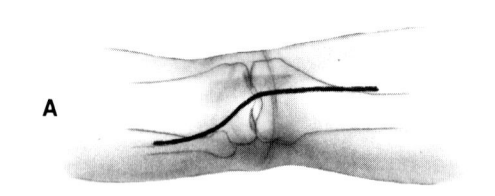

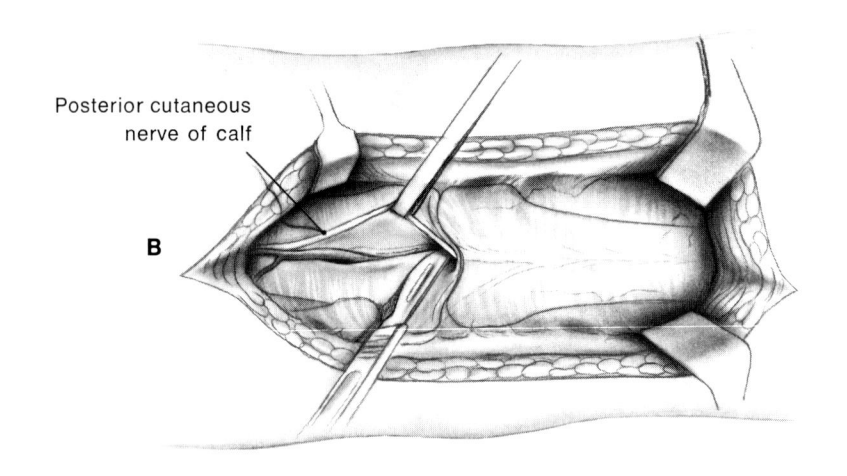

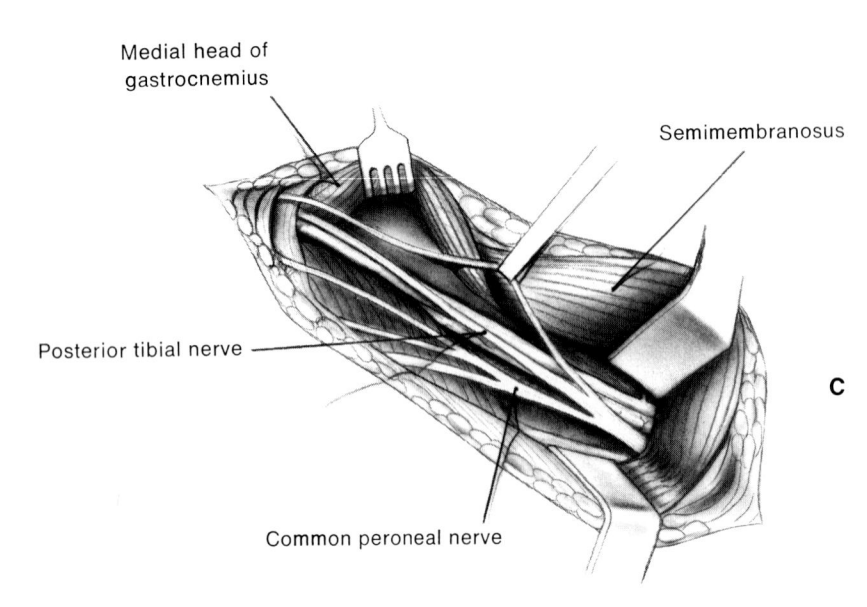

POSTERIOR CAPSULOTOMY OF KNEE (Plate 12-7)

GENERAL DISCUSSION. The posterior midline approach to the knee joint provides access to the posterior capsule of the knee joint, the posterior portions of the menisci, the posterior compartments of the knee, the posterior aspect of the femoral and tibial condyles, and the origin of the posterior cruciate ligament. This approach involves structures that, if damaged, may produce a permanent, serious disability; consequently, a thorough knowledge of the anatomy of the popliteal space is essential.

DETAILS OF PROCEDURE. The patient is positioned prone, and the knee is draped to allow free mobility of the knee during the procedure. A curvilinear incision is made from 10 cm above the knee joint to a level distal to the head of the fibula **(A)**. The iliotibial band is sectioned transversely just proximal to the lateral femoral condyle. The posterior cutaneous nerve of the calf and then the common peroneal nerve are identified, carefully mobilized, and retracted (**B** and **C**). The major popliteal vessels and nerves must be protected cautiously at all times.

(Plate 12-7) POSTERIOR CAPSULOTOMY OF KNEE

The tendon of origin of the medial head of the gastrocnemius is divided **(D)** and reflected laterally to expose the posterior capsule of the knee joint **(E)**. The capsule is opened, and the posterior structures of the knee joint are visualized **(F)**.

If posterior capsulotomy has been carried out to correct a fixed knee flexion contracture and the medial hamstrings are found to be severely contracted, they are lengthened by Z-plasty. Usually they are easily stretched out and are not a limiting factor in obtaining correction of any knee flexion contracture. The knee is passively extended without any excessive force. If the posterior cruciate ligament appears to impair extension of the knee, it is divided at its tibial attachment under direct vision. If indicated, the biceps tendon is lengthened by Z-plasty.

All divided tendons are resutured loosely with the knee extended as much as possible, and, if there is no problem with circulation, a well-padded long-leg cast is applied to maintain complete knee extension.

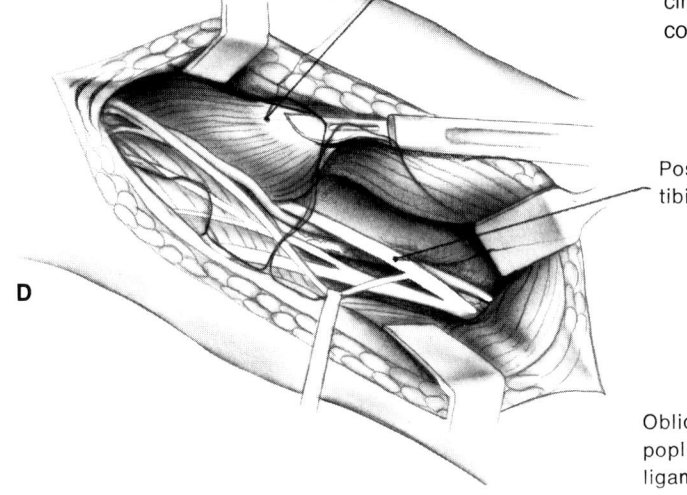

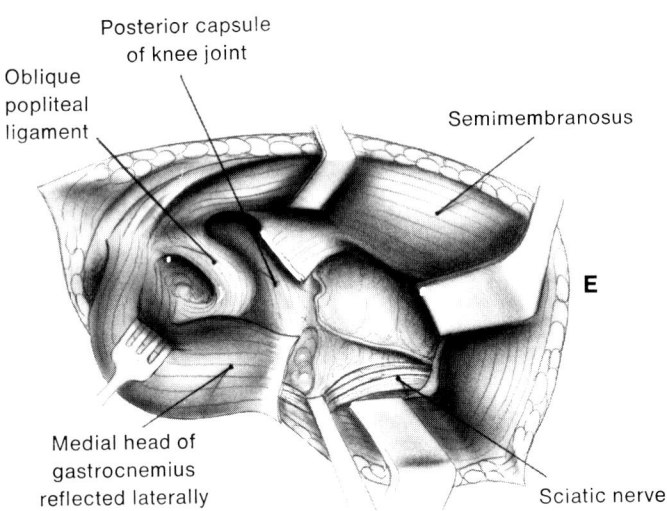

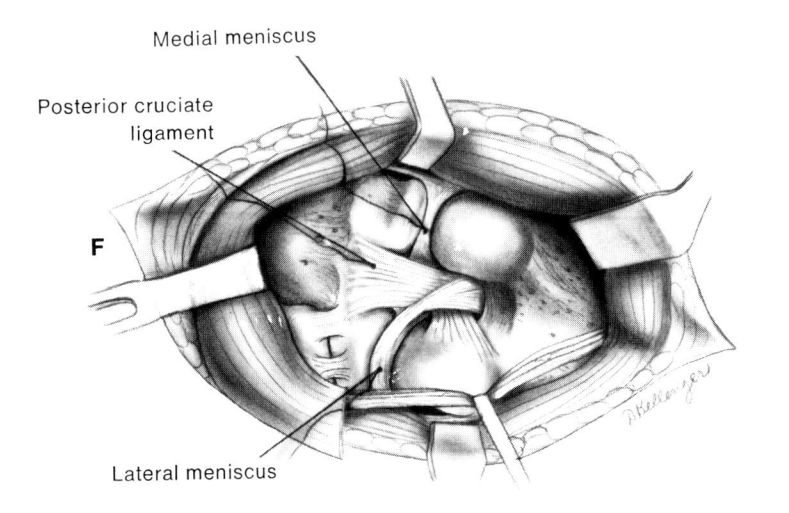

POSTOPERATIVE MANAGEMENT. The cast is bivalved 10 days postoperatively, and physical therapy is begun for knee mobility and quadriceps strengthening.

If the knee cannot be completely extended, hinges can be incorporated in the cast centered at the knee and the cast wedged postoperatively until full extension is obtained. A long-leg cast is then applied and bivalved; this is followed by the same physical therapy. A drop ring brace is used to hold the knee in full extension during walking until quadriceps redevelopment justifies the elimination of the brace. A posterior night splint is recommended for at least 6 months postoperatively.

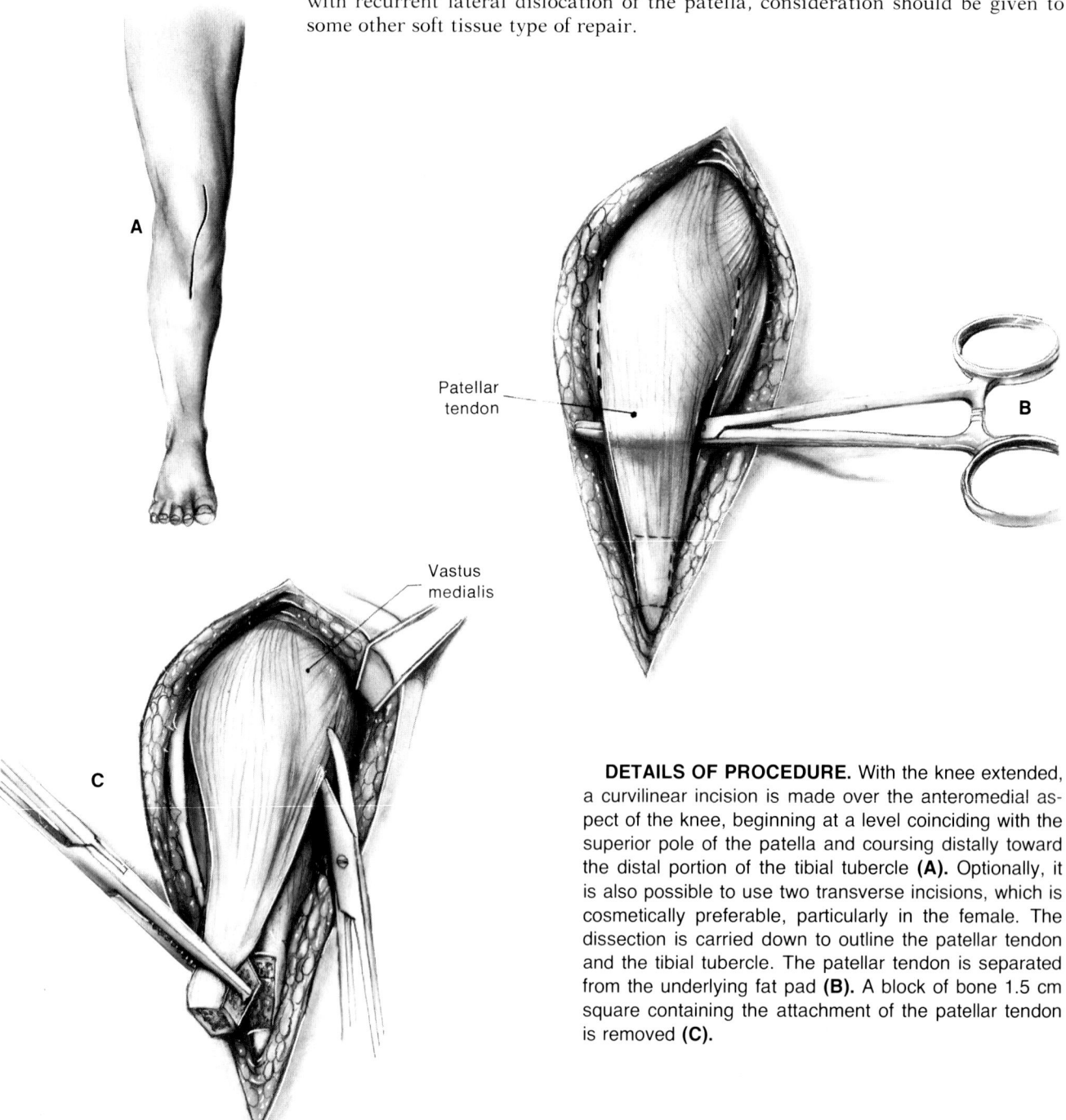

REPAIR FOR RECURRENT DISLOCATION OF PATELLA (HAUSER TECHNIQUE) (Plate 12-8)

GENERAL DISCUSSION. Dislocation of the patella almost always occurs in a lateral direction. Although some form of unusual stress to the knee may have occurred as a precipitating factor, there is often some predisposition to lateral dislocation of the patella related to laxity of the medial patellar retinaculum, flattening of the anterior prominence of the lateral femoral condyle, some degree of genu valgum, or a combination of these elements. An effective procedure to prevent recurrent lateral dislocation of the patella is transfer of the patellar tendon insertion. This is best reserved for the child whose bone growth is nearly complete to avoid the possibility of any growth disturbance at the proximal tibial epiphysis. For the younger child with recurrent lateral dislocation of the patella, consideration should be given to some other soft tissue type of repair.

DETAILS OF PROCEDURE. With the knee extended, a curvilinear incision is made over the anteromedial aspect of the knee, beginning at a level coinciding with the superior pole of the patella and coursing distally toward the distal portion of the tibial tubercle **(A)**. Optionally, it is also possible to use two transverse incisions, which is cosmetically preferable, particularly in the female. The dissection is carried down to outline the patellar tendon and the tibial tubercle. The patellar tendon is separated from the underlying fat pad **(B)**. A block of bone 1.5 cm square containing the attachment of the patellar tendon is removed **(C)**.

(Plate 12-8) REPAIR FOR RECURRENT DISLOCATION OF PATELLA (HAUSER TECHNIQUE)

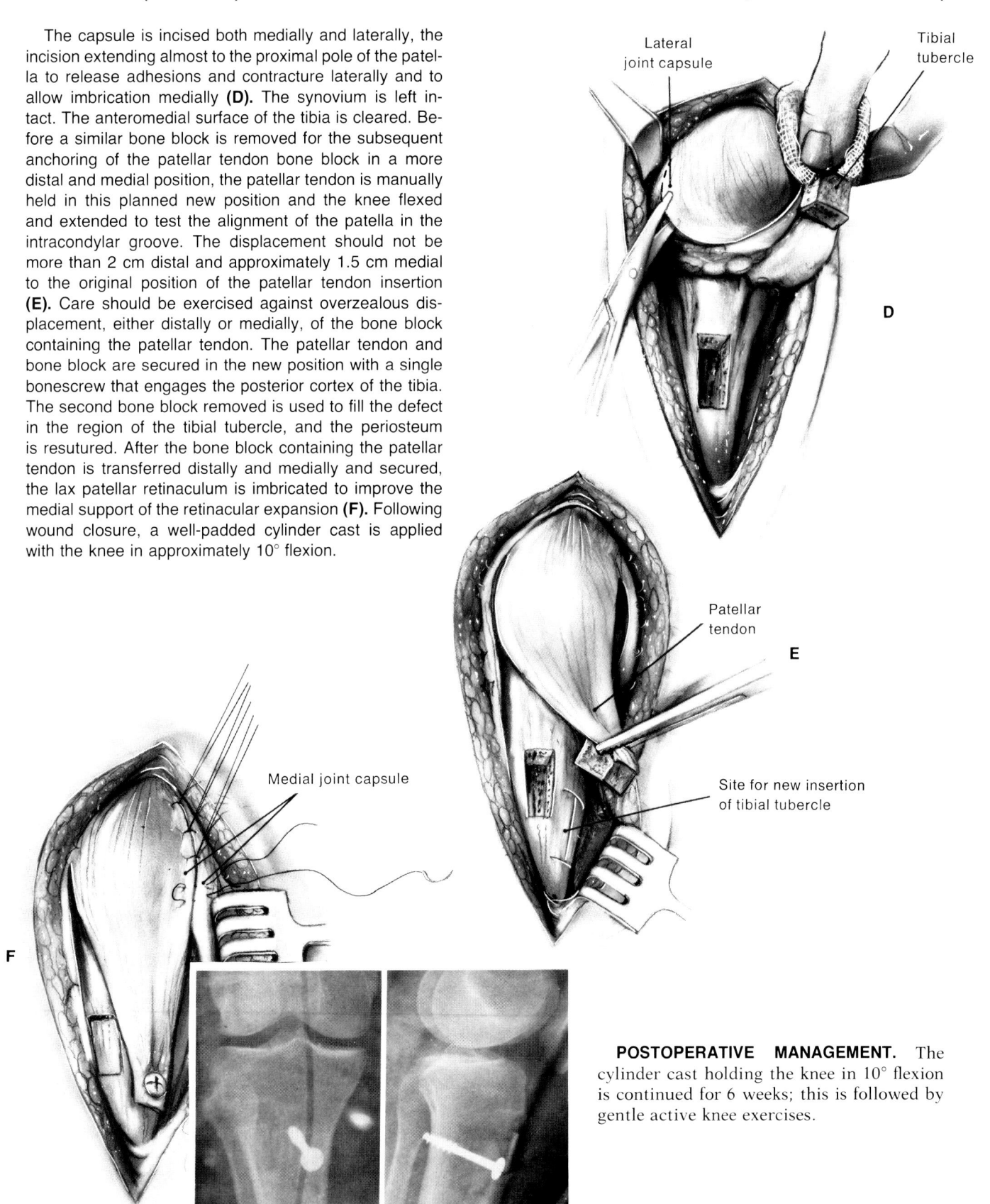

The capsule is incised both medially and laterally, the incision extending almost to the proximal pole of the patella to release adhesions and contracture laterally and to allow imbrication medially **(D)**. The synovium is left intact. The anteromedial surface of the tibia is cleared. Before a similar bone block is removed for the subsequent anchoring of the patellar tendon bone block in a more distal and medial position, the patellar tendon is manually held in this planned new position and the knee flexed and extended to test the alignment of the patella in the intracondylar groove. The displacement should not be more than 2 cm distal and approximately 1.5 cm medial to the original position of the patellar tendon insertion **(E)**. Care should be exercised against overzealous displacement, either distally or medially, of the bone block containing the patellar tendon. The patellar tendon and bone block are secured in the new position with a single bonescrew that engages the posterior cortex of the tibia. The second bone block removed is used to fill the defect in the region of the tibial tubercle, and the periosteum is resutured. After the bone block containing the patellar tendon is transferred distally and medially and secured, the lax patellar retinaculum is imbricated to improve the medial support of the retinacular expansion **(F)**. Following wound closure, a well-padded cylinder cast is applied with the knee in approximately 10° flexion.

POSTOPERATIVE MANAGEMENT. The cylinder cast holding the knee in 10° flexion is continued for 6 weeks; this is followed by gentle active knee exercises.

421

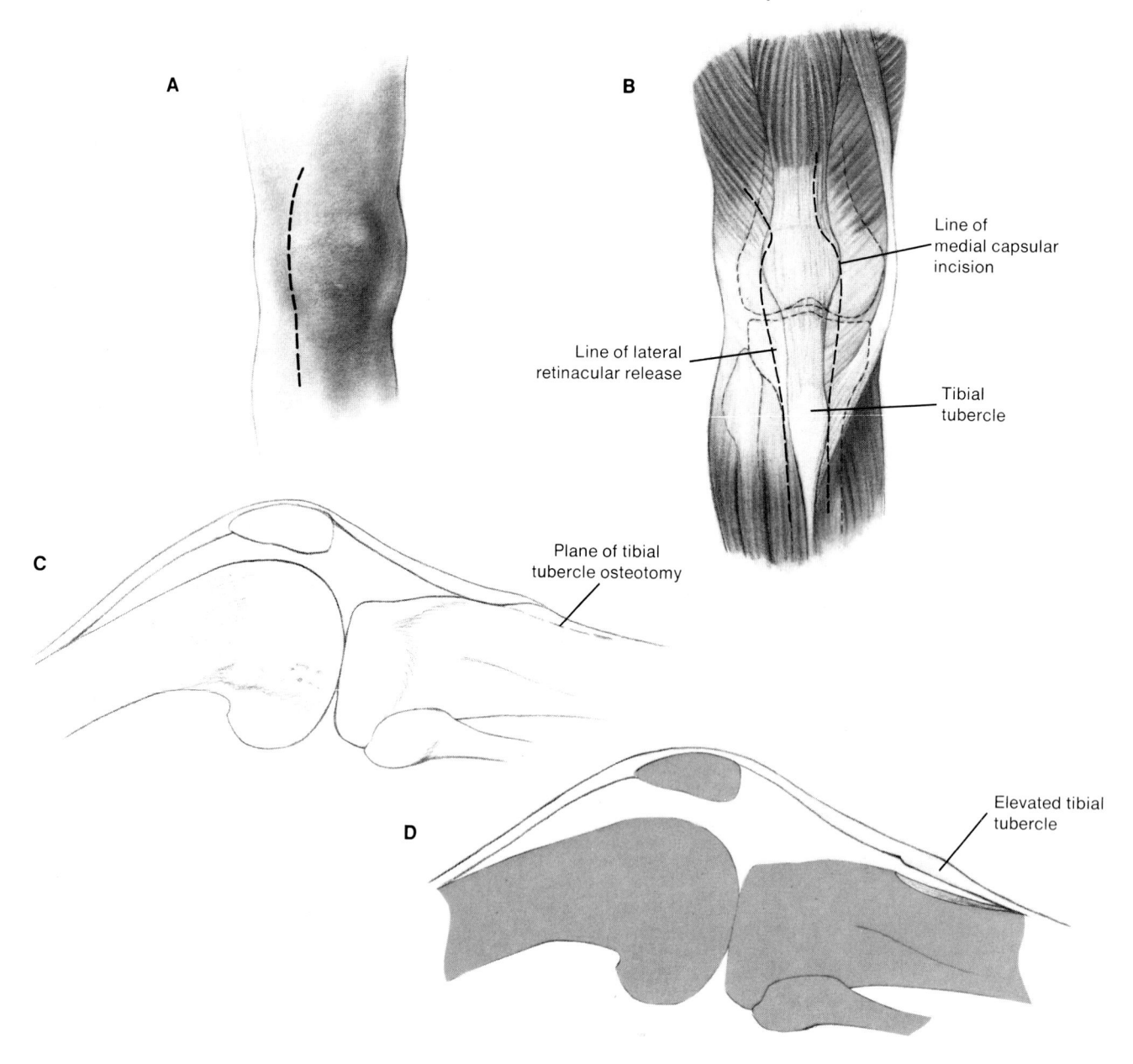

ELMSLIE-TRILLAT PATELLAR REALIGNMENT (Plate 12-9)

GENERAL DISCUSSION. An alternative method of proximal and distal extensor mechanism realignment has been attributed to Elmslie and popularized by Trillat. It can be considered for symptomatic patellofemoral instability with malalignment in the skeletally mature individual who has not responded to adequate conservative treatment.

DETAILS OF PROCEDURE. The knee is exposed through a long lateral parapatellar incision **(A)**. The plane of the prepatellar bursa is used to dissect the overlying soft tissues across the patella to the medial parapatellar region to provide adequate exposure for the procedure. A lateral retinacular release is carried out from the tibial tubercle up to and including the portion of the vastus lateralis attaching to the superolateral pole of the patella. A medial parapatellar capsular incision is made and extended proximally across the insertion of the vastus medialis and curved proximally in line with the fibers of the quadriceps tendon. The medial incision is also carried distally down to the tibial tubercle. The medial and lateral incisions are continued distally through the periosteum of the anterior tibia **(B)**. The patella is everted, and chondroplasty performed if there is significant chondromalacia of the patella.

The tibial tubercle is then osteotomized in a skiving fashion, becoming more and more superficial as it passes distally, eventually breaking through the cortex so that only a periosteal hinge remains intact distally. This step is shown schematically **(C and D)**. A sterile long-armed goniometer is used to accurately measure the correction, and the tibial

(Plate 12-9) ELMSLIE-TRILLAT PATELLAR REALIGNMENT

tubercle is hinged medially on its intact periosteal distal attachment so that the "Q-angle" is corrected down to the normal range of between 5° and 10° (**F** and **G**). A drill bit is used to hold the transferred tubercle in the selected position, and the knee is flexed well beyond 90° to be certain that the patellar tracking is satisfactory and that the tension is not excessive. If the selected position is not satisfactory, it can be altered before fixation. If the selected position is satisfactory, the transferred tubercle is then fixed with a cancellous lag screw (**E**).

The vastus medialis and medial capsule are then advanced laterally across the superomedial pole of the patella and distal quadriceps tendon, and plicating sutures are used (**H**). The knee is repeatedly flexed well beyond 90° to be certain that excessive tension is not being created. The tourniquet is then deflated and further hemostasis secured. The wound is closed over suction drainage and a standard sterile dressings and massive compression wrap with plaster shell are applied with the knee flexed 5°.

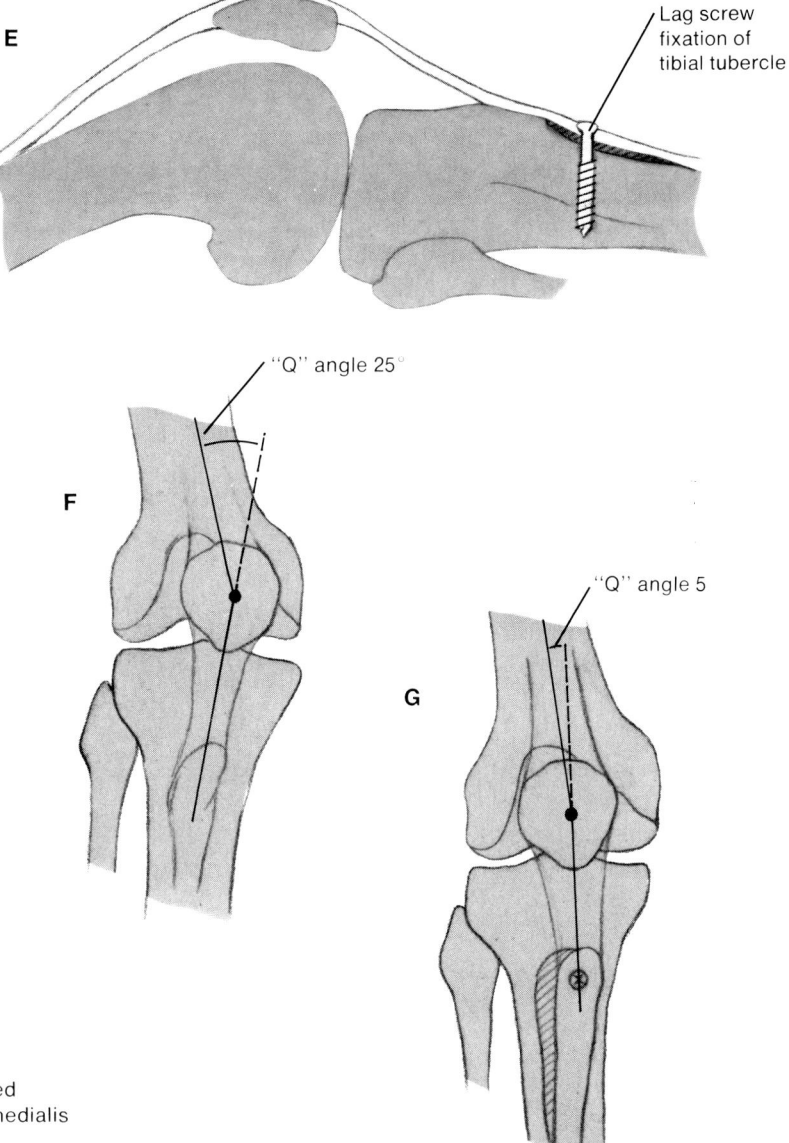

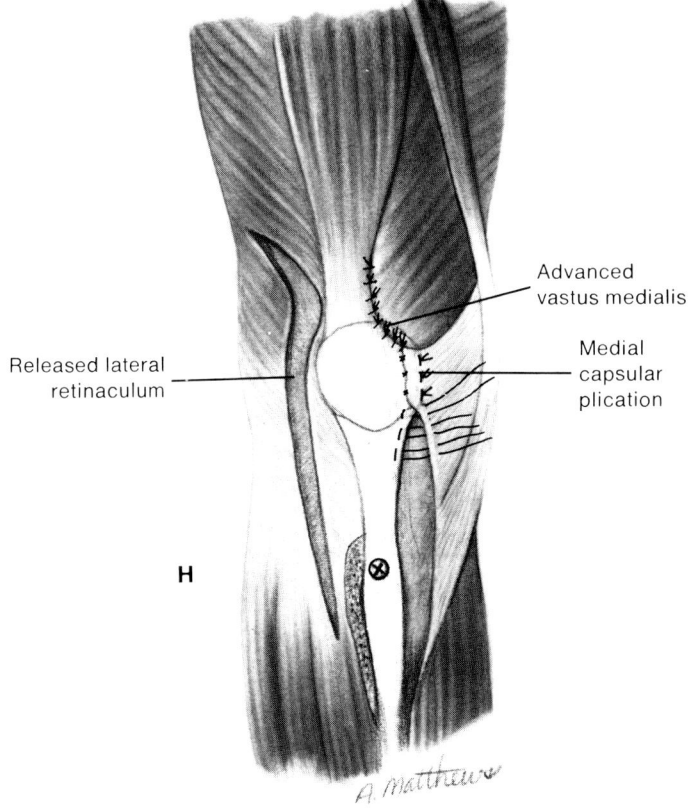

POSTOPERATIVE MANAGEMENT. At 48 hours the compression dressing is removed, as well as the suction drainage, and a removable knee extension splint applied. Intermittent passive flexion exercises with a knee sling exerciser are initiated, and the patient remains hospitalized until capable of flexing to 90°, which normally occurs by the fifth to seventh postoperative day. If adequate flexion is not occurring, gentle manipulation under anesthesia is carried out between 7 and 10 days postoperatively. Intermittent passive flexion exercises are continued throughout the first 6 weeks following surgery, with isometric quadriceps setting exercises beginning at 3 weeks, and straight leg raising at 4 weeks following surgery. Vigorous rehabilitation is initiated 6 weeks following surgery, after roentgenograms have demonstrated the occurrence of adequate healing of the transferred tibial tubercle.

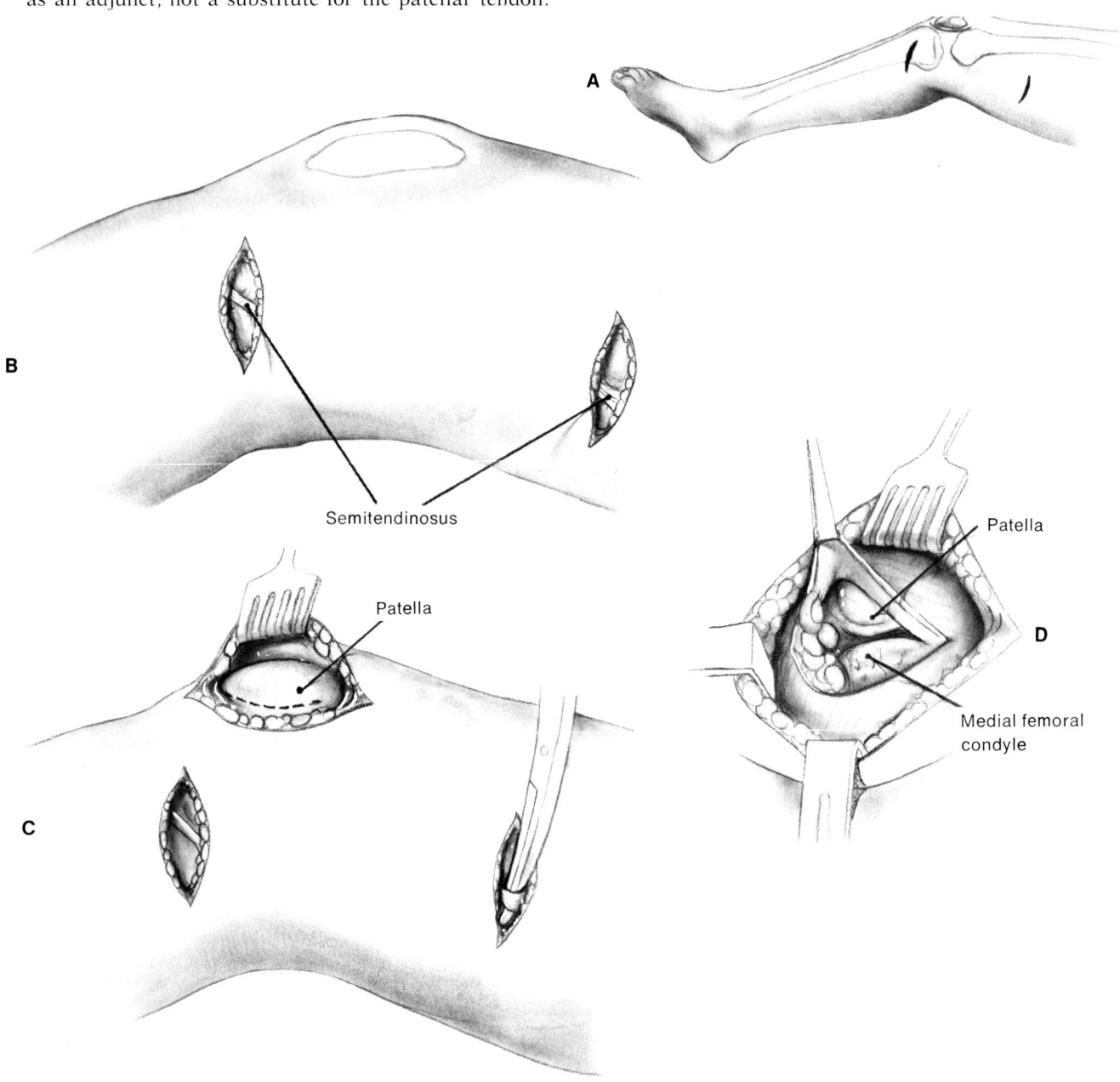

REPAIR FOR RECURRENT DISLOCATION OF PATELLA (SEMITENDINOSUS TENODESIS) (Plate 12-10)

GENERAL DISCUSSION. The repair described here for recurrent dislocation of the patella offers potential advantages compared with other types of repair. Specifically, this procedure, if correctly carried out, uses tenodesis with an expendable tendon to retain the patella in its normal position within the intracondylar groove of the femur without introducing and tilting or rotational change (inherent in certain other reparative procedures) that may accelerate degenerative changes within the patellofemoral compartment in subsequent years.

This procedure is suitable for recurrent dislocation of the patella before or after epiphyseal closure. Tenodesis with the semitendinosus tendon should be considered as an adjunct, not a substitute for the patellar tendon.

DETAILS OF PROCEDURE. The semitendinosus tendon is isolated at its insertion into the tibia and then at a point 12 to 14 cm proximal to its insertion. This may be accomplished through two separate incisions (**A** and **B**). The semitendinosus tendon is then divided 12 to 14 cm proximal to its insertion, its insertion into the tibia left intact (**C**). A medial parapatellar incision is made and extended down through the fascia approximately 1 cm from the medial border of the patella. A 3 cm longitudinal opening in the capsule is made along the medial border of the patella to permit visualization of the articular surface of the patella (**C** and **D**).

(Plate 12-10) REPAIR FOR RECURRENT DISLOCATION OF PATELLA (SEMITENDINOSUS TENODESIS)

A ³⁄₁₆-inch (0.48 cm) longitudinal hole is drilled from distal to proximal through the medial half of the patella with specific care to avoid any alteration of the articular surface of the patella **(E)**.

The loose end of the semitendinosus tendon is drawn distally into the incision over its insertion into the tibia, and it is then passed under the gracilis and sartorius toward the inferior and medial aspect of the patella and passed from distal to proximal through the hole in the medial portion of the patella **(F)**. As the patella is retained in normal position in the intracondylar groove, the loose end of the semitendinosus tendon is held under moderate tension and sutured back to itself or along the medial border of the patella as illustrated **(G)**.

Following closure of all wounds, a well-padded cylinder cast is applied with the knee in 0° to 10° flexion.

POSTOPERATIVE MANAGEMENT. Skin sutures may be removed through a window in the cast 10 to 14 days postoperatively. Protective plaster immobilization with the cylinder cast is continued for 6 weeks after surgery. Gradual active knee motion is encouraged in the following weeks. Return to normal activities should be possible by 3 months postoperatively.

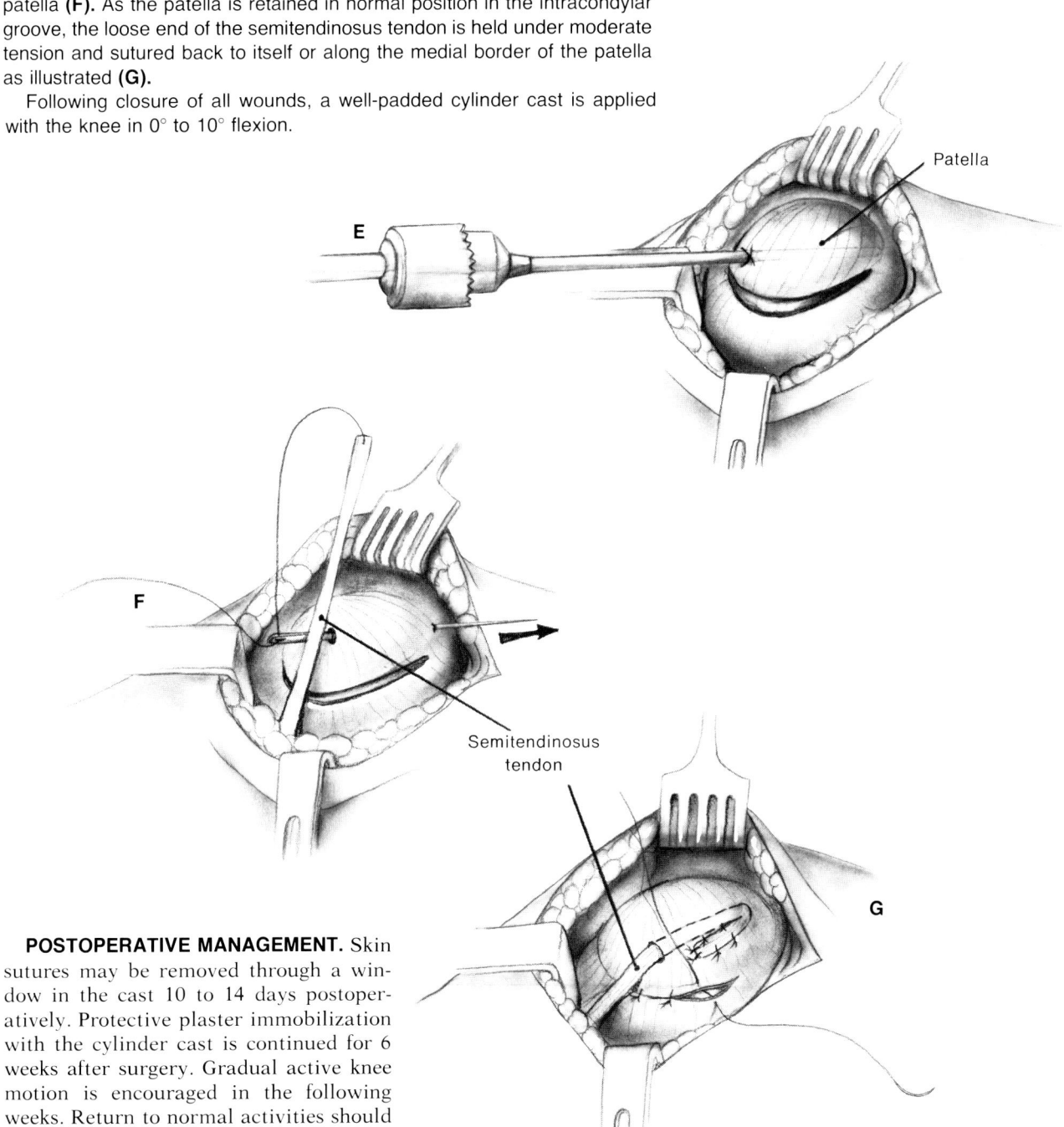

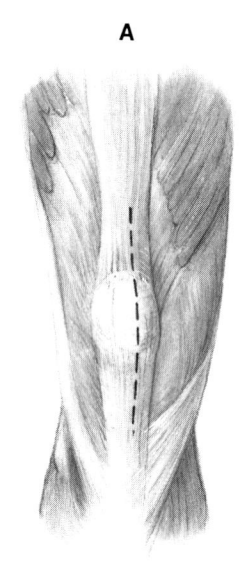

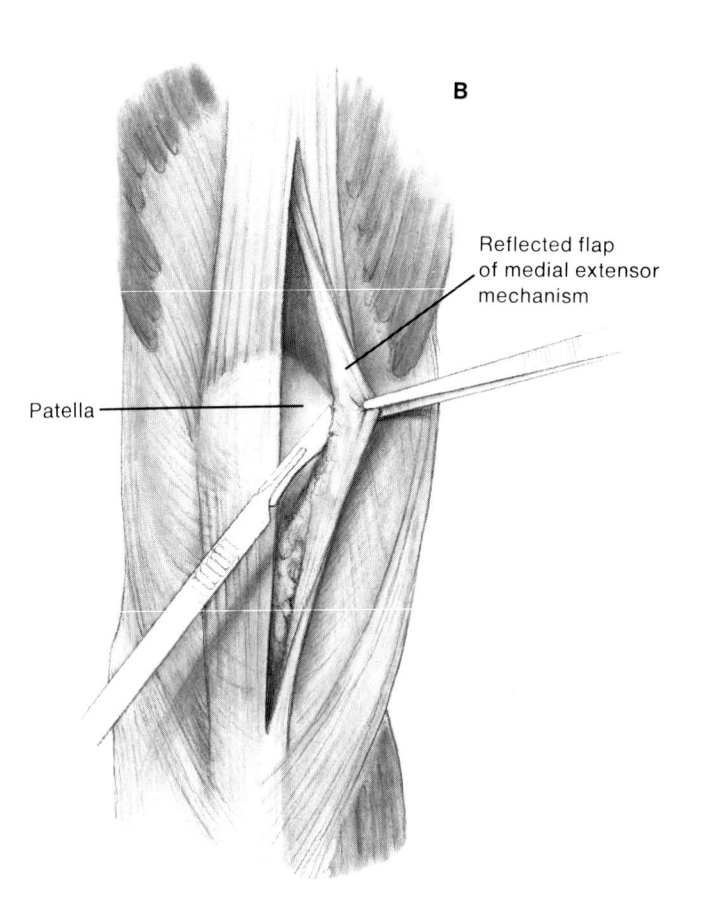

REPAIR FOR RECURRENT DISLOCATION OF PATELLA (INSALL TECHNIQUE) (Plate 12-11)

GENERAL DISCUSSION. Another soft tissue repair that is suitable for the skeletally immature child is the procedure described by Insall. It provides patellar stabilization while avoiding damage to the epiphyseal plates and can be a consideration for the younger child with recurrent dislocations of the patella.

DETAILS OF PROCEDURE. A midline, longitudinal incision or a long, lateral parapatellar longitudinal skin incision is made extending from well above the patella to slightly below the tibial tubercle. The subcutaneous tissues are dissected in the plane of the prepatellar bursa to expose the anterior aspect of the patella, the quadriceps and patellar tendons, and the medial and lateral retinaculum. A vertical incision is made through the quadriceps tendon in line with its fibers (separating the medial one third from the lateral two thirds of the tendon). The same line of incision is carried distally down the anterior surface of the patella and continues through the patellar tendon in line with its fibers to the level of the tibial tubercle **(A)**. A medial soft tissue flap is created by carefully dissecting the prepatellar tissue free from the anterior surface of the patella **(B)** so that the entire medial

426

(Plate 12-11) REPAIR FOR RECURRENT DISLOCATION OF PATELLA (INSALL TECHNIQUE)

flap can be advanced laterally over the remaining portion of the extensor mechanism **(C)**. A lateral retinacular release is then carried out from the level of the tibial tubercle to the vastus lateralis **(C)**. The procedure is completed by advancing the prepared medial soft tissue envelope laterally over the remainder of the extensor mechanism, securing the advancement with plicating sutures **(D)**. It is important that the medial advancement not be excessive, and the knee is repeatedly flexed beyond 90° to be certain that the tension is not too great. The tourniquet is released prior to wound closure and further hemostasis secured. The wound is closed over suction drainage. A well-padded compression dressing is applied to maintain the knee in 5° to 10° flexion.

POSTOPERATIVE MANAGEMENT. The postoperative management is the same as that described for the Elmslie-Trillat patellar realignment procedure (p. 423).

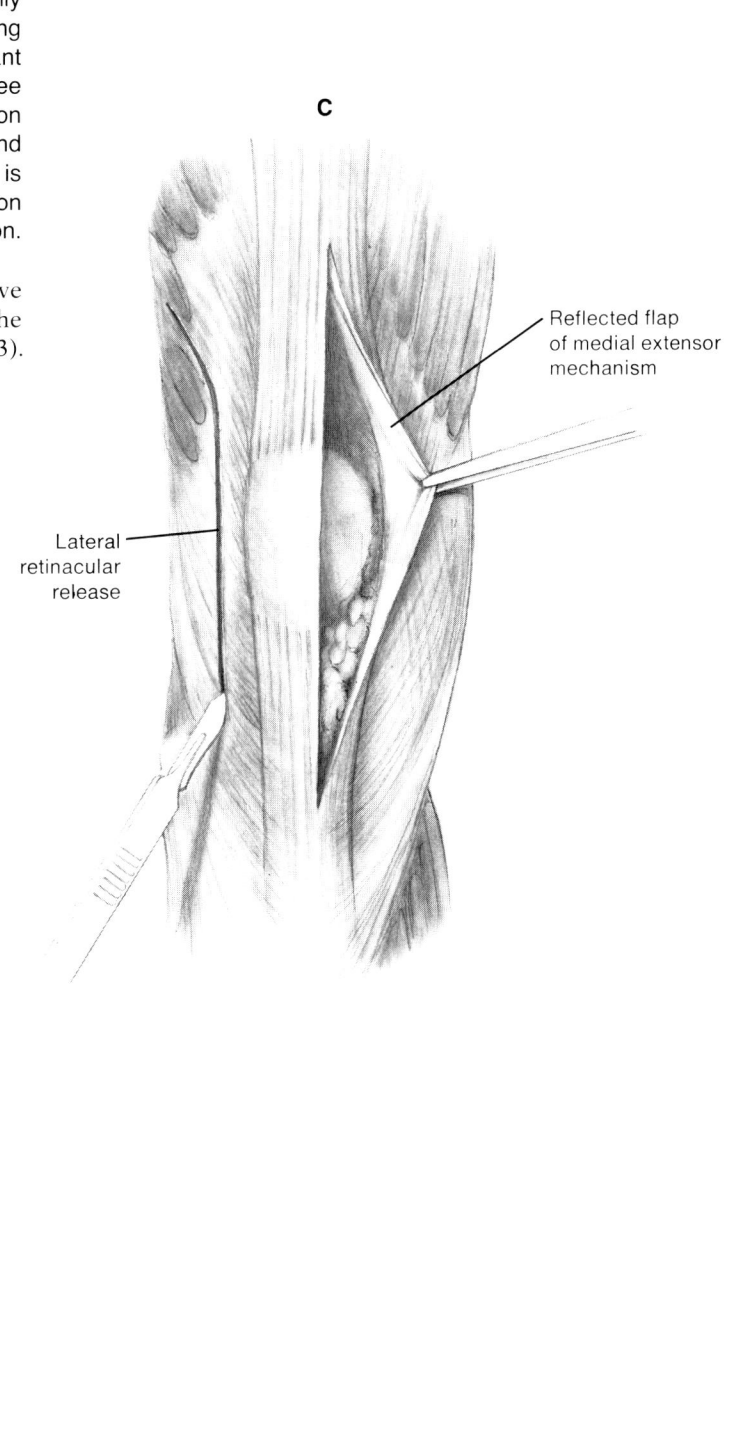

PATELLAR ADVANCEMENT (Plate 12-12)

GENERAL DISCUSSION. Advancement of the patella may be helpful if the patellar tendon has become elongated so the patella lies in a position more proximal than normal and if the knee has full passive extension but lacks ability for complete active extension. Patellar advancement should not be carried out if there is any uncorrected flexion contracture of the knee.

DETAILS OF PROCEDURE. The incision is made beginning anteromedially approximately 10 cm proximal to the knee joint and extended distally along the medial border of the patella and the patellar tendon **(A)**. The dissection is continued to outline the medial and lateral borders of the patellar tendon throughout its length from the inferior pole of the patella to the tibial tuberosity. The patellar tendon is freed from all soft tissue attachments, but the knee joint is not entered **(B)**. The distal end of the patellar tendon is freed from the tibial tuberosity **(C)** by either shaving off a thin layer of bone with a sharp osteotome or by sharp dissection with a scalpel.

The patella is mobilized by dividing the aponeurosis of the vastus medialis and vastus lateralis until the patellar tendon can be drawn distally to the desired level in the intracondylar groove of the femur. An osteoperiosteal flap, or trapdoor, is made in the anterior crest of the tibia as wide as the patellar tendon. The distal end of the patellar tendon is inserted beneath the osteoperiosteal flap and anchored under adequate tension to retain the patella in the desired position **(D)**. Interrupted sutures are placed on both sides of the repositioned patellar tendon and the previously divided patellar retinaculum on each side of the patella. A bone screw may be used to supplement the fixation.

Following wound closure, a well-padded cylinder cast is applied with the knee in 5° to 10° flexion.

POSTOPERATIVE MANAGEMENT. As soon as wound discomfort subsides, weight bearing in the cast is allowed. The external plaster immobilization is continued for 8 weeks postoperatively. Active and gentle passive exercises are continued thereafter until full mobility and quadriceps control of the knee have been obtained.

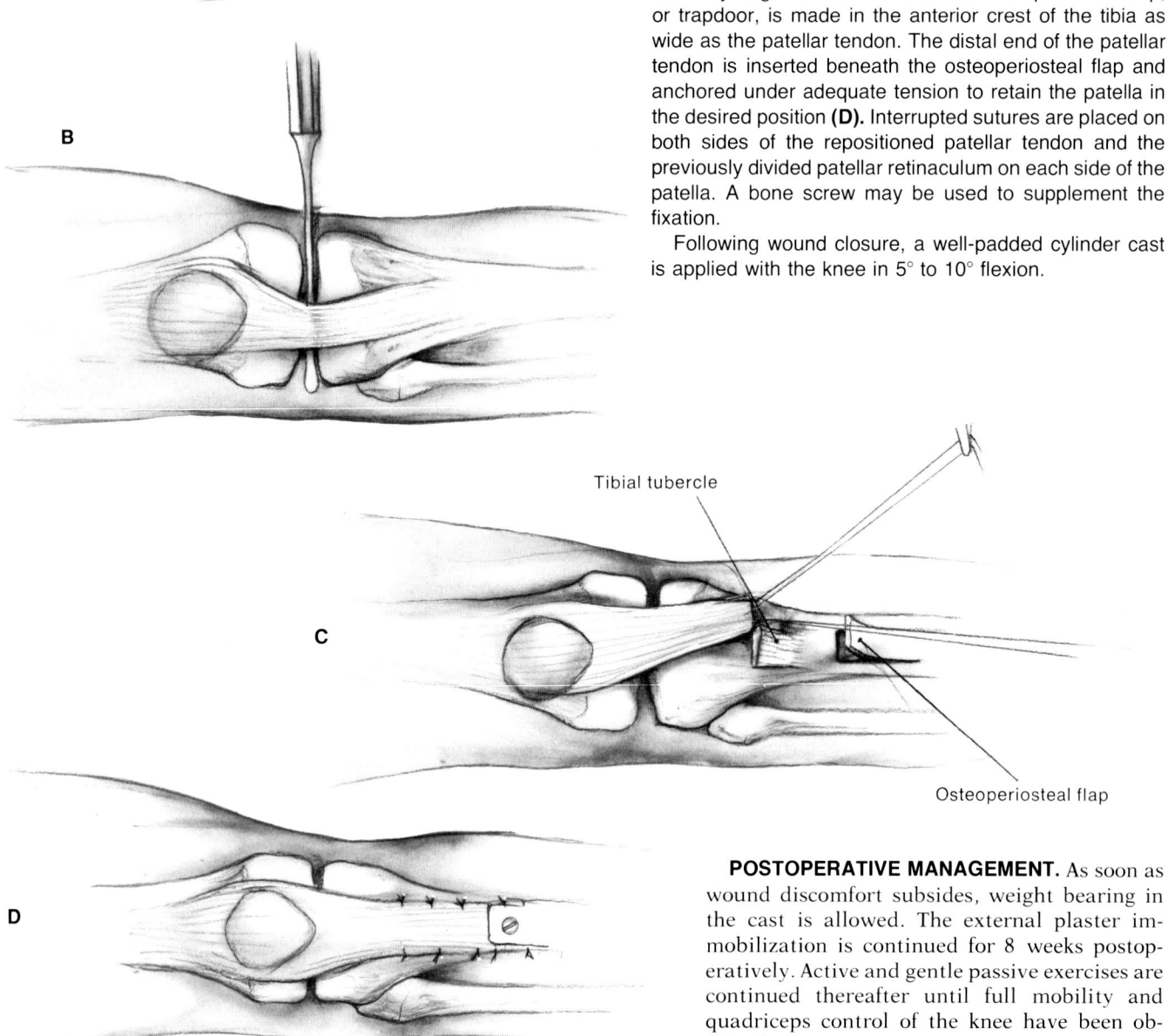

(Plate 12-13) REPAIR OF FRACTURE OF PATELLA

GENERAL DISCUSSION. If the patella is severely fragmented and separated following fracture, there may be no alternative except to remove all fragments of the patella; but if a proximal fragment constituting 50% or more of the patella remains intact, it should be preserved and the patellar tendon securely sutured to the remaining fragment. This should be considered particularly in young people. Similarly, if a distal fragment constituting 50% or more of the patella remains intact, the small proximal fragment should be excised, with repair of the quadriceps tendon to the remaining fragment of patella. Although the possibility of arthritis in the patellofemoral compartment remains, excision of the remaining portion of the patella can be carried out subsequently if this should become necessary.

DETAILS OF PROCEDURE. The fracture is exposed through a lateral parapatellar skin incision and a transverse incision through the fracture site **(A)**. The joint should be cleared of all loose fragments of bone and cartilage. The edges of the capsule and the patellar tendon are trimmed after excising the comminuted fragments **(A)**. If possible, a small fragment of the distal and anterior portion of the patella should be left in continuity with the patellar tendon to help in subsequently anchoring the patellar tendon to the intact proximal portion of the patella.

A

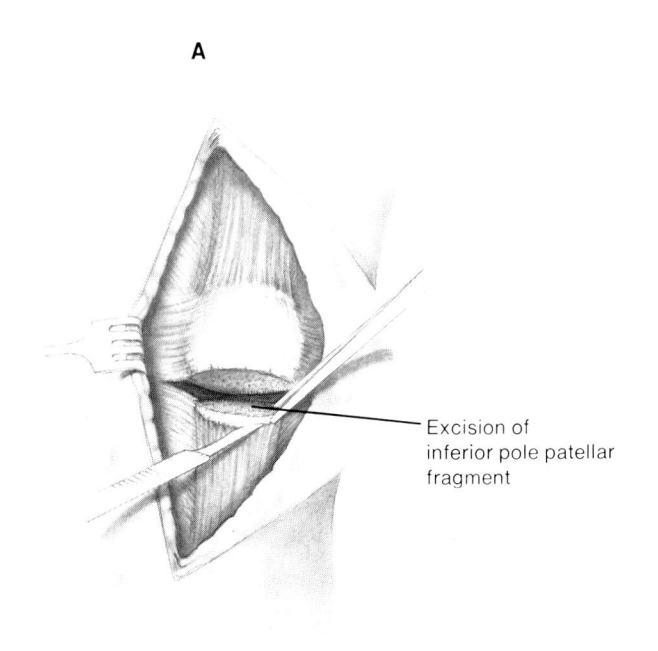

Excision of inferior pole patellar fragment

B

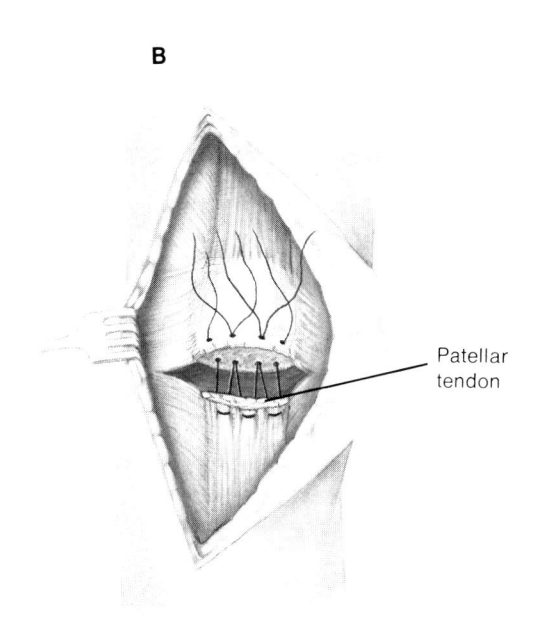

Patellar tendon

REPAIR OF FRACTURE OF PATELLA (Plate 12-13)

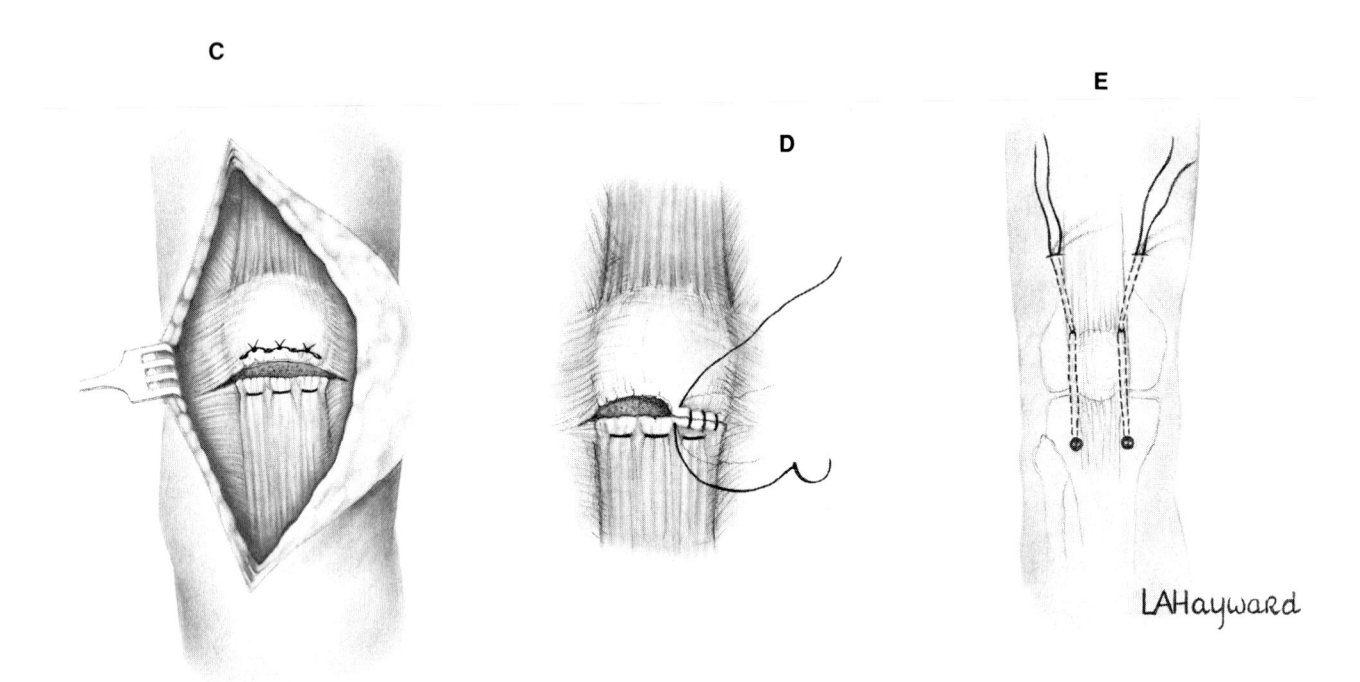

Four drill holes are prepared in the intact fragment of patella, beginning on the fracture surface immediately anterior to the articular cartilage. Three sutures are then placed appropriately through the patellar tendon distal to the small shell of attached bone, and the ends of the sutures are passed through the drill holes in the intact portion of the patella **(B)**. These sutures are then tied down, and if they have been placed correctly, the patellar tendon will come into contact with the deep surface of the fracture fragment near the articular edge **(C)**. This will prevent an abnormal tilt of the patellar fragment and the fracture surface from coming into contact with the femur. The repair is completed by suturing the soft tissues over the repair site **(D)**. Pull-out wires are used routinely to protect the repair from excessive tension in the postoperative period **(E)**. Following wound closure, a well-padded cylinder cast is applied with the knee in 5° to 10° flexion.

POSTOPERATIVE MANAGEMENT. The skin sutures are removed through a window in the cast at 2 weeks and the pull-out wires at 4 weeks following surgery, and isometric quadriceps setting exercises and passive flexion exercises are begun. A removable extension splint is used until 6 weeks following surgery, when more vigorous rehabilitation is initiated.

(Plate 12-14) PATELLECTOMY

GENERAL DISCUSSION. The patellofemoral compartment may be the source of distressing and disabling symptoms in the osteoarthritic knee. Osteoarthritis localized to the patellofemoral compartment of the knee may follow acute or chronic trauma to the knee. When the most significant source of symptoms is limited to the contiguous surfaces of the patella and femur, patellectomy can help the patient to be more comfortable and may improve the function of the knee joint.

The patella can be excised through an anteromedial or a transverse incision. If a transverse incision is made in the retinaculum, it will be better for regaining active extension of the knee but there may be more difficulty in regaining knee flexion postoperatively.

DETAILS OF PROCEDURE. A lateral parapatellar skin incision is used. After the skin and subcutaneous tissues are retracted medially and laterally through the plane of the prepatellar bursa, the contour of the patella is easily palpable. A transverse incision is made at the midpatella level, beginning in the lateral retinaculum, running across the anterior surface of the patella, and extending into the medial retinaculum **(A)**. The prepatellar tissue is dissected carefully from the anterior surface of the patella proximally and distally with care not to fragment the tissues. When the superior and inferior poles of the patella are reached, the quadriceps and patellar tendon are carefully released from the patella, the peripatellar synovium is also sectioned, and the patella is removed **(B)**.

The problem of securing adequate repair of the extensor mechanism is shown schematically **(C)**, with the arrow indicating the line of transverse incision at the midpatellar level, and illustrating that the prepatellar soft tissue is very thin compared to the thick, strong quadriceps and patellar tendon. After excision of the patella, there is a considerable gap between the ends of the quadriceps and the patellar tendons. If the extensor mechanism is simply mobilized to allow direct repair, the resultant shortening of the extensor mechanism may lead to difficulty in regaining flexion postoperatively.

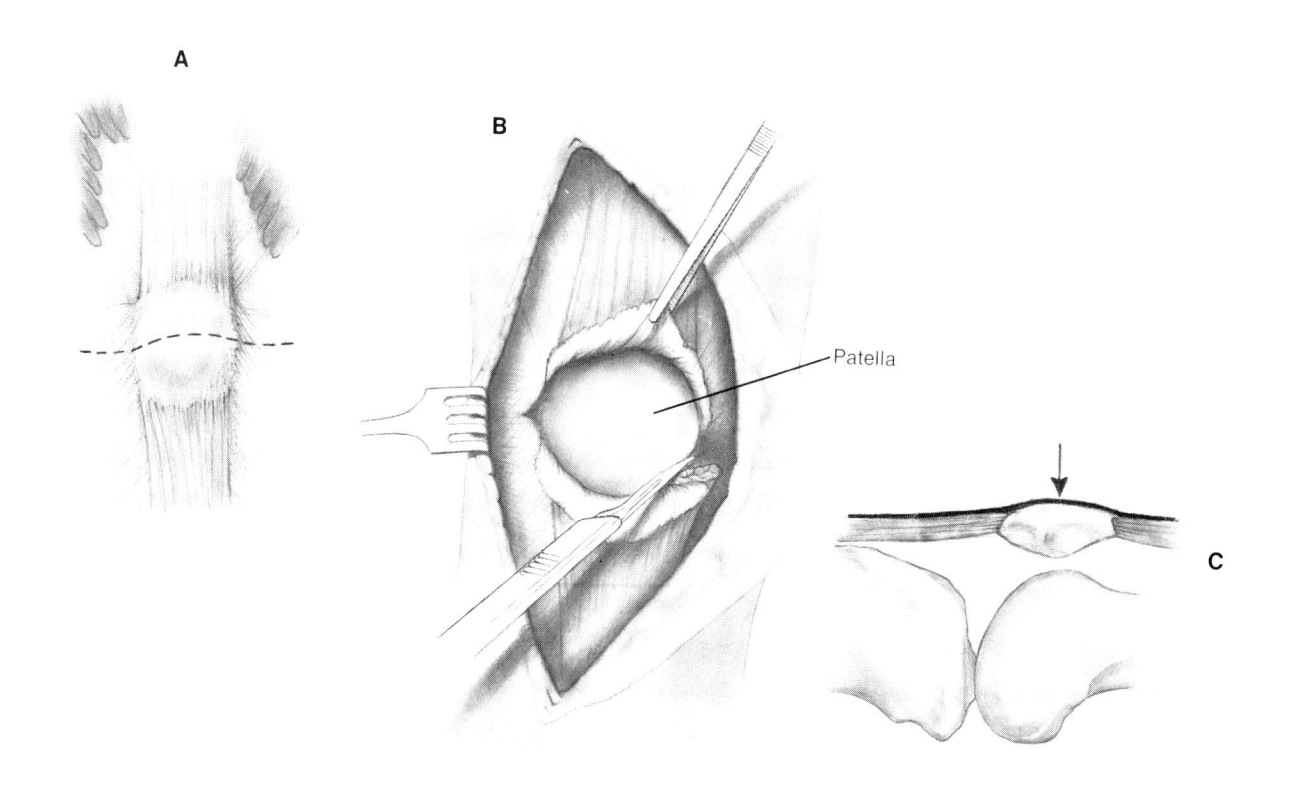

431

PATELLECTOMY (Plate 12-14)

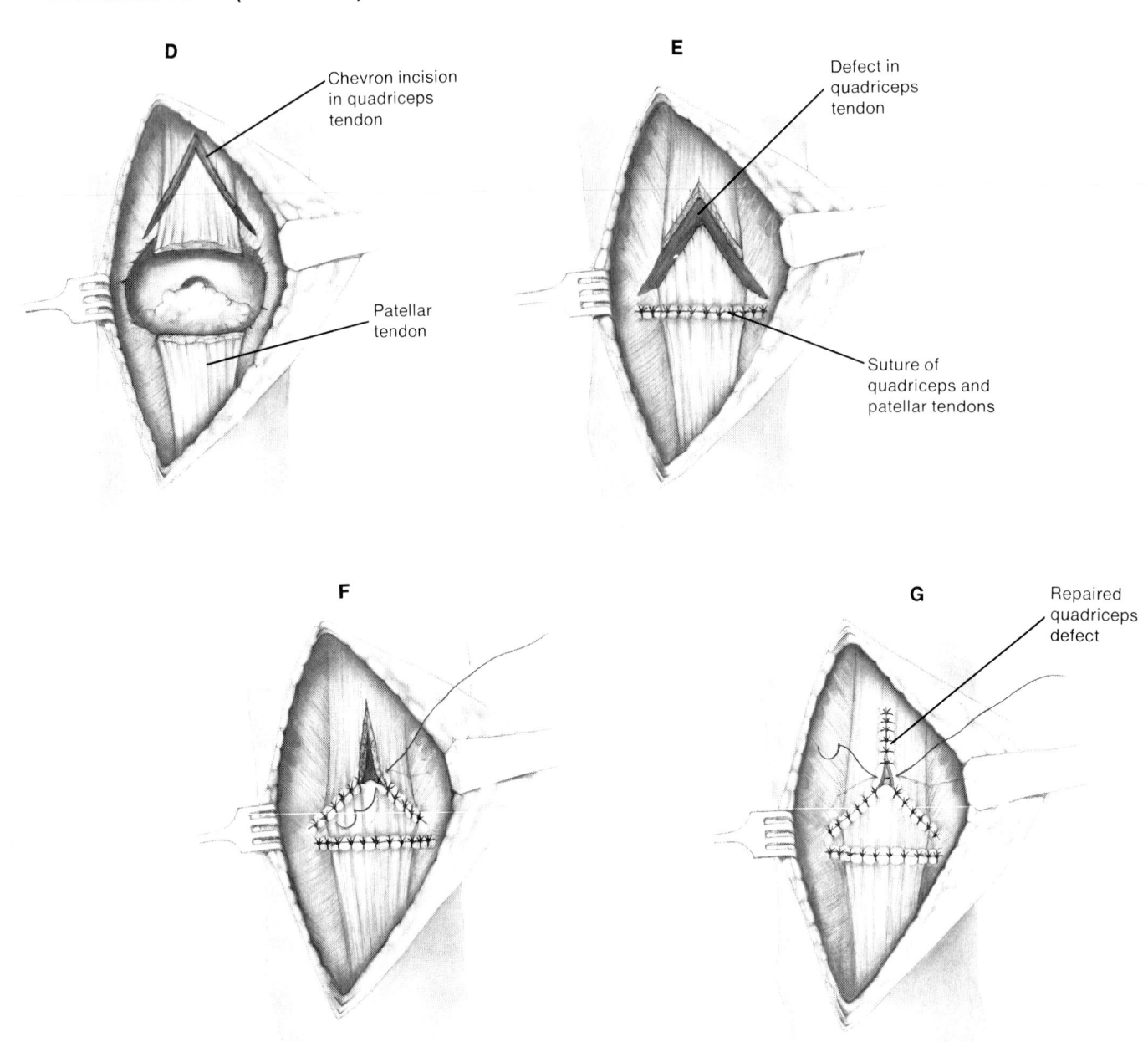

D — Chevron incision in quadriceps tendon; Patellar tendon

E — Defect in quadriceps tendon; Suture of quadriceps and patellar tendons

F

G — Repaired quadriceps defect

Repair of the extensor mechanism utilizing a Z-Y technique as proposed by Howe permits direct repair of the quadriceps tendon to the patellar tendon without necessitating advancement of the entire extensor mechanism. A chevron incision is made through the quadriceps tendon (**D**), which allows direct suture of the quadriceps tendon to the patellar tendon without tension (**E**). The resultant defect in the quadriceps tendon is closed by converting the V defect into a Y (**F** and **G**). The knee is repeatedly flexed beyond 90° to be certain that tension is not excessive on the sutures in the repair. The tourniquet is released prior to closure and a well-padded compression dressing applied to maintain the knee in 5° to 10° flexion.

POSTOPERATIVE MANAGEMENT. The compression dressing is removed 2 weeks postoperatively. The sutures are removed and intermittent passive flexion exercises are begun with the leg kept in a removable extension splint at all other times. Quadriceps setting exercises are begun 3 to 4 weeks after surgery and straight leg raising after 4 to 5 weeks. The intermittent passive flexion exercises are continued until 6 weeks postoperatively, when the splint is discontinued and vigorous rehabilitation is initiated.

(Plate 12-15) EPIPHYSEAL ARREST OF DISTAL FEMUR (EPIPHYSIODESIS)

GENERAL DISCUSSION. Epiphyseal arrest is the procedure of choice for leg length equalization prior to skeletal maturity. This can be accomplished either by the Phemister technique of obliterating the epiphyseal plate or by stapling as described by Blount. Green and Anderson have devised a graph that makes readily available the approximate shortening of the femur and tibia that may be expected from the arrest of the distal femoral and/or proximal tibial epiphyseal plates. Another formula for determining the time of epiphyseal arrest has been devised by White.

A good general rule of thumb regarding the anticipated potential growth from the distal femur or proximal tibia in a young child is to expect 1.3 cm of longitudinal growth per year from the distal femur and 0.9 cm of longitudinal growth from the proximal tibia until age 14 years in girls and 16 years in boys. One can then estimate the approximate age at which an epiphyseal arrest should be carried out, taking into consideration the fact that growth is slowed in the last year before full maturation. For specific determination of the age at which an epiphyseal arrest should be properly scheduled, one should refer to the most recent skeletal growth graphs by Green and Anderson.

DETAILS OF PROCEDURE. The operation is carried out under pneumatic tourniquet, and the leg is draped to permit subsequent flexion and extension of the knee. The knee is supported in slight flexion. Linear transverse or oblique incisions may be used, but the oblique incision is preferred **(A)**. The incisions are directed from anterior and proximal to posterior and distal. On the medial side the fascia is incised and the vastus medialis is retracted anteriorly, exposing the medial genicular vessels, which are ligated or cauterized (**B** and **C**). The epiphyseal plate can usually be seen glistening under the periosteum. The synovium, which overlaps the anterior portion of the epiphysis, can be gently reflected anteriorly. The anterior and posterior borders of the epiphyseal plate are identified to ensure proper anteroposterior placement of the bone block. A block of bone 1.5 by 3.0 cm is outlined. As the scalpel crosses the epiphyseal plate, the glistening white cartilage is noted. The incision is extended 1 cm distal to the epiphyseal plate **(D)**. Another incision 3.0 cm in length and 1.5 cm posterior and parallel with the first incision is then made. These two incisions are joined at the proximal and distal ends.

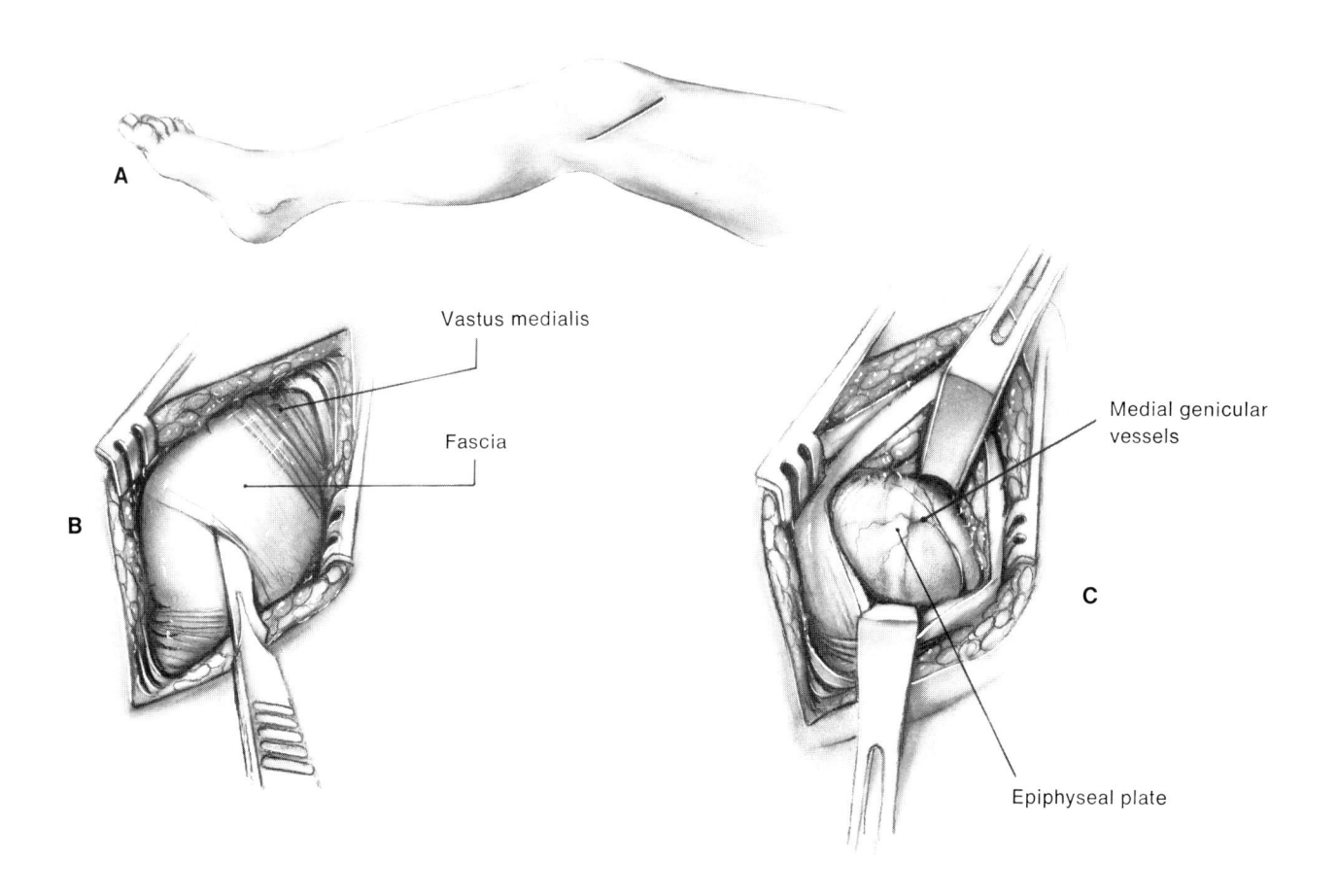

EPIPHYSEAL ARREST OF DISTAL FEMUR (EPIPHYSIODESIS) (Plate 12-15)

The rectangle of bone is removed with a thin-bladed osteotome (**E**). The epiphyseal plate is thoroughly curetted. Visualization of the epiphyseal plate during curettage is aided by use of a small suction tip or by frequent sponging (**F** and **G**). Only a thin rim of cartilage is left anterior and posterior. The bone block is reversed and reinserted (**H**). The periosteum is sutured over the reversed bone block (**I**).

(Plate 12-15) EPIPHYSEAL ARREST OF DISTAL FEMUR (EPIPHYSIODESIS)

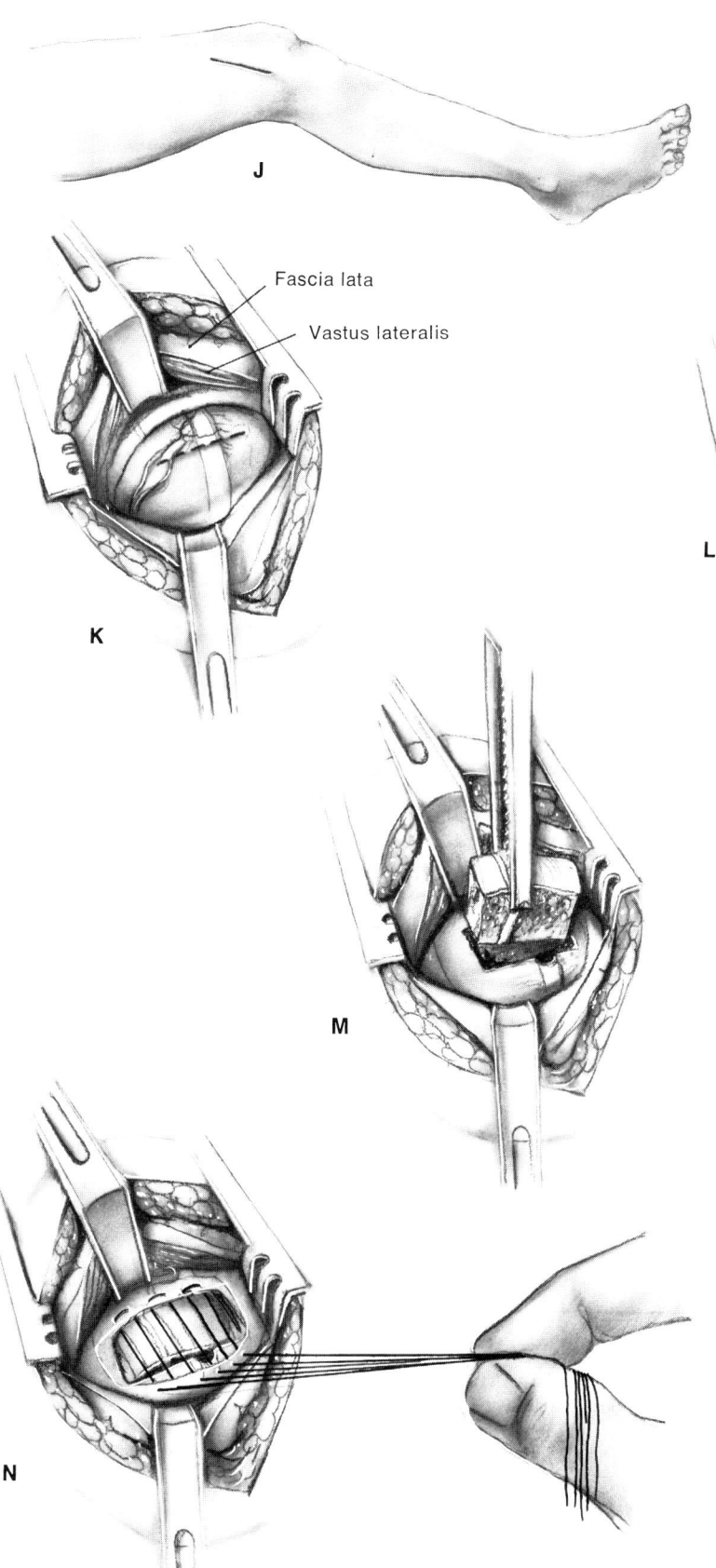

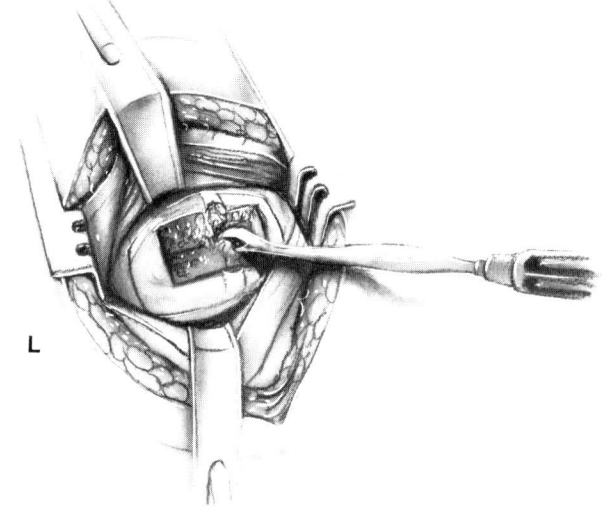

Attention is now directed to the lateral aspect of the knee. After the skin is incised and the fascia lata opened in line with its fibers, the lateral intermuscular septum is developed down to the femur and the vastus lateralis muscle is retracted anteriorly (**J** and **K**). The lateral genicular vessels, which lie just proximal to the epiphyseal plate, are cauterized. With wide retraction, as on the medial aspect of the femur, a bone block is outlined and removed in the same manner. The epiphyseal plate is thoroughly curetted (**L**) from the lateral side until the curetted area joins the defect created from the medial side of the femur. Cancellous bone is removed with a large curet from the distal femoral metaphysis and packed into the epiphyseal plate area before final reinsertion of the lateral bone block. The lateral bone block is also rotated 180° as it is replaced and secured with sutures placed through the periosteum (**M** and **N**). The tourniquet is removed, and the wounds are closed in layers. A circular plaster cast is applied from the toes to the groin with the knee in 10° to 15° flexion.

POSTOPERATIVE MANAGEMENT. The cast is removed after 6 weeks, and full weight bearing is usually possible by 8 weeks postoperatively.

435

EPIPHYSEAL ARREST OF DISTAL FEMUR (BY STAPLING) (Plate 12-16)

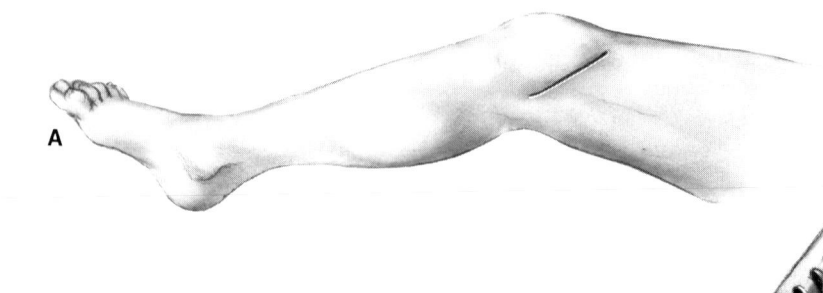

GENERAL DISCUSSION. An alternative method of epiphyseal arrest employs the use of staples placed across the growing epiphyseal plate. This method has been described by Blount and is effective in retarding epiphyseal growth. A small amount of longitudinal growth may continue after placement of the staples. Stapling may be used to arrest epiphyseal growth of the distal femur, the proximal tibia, or both. The timing of the surgery is based on available growth charts. It is possible that additional longitudinal growth may occur if the staples are removed before the epiphyseal plate is fused, but this recurrent growth after removal of staples is unpredictable. A distinct advantage of stapling to arrest epiphyseal growth is the fact that weight bearing can be permitted in the early postoperative period. Cast immobilization is not necessary, and the overall convalescence is shorter compared with that of a Phemister type epiphysiodesis.

Blount says that stapling retards epiphyseal growth 80% to 90% and causes a growth spurt at the other end of the bone. For severe valgus at the knees, Blount states that he would not hesitate to recommend medial stapling of the distal femoral epiphysis of one or both knees.

Epiphyseal stapling is most expedient soon after the patient has reached skeletal age of 8 years. As Blount would emphasize, a patient who cannot be followed closely should not undergo epiphyseal stapling. Many times the patient may have to have one or more staples removed or changed.

Epiphyseal stapling must be done carefully with roentgenogram control in two planes. Failure of epiphyseal stapling is most commonly caused by either improper placement or improper indications.

DETAILS OF PROCEDURE. For stapling of the distal femoral epiphysis, the exposure is the same as with Phemister epiphysiodesis with the principal exception that the periosteum is not incised or reflected from the distal femur. The leg is draped to permit passive movement of the knee into flexion and extension to facilitate exposure of the posterior and anterior aspects of the distal femur on each side.

On the medial side, the dissection is carried down through an oblique incision retracting the vastus medialis anteriorly (**A** to **C**). The epiphyseal plate can usually be seen and identified after the area has been wiped firmly with a dry sponge over the fingertips. Its location is checked with a straight needle. If there is no anticipation of removal of the staples in hope of further significant growth, one can readily identify the epiphyseal plate by incising the periosteum slowly until the glistening blue-white cartilage is seen.

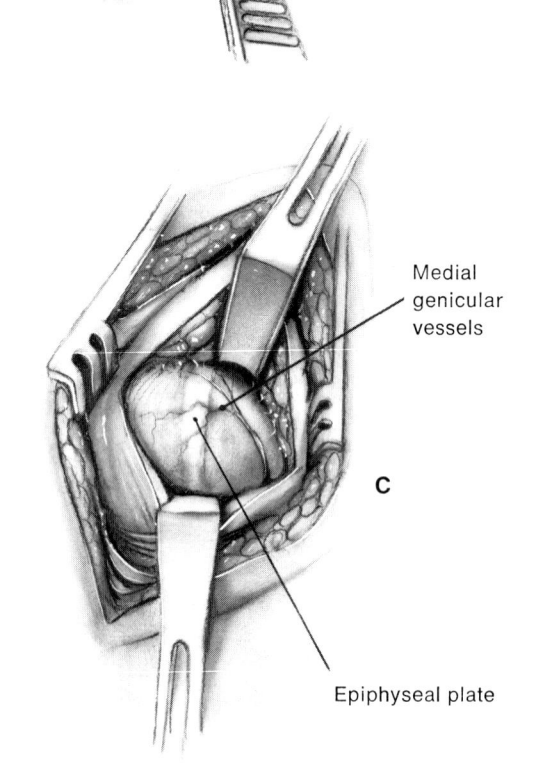

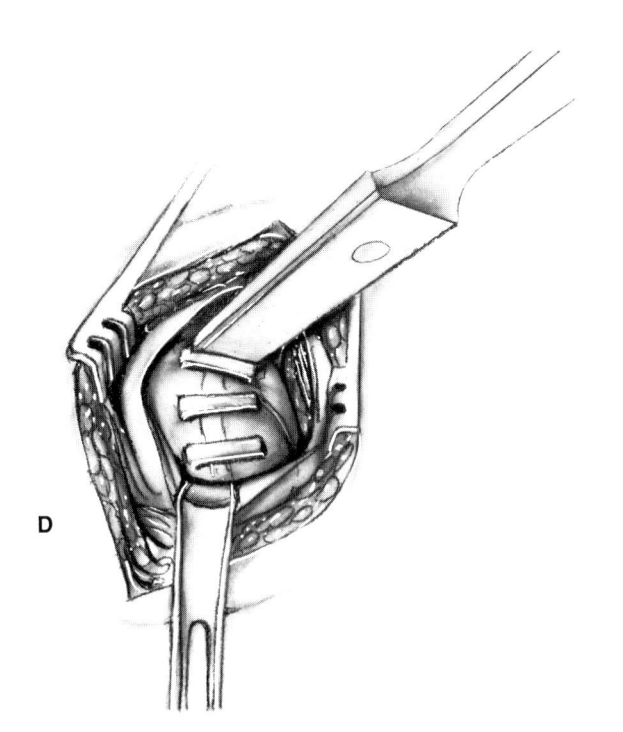

(Plate 12-16) EPIPHYSEAL ARREST OF DISTAL FEMUR (BY STAPLING)

Three staples are used on each side. These are placed perpendicular to the epiphyseal plate at equal distances from each other. Since the epiphyseal plate is curved, the proximal edges of the staples will approximate each other more closely than the distal edges. These staples are inserted through the periosteum **(D)**.

On the lateral side, skin and fascia lata are incised **(E)**. The biceps femoris and common peroneal nerve are retracted posteriorly. It is important that the cluster of staples on each side of the distal femur be placed equidistant from the anterior and posterior surfaces of the bone (**F** and **G**). After placement, the position of the staples relative to both the epiphyseal plate and to the anterior and posterior surfaces of the bone is checked by roentgenograms in the operating room (**H** and **I**). Any staples that are not correctly placed are removed and reinserted and again checked roentgenographically. When the desired position of each of the staples has been confirmed, they are tapped firmly into place and the wounds are closed.

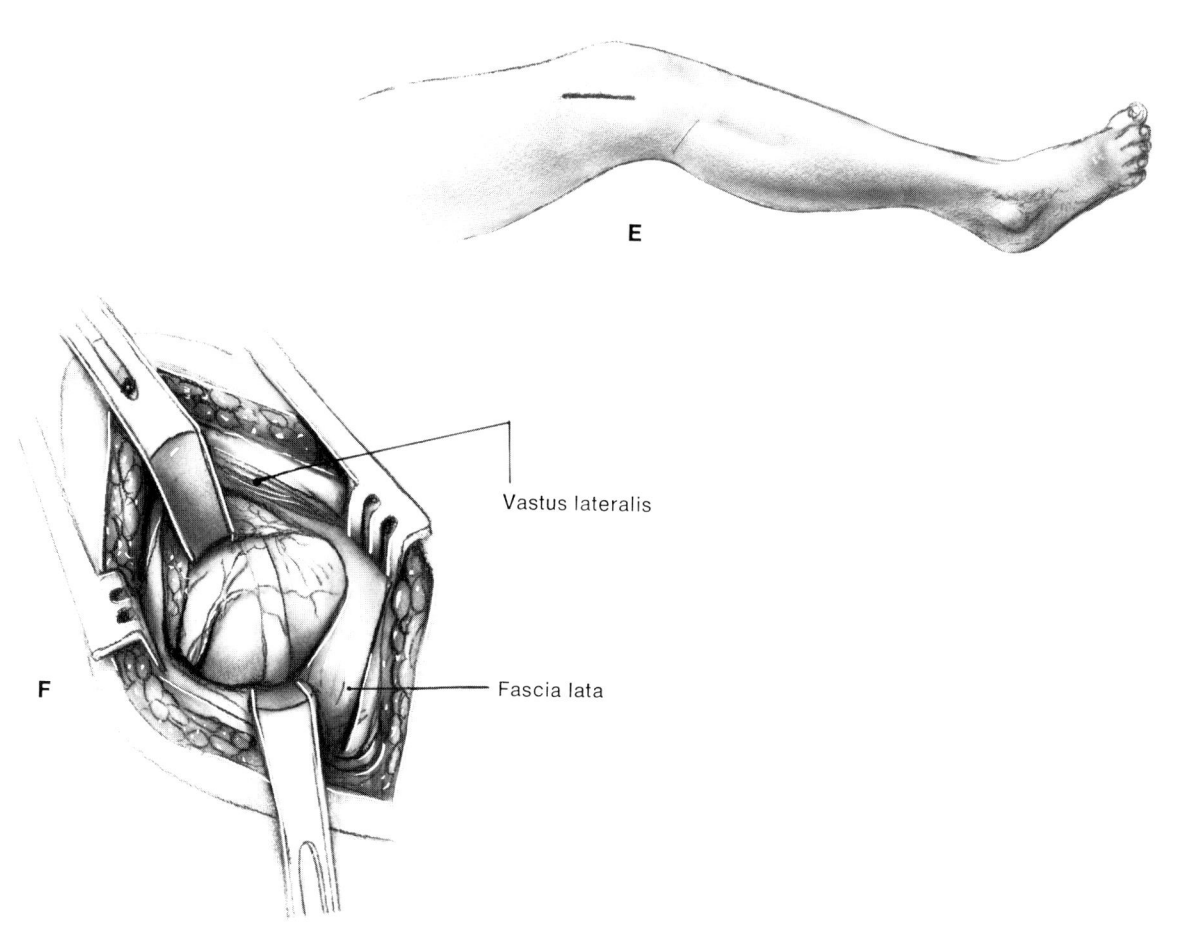

EPIPHYSEAL ARREST OF DISTAL FEMUR (BY STAPLING) (Plate 12-16)

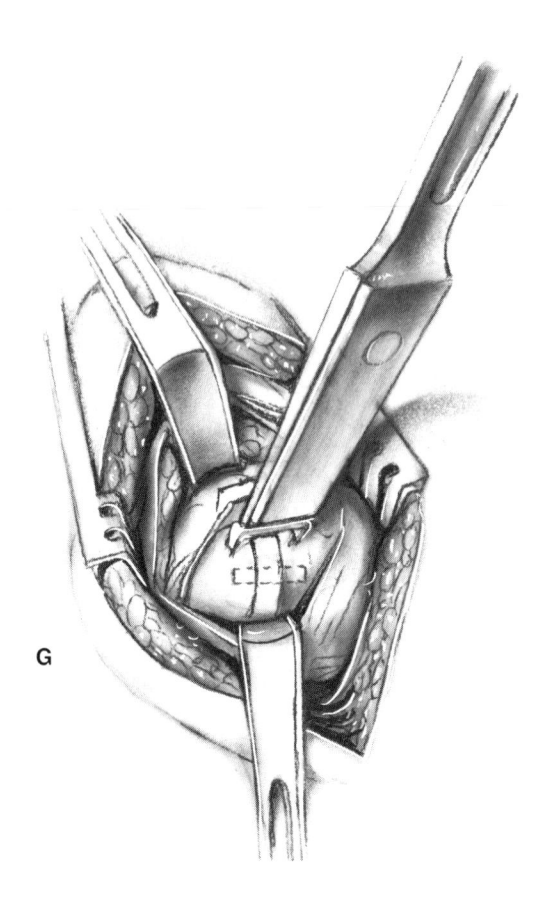

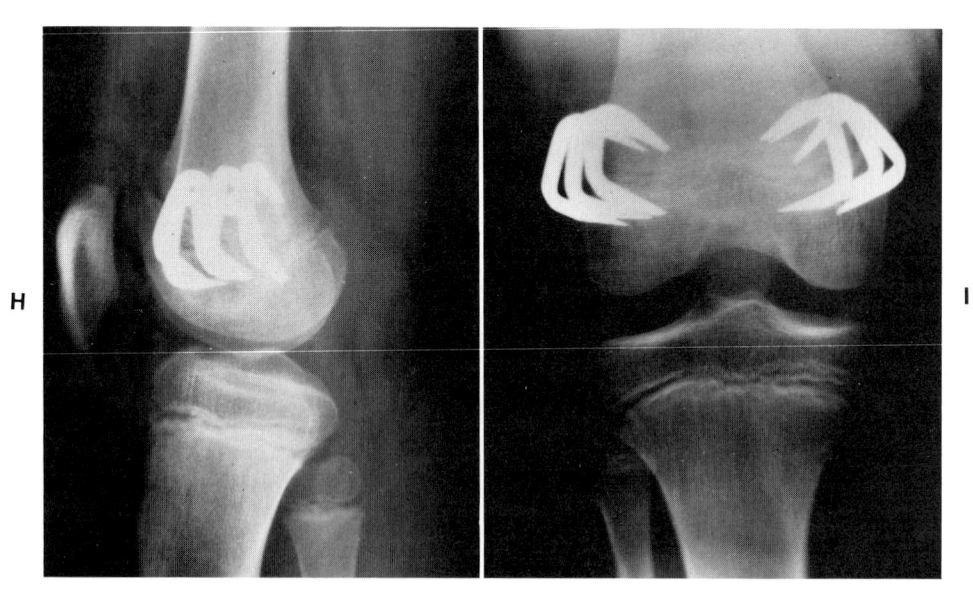

POSTOPERATIVE MANAGEMENT. No immobilization is necessary postoperatively. The patient is allowed to walk with crutches as soon as comfort permits. Full weight bearing without crutches is usually possible within 2 to 3 weeks.

(Plate 12-17) EPIPHYSIODESIS OF PROXIMAL TIBIA AND FIBULA

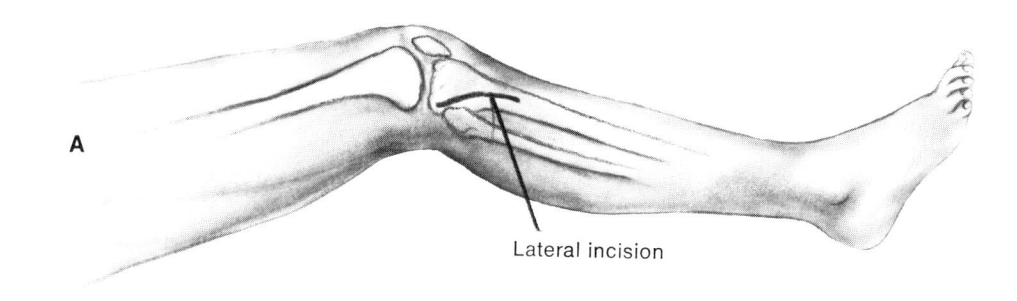

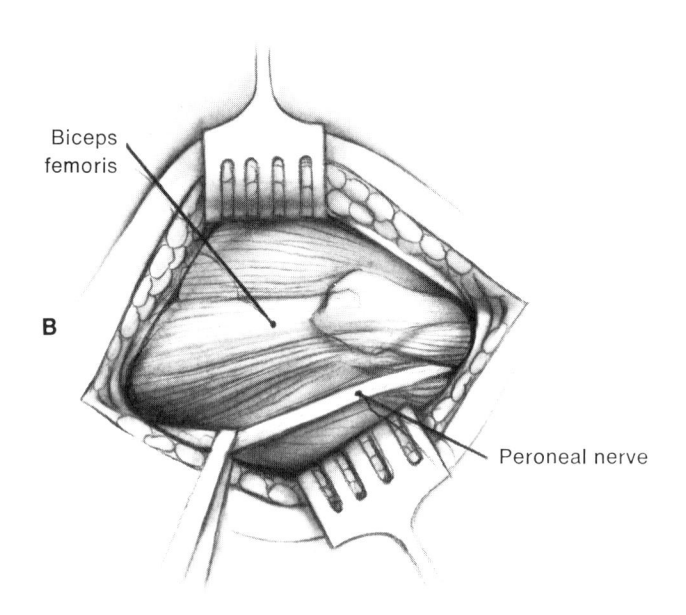

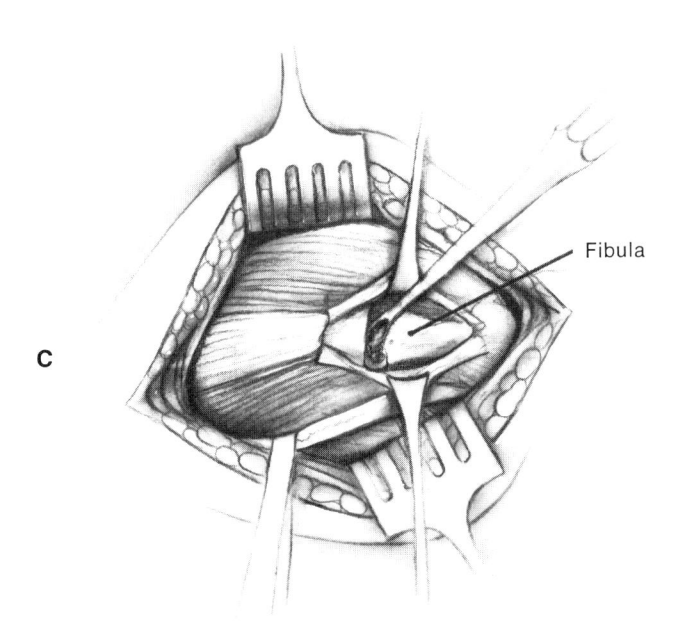

GENERAL DISCUSSION. The amount of leg length normally contributed by the proximal tibial and fibular epiphyseal plates is less than that contributed by the distal femoral epiphyseal plate, but occasionally it is desirable to produce a closure of the proximal tibial and fibular epiphyseal plates either in conjunction with, or subsequent to, distal femoral epiphysiodesis. The total amount of longitudinal growth contributed by the epiphyses of the proximal tibia and fibula is approximately two thirds of the measurable longitudinal length contributed by the distal femoral epiphyseal plate.

If consideration is being given to epiphysiodesis, it is best to obtain leg length roentgenograms and bone age films for accurate calculation of the proper time for epiphysiodesis based on available skeletal growth charts.

DETAILS OF PROCEDURE. The knee is supported in 30° flexion and, under pneumatic tourniquet, a curvilinear incision is made laterally so that the incision passes over the fibular head **(A)**. The peroneal nerve is identified and protected **(B)**. The epiphyseal plate of the proximal fibula is exposed subperiosteally and thoroughly curetted **(C)**.

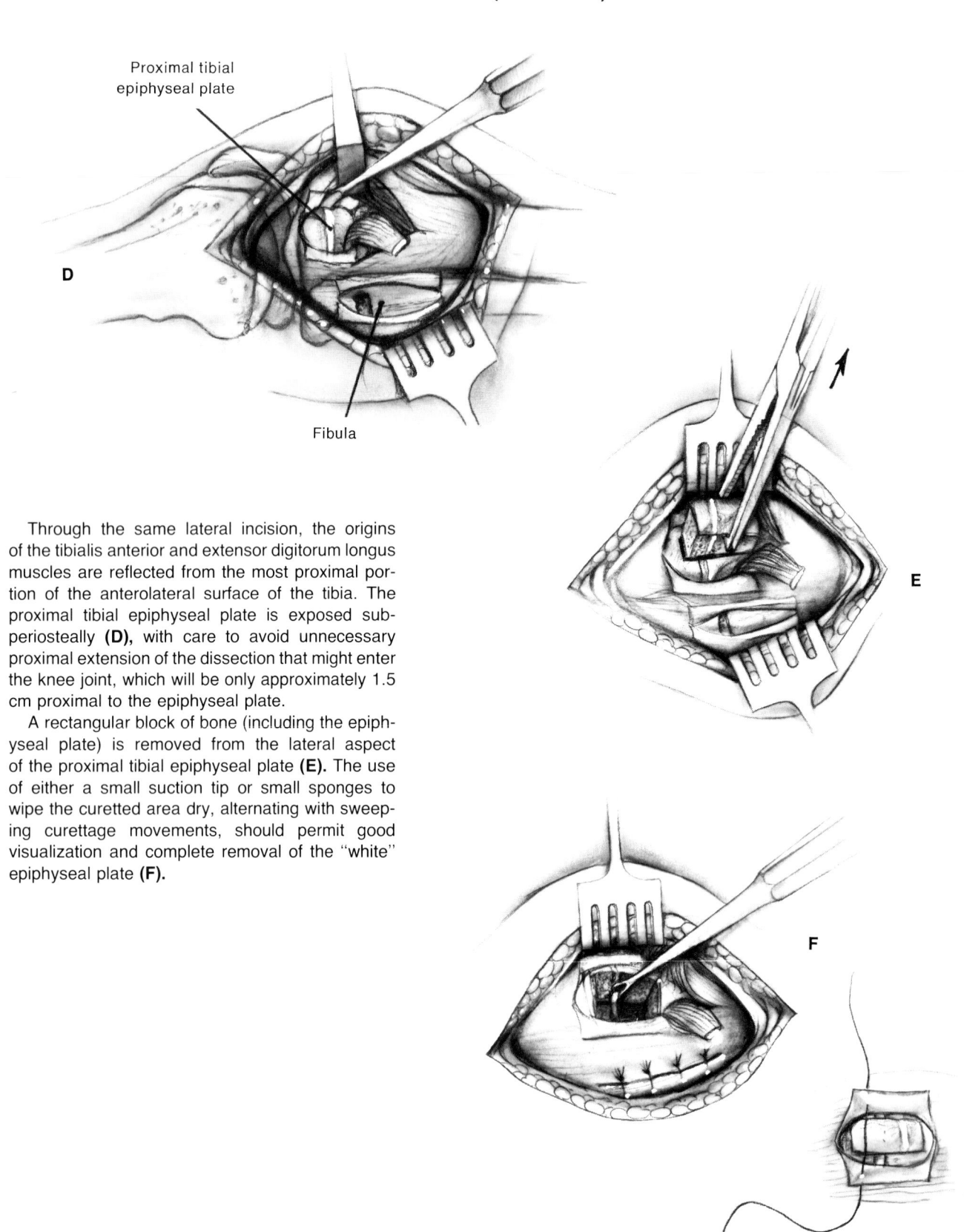

EPIPHYSIODESIS OF PROXIMAL TIBIA AND FIBULA (Plate 12-17)

Through the same lateral incision, the origins of the tibialis anterior and extensor digitorum longus muscles are reflected from the most proximal portion of the anterolateral surface of the tibia. The proximal tibial epiphyseal plate is exposed subperiosteally **(D)**, with care to avoid unnecessary proximal extension of the dissection that might enter the knee joint, which will be only approximately 1.5 cm proximal to the epiphyseal plate.

A rectangular block of bone (including the epiphyseal plate) is removed from the lateral aspect of the proximal tibial epiphyseal plate **(E)**. The use of either a small suction tip or small sponges to wipe the curetted area dry, alternating with sweeping curettage movements, should permit good visualization and complete removal of the "white" epiphyseal plate **(F)**.

440

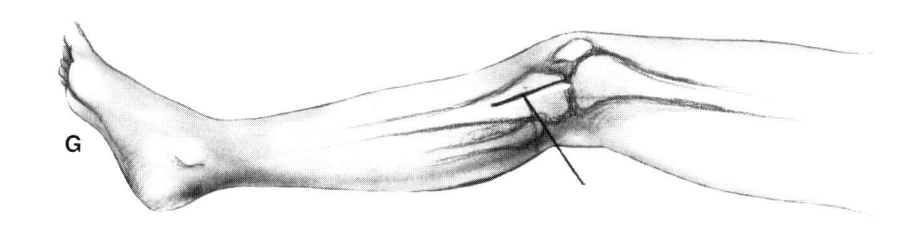

(Plate 12-17) EPIPHYSIODESIS OF PROXIMAL TIBIA AND FIBULA

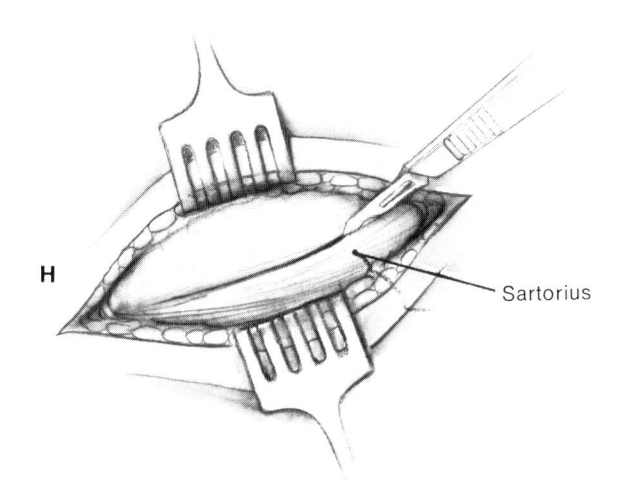

The medial aspect of the proximal tibia is then exposed by a similar longitudinal incision **(G)**. The thin medial fascia is incised **(H)**. The anterior margin of the sartorius muscle is subsequently retracted posteriorly, along with the anterior margin of the medial collateral ligament, for subperiosteal exposure of the tibial epiphyseal plate on the medial side **(I)**. Just as on the lateral side of the proximal tibia, a rectangular block of bone (including the epiphyseal plate) is removed from the medial side. Care must be taken through the medial and lateral exposures to obtain a "through-and-through" complete curettement of the epiphyseal plate extending to the anterior and posterior cortices of the tibia **(I)**.

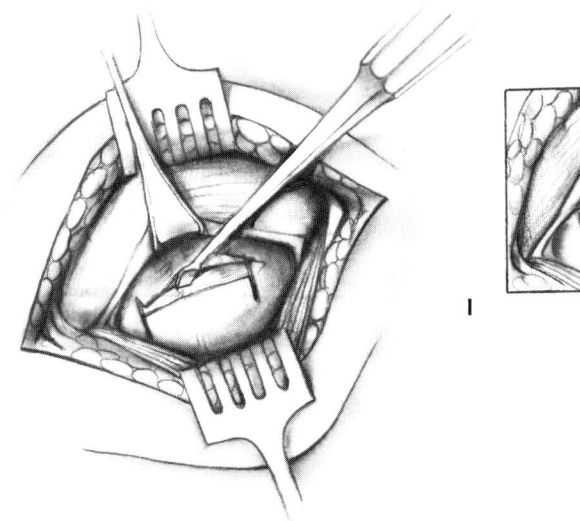

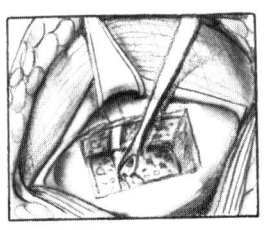

441

EPIPHYSIODESIS OF PROXIMAL TIBIA AND FIBULA (Plate 12-17)

When the epiphyseal plate has been completely removed, cancellous bone is curetted from the proximal tibial metaphysis to fill the defect left by the removed epiphyseal plate. The cortical rectangles from the medial and lateral aspects of the proximal tibia are replaced after rotating each 180° **(J)**. The periosteum and other soft tissues are closed **(K)**. The leg is placed in a long-leg cast with the knee in slight flexion.

POSTOPERATIVE MANAGEMENT. The long-leg cast is removed at the end of 6 weeks. This is followed by active mobilization of the knee and progressive weight bearing.

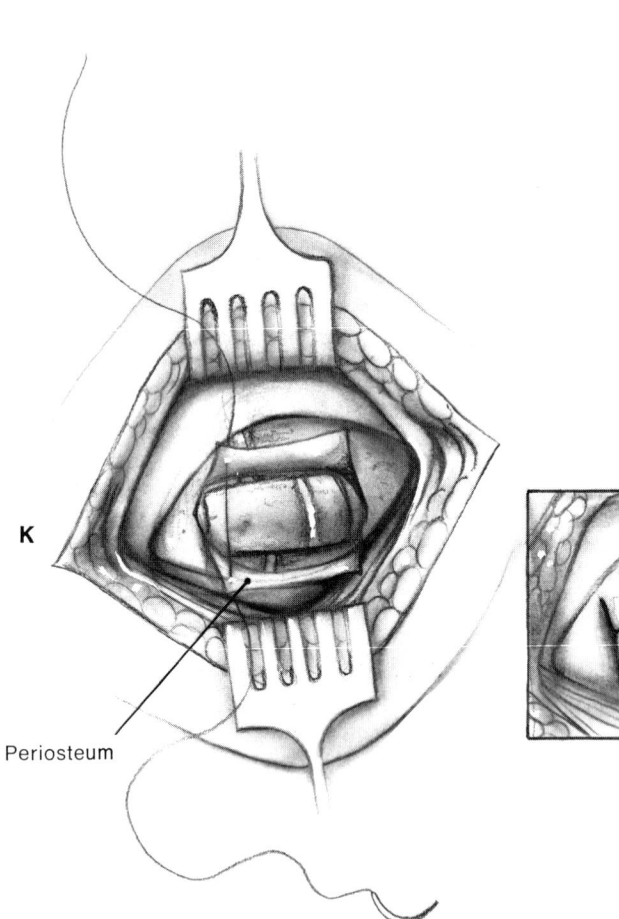

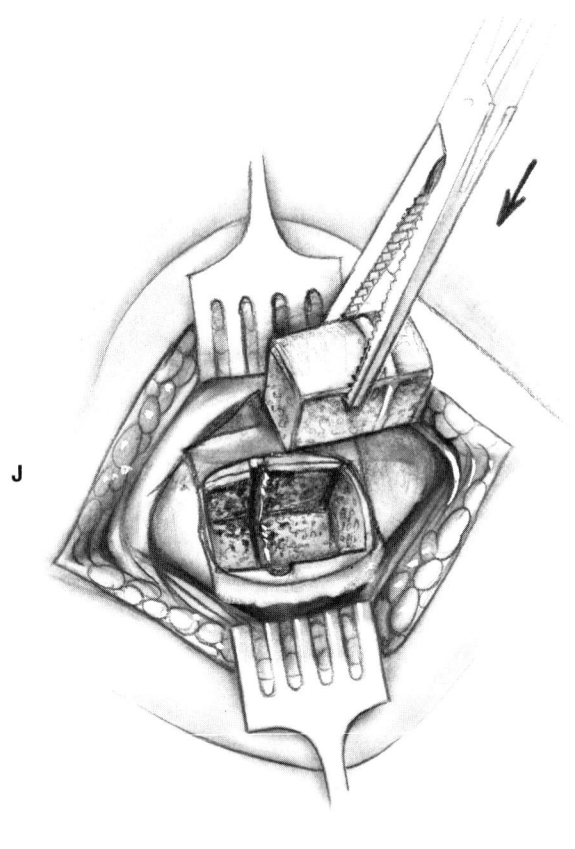

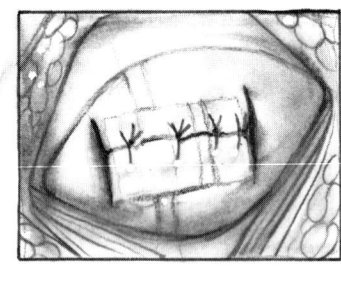

Periosteum

(Plate 12-18) REPAIR OF TORN MEDIAL COLLATERAL LIGAMENT

GENERAL DISCUSSION. To obtain optimal stability and functional recovery of the knee, early repair is recommended for complete tear of the medial collateral ligament. Unless the patient is examined immediately after injury, subsequent pain and muscle spasm may necessitate anesthesia for adequate examination of the injured knee when the mechanism of injury and the localization of pain and tenderness suggest the possibility of a complete tear of the medial collateral ligament.

Preoperative roentgenograms of the knee should always be obtained with particular attention to the possibility of a tibial plateau fracture or avulsion of a ligamentous bony attachment. Furthermore, if the patient is a child and the epiphyseal plates are still open, a valgus stress x-ray film should be obtained to rule out the possibility of an injured and unstable distal femoral or proximal tibial epiphyseal plate, either of which can simulate a complete tear of the medial collateral ligaments on clinical examination of the knee in a growing child. If stress films reveal instability of a child's knee to be at the distal femoral epiphyseal plate, the medial collateral ligament will be intact and no surgery will be indicated unless there is associated internal derangement. Since the superficial portion of the medial collateral ligament crosses the proximal tibial epiphyseal plate, if the stress x-ray film demonstrates instability at that level, the superficial medial collateral ligament will also be torn, and surgical treatment is recommended.

Injuries to the medial meniscus and anterior cruciate ligament are frequently associated with severe injuries of the medial collateral ligament.

DETAILS OF PROCEDURE. The knee is exposed through a medial utility approach (Plate 12-2, B). The deep fascial layer is initially opened in line with the course of the medial collateral ligament from the medial femoral epicondyle proximally to just above the level of the sartorius tendon of the pes anserinus distally. The proximal portion of the incision in the deep fascial layer is then extended posteriorly and the fascia carefully dissected from the underlying medial collateral ligament complex to provide adequate exposure including the posteromedial capsular region **(A)**. The details of the repair must be individualized for each case, depending on the pathology. The superficial portion of the medial collateral ligament should be thoroughly evaluated from its femoral origin to its tibial attachment beneath the pes anserinus. The trailing edge of the medial collateral ligament (tibial arm of the posterior oblique ligament) must also be carefully evaluated along with the posteromedial capsule (capsular arm of the posterior oblique ligament). The deep or capsular layer of the medial collateral ligament, which lies deep to the superficial portion of the ligament, may or may not be torn in the same area as the superficial portion. Preoperatively, precise localization of the points of maximum tenderness, along with palpation for soft tissue puffiness and edema, helps direct attention to a tear in the deep portion of the ligament, which lies beneath an intact portion of the superficial layer. This can be exposed by making a limited fiber-splitting incision through the superficial layer to expose the underlying deep layer, without compromising integrity of the superficial layer.

A medial parapatellar capsular incision is made to assess the status of the menisci and cruciate ligaments, so that concomitant surgical treatment of these structures can also be accomplished if they are torn.

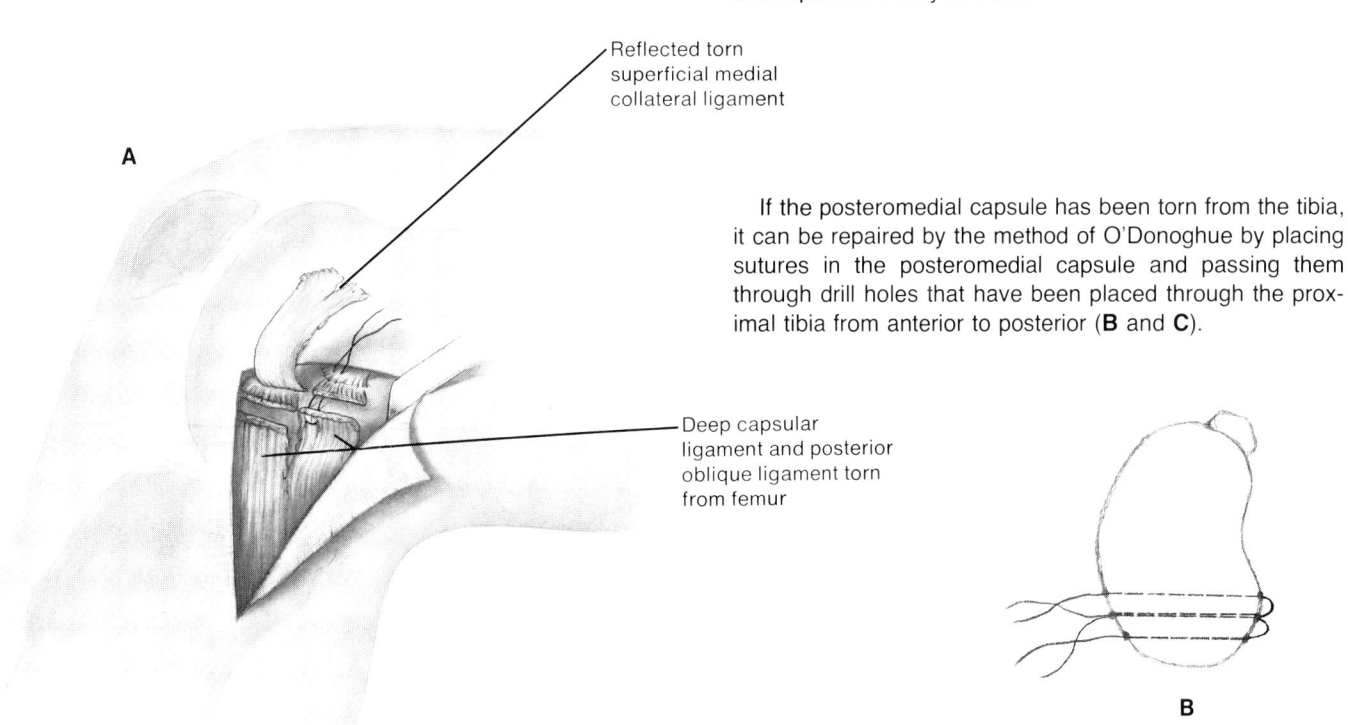

If the posteromedial capsule has been torn from the tibia, it can be repaired by the method of O'Donoghue by placing sutures in the posteromedial capsule and passing them through drill holes that have been placed through the proximal tibia from anterior to posterior (**B** and **C**).

443

REPAIR OF TORN MEDIAL COLLATERAL LIGAMENT (Plate 12-18)

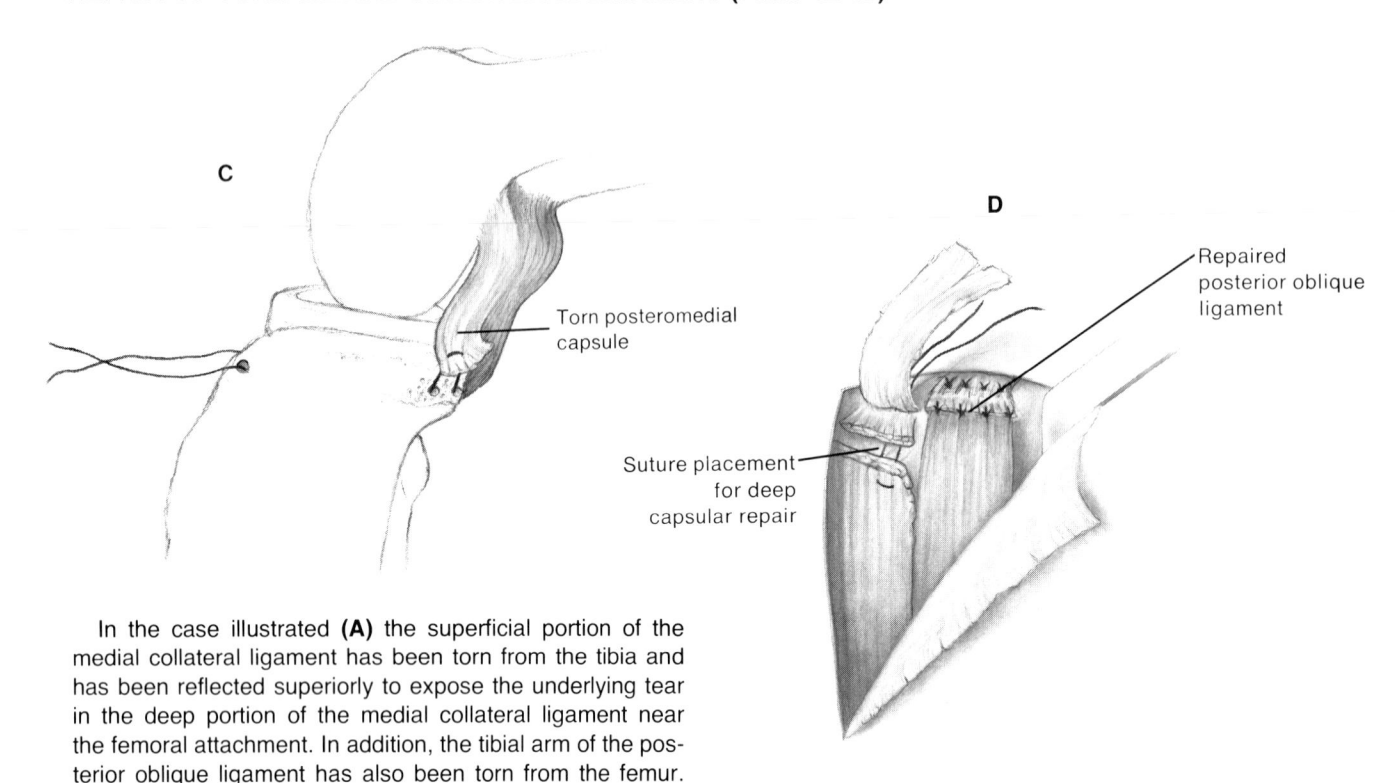

In the case illustrated (**A**) the superficial portion of the medial collateral ligament has been torn from the tibia and has been reflected superiorly to expose the underlying tear in the deep portion of the medial collateral ligament near the femoral attachment. In addition, the tibial arm of the posterior oblique ligament has also been torn from the femur.

The repair is accomplished by placing pants-over-vest plicating sutures to repair the tibial arm of the posterior oblique ligament back to the femoral origin (**A** and **D**). Similar sutures are then placed to repair the deep portion of the medial collateral ligament back to its femoral origin (**D**). At this point the knee should be checked gently for medial stability, and if instability remains, the sutures should be replaced so that adequate stability is achieved.

The superficial portion of the medial collateral ligament is then repaired by placing it back in its normal position, under mild tension, and fixing it in this position with a barbed staple and additional interrupted sutures (**E**). The knee is again checked gently for adequate stability. At this point the tourniquet is released and further hemostasis secured. The retinacular layer is repaired over the medial collateral ligament (**F**). The wound is closed in the routine fashion over suction drainage. A well-padded long-leg plaster cast is applied with the knee flexed 50° to 70° and with the tibia is slight internal rotation. If the anterior cruciate ligament has been repaired in addition to the medial collateral ligament, the knee is flexed only to approximately 40°.

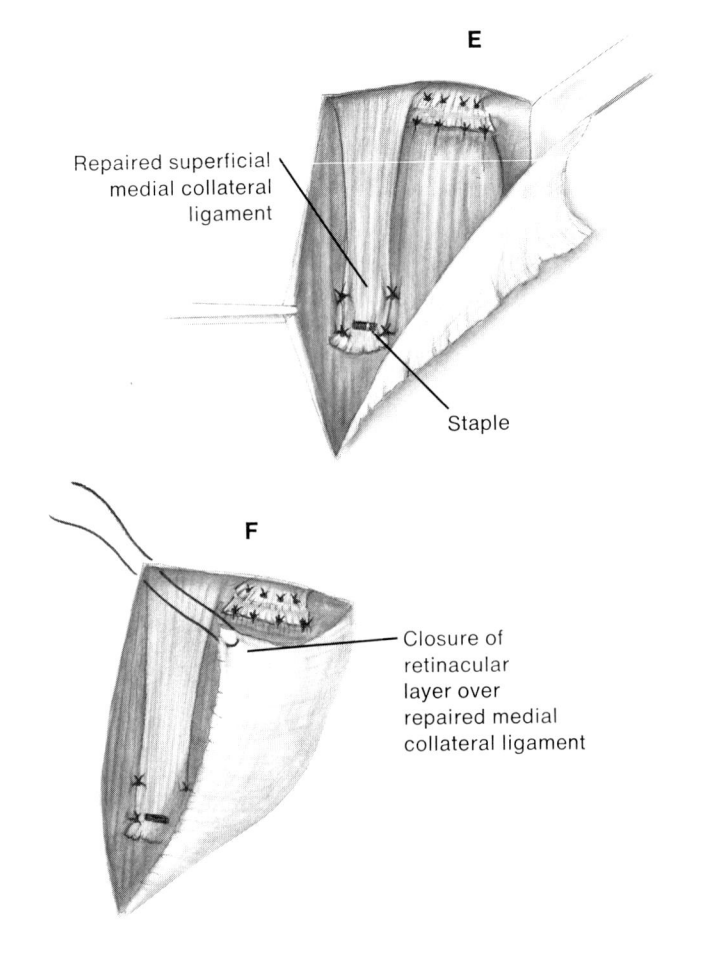

POSTOPERATIVE MANAGEMENT. Active quadriceps exercises are encouraged in the immediate postoperative period. The negative suction tubes are removed in 24 to 48 hours, and the patient ambulates on crutches as soon as possible with touch-down weight bearing. The knee is immobilized in the same position for a total of 5 weeks. Then it is placed in a cast brace with 30° to 60° hinges for an additional 3 weeks before removal of the cast brace, fitting with a protective knee brace, and initiation of vigorous rehabilitation.

(Plate 12-19) MEDIAL COLLATERAL LIGAMENT RECONSTRUCTION

GENERAL DISCUSSION. Every effort should be made to diagnose and treat acute tears of the medial collateral ligament so that chronic medial instabilities do not develop. However, when there is the history of a previous injury with valgus and external rotation mechanism, the history of functional instability, and the presence of significant straight medial and anteromedial rotatory instability on physical examination, surgical reconstruction of the medial collateral ligament complex may be considered. Before ligamentous reconstructive surgery is done, however, efforts should be made to control the functional instability with vigorous rehabilitative exercises and bracing for strenuous activities. Also, patient selection in terms of motivation and ability to participate in a vigorous postoperative rehabilitation program are of critical importance in the ultimate success or failure of the procedure. Ligamentous reconstructive procedures for a knee with advanced degenerative changes must be considered with great caution, since the ultimate result is frequently disappointing even though the knee is more stable postoperatively.

The procedure to be described combines features of medial collateral ligament reconstructive procedures described by Slocum and Larson, O'Donoghue, and Henning.

DETAILS OF PROCEDURE. The knee is exposed through a medial utility approach (Plate 12-2). The medial collateral ligament complex is exposed as described for medial collateral ligament repair (Plate 12-18). An anteromedial parapatellar capsular incision is made for inspection of the interior of the joint, and any coexisting internal derangements are treated as necessary. If the medial meniscus is normal, every effort should be made to tailor the reconstructive procedure so that adequate stability can be restored without sacrificing the medial meniscus. A posteromedial capsular incision is made obliquely in line with the trailing edge of the medial collateral ligament (tibial arm of the posterior oblique ligament). The first step in the reconstruction is to tighten the lax posteromedial capsule. If the medial meniscus has been removed, the posteromedial capsule is detached from its normal insertion to the posteromedial tibia. The posteromedial surface of the tibia is denuded of all soft tissues and freshened with a curet or a gouge. The posteromedial capsule is advanced distally and reattached with sutures placed through the posteromedial capsule and passed through drill holes to be tied on the anterior aspect of the tibia **(A)**. If the medial meniscus can be retained and the laxity in the capsule is in the menisco femoral portion, the posteromedial capsule can be tightened by detaching it proximally, advancing it in a proximal direction, and then reattaching it to its normal attachment site on the femur with sutures through drill holes or with the use of a barbed staple and sutures.

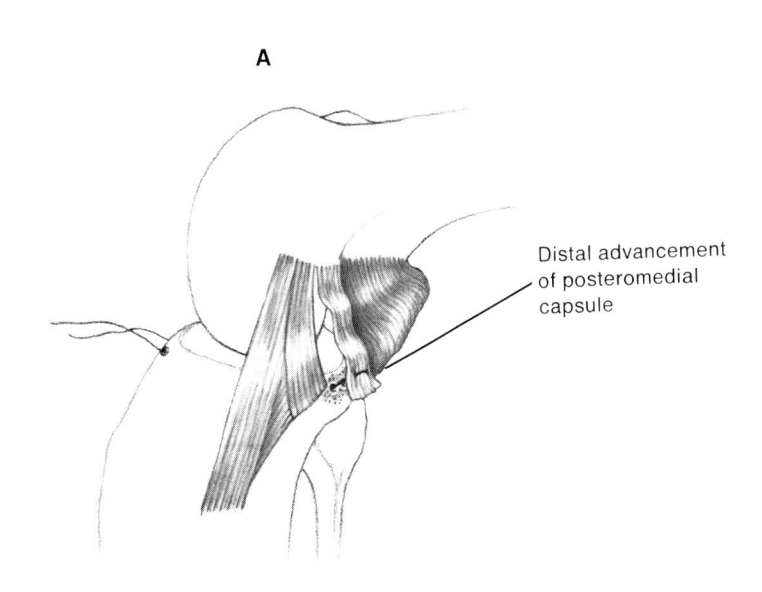

MEDIAL COLLATERAL LIGAMENT RECONSTRUCTION (Plate 12-19)

B

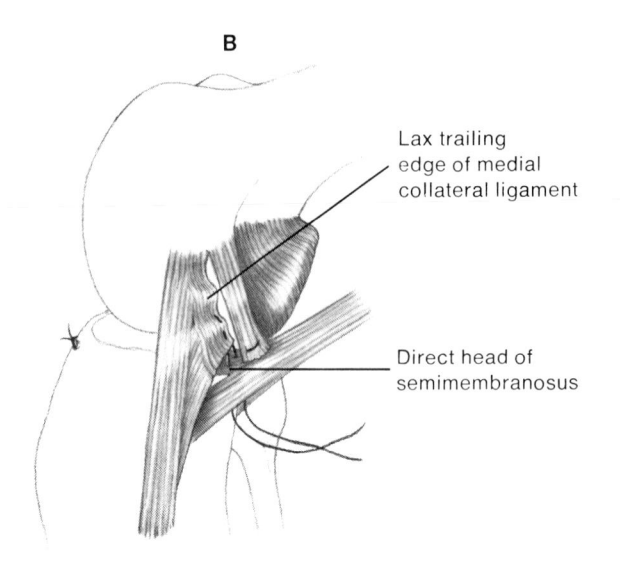

Lax trailing edge of medial collateral ligament

Direct head of semimembranosus

C

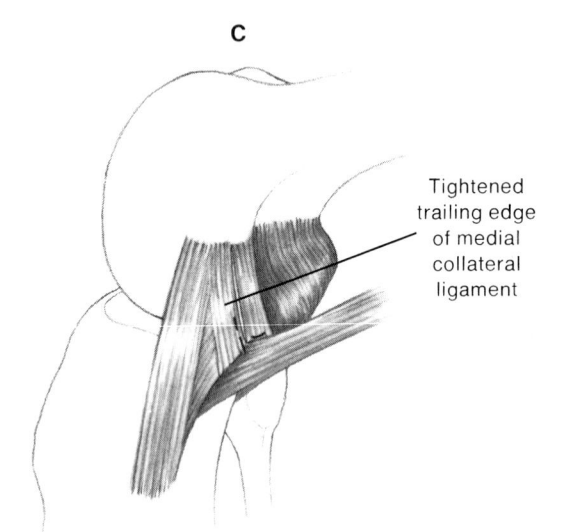

Tightened trailing edge of medial collateral ligament

The next step is to restore the normal tension in the trailing edge of the medial collateral ligament (tibial arm of the posterior oblique ligament). Sutures are placed through this structure and are carried down through the direct head of the semimembranosus tendon so that when the sutures are tied, the normal tension is restored to the trailing edge of the ligament (**B** and **C**). Posteromedial capsular advancement is then carried out by closing the previously made posteriomedial incision in a plicating fashion, overlapping the posterior edge of the capsule on the trailing edge of the medial collateral ligament, and advancing it as far as possible (**D**). This portion of the procedure should restore adequate straight medial stability and partially correct the anteromedial rotatory instability.

D

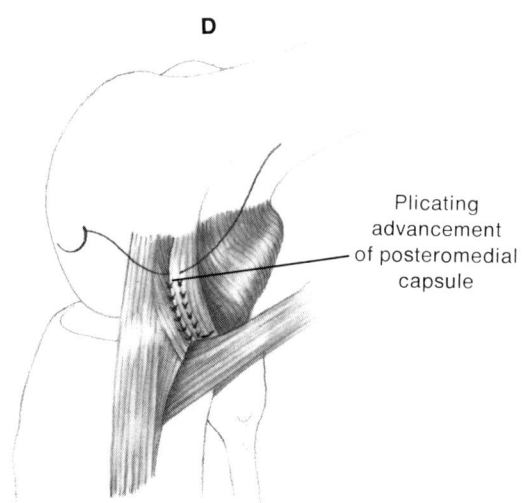

Plicating advancement of posteromedial capsule

(Plate 12-19) MEDIAL COLLATERAL LIGAMENT RECONSTRUCTION

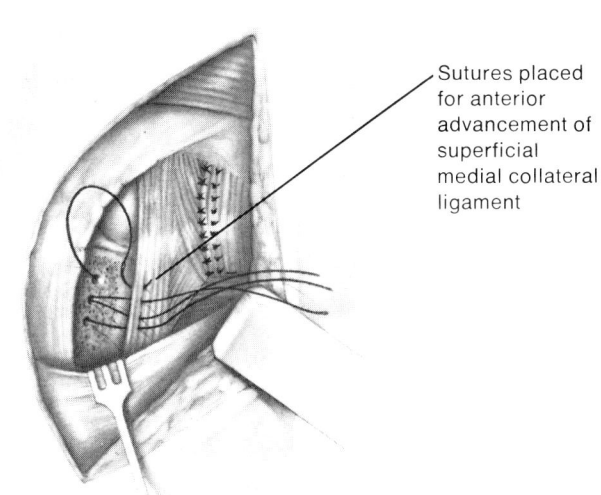

To obtain additional control of the anteromedial rotatory instability, the superficial portion of the medial collateral ligament is identified and dissected free from the underlying deep portion of the medial collateral ligament up to the level of the joint line, but without disturbing its normal attachment to the tibia beneath the pes anserinus (E). The anteromedial surface of the tibia below the joint line is denuded. Sutures are placed through drill holes and passed through the superficial portion of the medial collateral ligament (F) so that when the tibia is internally rotated beneath the superficial medial collateral ligament, the sutures will provide anchorage of the superficial portion of the medial collateral ligament to this area of the tibia (G). This step should provide more complete control of the anteromedial rotatory instability. The superficial portion of the medial collateral ligament tightens as the tibia is externally rotated, but it does not interfere with normal flexion.

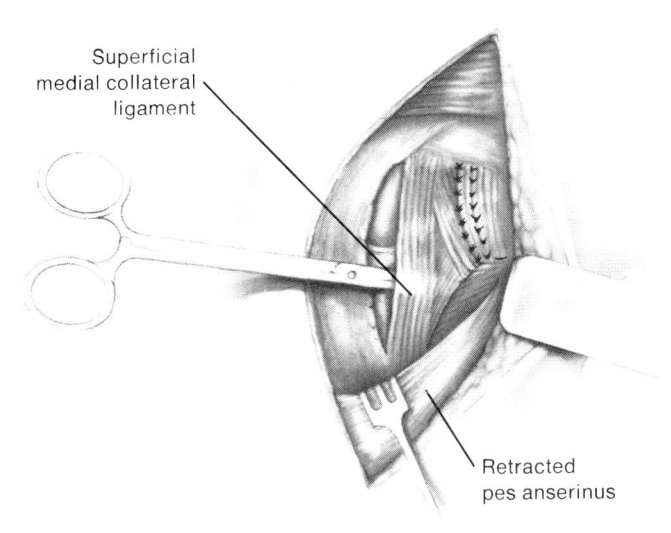

447

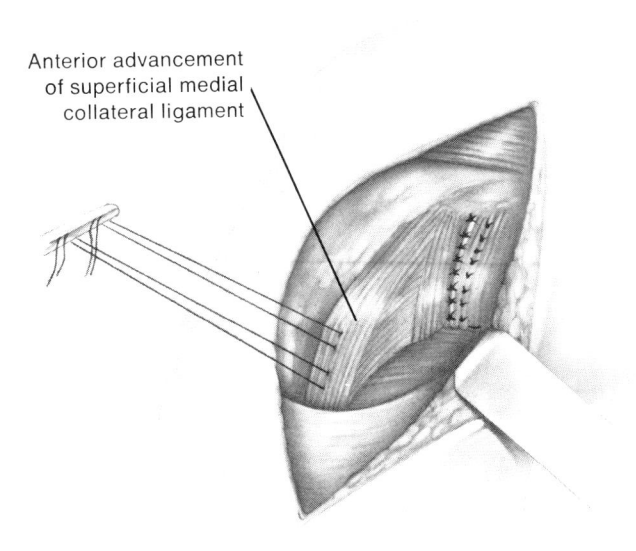

MEDIAL COLLATERAL LIGAMENT RECONSTRUCTION (Plate 12-19)

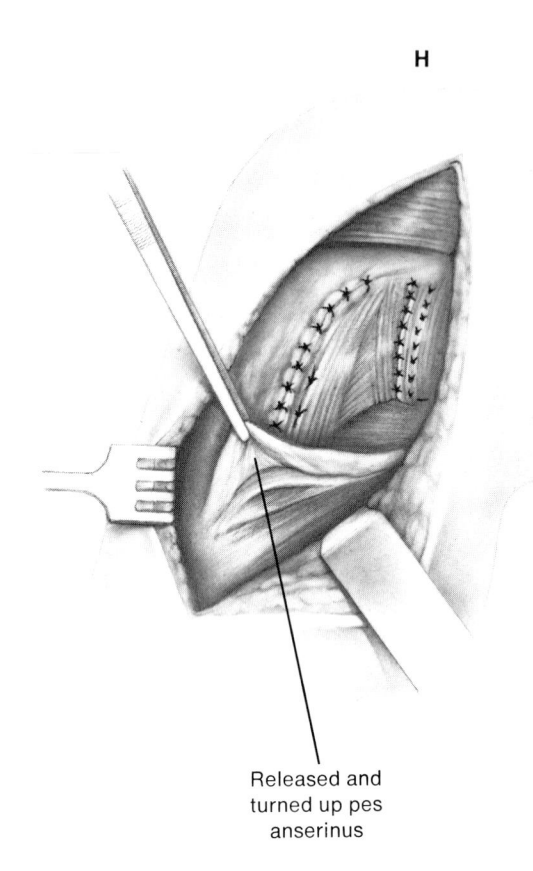

The final step in the procedure is to perform a pes anserinus transfer as described by Slocum and Larson. The inferior two thirds of the normal insertion of the pes anserinus is detached from the anteromedial face of the tibia with care to protect the insertion of the superficial medial collateral ligament and the sartorial branch of the saphenous nerve **(H)**. The pes anserinus is turned up, advanced as far anteriorly as possible, and sutured to the medial border of the patellar tendon and along the anteromedial capsule to enhance the internal rotation function of the pes anserinus **(I)**. The tourniquet is released, and further hemostasis secured. The wound is closed routinely over suction drainage. A well-padded long-leg cast is applied with the knee flexed 70° and the tibia internally rotated.

POSTOPERATIVE MANAGEMENT. Plaster immobilization in the same position is continued for 5 weeks. At that time a mold is taken for a derotation brace, and a cast brace is applied with 30° to 60° hinges for an additional 3 weeks. After removal of the cast brace the previously fabricated derotation brace is applied and the rehabilitation program initiated.

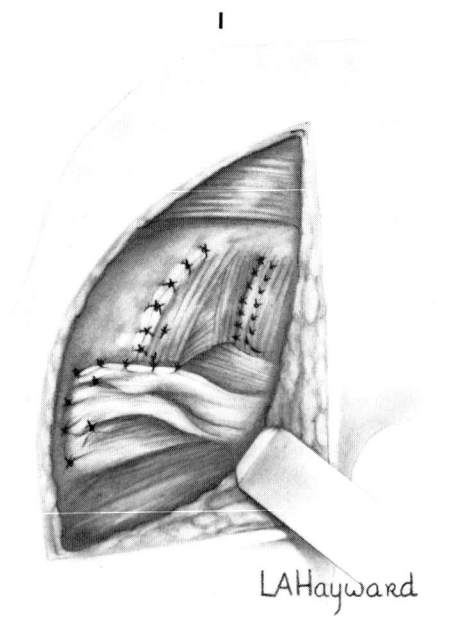

H

Released and turned up pes anserinus

I

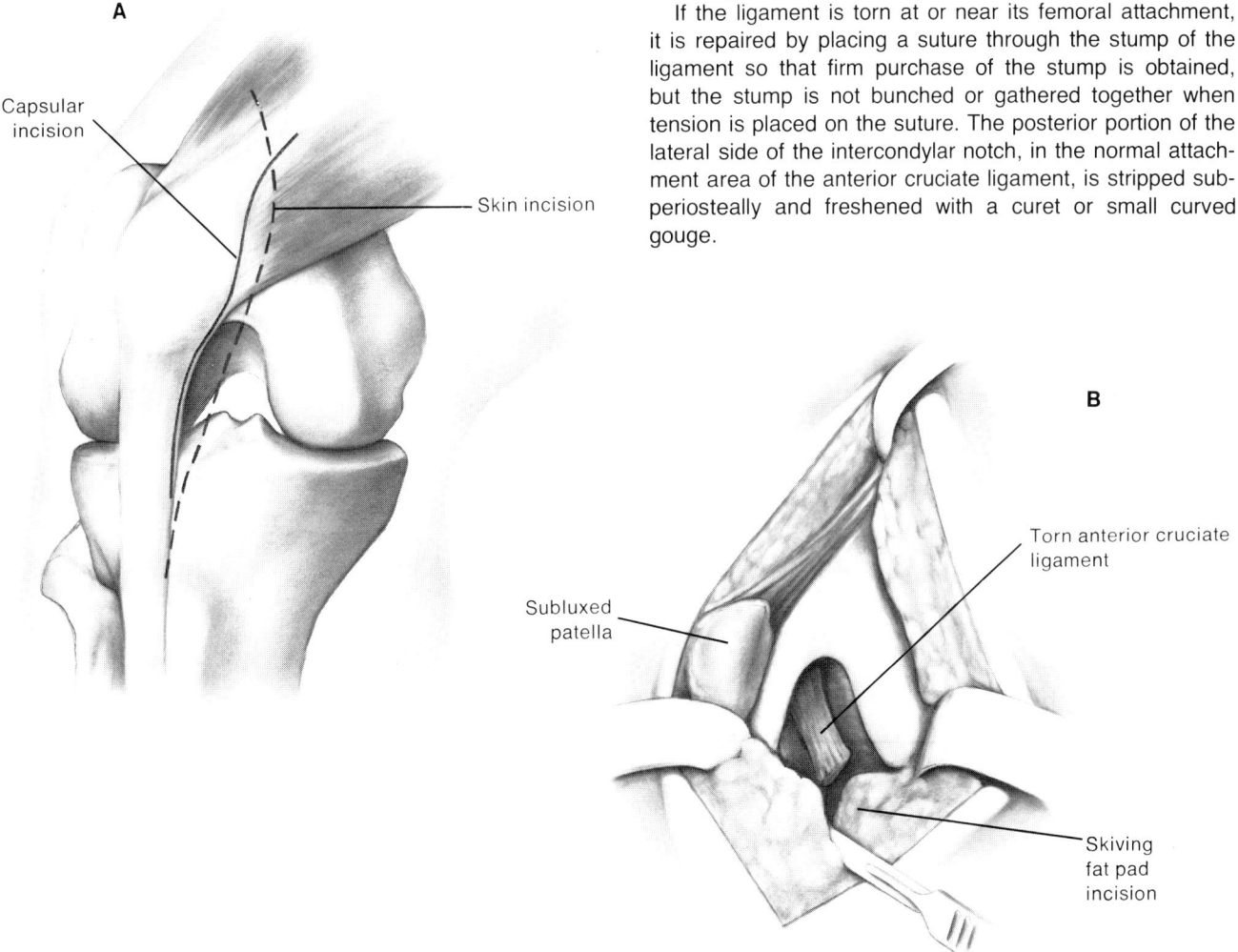

(Plate 12-20) ANTERIOR CRUCIATE LIGAMENT REPAIR

GENERAL DISCUSSION. Although primary repair of acute anterior cruciate ligament tears remains controversial, it is our preference to attempt primary repair whenever possible in younger individuals who are going to be placing strenous demands on their knees. Although it is true that clean tears of the ligament from the femoral attachment or the tibial attachment are unusual, usually the ligament ruptures near its femoral attachment. With the elongation that precedes actual rupture, there is sufficient length to permit repair back to the femur even though ligament shreds can be seen to be coming from the femoral attachment site. The techniques to be described can be used to repair lesions back to the femoral or tibial attachments, but are not suitable for true middle third tears. Marshall has described another technique for repair of middle third tears with satisfactory results.

DETAILS OF PROCEDURE. The knee is flexed over the end of the operating room table and placed on a bolster so that it can be flexed beyond 90°. The knee is initially exposed through a medial parapatellar approach (Plate 12-2). The interior of the knee is explored to be certain that a repairable anterior cruciate ligament tear exists and to examine for associated injury. If it is determined that anterior curciate repair is possible, the skin incision is then extended distally and proximally with a gentle curve toward the midline, as shown by the dotted line **(A)**. The capsular incision is then extended proximally along the vastus medialis tendon insertion, then in line with the quadriceps tendon, and then distally along the medial border of the patellar tendon, as shown by the solid line **(A)**. To further facilitate wide exposure of the intercondylar notch region, a skiving incision is made through the infrapatellar fat pad with care to avoid damaging the medial meniscus peripheral attachments **(B)**. This permits subluxation of the patella over the lateral femoral condyle and provides wide exposure of the intercondylar notch, which greatly facilitates anterior cruciate ligament repairs.

If the ligament is torn at or near its femoral attachment, it is repaired by placing a suture through the stump of the ligament so that firm purchase of the stump is obtained, but the stump is not bunched or gathered together when tension is placed on the suture. The posterior portion of the lateral side of the intercondylar notch, in the normal attachment area of the anterior cruciate ligament, is stripped subperiosteally and freshened with a curet or small curved gouge.

449

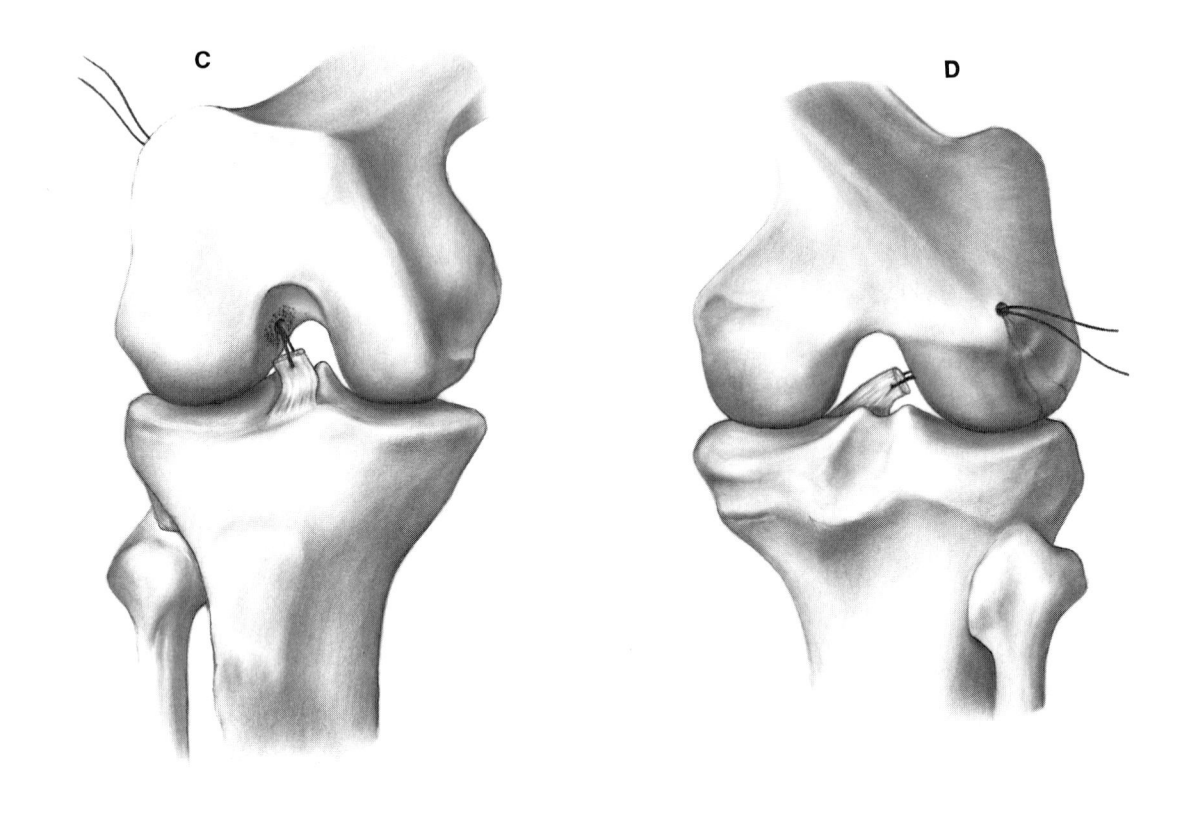

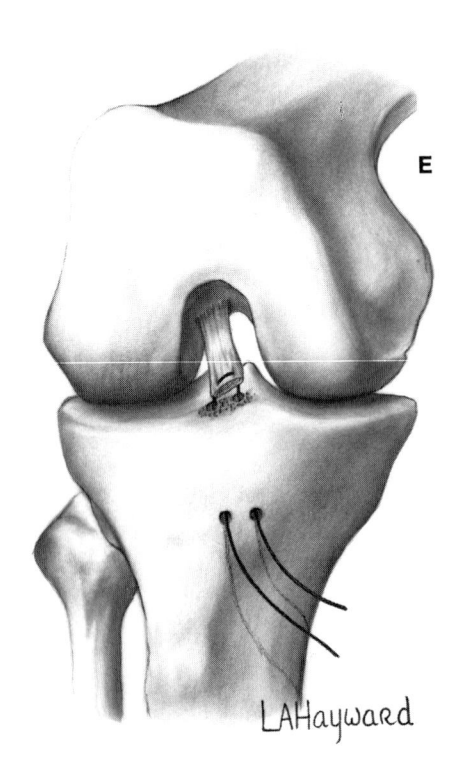

ANTERIOR CRUCIATE LIGAMENT REPAIR (Plate 12-20)

(Plate 12-20) ANTERIOR CRUCIATE LIGAMENT REPAIR

A single drill hole is placed through the posterior portion of the lateral femoral condyle. Special drill guides may be used so that the hole can be drilled from outside in. The hole can also be drilled from inside out, but great care must be taken that the hole is placed sufficiently posterior to permit the ligament to be pulled back into its normal anatomic relationship with the lateral femoral condyle. The exit site of the drill hole from the lateral femoral condyle is exposed through a separate lateral incision running proximally from the lateral femoral epicondyle and splitting the iliotibial tract in line with its fibers. The sutures are pulled through the drill hole as the knee is extended to approximately 30°, and the ligament is observed through the anterior incision to be certain that it is rotating properly and is coming into its normal position. The sutures are tied over a polypropylene button. This repair is shown semischematically from the anterior view **(C)** and the posterior oblique view **(D)**. An alternate method that is also proving to be satisfactory is to place two sutures in the stump of the anterior cruciate ligament, the first in the anteromedial portion of the ligament, and the second in the remaining posterolateral portion. The suture placed in the anteromedial portion of the ligament is passed posteriorly through the notch and brought "over the top" of the lateral femoral condyle as described by MacIntosh. The suture placed in the posterolateral portion of the ligament is passed through the drill hole, and the two sutures are tied together over the external surface of the lateral femoral condyle.

If the ligament is torn at or near its tibial attachment, the normal insertion site is first prepared by making a subperiosteal bed in the midst of any remaining fibers of the ligament still attached to the tibia. Two drill holes are made from the anteromedial surface of the tibia, and these emerge in the prepared site for reattachment **(E)**. A suture is placed through the stump of the anterior curciate ligament so that its ends are exiting from the opposite edges of the ligament. Each end of the suture is passed through one of the two drill holes **(E)** so that when the suture is pulled taut, the ligament is pulled down into its normal attachment site in the prepared bed on the tibia and tied over the anterior surface of the tibia after the knee has been brought to a position of 30° flexion.

The tourniquet is released and further hemostasis secured. The wound is closed over negative suction drainage. A well-padded long-leg plaster cast is applied with the knee flexed 30° and the tibia in neutral rotation. Primary repair of the anterior cruciate ligament is frequently accompanied by augmentation procedures. If the lateral meniscus has been torn, or if there is anterolateral rotatory instability of the pivot-shift type, an advancement of the long head of the biceps is performed (Plate 12-24). If the medial meniscus has been torn, or there is significant anteromedial rotatory instability, a pes anserinus transfer is performed (Plate 12-19). Intra-articular augmentation can also be considered.

POSTOPERATIVE MANAGEMENT. Cast immobilization in this position is continued for 5 weeks, when the cast is removed and a cast brace applied with 30° to 60° hinges. Straight leg-raising exercises are not used during the postoperative period because this may place undue stress on the repaired anterior cruciate ligament. However, vigorous isometric exercises are carried out in which the quadriceps and hamstring muscles are contracted simultaneously. At 8 weeks after surgery the cast brace is removed, a knee brace is applied, and vigorous rehabilitation is initiated. Progressive resistance exercises are done with only the hamstrings for the first 2 to 3 weeks. Quadriceps progressive resistance exercises are initiated, but are done in an isotonic fashion from 90° to 45° only for the first 6 months before full-range quadriceps progressive resistance exercises are begun.

ANTERIOR CRUCIATE LIGAMENT RECONSTRUCTION (Plate 12-21)

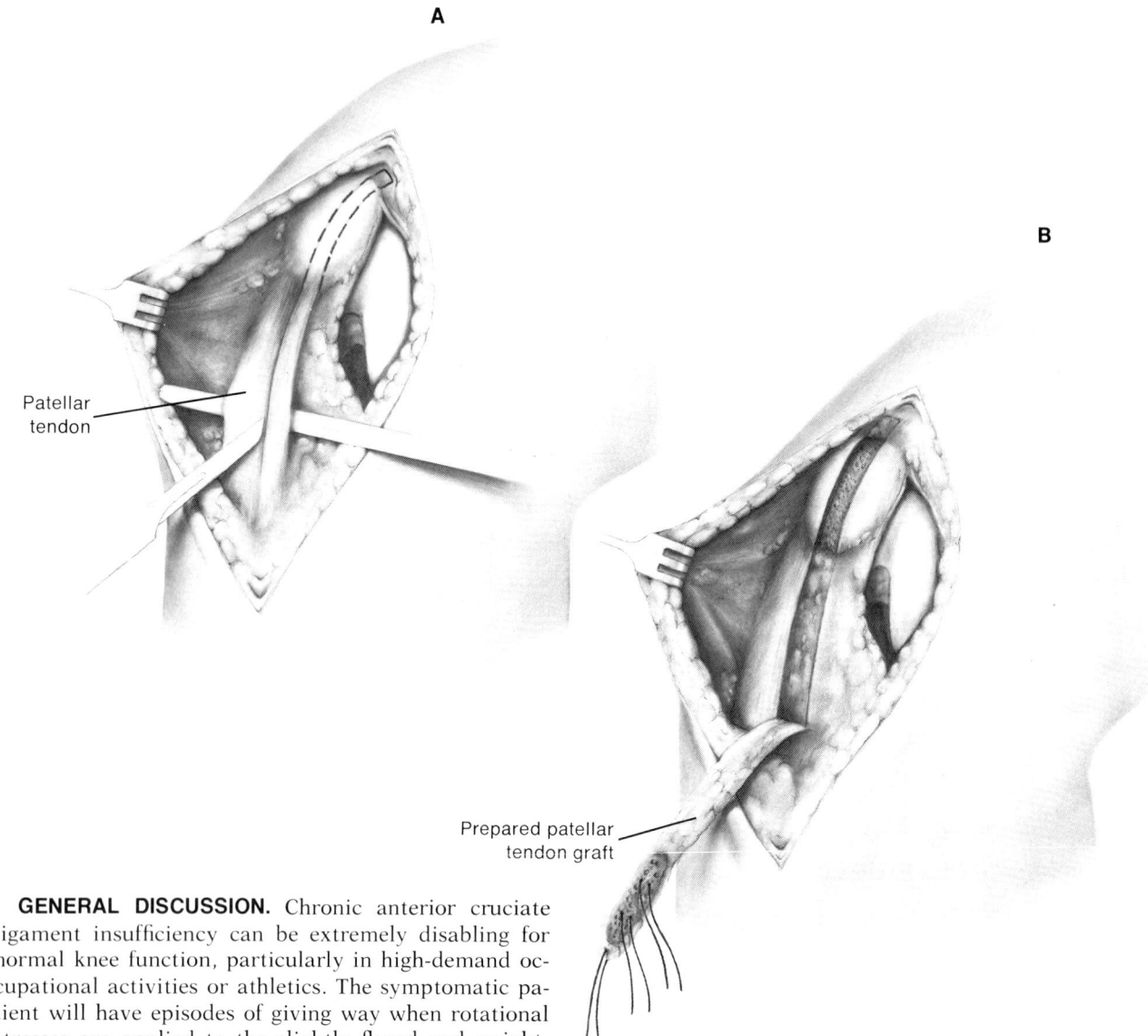

GENERAL DISCUSSION. Chronic anterior cruciate ligament insufficiency can be extremely disabling for normal knee function, particularly in high-demand occupational activities or athletics. The symptomatic patient will have episodes of giving way when rotational stresses are applied to the slightly flexed and weight-bearing knee. It can be a particularly devastating instability, not only from a functional standpoint, but also by leading to secondary tears of the menisci and degenerative changes of the medial and lateral compartments. When symptomatic functional instability from anterior cruciate ligament insufficiency is present, the physical examination will usually show a combined type of instability with abnormal anterior Drawer sign in neutral rotation, anteromedial rotatory instability, and anterolateral rotatory instability of the pivot shift type. Before anterior cruciate reconstructive surgery is considered, the same attempt at nonoperative treatment as described in Plate 12-17 for medial reconstruction should be undertaken, and the same patient selection factors are also important.

The procedure to be described uses the patellar tendon as described by Jones and modified by Eriksson and Clancy.

DETAILS OF PROCEDURE. The knee is exposed through a long medial parapatellar incision. An anteromedial capsular incision is made for inspection of the joint, and if other structures in addition to the anterior cruciate ligament are damaged, surgical treatment of these associated problems is carried out as indicated. The medial one third of the patellar tendon is identified (usually 1 cm) and incised in line with its fibers. The incision is continued proximally across the anterior patella and extended a short distance in continuity into the quadriceps tendon **(A)**. The anterior patellar bone is cut in the line of the incision with an oscillatory saw, and the tendon graft is carefully freed from the patella **(B)**. It is left attached distally to the tibial tubercle, and a thin sliver of anterior patellar bone is included. Drill holes are placed through the patellar bone portion of the graft for the passage of sutures that will be used later to secure the graft **(B)**.

(Plate 12-21) ANTERIOR CRUCIATE LIGAMENT RECONSTRUCTION

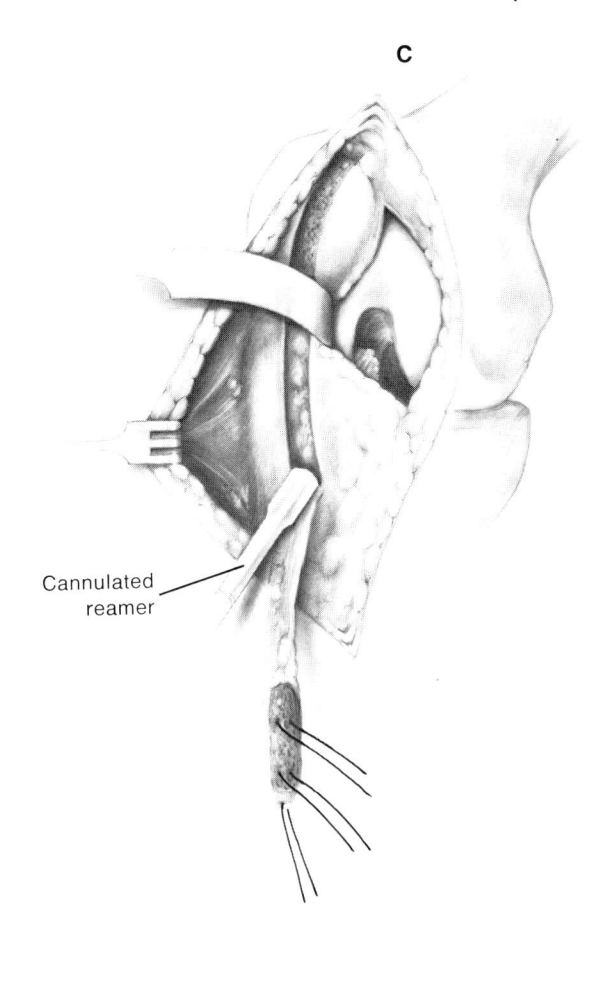

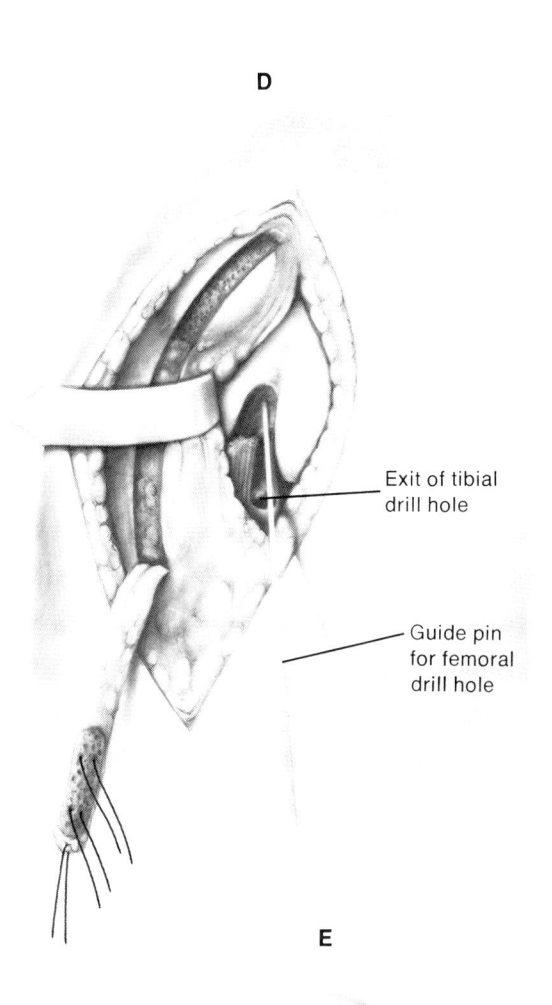

A guide wire is placed through the tibia from the tibial tubercle to the surface of the tibia where the anterior cruciate ligament normally inserts. It is important that the guide wire be placed anterior and medial to the anatomic center of attachment of the anterior cruciate ligament on the tibia. A cannulated reamer is then used to make the tibial drill hole with the aid of the previously placed guide wire (**C**). The posterior aspect of the lateral side of the intercondylar notch is then freshened with a periosteal elevator and curets, and a second guide wire is passed through the posterior portion of the lateral femoral condyle in the area of anatomic attachment of the anterior cruciate ligament.

453

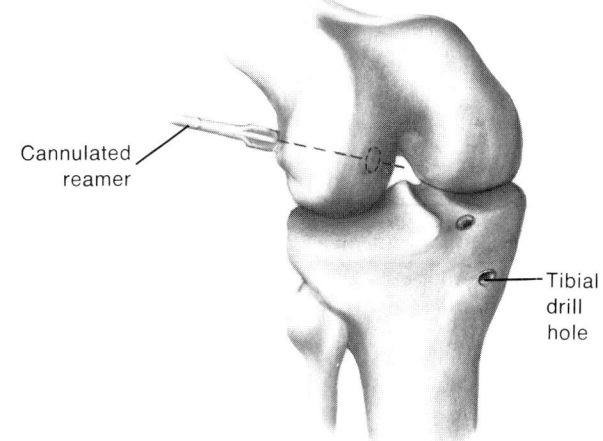

ANTERIOR CRUCIATE LIGAMENT RECONSTRUCTION (Plate 12-21)

A second incision is made laterally beginning at the lateral femoral epicondyle and proceeding proximally in line with the femur for approximately 5 cm. The iliotibial band is split in line with its fibers, and the vastus lateralis retracted to expose the exit point of the previously placed guide pin. The femoral drill hole is then made with a cannulated reamer from outside in, over the previously placed guide pin (**D** and **E**). The graft is then passed through the tibial drill hole **(F)**, and then into the femoral drill hole, while the graft is rotated 90° before it is pulled into the femoral drill hole, so that it is oriented similarly to the anterior cruciate ligament. It is important that the graft is pulled securely through the drill holes so that there is no slack. When the graft is observed coming through the tibial drill hole, it will be seen to lay against the posterior and lateral edge of the hole. The guide pin must be placed anterior and medial to the central point of attachment of the anterior cruciate ligament and the drill hole made eccentrically so that as the graft is lying against the posterolateral margin of the drill hole, it will be in anatomic position in regard to the tibia. With tension applied to the sutures pulling the graft up into the femoral drill hole, the knee should be checked through a range of motion, and for stability. If this is found to be satisfactory, then the sutures are passed through a sterile polypropylene button and securely tied over the button, which rests against the external surface of the lateral femoral condyle **(G).**

The tourniquet is then released and hemostasis secured. The incisions are then closed in a routine fashion with care to repair the quadriceps and medial parapatellar capsular and retinacular layers as carefully as possible, over closed suction drainage. A well-padded plaster cast is applied with the knee near full extension.

POSTOPERATIVE MANAGEMENT. Plaster immobilization is continued for approximately 5 weeks, at which time a 30° to 60° cast brace is applied for an additional 3 weeks before the rehabilitation program is initiated. The patient is protected with partial weight bearing on crutches and bracing for several weeks after the active rehabilitation process is initiated.

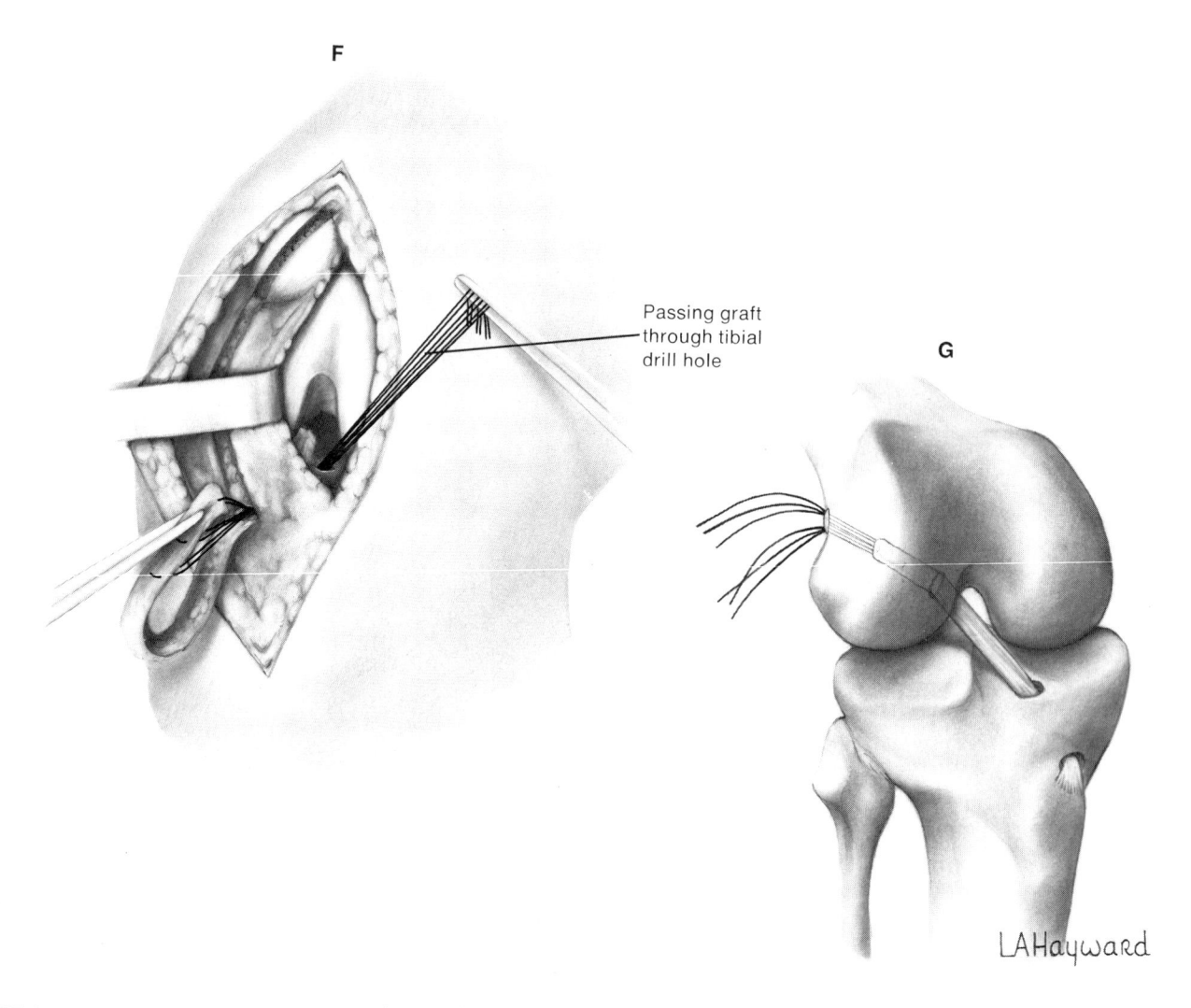

F

Passing graft through tibial drill hole

G

(Plate 12-22) REPAIR OF TORN POSTERIOR CRUCIATE LIGAMENT

GENERAL DISCUSSION. Repair of acute posterior cruciate ligament tears is not as controversial as repair of anterior cruciate ligament tears, since the vascularity and potential for successful healing is greater, and because of the critical importance of the posterior cruciate ligament to overall knee function. As with anterior cruciate ligament tears, the posterior cruciate ligament can tear at or near either bony attachment, or in the midsubstance. Because of the functional significance of the posterior cruciate ligament, it is our preference to attempt primary repair of all posterior cruciate ligament tears regardless of the site of the tear unless there are overriding contraindications to surgical intervention.

Occasionally the posterior cruciate ligament will be torn from the tibial attachment with a sizeable fragment of bone, which can be seen on routine x-ray pictures. This is best repaired through a classic posterior approach to the knee, the fragment of bone being reduced and fixed with a screw. The techniques to be described can be used to repair the posterior cruciate ligament back to either the femoral or the tibial attachment site when there is no fragment of bone, and midsubstance tears are repaired in both directions with a combination of the illustrated techniques.

DETAILS OF PROCEDURE. The knee is initially exposed through a medial parapatellar approach, as described in Plate 12-2, A. The knee is then explored, and the torn posterior cruciate ligament examined carefully to determine whether it is torn proximally from the femur, distally from the tibia, or in the midsubstance.

If the ligament is torn at or near the tibial insertion, the torn stump of the posterior cruciate ligament is delivered anteriorly into the incision, and sutures are placed through the distal stump of the ligament to achieve secure fixation without bunching the ligament together. A standard posteromedial approach is then carried out as described in Plate 12-2, A, and this will permit the tip of a finger to reach into the back of the knee and feel the depression in the intercondyle emminence of the posterior tibia where the posterior cruciate ligament should be attaching. This area of bone is roughened and freshened with the curet and periosteal elevator. Two parallel drill holes are then made through the proximal tibia from anterior to posterior, with both holes exiting posteriorly in the region of posterior cruciate attachment to the tibia. The posterior cruciate ligament stump with the previously placed suture is then placed back in its normal position in the posterior aspect of the intercondylar notch, and with suture passers, the suture ends are brought through the drill holes from posterior to anterior (**A** to **C**). Thus, when the sutures are pulled up tight, the posterior cruciate is pulled back into its normal position. The sutures are then tied over the anterior aspect of the tibia.

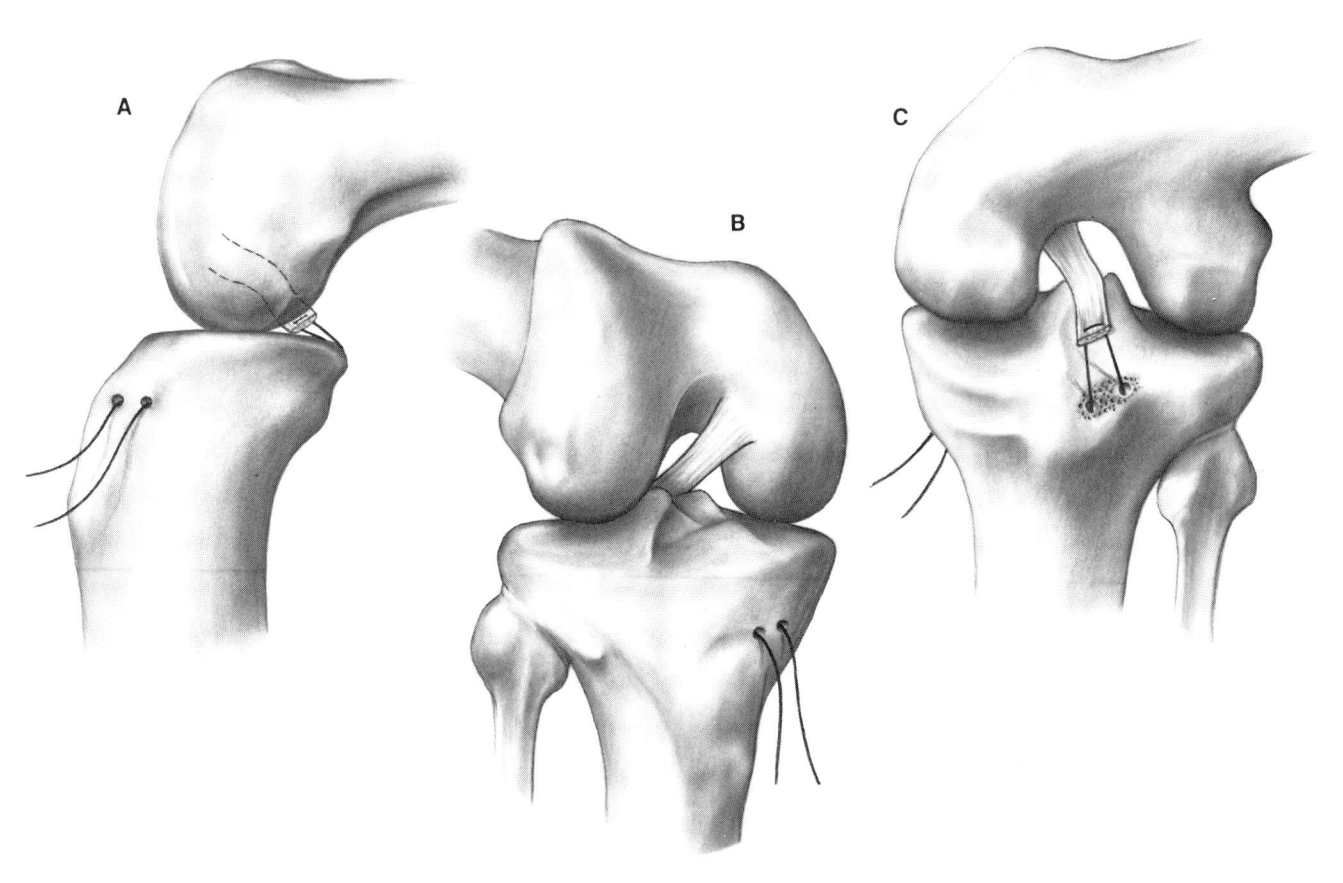

REPAIR OF TORN POSTERIOR CRUCIATE LIGAMENT (Plate 12-22)

If the posterior cruciate ligament is torn from the femoral end, then the repair can be carried out through the single anteromedial incision, by freshening the bony surface where the posterior cruciate ligament normally attaches. Then two drill holes are made from outside in through the medial femoral condyle so that sutures placed in the ligament stump can be passed through the drill holes to pull the ligament back into its normal position. The sutures are then tied over the external surface of the medial femoral condyle (**D** and **E**). If the ligament is torn in the middle one third, a combination of these two techniques is used so that the ligament is repaired both ways.

Prior to tying down the repaired sutures for posterior cruciate ligament repair, we prefer to insert a heavy transarticular fixation pin to ensure that there is no posterior subluxation of the tibia in the early postoperative period. Once the pin has been placed, the repaired sutures are tied down. The tourniquet is then released, further hemostasis is secured, and the incisions are closed in a routine fashion over suction drainage. A well-padded plaster cast is applied with the knee in 30° flexion.

POSTOPERATIVE MANAGEMENT. The plaster cast and transarticular pin are maintained for 5 weeks, when the pin is removed, and a 30° to 60° cast brace applied. The cast brace is maintained for 3 additional weeks. It is then removed, and the more vigorous rehabilitation program is initiated, during which brace protection is used for the first several weeks.

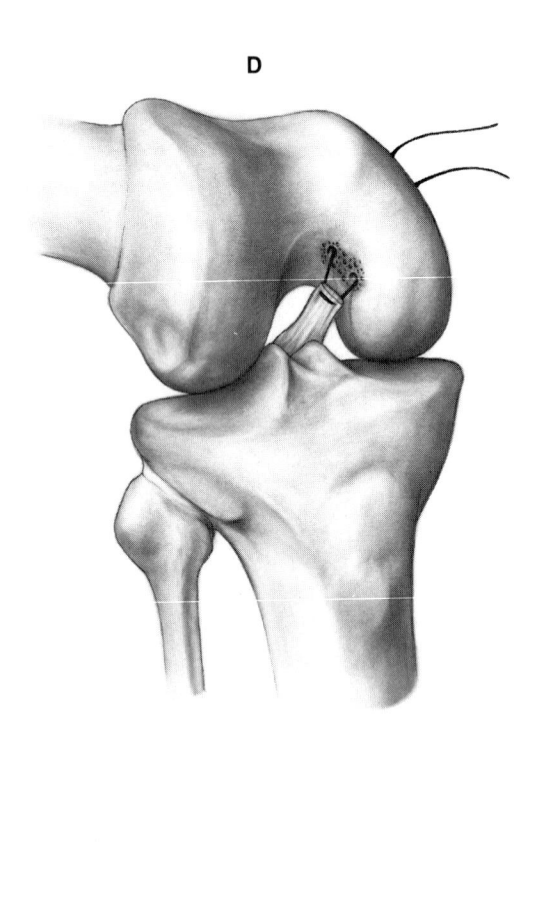

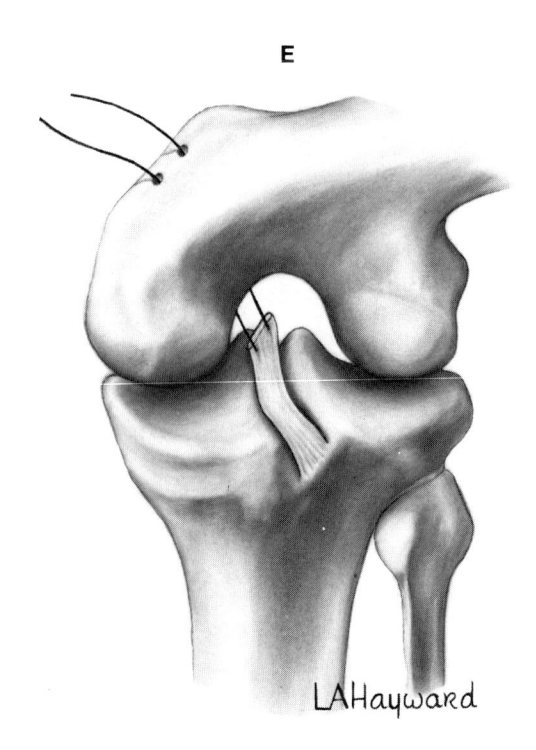

(Plate 12-23) REPAIR OF TORN LATERAL LIGAMENTS

GENERAL DISCUSSION. Disruption of the lateral collateral ligament complex is much less common than that of the medial, but promp diagnosis and early primary repair is just as important to obtain optimal stability and functional recovery. The one additional feature of concern with lateral side tears is injury to the common peroneal nerve, which occurs frequently. In addition to clinical evaluation for lateral stability, one should carefully assess the status of the common peroneal nerve.

DETAILS OF PROCEDURE. The lateral side of the knee is exposed through a lateral utility approach as described in Plate 12-2, and the lateral structures are carefully examined to determine the exact pathology. A frequent pattern of disruption is illustrated (**A**) in which the iliotibial tract is torn near its insertion to the tibia, the lateral capsular ligament is avulsed from the tibia, the popliteus tendon is avulsed from the lateral side of the femur, and the biceps, fibular collateral, and arcuate ligament complex are torn from the fibular head. The common peroneal nerve should be carefully explored to be certain that it is not disrupted. It is usually found to be in continuity, but swollen and hemorrhagic. It should be mobilized carefully and protected throughout the procedure.

Frequently there are additional lesions involving the lateral meniscus and one or both cruciate ligaments that should also be assessed with care, as well as the medial meniscus.

In some cases the posterior capsule will be avulsed from the tibia, and this should be repaired first by using sutures passed through drill holes as illustrated (**B** and **C**). The popliteus tendon should be repaired back to its normal attachment site on the lateral side of the femur and fixed with a small barbed staple and/or sutures through drill holes (**D**). The lateral capsule is then repaired back to the tibia with sutures placed through drill holes, after the bony surface of the tibia is freshened to help ensure satisfactory healing (**D**).

REPAIR OF TORN LATERAL LIGAMENTS (Plate 12-23)

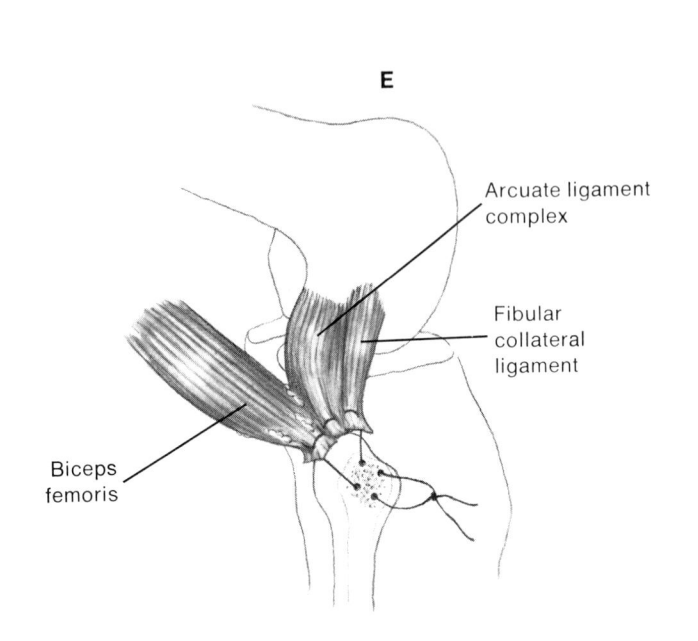

The arcuate ligament complex, fibular collateral ligament, and biceps femoris tendon are next reattached to the fibular head with properly placed sutures passed through drill holes, to reestablish the normal relationships and tension **(E)**. The posterolateral structures that attach to the fibula are then plicated and advanced anteriorly over the lateral capsule **(F)**. The knee must be frequently assessed for stability after each step of the procedure to make sure that there is no residual laxity. The iliotibial band is then repaired with direct sutures **(G)**, or if it has been avulsed from its tibial attachment, it can be reattached with a barbed staple.

The tourniquet is deflated and further hemostasis secured, and the wound closed in a routine fashion over closed suction drainage. A well-padded plaster cast is applied with the knee flexed approximately 70°. If it has been necessary to also repair one or both cruciate ligaments, the knee is flexed only 40° in the cast.

POSTOPERATIVE MANAGEMENT. The cast is maintained for 5 weeks and then replaced with a 30° to 60° cast brace. This is continued for 3 additional weeks before removal of the cast brace, fitting with a protective knee brace, and initiation of the rehabilitation program.

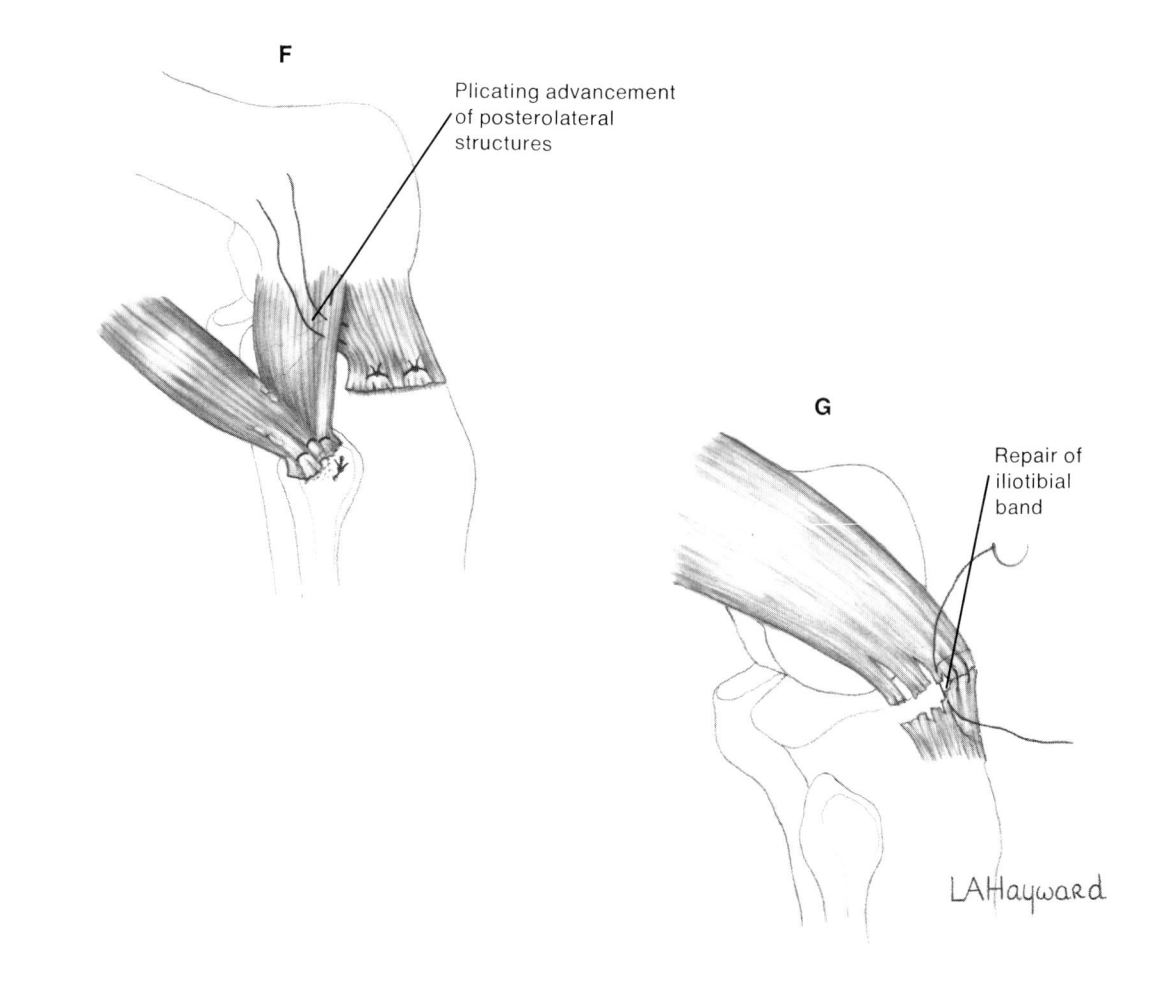

458

(Plate 12-24) MODIFIED MacINTOSH RECONSTRUCTION FOR CHRONIC ANTEROLATERAL ROTATORY INSTABILITY

GENERAL DISCUSSION. A common manifestation of chronic anterior cruciate ligament insufficiency is anterolateral rotatory instability, described as the "lateral pivot-shift" by MacIntosh and Galway. It is unusual for this instability to exist as an isolated entity; it is usually the anterolateral component of a combined type of instability associated with an old tear of the anterior cruciate ligament, which includes straight anterior instability and anteromedial rotatory instability. The procedure to be described is a slightly modified iliotibial band tenodesis as described by MacIntosh and Galway, augmented by advancement of the long head of the biceps femoris, to control the anterolateral component of chronic anterior cruciate ligament insufficiency.

DETAILS OF PROCEDURE. The lateral aspect of the knee is exposed through a lateral utility approach as described in Plate 12-2. The deep fascia and iliotibial band are widely exposed from the lateral border of the patella to Gerdy's tubercle of the tibia, to the fibular head, and as far proximaly as possible, to identify the important landmarks **(A)**.

A 10 cm strip of iliotibial band is then carefully dissected. The posterior 1.3 to 1.6 cm of the iliotibial band is used, and it is left attached to Gerdy's tubercle and detached proximally. The fibular collateral ligament is then identified, and the strip is passed beneath it with care to stay extrasynovial **(B)**. The strip is sutured to the fibular collateral ligament under tension. The strip is then passed through a partial-thickness tunnel in the arcuate ligament complex, and simi-

A

Iliotibial band

Biceps femoris

B

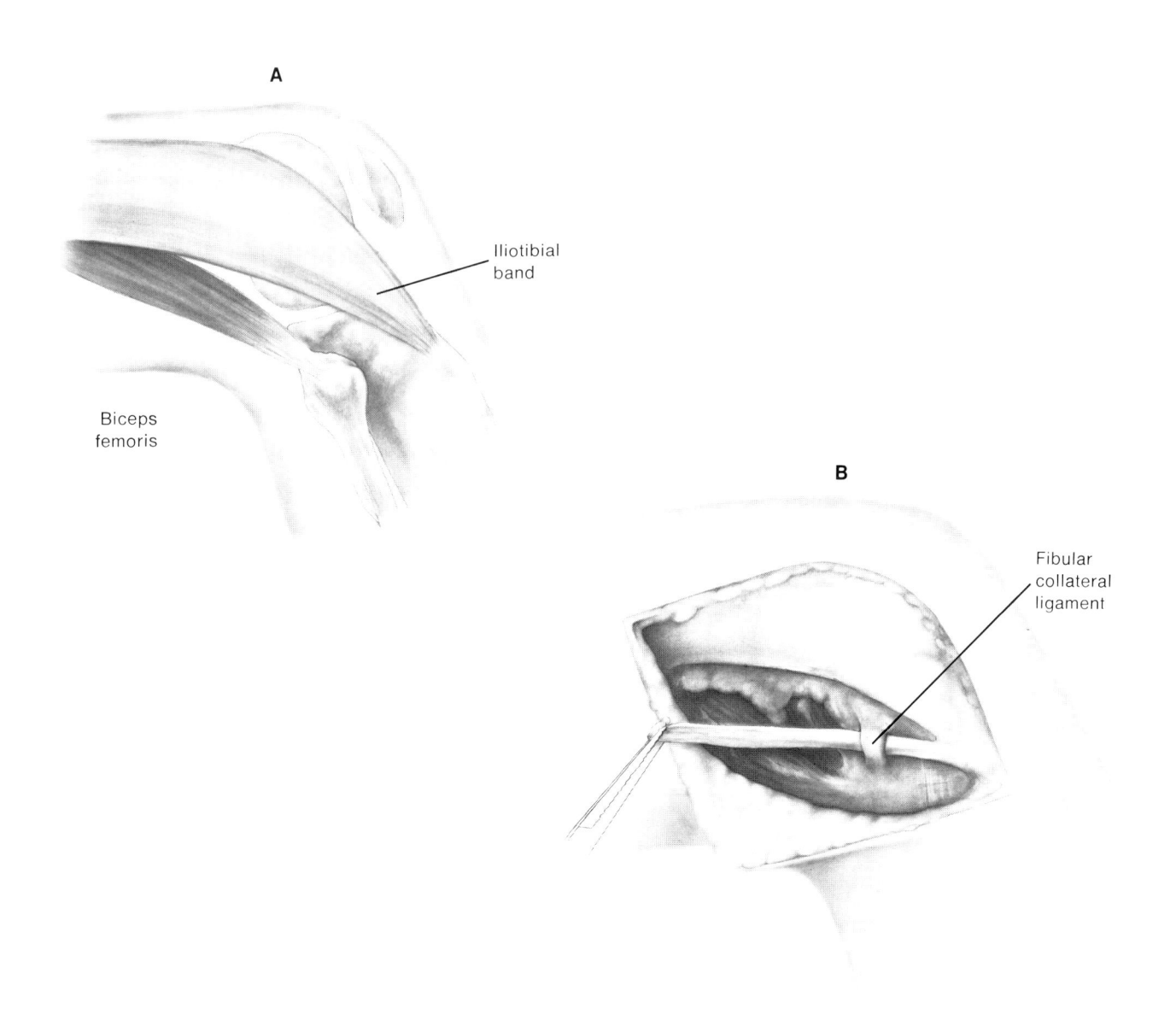

Fibular collateral ligament

459

MODIFIED MacINTOSH RECONSTRUCTION FOR CHRONIC ANTEROLATERAL ROTATORY INSTABILITY (Plate 12-24)

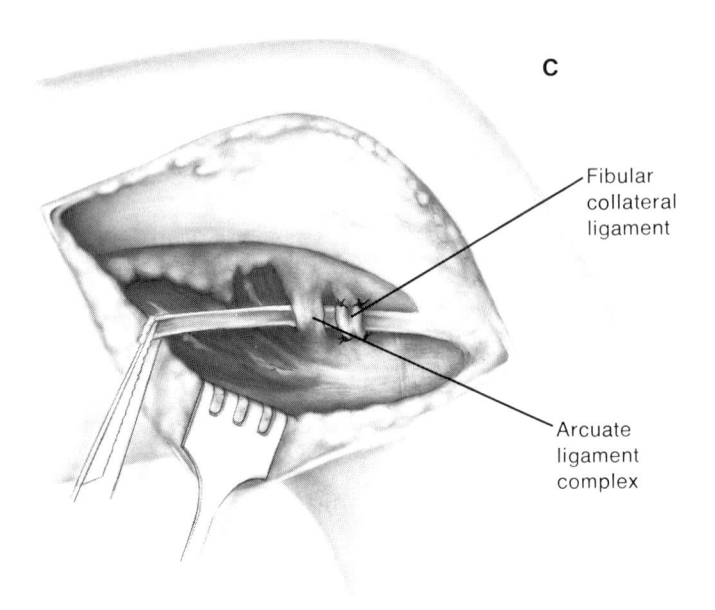

larly sutured to this structure under tension **(C)**. A subperiosteal tunnel is then created near the lateral femoral epicondyle at the confluence of the arcuate ligament complex, the lateral head of the gastrocnemius, and the fibular collateral ligament. The parallel incisions made to create this tunnel are placed in line with the fibers of these structures so that they are not divided or weakened. The fascial strip is then passed through the subperiosteal tunnel at the lateral femoral epicondyle and sutured into this area under tension **(D)**. The strip is then brought back down to the posterolateral corner and sutured on itself under tension **(E)**. The knee should be extended repeatedly at each step in this procedure to be certain that there is adequate tension and that the lateral pivot shift sign has been obliterated. Reefing sutures are then placed through the fibular collateral ligament, the fascial strip, the arcuate ligament complex, and the edge of the lateral gastrocnemius tendon to further reinforce the posterolateral corner of the capsule **(E)**. If there is sufficient length to the fascial strip, it is then brought anteriorly back toward Gerdy's tubercle and sutured into place to complete the iliotibial band tenodesis. Anterolateral rotatory instability of the pivot-shift type should be obliterated by check rein tightening of the fascial strip as the knee approaches full extension.

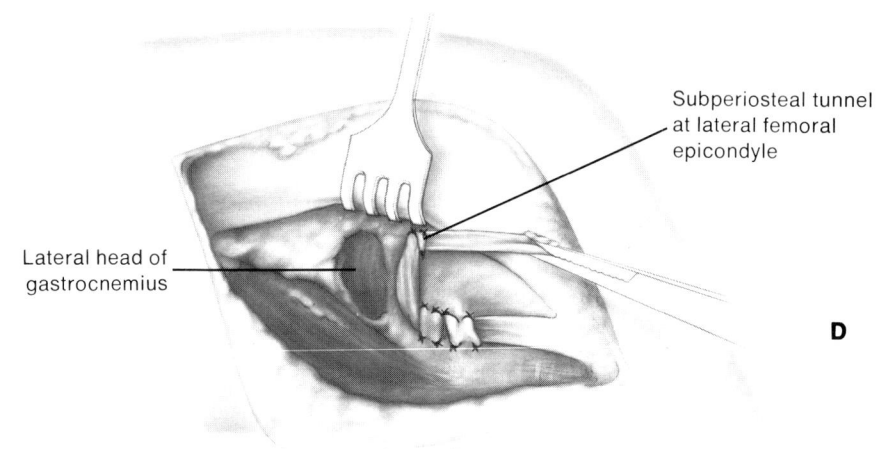

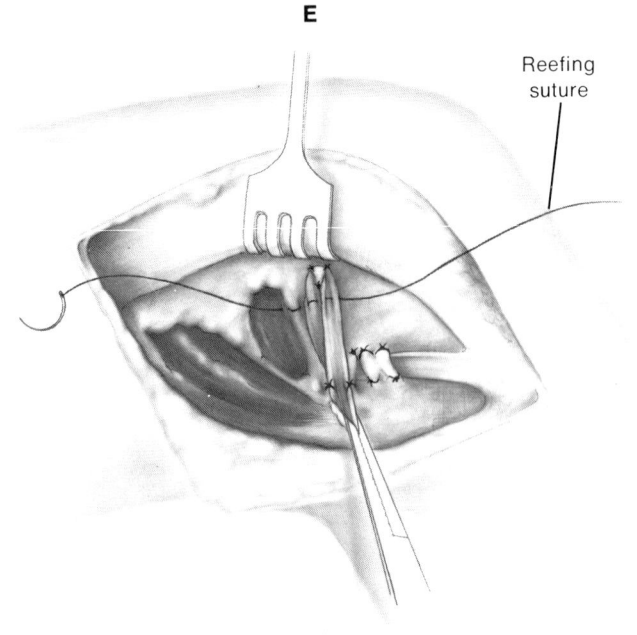

To add dynamic support for the reconstruction, the superficial portion of the biceps tendon (long head) is carefully dissected from its main insertion to the fibular head with great care to protect the fibular collateral ligament and the common peroneal nerve. The biceps tendon fibers that attach to the posterior border of the fibular collateral ligament and deep to this structure are not disturbed. The muscle belly of the biceps femoris is then separated in line with its

(Plate 12-24) MODIFIED MacINTOSH RECONSTRUCTION FOR CHRONIC ANTEROLATERAL ROTATORY INSTABILITY

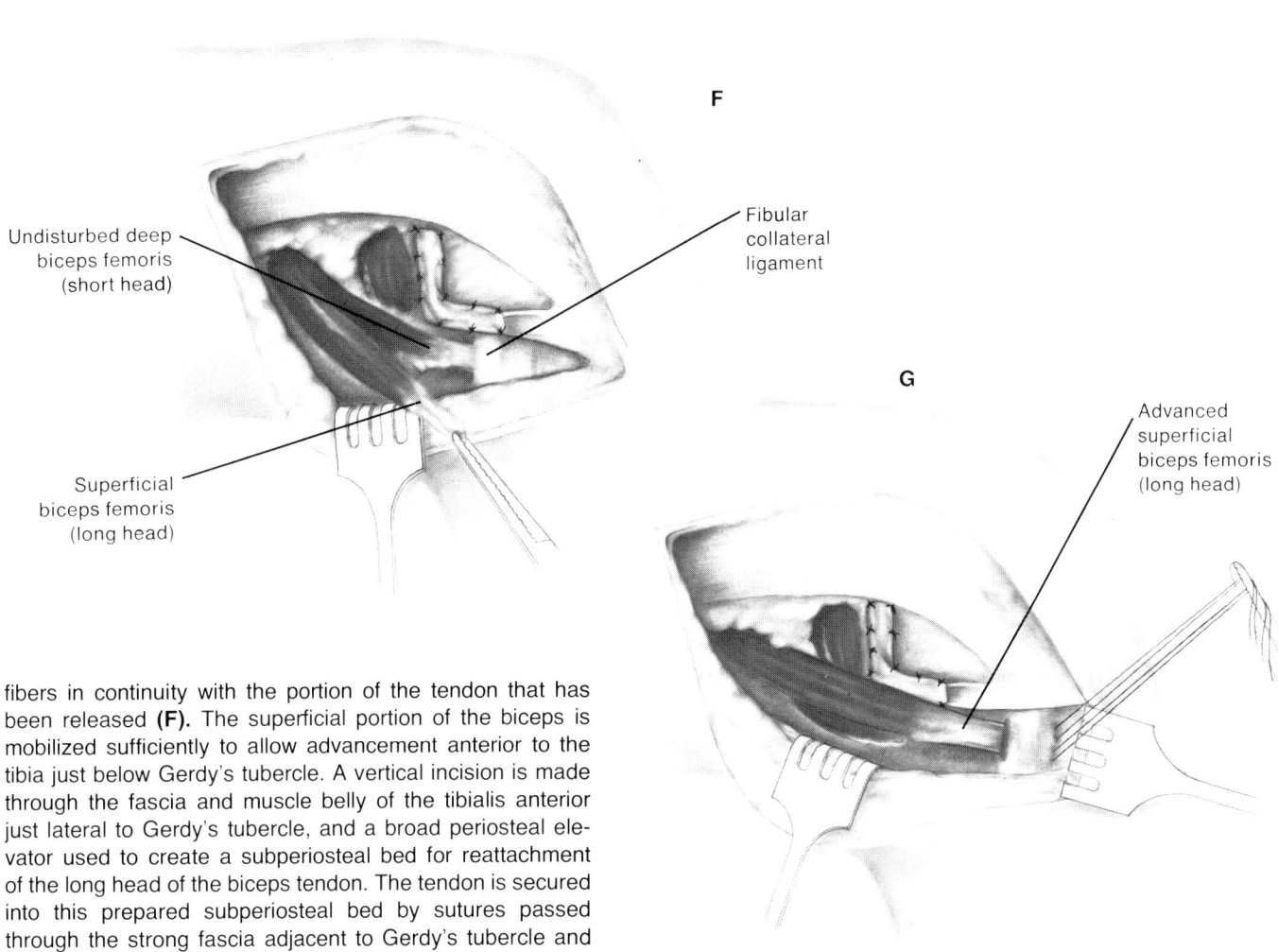

fibers in continuity with the portion of the tendon that has been released **(F)**. The superficial portion of the biceps is mobilized sufficiently to allow advancement anterior to the tibia just below Gerdy's tubercle. A vertical incision is made through the fascia and muscle belly of the tibialis anterior just lateral to Gerdy's tubercle, and a broad periosteal elevator used to create a subperiosteal bed for reattachment of the long head of the biceps tendon. The tendon is secured into this prepared subperiosteal bed by sutures passed through the strong fascia adjacent to Gerdy's tubercle and the lateral border of the patellar tendon **(G)**. Additional anchoring sutures are used to provide secure fixation. The deep fascia is sutured back to the remaining posterior border of the iliotibial band **(H)** over suction drainage, and the wound is closed in a routine fashion. This procedure frequently may be combined with other surgical procedures, including meniscectomy or meniscus reattachment, or additional ligament reconstruction procedures as appropriate in each individual patient. At the completion of the procedure, a well-padded long-leg cast is applied with the knee flexed 70° to 80° and the tibia slightly externally rotated. Prophylactic antibiotics are recommended.

POSTOPERATIVE MANAGEMENT. The cast is removed 2 weeks postoperatively, the sutures are removed, and a new long-leg cast is applied with an ankle-foot orthosis that allows ankle motion. At 5 weeks following the operation the patient is casted for a derotation brace and a 30° to 60° cast brace is applied. At 8 weeks postoperatively the cast brace is removed and the derotation brace is applied. More vigorous rehabilitation is initiated, beginning with only hamstring progressive resistance exercises for the first 2 weeks before quadriceps progressive resistance exercises are initiated.

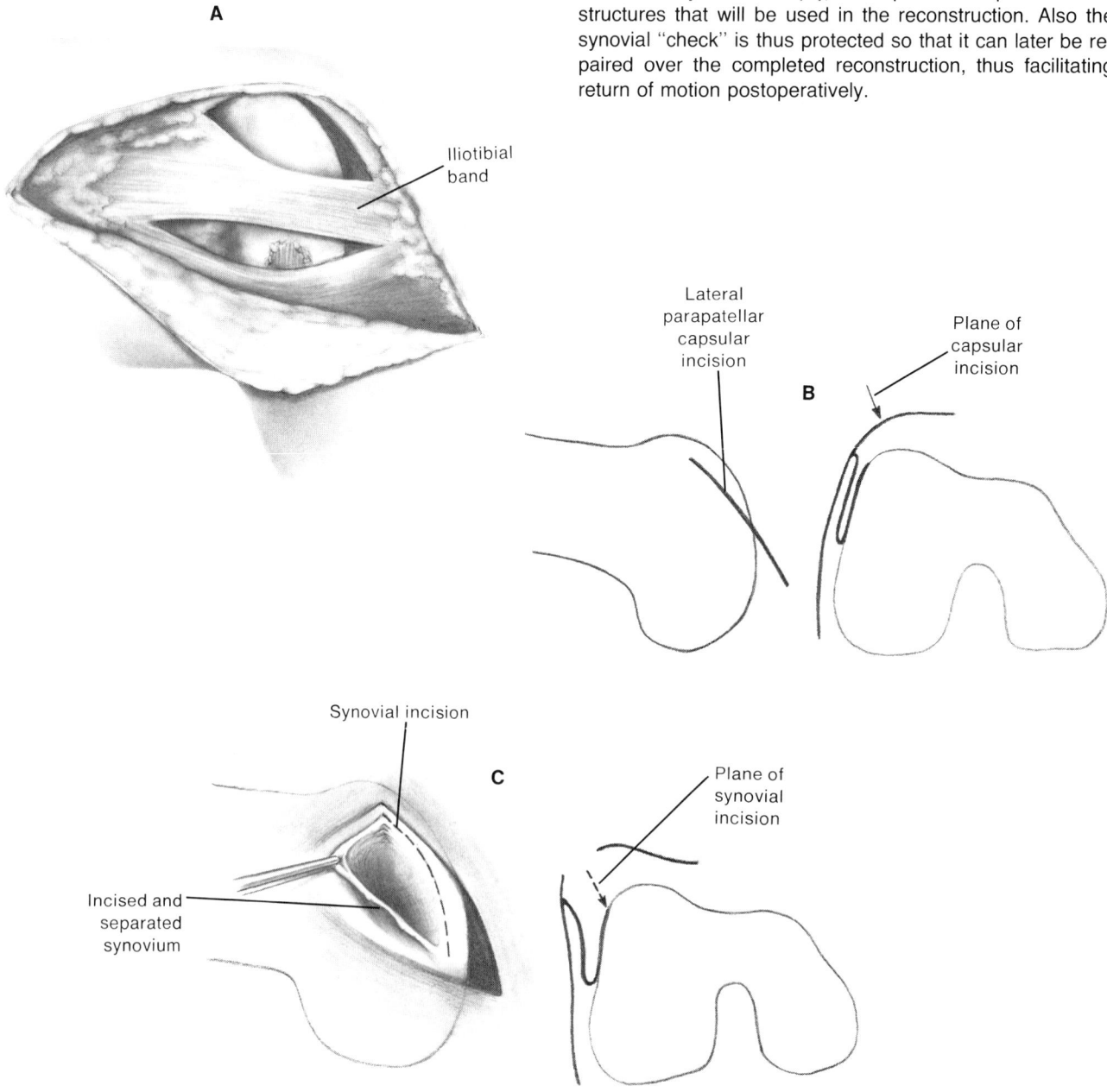

LATERAL LIGAMENT RECONSTRUCTION FOR LATERAL AND POSTEROLATERAL ROTATORY INSTABILITY (Plate 12-25)

GENERAL DISCUSSION. Significant trauma to the lateral ligament complex is much less common than to the medial collateral ligament, but when it does occur, it can lead to disabling instability. The general discussion of Plate 12-19 relating to medial collateral ligament reconstruction applies equally to consideration of reconstructive procedures for lateral instability. Posterolateral rotatory instability has been described by Hughston and Andrews, and the procedure described here is only slightly modified from the procedure they have described.

DETAILS OF PROCEDURE. The operation is carried out with the knee flexed to 90° over the end of the operating table and placed on a bolster. The lateral side of the knee is exposed through a lateral utility approach as described in Plate 12-2. Fiber-splitting incisions are made along the anterior and posterior borders of the iliotibial band, and a lateral parapatellar capsular incision is made **(A)**. The external surface of the lateral femoral condyle is exposed with care to preserve the synovial pocket described as the "cheek of the knee" by Trillat et al. The plane of the initial capsular incision is shown **(B)**, and the incision through the synovium along the femoral condyle is made so that it can be repaired later **(C)**. The layer of synovium adherent to the femur is then carefully dissected **(D)**, which provides exposure to the structures that will be used in the reconstruction. Also the synovial "check" is thus protected so that it can later be repaired over the completed reconstruction, thus facilitating return of motion postoperatively.

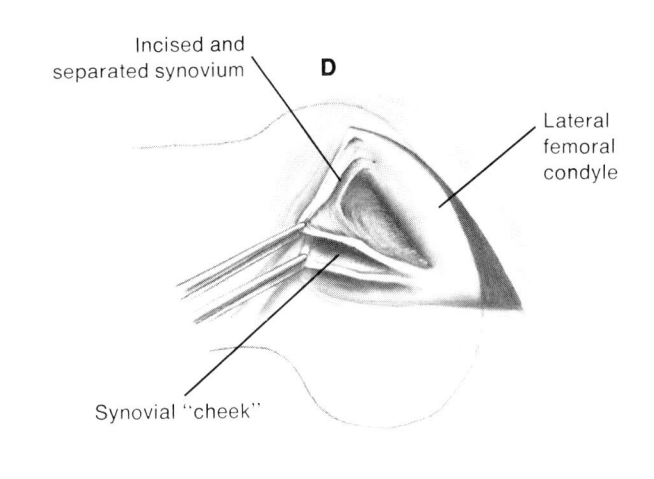

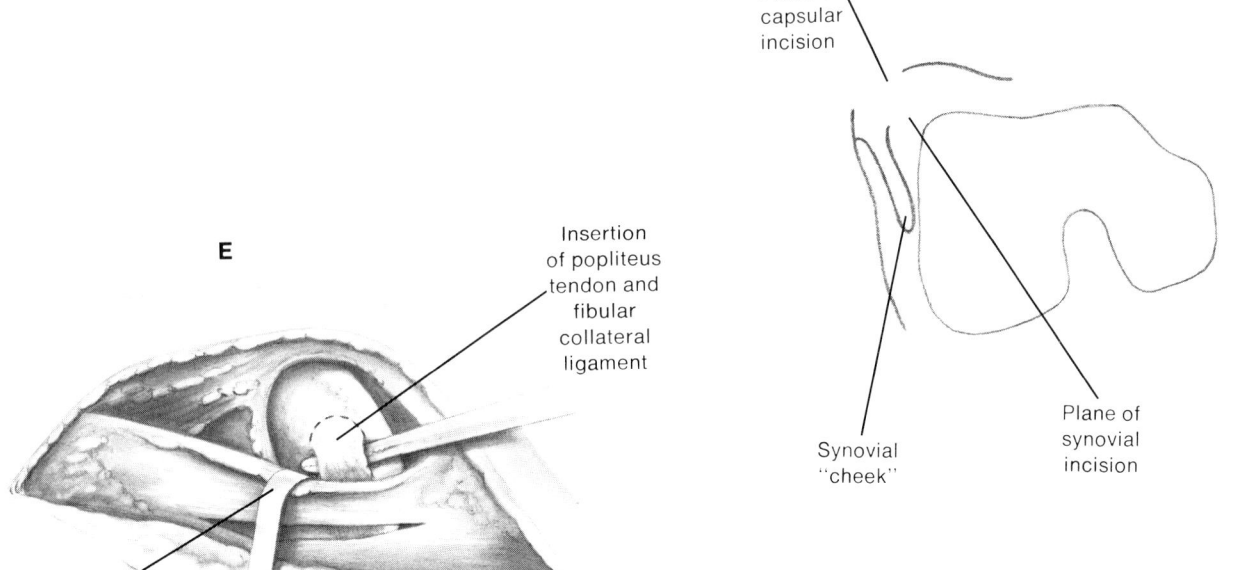

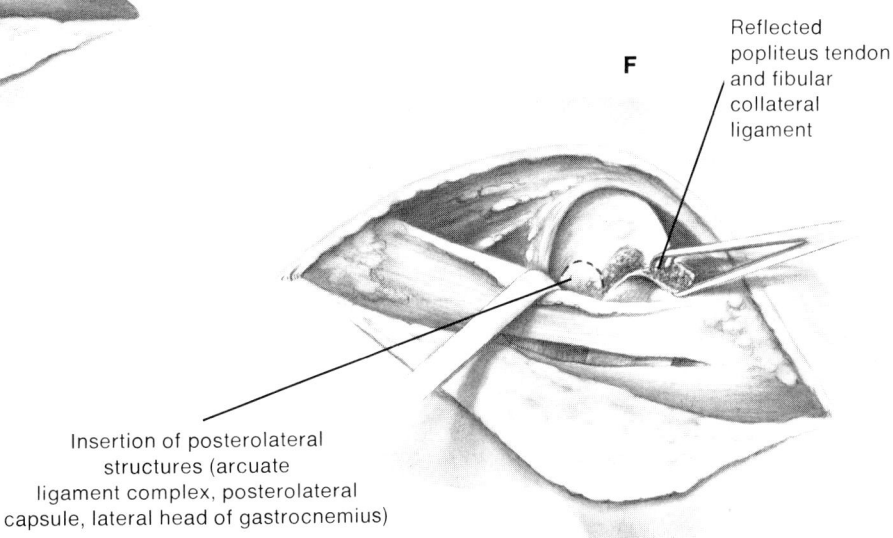

(Plate 12-25) LATERAL LIGAMENT RECONSTRUCTION FOR LATERAL AND POSTEROLATERAL ROTATORY INSTABILITY

The insertion of the popliteus tendon and fibular collateral ligament on the femur is identified and released from the femur with an osteotome so that a thin sliver of bone is left attached to the popliteus tendon and fibular collateral ligament **(E)**. A vertical incision is made along the posterior border of the fibular collateral ligament so that the released structures can be advanced proximally as far as necessary to control the straight lateral laxity. The arcuate ligament complex and lateral head of the gastrocnemius are then identified and similarly detached from the femur with a thin sliver of bone **(F)**. A fiber-splitting incision is made along the posterior margin of the released tissue distally toward the joint line to allow advancement anteriorly and proximally to control the posterolateral rotatory component of the instability. The flaps can be fashioned so that an intact lateral meniscus need not be sacrificed and yet adequate advancement to control the laxity is allowed.

463

LATERAL LIGAMENT RECONSTRUCTION FOR LATERAL AND POSTEROLATERAL ROTATORY INSTABILITY (Plate 12-25)

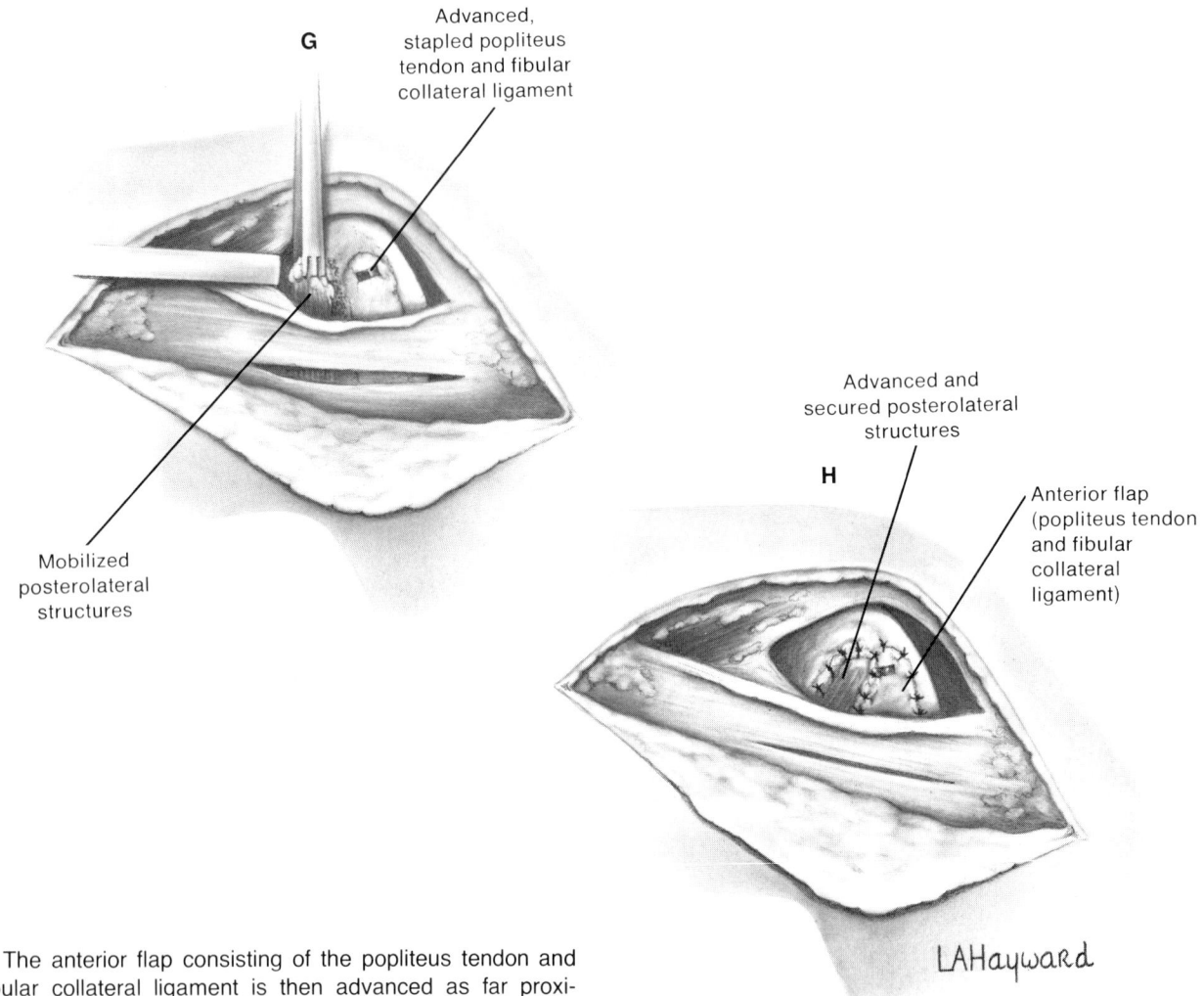

The anterior flap consisting of the popliteus tendon and fibular collateral ligament is then advanced as far proximally as necessary to control the straight lateral laxity and fixed in a prepared bony bed with a barbed staple **(G)**. The posterolateral flap is then advanced proximally and anteriorly over the top of the first flap as required to control the posterolateral rotatory instability, and fixed in a prepared bed with a second staple, and further secured with multiple interrupted sutures **(H)**. The knee should be gently tested for stability to be certain that adequate correction has been obtained. The synovial incision is then repaired with fine absorbable sutures to restore the lateral "cheek," and the remainder of the wound is closed in a routine fashion over suction drainage. This procedure is frequently combined with a pes anserinus transfer as described in Plate 12-19. A well-padded long-leg plaster cast is applied with the knee flexed 70° and the tibia in slight internal rotation. As recommended by Hughston and Andrews, an outrigger is applied to the cast to prevent external rotation of the lower extremity, which would place stress on the repair. When the patient is ready to be ambulated, the outrigger is replaced by a pelvic band with a free hip hinge, which will prevent external rotation during the period of cast immobilization.

POSTOPERATIVE CARE. Two weeks postoperatively the cast and the sutures are removed, and a new long-leg cast is applied with ankle-foot orthosis to allow ankle motion. The pelvic band and hip hinge are retained, however. At 5 weeks following surgery the cast is removed. The patient is fitted for a derotation brace, and a 30° to 60° cast brace is applied, the pelvic band and hip hinge being retained. At 8 weeks postoperatively the cast brace is removed, the prepared derotation brace is applied, and the vigorous rehabilitation program is initiated.

(Plate 12-26) OPEN REDUCTION AND INTERNAL FIXATION FOR TIBIAL PLATEAU FRACTURE

GENERAL DISCUSSION. Joint function following fracture of tibial articular surfaces will ultimately be proportionate to the accuracy of reduction. Open reduction for fractures of the tibial condyles may be indicated when the displacement is severe enough to produce varus or valgus deformities, instability, or gross irregularity of the articular surfaces. If open reduction is carried out, the interior of the joint should be exposed. Open reduction is technically easier if performed on the day of fracture or, if necessary, after the initial swelling has subsided or skin condition permits but within 10 to 14 days of the injury.

The extent of damage in a tibial plateau fracture is often more extensive than suggested by the roentgenograms. The procedure to be described is based on the method described by Hohl.

DETAILS OF PROCEDURE. For a displaced fracture of the lateral tibial plateau, the incision is made beginning 2.5 cm lateral to the superior pole of the patella and is extended distally to a point just lateral to the tibial tuberosity and then redirected distally and laterally to end approximately 6 cm distal to the joint line and just anterior to the fibula. The lateral edge of the wound is reflected until the proximal end of the fibula is visualized. The patellar retinaculum and the synovium of the knee joint are opened. Often the lateral meniscus is torn, traumatized, or displaced enough to require meniscectomy. If this should be necessary, the articular surface of the tibial plateau will be easier to inspect, but the undamaged lateral meniscus should not be removed merely for exposure. If the articular surface of the lateral tibial plateau is difficult to visualize, the lateral meniscus may be incised along its anterior and peripheral attachment and then retracted carefully. It should later be replaced and carefully resutured.

To expose the fracture of the lateral tibial plateau, the origin of the extensor muscles if reflected from the anterolateral aspect of the proximal tibia **(A)**. The depression of the articular surface involves the central portion of the tibial plateau, as indicated by the dashed line, and the peripheral shell of the tibial plateau may not be depressed. A window is created in the anterolateral surface of the tibia to permit access to the depressed articular fragments from below **(B)**, and the articular fragments are elevated back to their normal anatomic position under direct vision through the lateral parapatellar capsular incision. The position is checked by intraoperative x-ray pictures.

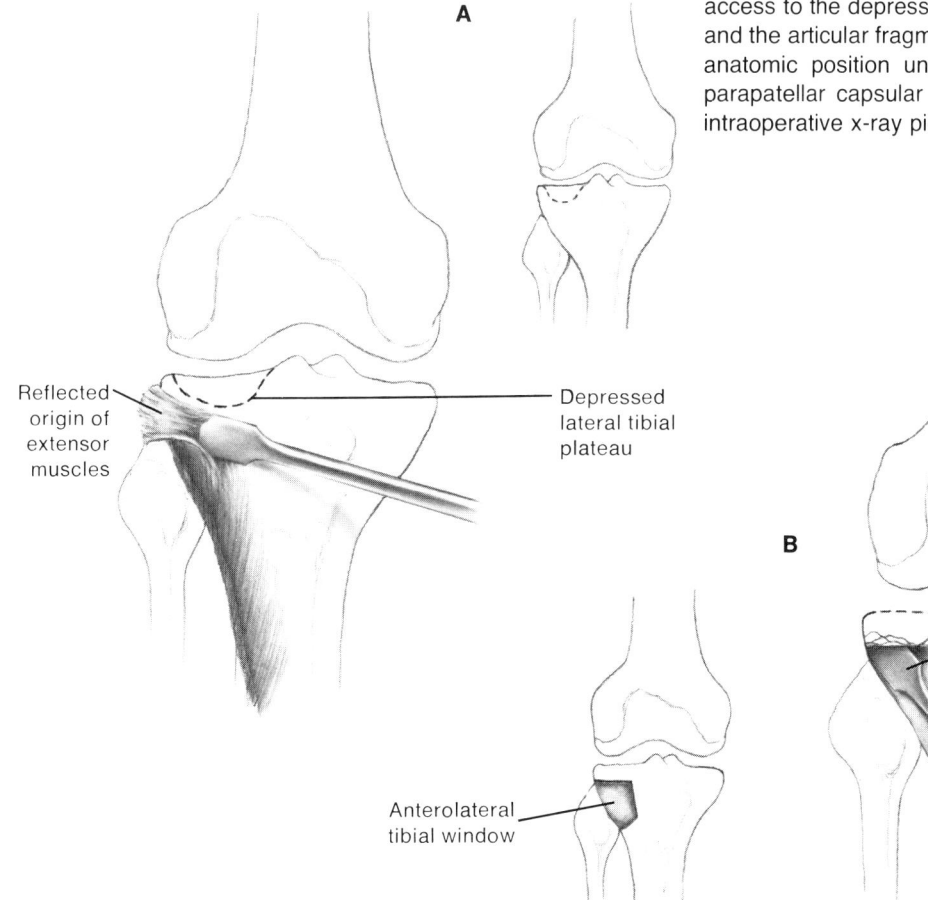

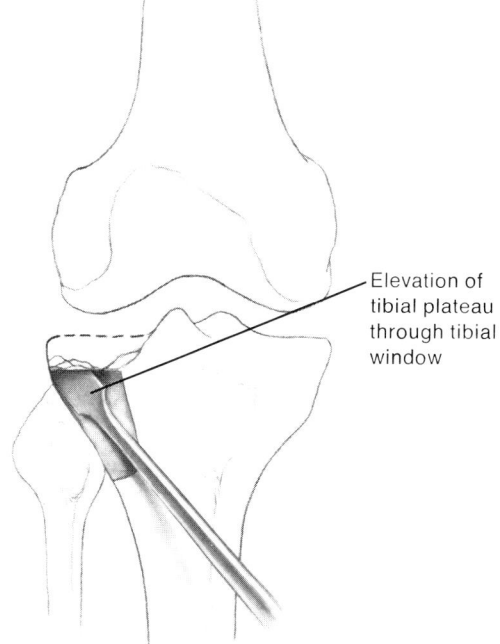

OPEN REDUCTION AND INTERNAL FIXATION FOR TIBIAL PLATEAU FRACTURE (Plate 12-26)

Once the articular surface has been restored to its normal position, there is inevitably a bony void in the subchondral region. An appropriately sized bicortical bone graft is obtained from the ipsilateral iliac crest **(C)**, as well as cancellous chips to use to fill the subarticular void, support the elevated articular surface, and help prevent settling and recurrence of deformity. The immediate subchondral area is packed with cancellous bone, and then the bicortical bone graft is trimmed to fit the space that is present and fixed in place with a tibial bolt that is passed through a lateral buttress plate and through the bone graft. Any remaining bony defect is packed with cancellous chips, and the bone screws are inserted to fix the buttress plate to the tibia (**D** and **E**). The accuracy of the reduction and the adequacy of the internal fixation are checked with intraoperative anteroposterior and lateral roentgenograms. The wound is closed in a routine fashion over suction drainage, and a compression dressing with plaster shell is applied.

POSTOPERATIVE MANAGEMENT. Early motion and delayed weight bearing are advocated following tibial plateau fractures unless prevented by associated injuries. At 48 hours after surgery the drainage tubes and dressing are removed, the patient is placed in balanced suspension with light skin traction, and passive flexion and extension exercises are initiated. When sufficient wound healing has occurred (10 to 14 days), the balanced suspension is discontinued and a long-leg cast brace applied with drop-lock hinges. The patient is ambulated with the hinges locked in full extension, which protects against any valgus stress, and weight bearing is avoided. However, in the seated position, the hinges can be unlocked for intermittent passive range of motion exercises three to five times daily. This process is continued until satisfactory bony healing has occurred. Gradual weight bearing can be initiated between the sixth and tenth week postoperatively, and usually the cast brace can be discontinued at 12 weeks. The rehabilitation process is continued with isometric quadriceps progressive resistance exercises and continuing motion exercises.

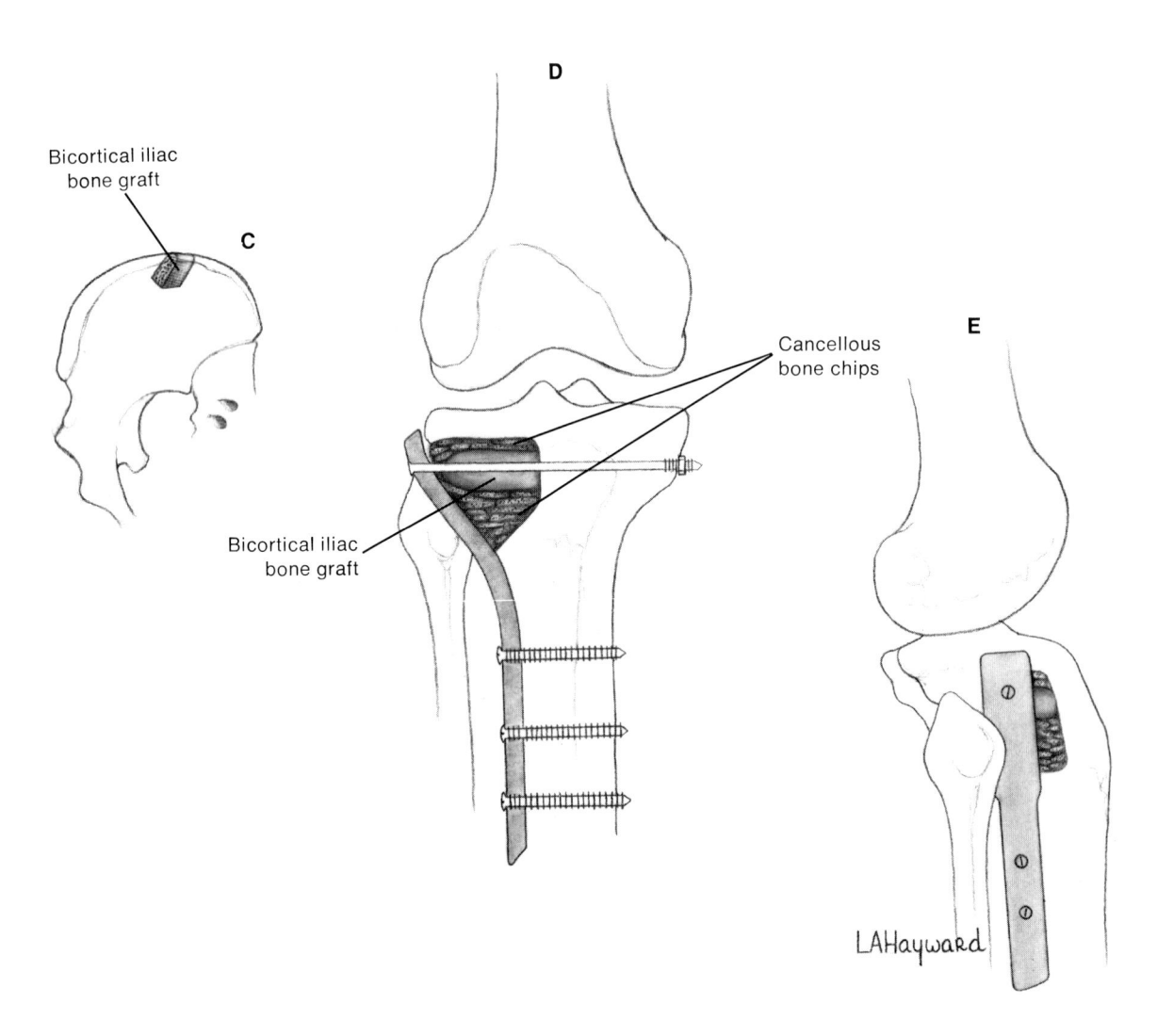

(Plate 12-27) DRAINAGE OF KNEE JOINT

GENERAL DISCUSSION. The primary indication for surgical drainage of the knee joint is acute septic arthritis. The need for drainage is determined by aspiration of the knee, and optimal results are obtained when the procedure is carried out soon after the onset of the infection, under the coverage of appropriate antibiotics.

DETAILS OF PROCEDURE. The knee is exposed through a standard anteromedial parapatellar incision as described in Plate 12-2. When the joint is first entered, specimens are obtained for cultures, which should be routinely checked for aerobic and anaerobic organisms, acid-fast bacteria, and fungi. The knee joint is then thoroughly irrigated with care to make sure that there are no areas of loculation or compartmentalization of the infectious process.

Through a separate stab wound, a sump tube is passed into the joint to be used for closed suction irrigation, as shown. The incision is then closed in a routine fashion and a bulky compression dressing applied.

POSTOPERATIVE MANAGEMENT. Appropriate systemic antibiotics are continued, with alterations made as appropriate when the results of the surgical cultures become available. The closed suction irrigation is maintained for 48 to 72 hours, with the small side tube used as the inflow channel and the large central lumen as the outflow. It is preferable to allow distention of the knee with intermittent drainage. This is done by clamping off the outflow to allow the knee to distend maximally, releasing the clamp on the outflow every 2 to 3 hours, and then reapplying the clamp to allow the knee to distend again. The intermittent distention hopefully will minimize synovial adhesions and facilitate return of knee motion.

After 48 to 72 hours the closed suction irrigation is discontinued, a removable knee splint is applied, and intermittent passive range of motion exercises are initiated. Systemic antibiotics are discontinued and oral antibiotics initiated when appropriate. Isometric exercises without weights are encouraged early, but progressive resistance exercises and weight bearing are delayed at least 6 weeks to avoid excessive stresses on the articular cartilage during the early postinfection period.

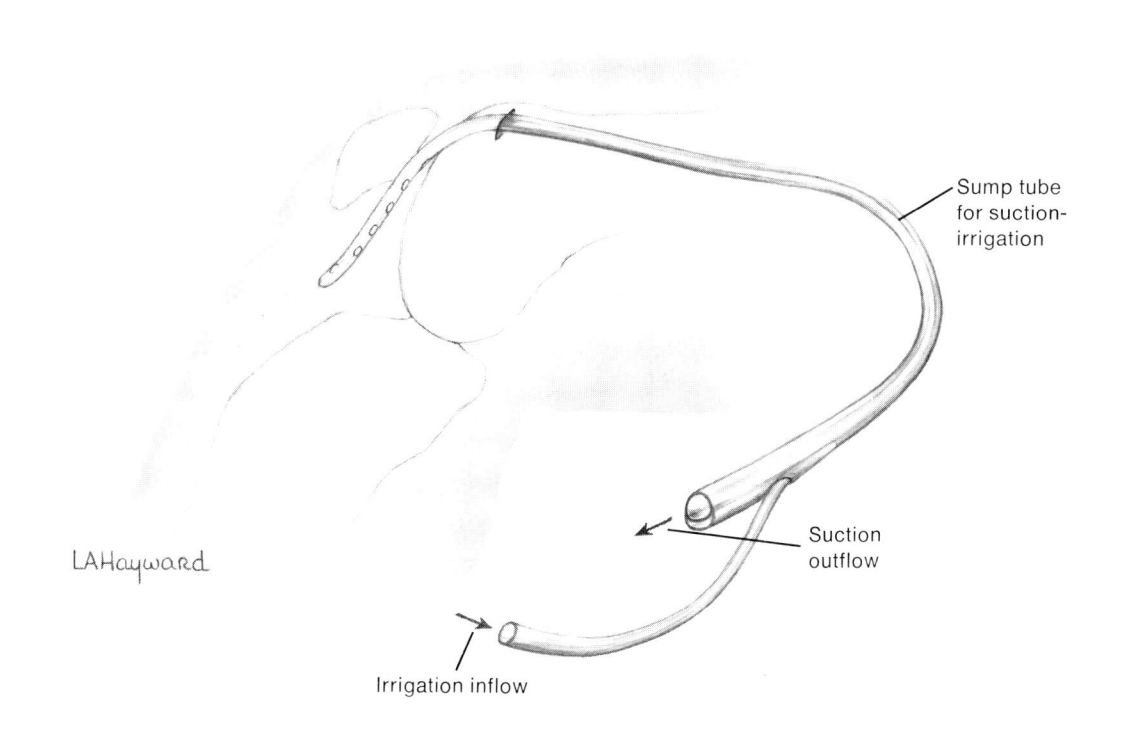

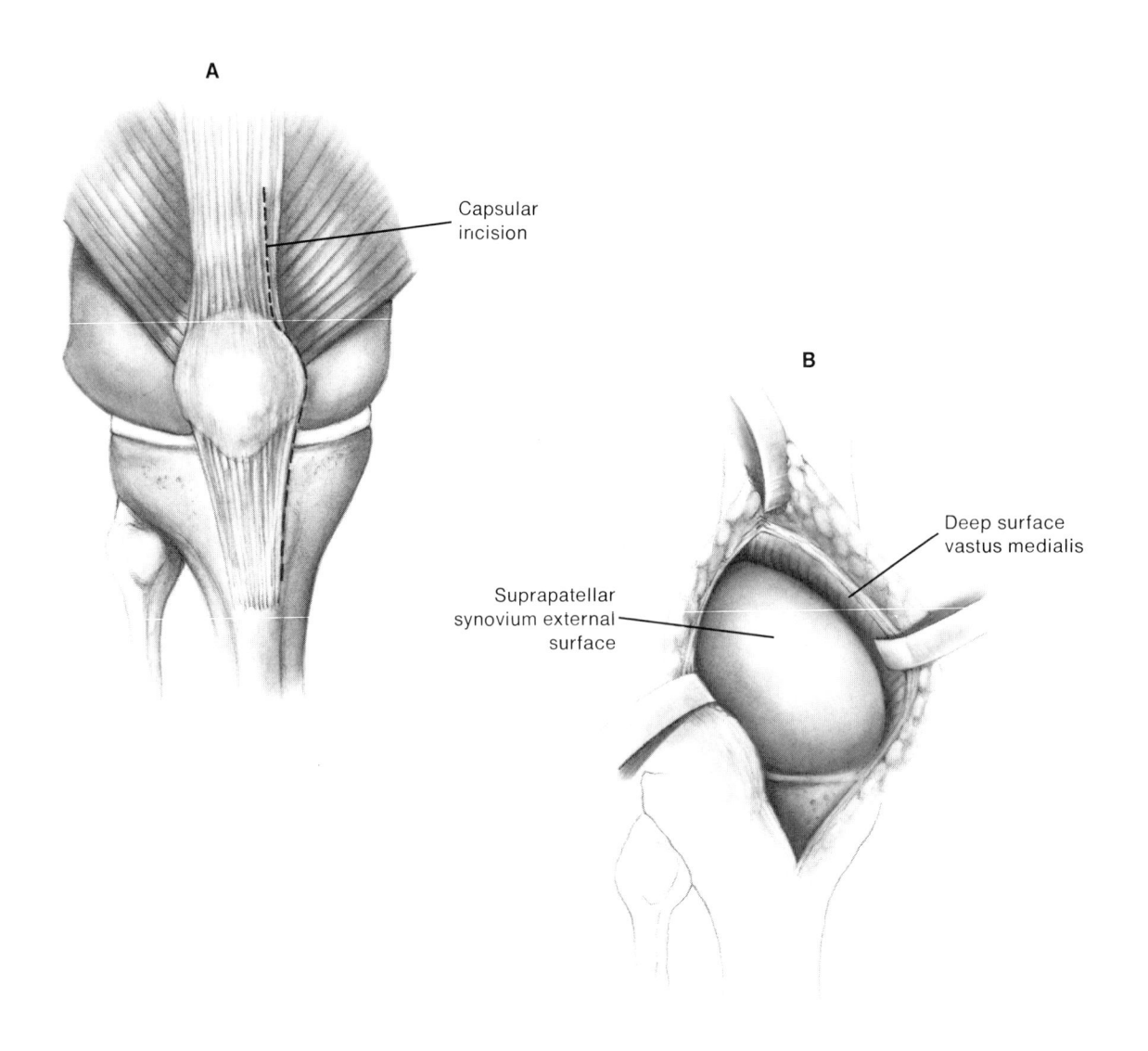

SYNOVECTOMY OF KNEE (Plate 12-28)

GENERAL DISCUSSION. Synovectomy of the knee joint in rheumatoid arthritis can aid in restoring function of the knee, and often improve the general condition of the patient as well, when the pathologic tissue is removed. The basic indication for synovectomy is failure to respond to medical management. The involvement of two or more joints and the presence of acute inflammation should not be considered as contraindications to synovectomy. Following synovectomy of the knee, joint motion should become equal or slightly better than before surgery, but marked improvement in knee motion should not be expected. Postoperatively, the knee joint should become sufficiently free of pain to allow a normal degree of walking with little or no discomfort. If pain beneath the patella is a prominent symptom preoperatively and the articular surface of the patella is found to be severely altered, excision of the patella should be combined with the synovectomy.

DETAILS OF PROCEDURE. The knee joint is exposed through a long anteromedial incision. The incision through the retinacular and capsular layer runs along the medial border of the patella, skirting the vastus medialis muscle belly proximally. It then extends considerably more proximally, in line with the fibers of the quadriceps tendon, and distally from the medial border of the patella adjacent to the patellar tendon **(A)**. The plane between the synovium and capsule of the knee joint is identified, and care is taken at this point not to penetrate the synovial layer. The extra synovial dissection is carried proximally, medially, and laterally in the suprapatellar pouch region until the area of synovial attachment to the femur is reached all around the articular margin of the femur **(B)**. At this point the knee joint is entered by incising the synovium around the margins of the patella, and the patella is dislocated laterally and everted over the flexed knee to allow wide exposure of the anterior aspect of the knee joint. En bloc excision of the synovium is car-

(Plate 12-28) SYNOVECTOMY OF KNEE

ried out by resecting the synovial attachments along the articular margin of the femur beginning laterally and then passing anteriorly and finally medially **(C)**. The large synovial mass has been released all around the femur except at its most medial point **(D)**. Following removal of the main mass of synovial tissue, any remaining synovium is removed with a rongeur, particularly in the intercondylar notch around the cruciate ligaments **(D)**. It is usually not necessary to invade the posterior compartment of the knee joint. The menisci are removed only when they are involved with the diseased process to a degree that they are no longer serviceable. Before wound closure the pneumatic tourniquet is released. A generalized ooze can be anticipated, but any vigorous bleeding must be brought under control. The wound is then closed in a routine fashion over suction drainage, and a bulky compression dressing is applied.

POSTOPERATIVE MANAGEMENT. The compression dressing and suction tubing are removed 48 hours postoperatively, and a removable extention knee splint applied. Intermittent passive range of motion with a knee-sling exerciser is initiated, and the range of knee flexion carefully followed. If 80° to 90° flexion has not been obtained by 10 days following surgery, gentle manipulation under anesthesia should be carried out, and the intermittent passive range of motion continued until at least 90° flexion is assured. Depending on the general condition of the patient, ambulation in the knee splint with touch-down partial weight bearing is initiated, along with isometric quadriceps and straight leg–raising exercises. The average hospitalization time is generally about 2 weeks. Isometric quadriceps progressive resistance exercises and increased weight bearing are delayed until approximately 6 weeks following surgery.

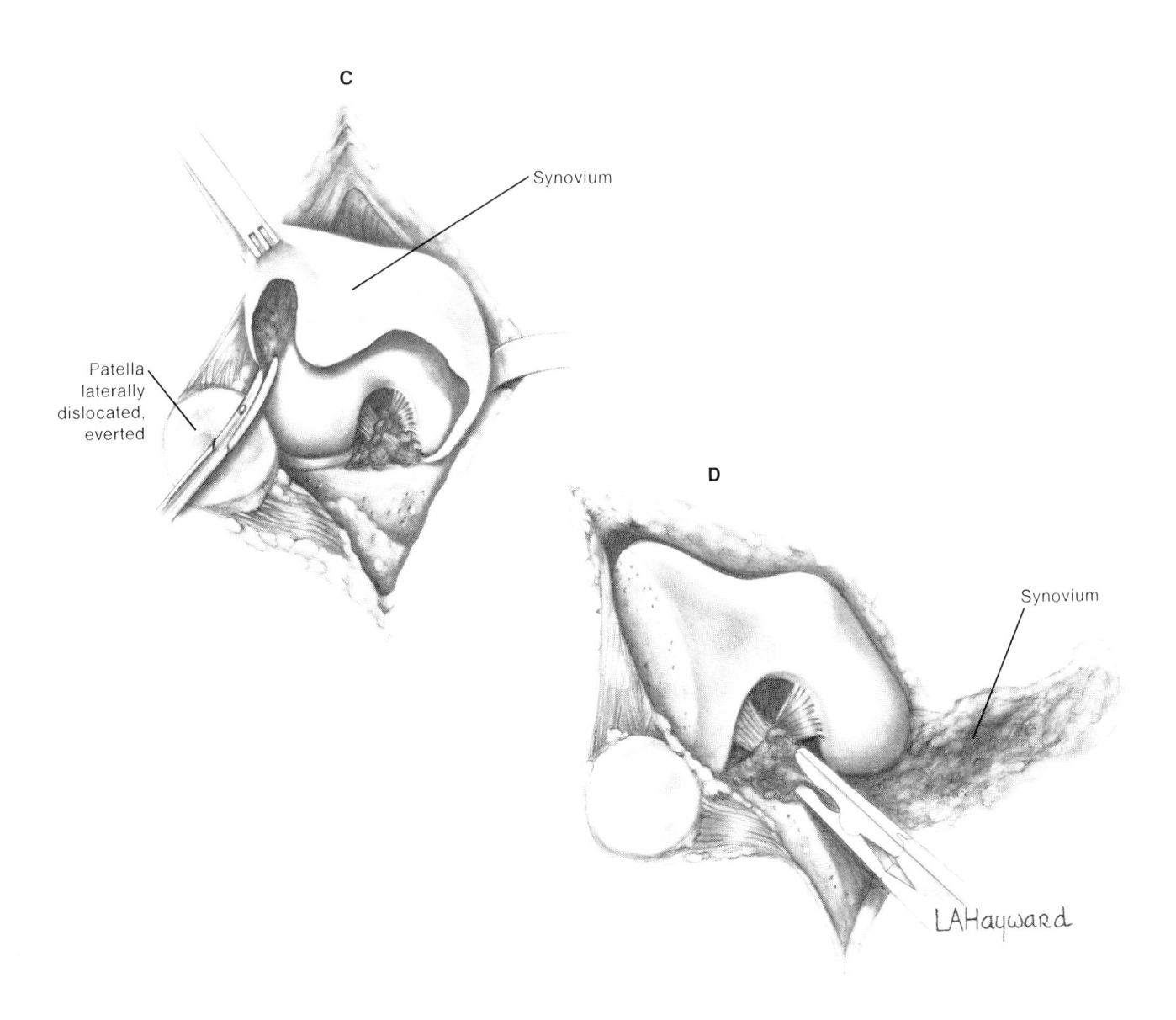

469

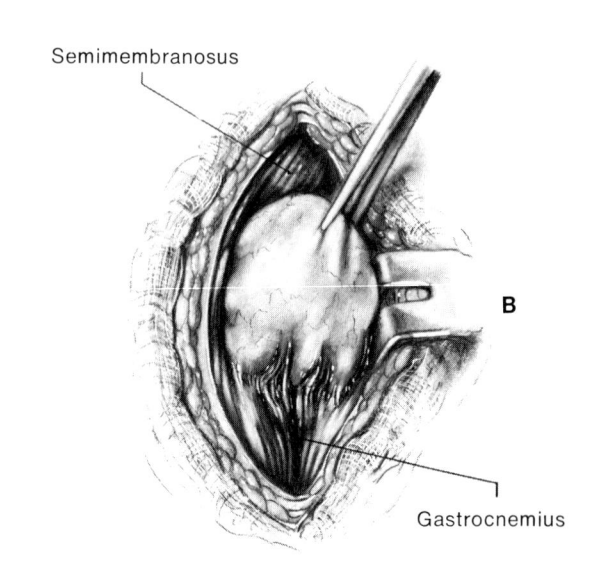

EXCISION OF POPLITEAL CYST (Plate 12-29)

GENERAL DISCUSSION. The presence of a popliteal, or Baker's, cyst may be encountered in children. If the cyst is large and symptomatic, it may warrant excision. The vast majority, if not all, of these popliteal cysts are distentions of the semimembranosus-gastrocnemius bursa. Communication with the knee joint is present in some but not all popliteal cysts. The diagnosis usually can be made by palpation and by transillumination of the cyst, but if there is any doubt, aspiration of normal synovial fluid will confirm the diagnosis.

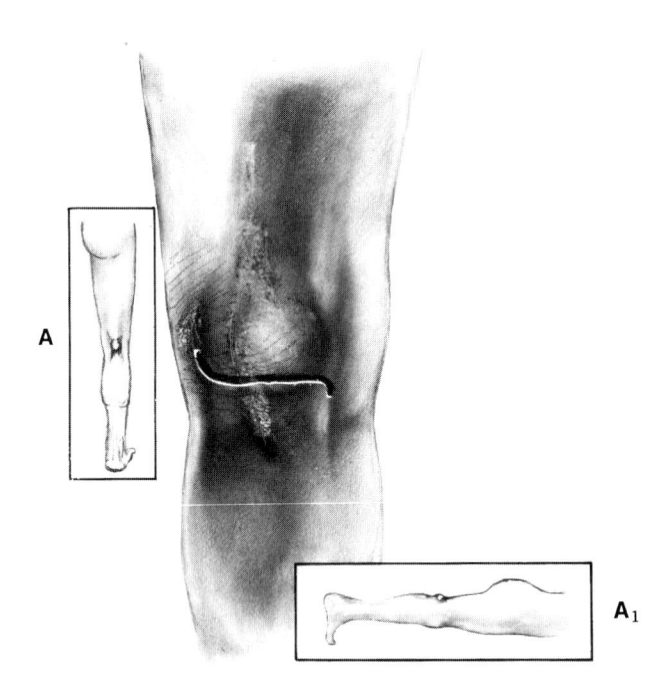

DETAILS OF PROCEDURE. A pneumatic tourniquet is applied high on the thigh, and the patient is placed in the prone position. A transverse skin incision is used **(A)**. Precaution must be taken to avoid injury to the popliteal vessels or the posterior tibial nerve located near the midline of the popliteal space. As the deep fascia is carefully incised, the thin-walled cystic mass will bulge into the wound. The semimembranosus muscle and tendon and the semitendinosus tendon are retracted medially. The medial head of the gastrocnemius is retracted laterally, widely exposing the cystic mass and any attachments of the cyst to the semimembranosus tendon and/or the gastrocnemius muscle and fascia **(B)**. The cyst wall is then carefully grasped, lifted, and freed by sharp dissection from its intimate attachment to the gastrocnemius muscle and fascia. Taking a thin layer of fascia and a few muscle fibers along with the cyst wall in this dissection makes it easier to mobilize the cyst without puncturing it. The cyst is attached to the gastrocnemius muscle and fascia distally and laterally.

(Plate 12-29) EXCISION OF POPLITEAL CYST

The cyst can now be lifted off its loose attachment to the underlying joint capsule. Sharp dissection of the cyst wall from its dense adherence to the semimembranosus muscle, again taking a few tendon fibers along with the cyst wall and finally separating the mass from fatty tissue superiorly, completely mobilizes the cyst. Now, by retracting the cyst superiorly, the pedicle, which may communicate with the knee joint over the medial femoral condyle, can be exposed. The pedicle is then sectioned **(C)** and the cyst is removed. The defect is usually small and can be closed with two or three interrupted plain catgut sutures **(D).** If the defect is large, because of a broad opening into the knee joint, it may be left open.

An alternative dissection technique is to expose the cyst wall in its superficial portion, then retract the medial head of the gastrocnemius and the semimembranosus as much as possible before incising the cyst. With the finger inside the cyst, as one might treat an inguinal hernia, the cyst wall is mobilized by sharp dissection from its attachments to the medial head of the gastrocnemius muscle and fascia and from the semimembranosus tendon to expose and divide the pedicle.

With either method, the tourniquet is released after the cyst has been removed and any active bleeding points are brought under control. The wound is closed by approximating the subcutaneous tissues and the skin. A bulky compression dressing is applied to the knee and leg.

POSTOPERATIVE MANAGEMENT. The patient is instructed in quadriceps exercises and allowed to flex the knee within the limitations of the dressing until it is removed 10 to 14 days postoperatively. Walking with crutches is started on the second or third day.

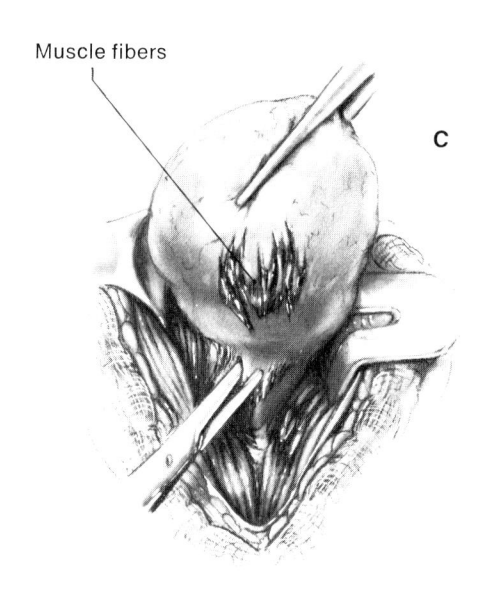

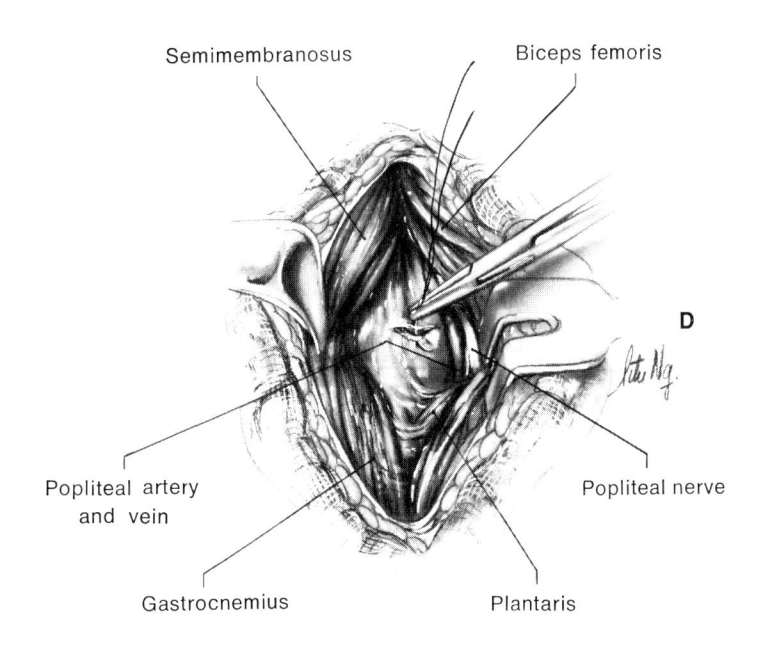

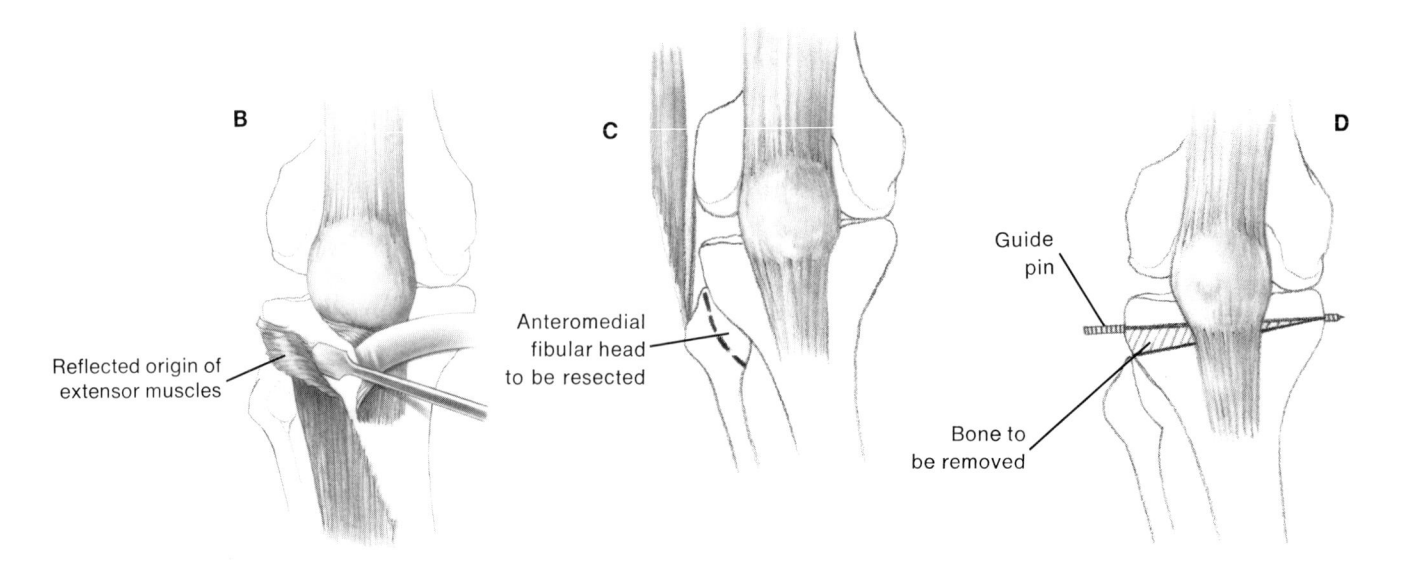

HIGH TIBIAL OSTEOTOMY FOR OSTEOARTHRITIS OF KNEE (Plate 12-30)

GENERAL DISCUSSION. The ideal indication for proximal tibial osteotomy (for osteoarthritis of the knee) is disabling knee pain and roentgenographic changes showing narrowing of the joint with resulting valgus or varus deformity but minimum degenerative changes in other respects. It is best if the patient is muscular and motivated enough to accomplish a good rehabilitation program. Bilateral knee involvement is not a contraindication. Coventry has described a closing wedge osteotomy made just distal to the knee joint. The advantages of a closing wedge osteotomy are that it is made near the deformity (that is, the knee), and it is made through cancellous bone, which heals rapidly (especially with early weight bearing).

As much as 20° of valgus deformity or 15° of varus deformity at the knee can be corrected by such an osteotomy. Routine bilateral weight-bearing anteroposterior roentgenograms of the knee should be included in the preoperative evaluation of the arthritic knee.

DETAILS OF PROCEDURE. For a lateral closing wedge osteotomy, the incision is slightly oblique, running from just above the fibular head laterally to just across the midline anteriorly, crossing the midline just proximal to the tibial tubercle **(A)**. The knee is kept slightly flexed throughout the procedure to relax tension in the neurovascular structures, which reduces the chance of inadvertent injury. The origin of the tibialis anterior is released from the anterolateral face of the tibia from the patellar tendon to the fibular head and retracted **(B)**. The anterior aspect of the fibular head is thus exposed, and the anteromedial portion of the fibular head is then osteotomized as described by Slocum et al., which obliterates the proximal tibia-fibular joint and provides wide access to the lateral and posterior aspect of the tibia **(C)**. A guide pin is then passed through the proximal tibia parallel to the joint line approximately 1 cm distal to the articular surface, and the position verified by intraoperative x-ray films **(D)**. With the guide pin as a landmark for the proximal cut, the amount of bone to be removed is determined and marked on the tibia with an osteotome. An approximate guideline is to make the height of the wedge 1 cm for every 10° correction to be obtained. Slocum et al. have described a detailed method to determine precisely the amount of bone to be removed. An oscillatory saw is used to begin the osteotomy, and care is taken to protect the posterior neurovascular structures with a retractor. The osteotomy is carefully carried to but not through the medial cortex. It is carried through the posterior cortex along the distal limb of the osteotomy only, which leaves a posterior shelf that helps stabilize the osteotomy after it has been closed **(E)**. The wedge of bone that is removed is saved for later use as a

(Plate 12-30) HIGH TIBIAL OSTEOTOMY FOR OSTEOARTHRITIS OF KNEE

bone graft. A wide flat osteotome is then used in the apex of the osteotomy to carry the osteotomy to but not completely through the medial cortex. The medial tibial cortex is then perforated with multiple drill holes **(F)**. When the osteotomy is ready to be closed, a slight increase in varus deformity will allow the osteotomy site to open easily. If this does not occur, there is most likely a strong bridge of bone remaining at the posteromedial cortex of the tibia, which should also be divided with the flat ostetome. The remaining medial cortex is then fractured by first increasing the varus deformity and then closing the osteotomy. The distal tibia should close inside the shelf of posterior cortex of the tibia described above, which helps stabilize the osteotomy by preventing posterior displacement. Alignment of the limb should be checked carefully both clinically and by intraoperative x-ray films, and more bone removed if adequate correction has not been achieved. The bone that was removed in the osteotomy is then used as graft to pack the defect between the partially osteotomized fibular head and the lateral surface of the tibia **(G)**.

The use of internal fixation in tibial osteotomy is controversial, since achieving rigid internal fixation is difficult because of the relatively small proximal fragment with thin cortex and cancellous bone. Another controversial issue is whether to perform arthrotomy to remove the badly degenerated and torn medial meniscus that is usually present and to perform a general debridement. If satisfactory internal fixation of the osteotomy site can be achieved, early joint motion can be initiated. This overcomes the objection to carrying out arthrotomy and joint debridement at the time of osteotomy for fear of losing joint motion because of immobilization necessary for osteotomy healing. The meniscus and articular debris can be removed by increasingly efficient techniques of operative arthroscopy, which obviates the need for open arthrotomy.

After the insertion of an internal fixation (and it certainly is not necessary to use internal fixation if adequate external immobilization and early weight bearing are instituted), the tourniquet is released and further hemostasis secured. The wound is closed in a routine fashion over suction drainage, and a bulky compression dressing with posterior plaster splint is applied with the knee in approximately 5° flexion.

POSTOPERATIVE MANAGEMENT. Quadriceps setting and straight leg-raising exercises are initiated as soon as possible. If satisfactory internal fixation has been used, then early passive motion exercises can be initiated and an extension knee splint used between exercise periods. If no internal fixation has been used, then it is necessary to maintain external fixation, and after 48 to 72 hours the bulky compression dressing is removed and a well-molded cylinder or long-leg cast is applied. The patient is ambulated as soon as possible, with encouragement of weight bearing as tolerated. The immobilization is continued for 4 to 6 weeks until adequate healing has occurred, when knee motion can be instituted, as well as isometric quadriceps progressive resistance exercises.

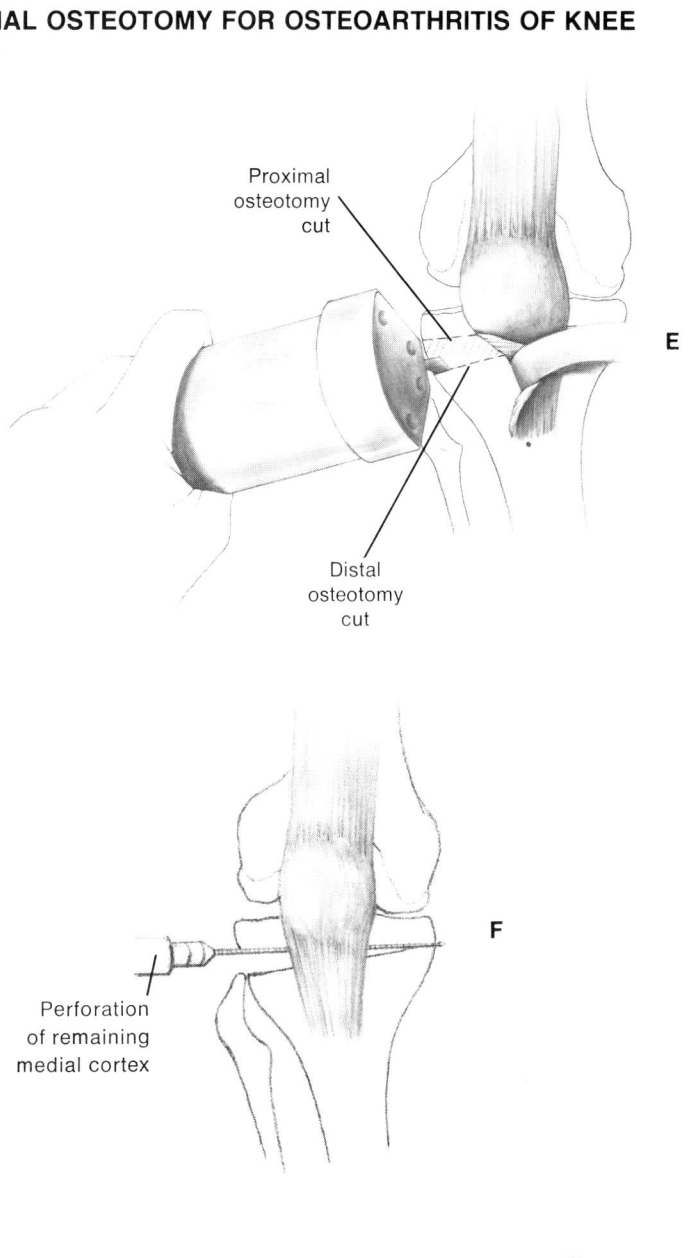

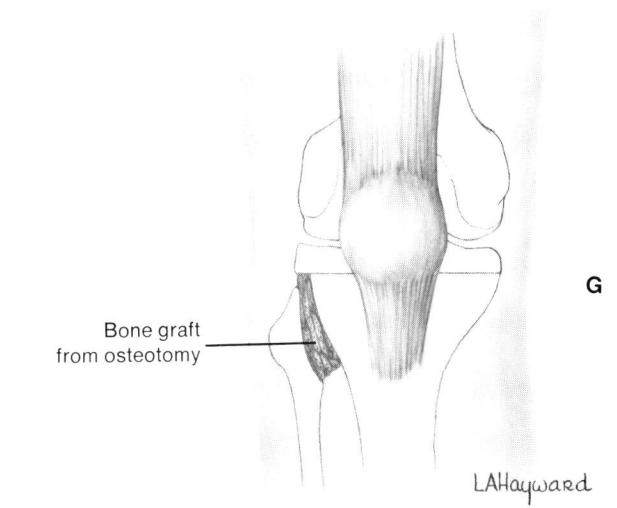

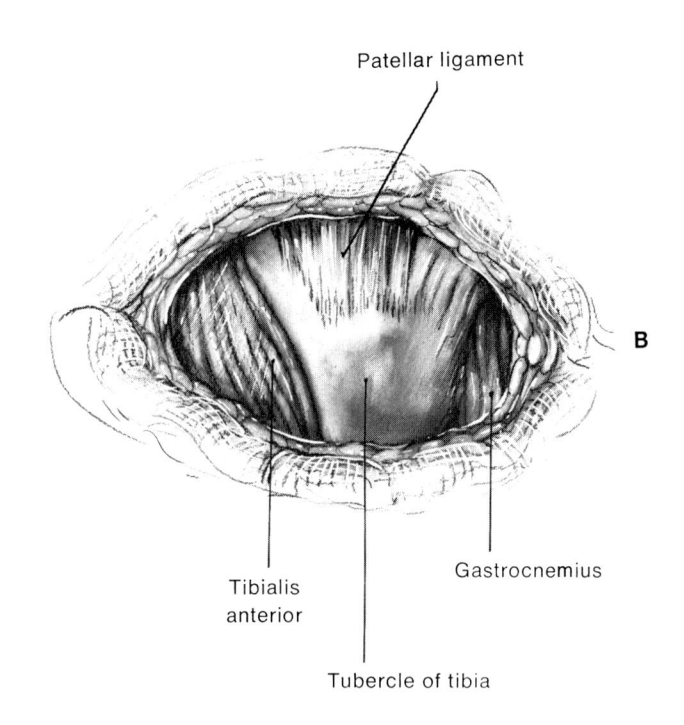

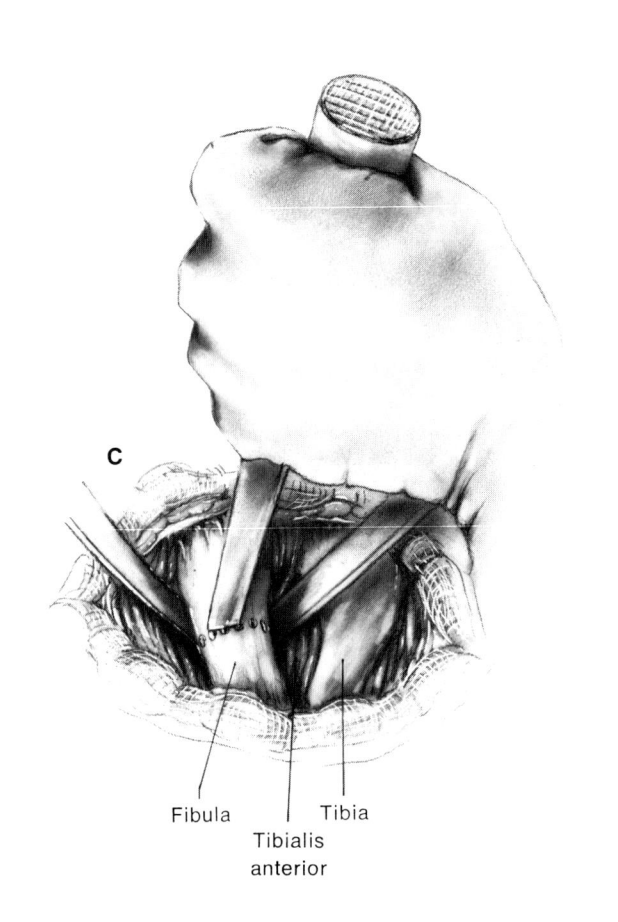

PROXIMAL TIBIAL OSTEOTOMY FOR GENU RECURVATUM (Plate 12-31)

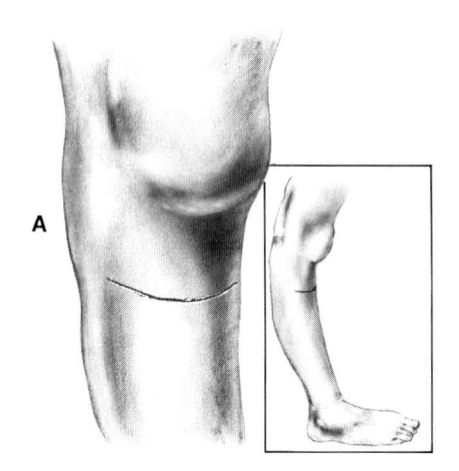

GENERAL DISCUSSION. Genu recurvatum can be a distressing deformity. It is not only unsightly (see insert, Plate 12-29, *A*), but causes easy fatigue and pain and decreases tolerance for weight-bearing activity. In the past the deformity has been most commonly seen as an aftereffect of paralytic poliomyelitis. Its inception is in the acute stage of poliomyelitis, and it is usually caused by inadequate support to the back of the knee in the first 2 to 3 weeks of the disease. Once the structures over the back of the knee have been stretched, it is extremely difficult to prevent progressive recurvatum after weight-bearing activity is started.

In the presence of a mild degree of recurvatum in the very young child, protection of the knee in a caliper "back-knee" brace that blocks the knee at 10° short of normal extension is the only effective measure to discourage progression of the deformity. If there is useful quadriceps power, free motion is allowed at the knee except for the block in extension. The knee may require protection for years, but the effort will be worth it. Prevention of a progressive recurvatum deformity when a patient convalescing from paralytic poliomyelitis begins to walk is a major accomplishment of conservative management.

Osteotomy of the proximal tibia and fibula is the best single procedure for the management of marked genu recurvatum if operation correction becomes necessary.

DETAILS OF PROCEDURE. With the patient supine on the fracture table, the proximal tibia and fibula are approached through a transverse incision placed about 2.5 cm distal to the tibial tubercle (**A** and **B**). The lateral angle of the incision is retracted distally. The muscle fibers over the proximal 3 cm of the fibula are carefully separated with a blunt instrument in a proximal to distal direction. The exposure is carried down to the periosteum of the fibula anteriorly. A short segment of fibula can then be exposed safely by subperiosteal reflection without danger of injury to the peroneal nerve. Drill holes are made, and the fibula is osteotomized with a thin, sharp osteotome (**C**). The periosteum and fascia are then reapproximated over the fibula.

(Plate 12-31) PROXIMAL TIBIAL OSTEOTOMY FOR GENU RECURVATUM

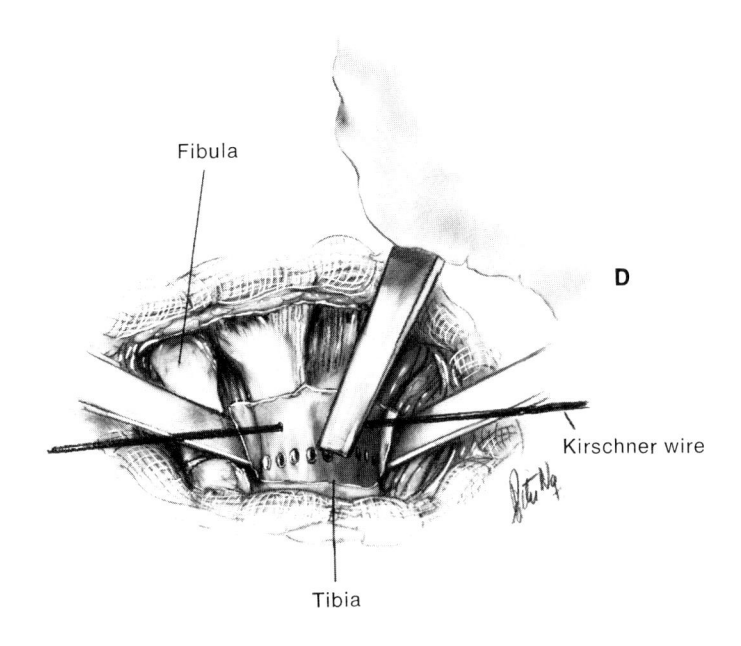

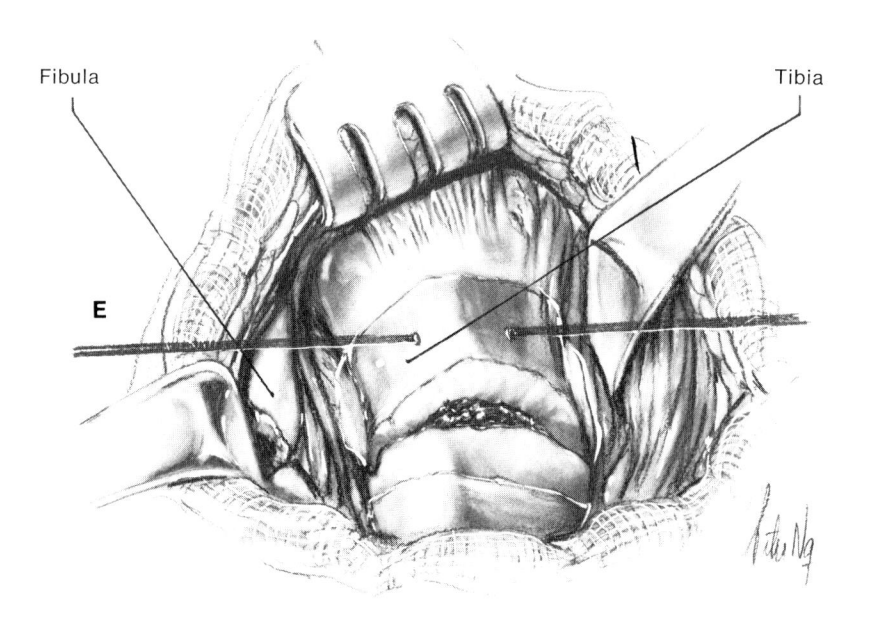

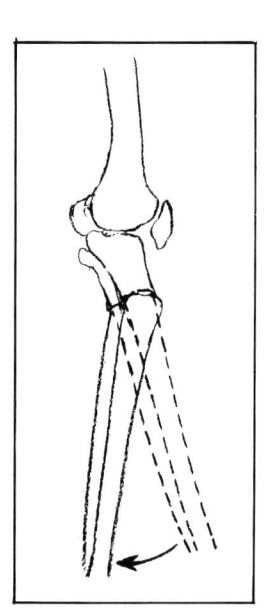

A linear longitudinal incision is made through the periosteum over the crest of the tibia from the tibial tubercle distally. This is converted to an "H" by short, transverse incisions, and the proximal tibia is exposed subperiosteally. An inverted-V or dome-shaped osteotomy is outlined with drill holes through both cortices of the tibia distal to the patellar tendon attachment. A heavy Kirschner wire is placed transversely through the distal portion of the proximal fragment of the tibia, and a traction bow is applied to the wire. The tibia is then divided with an osteotome (D).

While the proximal fragment is supported with the traction bow, the distal tibia is allowed to drop, creating anterior angulation at the osteotomy site (E). If necessary, the proximal end of the distal tibial fragment is trimmed with a rongeur to create a stable seating of the pointed distal fragment in the concavity of the proximal fragment. Valgus and rotational malalignment can be corrected at the same time.

475

PROXIMAL TIBIAL OSTEOTOMY FOR GENU RECURVATUM (Plate 12-31)

An assistant continues to hold the traction bow supporting the proximal tibia while the subcutaneous tissue and skin are closed. Dressing and sterile sheet-wadding are applied to the leg. The drapes are removed, and the alignment of the leg in all planes is adjusted. An attempt is made to maintain the knee joint in the recurvatum position by forward pull on the traction bow. If the Kirschner wire is in the distal portion of the proximal tibial fragment, this is effective; but if the pin is in the middle of the proximal fragment, a toggle effect can neutralize the effectiveness of the wire. A circular plaster cast is first applied to the leg from the upper thigh to the ankle, maintaining the desired position and alignment and incorporating the Kirschner wire. The cast is then extended to include the foot.

Anteroposterior and lateral roentgenograms are obtained before the patient is removed from the operating table. If the position and alignment are not as planned, cast wedging in one or two planes as necessary can be done either immediately or in the first few days postoperatively.

POSTOPERATIVE MANAGEMENT. The Kirschner wire is removed after 6 to 8 weeks. Further immobilization in a long-leg cast is continued until the osteotomy shows roentgenographic evidence of bony union. This may require 12 to 16 weeks. Preoperative (**F** and **G**) and postoperative (**H** and **I**) views are shown.

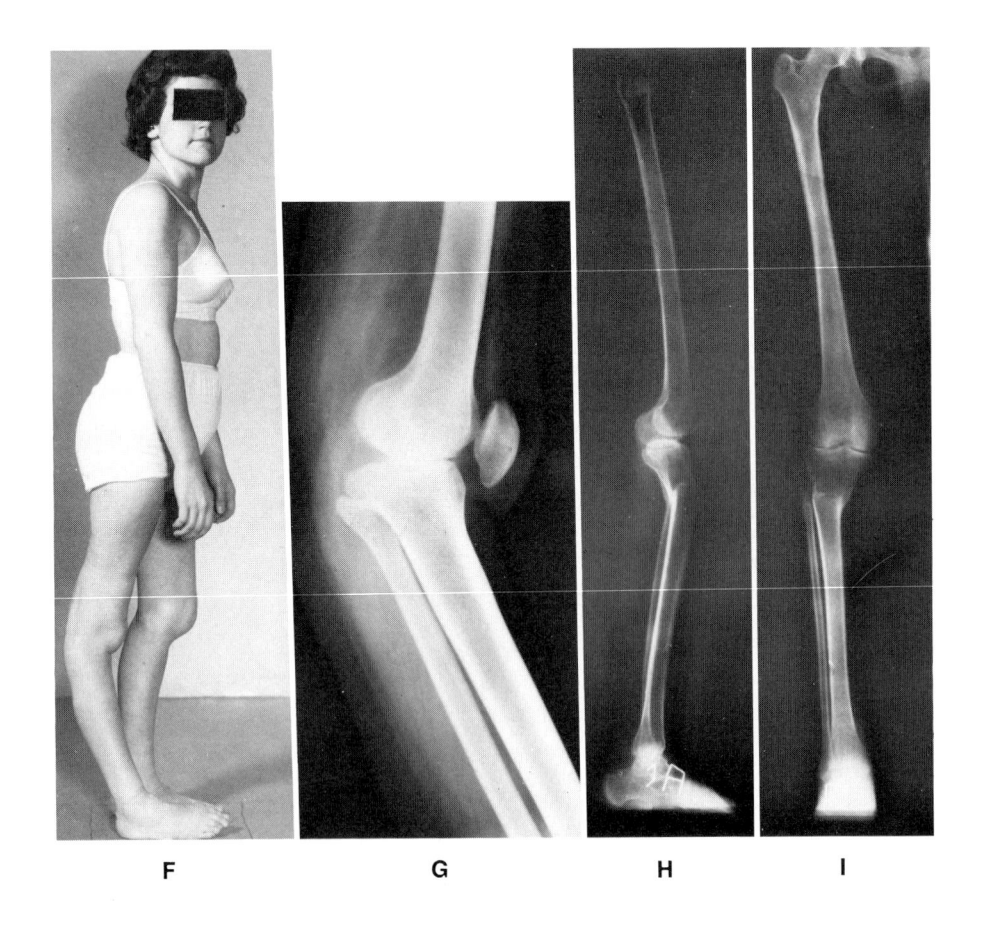

F G H I

(Plate 12-32) ANIMETRIC TOTAL KNEE REPLACEMENT (NONCONSTRAINED)

GENERAL DISCUSSION. Total knee joint reconstruction may be indicated for the patient with a painful and disabled knee. Specific indications for the use of a nonconstrained knee joint prosthesis include pain, instability, deformity, and loss of function.

The animetric total knee prosthesis is used for the patient with pain because of bicompartmental bony destruction of the knee joint. It is a nonconstrained prosthesis and is dependent on tissue tension for its stability.

DETAILS OF PROCEDURE. A midline incision is used to expose the knee joint **(A)**. After the skin flaps are reflected, a median parapatellar incision is made and the patellar tendon is exposed on its medial aspect. The patellar retinaculum is divided, allowing entry of the knee joint along the entire length of the incision. The patella itself can then be everted laterally with flexion of the knee joint **(B)**.

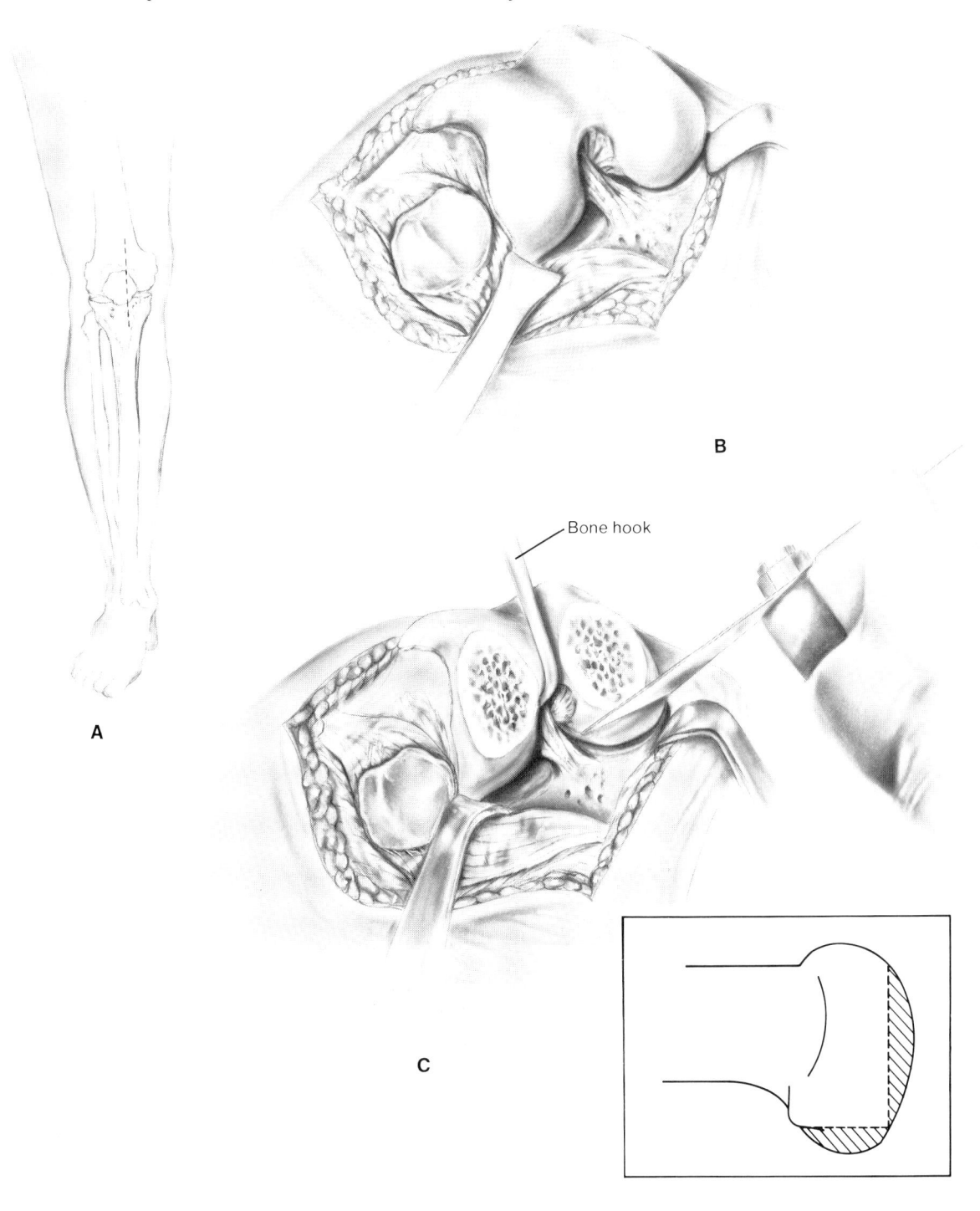

477

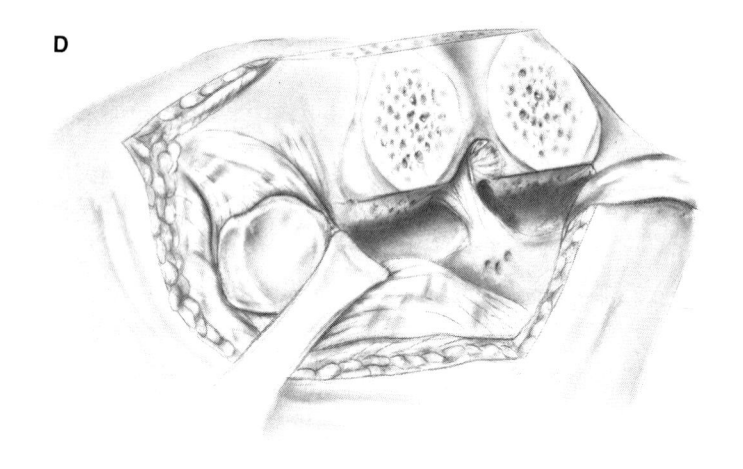

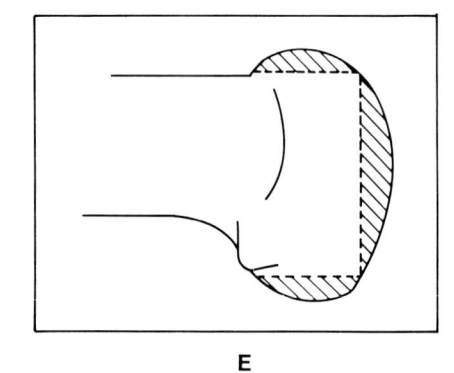

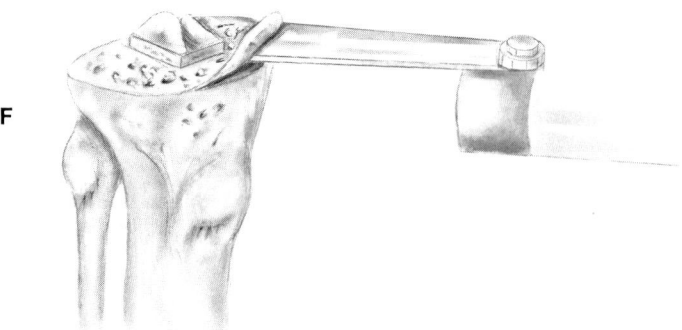

ANIMETRIC TOTAL KNEE REPLACEMENT (NONCONSTRAINED) (Plate 12-32)

Attention is directed toward preparation of the femur to accommodate the prosthesis. The initial cut on the distal femur is made perpendicular to the long axis of the femur. Then the posterior condyles are divided **(C),** and finally an anterior parallel cut is made (**D** and **E**).

Following preparation of the femoral condyles, the tibial condyles are prepared to accommodate the prosthesis. The cruciate ligaments are preserved while the tibial plateaus are divided in a transverse manner with either a saw or an osteotome **(F).** A trial prosthesis is used to estimate the fit and alignment. Drill holes are made in the distal femoral condyles to accommodate the femoral prosthesis (**G** and **H**). The final cuts are created to accommodate the runners of the plastic tibial component, allowing for accurate placement of this component **(I).**

(Plate 12-32) ANIMETRIC TOTAL KNEE REPLACEMENT (NONCONSTRAINED)

G

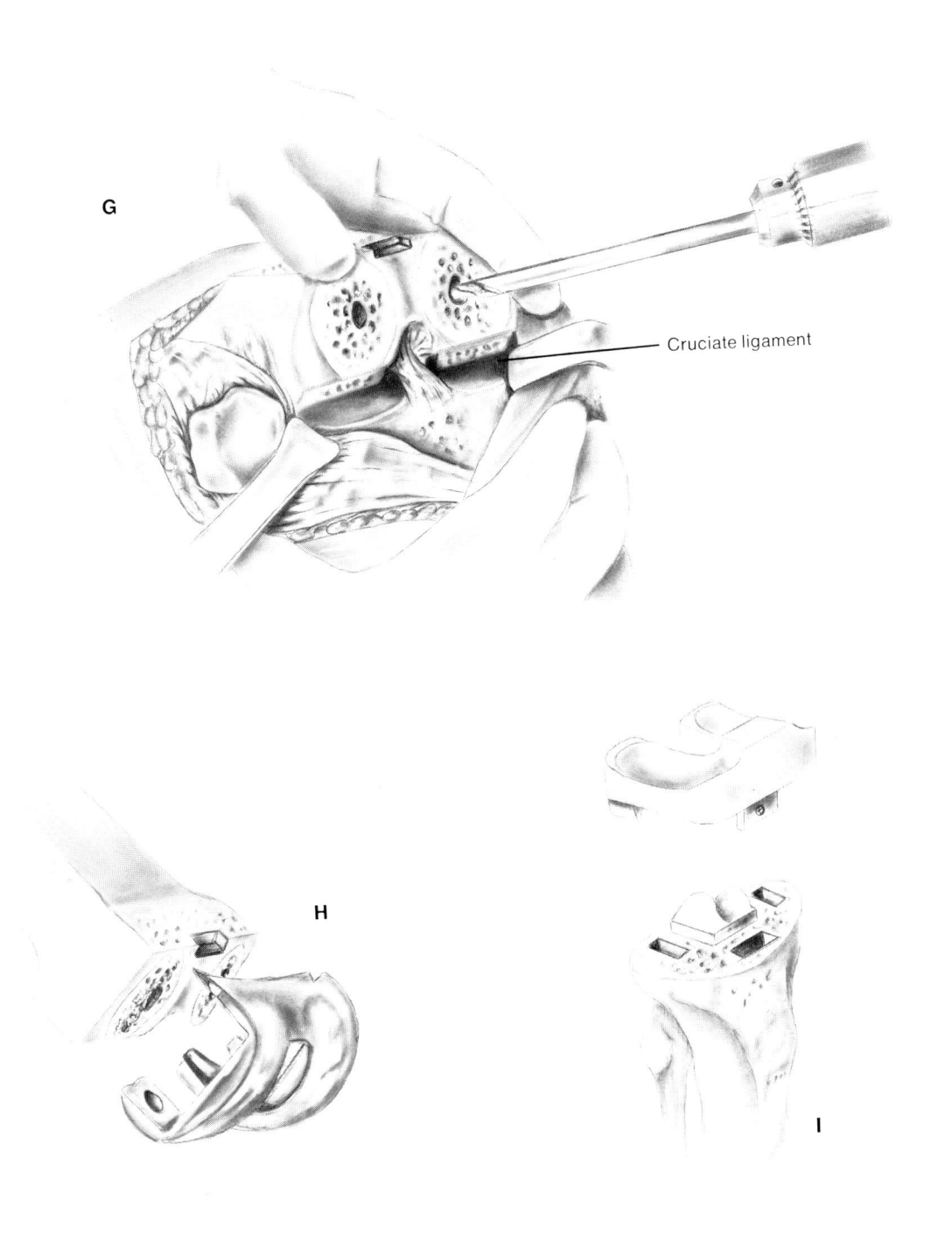

Cruciate ligament

H

I

479

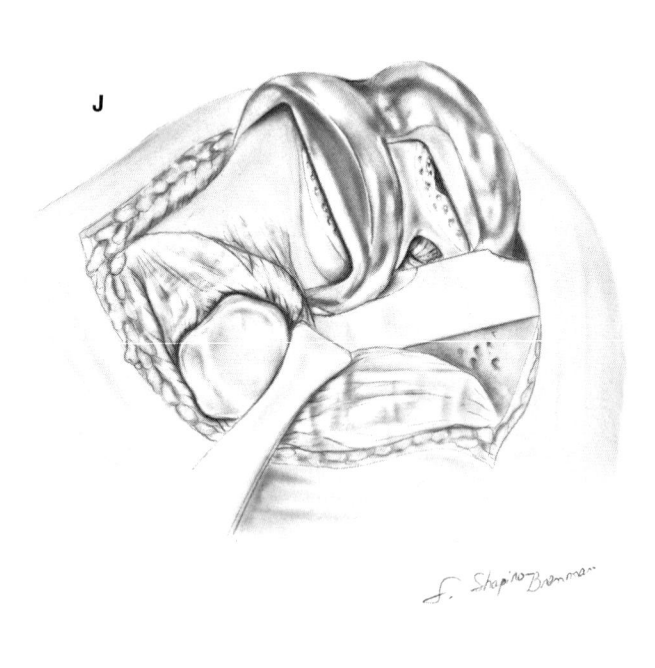

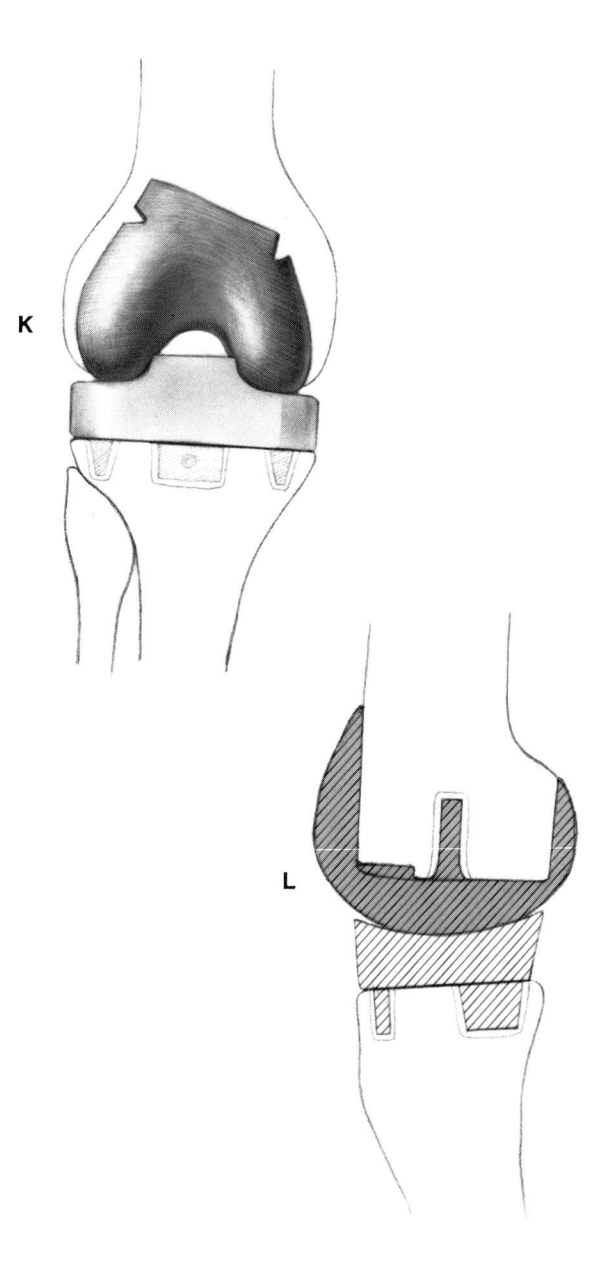

ANIMETRIC TOTAL KNEE REPLACEMENT (NONCONSTRAINED) (Plate 12-32)

Care is taken during the procedure to preserve both medial and lateral collateral ligaments and the cruciate ligaments. A trial reduction allows for an evaluation of the overall alignment and stability of the knee joint. Angular deformities and instability of the knee can be corrected by selecting proper thickness of the tibial prosthesis. The tissue tension on the collateral ligaments allows for extension and flexion to at least 90° and must occur without subluxation of the prosthesis (**J**).

After the appropriate sized tibial prosthesis is selected, the femoral component is cemented following cleansing of the condylar surfaces with a Water Pic spray. The bone cement is applied under pressure, and all excessive cement is trimmed from the periphery of the femoral prosthesis. The tibial component is placed with particular attention to removing all cement posteriorly and from the intercondylar notch area. As the bone cement hardens, the knee is placed in full extension (**K** and **L**). Closure is accomplished in layers over an indwelling suction catheter, and the skin is closed with staples. A Robert Jones compression dressing with an outer shell of plaster of paris is applied with the knee in full extension.

POSTOPERATIVE MANAGEMENT. The Robert Jones compression dressing is removed 5 days postoperatively, and a roentgenogram of the knee is obtained. Active quadriceps motion and flexion and extension exercises are begun under the supervision of a physical therapist. The patient is encouraged to begin partial weight bearing, using crutches or a walker for support. The stitches are removed at 2 weeks postoperatively, and vigorous physical therapy is pursued to attain at least 90° flexion and full extension. The patient is maintained on partial weight bearing for 8 weeks following the operation.

(Plate 12-33) SPHEROCENTRIC TOTAL KNEE REPLACEMENT (SEMICONSTRAINED)

GENERAL DISCUSSION. Total knee reconstruction may be indicated for the patient with a painful and disabled knee. Specific indications for its use include pain, instability, and loss of function. If all the compartments of the knee joint are severely involved with arthritic changes, then knee joint reconstruction should be considered. If a patient with rheumatoid arthritis or osteoarthritis has multiple joint involvement, restoration of knee joint function will enhance the ability to remain active.

The spherocentric semiconstrained total knee prosthesis is reserved for the patient with pain, angular deformity, and bicompartmental destruction. The total knee replacement prosthesis illustrated has been developed by the University of Michigan and is dependent on triaxial motion for its function. It is a useful prosthesis for the patient with an involved knee joint. In addition, there are many other designs on nonconstrained and semiconstrained knee joint prostheses currently in use.

DETAILS OF PROCEDURE. A midline incision is used to expose the knee joint **(A)**. After the skin flaps are reflected, a medial parapatellar incision is made adjacent to the patella **(B)**. The patellar tendon is exposed on the medial aspect, and the patellar retinaculum is divided so that the knee joint is entered along the entire length of the incision. After wide release of the capsule and superior patellar tendon, the patella itself can be everted laterally with flexion of the knee joint. The cruciate ligaments are divided at the femoral sites and both medial and collateral ligaments are divided at the femoral attachments, allowing for a complete exposure of the knee joint. With the knee at 90° a transverse tibial cut is made at right angles to the tibia, and the proximal 1 cm of the tibia is removed en bloc **(C)**.

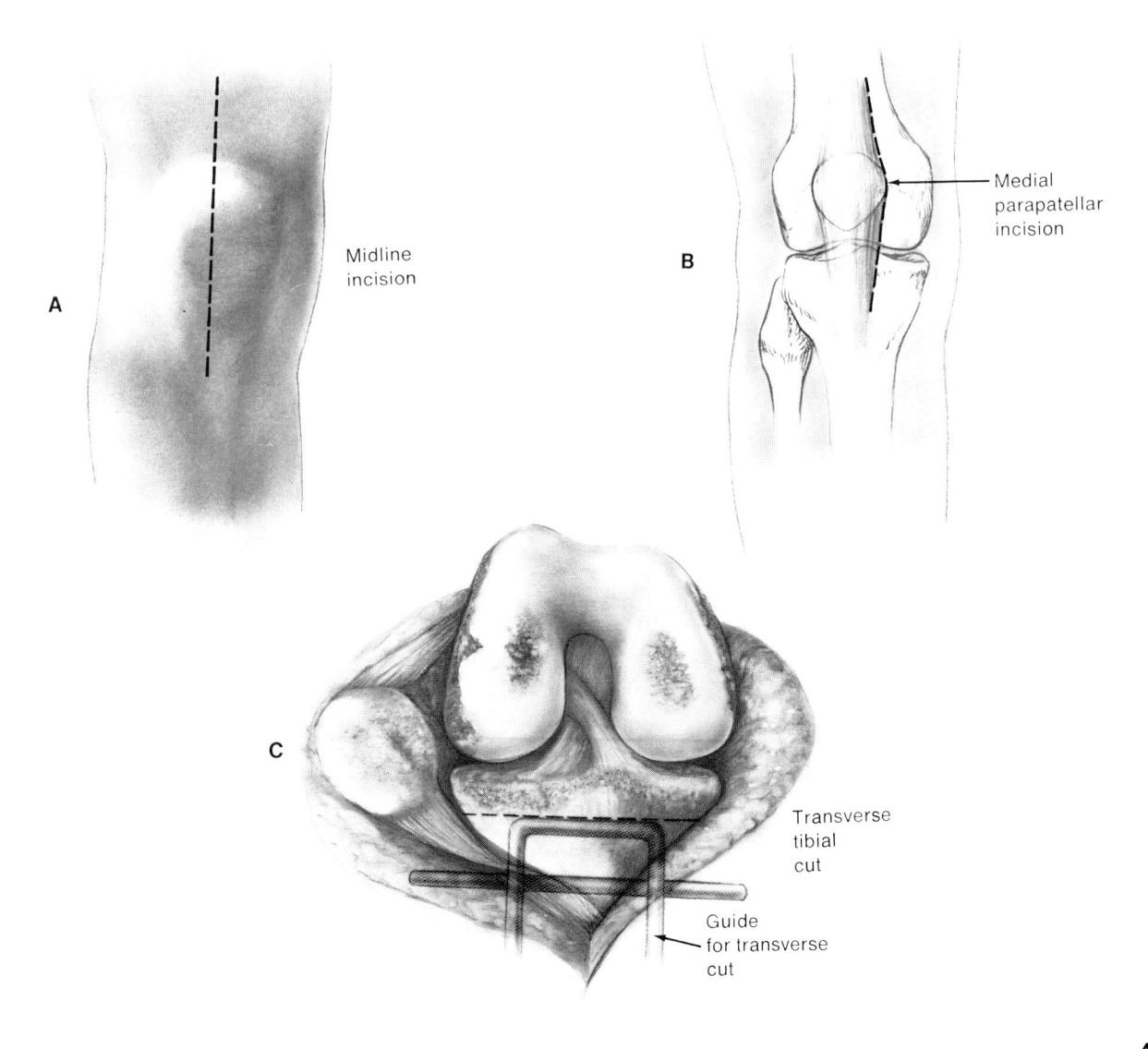

SPHEROCENTRIC TOTAL KNEE REPLACEMENT (SEMICONSTRAINED) (Plate 12-33)

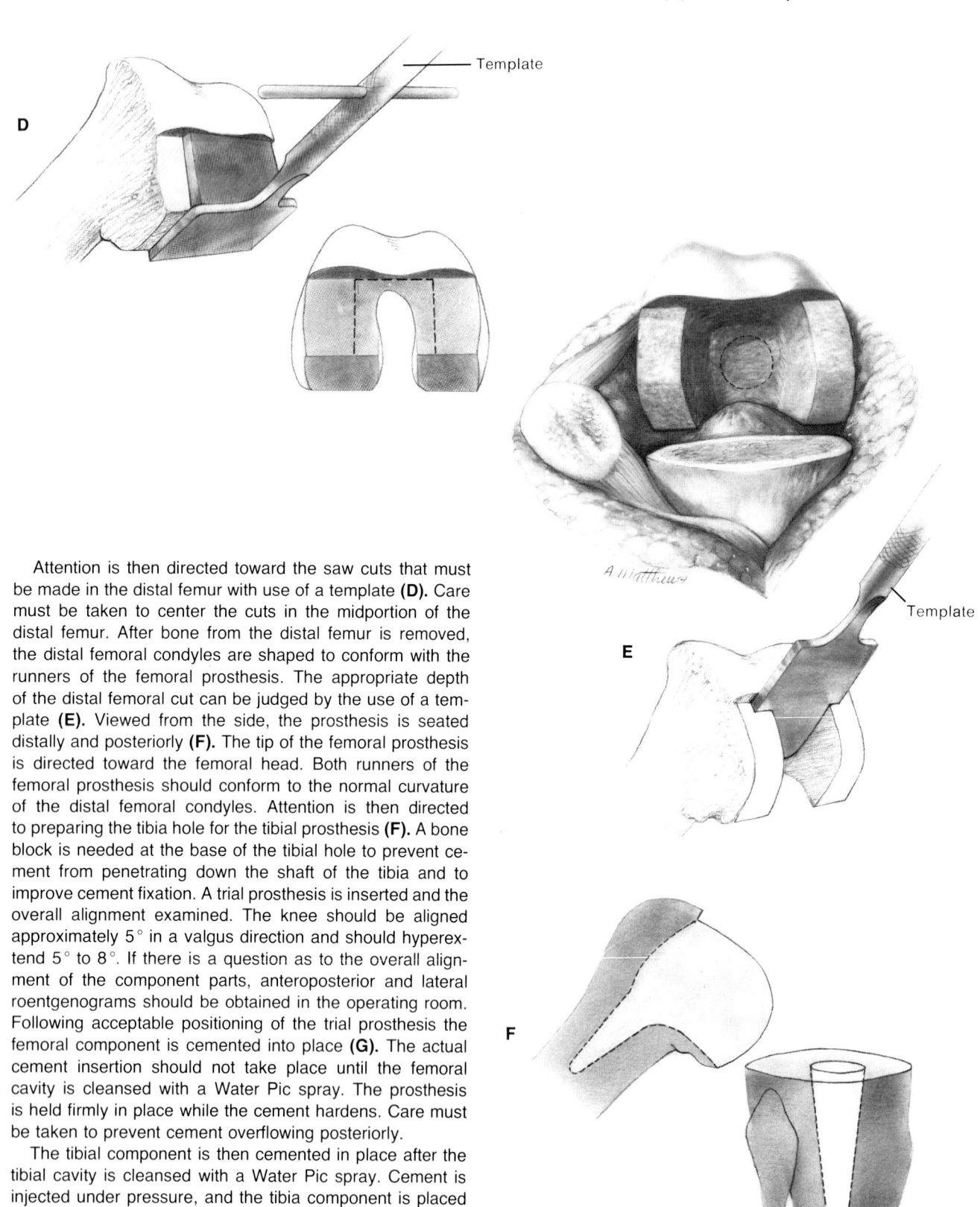

Attention is then directed toward the saw cuts that must be made in the distal femur with use of a template **(D)**. Care must be taken to center the cuts in the midportion of the distal femur. After bone from the distal femur is removed, the distal femoral condyles are shaped to conform with the runners of the femoral prosthesis. The appropriate depth of the distal femoral cut can be judged by the use of a template **(E)**. Viewed from the side, the prosthesis is seated distally and posteriorly **(F)**. The tip of the femoral prosthesis is directed toward the femoral head. Both runners of the femoral prosthesis should conform to the normal curvature of the distal femoral condyles. Attention is then directed to preparing the tibia hole for the tibial prosthesis **(F)**. A bone block is needed at the base of the tibial hole to prevent cement from penetrating down the shaft of the tibia and to improve cement fixation. A trial prosthesis is inserted and the overall alignment examined. The knee should be aligned approximately 5° in a valgus direction and should hyperextend 5° to 8°. If there is a question as to the overall alignment of the component parts, anteroposterior and lateral roentgenograms should be obtained in the operating room. Following acceptable positioning of the trial prosthesis the femoral component is cemented into place **(G)**. The actual cement insertion should not take place until the femoral cavity is cleansed with a Water Pic spray. The prosthesis is held firmly in place while the cement hardens. Care must be taken to prevent cement overflowing posteriorly.

The tibial component is then cemented in place after the tibial cavity is cleansed with a Water Pic spray. Cement is injected under pressure, and the tibia component is placed in proper alignment and rotation **(H)**.

(Plate 12-33) SPHEROCENTRIC TOTAL KNEE REPLACEMENT (SEMICONSTRAINED)

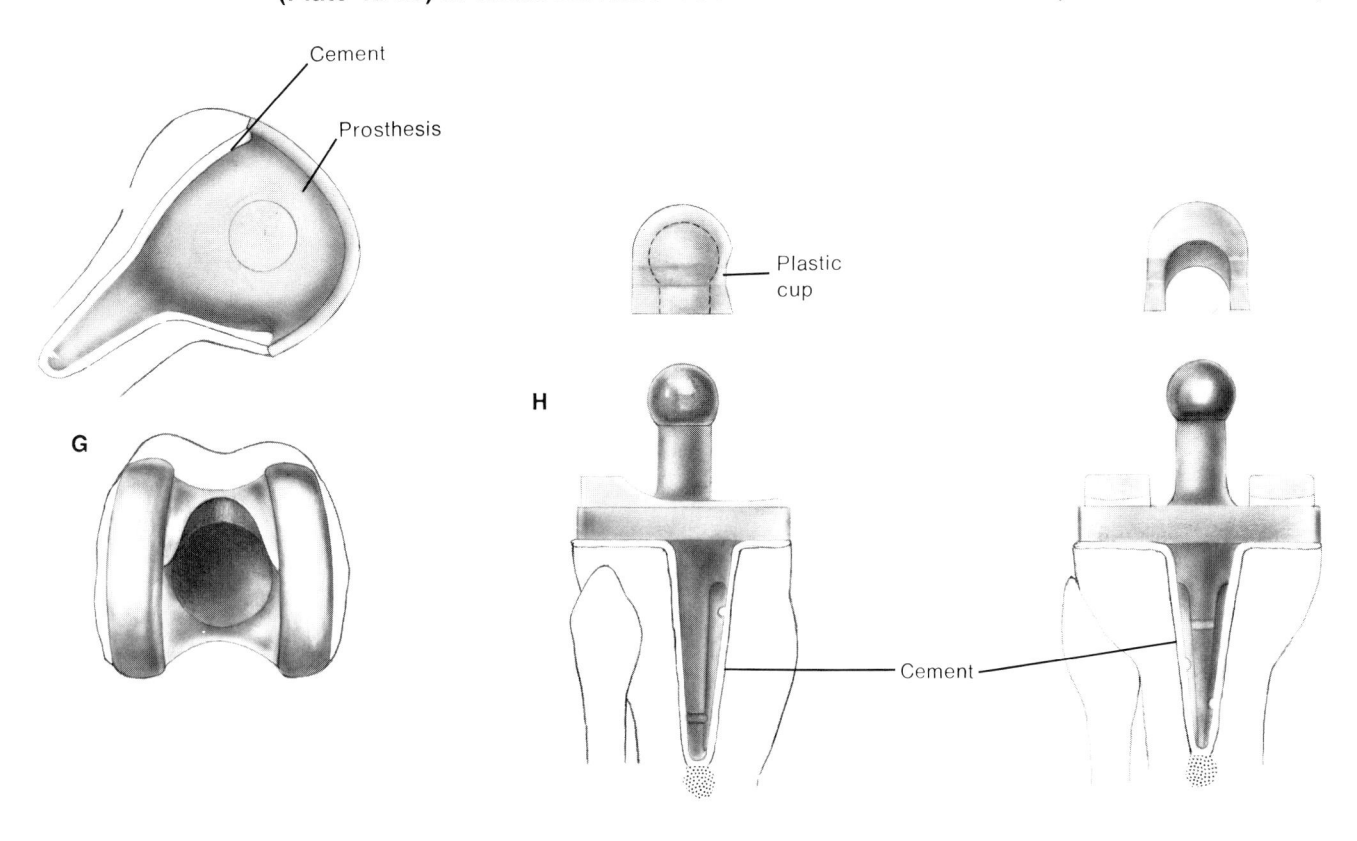

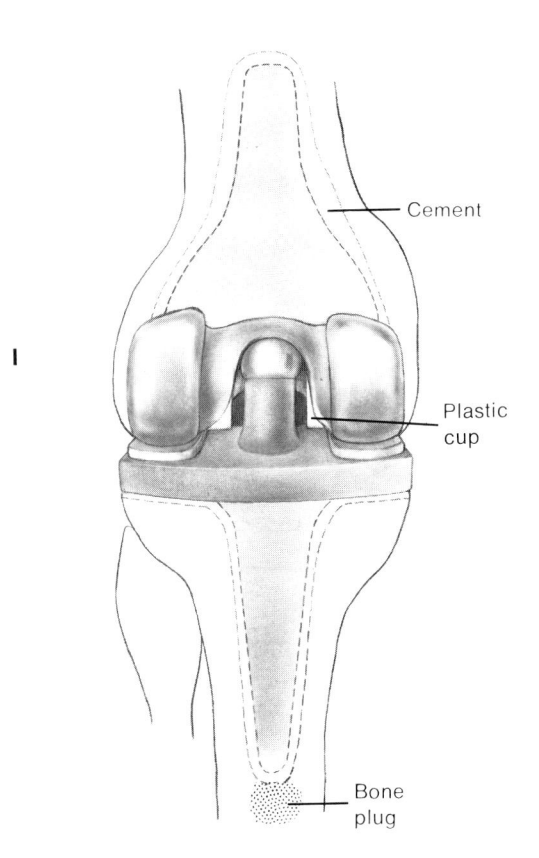

After this step the tourniquet should be released and all major bleeding controlled. This will allow for examination of posterior vessel bleeding from the posterior capsular area. After the bleeding has been controlled, the plastic cup is placed over the tibial ball and inserted into the femoral component (**H** and **I**). This can be accomplished with the insertion clamp.

Closure is accomplished in layers with staples for skin. The wound is closed over an indwelling suction catheter. A Robert Jones compression dressing with an outer shell of plaster of paris is applied with the knee in full extension.

POSTOPERATIVE MANAGEMENT. The Robert Jones compression dressing is removed 5 days postoperatively, and a roentgenogram is obtained of the knee. Active quadriceps motion and flexion and extension exercises are begun under the supervision of a physical therapist. The patient is encouraged to begin partial weight bearing using crutches or a walker. The patient is kept in the partial weight-bearing mode for 8 weeks following the operation. Stitches are removed at 2 weeks postoperatively, and vigorous physical therapy is pursued to attain at least 95° flexion and full extension.

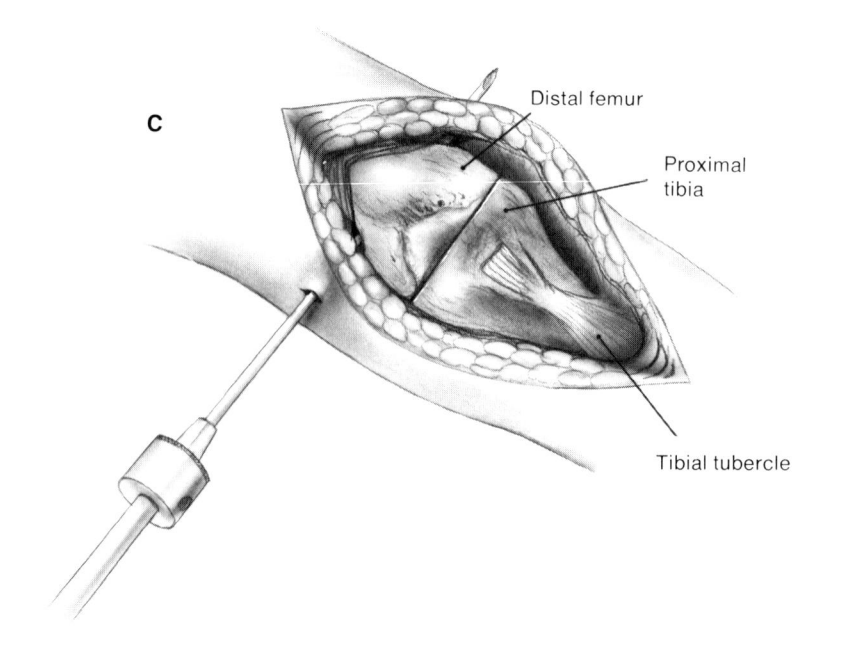

COMPRESSION ARTHRODESIS OF KNEE (Plate 12-34)

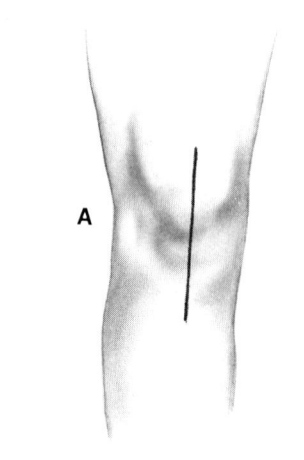

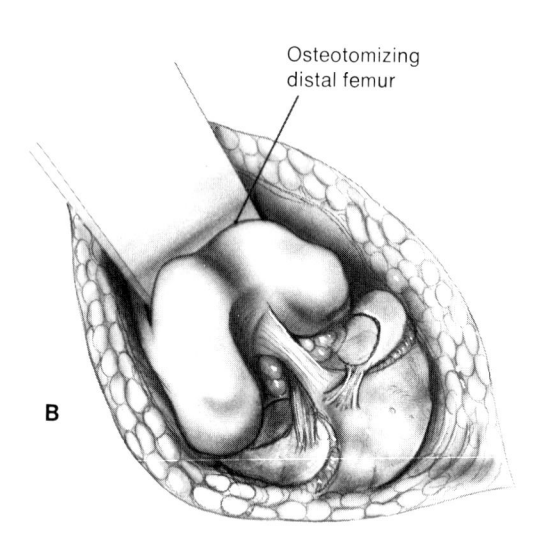

GENERAL DISCUSSION. Arthrodesis of the knee may be indicated in a tuberculous knee joint or in an arthritic knee if the articular surfaces are so severely damaged that satisfactory function cannot be expected with other treatment measures. It may be necessary following failed total knee replacement. When arthrodesis of the knee is necessary, the relief of pain will more than compensate for the residual disability of a stiff knee. Relaxation of the hamstring muscles and sciatic nerve after resection of 2 to 4 cm of the knee joint increases the ability for straight leg raising 30° to 40°. This, combined with the shortening of the extremity, enables the patient to put on shoes and socks. The average patient quickly learns to get in and out of chairs and to get up from the floor.

Charnley recommends that compression arthrodesis be avoided for any patient younger than 10 years of age. Bilateral arthrodesis of the knee should not be considered under most circumstances.

DETAILS OF PROCEDURE. A longitudinal incision is made over the anterior aspect of the knee joint **(A)**. The quadriceps and patellar tendons are divided, and the patella is excised. The joint capsule and synovium are opened transversely back to the collateral ligaments. Both medial and lateral collateral ligaments are divided. The knee is then flexed, and all available synovium is completely excised along with the menisci, cruciate ligaments, and the infrapatellar fat pad. The posterior compartment is exposed by subluxing the tibia forward on the femur with a large periosteal elevator or bone lever placed in the intracondylar notch of the femur.

(Plate 12-34) COMPRESSION ARTHRODESIS OF KNEE

A broad osteotome or bone saw is used to divide the superior surface of the tibia exactly perpendicular to the longitudinal axis of the tibia to remove a thin portion of bone and cartilage (at least 1 cm thick). A segment of bone of similar thickness is removed from the distal end of the femur **(B)** so that contiguous cancellous surfaces will be in apposition when the knee is placed in the desired position. This position is generally with the knee in approximately 5° flexion. If a varus or a valgus deformity is to be corrected, the plane of bone that is excised from the distal end of the femur is adjusted accordingly. Strong Steinmann pins are inserted transversely through the distal end of the femur **(C)**.

The compression clamps are now used as a guide in locating the correct position for insertion of heavy Steinmann pins through the proximal end of the tibia. With the Steinmann pins in place through the tibia and femur, the Charnley compression clamps are applied and tightened with the cancellous bone surfaces in complete contact **(D)**. A compression load of approximately 100 pounds is obtained. The wound is closed and a well-padded long-leg cast is applied incorporating the Steinmann pins **(E)**.

POSTOPERATIVE MANAGEMENT. Weight bearing between crutches is allowed as soon as the wound discomfort permits. At 4 weeks postoperatively, the long-leg cast and the femoral and tibial pins and clamps are carefully removed. A well-molded cylinder cast is then reapplied, and continued weight bearing is encouraged. The cylinder cast is continued an additional 4 or more weeks until there is clinical and roentgenographic evidence that the arthrodesis is solid.

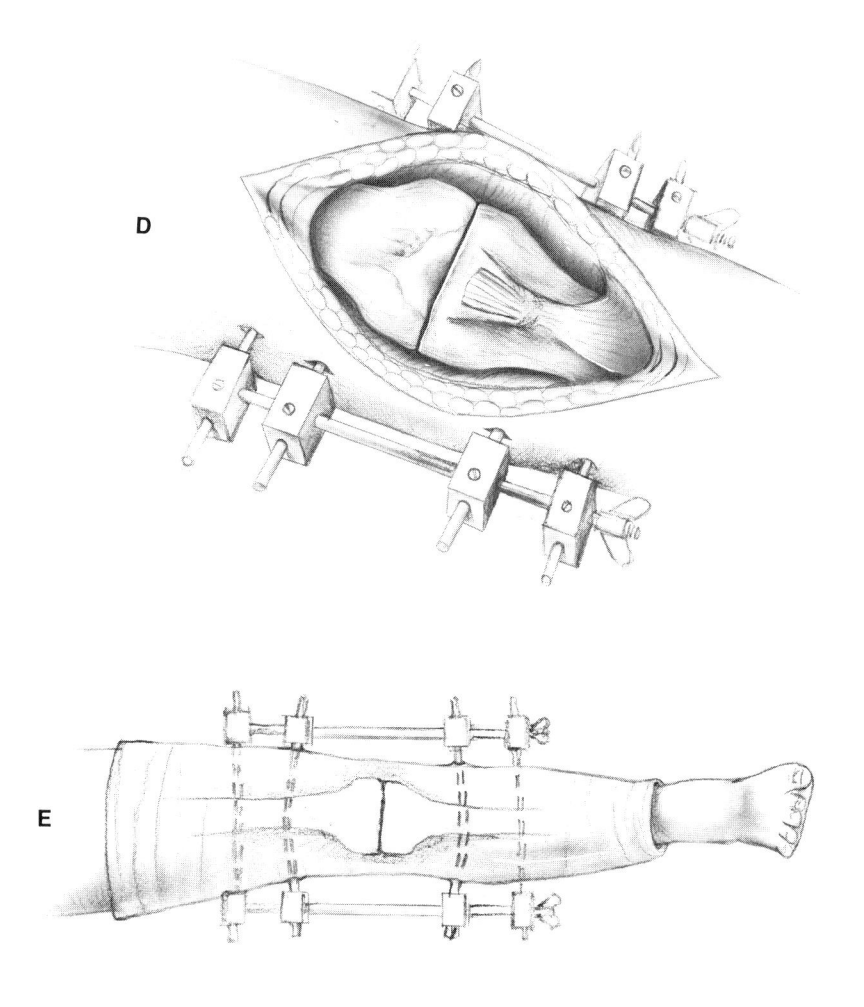

REFERENCES

Abbott, L. C., and Carpenter, W. F.: Surgical approaches to the knee joint, J. Bone Joint Surg. **27**:277, 1945.

Abbott, L. C., and Gill, G.G.: Surgical approaches to the epiphyseal cartilages of the knee and ankle joints, Arch. Srug. **46**:591, 1943.

Abbott, L. C., Saunders, J. B. deC. M., Bost, F. C., and Anderson, C. E.: Injuries to the ligaments of the knee joint, J. Bone Joint Surg. **26**:503, 1944.

Ackroyd, C. E., and Polyzoides, A. J.: Patellectomy for osteoarthritis, J. Bone Joint Surg. **60-B**:353, 1978.

Ahlberg, A., Scham, S., and Unander-Scharin, L.: Osteotomy in the degenerative and rheumatoid arthritis of the knee joint, Acta Orthop. Scand. **39**:379, 1968.

Ahstrom, J. P.: Osteochondral fracture in the knee joint associated with hypermobility and dislocation of the patella. Report of 18 cases, J. Bone Joint Surg. **47-A**:1491, 1965.

Anderson, M., Green, W. T., and Messner, M. B.: Growth and predictions of growth in the lower extremities, J. Bone Joint Surg. **45-A**:1, 1963.

Anderson, M., Messner, M. B., and Green, W. T.: Distribution of length of the normal femur and tibia n children from one to eighteen years of age, J. Bone Joint Surg. **46-A**:1197, 1964.

Andrews, J. R., and Hughston, J. C.: Treatment of patellar fractures by partial patellectomy, South. Med. J. **70**:809, 1977.

Appel, H.: Late results after meniscectomy in the knee joint. A clinical and roentgenologic follow-up investigation, Acta Orthop. Scand. (Suppl.) 133, 1970.

Arden, H. P., and Baber, L. D.: Synovectomy of knee joint in rheumatoid arthritis, J.A.M.A. **187**:4, 1964.

Aufranc, O. E.: Approach to the knee joint by release of the lateral ligaments, Clin. Orthop. **55**:97, 1967.

Baker, W. M.: On the formation of the synovial cyst in the leg in connection with disease in the knee joint, St. Barth. Hosp. Repts, **13**:245, 1875.

Bardenheier, J. A., III, Morgan, H. C., and Stamp, W. G.: Treatment and sequelae of experimentally produced septic arthritis, Surg. Gynecol. Obstet. **122**:249, 1966.

Bargen, J. H., Day, W. H., Freeman, M. A. R., and Swanson, S. A. V.: Mechanical tests on the tibial components of nonhinged knee prostheses, J. Bone Joint Surg. **60-B**:256, 1978.

Barr, J. S.: The treatment of fracture of the external tibial condyle (bumper fracture), J.A.M.A. **115**:1683, 1940.

Bauer, G. C. H., Insall, J., and Koshino, T.: Tibial osteotomy in gonarthrosis (osteo-arthritis of the knee), J. Bone Joint Surg. **51-A**:1545, 1969.

Becton, J. L., and Young, H. H.: Cysts of semilunar cartilage of the knee, Arch. Surg. **90**:708, 1965.

Bentley, G.: The surgical treatment of chondromalacia patellae, J. Bone Joint Surg. **60-B**:74, 1978.

Blazina, M. E.: Classification of injuries to the articular cartilages of the knee in athletics, American Academy of Orthopaedic Surgeons: Symposium on sports medicine, St. Louis, 1969, The C. V. Mosby Co., p. 118.

Blount, W. P.: Tibia vara, J. Bone Joint Surg. **19**:1, 1937.

Blount, W. P.: Unequal leg length, American Academy of Orthopaedic Surgeons Instructional Course Lectures, vol. 17, St. Louis, 1960, The C. V. Mosby Co.

Blount, W. P.: A mature look at epiphyseal stapling, Clin. Orthop. **77**:158, 1971.

Blount, W. P., and Clark, G. R.: Control of bone growth by epiphyseal stapling, preliminary report, J. Bone Joint Surg. **31-A**:464, 1949.

Blount, W. P., and Zeier, F.: Control of bone length, J.A.M.A. **148**:451, 1952,

Blum, B., Mowat, A. G., Bentley, G., and Morris, J. R.: Knee arthroplasty in patients with rheumatoid arthritis, Ann. Rheum. Dis. **33**:1, 1974.

Bost, F. C., Schottstaedt, E. R., and Larsen, L. J.: Surgical approaches to the knee joint, American Academy of Orthopaedic Surgeons Instructional Course Lectures, vol. 2, Ann Arbor, Mich., 1954, J. W. Edwards.

Bowker, J. H., and Thompson, E. B.: Surgical treatment of recurrent dislocation of the patella. A study of 48 cases, J. Bone Joint Surg. **46-A**:1451, 1964.

Boyd, H. B.: Surgical approaches. In Crenshaw, A. H., editor: Campbell's Operative orthopaedics, vol. 1, ed. 5, St. Louis, 1971, The C. V. Mosby Co.

Boyd, H. B., and Hawkins, B. L.: Patellectomy. A simplified technique, Surg. Gynecol. Obstet. **86**:357, 1948.

Brantigan, O. C., and Voshell, A. F.: Ligaments of the knee joint, J. Bone Joint Surg. **28**:66, 1946.

Brantigan, O. C., and Voshell, A. F.: The mechanics of the ligaments and menisci of the knee joint, J. Bone Joint Surg. **23**:44, 1941.

Bristow, W. R.: Internal derangement of the knee joint, Am. J. Surg. **43**:458, 1939.

Broderson, M. P., Fitzgerald, R. H., Peterson, L. F. A., Coventry, M. B., and Bryan, R. S.: Arthrodesis of the knee following failed total knee arthroplasty, J. Bone Joint Surg. **61-A**:181, 1979.

Bruce, J., and Walmsley, R.: Excision of the patella. Some experimental and anatomical observations, J. Bone Joint Surg. **24**:311, 1942.

Bryan, R. S., Dickson, J. H., and Taylor, W. F.: Recovery of the knee following meniscectomy. An evaluation of suction drainage and cast immobilization, J. Bone Joint Surg. **51-A**:973, 1969.

Burleson, R. J., Bickel, W. H., and Dahlin, D. C.: Popliteal cyst. A clinicopathological survey, J. Bone Joint Surg. **38-A**:1265, 1956.

Butt, W. P., and McIntyre, J. L.: Double-contrast arthrography of the knee, Radiology **92**:487, 1969.

Byers, P. D., et al.: The diagnosis and treatment of pigmented villonodular synovitis, J. Bone Joint Surg. **50-B**:290, 1968.

Campbell, W. C.: Arthroplasty of the knee; report of cases, J. Orthop. Surg. **3**:430, 1921.

Campbell, W. C.: Interposition of Vitallium plates in arthroplasties of the knee, Am. J. Surg. **47**:639, 1940.

Cargill, A. O'R., and Jackson, J. P.: Bucket-handle tear of the medial meniscus. A cast for conservative surgery, J. Bone Joint Surg. **58-A**:248, 1976.

Carpenter, E. B., and Dalton, J. B., Jr.: A critical evaluation of epiphyseal stimulation, J. Bone Joint Surg. **38-A**:1089, 1956.

Cave, E. F., and Rowe, C. R.: The patella, its importance in derangements of the knee, J. Bone Joint Surg. **32-A**:542, 1950.

Cave, E. F., Rowe, C. R., and Yee, L. B. K.: Chondromalacia of the patella, Surg. Gynecol. Obstet. **81**:446, 1965.

Chandler, F. A.: Patellar advancement operation. A revised technic, J. Int. Surg. **3**:433, 1940.

Charif, P., and Reichelderfer, T. E.: Genu recurvation congenitum in the newborn: its incidence, course, treatment, prognosis, Clin. Pediatr. **4**:587, 1965.

Charnley, J.: Horizontal approach to the medial semilunar cartilage, J. Bone Joint Surg. **30-B**:659, 1948.

Charnley, J.: Positive pressure in arthrodesis of the knee joint, J. Bone Joint Surg. **30-B**:478, 1948.

Charnley, J.: Arthrodesis of the knee, Clin. Orthop. **18**:37, 1960.

Charnley, J., and Baker, S. L.: Compression arthrodesis of the knee. A clinical and histological study, J. Bone Joint Surg. **34-B**:187, 1952.

Charnley, J., and Lowe, H. G.: A study of the end results of compression arthrodesis of the knee, J. Bone Joint Surg. **40-B**:633, 1958.

Childress, H. M.: Popliteal cysts associated with undiagnosed posterior lesions of the medial meniscus, J. Bone Joint Surg. **36-A**:1233, 1954.

Childress, H. M.: Popliteal cyst associated with undiagnosed posterior lesions of the medial meniscus. The significance of age in diagnosis and treatment, J. Bone Joint Surg. **52-A**:1487, 1970.

Clancy, W. J.: Reconstruction of the anterior cruciate ligament using the patella tendon, presented at the annual meeting, American Orthopaedic Society for Sports Medicine, San Diego, 1977.

Clayton, M. L.: Surgery of the lower extremity in rheumatoid arthritis, J. Bone Joint Surg. **45-A**;1517, 1963.

Cleveland, M.: Operative fusion of the unstable of flail knee due to anterior poliomyelitis. A study of late results, J. Bone Joint Surg. **14**:525, 1932.

Cleveland, M., and Bosworth, D. M.: Surgical correction of flexion deformity of knees due to spastic paralysis, Surg. Gynecol. Obstet. **63**:659, 1936.

Cohen, S. H., Ehrlich, G. E., Kauffman, M. S., and Cope, C.: Thrombophlebitis following knee surgery, J. Bone Joint Surg. **55-A**:106, 1973.

Coker, T. P., and Kent, M.: Peroneal-nerve irritation associated with cystic lateral meniscus of the knee. A report of 2 cases, J. Bone Joint Surg. **49-A**:362, 1967.

Compere, C. L., Hill, J. A., Lewinnek, G. E., and Thompson, R. G.: A new method of patellectomy for patellofemoral arthritis, J. Bone Joint Surg. **61-A**:714, 1979.

Coventry, M. D.: Osteotomy of the upper portion of the tibia for degenerative arthritis of the knee. A preliminary report, J. Bone Joint Surg. **47-A**:984, 1965.

Coventry, M. B.: Stepped staple for upper tibial osteotomy, J. Bone Joint Surg. **51-A**:1011, 1969.

Coventry, M. B.: Osteotomy about the knee for degenerative and rheumatoid arthritis. Indications, operative technique, and results, J. Bone Joint Surg. **55-A**:23, 1973.

Cowan, D. J.: Reconstruction of the anterior cruciate ligament by the method of Kenneth Jones (1963). Proc. R. Soc. Med. **58**:336, 1965.

Cracchiolo, A., III, Blazina, M. E., and Marmor, L.: Masses at the medial side of the knee joint, Clin. Orthop. **62**:167, 1969.

Crauener, E. K.: Hernia of the knee joint (Baker's cyst), J. Bone Joint Surg. **14**:186, 1932.

Dandy, D. J.: Recurrent subluxation of the patella on extension of the knee, J. Bone Joint Surg. **53-B**:483, 1971.

D'Arcy, J.: Pes anserinus transposition for chronic anteromedial rotational instability of the knee, J. Bone Joint Surg. **60-B**:66, 1978.

DeHaven, K. B., and Collins, H. R.: Diagnosis of internal derangements of the knee. The role of arthroscopy, J. Bone Joint Surg. **57-A**:802, 1975.

Denham, R. A., and Bishop, R. E. D.: Mechanics of the knee and problems in reconstructive surgery, J. Bone Joint Surg. **60-B**:345, 1978.

Devas, M. B.: High tibial osteotomy for arthritis of the knee. A method specially suitable for the elderly, J. Bone Joint Surg. **51-B**:95, 1969.

Drennan, D. B., Fahey, J. J., and Maylahn, D. J.: Important factors in achieving arthrodesis of the Charcot knee, J. Bone Joint Surg. **53-A**:1180, 1971.

Duthie, H. L., and Hutchinson, J. R.: The results of partial and total excision of the patella, J. Bone Joint Surg. **40-B**:75, 1958.

Ellison, A. E.: Distal iliotibial-band transfer for anterolateral rotatory instability of the knee, J. Bone Joint Surg. **61-A**:330, 1979.

Eriksson, E.: Reconstruction of the anterior cruciate ligament, Orth. Clin. North Am. **7**:309, 1976.

Evarts, C. M.: Thromboembolism following reconstructive surgery of the knee. In Symposium on reconstructive surgery of the knee, American Academy of Orthopaedic Surgeons, St. Louis, 1978, The C. V. Mosby Co., pp. 337.339.

Evarts, C. M., and DeHaven, K.: Proximal tibial osteotomy, Ortho. Clin. North Am. **2**:1:231, 1971.

Evarts, C. M., DeHaven, K. E., and Nelson, C. L., Jr.: Proximal tibial osteotomy for degenerative arthritis of the knee, Orthop. Clin. North Am. **2**:231-243, 1971.

Fairbank, H. A. T.: Osteo-chondritis dissecans, Br. J. Surg. **21**:67, 1933.

Fairbank, T. J.: Knee joint changes after meniscectomy, J. Bone Joint Surg. **30-B**:664, 1948.

Ferguson, A. B., Jr., Brown, T. D., Fu, F. H., and Rutkowski, R.: Relief of patellofemoral contact stress of anterior displacement of the tibial tubercle, J. Bone Joint Surg. **61-A**:159, 1979.

Frankel, V. H., Burstein, A. H., and Brooks, D. B.: Biomechanics of internal derangement of the knee. Pathomechanics as determined by analysis of the instant centers of motion, J. Bone Joint Surg. **53-A**:945, 1971.

Frantz, C. H.: Epiphyseal stapling: a comprehensive review, Clin. Orthop. **77**:149, 1971.

Freiberg, A. H.: The removal of the meniscus from the knee joint, J. Bone Joint Surg. **3**:697, 1921.

Gallo, G. A., and Bryan, R. S.: Cysts of the semilunar cartilages of the knee. A report of sixteen cases including arthrographic study, Am. J. Surg. **116**:65, 1968.

Galway, R. D., Beaupre, A., and MacIntosh, D. L.: Pivot-shift: a clinical sign of symptomatic anterior cruciate instability, J. Bone Joint Surg. **54-B**:763-764, 1972.

Garcia, A., and Neer, C. S., II: Isolated fractures of the intercondylar eminence of the tibia, Am. J. Surg. **95**:593, 1958.

Gariépy, R.: Genu varum treated by high tibial osteotomy (in proceedings of the joint meeting of the orthopaedic associations), J. Bone Joint Surg. **46-B**:783, 1964.

Gariépy, R.: Ostéotomie tibiale transpéroniere (in symposium: les gonarthroses d'origine statique), Rev. Chir. Orthop. **53**:180, 1967.

Gear, M. W. L.: The late results of meniscectomy, Br. J. Surg. **54**:270, 1967.

Geens, S.: Synovectomy and debridement of the knee in rheumatoid arthritis. I. Historical review, J. Bone Joint Surg. **51-A**:617, 1969.

Geens, S., et al.: Synovectomy and debridement of the knee in rheumatoid arthritis. II. Clinical and roentgenographic study of thirty-one cases, J. Bone Joint Surg. **51-A**:626, 1969.

Ghormley, R. K.: Late joint changes as a result of internal derangements of the knee, Am. J. Surg. **76**:496, 1948.

Gillies, H., and Seligson, D.: Precision in the diagnosis of meniscal lesions: a comparison of clinical evaluation, arthrography and arthroscopy, J. Bone Joint Surg. **61-A**:343, 1979.

Girzadas, D. V., Geens, S., Clayton, M. L., and Leidholt, J. D.: Performance of a hinged metal knee prosthesis. A case report with a follow-up of three and one-half years and histological and metallurgical data, J. Bone Joint Surg. **50-A**:355, 1968.

Goldie, I., and Schlossman, D.: Radiologic changes in rheumatoid knee-joint before and after synovectomy, Clin. Orthop. **64**:98, 1969.

Goldthwait, J. E.: Dislocation of the patella, Trans. Am. Orthop. Assoc. **8**:237, 1895.

Goldthwait, J. E.: Permanent dislocation of the patella, Ann. Surg. **29**:62, 1899.

Goldthwait, J. E.: Slipping or recurrent dislocation of the patella. With the report of eleven cases, Boston Med. Surg. J. **150**:169, 1904.

Green, D. P., Parkes, J. C., II, and Stinchfield, F. E.: Arthrodesis of the knee. A follow-up up study, J. Bone Joint Surg. **49-A**:1065, 1967.

Green, J. P.: Osteochondritis dissecans of the knee, J. Bone Joint Surg. **48-B**:82, 1966.

Green, J. P., and Waugh, W.: Congenital lateral dislocation of the patella, J. Bone Joint Surg. **50-B**:285, 1968.

Green, W. T., and Anderson, M.: Epiphyseal arrest for the correction of discrepancies in length of the lower extremities, J. Bone Joint Surg. **39-A**:853, 1957.

Green, W. T., and Anderson, M.: Experiences with epiphyseal arrest in correcting discrepancies in length of the lower extremities in infantile paralysis. A method of predicting the effect, J. Bone Joint Surg. **29**:659, 1947.

Green, W. T., and Banks, H. H.: Osteochondritis dissecans in children, J. Bone Joint Surg. **35-A**:26, 1953.

Green, W. T., Wyatt, G. M., and Anderson, M.: Orthoroentgenography as a method of measuring the bones of the lower extremities, Clin. Orthop. **61**:10, 1968.

Greulich, W. W., and Pyle, S. I.: Radiographic atlas of skeletal development of the hand and wrist, Stanford, Cal., 1950, Stanford University Press.

Groves, E. W. H.: Operation for the repair of the crucial ligaments, Lancet **2**:674, 1917.

Groves, E. W. H.: The cruciate ligaments of the knee joints: their function, rupture, and the operative treatment of the same, Br. J. Surg. **7**:505, 1920.

Gunn, A. L.: High tibial osteotomy for arthritis of the knee, J. Bone Joint Surg. **48-B**:389, 1966.

Gunn, D. R.: Contracture of the quadriceps muscle. A discussion on the etiology and relationship to recurrent dislocation of the patella, J. Bone Joint Surg. **46-B**:492, 1964.

Hagemann, W. F., Woods, G. W., and Tullos, H. S.: Arthrodesis in failed total knee replacement, J. Bone Joint Surg. **60-A**:790, 1978.

Hampton, O. P., Jr.: Observations on the management of suppurative arthritis of the knee joint, Am. J. Surg. **74**:631, 1947.

Harris, W. R., and Kostuik, J. P.: High tibial osteotomy for osteoarthritis of the knee, J. Bone Joint Surg. **52-A**:330, 1970.

Harty, M.: Anatomic features of the lateral aspect of the knee joint, Surg. Gynecol. Obstet. **130**:11, 1970.

Hauser, E. D. W.: Total tendon transplant for slipping patella. New operation for recurrent dislocation of the patella, Surg. Gynecol. Obstet. **66**:199, 1938.

Haverson, S. B., and Rein, B. I.: Lateral discoid meniscus of the knee: arthrographic diagnosis, Am. J. Roentgenol. Radium Ther. Nucl. Med. **109**:581, 1970.

Helfet, A. J.: Mechanism of derangements of the medial semilunar cartilage and their management, J. Bone Joint Surg. **41-B**:319, 1959.

Helfet, A. J.: The management of internal derangements of the knee, Philadelphia, 1963, J. B. Lippincott Co.

Henderson, M. S.: Posterolateral incision for the removal of loose bodies from the posterior compartment of the knee joint, Surg. Gynecol. Obstet. **33**:698, 1921.

Henderson, M. S.: Bucket-handle fractures of the semilunar cartilages, J.A.M.A. **90**:1359, 1928.

Henderson, M. S., and Jones, H. T.: Loose bodies in joints and bursae due to synovial osteochondromatosis, J. Bone Joint Surg. **5**:400, 1923.

Henning, C. E.: Personal communication, 1976.

Hodgen, J. T., and Frantz, C. H.: Arrest of growth of the epiphyses, Arch. Surg. **53**:664, 1946.

Hohl, M.: Tibial condylar fractures, J. Bone Joint Surg. **49-A**:1455, 1967.

Hohl, M., and Luck, J. V.: Fractures of the tibial condyle. A clinical and experimental study, J. Bone Joint Surg. **38-A**:1001, 1956.

Høstrup, H., and Pilgaard, S.: Epiphyseodesis and epiphyseal stapling on the lower limb, Acta Orthop. Scand. **40**:130, 1969.

Howe, W. M.: Personal communication, 1976.

Howorth, B.: Knock knees. With special reference to the stapling operation, Clin. Orthop. **77**:233, 1971.

Hughston, J. C.: Acute knee injuries to athletes, Clin. Orthop. **23**:114, 1962.

Hughston, J. C.: Subluxation of the patella, J. Bone Joint Surg. **50-A**:1003, 1968.

Hughston, J. C., Andrews, J. R., Corss, M. J., and Moschi, A.: Classification of knee ligament instabilities. I. The medial compartment and cruciate ligaments, J. Bone Joint Surg. **58-A**:159, 1976.

Hughston, J. C., Andrews, J. R., Cross, M. J., and Moschi, A.: Classification of knee ligament instabilities. II. The lateral compartment, J. Bone Joint Surg. **58-A**:173, 1976.

Hughston, J. C., Andrews, J. R., Regan, T., McLeod, W. D., and Uthus, D.: Posterolateral instability of the knee, presented at the annual meeting of the American Academy of Orthopaedic Surgeons, New Orleans, 1976.

Hughston, J. C., and Eilers, A. F.: The role of the posterior oblique ligament in repairs of acute medial (collateral) ligament tears of the knee, J. Bone Joint Surg. **55/A**:923, 1973.

Inge, G.: Eighty-six cases of chronic synovitis of knee joint treated by synovectomy, J.A.M.A. **111**:2451, 1938.

Insall, J.: A midline approach to the knee, J. Bone Joint Surg. **53-A**:1584, 1971.

Insall, J., Falvo, K. A., and Wise, D. W.: Chondromalacia patellae, J. Bone Joint Surg. **58-A**:1, 1976.

Insall, J. N., Ranawat, C. S., Aglietti, P., and Shine, J.: A comparison of four models of total knee-replacement prostheses, J. Bone Joint Surg. **58-A**:754, 1976.

Insall, J., Scott, W. N., and Ranawat, C. S.: The total condylar knee prosthesis. A report of two hundred and twenty cases, J. Bone Joint Surg. **61-A**:174, 1979.

Insall, J., Shoji, H., and Mayer, V.: High tibial osteotomy. A five-year evaluation, J. Bone Joint Surg. **56-A**:1397, 1874.

Irwin, C. E.: Genu recurvatum following poliomyelitis; controlled method of operative correction, J.A.M.A. **120**:1942.

Jack, E. A.: Experimental rupture of the medial collateral ligament of the knee, J. Bone Joint Surg. **32-B**:396, 1950.

Jackson, J. P.: Degenerative changes in the knee after meniscectomy, Br. Med. J. **2**:525, 1968.

Jackson, J. P., and Waugh, W.: Tibial osteotomy for osteoarthritis of the knee, J. Bone Joint Surg. **42-B**:746, 1961.

Jackson, J. P., Waugh, W., and Green, J. P.: High tibial osteotomy for osteoarthritis of the knee, J. Bone Joint Surg. **51-B**:88, 1969.

Jackson, R. W., and Dandy, D. J.: Arthroscopy of the knee, New York, 1976, Grune & Stratton.

Johnson, E. W., Jr.: Contractures of the iliotibial band, Surg. Gynecol. Obstet. **96**:599, 1953.

Johnson, J. T. H.: Neuropathic fractures and joint injuries. Pathogenesis and rationale of prevention and treatment, J. Bone Joint Surg. **49-A**:1, 1967.

Johnson, L. L.: Comprehensive arthroscopic examination of the knee, St. Louis, 1977, The C. V. Mosby Co.

Johnson, R. J., Kettelkamp, D. B., Clark, W., and Leaverton, P.: Factors affecting late results meniscectomy, J. Bone Joint Surg. **56-A**:719, 1974.

Jones, J. B., Francis, K. C., and Mahoney, J. R.: Recurrent dislocating patella; etiology and treatment, Clin. Orthop. **20**:230, 1961.

Jones, K. G.: Reconstruction of the anterior cruciate ligament. A technique using the central one-third of the patellar ligament, J. Bone Joint Surg. **45-A**:925, 1963.

Jones, R. E., Smith, E. C., and Reisch, J. S.: Effects of medial meniscectomy in patients older than forty years, J. Bone Joint Surg. **60-A**:783, 1978.

Jordan, H. H.: Hemophilic arthropathies; the principles and practice or orthopaedic treatment, Springfield, Ill., 1958, Charles C Thomas, Publisher.

Katz, M. P., Grogono, B. J. S., and Soper, K. P.: Etiology and treatment of congenital dislocation of the knee, J. Bone Joint Surg. **49-B**:112, 1967.

Kaufer, H.: Mechanical function fo the patella, J. Bone Joint Surg. **53-A**:1551, 1971.

Kelikian, H.: Posterior approach to the knee, Surg. Clin. North Am. **27**:157, 1947.

Kennedy, J. C.: Complete dislocation of the knee joint, J. Bone Joint Surg. **45-A**:889, 1963.

Kennedy, J. C., and Bailey, W. H.: Experimental tibialplateau fractures. Studies of the mechanism and a classification, J. Bone Joint Surg. **50-A**:1522, 1968.

Kennedy, J. C., and Fowler, P. J.: Medial and anterior instability of the knee. An anatomical and clinical study using stress machines, J. Bone Joint Surg. **53-A**:1257, 1971.

Kennedy, J. C., Stewart, R., and Walker, D. M.: Anterolateral rotatory instability of the knee joint. An early analysis of the Ellison procedure, J. Bone Joint Surg. **60-A**:1031, 1978.

Kennedy, J. C., Weinberg, H. W., and Wilson, A. S.: The anatomy and function of the anterior cruciate ligament. As determined by clinical and morphological studies, J. Bone Joint Surg. **56-A**:223, 1974.

Key, J. A.: Positive pressure in arthrodesis for tuberculosis of the knee joint, South. Med. J. **25**:909, 1932.

Krida, A.: Anterior crucial and internal lateral ligament reconstruction, American Academy of Orthopaedic Surgeons Instructional Course Lectures, vol. 2, Ann Arbor, Mich., 1944, J. W. Edwards, p. 416.

Lam, S. J. S.: Reconstruction of the anterior cruciate ligament using the Jones Procedure and its Guy Hospital modification, J. Bone Joint Surg. **50-A**:1213, 1968.

Langenskiöld, A., and Riska, E. B.: Tibia vara (osteochondrosis deformans tibiae). A survey of seventy-one cases, J. Bone Joint Surg. **46-A**:1405, 1964.

Last, R. J.: The popliteus muscle and the lateral meniscus, J. Bone Joint Surg. **32-B**:93, 1950.

Laurin, C. A., et al.: Long-term results of synovectomy of the knee in rheumatoid patients, J. Bone Joint Surg. **56-A**:521, 1974.

Leach, R. E., Gregg, T., and Siber, F. J.: Weight-bearing radiography in osteoarthritis of the knee, Radiology **97**:265, 1970.

Leach, R. E., Stryker, W. S., and Zohn, D. A.: A comparative study of isometric and isotonic quadriceps exercise programs, J. Bone Joint Surg. **47-A**:1421, 1965.

Lidge, R. T.: Medial meniscectomy in the osteoarthritic knee, Clin. Orthop. **68**:63, 1970.

Liljedahl, S., Lindvall, N., and Wetterfors, J.: Early diagnosis and treatment of acute ruptures of the anterior cruciate ligament. A clinical and arthrographic study of 48 cases, J. Bone Joint Surg. **47-A**:1503, 1965.

Lipscomb, P. R., and Henderson, M. S.: Internal derangements of the knee, J.A.M.A. **135**:827, 1947.

Lipscomb, P. R., Jr., Lipscomb, P. R., Sr., and Bryan, R. S.: Osteochondritis dissecans of the knee with loose fragments. Treatment by replacement and fixation with readily removed pins, J. Bone Joint Surg. **60-A**:235, 1978.

Litchman, H., Silver, C., and Simon, S.: Injuries to the medial meniscus in the aging patient, J.A.M.A. **196**:164, 1966.

Losee, R. E., Johnson, T. R., and Southwick, W. O.: Anterior subluxation of the lateral tibial plateau. A diagnostic test and operative repair, J. Bone Joint Surg. **60-A**:1015, 1978.

MacIntosh, D. L., and Tregunning, R. J.: A follow-up study of 'over-the-top' repair of acute tears of the anterior cruciate ligament, J. Bone Joint Surg. **59-B**:511, 1976.

Macnab, I.: Recurrent dislocation of the patella, J. Bone Joint Surg. **34-A**:957, 1952.

Magnuson, P. B.: Technic of debridement of the knee joint for arthritis, Surg. Clin. North Am. **26**:249, 1946.

Makin, M., Ben-Hur, N., and Weinberg, H.: Partial patellectomy for transverse fracture of the patella, Isr. Med. J. **21**:79, 1962.

Mallock, J. D.: Popliteal cysts in children, Br. J. Surg. **57**:616, 1970.

Marmor, L.: Synovectomy of the rheumatoid knee. Clin. Orthop. **44**:151, 1966.

Marmor, L.: Surgery of the rheumatoid knee. Synovectomy and debridement, J. Bone Joint Surg. **55-A**:535, 1973.

Mather, C.: Injuries of the knee joint. In Orthopaedic Surgery in the European Theater of Operations, Washington, D.C., 1956, Office of the Surgeon General.

Mauck, H. P.: Severe acute injuries of the knee, Am. J. Surg. **56**:54, 1942.

Mayer, L.: Congenital anterior subluxation of the knee, Am. J. Orthop. **10**:411, 1913.

Mazet, R., Jr., and Hennessy, C. A.: Knee disarticulation. A new technique and a new knee-joint mechanism, J. Bone Joint Surg. **48-A**:126, 1966.

McFarland, B.: Excision of patella for recurrent dislocation, J. Bone Joint Surg. **30-B**:158, 1948.

McGinty, J. B., Geuss, L. F., and Marrin, R. A.: Partial or total meniscectomy. A comparative analysis, J. Bone Joint Surg. **59-A**:763, 1977.

McKeever, D. C.: Transplantation of the tibial tubercle, J. Bone Joint Surg. **33-A**:478, 1951.

McKeever, D. C.: Recurrent dislocation of the patella, Clin. Orthop. **3**:55, 1954.

McKenna, R., Bachmann, F., Kaushal, S. P., and Galante, J. O.: Thromboembolic disease in patients undergoing total knee replacement, J. Bone Joint Surg. **58-A**:928, 1976.

Medbö, I.: Tibia vara (osteochondrosis deformans tibiae or Blount's disease). Treatment and follow-up examination, Acta Orthop. Scand. **34**:323, 1964.

Menelaus, M. B.: Correction of leg length discrepancy by epiphyseal arrest, J. Bone Joint Surg. **48-B**:336, 1966.

Meyerding, H. W., and VanDemark, R. E.: Posterior hernia of the knee (Baker's cyst, popliteal cyst, semimembranosus bursitis and popliteal bursitis), J.A.M.A. **122**:858, 1943.

Milgram, J. E.: Arthrodesis of the knee, American Academy of Orthopaedic Surgeons Instructional Course Lectures, vol. 2, Ann Arbor, Mich., 1944, J. W. Edwards, p. 315.

Miller, J. A., Jr.: Joint paracentesis from an anatomic point of view. II. Hip, knee, ankles, and foot, Surgery **41**:999, 1957.

Mochizuki, R. M., and Schurman, D. J.: Patellar complications following total knee arthroplasty, J. Bone Joint Surg. **61-A**:879, 1979.

Moore, F. H., and Smillie, I. S.: Arthrodesis of the knee joint, Clin. Orthop. **13**:215, 1959.

Neibauer, J. J., and King, D. E.: Congenital dislocation of the knee, J. Bone Joint Surg. **42-A**:207, 1960.

Nelson, C. L., Jr., and Evarts, C. M.: Arthroplasty and arthrodesis of the knee joint, Orthop. Clin. North Am. **2**:245, 1971.

Neviaser, J. S.: Division of the tibial collateral ligament for removal of the medial meniscus. A long-term follow-up study, Clin. Orthop. **55**:105, 1967.

Nicholas, J. A.: Internal derangement of the knee: diagnosis and management, American Academy of Orthopaedic Surgeons Symposium on sports medicine, St. Louis, 1969, The C. V. Mosby Co., p. 152

Nicholas, J. A.: The five-one reconstruction for anteromedial instability of the knee. Indications, technique and the results in fifty-two patients, J. Bone Joint Surg. **55-A**:899, 1973.

Norwood, L. A., Jr., Andrews, J. R., Meisterling, R. C., and Clancy, G. L.: Acute anterolateral instability of the knee, J. Bone Joint Surg. **61-A**:704, 1979.

Noyes, F. R., and Sonstegard, D. A.: Biomechanical function of the pes anserinus at the knee and the effect of its transplantation, J. Bone Joint Surg. **55-A**:1225, 1973.

O'Donoghue, D. H.: Surgical treatment of fresh injuries, J. Bone Joint Surg. **32-A**:721, 1950.

O'Donoghue, D. H.: An analysis of end results of surgical treatment of major injuries to the ligaments of the knee, J. Bone Joint Surg. **37-A**:1, 1955.

O'Donoghue, D. H.: Treatment of injuries to athletes, Philadelphia, 1962, W. B. Saunders Co.

O'Donoghue, D. H.: A method for replacement of the anterior cruciate ligament of the knee. Report of twenty cases, J. Bone Joint Surg. **45-A**:905, 1963.

O'Donoghue, D. H.: Reconstruction for medial instability of the knee. Technique and results in sixty cases, J. Bone Joint Surg. **55-A**:941, 1973.

O'Donoghue, D. H., Thompkins, F., and Hays, M. B.: Strength of quadriceps function after patellectomy, West. J. Surg. **60**:159, 1952.

Orr, H. W.: A review of the surgical treatment of congenital dislocation, recurrent dislocation, or slipping patella, Clin. Orthop. **3**:3, 1954.

Ouellet, R., Lévesque, H. P., and Laurin, C. A.: The ligamentous stability of the knee: an experimental investigation, Can. Med. Assoc. J. **100**:45, 1969.

Paradies, L. H.: Synovectomy of the knee. In Higmans, W., Paul, W. D., and Herschel, H., editors: Early synovectomy in rheumatoid arthritis. Proceedings of the Symposium on early synovectomy in rheumatoid arthritis, Amsterdam, April, 1967, Amsterdam, 1969, Excerpta Medica Foundation, p. 129.

Pardee, M. L.: Synovectomy of the knee joint. A review of the literature and presentation of cases, J. Bone Joint Surg. **30-A**:908, 1948.

Patrick, J.: Aneurysm of the popliteal vessels after meniscectomy, J. Bone Joint Surg. **45-B**:570, 1963.

Peterson, L. F. A.: Surgery for rheumatoid arthritis—timing and techniques the lower extremity, J. Bone Joint Surg. **50-A**:587, 1968.

Peterson, L. F. A.: Current status of total knee arthroplasty, Arch. Surg. **112**:1099, 1977.

Phemister, D. B.: Operative arrestment of longitudinal growth of bones, in the treatment of deformities, J. Bone Joint Surg. **15**:1, 1933.

Pilcher, M. F.: Epiphyseal stapling: thirty-five cases followed to maturity, J. Bone Joint Surg. **44-B**:82, 1962.

Pistevos, G., and Duckworth, T.: The correction of genu valgum by epiphyseal stapling, J. Bone Joint Surg. **59-B**:72, 1977.

Poirier, H.: Epiphyseal stapling and leg equalization, J. Bone Joint Surg. **50-B**:61, 1968.

Porter, B. B.: Crush fractures of the lateral tibial table. Factors influencing the prognosis, J. Bone Joint Surg. **52-B**:676, 1970.

Potter, T. A., Weinfeld, M.S., and Thomas, W. H.: Arthroplasty of the knee in rheumatoid arthritis and osteoarthritis. A follow-up study after implantation of the McKeever and MacIntosh prostheses, J. Bone Joint Surg. **54-A**:1, 1972.

Quigley, T. B.: The treatment of avulsion of the collateral ligaments of the knee, Am. J. Surg. **78**:574, 1949.

Ray, R. L., and Ehrlich, M. G.: Lateral hamstring transfer and gait improvement in the cerebral palsy patient, J. Bone Joint Surg. **61-A**:719, 1979.

Reckling, F. W., Asher, M. A., Mantz, F. A., and Helton, D. O.: Performance analysis of the ex vivo geometric total knee prosthesis, J. Bone Joint Surg. **57-A**:108, 1975.

Reynolds, F. C.: Diagnosis of ligamentous injuries of the knee In Symposium on sports medicine, American Academy of Orthopaedic Surgeons, St. Louis, 1969, The C. V. Mosby Co., p. 178.

Riley, L. H., Jr., and Hungerford, D. S.: Geometric total knee replacement for treatment of the rheumatoid knee, J. Bone Joint Surg. **60-A**:523, 1978.

Roberts, J. M.: Fractures of the condyles of the tibia. An anatomical and clinical end-result study of one hundred cases, J. Bone Joint Surg. **50-A**:1505, 1968.

Rosenberg, N. J.: Osteochondral fractures of the lateral femoral condyle, J. Bone Joint Surg. **46-A**:1013, 1964.

Roux, D.: Luxation habituelle de la rotule; traitement operatoire, Rev. Chir. (Paris) **8**:682, 1888.

Russell, E., et al.: Some normal variations of knee arthrograms and their anatomical significance, J. Bone Joint Surg. **60-A**:66, 1978.

Scal, P. V., and Chan, R. N. W.: Tibial osteotomy for osteoarthrosis of the knee: 5- to 10-year follow-up study, Acta Orthop. Scand. **46**:141, 1975.

Shoji, H., and Insall, J.: High tibial osteotomy for osteoarthritis of the knee with valgus deformity, J. Bone Joint Surg. **55-A**:963, 1973.

Sideman, S., and Siegel, I.: Meniscal derangement in the osteoarthritis knee joint, J.A.M.A. **192**:626, 1962.

Slocum, D. B., and Larson, R. L.: Pes anserinus transplantation. A surgical procedure for control of rotary instability of the knee, J. Bone Joint Surg. **50-A:**226, 1968.

Slocum, D. B., and Larson, R. L.: Rotarty instability of the knee. Its pathogenesis and a clinical test to demonstrate its presence, J. Bone Joint Surg. **50-A:**211, 1968.

Slocum, D. B., Larson, R. L., and James, S. L.: Late reconstruction of the medial compartment of the knee, Clin. Orthop. **100:**23, 1974.

Smillie, I. S.: Observations on the regeneration of the semilunar cartilages in man, Br. J. Surg. **31:**398, 1944.

Smillie, I. S.: Treatment after-treatment and complications of injuries of menisci. In Smillie, I. S.: Injuries of the Knee Joint, ed. 2, Baltimore, 1951, The Williams & Wilkins Co.

Smillie, I. S.: Treatment of osteochondritis dissecans, J. Bone Joint Surg. **39-B:**248, 1957.

Smillie, I. S.: Osteochondritis dissecans: loose bodies in joints; etiology, pathology, treatment, 1960, The Williams & Wilkins Co. Baltimore.

Smillie, I. S.: Injuries of the knee joint, ed. 3, Baltimore, 1962, The Williams & Wilkins Co.

Smillie, I. S.: The current pattern of internal derangements of the knee joint relative to the menisci, Clin. Orthop. **51:**117, 1967.

Smith, B., and Blair, H.: Tibial collateral ligament strain due to occult derangement of medial meniscus confirmed by operation in 30 cases, J. Bone Joint Surg. **36-A:**88, 1954.

Sonstegard, D. A., Kaufer, H., and Matthews, L. S.: The spherocentric knee. Biomechanical testing and clinical trial, J. Bone Joint Surg. **59-A:**602, 1977.

Soto-Hall, R.: Traumatic degeneration of the articular cartilage of the patella, J. Bone Joint Surg. **27:**426, 1945.

Southwick, W. O., Becker, G. E., and Albright, J. A.: Dovetail patella tendon transfer for recurrent dislocating patella, J.A.M.A. **204:**665, 1968.

Speed, J. S.: Synovectomy of the knee joint, J.A.M.A. **83:**1814, 1924.

Speed, J. S., and Trout, P. C.: Arthroplasty of the knee. A follow-up study, J. Bone Joint Surg. **31-B:**53, 1949.

Stamp, W. G., and Lansche, W. E.: Treatment of discrepancy in leg length, South. Med. J. **53:**764, 1960.

Starr, D. E.: Repair of old ligamentous injuries of the knee; Clin. Orthop. **23:**162, 1962.

Stevens, J., and Whitefield, G. A.: Synovectomy of the knee in rheumatoid arthritis, Ann. Rheum. Dis. **25:**214, 1966.

Stewart, M.: Unusual athletic injuries, American Academy of Orthopaedic Surgeons Instructional Course Lectures, vol. 17, St. Louis, 1960, The C. V. Mosby Co., p. 377.

Stewart, M., and Bland, W. G.: Compression in arthrodesis. A comparative study of methods of fusion of the knee in ninety-three cases, J. Bone Joint Surg. **40-A:**585, 1958.

Stougård, J.: Patellectomy, Acta Orthop. Scand. **41:**110, 1970.

Straub, L. R., Thompson, T. C., and Wilson, P. D.: The results of epiphyseodesis and femoral shortening in relation to equalization of limb length, J. Bone Joint Surg. **27:**254, 1945.

Sutton, F. S., Jr., Thompson, C. H., Lipke, J., and Kettelkamp, D. B.: The effect of patellectomy on knee function, J. Bone Joint Surg. **58-A:**537, 1976.

Tapper, E. M., and Hoover, N. W.: Late results after meniscectomy, J. Bone Joint Surg. **51-A:**517, 1969.

Todd, T. W.: Atlas of skeletal maturation, St. Louis, 1937, The C. V. Mosby Co.

Torgerson, W. R.: Tibial osteotomy in the treatment of osetoarthritis of the knee, Surg. Clin. North Amer. **45:**779, 1965.

Trillat, A., De Jour, J., and Coutte, A.: Diagnosticet traitment des subluxations rescindivent es de la rotule, Rev. Chir. Orth. **50:**813, 1964.

Trueta, J.: The influence of the blood supply in controlling bone growth, Bull. Hosp. Joint Dis. **14:**147, 1953.

Van Gorder, G. W., and Chen, C. M.: The central graft operation for fusion of tuberculous knees, ankles, and elbows, J. Bone Joint Surg. **41-A:**1029, 1959.

Venable, C. S., Stuck, W. G., and Beach, A.: Effects of bone of presence of metals; based upon electrolysis; experimental study, Ann. Surg. **105:**917, 1937.

Warren, L. F., and Marshall, J. L.: The supporting structures and layers on the medial side of the knee. An anatomical analysis, J. Bone Joint Surg. **61-A:**56, 1979.

Watanabe, M.: Present state of arthroscopy, Int. Orthop. **2:**101, 1978.

Wentworth, E. T.: Gradual reduction of congenital anterior dislocated knees, J. Bone Joint Surg. **10:**585, 1928.

West, F. E.: Fractures of the patella, American Academy of Orthopaedic Surgeons Instructional Course Lectures, vol. 18, St. Louis, 1961, The C. V. Mosby Co., p. 84.

West, F. E.: End results of patellectomy, J. Bone Joint Surg. **44-A:**1089, 1962.

West, F. E., and Soto-Hall, R.: Recurrent dislocation of the patella in the adult. End results of patellectomy with quadricepsplasty, J. Bone Joint Surg. **40-A:**386, 1958.

Whipple, T. L., and Bassett, F. H.: Arthroscopic examination of the knee. Polypuncture technique with percutaneous intra-articular manipulation, J. Bone Joint Surg. **60-A:**444, 1978.

Wiberg, G.: Roentgenographic and anatomic studies on the femoropatellar joint. With special reference to chondromalacia patellae, Acta Orthop. Scand. **12:**319, 1941.

Wilde, A. H., Collins, H. R., Evarts, C. M., and Nelson, C. L., Jr.: Geometric knee replacement arthroplasty: indications for operation and preliminary experience. Orthop. Clin. North Am. **4:**547, 1973.

Wilde, A. H., Collins, H. R., Evarts, C. M., Nelson, C. L., Jr., DeHaven, K. E., and Bergfeld, J. A.: Current use of geometric knee-replacement arthroplasty, Orthop. Review **3:**25, 1974.

Wiles, P., Andrews, P. S., and Bremner, R. A.: Chondromalacia of the patella. A study of the later results of excision of the articular cartilage, J. Bone Joint Surg. **42-B:**65, 1960.

Wilkinson, J.: Fracture of patella treated by total excision, J. Bone Joint Surg. **59-B:**352, 1977.

Wilkinson, M. C., and Lowry, J. H.: Synovectomy for rheumatoid arthritis, J. Bone Joint Surg. **47-B:**482, 1965.

Willner, P.: Recurrent dislocation of the patella, Clin. Orthop. **69:**213, 1970.

Wilson, J. N.: A diagnostic sign in osteochondritis dissecans of the knee, J. Bone Joint Surg. **49-A:**477, 1967.

Wilson, P. D., Eyre-Brook, A. L., and Francis, J. D.: A clinical and anatomical study of the semimembranosus bursa in relation to popliteal cyst, J. Bone Joint Surg. **20:**963, 1938.

Wynn, P. C. B., Nichols, P. J. R., and Lewis, N. R.: Meniscectomy. A review of 1723 cases, Ann. Phys. Med. **4:**201, 1958.

Yamada, K., and Shinno, N.: Arthroplasty of the knee. A follow-up of fifty-four cases treated by operative reconstruction of the sliding apparatus in the stiffened knee, J. Bone Joint Surg. **51-A:**1480, 1969.

Young, H. H., and Regan, J. M.: Total excision of the patella for arthritis of the knee, Minn. Med. **28:**909, 1945.

Zuege, R. C., Kempken, T. G., and Blount, W. P.: Epiphysilateral stapling for angular deformity at the knee, J. Bone Joint Surg. **61-A:**320, 1979.

13

LOWER LEG

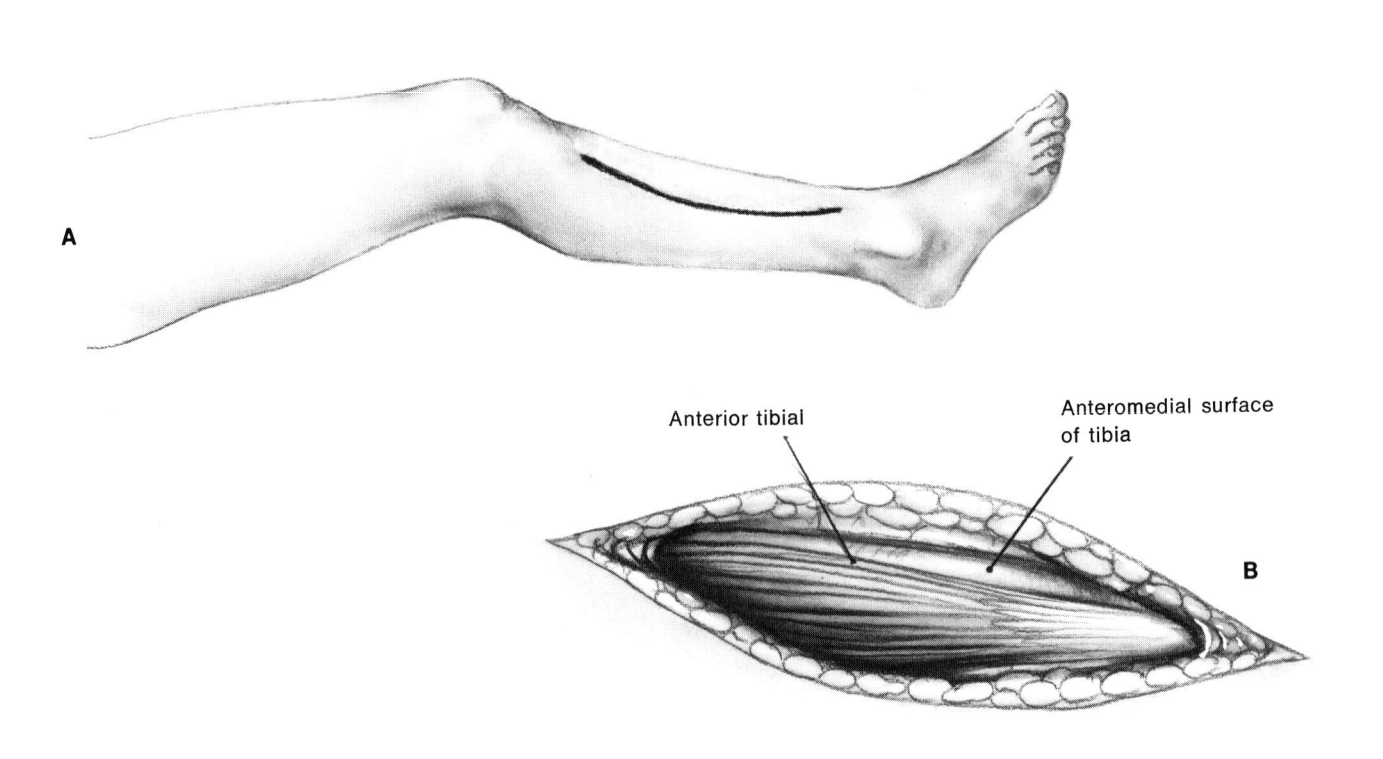

OPEN REDUCTION FOR TIBIAL SHAFT FRACTURE (ANTEROLATERAL APPROACH) (Plate 13-1)

GENERAL DISCUSSION. The anterolateral is one approach that may be used for exposure and internal fixation of a fracture of the shaft of the tibia. However, when internal fixation is required, exposure of the tibial shaft through a posterolateral approach is often a preferable alternative approach for internal fixation of tibial shaft fractures.

Plate fixation for short oblique or transverse fractures of the tibia, using either a compression plate or a standard Lane plate, can provide good stabilization of the fractured tibial shaft. If a standard Lane plate is used, its length should be at least five times the diameter of the bone. If the fracture of the tibia is a long oblique or spiral fracture and requires internal fixation, transfixion screws at 90° to the longitudinal axis of the bone may be sufficient for internal fixation of these fractures rather than internal fixation with a plate and transfixion screws.

If the open reduction of the tibia is being carried out for delayed union or nonunion of a tibial fracture, the shaft of the fibula should be osteotomized as part of the procedure.

DETAILS OF PROCEDURE. With the patient supine, a curvilinear incision is made over the anterior compartment of the lower leg and centered at the level of the fracture so the incision is convex laterally and the proximal and distal ends of the incision are located approximately 1 cm lateral to the anterior crest of the tibia **(A)**. While the skin incision is being made, care should be taken to avoid injury to the superficial branch of the peroneal nerve, which becomes subcutaneous in the lateral aspect of the lower leg just above its midportion. After supplying the peroneus longus and peroneus brevis muscles, this nerve is located in the subcutaneous tissue over the lower portion of the leg and anterior aspect of the ankle, providing the major sensory innervation to the skin on the anterolateral aspect of the lower leg and to the dorsum of the foot. The fascia of the anterior compartment is opened in line with the skin incision **(B)**, and the muscles of the anterior compartment are reflected laterally from the anterolateral surface of the tibia. This lateral reflection of the anterior compartment muscles for exposure of the shaft of the tibia can be accomplished easily inasmuch as the anterior tibial muscle, which takes partial origin from the upper one quarter of the anterolateral surface of the tibia and from along the interosseous border of the upper two thirds of the tibia, is only muscle that has a bony attachment to the anterolateral surface of the tibia.

(Plate 13-1) OPEN REDUCTION FOR TIBIAL SHAFT FRACTURE (ANTEROLATERAL APPROACH)

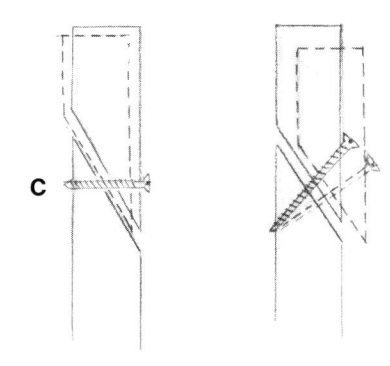

As the anterior compartment muscles are reflected laterally, the interosseous membrane may be visualized with its fibers directed obliquely distally from tibia to fibula. It should be remembered that the anterior tibial artery, with the deep branch of the peroneal nerve located to its lateral side, lies on the interosseous membrane after the extensor compartment is entered above the upper border of the interosseous membrane. These important structures course vertically downward on the interosseous membrane with companion veins and, at the lower end of the tibia, cross the ankle joint midway between the malleoli underneath the extensor retinaculum. Throughout its course the anterior tibial artery is located in the interval between the anterior tibial muscle and the extensor digitorum longus muscle.

The periosteum is incised along the anterolateral surface of the tibia, away from the anterior crest, and is preserved **(C)**. If one or more screws are sufficient for internal fixation, they should be inserted perpendicular to the shaft of the tibia (**D** and **E**) and not perpendicular to the fracture line.

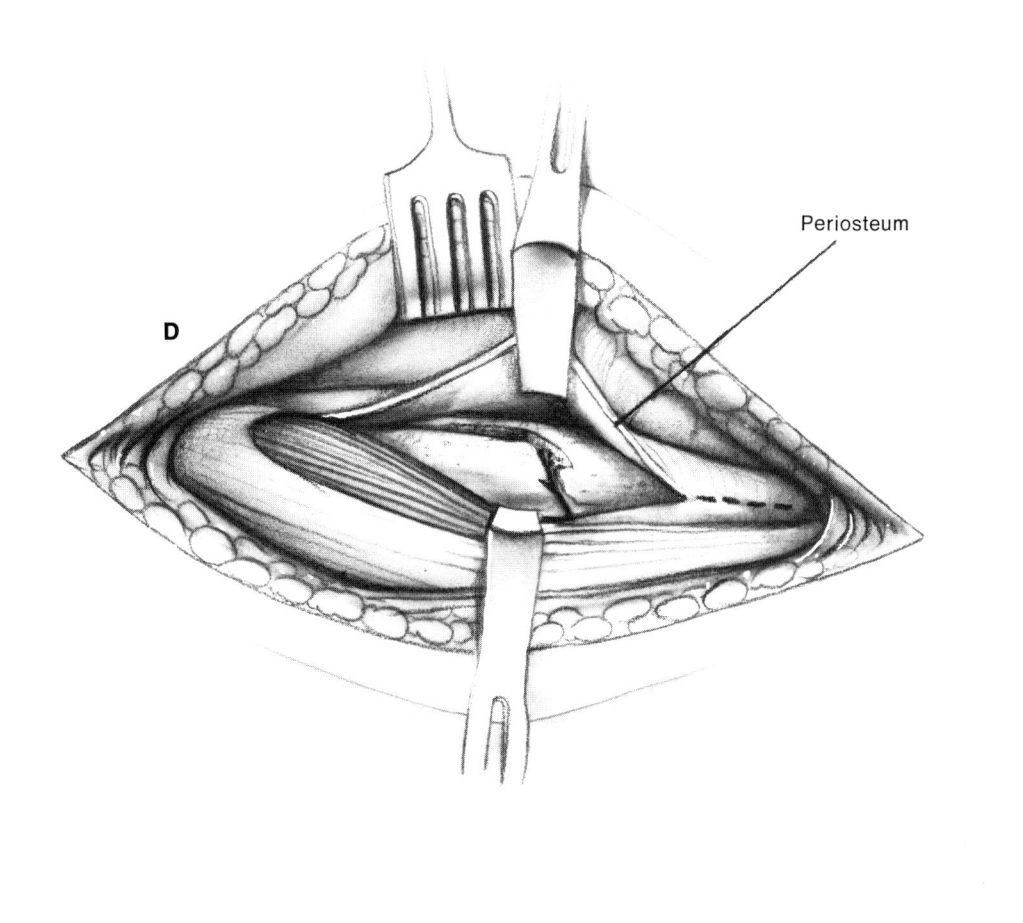

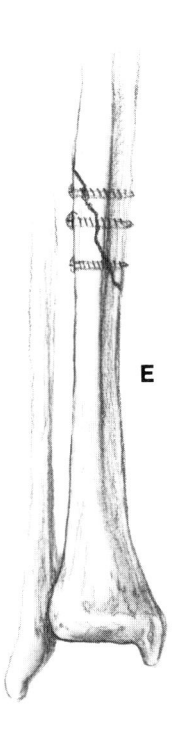

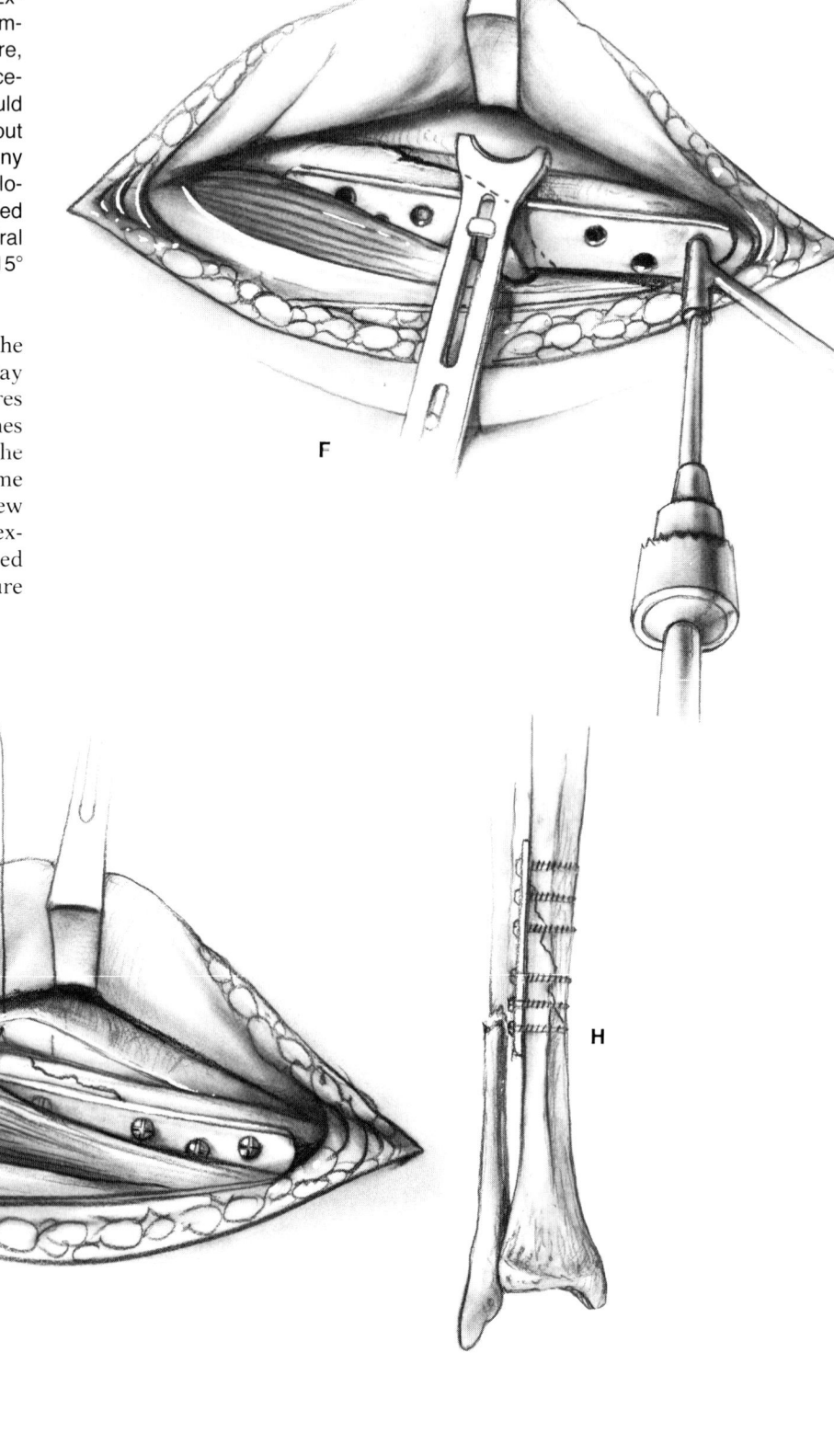

OPEN REDUCTION FOR TIBIAL SHAFT FRACTURE (ANTEROLATERAL APPROACH) (Plate 13-1)

Bone forceps may be required to obtain reduction of the fracture in terms of rotation, alignment, and apposition of the fracture fragments as a selected plate and screws are applied (**F** to **H**). If bone graft is to be added simultaneously with internal fixation, it must be judiciously applied across the fracture area. Excessive volume of bone graft in this tight compartment can jeopardize soft tissue closure, thereby, in turn, jeopardizing the entire procedure and ultimate outcome. The wound should be closed without undue tension and without resorting to a lateral relaxing incision or any other compromise with good soft tissue closure. Following wound closure, a well-padded long-leg cast is applied with the ankle in neutral position and the knee in approximately 15° flexion.

POSTOPERATIVE MANAGEMENT. The wound may be inspected after the first day through a window in the cast and sutures removed 2 weeks postoperatively. Crutches are used without weight bearing on the involved leg for 2 to 4 weeks, at which time the initial cast is replaced by a snug new long-leg cast with the knee in 0° to 5° flexion. Progressive weight bearing is permitted subsequently in this cast until fracture union is complete.

(Plate 13-2) OPEN REDUCTION FOR TIBIAL SHAFT FRACTURE (POSTEROLATERAL APPROACH)

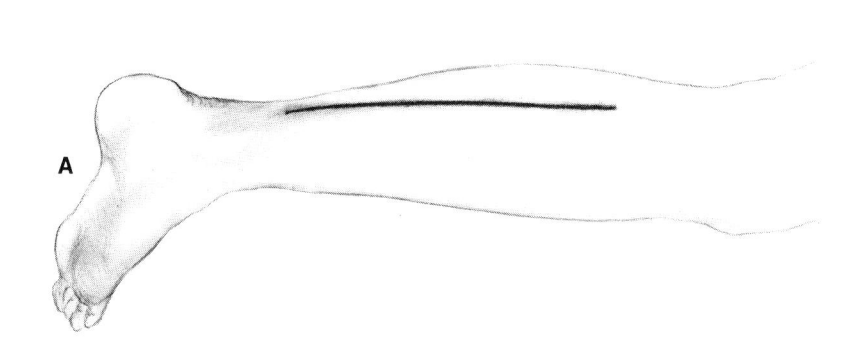

GENERAL DISCUSSION. The posterolateral approach to the tibia is especially applicable for tibial fractures requiring open reduction when there is compromised skin over the anterior aspect of the lower leg. Implantation of bone graft entails less danger of sequestration when introduced behind the interosseous membrane through this approach. For infected fractures of the bones of the lower leg needing open reduction but complicated by anterior drainage, an attempt should be made to place any bone graft posteriorly so contact is made between both the tibia and fibula; that is, under these circumstances, cross union of these bones is desirable.

This posterolateral approach is particularly valuable in the middle two thirds of the tibial shaft.

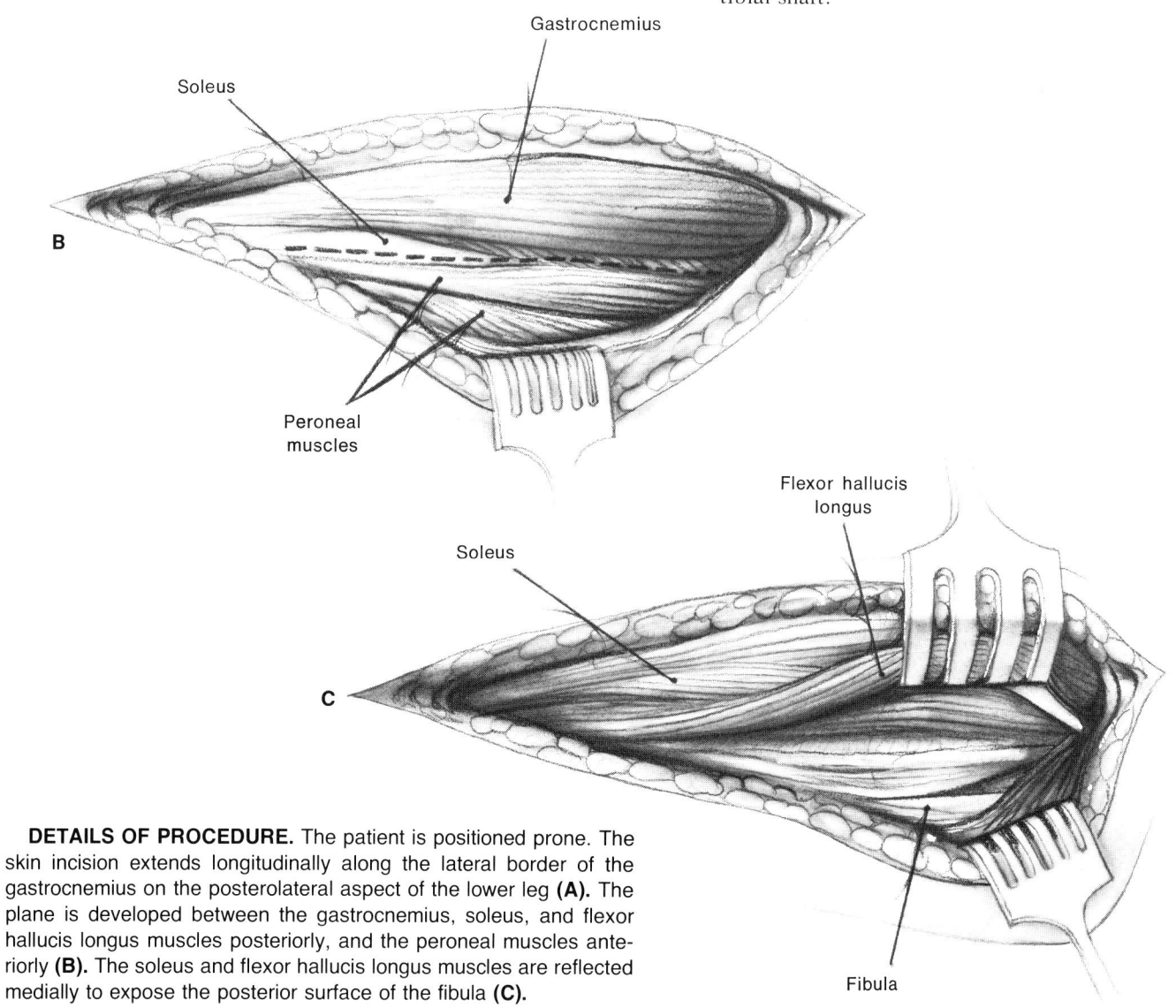

DETAILS OF PROCEDURE. The patient is positioned prone. The skin incision extends longitudinally along the lateral border of the gastrocnemius on the posterolateral aspect of the lower leg **(A)**. The plane is developed between the gastrocnemius, soleus, and flexor hallucis longus muscles posteriorly, and the peroneal muscles anteriorly **(B)**. The soleus and flexor hallucis longus muscles are reflected medially to expose the posterior surface of the fibula **(C)**.

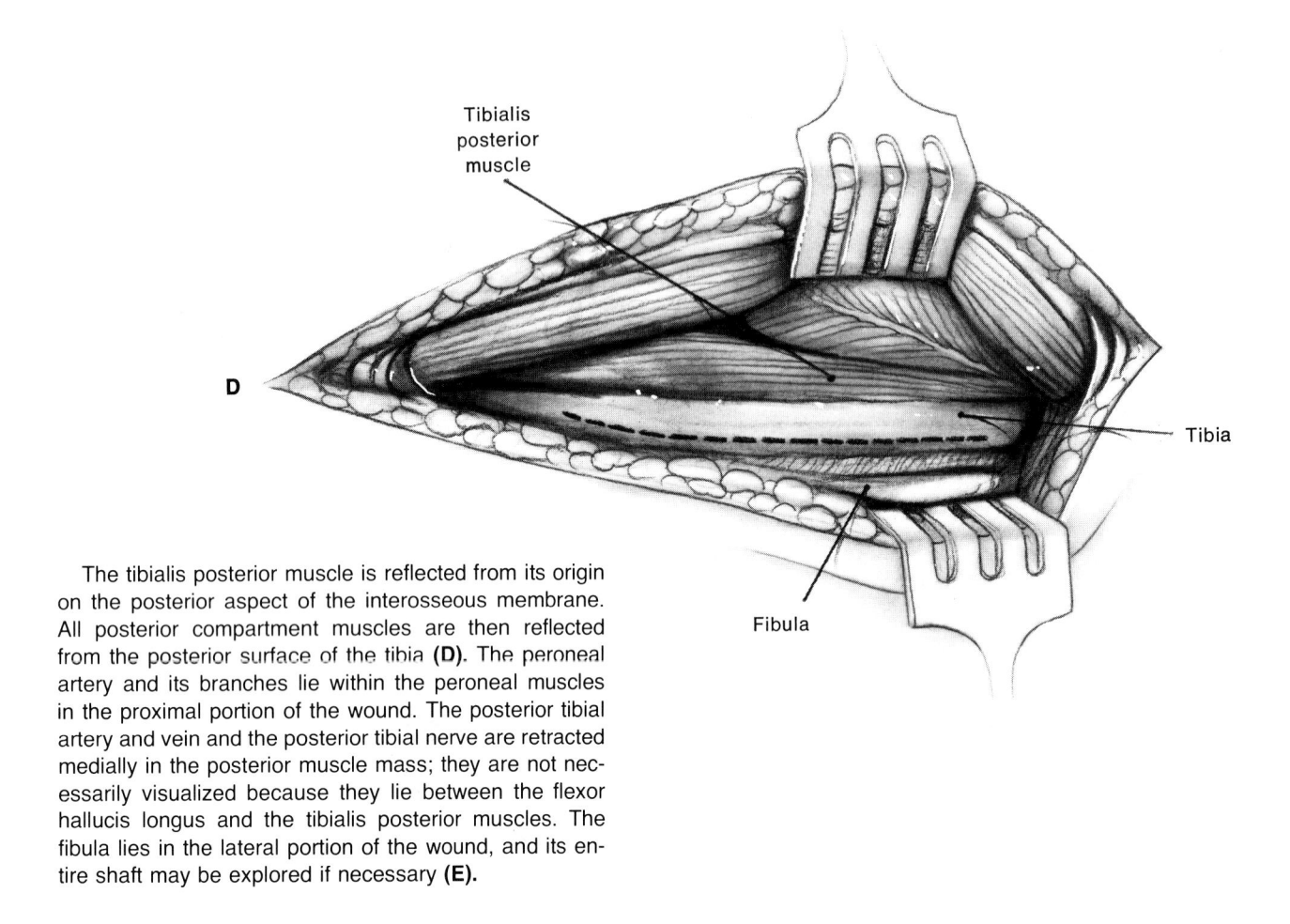

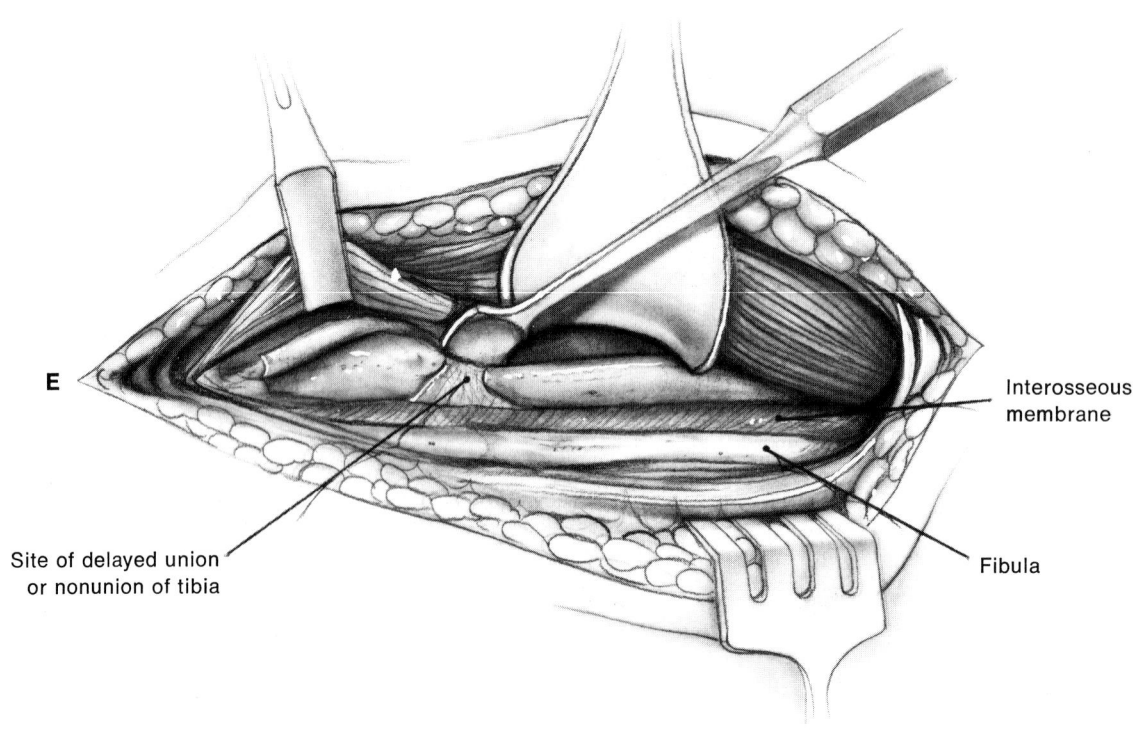

OPEN REDUCTION FOR TIBIAL SHAFT FRACTURE (POSTEROLATERAL APPROACH) (Plate 13-2)

The tibialis posterior muscle is reflected from its origin on the posterior aspect of the interosseous membrane. All posterior compartment muscles are then reflected from the posterior surface of the tibia **(D)**. The peroneal artery and its branches lie within the peroneal muscles in the proximal portion of the wound. The posterior tibial artery and vein and the posterior tibial nerve are retracted medially in the posterior muscle mass; they are not necessarily visualized because they lie between the flexor hallucis longus and the tibialis posterior muscles. The fibula lies in the lateral portion of the wound, and its entire shaft may be explored if necessary **(E)**.

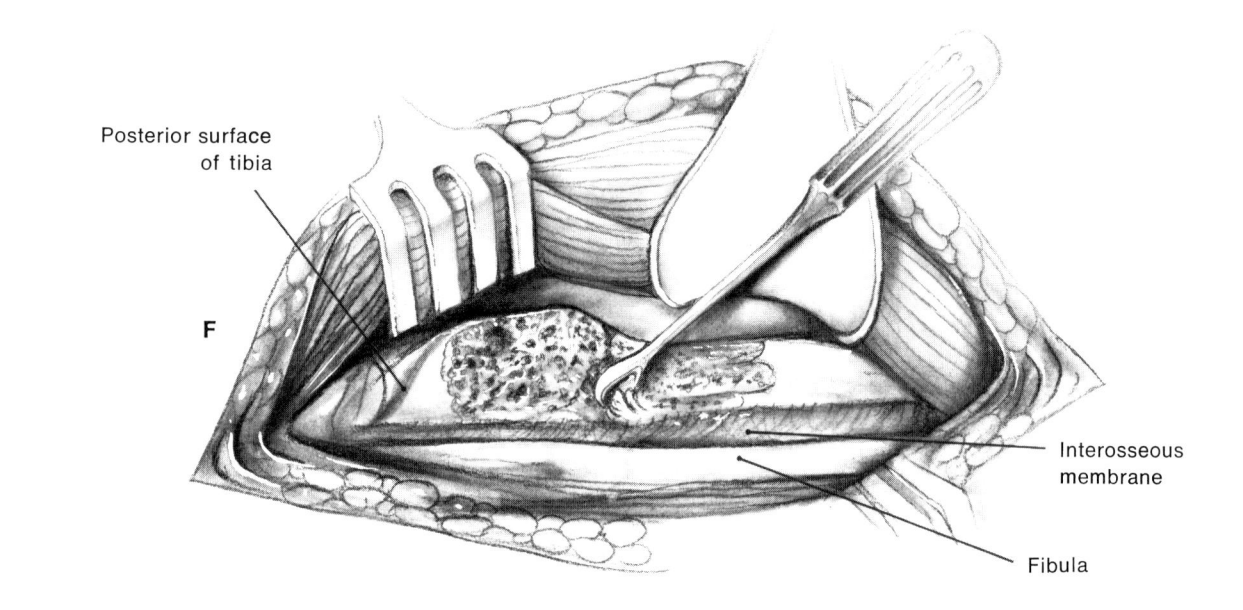

(Plate 13-2) OPEN REDUCTION FOR TIBIAL SHAFT FRACTURE (POSTEROLATERAL APPROACH)

The relatively flat posterior surface of the tibial shaft may be completely exposed through this approach, except for the proximal one fourth where the popliteus muscle has its origin and where the proximal portions of the posterior tibial vessels and the posterior tibial nerve are not protected within the reflected posterior compartment muscles. The site of a nonunion of the tibia can be prepared and supplemented with bone graft (**F** and **G**).

For the wound closure, the posterior compartment muscle mass is allowed to fall back into place. The deep fascia on the lateral side of the leg is closed with interrupted sutures. A long-leg cast is applied following completion of the wound closure.

POSTOPERATIVE MANAGEMENT. Management after surgery will depend on the individual circumstances and the specific procedure that is carried out through the posterolateral approach to the tibia.

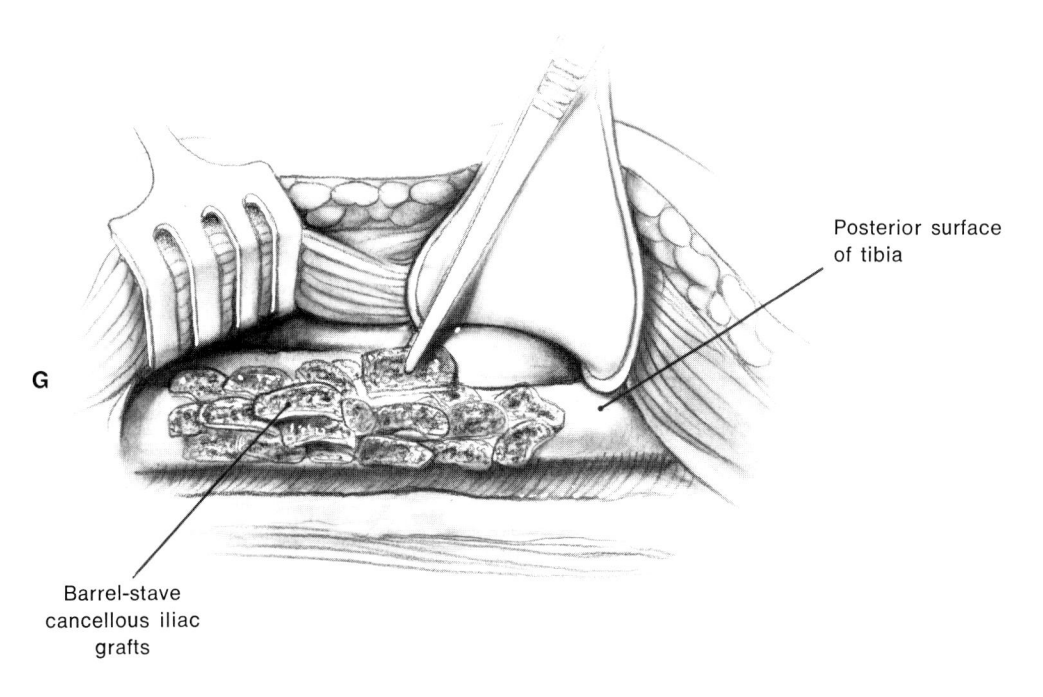

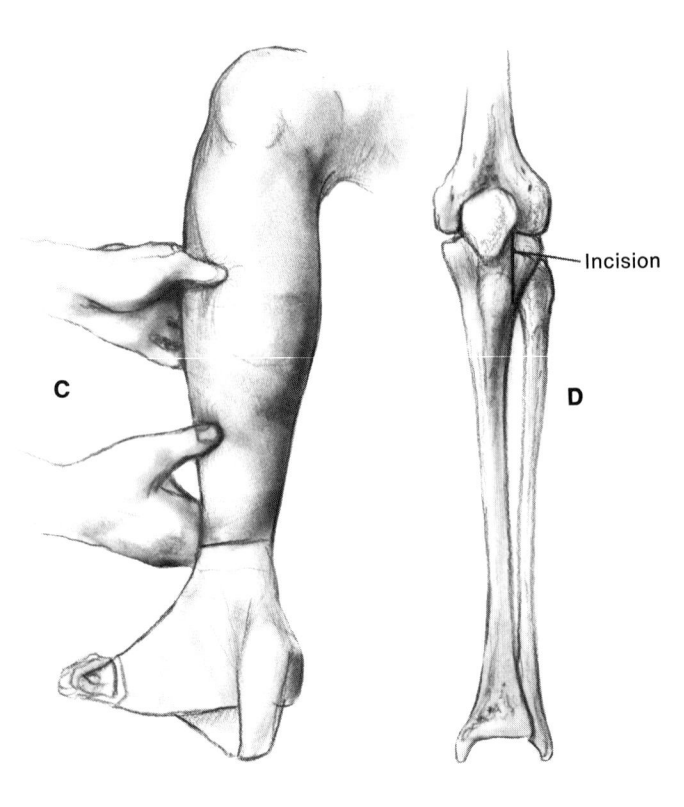

INTRAMEDULLARY NAILING FOR TIBIAL SHAFT FRACTURE (Plate 13-3)

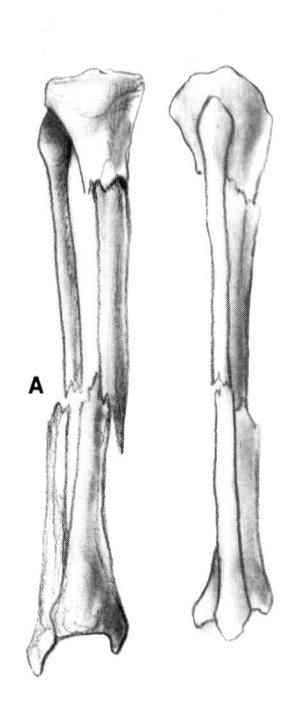

GENERAL DISCUSSION. Intramedullary fixation for fractures of the shaft of the tibia can be used for any fracture of the tibial shaft from the junction of the upper and middle thirds to within 8 cm of the ankle joint. This method of internal fixation is most effective in fractures of the middle third of the tibia. It can be particularly helpful in segmental fractures of the shaft of the tibia (**A**). There is no advantage for using this method in isolated fractures of the upper third or the distal end of the tibia.

Fixation of fractures of the tibia by intramedullary fixation is seldom firm enough to prevent rotational motion at the fracture site and, consequently, external immobilization must usually be supplemented. This eliminates one of the chief advantages of intramedullary fixation—that is, early mobilization of adjacent joints—but it can make early weight bearing possible.

When an intramedullary nail is inserted for internal fixation of a fracture of the tibia, the nail should be inserted, if possible, without exposing the fracture. This minimizes the likelihood of infection, and the periosteal blood supply is better preserved.

The Lottes nail can be inserted by entering the tibia in the region of the tibial tubercle as illustrated. Some surgeons prefer a straight Küntscher nail inserted in the region of the tibial spines. For determination of the length of the nail that should be used, a tape or ruler is used preoperatively to measure the distance from the medial malleolus to the tibial tuberosity on the unaffected leg.

Intramedullary nailing of the tibia by the Lottes technique requires only a small array of equipment, but it should not be attempted without a complete set of these intramedullary tibial nails of various lengths and the few special instruments. Later, postoperative removal of the nail can be a formidable procedure if the medullary canal of the tibia is small and if the intramedullary tibial nail is deeply embedded in the bone.

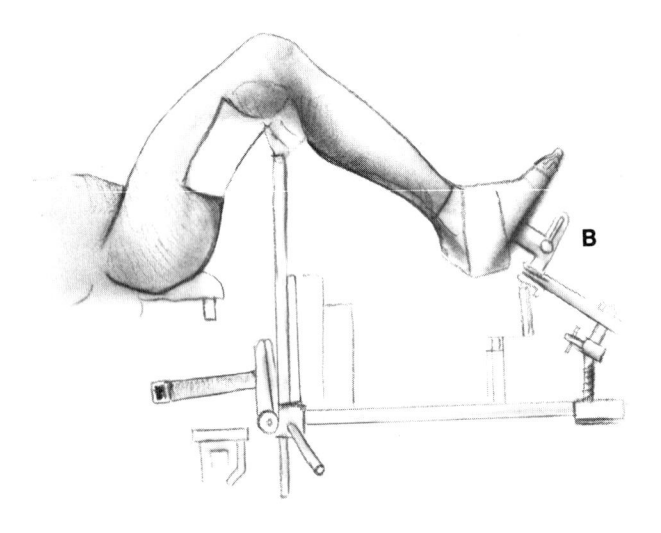

DETAILS OF PROCEDURE. Intramedullary nailing for tibial shaft fracture (or fractures) may be carried out with the patient suprine and with the patient's legs over the end of the operating table (or on a fracture table with the hip flexed at approximately 50° and the knee in a position of 90° flexion) (**B** and **C**). A longitudinal incision is made in a distal direction from the medial side of the patella to a point 1 cm medial to the most prominent portion of the tibial tubercle (**D**). The tibia is exposed by subperiosteal dissection in the distal portion of the wound with care to avoid entering the knee joint.

(Plate 13-3) INTRAMEDULLARY NAILING FOR TIBIAL SHAFT FRACTURE

A ⅜-inch drill is used to make a hole through the proximal tibial cortex on the medial side of the tibial tubercle. The drill is first directed transversely and then in a distal direction **(E)**. A retractor or shield should be used to protect the soft tissues proximally. When a longitudinal drill hole has been prepared in this area of the proximal tibia, the driver is attached to the Lottes nail (of predetermined length). The Lottes nail is placed into the drill hole in the proximal tibia so the single fin on the concave surface of the nail is directed anteriorly **(F)**. Again with the soft tissues protected proximally, the proximal portion of the nail is held in a manner to keep the nail parallel with the longitudinal axis of the tibia, and the nail is driven into the tibia to the level of the fracture. The two posterior fins on the convex surface of the nail should rest against the posterior cortex of the tibia. When the nail has been driven to the level of the fracture, the fracture reduction (in terms of displacement, alignment, and rotation) is checked clinically, and the nail is then driven several centimeters across the fracture site **(G)**. At this time, the stability of the fracture must be checked. If the fracture is still unstable, the nail has probably not entered the distal segment of the tibia and should be withdrawn and reinserted.

Prior to final seating of the nail, reduction of the fracture should be checked roentgenographically in two planes to be certain that the placement of the Lottes nail and position of the fracture are satisfactory. When the Lottes nail is in its final position, a portion of the threaded proximal end of the nail will protrude slightly in the area of the tibial tubercle for subsequent extraction if necessary **(H)**. Following wound closure, a well-padded long-leg cast is applied.

POSTOPERATIVE MANAGEMENT. Two weeks postoperatively the sutures are removed, the fracture is checked roentgenographically, and a new long-leg cast is applied with the knee in 5° to 10° flexion. If there is need to alter rotation at the fracture site, this can be done to a limited degree during application of the new cast at this time. With maximum stability and contact of the tibial fracture fragments, full weight bearing can be permitted as tolerated. If the tibial fracture is comminuted, weight bearing may need to be delayed until there is roentgenographic evidence of early bridging callus. The intramedullary tibial nail should not be removed until the tibial fracture line is obliterated with roentgenographic evidence of solid union.

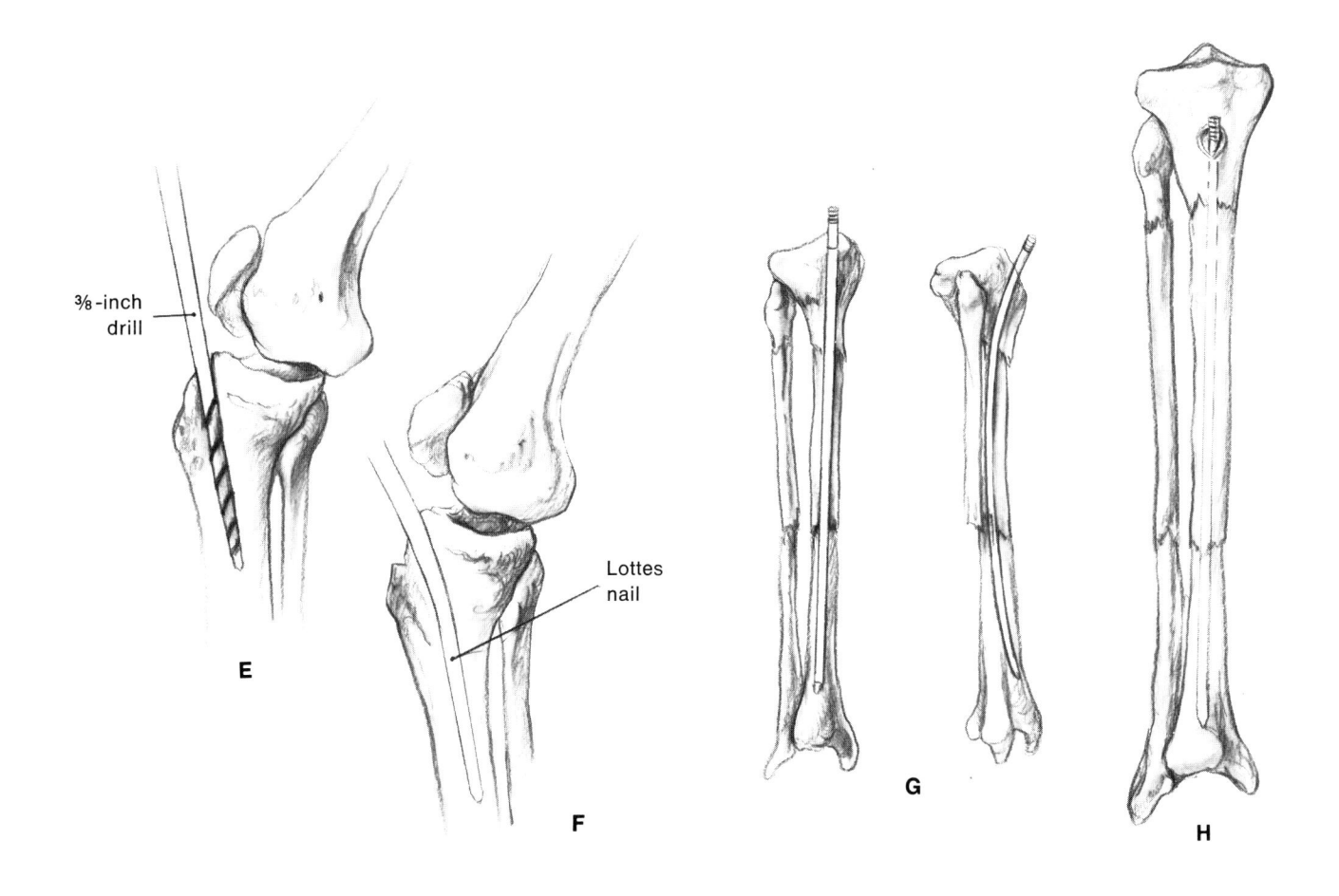

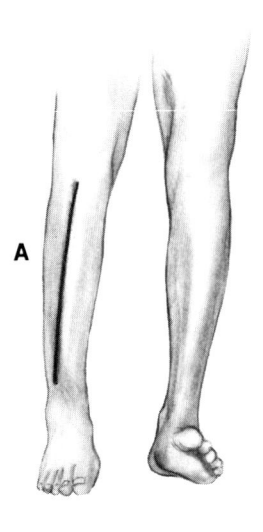

FASCIOTOMY OF ANTERIOR TIBIAL COMPARTMENT (Plate 13-4)

GENERAL DISCUSSION. The anterior tibial compartment is an inelastic compartment formed by the tibia, fibula, interosseous membrane, and the anterior crural fascia. Increased pressure, by edema or hematoma within this compartment, can cause tissue ischemia by arterial compression. Prodromal symptoms include pain over the anterior aspect of the lower leg or severe pain when active dorsiflexion of the foot is attempted. Erythema and edema will follow. In the chronic stage of this syndrome, without treatment there will be paralysis of the extensor hallucis longus and usually the anterior tibial as well. The peroneal nerve is almost always damaged. Finally, the anterior compartment muscles become fibrotic with a "silent" electromyogram (EMG), and the foot becomes fixed at a right angle.

The anterior tibial compartment syndrome may be encountered in patients who have primary vascular disease in a lower extremity, in younger patients who have overused the lower leg muscles, in patients who have had trauma to the lower leg, or in patients who have had surgery of the lower leg.

In the acute anterior tibial compartment syndrome there will be marked tenderness to palpation over the anterior compartment muscles. Erythema, swelling, increased local temperature, and a glossy appearance of the skin over the anterior compartment will be present. The dorsalis pedis pulse may or may not be absent, but its presence does not preclude an anterior tibial compartment syndrome. The occurrence of weakness or paralysis of the muscles of the anterior compartment along with these other clinical findings confirms the diagnosis. The motor paralysis may occur with startling rapidity usually involving the extensor hallucis longus or anterior tibial muscle initially. Because of the severity of pain in the leg, the patient may not want to contract his peroneal or posterior compartment muscles, and these muscles may appear to be weak or paralyzed. Sensation is often lost between the great toe and the second toe in the area innervated by the deep branch of the peroneal nerve.

With the onset of tissue ischemia, a low-grade fever may be present and the white blood cell count is frequently elevated. However, the diagnosis should be made on the basis of the history and the physcial examination without delay or need for supplemental laboratory tests. Time must not be wasted in accumulating laboratory data if the patient is to recover function.

The differential diagnosis may include cellulitis, osteomyelitis, stress fracture of the tibia, thrombophlebitis, intermittent claudication, and an ill-defined condition common to athletes called "shin splints." A history of strenuous physical activity is associated with stress fracture and shin splints, but the tenderness of stress fracture is limited to the fracture site (the proximal tibial shaft) and the immediately surrounding area. With shin splints, muscle paralysis is not present and there is no inflammatory reaction. Cellulitis and, to a lesser degree, thrombophlebitis may be confused with the advanced stage of an acute anterior tibial compartment syndrome. However, the critical finding in anterior tibial compartment syndrome is weakness or paralysis of the anterior compartment muscles. This does not occur in other conditions to be considered in differential diagnosis.

Once the diagnosis of an acute anterior tibial compartment syndrome is made, mandatory treatment is emergency fasciotomy of the anterior compartment of the lower leg. It is not known after what exact duration of time the regenerative ability of the muscle is irreversibly damaged, but it may be approximately 6 hours. If the ischemia lasts longer than 12 hours, extensive necrosis occurs in muscle fibers. Therefore the relief of the anterior compartment pressure by dividing the tibial fascia longitudinally is an urgent matter. This treatment is of little or no benefit after 3 days.

DETAILS OF PROCEDURE. A single longitudinal incision **(A)** or several short longitudinal incisions are made over the anterior compartment of the lower leg **(B)**. The crural fascia covering the anterior compartment muscles of the lower leg should be opened from just below the level of the tibial tubercle to just above the level of the superior extensor retinaculum of the ankle **(C)**. The skin incision does not need to be as long as the longitudinal opening in the fascia. However, the skin incision must be long enough to allow the complete fasciotomy to be carried out with either scissors or a fasciatome at each end of the skin incision, and the skin incision must be sufficiently long to release potential constricting or compressing force of the skin itself over the anterior compartment muscles. The procedure should be done without tourniquet.

In the acute anterior tibial comparement syndrome, muscle will bulge through the surgically created defect as the fascia is opened. When the operation is carried out early, the muscle may be observed to be pinkish white immediately on opening of the fascia, and the color of the muscle may

(Plate 13-4) FASCIOTOMY OF ANTERIOR TIBIAL COMPARTMENT

gradually become deep red after fasciotomy. In later operations the muscle may appear grayish white and may not respond to either mechanical or electrical stimuli. Only the subcutaneous tissue and skin are closed, and the skin must not be closed under tension **(D)**. If necessary, a split skin graft is used to complete the wound closure without tension. A posterior plaster splint, holding the ankle in neutral position, is applied following wound closure and the patient is placed in bed with the leg elevated slightly to aid the venous and lymphatic return from the limb.

POSTOPERATIVE MANAGEMENT. Application of ice packs to the lower leg, following surgery, decreases the need of the involved muscles for oxygen. Heat is contraindicated. After the second or third postoperative day, subsequent treatment depends on the extent of functional return of the anterior compartment muscles. The prognosis for muscle recovery will be related to the time interval between the onset of acute symptoms and the surgical fasciotomy. Any muscles that at operation were observed to be white and unresponsive to external mechanical or electrical stimulation will probably not demonstrate functional recovery postoperatively. Any functional muscle recovery that has not returned within 3 weeks following fasciotomy for an acute anterior tibial compartment syndrome is not likely to occur subsequently.

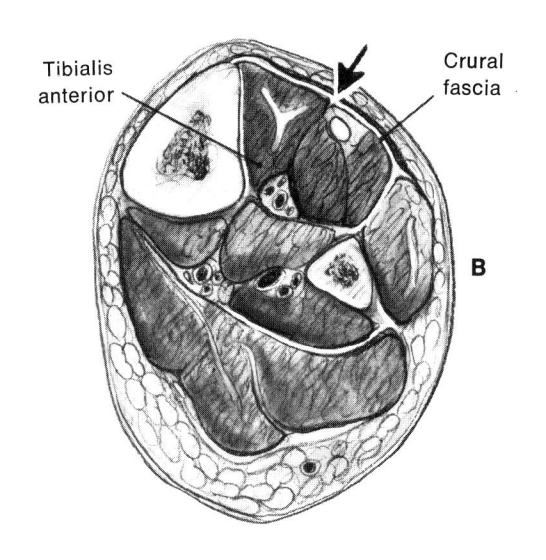

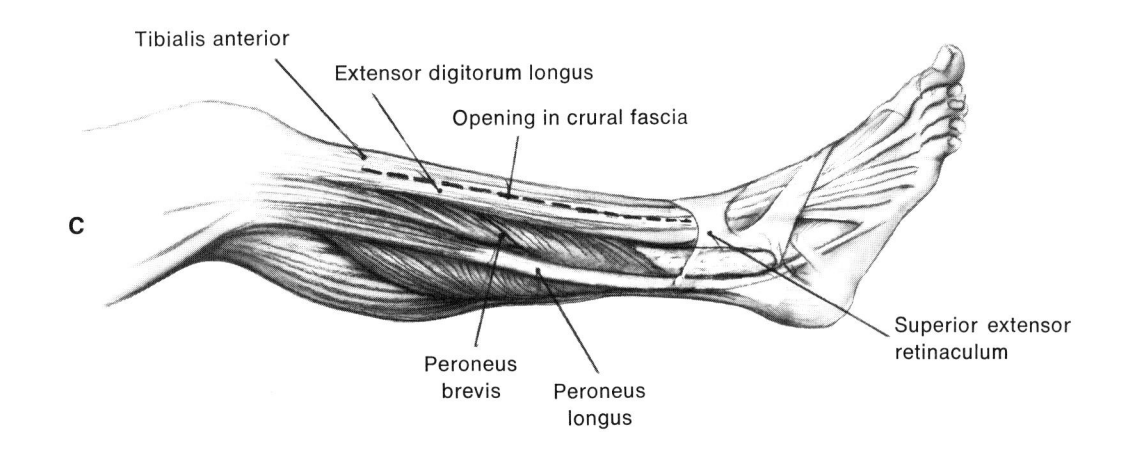

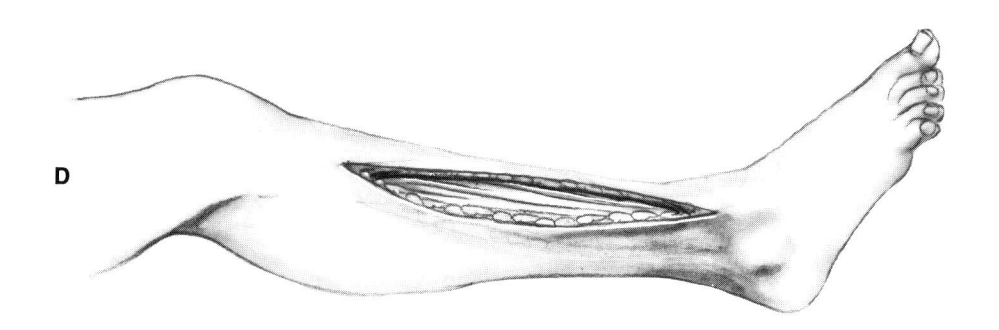

503

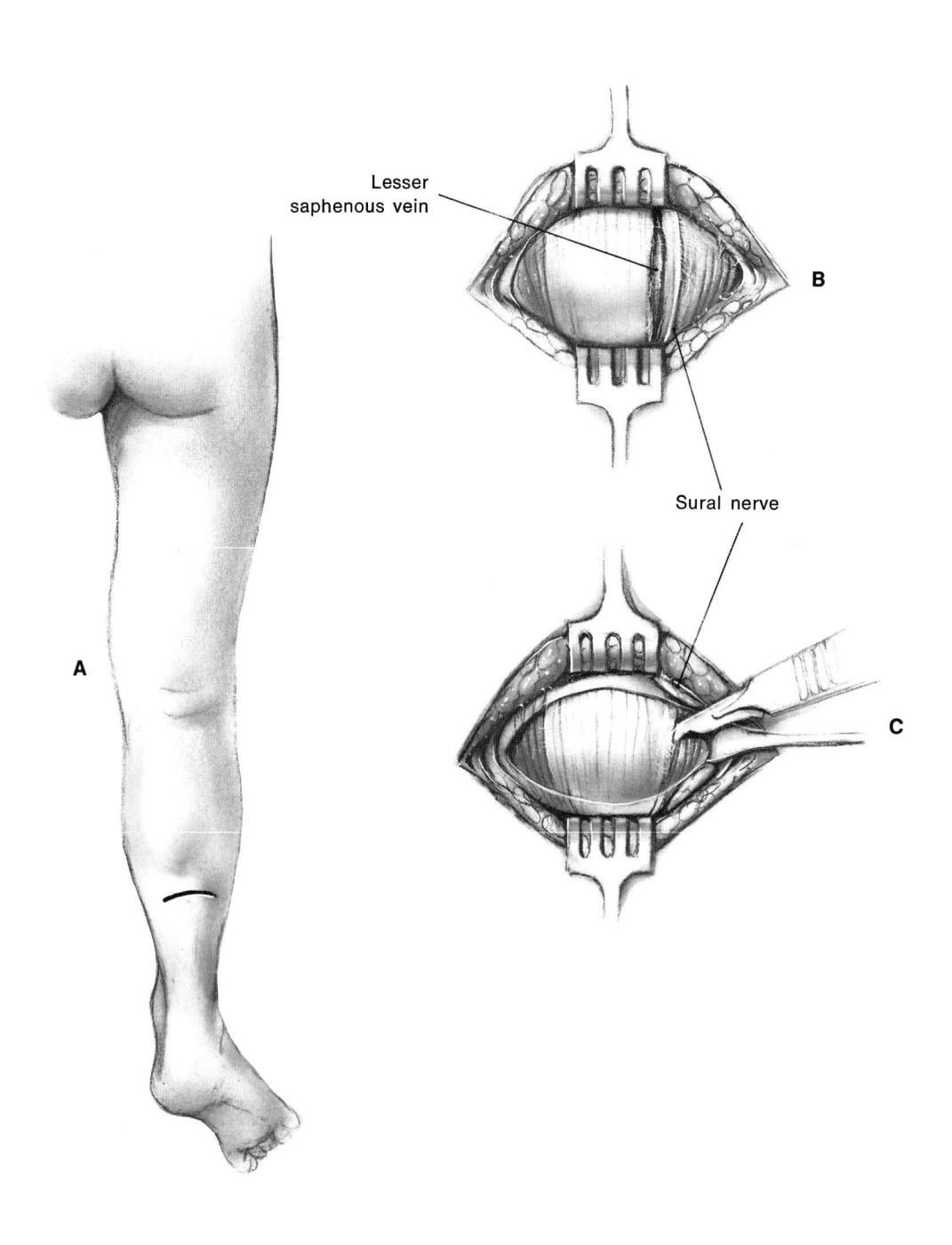

RECESSION OF GASTROCNEMIUS (STRAYER) (Plate 13-5)

GENERAL DISCUSSION. For the child with a spastic equinus deformity, recession of the gastrocnemius is a useful alternative to tendo Achillis lengthening, particularly if the equinus is found to be less pronounced when the knee is flexed to 90° as compared with full extension of the knee. Continuity of the tendo Achillis is maintained. The postoperative gait improvement is probably related at least partially to a diminution of the stretch reflex by way of the gastrocnemius, which in turn relieves heel cord tension in these patients.

DETAILS OF PROCEDURE. With the patient prone, the operation is carried out through a transverse incision **(A)**. The proper level of the incision is determined by visualizing and by palpating the level where the muscle belly of the gastrocnemius changes to tendon at approximately the middle of the calf. The fascia is divided transversely with care to protect the sural nerve and the lesser saphenous vein, which are retracted (**B** and **C**).

(Plate 13-5) RECESSION OF GASTROCNEMIUS (STRAYER)

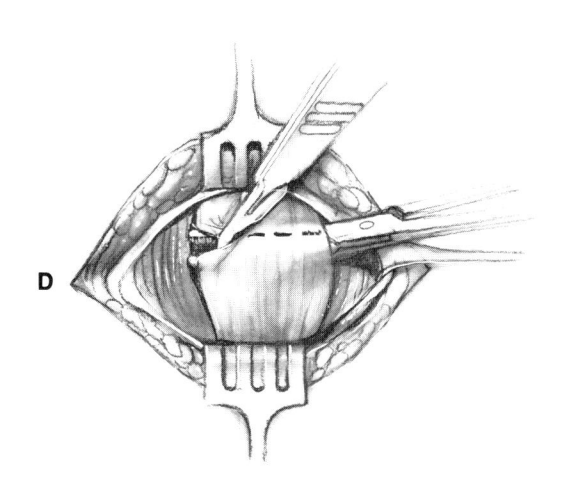

The aponeurosis of the gastrocnemius is mobilized at the musculotendinous junction from the underlying soleus, and a clamp is placed transversely between the two muscles where the gastrocnemius joins the common tendon. Care must be taken to avoid the superficial peroneal nerve on the lateral aspect of these muscles. With the sural nerve and lesser saphenous vein safely retracted, the gastrocnemius aponeurosis is divided transversely **(D)**. The plantaris tendon, which is found medially at this level, is also divided. The proximal portion of the divided gastrocnemius is mobilized by dividing any remaining fibrous attachments at its edge or to the underlying soleus. The ankle is then dorsiflexed **(E)**, and this should allow at least 2.5 cm of separation where the gastrocnemius aponeurosis has been divided. The proximal portion of the gastrocnemius aponeurosis is sutured in this separated position to the underlying soleus **(F)**.

Only subcutaneous tissue and skin are closed. A long-leg cast is applied with the knee in slight flexion and the ankle in 5° to 10° dorsiflexion.

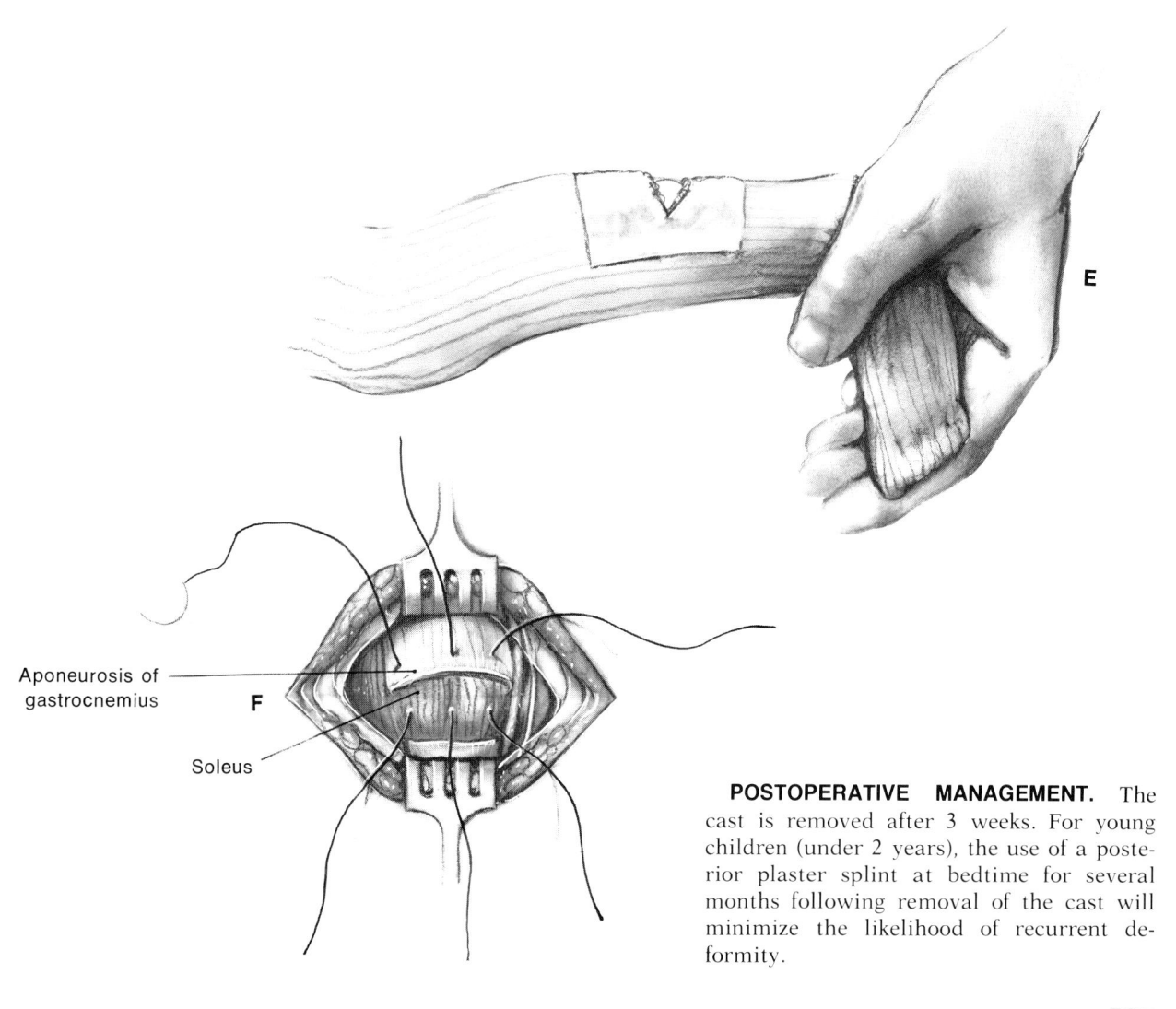

POSTOPERATIVE MANAGEMENT. The cast is removed after 3 weeks. For young children (under 2 years), the use of a posterior plaster splint at bedtime for several months following removal of the cast will minimize the likelihood of recurrent deformity.

BELOW-KNEE AMPUTATION (Plate 13-6)

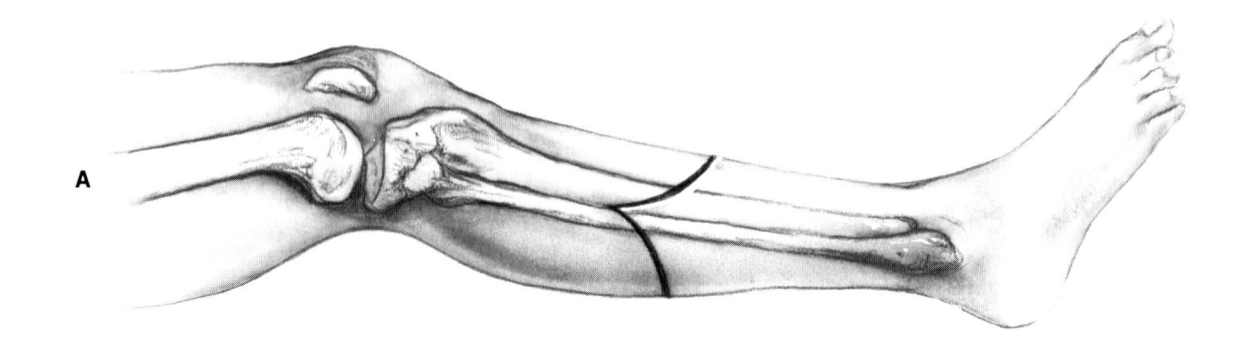

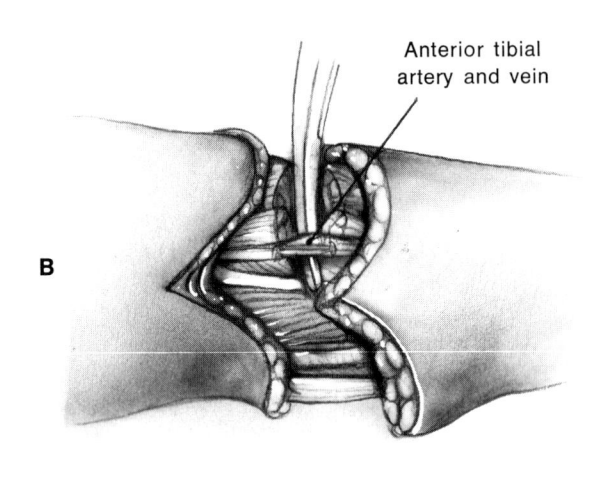

GENERAL DISCUSSION. The most common indication for below-knee amputation is serious circulatory impairment in the distal portion of the lower extremity. Below-knee amputation may occasionally be indicated for congenital, traumatic, infectious, or neoplastic conditions involving the distal portion of the lower extremity when assessment of all factors indicates that the patient will be able to manage better without the distal portion of the leg. For a person of average height, amputation at a level 15 to 16 cm below the medial tibial plateau permits good prosthetic accommodation.

DETAILS OF PROCEDURE. The procedure is carried out with the patient supine. The use of a tourniquet is avoided if the amputation is being done for peripheral vascular disease. The anterior and posterior skin flaps are carefully mapped out with the anterior flap slightly longer **(A)**. This will allow the closed wound to be slightly posterior to the divided tibia. In outlining the anterior and posterior skin flaps, the proximal end of the skin incision on the medial and lateral aspects of the leg should end at the level planned for division of the tibia. After the incision has been completed for both flaps, extending down through subcutaneous tissue and fascia, the anterior and posterior flaps are reflected proximally.

The anterior compartment muscles are divided first, and this is done at a level 1 to 2 cm distal to the level planned for transection of the tibia in order to allow for retraction of these muscles. As these anterior compartment muscles are divided, the superficial peroneal nerve is identified between the extensor hallucis longus and the tibialis anterior muscle, sharply transected, and allowed to retract. The anterior tibial artery and vein will be located in close proximity adjacent to the interosseous membrane, and these are doubly ligated proximally and divided **(B)**. The posterior tibial neurovascular bundle is isolated at this time from the medial side of the leg (between the soleus muscle and the flexor digitorum longus) and divided in the same manner.

The level for bone transection is again identified. Prior to transverse division of the bone, a bevel is created in the anterior crest of the tibia by placing the saw 2 cm proximal to the planned level of bone transection, and a 45° oblique cut is made in the anterior crest of the tibia extending to the ultimate transection level. The tibia and fibula are divided transversely at the same level at this time **(C)**. The posterior muscles are divided with a large amputation knife beginning 1 to 2 cm distal to the level of bone transection.

(Plate 13-6) BELOW-KNEE AMPUTATION

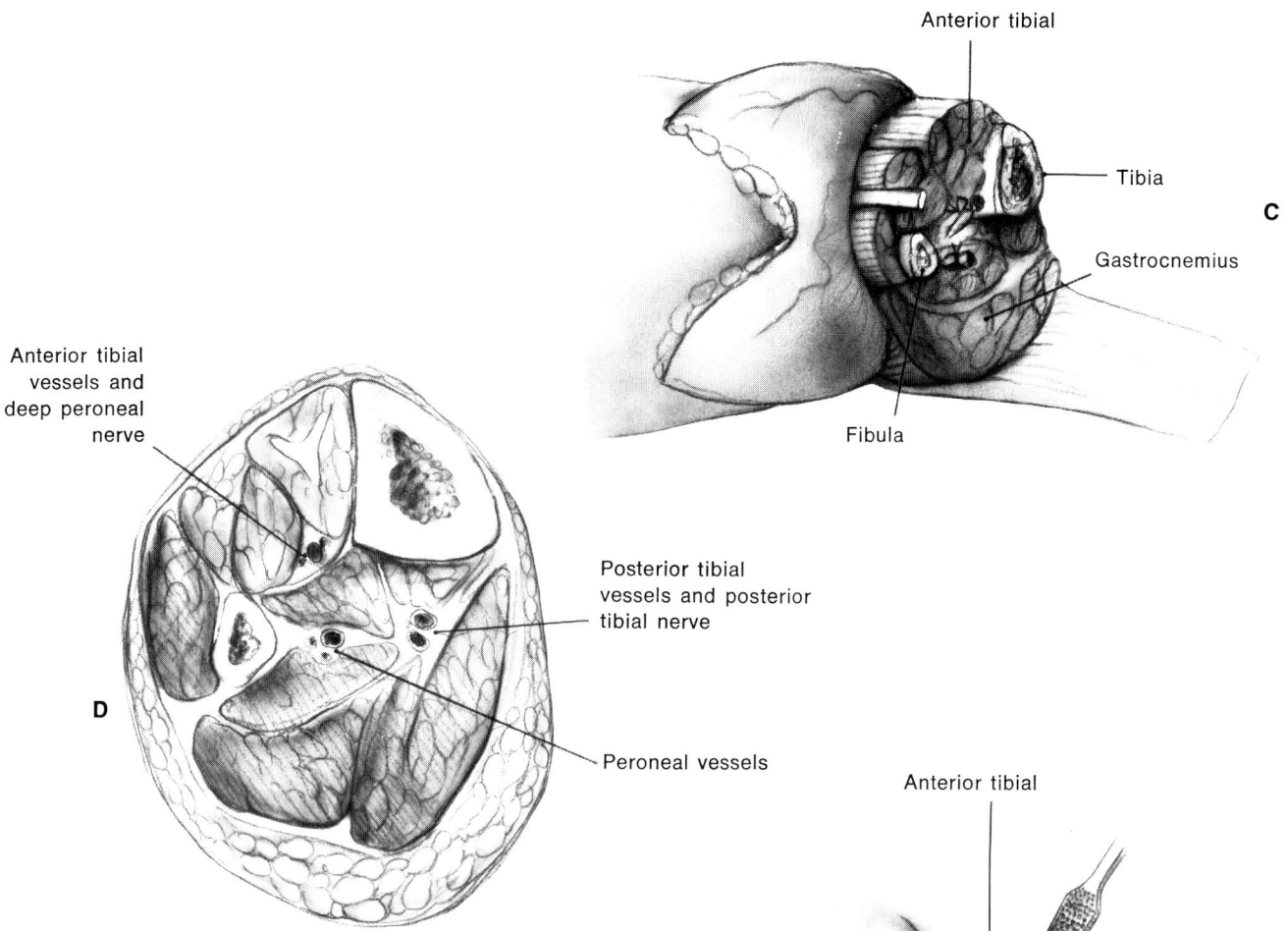

The peroneal vessels will be encountered just medial to the fibula between the tibialis posterior and flexor hallucis longus muscles (D) and should be ligated. The divided end of the fibula is now exposed subperiosteally and divided with bone cutters or a Gigli saw at a level 3 cm proximal to the distal end of the transected tibia (E).

The fascia, subcutaneous tissue, and skin are closed successively with interrupted sutures with care to avoid any triangular "dog ears" at the edges of the wound. A Penrose drain is left under the fascia (F).

A thin elastic compression bandage is applied to the stump, which is then placed in a posterior molded plaster splint with the knee joint in full extension unless immediate prosthetic fitting in the operating room has been planned.

POSTOPERATIVE MANAGEMENT. The Penrose drain is removed on the first postoperative day. The posterior plaster splint is removed 3 to 5 days postoperatively. The patient should be encouraged to do active knee exercises. Sutures are removed 2 weeks postoperatively. Elastic bandaging of the stump is continued until all postoperative edema has subsided or until the initial prosthesis is available.

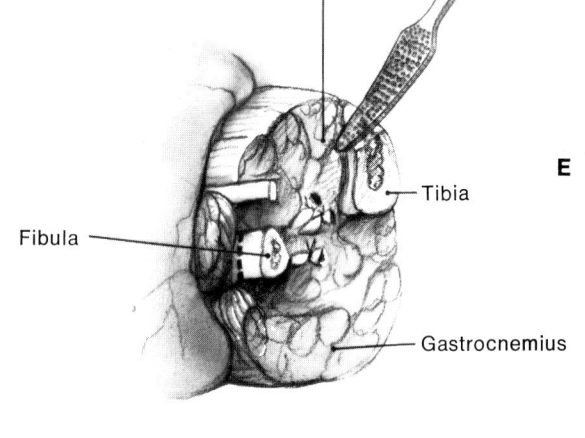

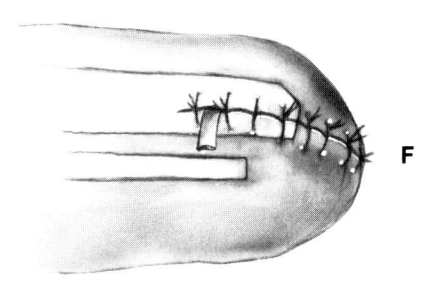

507

REFERENCES

Aitken, G. T.: Surgical amputation in children, J. Bone Joint Surg. **46-A:**1735, 1963.

Allgower, M., and Krupp, S.: External fixation as adjunct to use of flaps to the lower extremity, Chir. Plast. **3:**271, 1976.

Alms, M.: Medullary nailing for fracture of the shaft of the tibia, J. Bone Joint Surg. **44-B:**328, 1962.

Arzimanoglou, A., and Skiadaressis, G.: Study of internal fixation by screws of oblique fractures in long bones, J. Bone Joint Surg. **34-A:**219, 1952.

d'Aubigne, R. M.: Surgical treatment of non-union of long bones, J. Bone Joint Surg. **31-A:**256, 1949.

Blandy, J. P., and Fuller, R.: March gangrene. Ischaemic myositis of the leg muscles from exercise, J. Bone Joint Surg. **39-B:**679, 1957.

Bleck, E. E., Canty, T. J., and Doolittle, R. C.: Below-the-knee, closed-end, soft socket, J. Bone Joint Surg. **45-A:**967, 1963.

Blount, W. P.: Unequal leg length, American Academy of Orthopaedic Surgeons Instructional Course Lectures, vol. 17, St. Louis, 1960, The C. V. Mosby Co., p. 218.

Boyd, H. B., and Lipinski, S. W.: Causes and treatment of non-union of the shafts of the long bones with a review of 741 patients, American Academy of Orthopaedic Surgeons Instructional Course Lectures, vol. 17, St. Louis, 1960, The C. V. Mosby Co., p. 165.

Boyd, H. B., Lipinski, S. W., and Wiley, J. H.: Observations on non-union of the shafts of the long bones: with a statistical analysis of 842 patients, J. Bone Joint Surg. **43-A:**159, 1961.

Brantigan, O., and Voshell, A. F.: The tibial collateral ligament: its function, its bursae, and its relation to the medial meniscus, J. Bone Joint Surg. **25:**121, 1943.

Burgess, E. M.: Sites of amputation election according to modern practice, Clin. Orthop. **37:**17, 1964.

Burgess, E. M., and Marsden, F. W.: Major lower extremity amputations following arterial reconstruction, Arch. Surg. **108:**665, 1974.

Burgess, E. M., and Romano, R. L.: The management of lower extremity amputees using immediate postsurgical prostheses, Clin. Orthop. **57:**137, 1968.

Burgess, E. M., Romano, R. L., and Traub, J. E.: Immediate post-surgical prosthetic fitting. Prosthetic research study report, Bull. Prosthet. Res. **10-4:**42, 1965.

Burgess, E. M., Romano, R. L., and Zettl, J. H.: The management of lower extremity amputations, TR 10-6, Washington, D.C., 1969, Veterans Administration.

Burgess, E. M., Romano, R. L., Zettl, J. H., and Schrock, R. D., Jr.: Amputations of the leg for peripheral vascular insufficiency, J. Bone Joint Surg. **53-A:**874, 1971.

Burgess, E. M., Traub, J. E., and Wilson, A. B.: Immediate postsurgical prosthesis in the management of lower extremity amputees, TR 10-5, Washington, D.C., 1967, Veterans Administration.

Burkhalter, W. E., and Protzman, R.: Tibial shaft fractures, J. Trauma **15:**785, 1975.

Burwell, H. N.: Plate fixation of tibial shaft fractures, J. Bone Joint Surg. **53-B:**258, 1971.

Campbell, R. E., and Van Wagoner, F. H.: Ischemic necrosis of the anterior tibial compartment musculature, Arch. Surg. **71:**662, 1955.

Carpenter, E. B.: Management of fractures of the shaft of the tibia and fibula, J. Bone Joint Surg. **48-A:**1640, 1966.

Carpenter, E. B., Doobie, J. J., and Siewers, C. F.: Fractures of the shaft of the tibia and fibula. Comparative end results from various types of treatment in a teaching hospital, Arch. Surg. **64:**443, 1952.

Carter, A. B., Richards, R. L., and Zachary, R. B.: The anterior tibial syndrome, Lancet **2:**928, 1949.

Cave, E. F., editor: Fractures and other injuries, Chicago, 1958, Year Book Medical Publishers, Inc.

Chrisman, O. D., and Snook. G. A.: The problem of refracture of the tibia, Clin. Orthop. **60:**217, 1968.

Compere, C.: Early fitting of prosthesis after amputation, Surg. Clin. North Am. **48:**215, 1968.

Dehne, E.: Healing of clinical fractures of the tibia without internal fixation. In Robinson, R. A., editor: The healing of osseous tissue, National Academy of Sciences National Research Council, 1965, p. 71.

Dehne, E.: Treatment of fractures of the tibial shaft, Clin. Orthop. **66:**159, 1969.

Dehne, E., Deffer, P. A., Hall, R. M., Brown, P. W., and Johnson, E. V.: The natural history of the fractured tibia, Surg. Clin. North Am. **41:**1495, 1961.

Dehne, E., Metz, C. W., Deffer, P. A., and Hall, R. M.: Nonoperative treatment of the fractured tibia by immediate weight bearing, J. Trauma **1:**514, 1961.

Dickson, F. D.: The treatment of cerebral spastic paralysis with specific reference to the Stöffel operation, J.A.M.A. **83:**1236, 1924.

Dietrichson, G. J. F., and Stören, G.: Posterolateral approach—a back-door to infected tibial shaft fractures, Acta Chir. Scand. **120:**471, 1965.

Edwards, P.: Fracture of the shaft of the tibia: 492 consecutive cases in adults. Importance of soft tissue injury, Acta Orthop. Scand. (Suppl.) 76, 1965.

Eggers, G. W. N.: Internal contact splint, J. Bone Joint Surg. **30-A:**40, 1948.

Eggers, G. W. N.: Effect of contact compression on osteogenesis, American Academy of Orthopaedic Surgeons Instructional Course Lectures, vol. 9, Ann Arbor, Mich., 1952, J. W. Edwards.

Eggers, G. W. N., Shindler, T. O., and Pomerat, C. M.: The influence of the contact-compression factor on osteogenesis in surgical fractures, J. Bone Joint Surg. **31-A:**693, 1949.

Ellis, H.: The speed of healing after fractures of the tibial shaft, J. Bone Joint Surg. **40-B:**42, 1958.

Freeland, A. E., and Mutz, S. B.: Posterior bone-grafting for infected ununited fracture of the tibia, J. Bone Joint Surg. **58-A:**653, 1976.

Freeman, A. W., and Garnes, A. L.: Open tibial shaft fractures—immediate soft tissue closure, Am. J. Surg. **95:**415, 1958.

Friedenberg, Z. B., and French, G.: The effects of known compression forces on fracture healing, Surg. Gynecol. Obstet. **94:**743, 1952.

Ganguli, S., Bose, K. S., and Datta, S. R.: Performance of BK amputees using PTB prostheses, Acta Orthop. Scand. **46:**123, 1975.

Ganosa, A. C., Lozano, J. C., and Rogers, S. P.: Straight nails in tibial fractures. Technique and report of 30 cases, J. Bone Joint Surg. **49-A:**280, 1967.

Ger, R.: The management of pretibial skin loss, Surgery **63:**757, 1968.

Ger, R.: Muscle transposition for treatment and prevention of chronic post-traumatic osteomyelitis of the tibia, J. Bone Joint Surg. **59-A:**784, 1977.

Golbranson, F. L., et al.: Immediate postsurgical fitting and early ambulation, Clin. Orthop. **56:**119, 1968.

Gonzalez, E. G., Corcoran, P. J., and Reyes, R. L.: Energy expenditure in below-knee amputees. Correlation with stump strength, Arch. Phys. Med. Rehab. **55**:111, 1974.

Gothman, L.: Local arterial changes associated with experimental fractures of the rabbit's tibia treated with encircling wires (cerclage). A microangiographic study, Acta Chir. Scand. **123**:17, 1962.

Greenbaum, E. I., and O'Loughlin, B. J.: Value of delayed filming in the anterior tibial compartment syndrome secondary to trauma, Radiology **93**:373, 1969.

Griffiths, J. C.: Tendon injuries around the ankle, J. Bone Joint Surg. **47-B**:686, 1965.

Grunwald, A., and Siberman, Z.: Anterior tibial syndrome, J.A.M.A. **171**:2210, 1959.

Harmon, P. H.: A simplified surgical approach to the posterior tibia for bone-grafting and fibular transference, J. Bone Joint Surg. **27**:496, 1945.

Hicks, J. H.: Amputation in fractures of the tibia, J. Bone Joint Surg. **46-B**:388, 1964.

Hoaglund, F. T., and States, J. D.: Factors influencing the rate of healing in tibial shaft fractures, Surg. Gynecol. Obstet. **124**:71, 1967.

Horn, C. E.: Acute ischemia of the anterior tibial muscle and the long extensor muscles of the toes, J. Bone Joint Surg. **27-A**:615, 1945.

Hughes, J. R.: Ischaemic necrosis of the anterior tibial muscles due to fatigue, J. Bone Joint Surg. **30-B**:581, 1948.

Jones, K. G., and Barne, H. C.: Cancellous bone grafting for nonunion of the tibia through the posterolateral approach, J. Bone Joint Surg. **37-A**:1550, 1955.

Kendrick, R. R.: Below-knee amputation in arteriosclerotic gangrene, Br. J. Surg. **44**:13, 1956.

Kennelly, B. M., and Blumberg, L.: Bilateral anterior tibial claudication. Report of two cases in which the patients were cured by bilateral fasciotomy, J. A. M. A. **203**:487, 1968.

King, T.: Compression of the bone ends as an aid to union in fractures. A report on 49 ununited and four recent fractures, J. Bone Joint Surg. **39-A**:1238, 1957.

Knutsson, B., and Stahl, F.: Immediate postoperative fitting of prosthesis for lower limbs, Acta Orthop. Scand. **36**:459, 1965.

Lamb, R. H.: Posterolateral bone graft for nonunion of the tibia, Clin. Orthop. **64**:114, 1969.

Leach, R. E., Hammond, G., and Stryker, W. S.: Anterior tibial compartment syndrome. Acute and chronic, J. Bone Joint Surg. **49-A**:451, 1967.

Lim, R. C., Jr., et al.: Below-knee amputation for ischemic gangrene, Surg. Gynecol. Ostet. **125**:493, 1967.

Lottes, J. O.: Blind-nailing technique for insertion of the triflange medullary nail, J.A.M.A. **155**:1039, 1954.

Lottes, J. O., Hill, L. J., and Key, J. A.: Closed reduction, plate fixation and medullary nailing of fractures of both bones of the leg. A comparative end-result study, J. Bone Joint Surg. **34-A**:861, 1952.

Lottes, J. O., and Key, J. A.: Complications and errors in technic in medullary nailing for fractures of the femur, Clin. Orthop. **2**:38, 1953.

Marmor, L., and Sollars, R.: Lower extremity amputations and their appropriate prosthesis, J. Trauma **4**:435, 1964.

Mavor, G. E.: The anterior tibial syndrome, J. Bone Joint Surg. **38-B**:513, 1956.

McCarroll, H. R.: The surgical management of ununited fractures of the tibia, J.A.M.A. **175**:578, 1961.

Mooney, V., Harvey, J. P., McBride, E., and Snelson, R.: Comparison of postoperative stump management: plaster vs. soft dressings, J. Bone Joint Surg. **53-A**:241, 1971.

Mooney, V., Wagner, F. W., Jr., Waddell, Jr., and Ackerson, T.: The below-the-knee amputation for vascular disease, J. Bone Joint Surg. **58-A**:365, 1976.

Moretz, W. H.: The anterior compartment (anterior tibial) ischemia syndrome, Am. Surg. **19**:728, 1953.

Morton, K. S., and Starr, D. E.: Closure of the anterior portion of the upper tibial epiphysis as a complication of tibial-shaft fracture, J. Bone Joint Surg. **46-A**:570, 1964.

Mozes, M., Ramon, Y., and Jahr, J.: The anterior tibial syndrome, J. Bone Joint Surg. **44-A**:730, 1962.

Mumenthaler, M., Mumenthaler, A., and Medici, V.: Das tibialis anterior-Syndrom nach Operationen am Unterschenkel Seine Fehldiagnose als Peronaeusparese, Arch. Orthop. Unfallchir. **66**:201, 1969.

Nicoll, E. A.: Fractures of the tibial shaft. A survey of 705 cases, J. Bone Joint Surg. **46-B**:373, 1964.

Owen, R., and Tsimboukis, B.: Ischaemia complicating closed tibial and fibular shaft fractures, J. Bone Joint Surg. **49-B**:268, 1967.

Pedersen, H. E., LaMont, R. L., and Ramsey, R. H.: Below-knee amputation for gangrene, South. Med. J. **57**:820, 1964.

Record, E. E.: Surgical amputation in the geriatric patient, J. Bone Joint Surg. **45-A**:1742, 1963.

Rhinelander, F. W., and Bargary, R. A.: Microangiography in bone healing. I. Undisplaced closed fractures, J. Bone Joint Surg. **44-A**:1273, 1962.

Rhinelander, F. W.: Tibial blood supply in relation to fracture healing, Clin. Orthop. **105**:34, 1974.

Roon, A. J., Moore, W. S., and Goldstone, J.: Below knee amputation: a modern approach, Am. J. Surg. **134**:153, 1977.

Rush, L. V.: Atlas of Rush pin technics. A system of fracture treatment, Meridian, Miss., 1955, The Berivon Co.

Sakillarides, H. T., Freeman, P. A., and Grant, B. D.: Delayed union and non-union of tibial-shaft fractures, J. Bone Joint Surg. **46-A**:557, 1964.

Sarmiento, A.: A functional below-the-knee case for tibial fractures, J. Bone Joint Surg. **49-A**:855, 1967.

Sarmiento, A.: Recent trends in lower extremity amputation. Surgery and rehabilitation, Nurs. Clin. North Am. **2**:399, 1967.

Sarmiento, A.: A functional below-the-knee brace for tibial fractures. A report on its use in one hundred thirty-five cases, J. Bone Joint Surg. **52-A**:295, 1970.

Sarmiento, A., Uricchio, J. V., Jr., and May, B. J.: Experiences with patella tendon-bearing prostheses in geriatric amputees, Clin. Orthop. **50**:181, 1967.

Sarmiento, A., and Warren, W. D.: A re-evaluation of lower extremity amputations, Surg. Gynecol. Obstet. **129**:799, 1969.

Sarmiento, A., et al.: Lower extremity amputation: The impact of immediate postsurgical prosthetic fitting, Clin. Orthop. **68**:22, 1970.

Schrock, R. D., Jr.: Peroneal nerve palsy following derotation osteotomies for tibial torsion, Clin. Orthop. **62**:172, 1969.

Slätis, P., and Rokkanen, P.: Closed intramedullary nailing of tibial shaft fractures. A comparison with conservatively treated cases, Acta Orthop. Scand. **38**:88, 1967.

Slocum, D. B.: The shin splint syndrome, medical aspects and differential diagnosis, Am. J. Surg. **114**:875, 1967.

Sofield, H. A.: Congenital pseudarthrosis of the tibia, Clin. Orthop. **76**:33, 1971.

Sofield, H. A., and Millar, E. A.: Fragmentation, realignment and intramedullary rod fixation of deformities of the long bones in children. A ten-year appraisal, J. Bone Joint Surg. **41-A:**1371, 1959.

Spademan, R.: Lower-extremity injuries as related to the use of ski safety bindings, J.A.M.A. **203:**445, 1968.

Spencer, G. E., Jr.: Intramedullary fixation in fractures of the shaft of the tibia, Surg. Clin. North Am. **41:**1531, 1961.

Stark, W. A.: Anterior compartment syndrome, Clin. Orthop. **62:**180, 1969.

Still, J. M., Jr., Wray, C. H., and Moretz, W. H.: Selective physiologic amputation: A valuable adjunct in preparation for surgical operation, Ann. Surg. **171:**143, 1970.

Stöffel, A.: The treatment of spastic contracture, Am. J. Orthop. Surg. **10:**611, 1912-1913.

Strayer, L. M., Jr.: Recession of the gastrocnemius. An operation to relieve spastic contracture of the calf muscles, J. Bone Joint Surg. **32-A:**671, 1950.

Strayer, L. M., Jr.: Gastrocnemius recession. Five-year report of cases, J. Bone Joint Surg. **40-A:**1019, 1958.

Stuck, W. G., and Dunlop, K.: End results of treatment of compound fractures of the tibia, Milit. Surg. **105:**282, 1949.

Swanson, A. B., Hotchkiss, B., and Meadows, V.: Improving end-bearing characteristics of lower-extremity amputation stumps, Inter-Clin. Imform. Bull. **7:**11, 1967.

Thompson, R. G.: Amputation in the lower extremity, J. Bone Joint Surg. **45-A:**1723, 1963.

Tosberg, W. A.: Immediate post-operative prosthetic fitting, Orthop. Prosth. Appliance J. **19:**30, 1965.

Van Der Linden, W., Sunzel, H., and Larsson, K.: Fractures of the tibial shaft after skiing and other accidents, J. Bone Joint Surg. **57-A:**321, 1975.

Van Nes, C. P.: Congenital pseudarthrosis of the leg, J. Bone Joint Surg. **48-A:**1467, 1966.

Vitale, M., and Redhead, R. G.: The modern concept of the general management of amputee rehabilitation including immediate post-operative fitting, Ann. R. Coll. Surg. Engl. **40:**251, 1967.

Waddell, J. P.: Anterior tibial compartment syndrome, Can. Med. Assoc. J. **116:**653, 1977.

Wade, P. A., and Campbell, R. D., Jr.: Open versus closed methods in treating fractures of the leg, Am. J. Surg. **95:**599, 1958.

Warren, R., and Kihn, R. B.: A survey of lower extremity amputations for ischemia, Surgery **63:**107, 1968.

Warren, R., and Moseley, R. V.: Immediate post-operative prosthesis for below-the-knee amputations. A preliminary report, Am. J. Surg. **116:**429, 1968.

Watson-Jones, R.: Fractures and joint injuries, vols. 1 and 2, ed. 4, Baltimore, 1957, The Williams and Wilkins Co.

Wood, W. L., Zlotsky, N., and Westin, G. W.: Congenital absence of the fibula. Treatment by Syme amputation—indications and techniques, J. Bone Joint Surg. **47-A:**1159, 1965.

Wray, J. B.: Acute changes in femoral arterial blood flow after closed tibial fracture in dogs, J. Bone Joint Surg. **46-A:**1262, 1964.

14

ANKLE

TENDO ACHILLIS LENGTHENING (Plate 14-1)

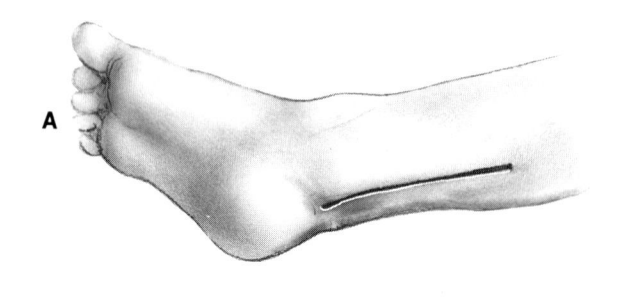

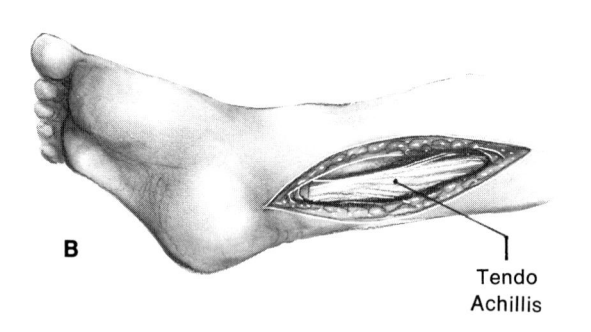

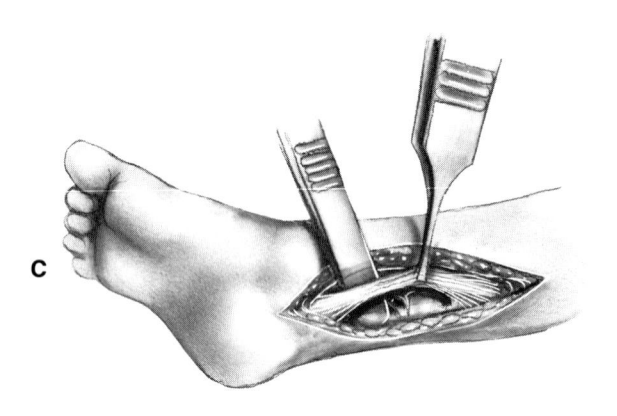

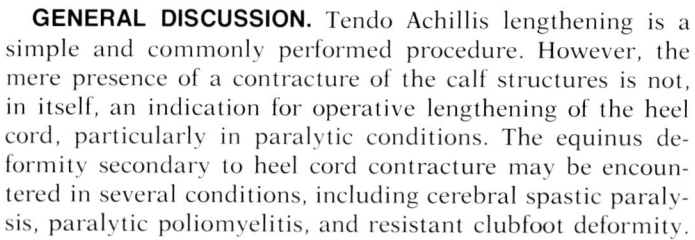

GENERAL DISCUSSION. Tendo Achillis lengthening is a simple and commonly performed procedure. However, the mere presence of a contracture of the calf structures is not, in itself, an indication for operative lengthening of the heel cord, particularly in paralytic conditions. The equinus deformity secondary to heel cord contracture may be encountered in several conditions, including cerebral spastic paralysis, paralytic poliomyelitis, and resistant clubfoot deformity.

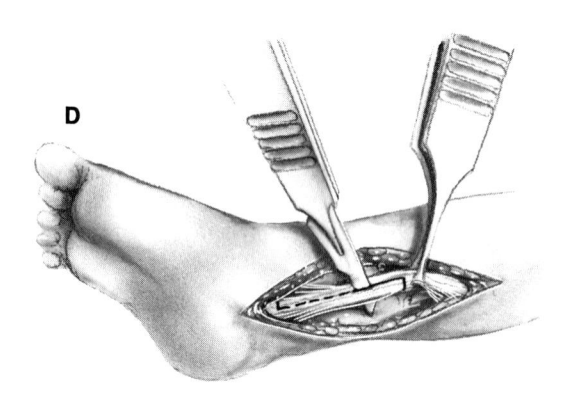

In paralytic conditions, lengthening of the heel cord in the presence of a heel cord contracture should be done only after detailed analysis of the disability, since the overall disability may potentially be worsened rather than improved by the operation. If the calf muscles are weak, the heel cord contracture may be an advantage; it may be responsible for a better gait and increased tolerance for walking and running activities that will suffer if the heel cord is lengthened. A tight heel cord may also be useful in stabilizing a knee that has poor quadriceps control. In most cases, adequate lengthening of the heel cord can be brought about by cast changes or wedging with no ill effect on the functional strength of the calf muscles.

Several techniques for tendo Achillis lengthening are widely used. If there has been a previous surgical lengthening of the heel cord, a Z-plasty will be necessary for lengthening the tendon. Posterior capsulotomy of the ankle joint will be necessary if there is associated capsular contracture.

DETAILS OF PROCEDURE. A posteromedial incision approximately 10 cm long is made and carried down to the tendo Achillis (**A** and **B**). The tendon sheath is opened, and the tendon is divided longitudinally from side to side. The anterior half is carefully sectioned just above the calcaneus. The posterior half is then sectioned about 10 cm proximally, thereby leaving a posterior flap attached to the calcaneus and an anterior flap attached to the gastrocnemius and soleus (**C** and **D**). The ankle is dorsiflexed, and the ends of the tendon are sutured without tension **(E)**. The wound is closed in layers, and a long-leg cast is applied with the ankle in slight dorsiflexion and the knee in slight flexion.

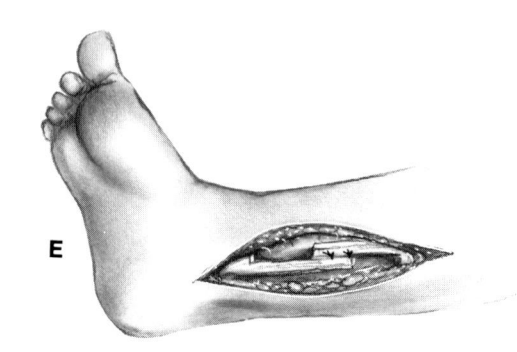

(Plate 14-1) TENDO ACHILLIS LENGTHENING

When there has been no previous surgery, an alternative method is recommended for tendo Achillis lengthening in the young child. Through the same incision the tendon sheath is opened (**F** and **G**). The anterior two thirds of the tendon is sectioned near its insertion into the calcaneus (**H**). Then the medial two thirds of the tendon is sectioned at the proximal end of the wound (**I**). Moderate dorsiflexion force is applied to the ankle and the spiraling fibers of the tendon slide on each other (**J**). No suturing of the tendon is necessary with this method unless to minimize any residual prominence at the ends of tendon postions that have been sectioned and displaced during the lengthening. The plantaris tendon, if present, is divided. The wound is closed in layers, and a long-leg cast is applied, holding the ankle in slight dorsiflexion and the knee in slight flexion.

POSTOPERATIVE MANAGEMENT. In young children (under 3 years), the cast and sutures can generally be removed 3 weeks postoperatively. For children under 2 years, the subsequent use of a posterior plaster splint at bedtime will minimize the likelihood of recurrent plantar flexion deformity.

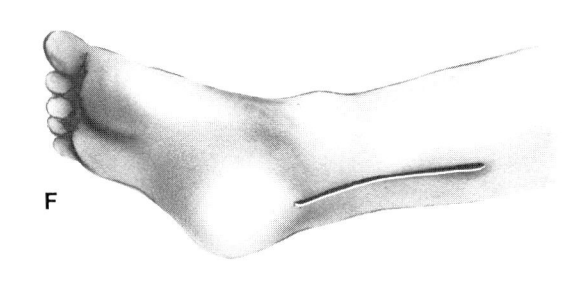

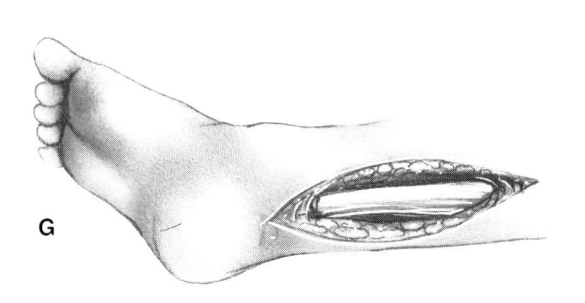

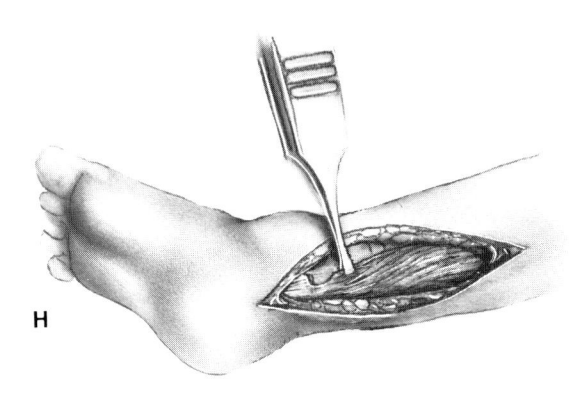

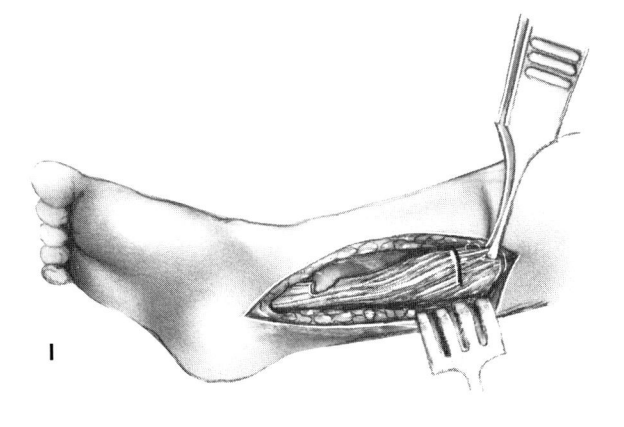

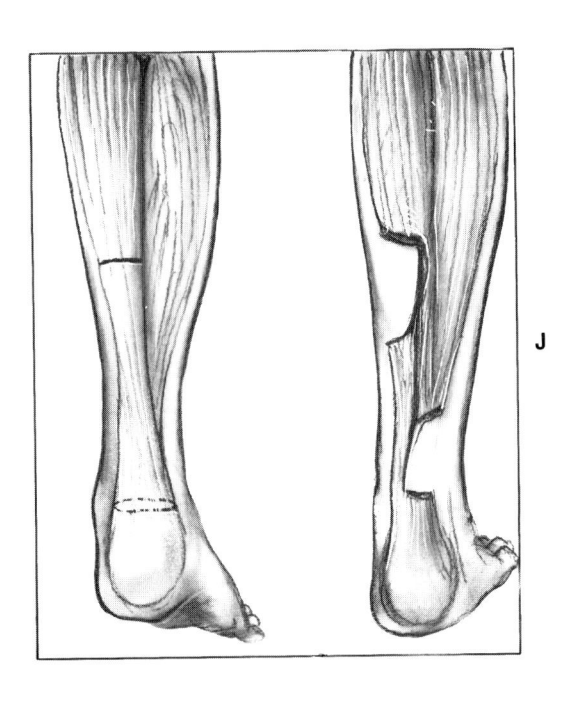

513

TENODESIS OF TENDO ACHILLIS (Plate 14-2)

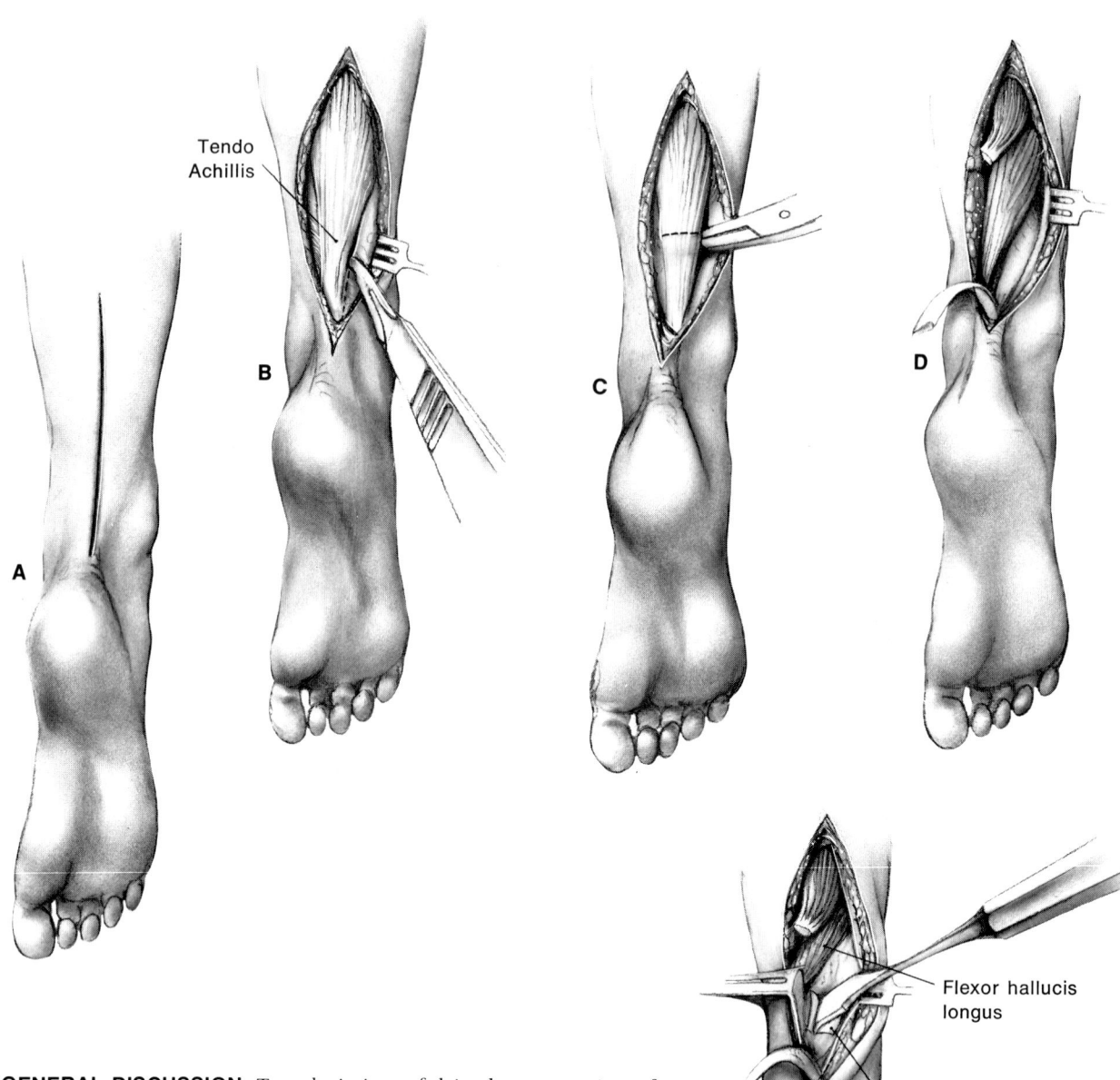

GENERAL DISCUSSION. Tenodesis is useful in the prevention of a progressive calcaneus deformity when sufficient muscle power is not available to consider posterior tendon transfers to the calcaneus. Tenodesis of the tendo Achillis is also helpful, on occasion, to reinforce a posterior tendon transfer that is not providing enough muscle power for a good "push off" during gait.

DETAILS OF PROCEDURE. The patient is placed in a prone position, and the pneumatic tourniquet is used. It is helpful to have a linen bundle under the ankle. A posterior longitudinal incision approximately 15 cm in length is made along the tendo Achillis, ending distally at the level of the medial malleolus (**A**). The tendon sheath is opened, and the tendo Achillis is divided transversely just below the musculotendinous junction (**B** to **D**). The distal portion of the Achilles tendon is then mobilized. The posterior surface of the tibia is exposed by retracting the flexor hallucis longus and the neurovascular bundle medially (**E**). It is best to locate the neurovascular bundle early and then protect it along with the flexor hallucis longus by gentle retraction.

514

(Plate 14-2) TENODESIS OF TENDO ACHILLIS

A point of insertion into the tibia is selected according to the length of the available tendon so it will be possible to insert the tendon well into the bone marrow and under the superior lip of the entry hole through the posterior cortex. Two drill holes, drilled obliquely distally in the posterior surface of the tibia, are then made proximal to the entry hole. A hole of appropriate size is then made in the posterior cortex of the tibia at the selected point to receive the entire circumference of the Achilles tendon **(F)**. The tendon that will be within bone is scarified, and a Bunnell stainless-steel wire suture is placed in the tendon at the appropriate level with the suture ends going out the corners of the tendon. Each end of the wire suture is passed into the medullary space of the tibia and out one of the small drill holes proximally. The end of the tendon is carefully placed into the marrow cavity of the tibia, and the ends of the wire sutures are pulled proximally to bring the full thickness of the tendo Achillis well into the medullary space of the tibia **(G)**. With the ankle held in 5° to 10° of plantar flexion **(H)**, the wire suture is securely tied over the bony bridge proximally. Leaving a loose tongue of tendon proximally makes it easier to bring the full thickness of tendon into the tibia. Care is now taken to avoid dorsiflexion of the foot until the wound has been closed by approximation of subcutaneous tissue and skin and a cast has been applied from toes to tibial tubercle with the foot in moderate equinus.

POSTOPERATIVE MANAGEMENT. Crutches are used and weight bearing is not permitted until the cast is removed after 8 weeks. The tenodesis is protected in a brace with the ankle blocked so dorsiflexion of the ankle is limited at 5° of plantar flexion for an additional 2 to 3 months as full weight bearing is resumed.

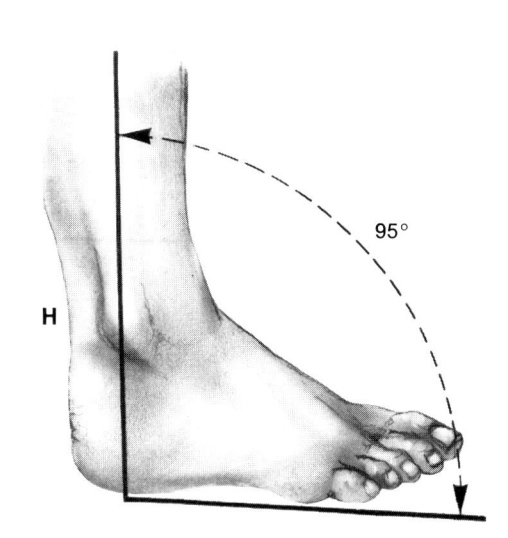

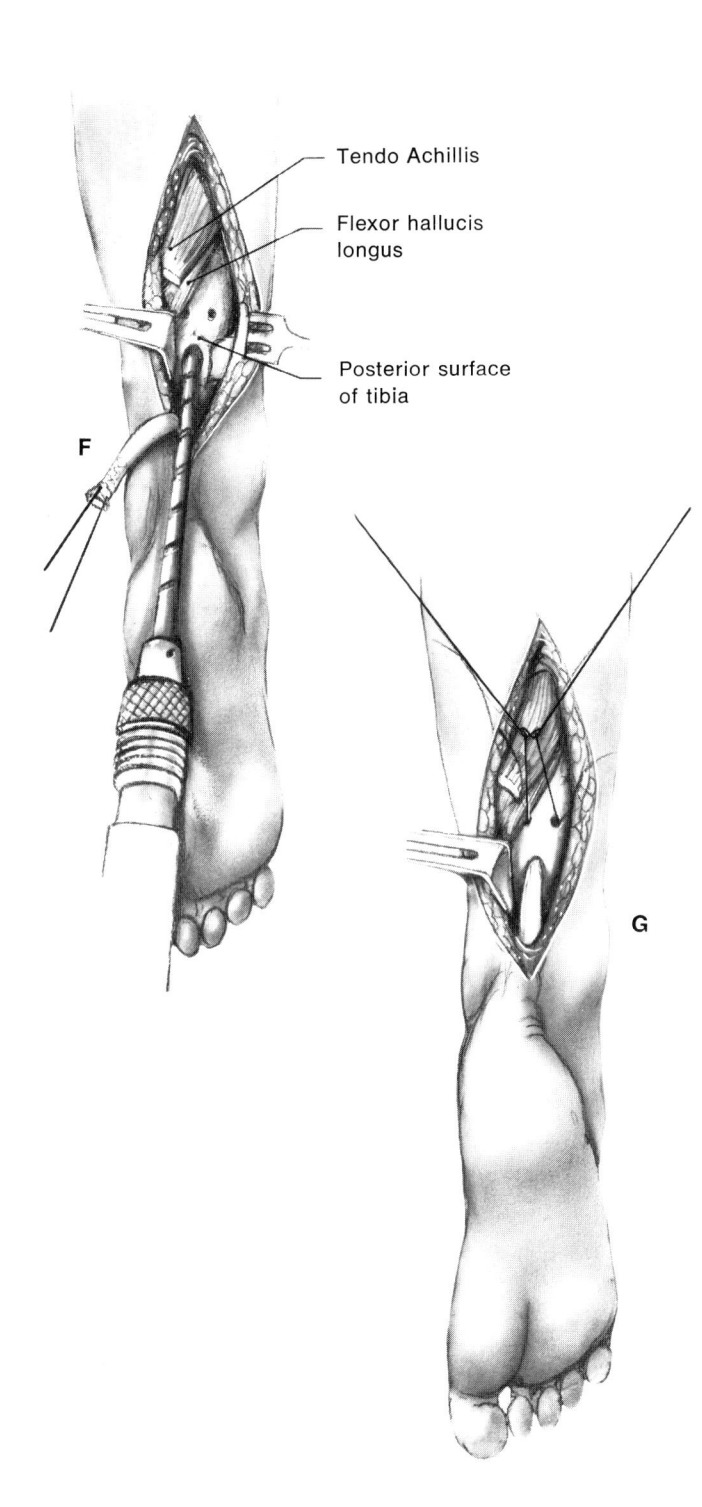

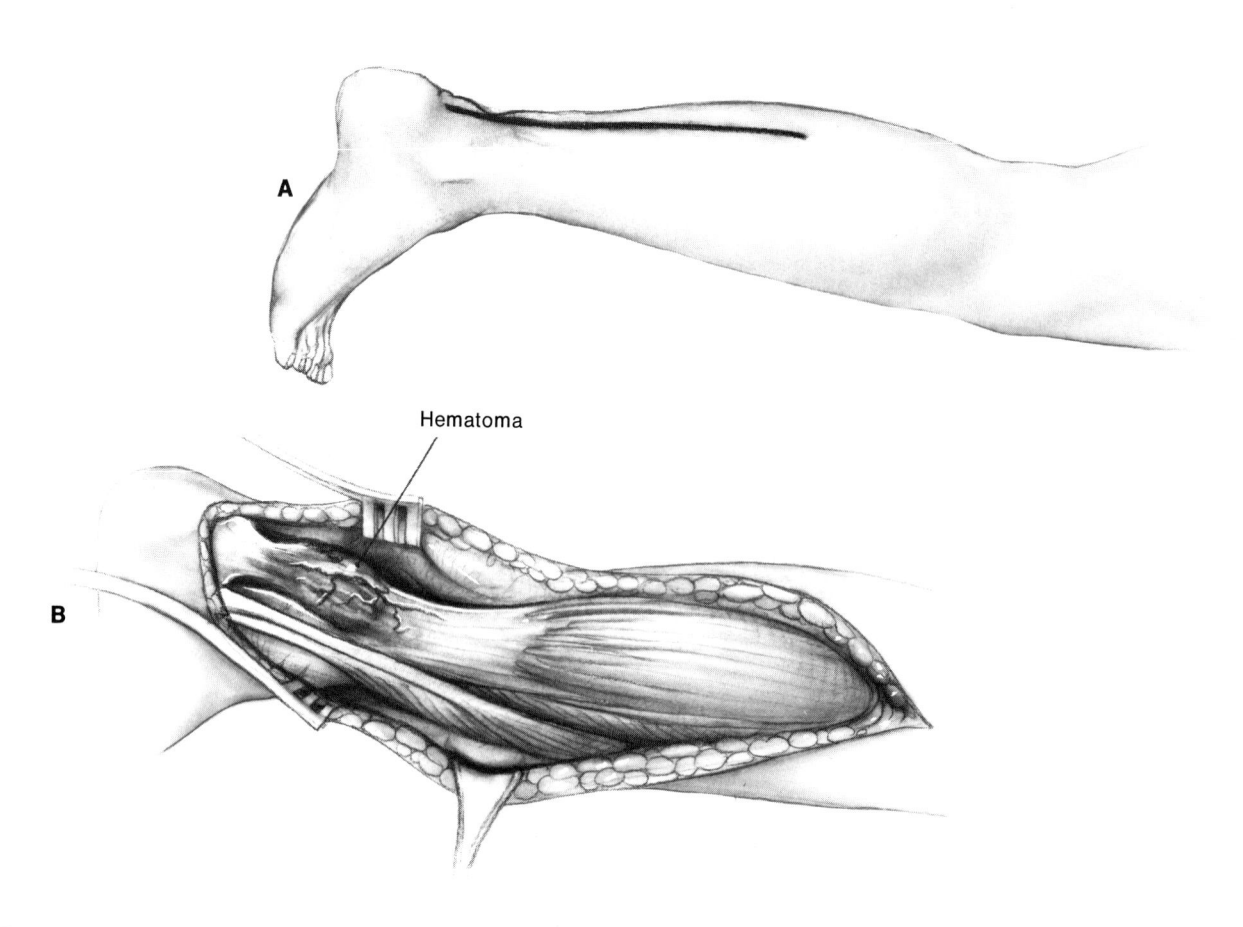

REPAIR OF RUPTURED TENDO ACHILLIS (Plate 14-3)

GENERAL DISCUSSION. When the tendo Achillis ruptures, the tendon fibers are usually torn into irregular longitudinal strips near its insertion into the calcaneus. Rupture may occur near the musculotendinous junction, particularly in young individuals, but rupture near its insertion into the calcaneus is more common in middle-aged people. In both locations the ruptured tendo Achillis may be difficult to repair.

At the time of injury the patient usually has sudden intense pain in the region of the distal portion of the tendo Achillis. There is inability to walk normally or even support the body on the foot. If pain is slight, the patient may be able to walk on the foot but will be unable to stand on the toes. Examination will reveal swelling of the soft tissues immediately above the calcaneus. There is usually a visible and palpable depression in the tendo Achillis 2 to 6 cm proximal to the calcaneus. The patient may be able to actively move the foot in a plantar direction without resistance, but against resistance a marked loss of power will be noted. Fresh rupture of the tendo Achillis is occasionally overlooked or the diagnosis delayed because the foot can be actively plantar flexed.

Thompson describes a test to aid in diagnosis. With the patient prone and with both feet extending past the end of the examining table, the calf muscles on the affected side are squeezed by the examiner; if the tendon is intact, the foot will plantar flex, and, conversely, if the tendon is ruptured, the foot will not. This test is reliable to demonstrate complete rupture of the tendo Achillis.

DETAILS OF PROCEDURE. With the patient in the prone position and with a linen roll or other support anterior to the ankle to allow the foot to rest in a protected position, a posterior longitudinal incision is used **(A)**. The incision extends over the posterior aspect of the calf from the midcalf level to the level of the posterosuperior margin of the calcaneal tuberosity. When the injury has been recent, the location of the rupture will be apparent by the hematoma that will be found subcutaneously **(B)**. The ends of the ruptured tendon are usually shredded and irregular **(C)**. The adjacent plantaris tendon, if present, may remain intact.

The divided ends of the ruptured Achilles tendon are reapproximated with interrupted mattress sutures circumferentially with the foot in 5° to 10° plantar flexion **(D and E)**.

A long tongue of fascia overlying the posterior surface of the gastrocnemius is then outlined in such a manner that its base (distally) can remain intact and it can be reversed back over the initial end-to-end suture of the ruptured Achilles tendon **(F)**.

(Plate 14-3) REPAIR OF RUPTURED TENDO ACHILLIS

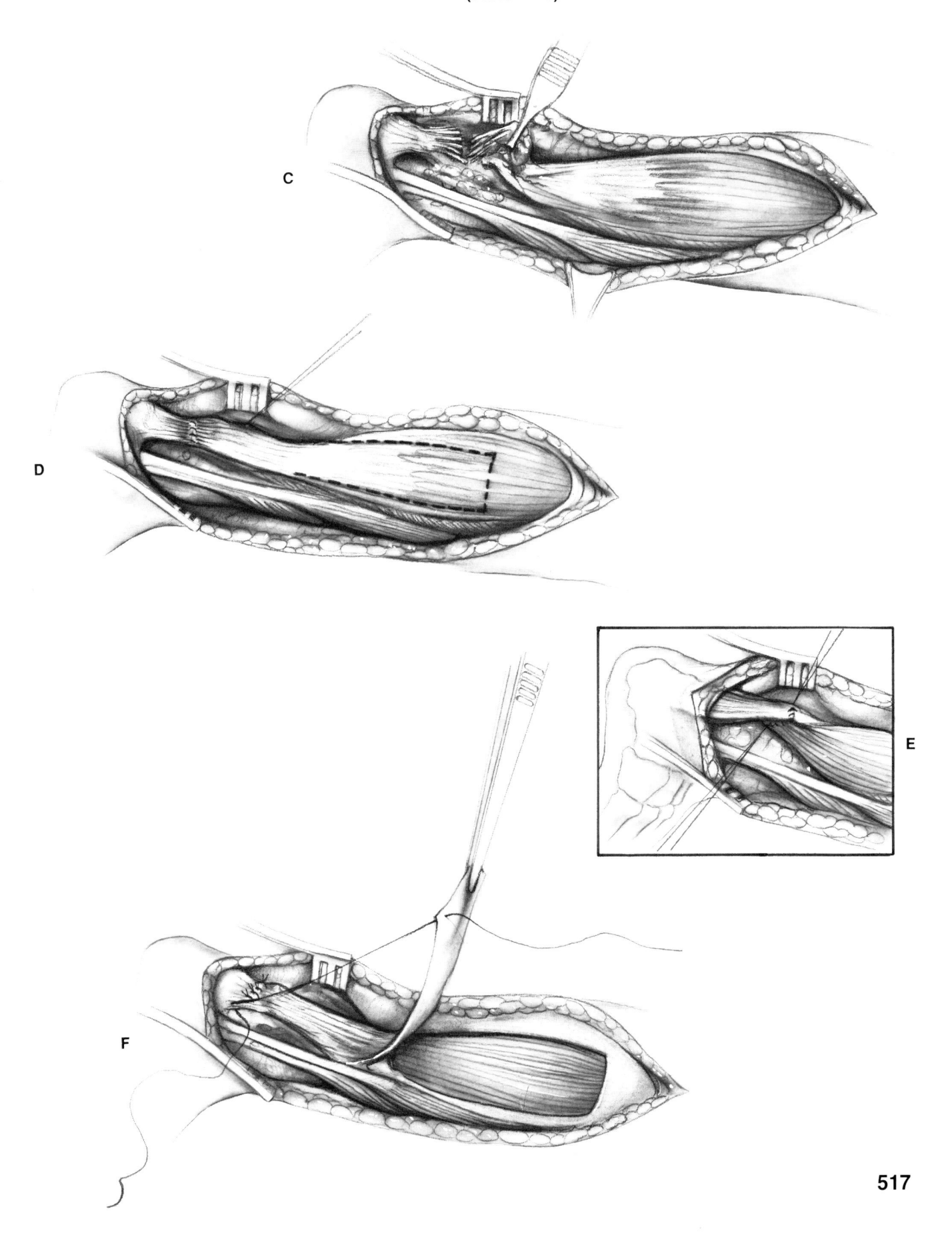

REPAIR OF RUPTURED TENDO ACHILLIS (Plate 14-3)

This fascia is sutured on both sides of the end-to-end suture of the ruptured tendon with multiple sutures and in a manner to provide supplemental reinforcement of the direct end-to-end repair of the ruptured Achilles tendon **(G)**. The surgically created defect where fascia has been removed over the gastrocnemius muscle may be left open or partially closed as far as this is possible without tension or constriction of the underlying posterior calf muscles. Subcutaneous tissues and skin are reapproximated in layers with particular attention to the distal portion of the wound where subcutaneous tissue is minimal and where postoperative wound breakdown is most likely to occur whenever there is postoperative difficulty with wound healing. Following wound closure, a long-leg cast is applied extending from midthigh to the toes with the ankle in a position of 5° to 10° plantar flexion **(H)**.

POSTOPERATIVE MANAGEMENT. Protection in a long-leg cast is continued for 6 weeks followed by use of a short-leg walking cast or a brace with an ankle stop to prevent passive dorsiflexion of the ankle above neutral for an additional 6 weeks. Thereafter, weight-bearing activities are gradually resumed without external protection, but activities involving forceful or potential sudden stress on the repaired Achilles tendon should be avoided until at least 4 months postoperatively.

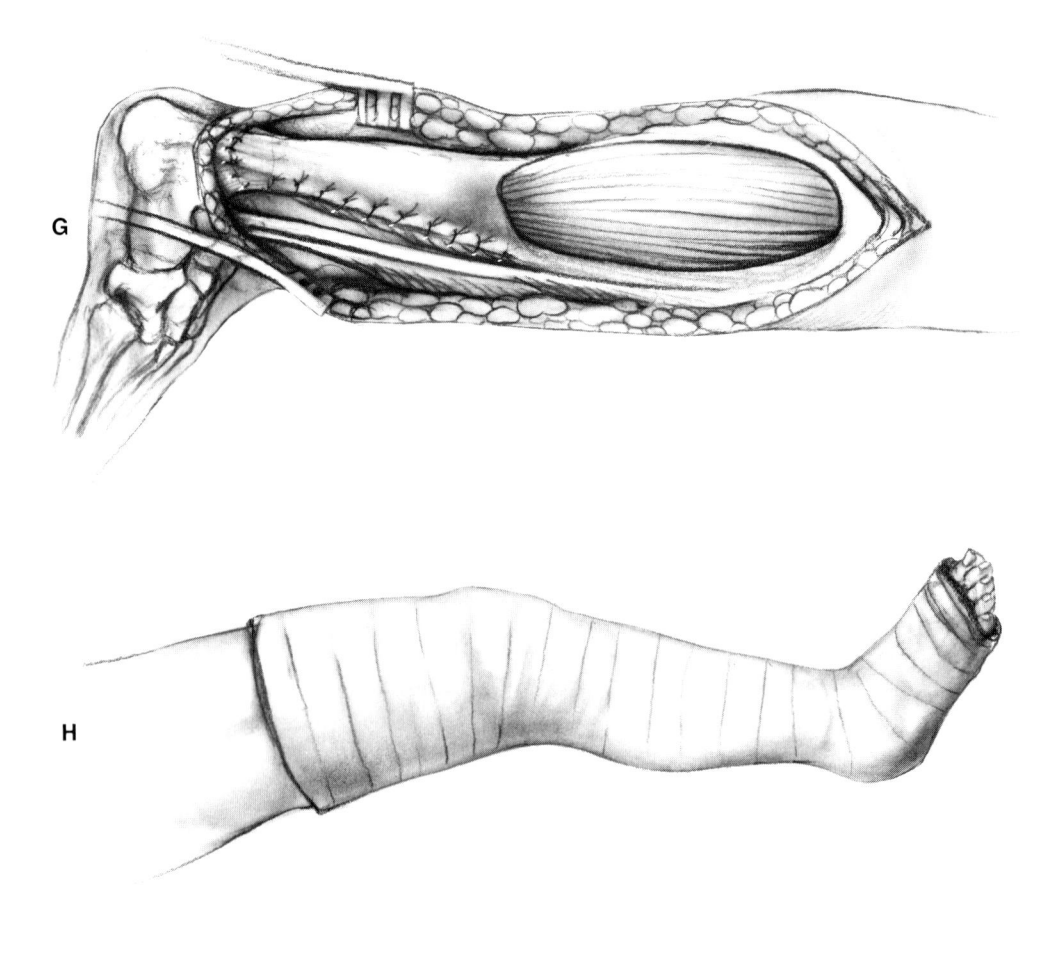

(Plate 14-4) REPAIR OF RUPTURE OF ANTERIOR TIBIAL TENDON

GENERAL DISCUSSION. Although traumatic avulsion or rupture of tendons in the anterior compartment of the leg or in the foot is uncommon, occasional rupture of the anterior tibial tendon may be encountered.

Trauma causing a rupture of the anterior tibial tendon may be powerful or mild. It may be caused by a fall or twisting of the ankle especially when extreme plantar flexion is exerted. Possibly, the same area may have been previously injured with residual fraying or degeneration of a portion of a tendon, predisposing it to complete rupture. When there is complete rupture of the anterior tibial tendon, symptoms will include immediate pain and early swelling, perhaps over the navicular or the first cuneiform bone, accompanied by an inability to coordinate normal foot motion. Dorsiflexion of the foot may be difficult, and there may be a tendency to stub the toes. A few days after injury, extensive ecchymosis may appear over the distal portion of the tendon. There may be a palpable defect along the course of the anterior tibial tendon at its distal end. When the soft tissue edema subsides, this defect may become visible as well. The distal end of the ruptured tendon will feel like a bulbous mass.

When the diagnosis of complete rupture of the anterior tibial tendon is made, early surgical repair should be performed.

DETAILS OF PROCEDURE. With the patient in the supine position and with pneumatic tourniquet control, a longitudinal incision is made over the site of rupture of the anterior tibial tendon **(A)**, which may be near its insertion into the first cuneiform bone and the first metatarsal. The proximal portion of the tendon is withdrawn into the wound **(B)**.

Careful attention should be taken to preserve the thickened portion of the deep fascia, which serves functionally as the superior and inferior extensor retinaculum, unless it is evident that the site of tendon rupture and normal excursion of this tendon might be impaired by a portion of the extensor retinaculum. There is generally no need to divide the transverse crural ligament (that is, the superior extensor retinaculum), but a portion of this ligament may be released if it appears necessary to allow unhampered excursion of the repaired tendon postoperatively.

REPAIR OF RUPTURE OF ANTERIOR TIBIAL TENDON (Plate 14-4)

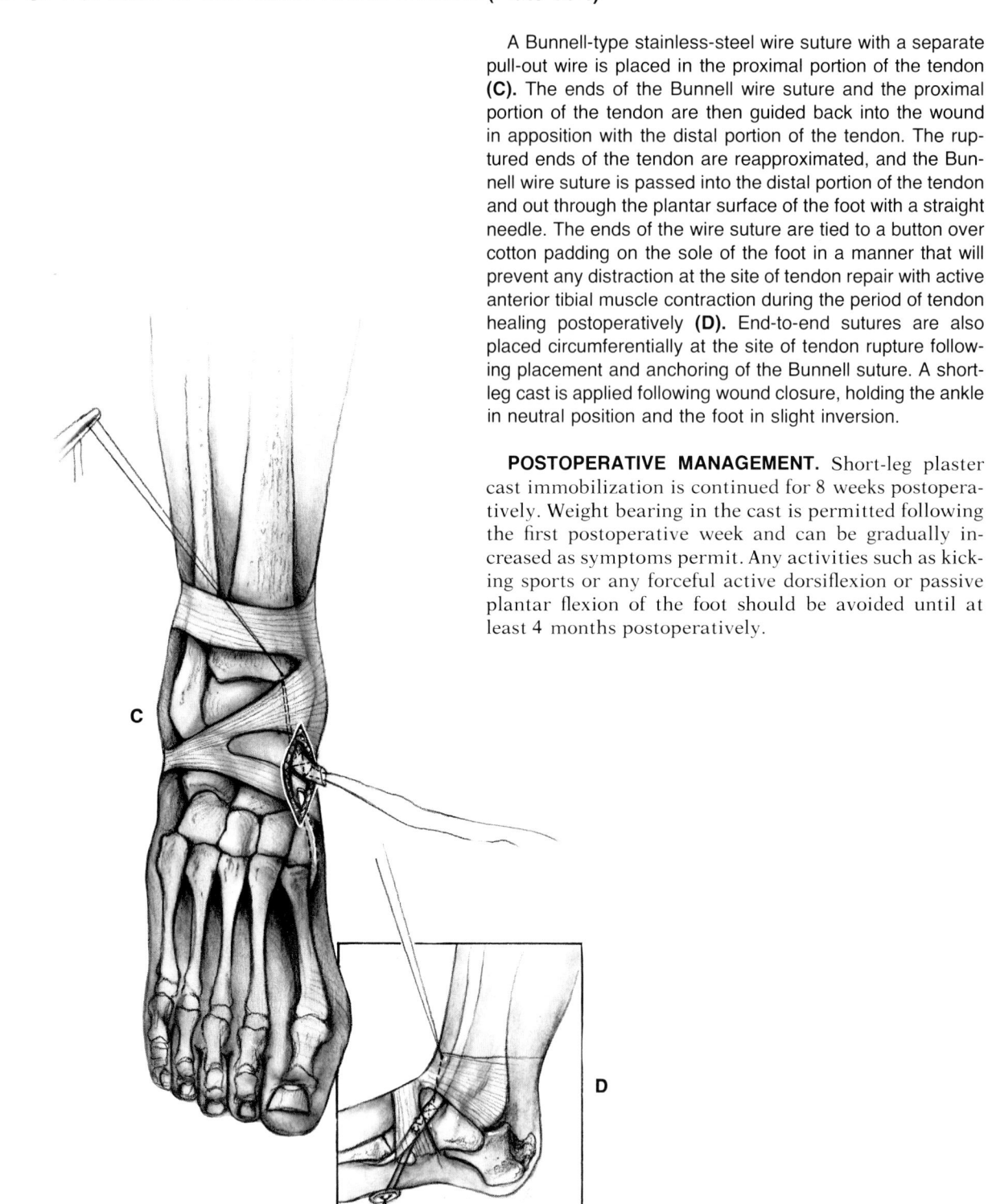

A Bunnell-type stainless-steel wire suture with a separate pull-out wire is placed in the proximal portion of the tendon **(C)**. The ends of the Bunnell wire suture and the proximal portion of the tendon are then guided back into the wound in apposition with the distal portion of the tendon. The ruptured ends of the tendon are reapproximated, and the Bunnell wire suture is passed into the distal portion of the tendon and out through the plantar surface of the foot with a straight needle. The ends of the wire suture are tied to a button over cotton padding on the sole of the foot in a manner that will prevent any distraction at the site of tendon repair with active anterior tibial muscle contraction during the period of tendon healing postoperatively **(D)**. End-to-end sutures are also placed circumferentially at the site of tendon rupture following placement and anchoring of the Bunnell suture. A short-leg cast is applied following wound closure, holding the ankle in neutral position and the foot in slight inversion.

POSTOPERATIVE MANAGEMENT. Short-leg plaster cast immobilization is continued for 8 weeks postoperatively. Weight bearing in the cast is permitted following the first postoperative week and can be gradually increased as symptoms permit. Any activities such as kicking sports or any forceful active dorsiflexion or passive plantar flexion of the foot should be avoided until at least 4 months postoperatively.

(Plate 14-5) TARSAL TUNNEL RELEASE

GENERAL DISCUSSION. The characteristic symptoms of the tarsal tunnel syndrome are diffuse intermittent, sharp, distressing pain in the plantar aspect of the foot and paresthesia in the toes. These symptoms are produced by compression of the posterior tibial nerve within the fibro-osseous tunnel lying beneath the flexor retinaculum on the medial side of the ankle. Decompression of the posterior tibial nerve can provide prompt and lasting relief.

Just as with compression neuropathy of the median nerve within the carpal tunnel, symptoms may be more bothersome at night. There may be tenderness along the course of the posterior tibial nerve posterior to the medial malleolus and beneath the flexor retinaculum. Percussion of the nerve in the same area on the posteromedial aspect of the ankle may reproduce the symptoms in the foot and toes. In long-standing cases, muscle atrophy may develop in the distally innervated muscles just as with long-standing compression of combined motor and sensory nerves elsewhere as, for example, with the median nerve at the wrist. Sensory symptoms precede any muscle changes. There is experimental evidence suggesting that the principal factor in the production of sensory symptoms in nerve compression syndromes is arterial insufficiency (Fullerton, 1963). The more slowly occurring muscle atrophy, thought to be secondary to later structural changes produced within the nerve, is less likely than the associated sensory symptoms to benefit from nerve decompression. Although symptoms may spread proximally up the lower leg, the greatest intensity of discomfort will be in the foot when the posterior tibial nerve or either one of its terminal branches, that is, the medial and lateral plantar nerves, is compressed along its course on the medial aspect of the ankle and foot.

TARSAL TUNNEL RELEASE (Plate 14-5)

DETAILS OF PROCEDURE. A curvilinear incision is made posteromedially beginning at a point several centimeters proximal to the medial malleolus and extending distally along the course of the posterior tibial nerve behind and below the medial malleolus **(A)**. The posterior tibial nerve is identified above the flexor retinaculum (which is a thickening of the deep fascia bridging the long flexor tendons and the neurovascular bundle behind and below the medial malleolus). The fascia is opened in line with the skin incision. The posterior tibial nerve about the ankle will be found posterior to the tendons of the flexor digitorum longus and posterior tibial muscles, and along with the posterior tibial artery and veins immediately on the medial side of the tendon of flexor hallucis longus (**B** and **C**).

The posterior tibial nerve should be isolated throughout its course behind and below the medial malleolus with care to protect its distal branches **(D)**. The posterior tibial nerve may divide into its terminal branches, the medial and lateral plantar nerves, at the level of the ankle joint or distally where this nerve enters the foot between the abductor hallucis muscle and the quadratus plantae muscle (that is, flexor accessorius muscle). Unlike the flexor retinaculum at the wrist, there may be deep extensions of fibrous bands from the flexor retinaculum at the ankle that may contribute to compression of the posterior tibial nerve or its branches. Any deep fibrous bands constricting the nerve along its course should be released. There may be visible evidence of definite compression of the nerve at some point and enlargement of the nerve proximally. Also, it is possible that the nerve may appear grossly normal at the time of surgery and symptoms may still be relieved following decompression.

The narrowest part of the tarsal tunnel is likely to be at the anterior end of the tunnel below the medial malleolus. Decompression of the nerve should be continued approximately 2 cm beyond the point where the posterior tibial nerve or each plantar nerve passes deep to the abductor hallucis muscle into the sole of the foot. When the flexor retinaculum has been opened throughout its length and the posterior tibial nerve freed of any possible constricting bands throughout its course behind and below the ankle (including the area of its entry into the intrinsic foot muscles on the medial side of the foot), the nerve and its branches are allowed to remain in their normal anatomical position. No attempt is made to close the deep fascia. Subcutaneous tissue and skin are closed, and a soft dressing is applied.

POSTOPERATIVE MANAGEMENT. Elevation of the foot combined with active ankle and foot motion as tolerated in the first few postoperative days is followed by progressive return to full weight bearing and normal activities within the following 10 days to 2 weeks. If the diagnosis has been correct, the patients will notice, and often within 24 hours, a significant relief of symptoms following tarsal tunnel release.

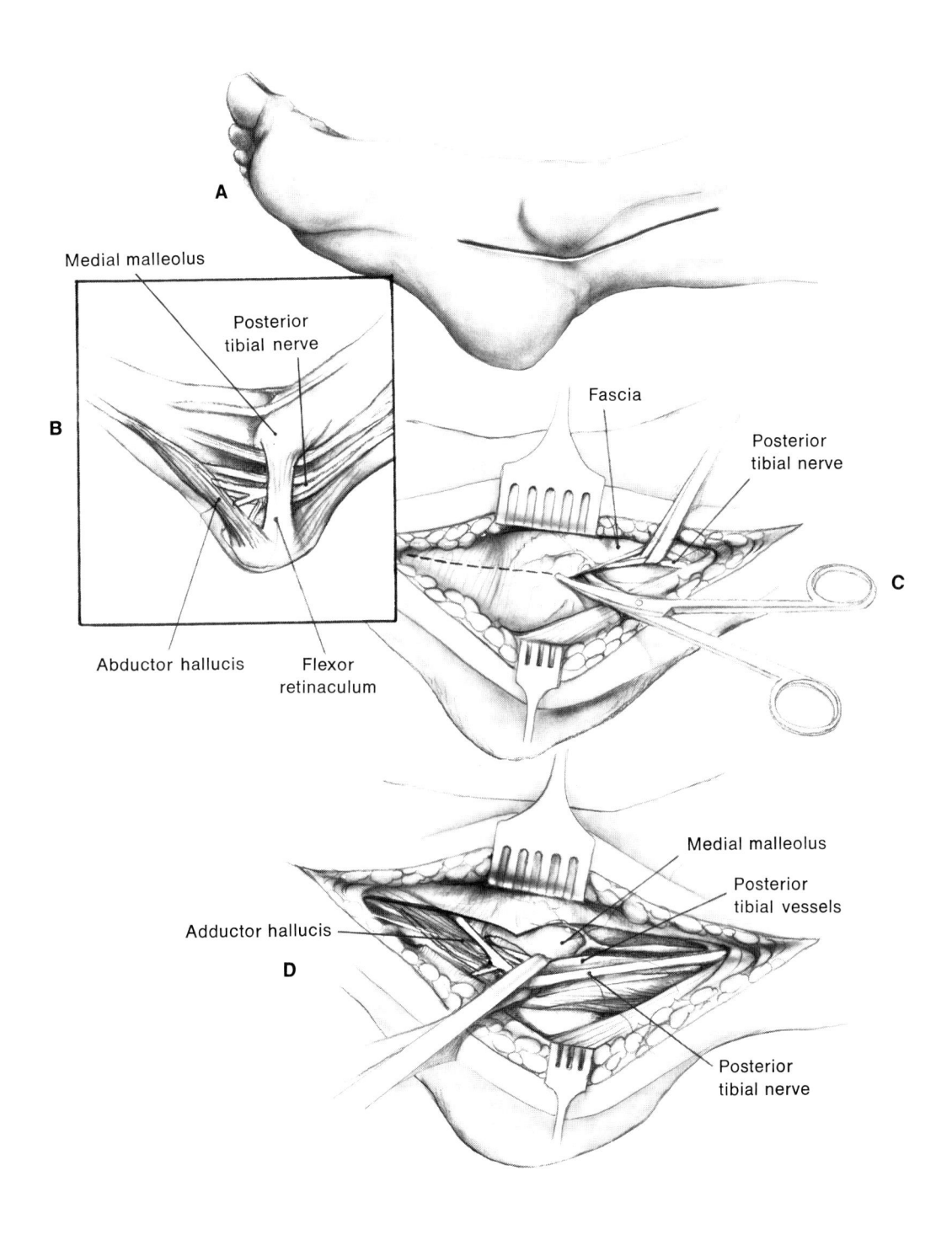

(Plate 14-5) TARSAL TUNNEL RELEASE

523

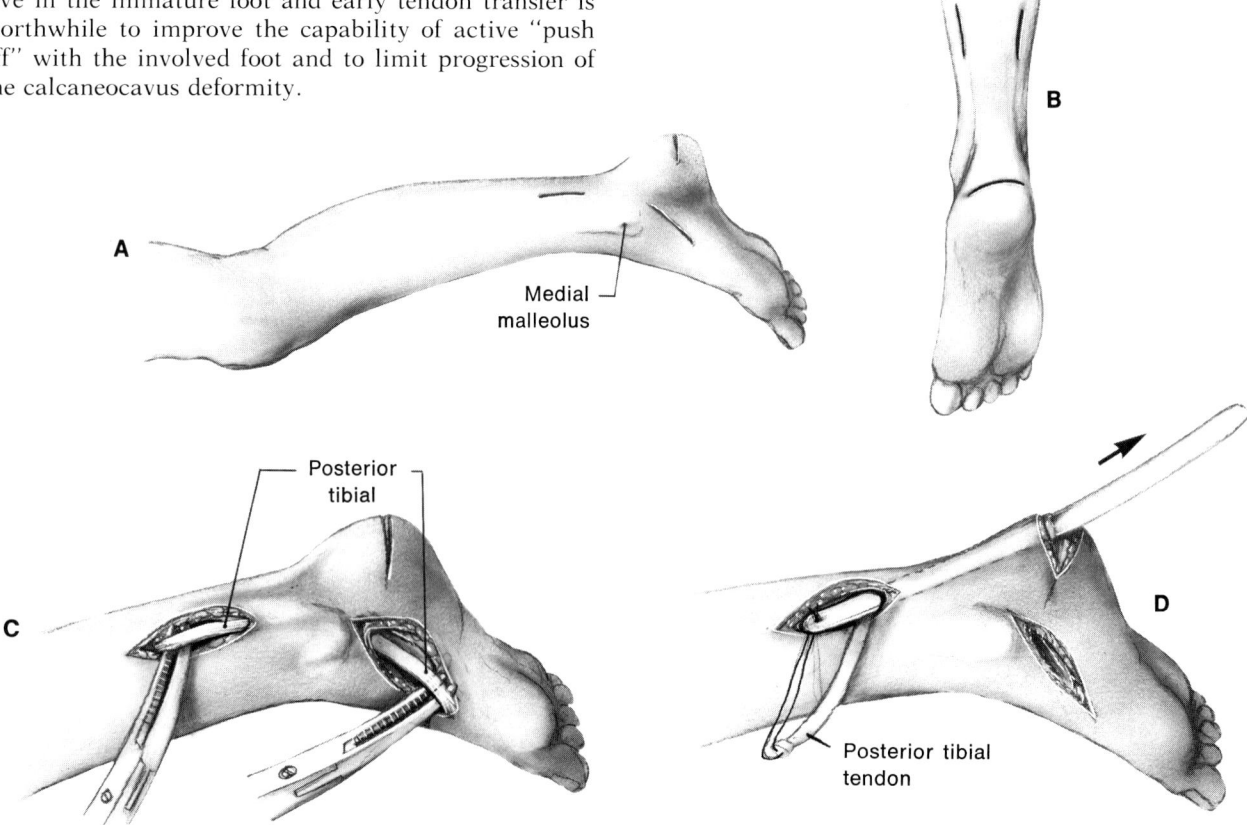

TRANSFER OF POSTERIOR TIBIAL AND PERONEUS BREVIS TENDONS TO CALCANEUS (Plate 14-6)

GENERAL DISCUSSION. Progressive calcaneus deformity in the young child caused by paralysis of the triceps surae muscles is a deformity difficult to control. If there is no adequate muscle power for posterior transfer, a tendo Achillis tendodesis with subtalar stabilization can be helpful.

However if the only function lost is in the posterior calf muscles, a posterior transfer of the peroneus brevis and posterior tibial tendons into the calcaneus, preceded by an extra-articular stabilization of the subtalar joint (Grice), can be useful. The peroneus longus tendon may be used for posterior transfer if this stronger peroneal muscle is needed, but, if this is done, the peroneus brevis tendon must be sectioned and sutured to the remaining distal stump of the peroneus longus tendon.

This procedure is one of the more useful operations in the treatment of the paralytic calcaneus deformity in a child. The calcaneus deformity is initiated by loss of effective function of the gastrocnemius-soleus complex. As the foot goes into dorsiflexion, the remaining intrinsic and extrinsic muscles about the foot frequently act secondarily to produce plantar flexion of the forefoot and an associated cavus deformity of the foot. With the talus and calcaneus dorsiflexed, the posterior tibial tendon and peroneal muscles tend to augment the intrinsic muscles to increase this element of cavus deformity. In spite of shoe modifications, bracing, and exercises, the calcaneocavus deformity is frequently progressive in the immature foot and early tendon transfer is worthwhile to improve the capability of active "push off" with the involved foot and to limit progression of the calcaneocavus deformity.

DETAILS OF PROCEDURE. The posterior tibial tendon and peroneus brevis tendon are divided as far distally as possible through separate medial and lateral foot incisions. Incisions are then made on the medial and lateral sides of the tendo Achillis above the malleoli and another incision is made transversely across the back of the heel **(A to C)**. The posterior tibial tendon is pulled through the medial incision and redirected subcutaneously to the wound over the back of the heel **(D)**. The peroneus brevis is isolated near its insertion into the base of fifth metatarsal and also proximal to the ankle through separate longitudinal incisions **(E)**.

The peroneus brevis is likewise drawn into the proximal wound **(F)**. It is then redirected subcutaneously to the heel **(G)**.

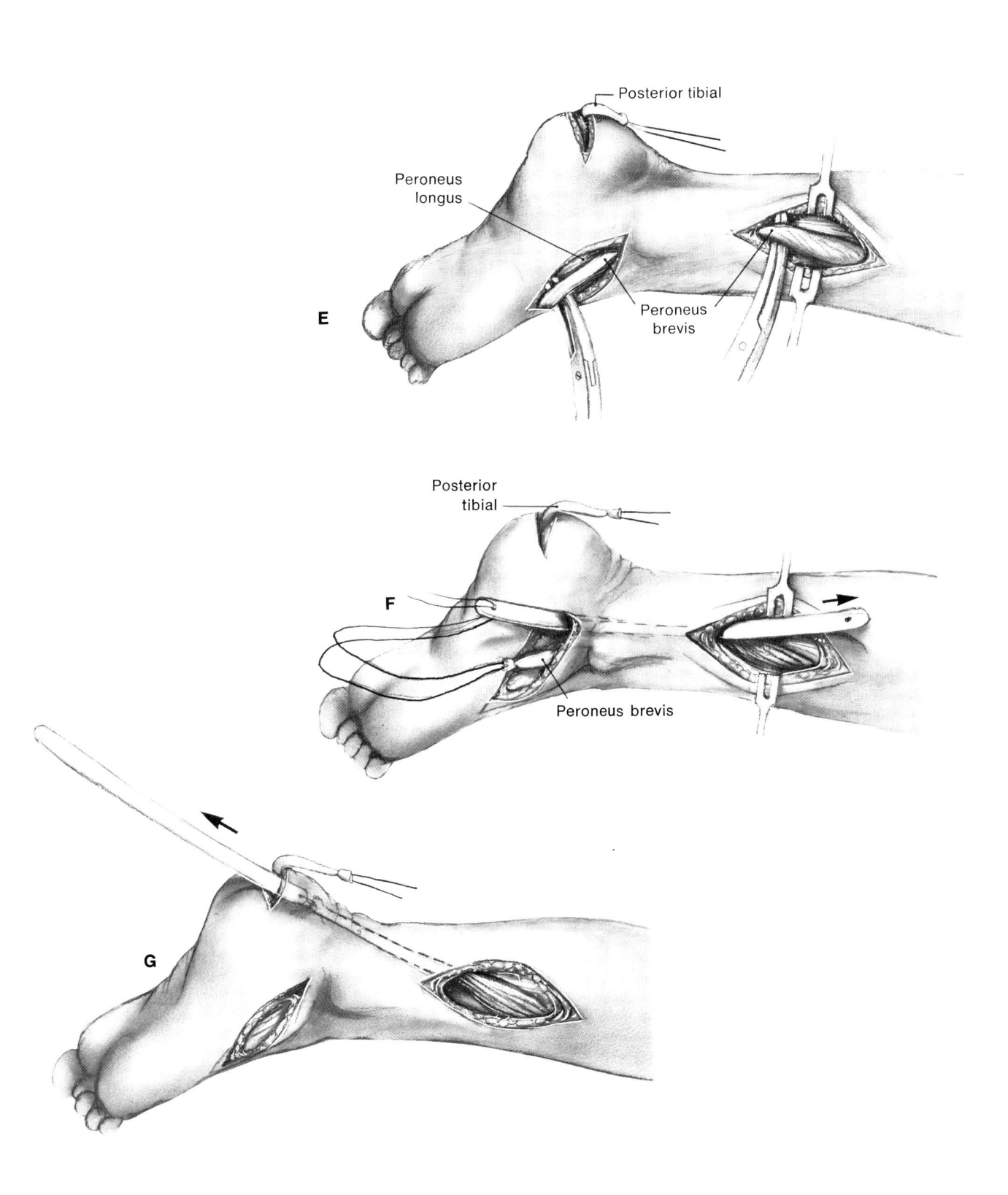

(Plate 14-6) TRANSFER OF POSTERIOR TIBIAL AND PERONEUS BREVIS TENDONS TO CALCANEUS

TRANSFER OF POSTERIOR TIBIAL AND PERONEUS BREVIS TENDONS TO CALCANEUS (Plate 14-6)

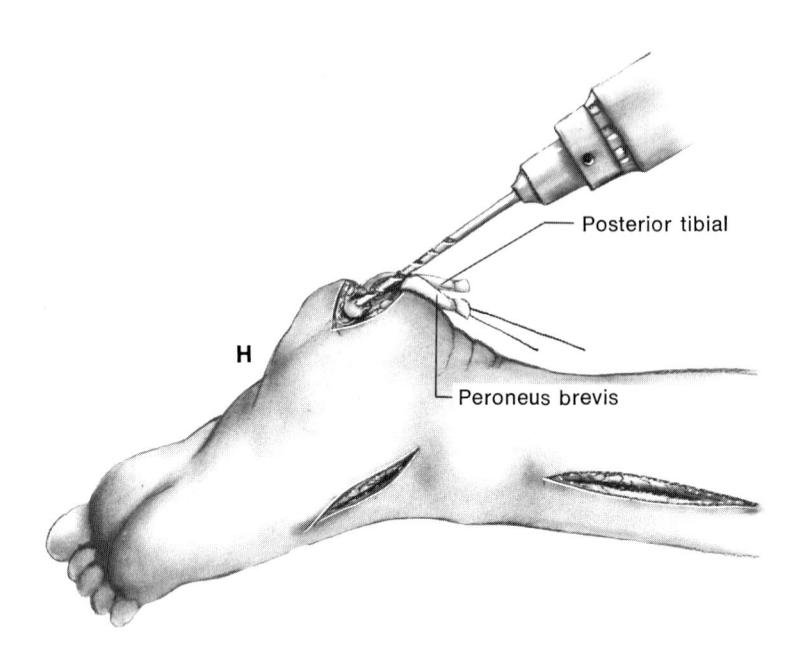

A large drill hole is made through the center of the apophysis of the calcaneus (**H**). The drill hole is directed forward and laterally. With a curet, the drill hole is then enlarged to accept both tendons easily. A Bunnell stainless-steel pull-out suture is placed in both tendons, and the wire suture is pulled through the hole in the calcaneus. The ankle is placed in complete plantar flexion and the tendons are pulled firmly into the bony bed in the calcaneus under moderate tension; the wire suture is tied over a padded button on the sole of the foot (**I**). The pull-out wire exits through the skin over the lower leg posteriorly. The incisions are closed in routine fashion, and a circular plaster cast is applied from the toes to the tibial tubercle, with the foot in complete equinus.

POSTOPERATIVE MANAGEMENT. The cast is removed after 8 weeks. Plantar-flexion exercises are carried out and the ankle is protected for 6 months in a calcaneus brace with a calf strap to prevent dorsiflexion of the ankle above a neutral position during walking.

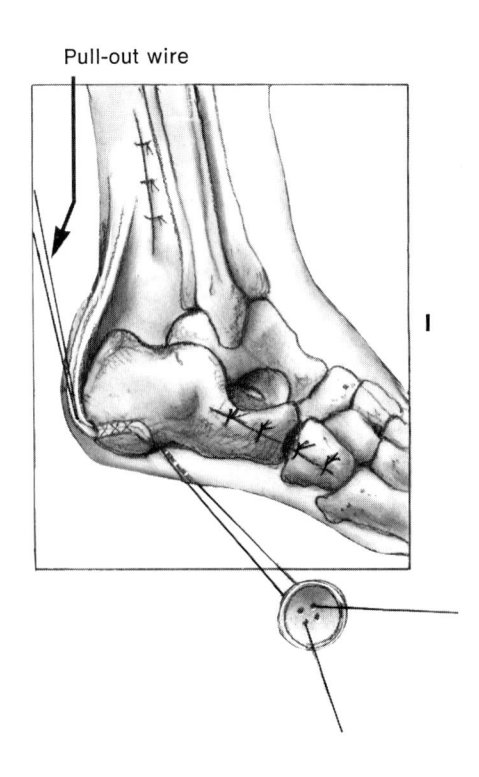

(Plate 14-7) OPEN REDUCTION AND INTERNAL FIXATION FOR FRACTURE OF MEDIAL MALLEOLUS

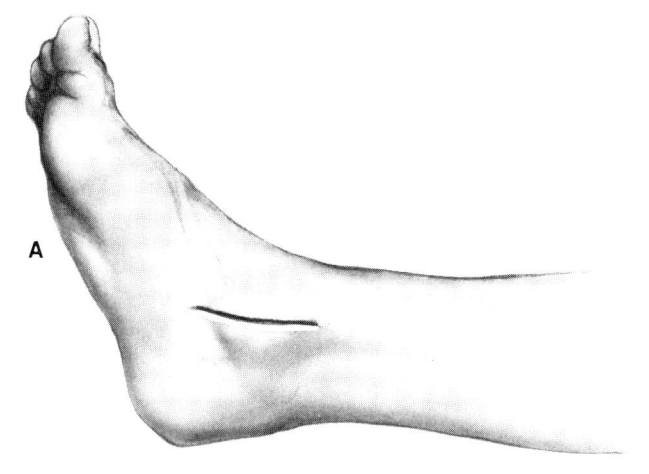

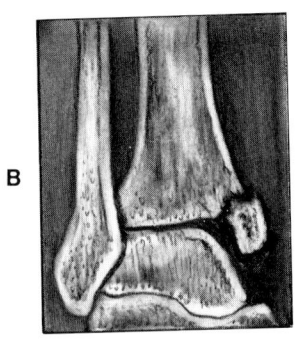

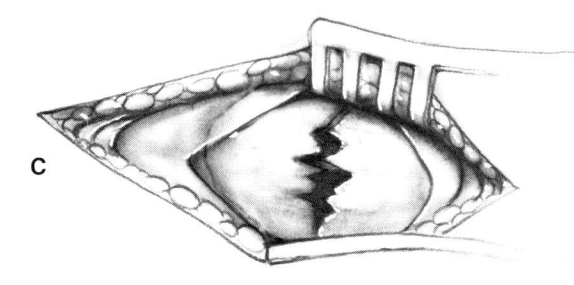

GENERAL DISCUSSION. Following fractures of the ankle, only slight variations from normal are compatible with good joint function. Roentgenograms following any closed reduction should be reviewed with the consideration that the normal relation of the ankle mortise and the contours of the articular surfaces should be anatomically reduced.

For most displaced bimalleolar fractures (**B**), open reduction and internal fixation of the medial malleolus should be considered unless anatomic closed reduction is possible or unless the age and/or general condition of the patient makes operative repair inadvisable. Fixation of the medial malleolus alone is frequently sufficient to obtain good restoration of the ankle mortise and reduction of associated fractures.

DETAILS OF PROCEDURE. With the patient in the semilateral position on the affected side, a longitudinal curvilinear incision is made centered over the medial malleolus (**A** and **C**). The distal fragment of the medial malleolus is often displaced anteriorly. Frequently a small portion of periosteum and/or the posterior tibial tendon may be found interposed between the fracture surfaces. A bone-holding clamp is used to hold the detached medial malleolus in normal position after the hematoma is carefully suctioned and the fracture surfaces visualized. The distal portion of the medial malleolus is held securely in anatomic position as a drill hole is made through its distal tip in a proximal and lateral direction toward the metaphysis of the tibia (this drill hole and the subsequent bone screw must not violate the ankle mortise) (**D**).

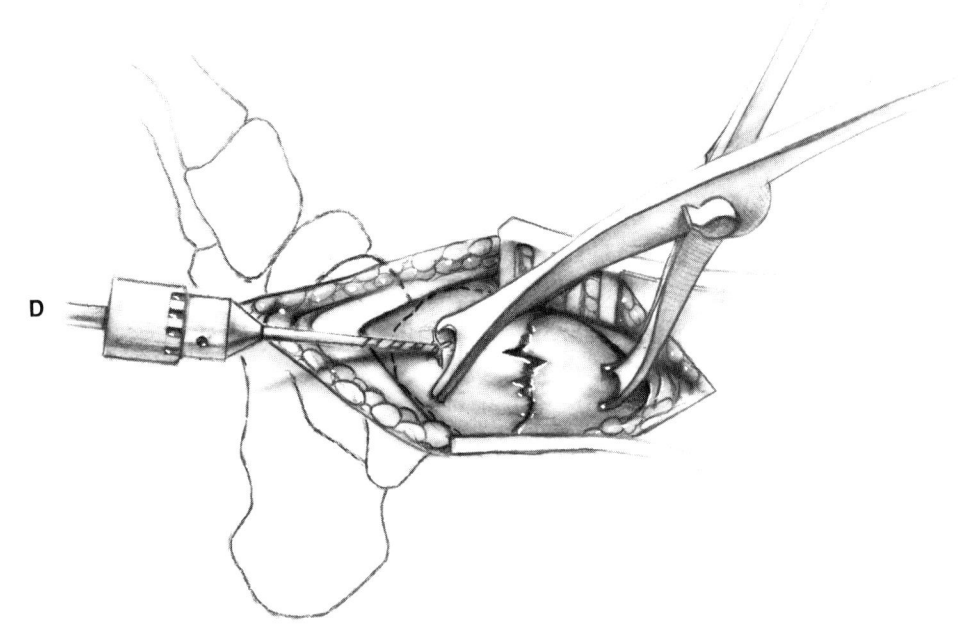

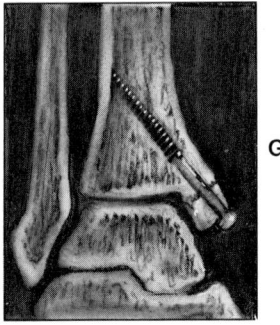

OPEN REDUCTION AND INTERNAL FIXATION FOR FRACTURE OF MEDIAL MALLEOLUS (Plate 14-7)

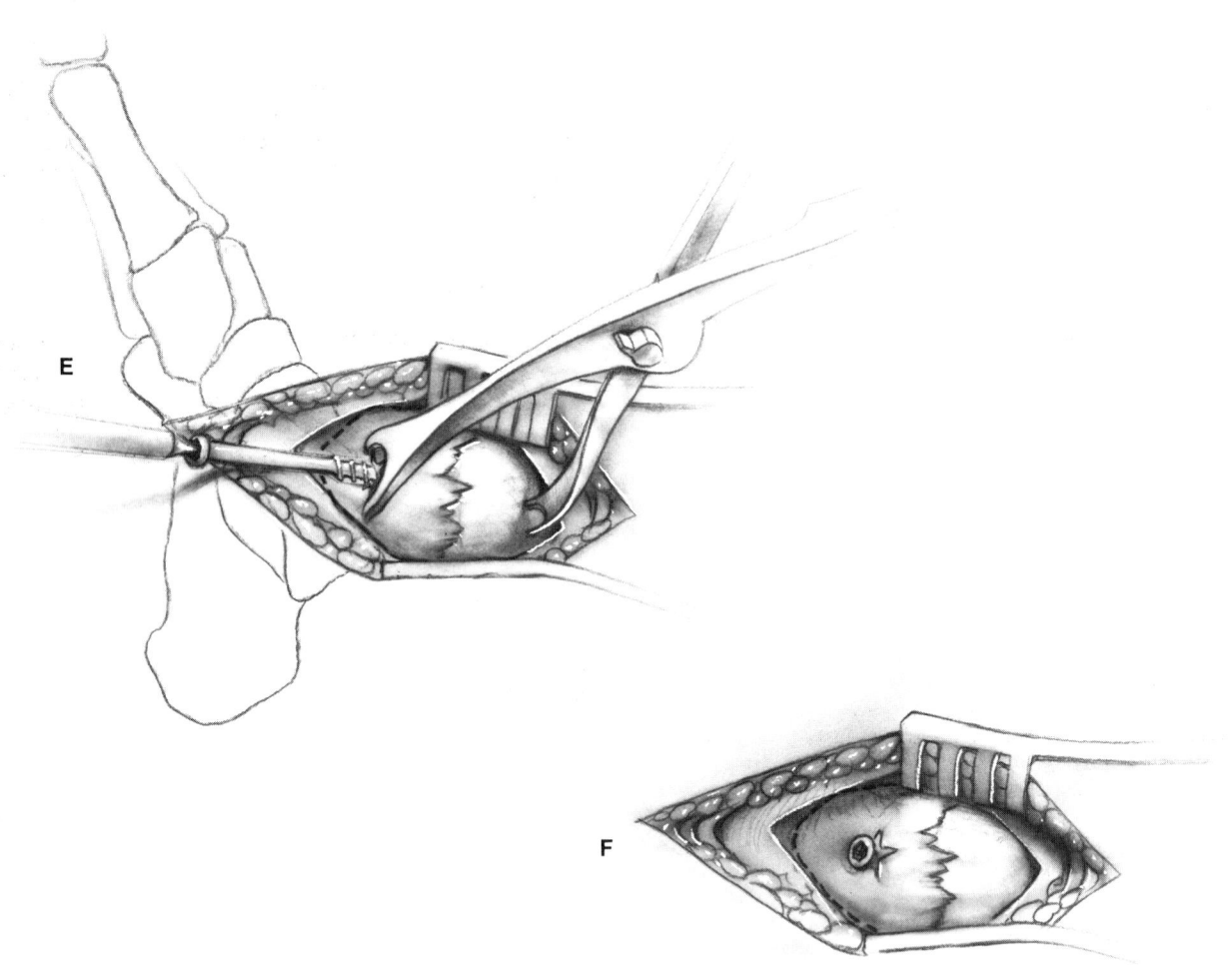

A screw approximately 5 cm long (either a standard bone screw or optionally a compression-type screw) is inserted (**E** and **F**). Roentgenograms must be taken in the operating room prior to final wound closure, or following manipulation of the ankle mortise, to confirm satisfactory position of all fracture fragments, the ankle mortise, and the screw used for internal fixation (**G**). A well-padded external plaster cast should extend from the toes to at least the midthigh level.

POSTOPERATIVE MANAGEMENT. The duration of plaster immobilization is determined by the nature and extent of injuries to the ankle. If the medial malleolus has been an isolated bony injury, plaster immobilization can be discontinued 6 weeks postoperatively. If the medial malleolus is only one of several fractures (for example, a trimalleolar fracture), the top portion of the long-leg cast is removed 10 weeks postoperatively and the remainder of the plaster is generally removed 2 weeks later. Gradual weight bearing is allowed depending on clinical and roentgenographic findings.

(Plate 14-8) OPEN REDUCTION AND INTERNAL FIXATION FOR FRACTURE OF POSTERIOR LIP OF TIBIA

GENERAL DISCUSSION. Among fractures about the ankle joint, trimalleolar-type fractures most frequently require open operative repair. The indications for open reduction of the posterior tibial fragment depend largely on the size of the posterior fragment. If the fragment consists of less than one third of the articular surface, open reduction of the posterior fragment is usually not necessary. The displaced posterior fragment **(B)** will remain in a slightly proximal position unless it is reduced and stablized operatively. If there is even slight posterior subluxation of the talus, this should not be accepted. Proximal displacement of the posterior tibial fragment creates an offset at the fracture. With the foot displaced posteriorly, this irregularity in the articular surface of the tibia is brought against the weight-bearing surface of the talus, shaving and eroding it with motion and weight bearing until traumatic arthritis ultimately develops.

If concomitant open reduction and internal fixation of the medial malleolus is necessary, the posterior tibial fragment should be replaced and fixed internally initially.

DETAILS OF PROCEDURE. The patient is placed in the prone position, and the ankle is supported with folded towels under the anterior aspect of the ankle. A longitudinal incision is made along the lateral border of the tendo Achillis **(A)**. The dissection is continued down to the posterior capsule of the ankle joint by retracting the tendo Achillis and the flexor hallucis longus tendon medially. The flexor hallucis longus tendon will be noted to cross the posterior capsule somewhat obliquely from the superior portion of the wound toward the medial malleolus **(C)**. The entire superior portion of the fracture of the posterior lip of the tibia should be clearly exposed.

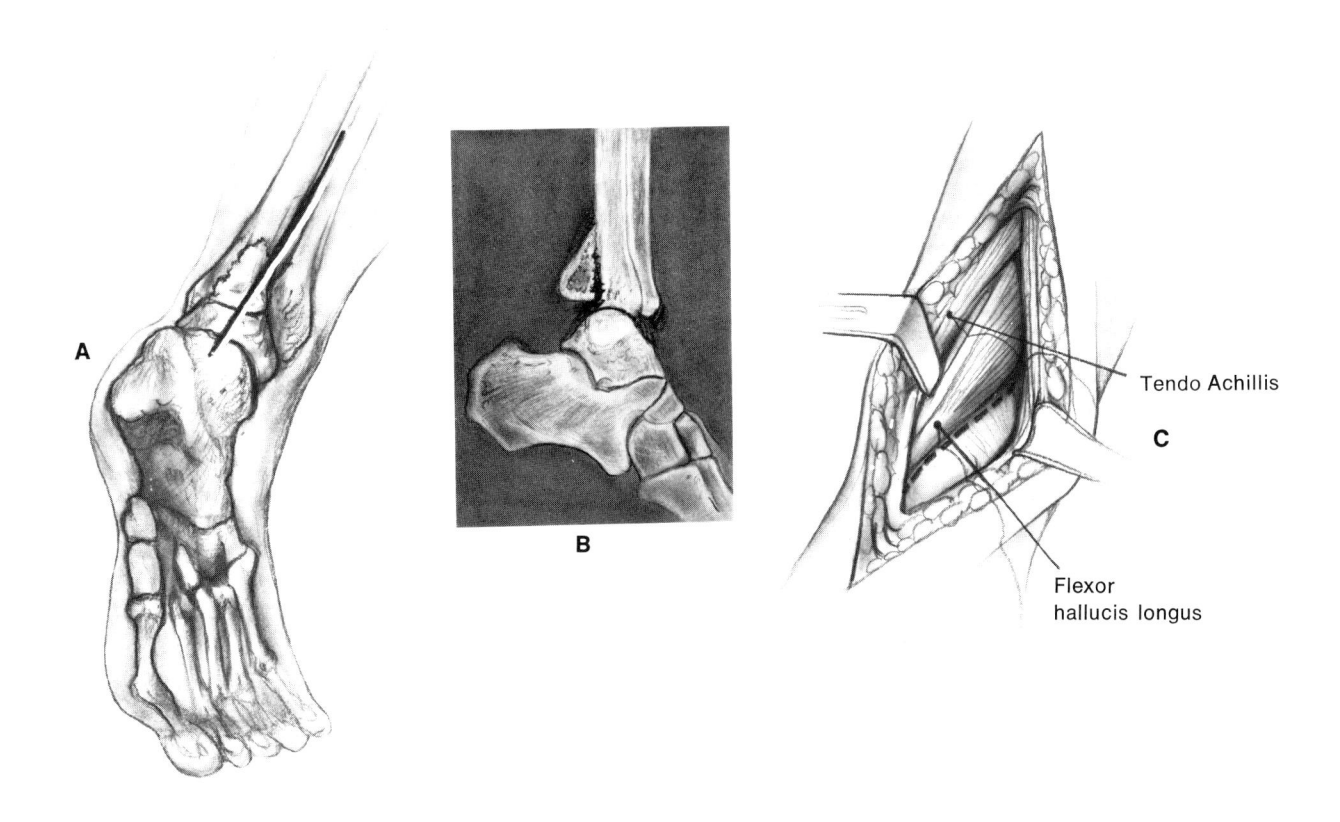

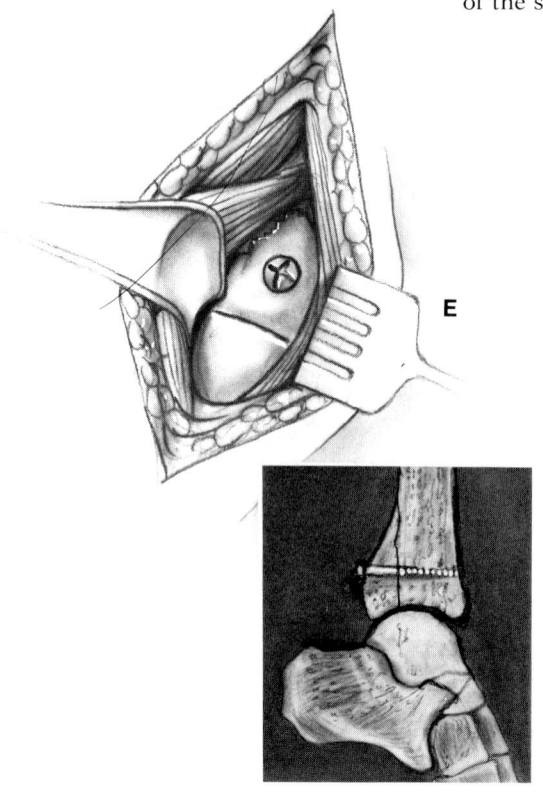

OPEN REDUCTION AND INTERNAL FIXATION FOR FRACTURE OF POSTERIOR LIP OF TIBIA (Plate 14-8)

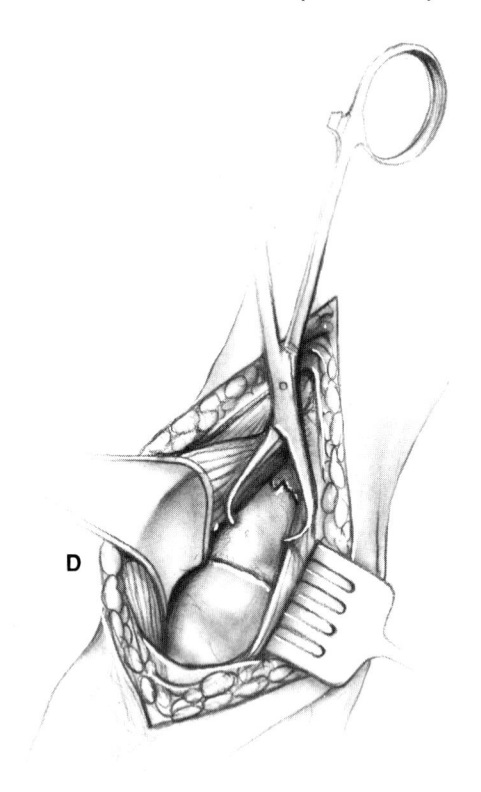

After normal relationship has been established between the talus and tibia by forward traction on the foot and, generally, inversion of the foot as well, the proximal displacement of the posterior lip of the tibia is corrected and held in the reduced position with a suitable bone clamp or pressure bar **(D)**. This fragment should be held firmly in anatomic position while one or two screws are inserted through it into the diaphysis of the tibia **(E)**. The normal concavity of the distal articular surface of the tibia from posterior to anterior must be considered in the placement of any transfixing screw to avoid encroachment on the articular surface of the ankle joint with the transfixing screw. The position of the fracture and the tibiotalar relationship should be checked by roentgenograms before the wound is closed **(F)**. If a closed manipulation is necessary in addition to fixation of the posterior lip of the tibia, additional roentgenograms must be obtained to confirm the position of all fragments following application of the long-leg plaster cast.

POSTOPERATIVE MANAGEMENT. Repeat roentgenograms of the ankle should be obtained 1 week postoperatively. The wound can be examined and sutures removed through a window in the posterior portion of the cast 10 to 14 days postoperatively. Depending on the nature of the total ankle injury, plaster immobilization may be discontinued 10 to 12 weeks postoperatively. The top portion of the cast is removed 2 weeks prior to removal of the lower leg portion of the cast to allow the patient to regain free knee motion. Gradual weight bearing is resumed subsequently depending on the nature of the specific injury and the degree of overall stability.

(Plate 14-9) INTERNAL FIXATION FOR TIBIOFIBULAR DIASTASIS

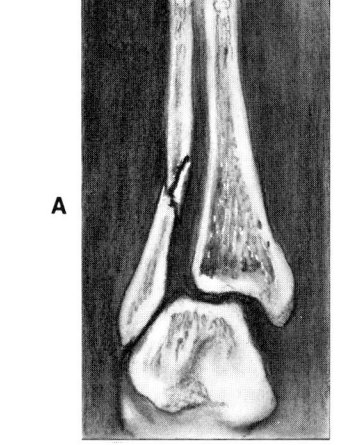

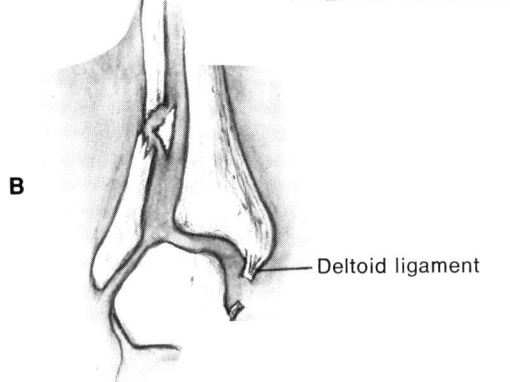

GENERAL DISCUSSION. The tibiofibular ligaments retaining the distal ends of the tibia and fibula in approximation are often damaged by forces transmitted through the ankle. There may be associated fractures of the malleoli or fibular shaft and subluxation or dislocation of the ankle. In most instances of disruption of the normal inferior tibiofibular relationship, there is a fracture of the fibula 5 to 15 cm proximal to the distal end of the fibula, frequently with a triangular segment of fibular cortex on the medial or lateral side, fracture of the medial malleolus or complete tear of the deltoid ligament, and lateral displacement of the talus (**A** and **B**).

The tibiofibular ligaments are located in the coronal plane and constitute the tibiofibular syndesmosis. They are necessary for stability of the ankle mortise. When there has been disruption of the tibiofibular ligaments with or without associated fractures, the goal should be perfect anatomic reduction. If this cannot be obtained by closed manipulation, open reduction and internal fixation of the tibiofibular diastasis are indicated.

DETAILS OF PROCEDURE. A longitudinal incision is made laterally over the distal fibula **(C)**. The ankle mortise is reduced, and while the foot is held in neutral position (specifically, no plantar flexion), a transfixing screw or Barr bolt is inserted through the fibula and into the tibia to retain the reduced anatomic position of the inferior tibiofibular relationship and the ankle mortise **(D)**. Position of the ankle mortise and the screw (or bolt) used for internal fixation should be checked roentgenographically prior to wound closure **(E)**. A long-leg cast is applied following closure of the wound.

POSTOPERATIVE MANAGEMENT. The cast is removed and weight bearing is started when bone healing and mortise stability are anticipated clinically and roentgenographically, usually 8 to 12 weeks postoperatively.

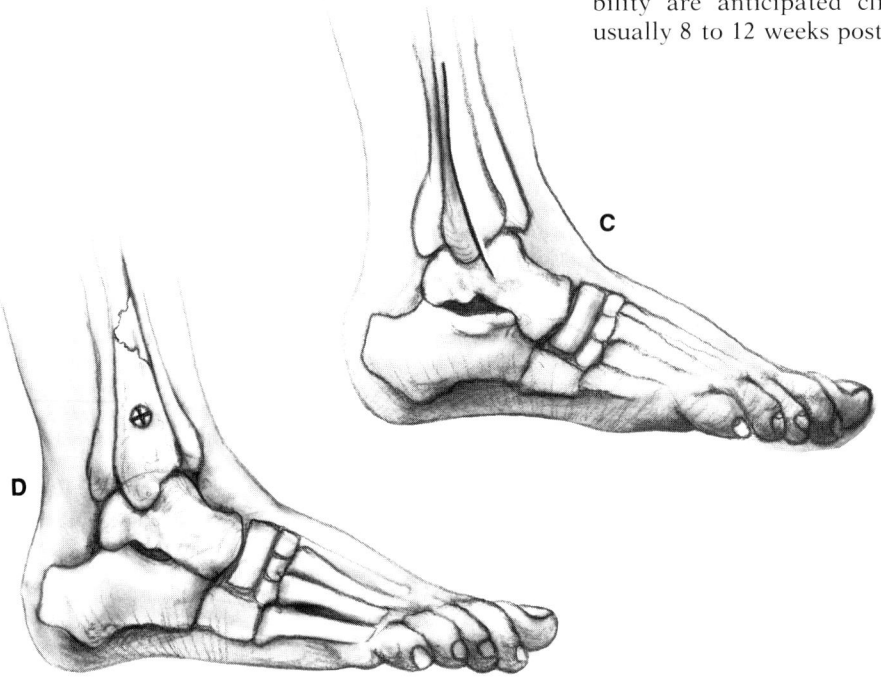

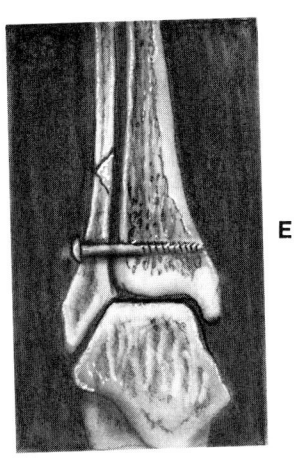

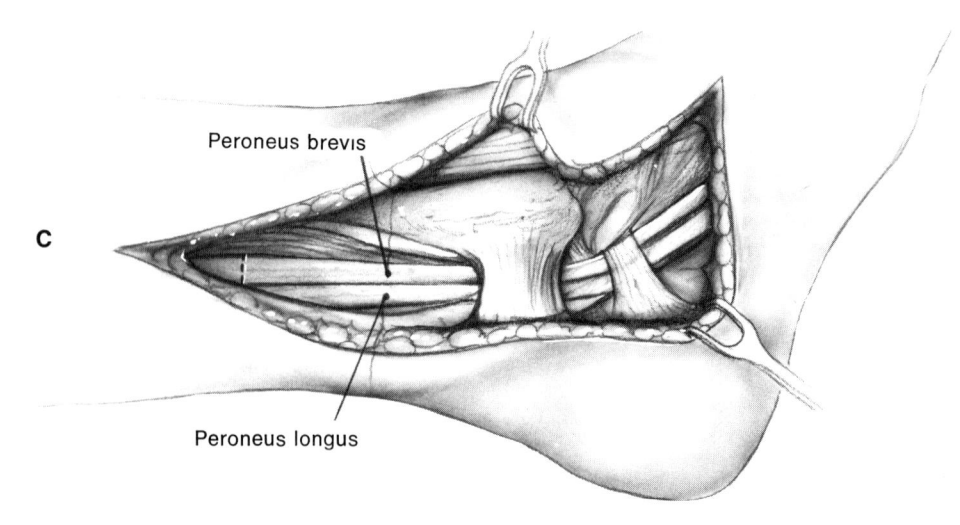

RECONSTRUCTION OF LATERAL LIGAMENTS OF ANKLE (Plate 14-10)

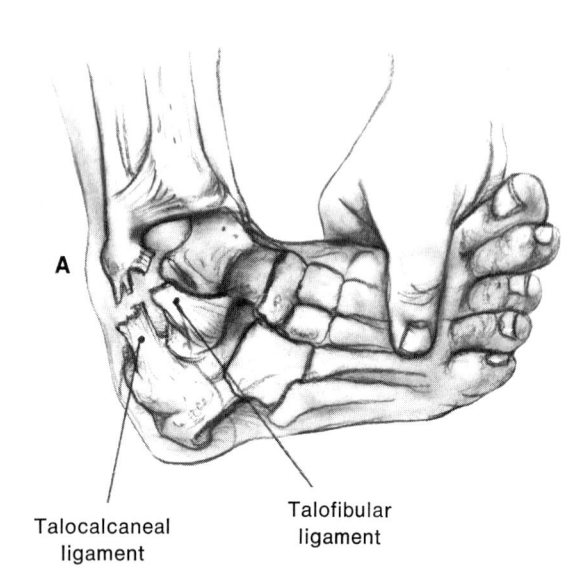

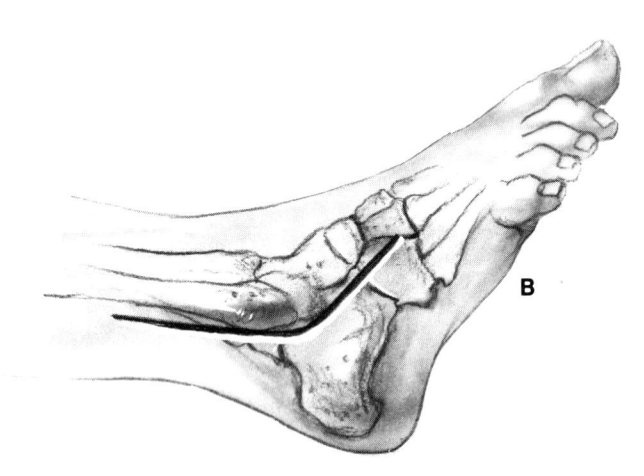

GENERAL DISCUSSION. If there is recurrent instability of the ankle following old rupture of the lateral ligaments of the ankle or occasionally after acute injury involving combined rupture of the anterior talofibular and talocalcaneal ligaments (associated with demonstrable talar tilt exceeding 15°) **(A)**, the lateral ligaments of the ankle can be reconstructed with the tendon of the peroneus brevis.

DETAILS OF PROCEDURE. A lateral incision is made beginning at the junction of the middle and distal thirds of the fibula, extending along the posterior border of the shaft of the distal fibula, and then curving forward to end 5 cm anterior to the tip of the lateral malleolus **(B)**. The peroneus brevis tendon is divided from its muscle (**C** and **D**) as far proximally as possible, and the proximal end of the divided peroneus brevis is sutured to the peroneus longus tendon.

A tunnel large enough to receive the tendon of the peroneus brevis is then drilled through the fibula, beginning at the tip of the lateral malleolus and emerging posteriorly 3 cm proximal to the distal end of the fibula.

The tendon of the peroneus brevis, withdrawn distally from beneath the peroneal retinaculum, is passed through this tunnel in the fibula from distal to proximal and sutured under tension to the adjacent soft tissue at both ends of the tunnel while the foot is held in slight eversion **(E)**. Following wound closure, a short-leg cast is applied holding the ankle and subtalar joints in neutral position.

An alternative technique **(F)** is to pass the tendon of peroneus brevis through drill holes in the fibula and talus in the manner described by Watson-Jones.

POSTOPERATIVE MANAGEMENT. Weight bearing is allowed on the involved ankle in the short-leg cast beginning 2 to 3 weeks postoperatively. The cast is removed 8 weeks postoperatively, and unlimited activity is allowed subsequently.

(Plate 14-10) RECONSTRUCTION OF LATERAL LIGAMENTS OF ANKLE

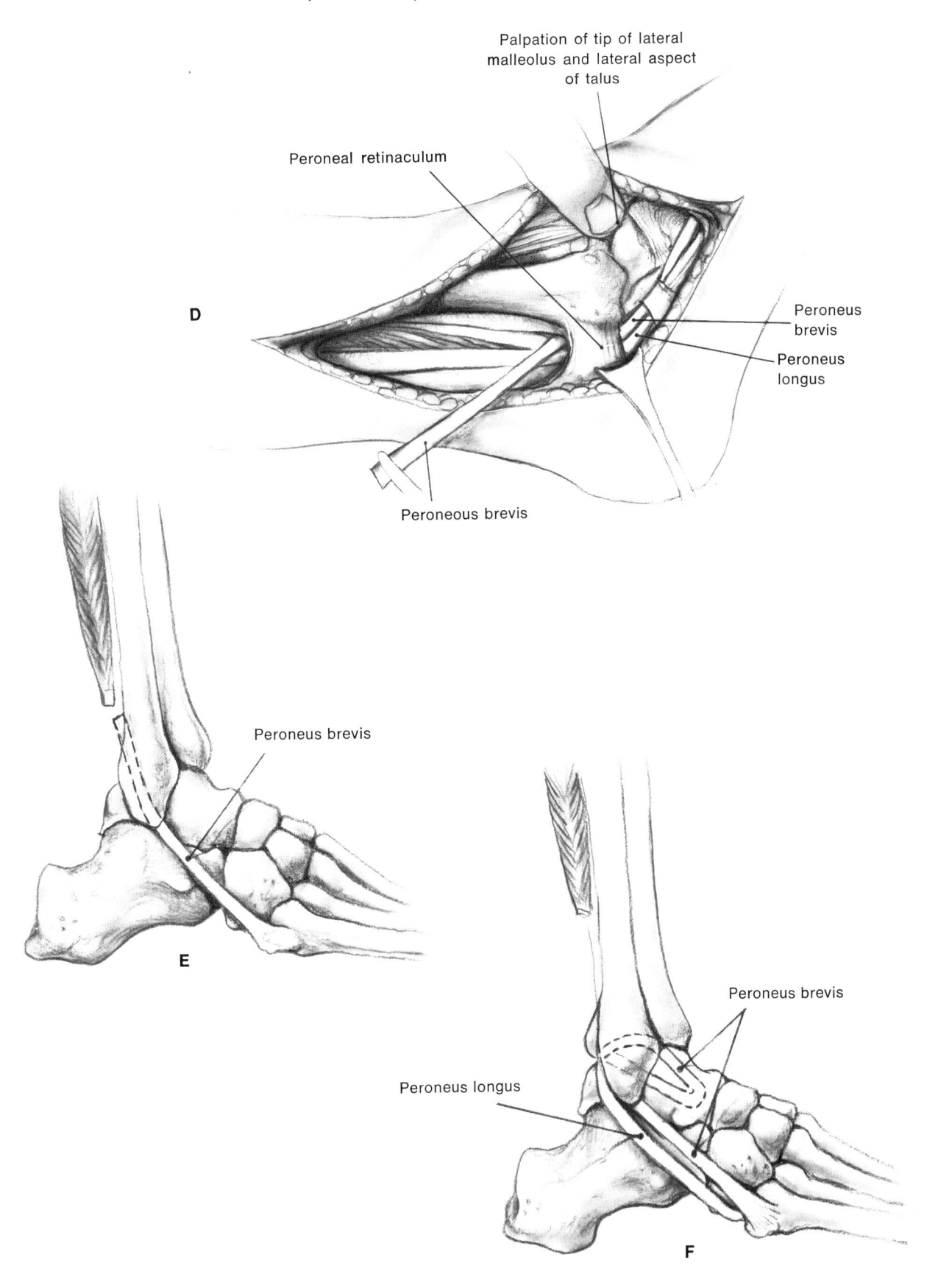

DRAINAGE OF ANKLE JOINT (Plate 14-11)

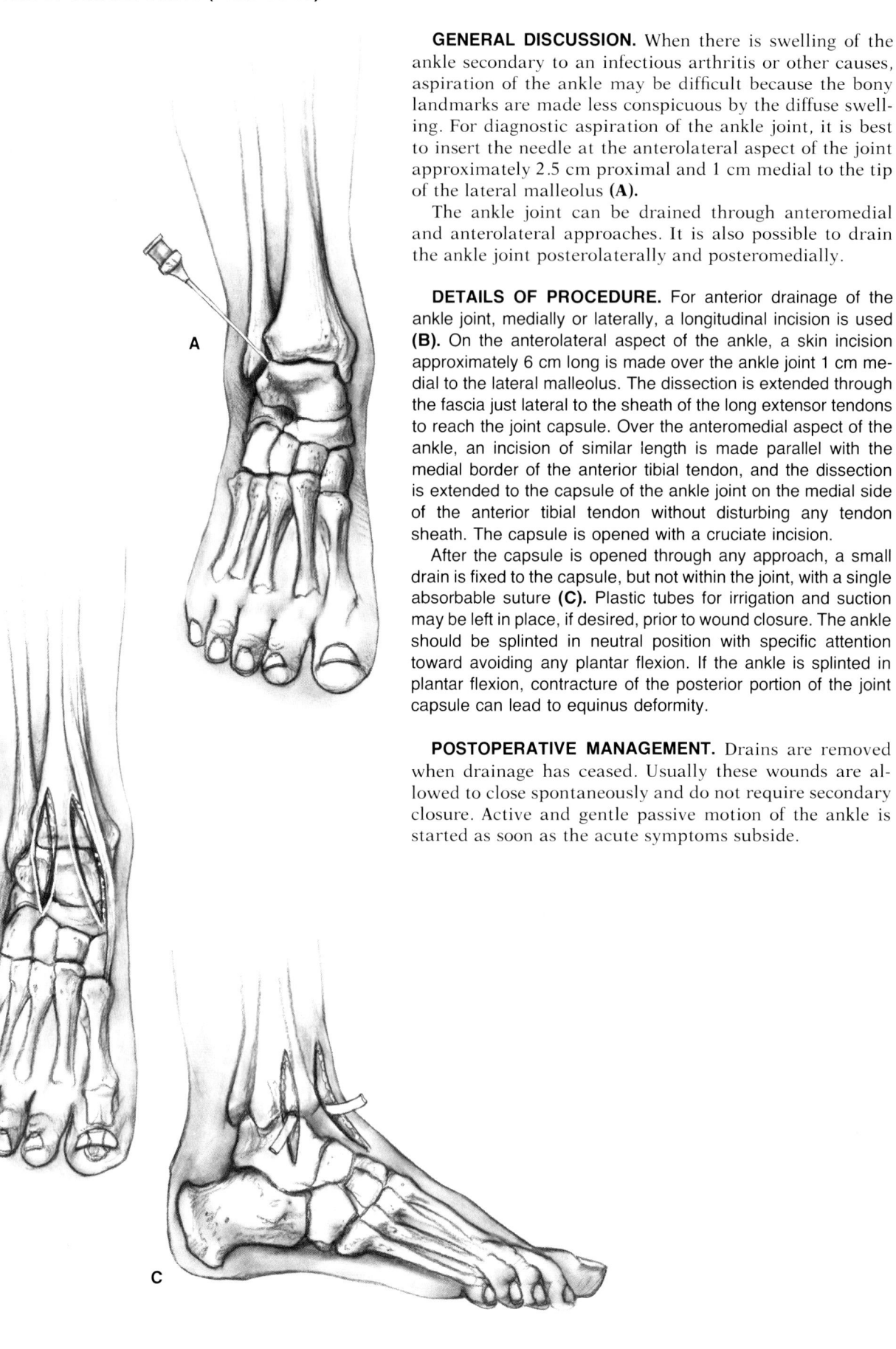

GENERAL DISCUSSION. When there is swelling of the ankle secondary to an infectious arthritis or other causes, aspiration of the ankle may be difficult because the bony landmarks are made less conspicuous by the diffuse swelling. For diagnostic aspiration of the ankle joint, it is best to insert the needle at the anterolateral aspect of the joint approximately 2.5 cm proximal and 1 cm medial to the tip of the lateral malleolus (**A**).

The ankle joint can be drained through anteromedial and anterolateral approaches. It is also possible to drain the ankle joint posterolaterally and posteromedially.

DETAILS OF PROCEDURE. For anterior drainage of the ankle joint, medially or laterally, a longitudinal incision is used (**B**). On the anterolateral aspect of the ankle, a skin incision approximately 6 cm long is made over the ankle joint 1 cm medial to the lateral malleolus. The dissection is extended through the fascia just lateral to the sheath of the long extensor tendons to reach the joint capsule. Over the anteromedial aspect of the ankle, an incision of similar length is made parallel with the medial border of the anterior tibial tendon, and the dissection is extended to the capsule of the ankle joint on the medial side of the anterior tibial tendon without disturbing any tendon sheath. The capsule is opened with a cruciate incision.

After the capsule is opened through any approach, a small drain is fixed to the capsule, but not within the joint, with a single absorbable suture (**C**). Plastic tubes for irrigation and suction may be left in place, if desired, prior to wound closure. The ankle should be splinted in neutral position with specific attention toward avoiding any plantar flexion. If the ankle is splinted in plantar flexion, contracture of the posterior portion of the joint capsule can lead to equinus deformity.

POSTOPERATIVE MANAGEMENT. Drains are removed when drainage has ceased. Usually these wounds are allowed to close spontaneously and do not require secondary closure. Active and gentle passive motion of the ankle is started as soon as the acute symptoms subside.

(Plate 14-12) MODIFIED SYME AMPUTATION

GENERAL DISCUSSION. This procedure may occasionally be indicated for a deformed, diseased, or severely injured foot.

DETAILS OF PROCEDURE. With the foot and ankle in neutral position, the incision is outlined with a marking pen. The anterior portion of the incision begins at a point below the tip of the medial malleolus and extends across the anterior aspect of the ankle joint to a point below the tip of the lateral malleolus. The other portion of the incision extends vertically downward from the medial malleolus, across the plantar aspect of the foot, and up to meet the lateral end of the initial incision **(A)**. All structures are divided in line with the skin incisions down to bone **(B)**. The anterior capsule of the ankle joint is opened completely. The medial and lateral collateral ligaments are divided. When these ligaments have been divided, inferior dislocation of the talus can be accomplished. With maximum plantar flexion of the foot, the posterior structures can be dissected off the talus and the calcaneus. The tendo Achillis is divided at its insertion. As the talus is plantar flexed and dislocated from the ankle joint, the soft tissue on the plantar surface of the calcaneus is dissected subperiosteally. This subperiosteal dissection is important to preserve intact the specialized subcutaneous tissue in the heel flap for the ultimate end bearing stump. When the calcaneus has been mobilized subperiosteally to the level of the plantar skin incision, the periosteum is divided at this level, and the foot, including the talus and calcaneus, is entirely removed. In the plantar flap, arteries are ligated only at the cut edge of the skin flap. The calcaneal arteries form the most important blood supply to the plantar flap and, if injured, can cause loss of the skin flap. These arteries can be avoided by dissecting only subperiosteally. Nerves are divided sharply at the level of the skin incision. The muscles in the plantar flap are not removed or dissected. If "dog ears" persist with the plantar flap, these should not be trimmed, since this might impair the circulation. The distal end of the tibia is removed to make a level surface. In children, this may be a matter of removing the cartilage of the joint surface. In older patients, a transverse cut is made through the bone just above the tibial articular surface. The fibula is divided simultaneously at the same level **(C)**.

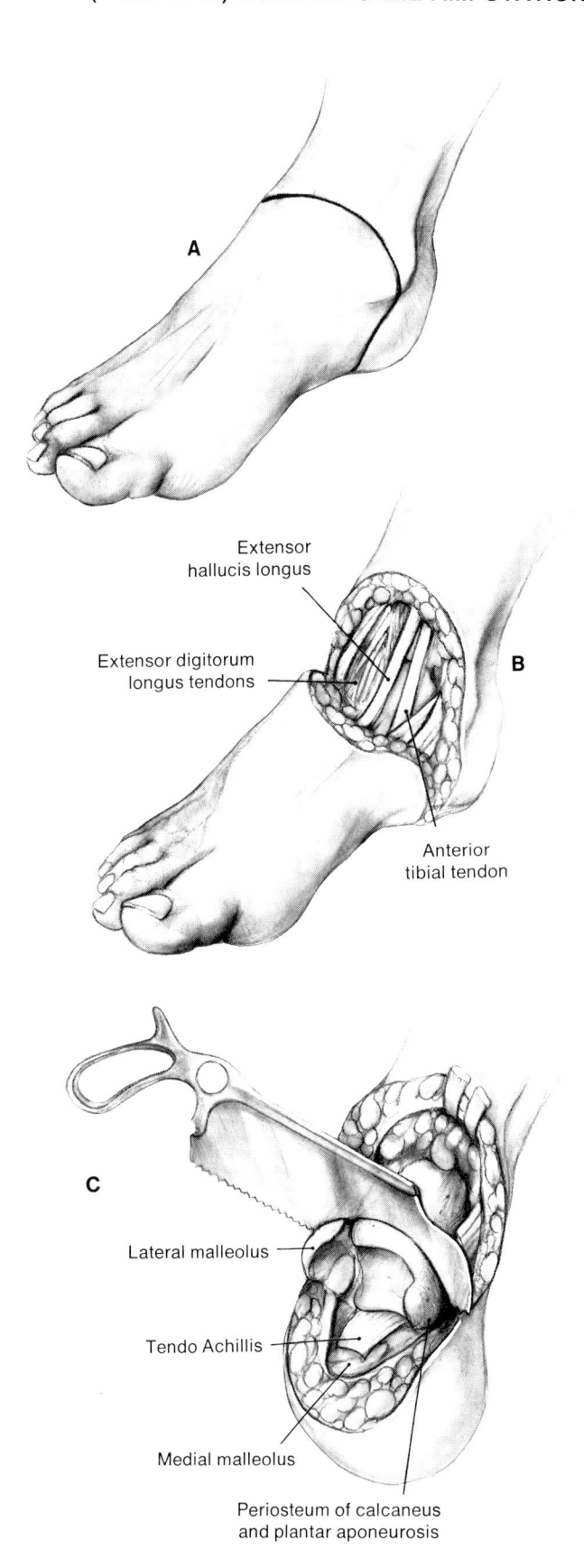

MODIFIED SYME AMPUTATION (Plate 14-12)

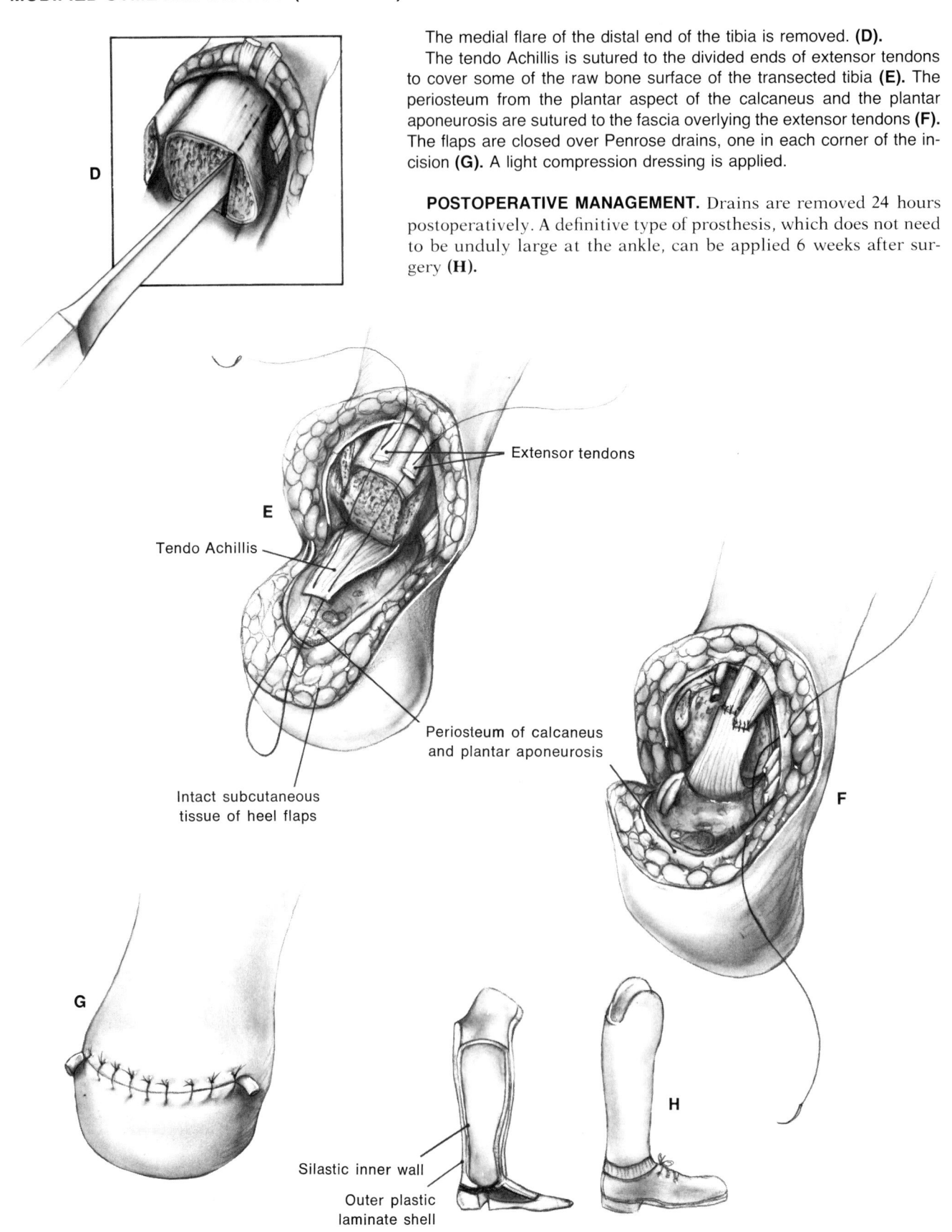

The medial flare of the distal end of the tibia is removed. **(D)**.

The tendo Achillis is sutured to the divided ends of extensor tendons to cover some of the raw bone surface of the transected tibia **(E)**. The periosteum from the plantar aspect of the calcaneus and the plantar aponeurosis are sutured to the fascia overlying the extensor tendons **(F)**. The flaps are closed over Penrose drains, one in each corner of the incision **(G)**. A light compression dressing is applied.

POSTOPERATIVE MANAGEMENT. Drains are removed 24 hours postoperatively. A definitive type of prosthesis, which does not need to be unduly large at the ankle, can be applied 6 weeks after surgery **(H)**.

(Plate 14-13) ARTHRODESIS OF ANKLE (LATERAL APPROACH)

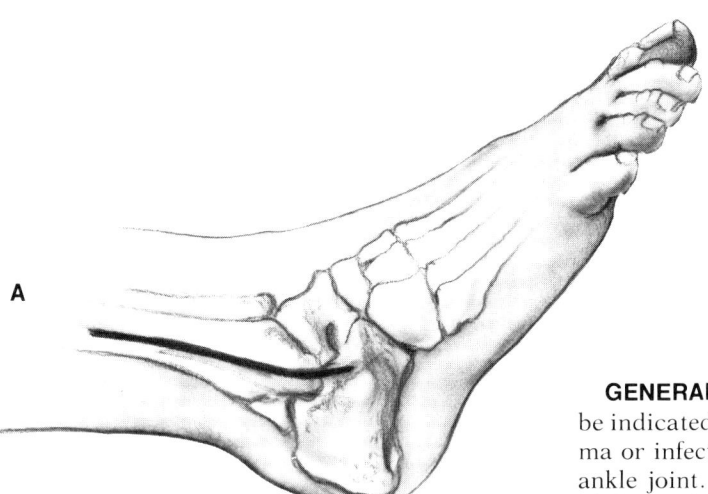

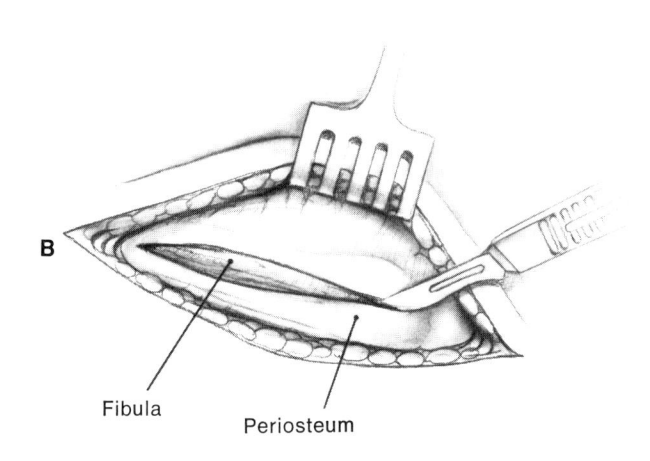

GENERAL DISCUSSION. Arthrodesis of the ankle may be indicated for stabilization of the ankle following trauma or infection or for paralytic conditions affecting the ankle joint. Generally, the best position for arthrodesis of the ankle is in neutral position with respect to dorsiflexion and plantar flexion. One alternative method for arthrodesis of the ankle is carried out through a lateral or transfibular approach.

DETAILS OF PROCEDURE. A longitudinal incision is made along the subcutaneous surface of the distal fibula. The distal end of the incision should curve gently forward below the tip of the lateral malleous **(A)**. This incision allows exposure of the distal 10 cm of the fibula and the lateral aspect of the talus. The distal fibula is exposed subperiosteally **(B)**, and drill holes are made in preparation for osteotomy of the fibula **(C)**. The fibula is osteotomized obliquely to minimize the prominence of the remaining proximal fibula.

537

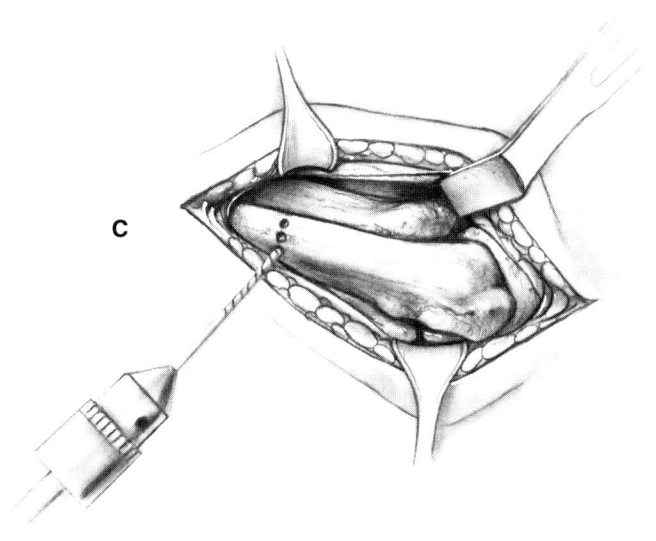

ARTHRODESIS OF ANKLE (LATERAL APPROACH) (Plate 14-13)

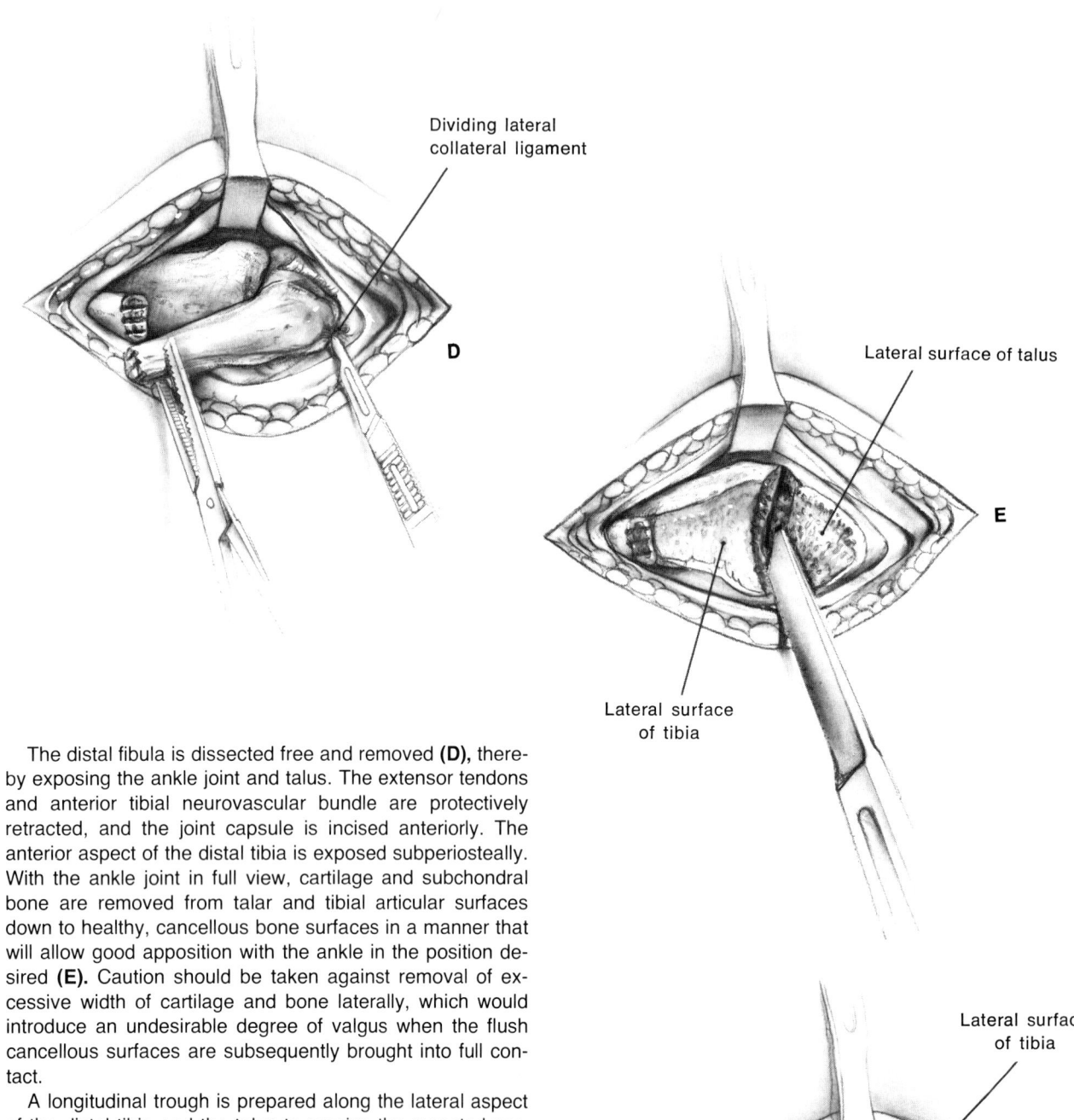

The distal fibula is dissected free and removed **(D)**, thereby exposing the ankle joint and talus. The extensor tendons and anterior tibial neurovascular bundle are protectively retracted, and the joint capsule is incised anteriorly. The anterior aspect of the distal tibia is exposed subperiosteally. With the ankle joint in full view, cartilage and subchondral bone are removed from talar and tibial articular surfaces down to healthy, cancellous bone surfaces in a manner that will allow good apposition with the ankle in the position desired **(E)**. Caution should be taken against removal of excessive width of cartilage and bone laterally, which would introduce an undesirable degree of valgus when the flush cancellous surfaces are subsequently brought into full contact.

A longitudinal trough is prepared along the lateral aspect of the distal tibia and the talus to receive the resected portion of fibula. The resected fibula is likewise rongeured superficially on its contact surface. When everything is ready, the ankle is carefully held in the desired position, and two staples are placed across the joint (posterolaterally and anterolaterally) to stabilize it in the selected position **(F)**.

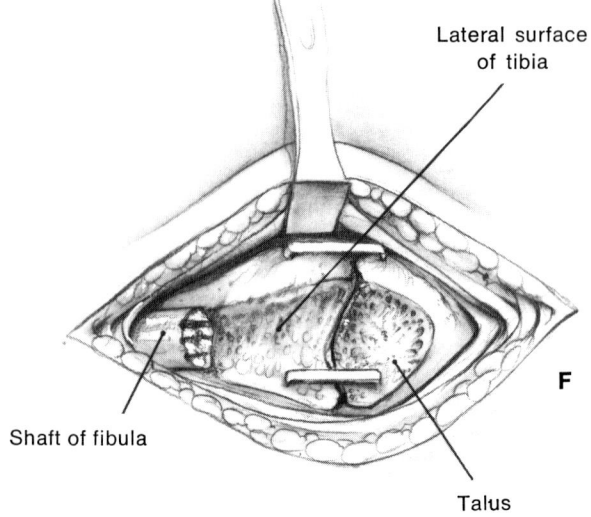

538

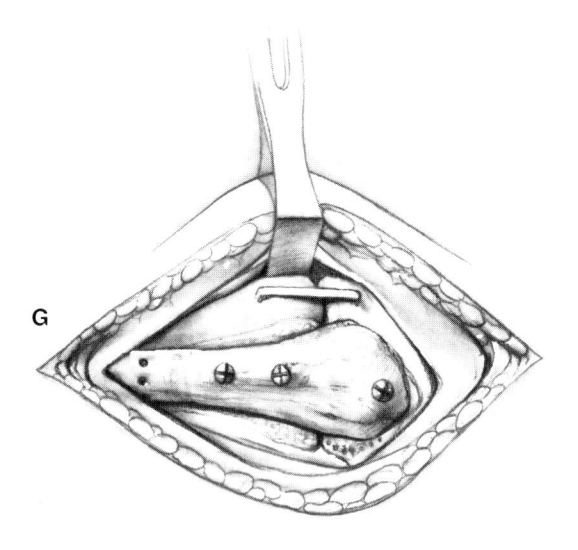

(Plate 14-13) ARTHRODESIS OF ANKLE (LATERAL APPROACH)

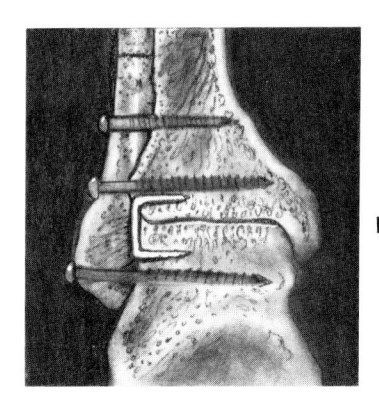

The prepared fibular graft is then placed across the joint and secured in that position with two or three screws (**G** to **I**). The cancellous surfaces of the distal tibia and superior aspect of the talus should be in firm apposition with the foot at 90° to the longitudinal axis of the tibia. The wound is closed in layers by reapproximation of the periosteofascial flap over the fibula, subcutaneous tissue, and skin. A well-molded circular cast is applied up to the knee.

POSTOPERATIVE MANAGEMENT. Immobilization is maintained for 3 months or until a solid fusion is evident roentgenographically. Weight bearing in the cast may be allowed at 6 weeks.

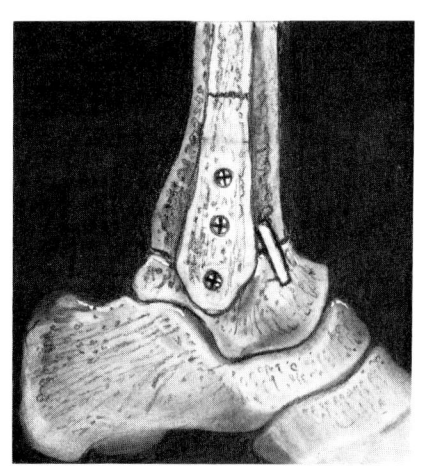

539

COMPRESSION ARTHRODESIS OF ANKLE (ANTERIOR APPROACH) (Plate 14-14)

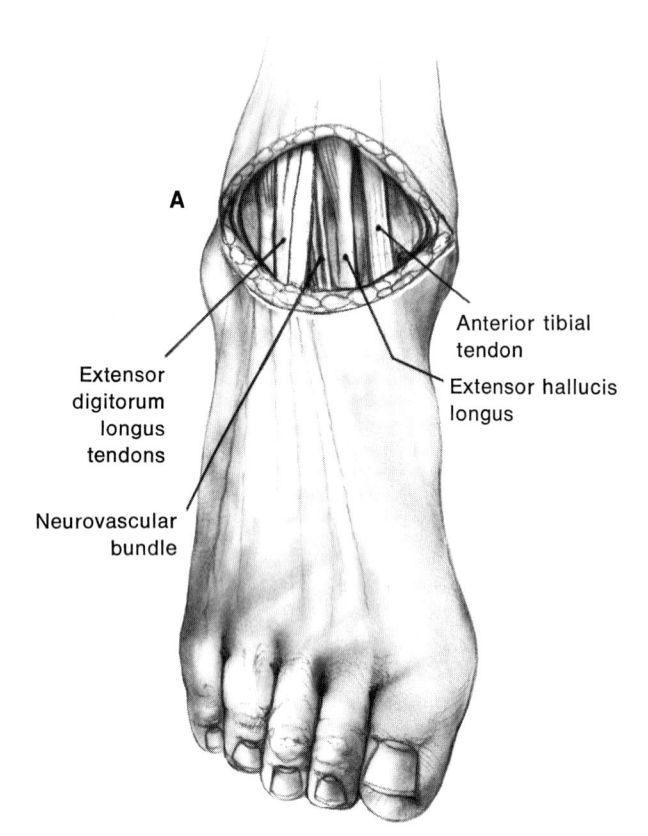

GENERAL DISCUSSION. The compression principle is specifically helpful in arthrodesis procedures, the knee and ankle joints being more suitable than other major joints. Charnley has pointed out that fusion can be obtained more readily by compression arthrodesis than by other methods. The technique is useful for malunited fractures of the ankle; equinus and medial and lateral angular deformities can be readily corrected. Compression arthrodesis is also a potential method for fusing the ankle of a growing child without damaging the distal tibial epiphyseal plate.

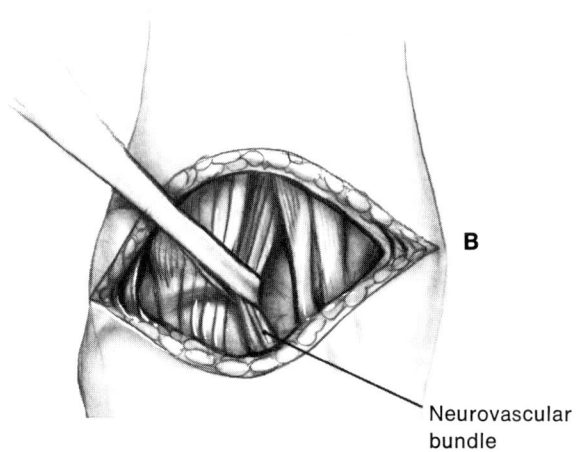

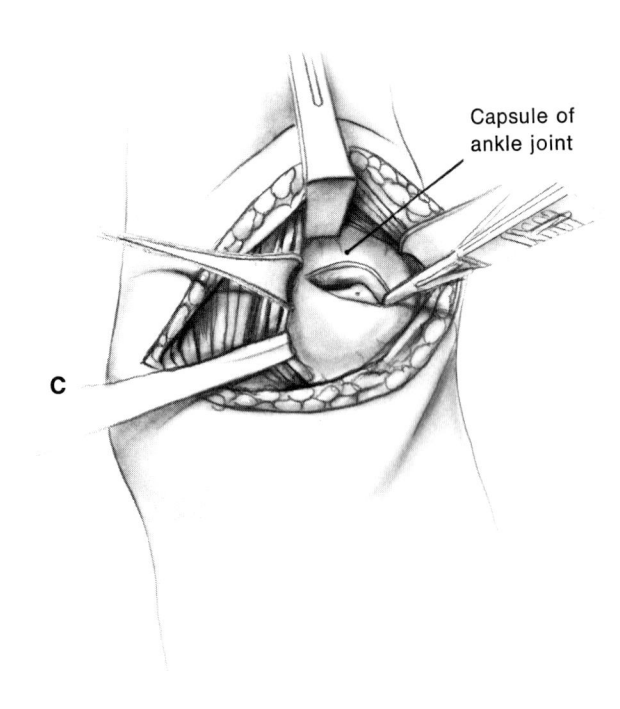

DETAILS OF PROCEDURE. The incision is made across the anterior aspect of the ankle joint extending from a point 1 cm proximal to the tip of the medial malleolus to a comparable position over the lateral malleolus. The incision should be curved distally at its midportion so the line of division of the extensor tendons will not be directly beneath the skin incision **(A)**. Skin and subcutaneous tissues are dissected proximally to form a thick flap and to expose the extensor tendons. Although Charnley divides all extensor tendons and the neurovascular bundle anteriorly, it is possible to accomplish compression arthrodesis of the ankle by mobilizing and retracting the extensor tendons and the neurovascular bundle **(B)**. The soft tissues are mobilized so that a periosteal elevator can be placed posterior to each malleolus in conjunction with exposure of the distal tibia. The capsule of the ankle joint is opened anteriorly **(C)**.

(Plate 14-14) COMPRESSION ARTHRODESIS OF ANKLE (ANTERIOR APPROACH)

The collateral ligaments are divided **(D)** on both sides of the ankle, and the foot is plantar flexed. As the extensor tendons and neurovascular bundle are retracted medially or laterally as necessary for exposure, the articular surfaces of the distal tibia and fibula are removed **(E)**. With the foot in the desired position, a section of bone approximately 6 mm thick is removed from the superior surface of the talus **(F)**.

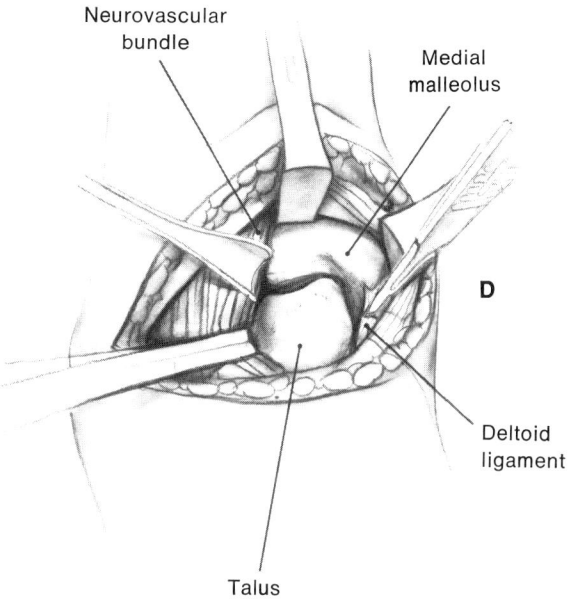

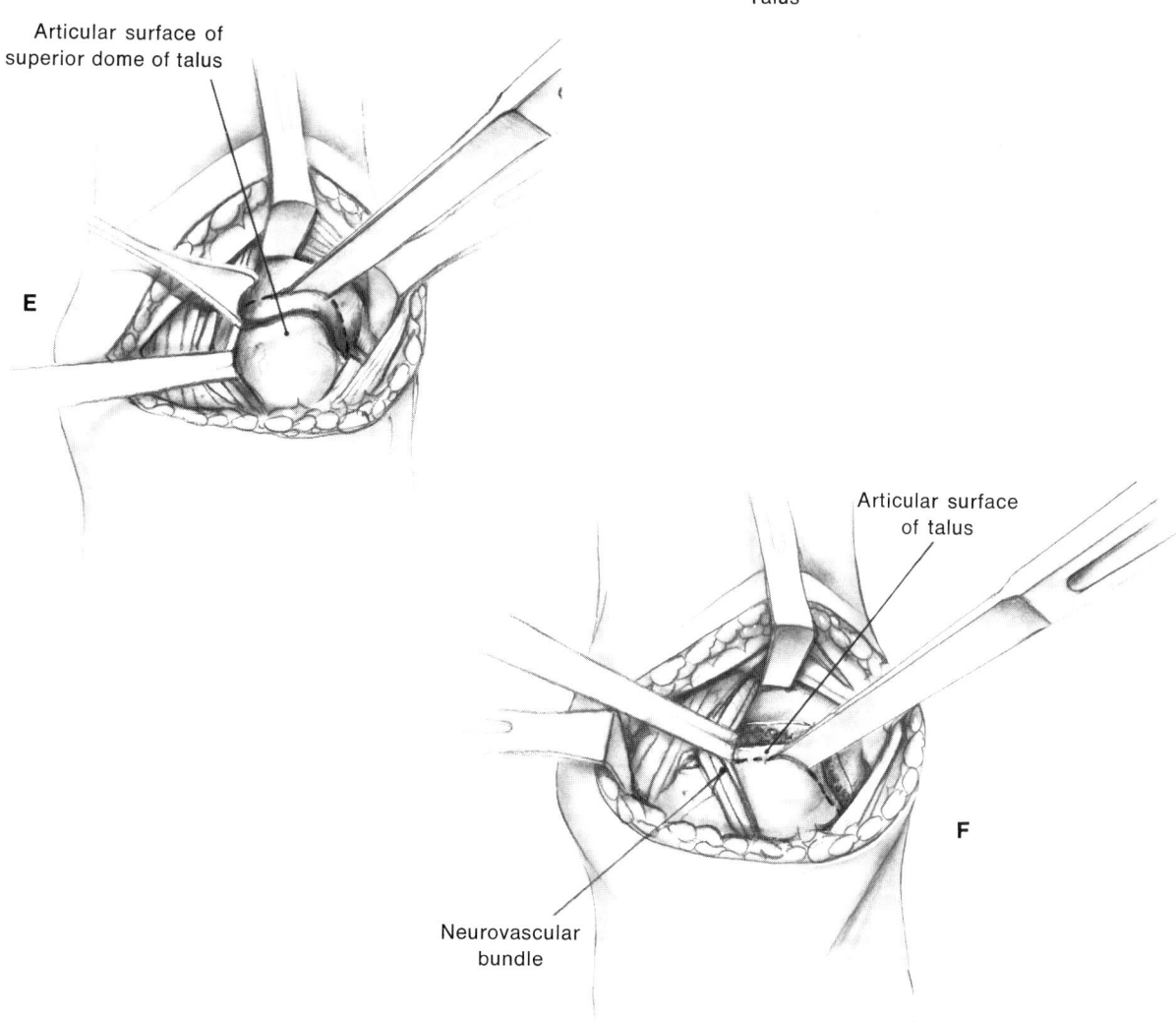

COMPRESSION ARTHRODESIS OF ANKLE (ANTERIOR APPROACH) (Plate 14-14)

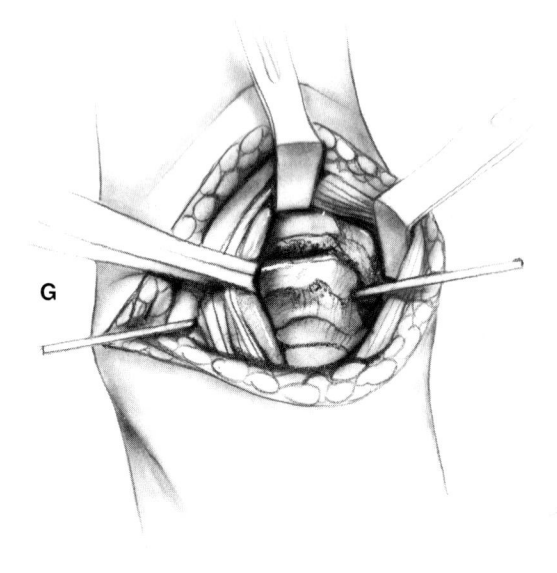

A Steinmann pin is passed through the talus well anterior to the axis of the talus so the pull of the pin will counterbalance the pull of the tendo Achillis posteriorly (**G** and **I**). Care should be taken to avoid penetrating the subtalar joint with this distal pin. The compression clamp should then be applied to the distal pin to serve as a guide for locating the proper level to insert the proximal pin through the shaft of the tibia. With both Steinmann pins in place, the compression clamps are applied and tightened (**H**). Any rotatory deformity is corrected simultaneously. Following wound closure, a well-padded short-leg cast incorporating the two Steinmann pins is applied.

POSTOPERATIVE MANAGEMENT. The initial cast and the two Steinmann pins are removed 4 to 6 weeks postoperatively, and a well-molded walking short-leg cast is immediately reapplied. Below-knee plaster immobilization is continued for an additional 4 weeks or until there is roentgenographic and clinical evidence that the fusion is solid.

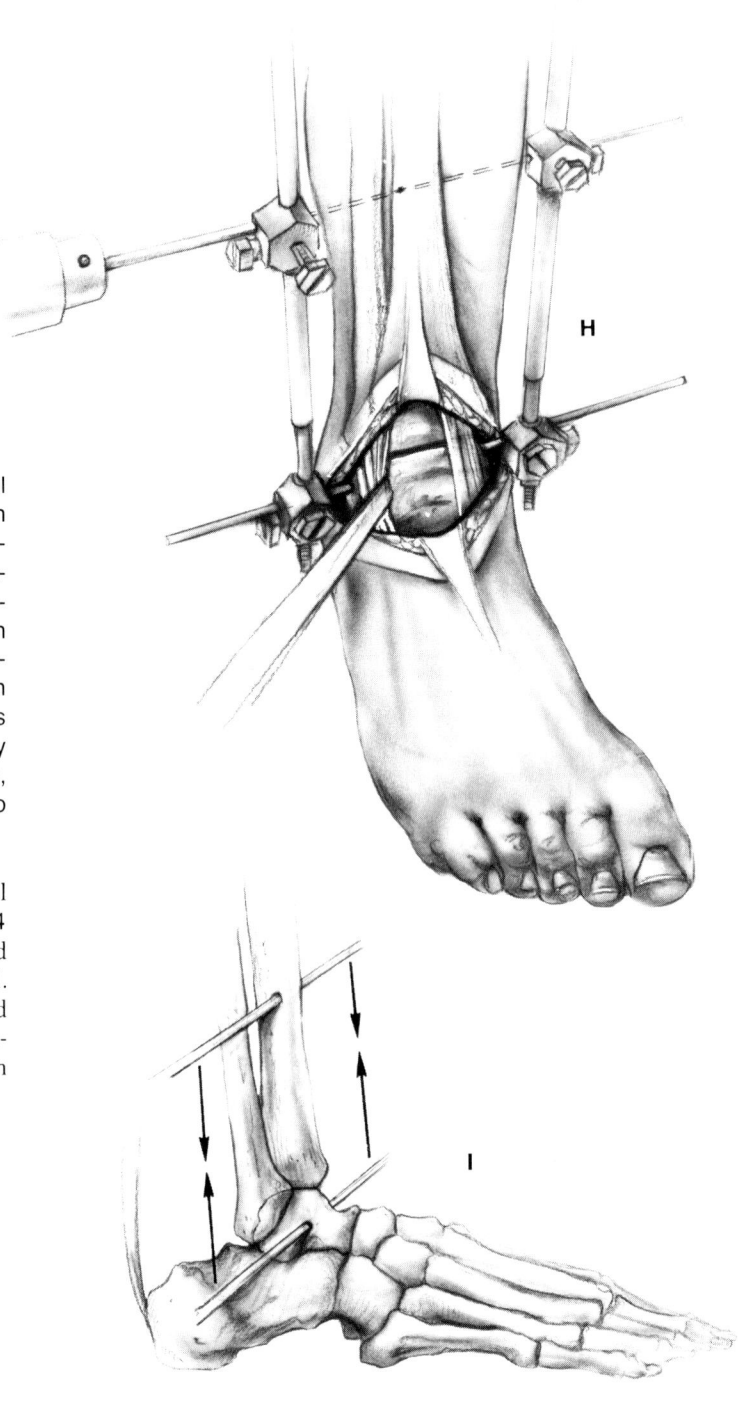

REFERENCES

Adams, J. C.: Arthrodesis of the ankle joint. Experiences with the transfibular approach, J. Bone Joint Surg. **30-B**:506, 1948.

Aitken, G. T.: Amputation as a treatment for certain lower-extremity congenital abnormalities, J. Bone Joint Surg. **41-A**:1267, 1959.

Aitken, G. T.: Surgical amputation in children, J. Bone Joint Surg. **45-A**:1735, 1963.

Albee, F. H.: Orthopaedic and reconstructive surgery, Philadelphia, 1919, W. B. Saunders Co.

Alldredge, R. H.: Diastasis of the distal tibiofibular joint and associated lesions, J.A.M.A. **115**:2136, 1940.

Anderson, K. J., and LeCocq, J. F.: Operative treatment of injury to the fibular collateral ligament of the ankle, J. Bone Joint Surg. **36-A**:825, 1954.

Anderson, K. J., LeCocq, J. F., and Clayton, M. L.: Athletic injury to the fibular collateral ligament of the ankle, Clin. Orthop. **23**:146, 1962.

Arner, O., and Lindholm, A.: Subcutaneous rupture of the Achilles tendon. A study of 92 cases, Acta Chir. Scand. (Suppl.) 239, 1959.

Baker, G. C. W., and Stableforth, P. G.: Syme's amputation. A review of sixty-seven cases, J. Bone Joint Surg. **51-B**:482, 1969.

Baker, L. .D: A rational approach to the surgical needs of the cerebral palsy patient, J. Bone Joint Surg. **38-A**:313, 1956.

Banks, H. H., and Green, W. T.: The correction of equinus deformity in cerebral palsy, J. Bone Joint Surg. **40-A**:1359, 1958.

Barr, J. S., and Record, E. E.: Arthrodesis of the ankle for correction of foot deformity, Surg. Clin. North Am. **27**:1281, 1947.

Barr, J. S., and Record, E. E.: Arthrodesis of the ankle joint, N. Engl. J. Med. **248**:53, 1953.

Bingold, A. C.: Ankle and subtalar fusion by a transarticular graft, J. Bone Joint Surg. **38-B**:862, 1956.

Burwell, H. N., and Charnley, A. D.: The treatment of displaced fractures at the ankle by rigid internal fixation and early joint movement, J. Bone Joint Surg. **47-B**:634, 1965.

Campbell, C. J., Rinehard, W. T., and Kalenak, A.: Arthrodesis of the ankle. Deep autogenous inlay grafts with maximum cancellous-bone apposition, J. Bone Joint Surg. **56-A**:63, 1974.

Catterall, R. C. F.: Syme's amputation by Joseph Lister after sixty-six years, J. Bone Joint Surg. **49-B**:144, 1967.

Charnley, J.: Compression arthrodesis of the ankle and shoulder, J. Bone Joint Surg. **33-B**:180, 1951.

Childress, H. M.: Vertical transarticular-pin fixation for unstable ankle fractures, J. Bone Joint Surg. **47-A**:1323, 1965.

Chrisman, O. D., and Snook, G. A.: Reconstruction of lateral ligament tear of the ankle. An experimental study and clinical evaluation of seven patients treated by a new modification of the Elmslie procedure, J. Bone Joint Surg. **51-A**:904, 1969.

Chuinard, E. G., and Peterson, R. E.: Distraction-compression bone-graft arthrodesis of the ankle. A method especially applicable in children, J. Bone Joint Surg. **45-A**:481, 1963.

Clark, B. L., Derby, A. C., and Power, G. R. I.: Injuries of the lateral ligament of the ankle. Conservative versus operative repair, Can. J. Surg. **8**:358, 1965.

Clayton, M. L., Trott, A. W., and Ulin, R.: Recurrent subluxation of the ankle, J. Bone Joint Surg. **33-A**:502, 1951.

Colton, C. L.: Fracture-diastasis of the inferior tibiofibular joint, J. Bone Joint Surg. **50-B**:830, 1968.

Colton, C. L.: The treatment of Dupuytren's fracture-dislocation of the ankle, J. Bone Joint Surg. **53-B**:63, 1971.

Cotton, F. J.: A new type of ankle fracture, J.A.M.A. **64**:318, 1915.

Cubbins, W. R., Callahan, J. J., and Scuderi, C. S.: Cruciate ligaments: a resume of operative attacks and results obtained, Am. J. Surg. **43**:481, 1939.

Dale, G. M.: Syme's amputation for gangrene from peripheral vascular disease, Artif. Limbs **6**:44, 1961.

Demottaz, J. D., Mazur, J. M., Thomas, W. H., Sledge, C. B., and Simon, S. R.: Clinical study of total ankle replacement with gait analysis. A preliminary report, J. Bone Joint Surg. **61-A**:976, 1979.

Denham, R. A.: Internal fixation for unstable ankle fractures, J. Bone Joint Surg. **46-B**:206, 1964.

Dupuytren, G.: Mémoire sur la fracture de l'extrémité inférieure du péroné, les luxations et les accidents qui en sont la suite. Annuaire médico-chirurgical des Hôpitaux et Hospices Civils de Paris **1**:1, 1819.

Edwards, W. G., et al.: The tarsal tunnel syndrome. Diagnosis and treatment, J.A.M.A. **207**:716, 1969.

Elmslie, R. C.: Recurrent subluxation of the ankle joint, Ann. Surg. **100**:364, 1934.

Evans, D. L.: Recurrent instability of the ankle. A method of surgical treatment, Proc. R. Soc. Med. **46**:343, 1953.

Freeman, M. A. R.: Instability of the foot after injuries to the lateral ligament of the ankle, J. Bone Joint Surg. **47-B**:669, 1965.

Freeman, M. A. R.: Treatment of ruptures of the lateral ligament of the ankle, J. Bone Joint Surg. **47-B**:661, 1965.

Fullerton, P. M.: The effect of ischemia on nerve conduction in the carpal tunnel syndrome, J. Neurol. Neurosurg. Psychiatry **26**:385, 1963.

Gallie, W. E.: Tendon fixation in infantile paralysis, Am. J. Orthop. Surg. **14**:18, 1916.

Gatellier, J.: The juxtaretroperoneal route in the operative treatment of fracture of malleolus with posterior marginal fragment, Surg. Gynecol. Obstet. **52**:67, 1931.

Gillespie, H. S., and Boucher, P.: Watson-Jones repair of lateral instability of the ankle, J. Bone Joint Surg. **53-A**:920, 1971.

Gillies, H., and Chalmers, J.: The management of fresh ruptures of the tendo achillis, J. Bone Joint Surg. **52-A**:337, 1970.

Goergen, T. G., Danzig, L. A., Resnick, D., and Owen, C. A.: Roentgenographic evaluation of the tibiotalar joint, J. Bone Joint Surg. **59-A**:874, 1977.

Goodgold, J., Kopell, H. P., and Spielholz, N. I.: The tarsal-tunnel syndrome. Objective diagnostic criteria, N. Engl. J. Med. **273**:742, 1965.

Gordon, S. L., Dunn, E. J., and Malin, T. H.: Lateral collateral ligament ankle injuries in young athletic individuals, J. Trauma **16**:225, 1976.

Graham, C. E.: A new method for arthrodesis of the ankle joint, Clin. Orthop. **68**:75, 1970.

Green, W. T., and Grice, D. S.: The management of calcaneus deformity, American Academy of Orthopaedic Surgeons Instructional Course Lectures, vol. 13, Ann Arbor, Mich., 1956, J. W. Edwards, p. 135.

Harris, R. I.: Syme's amputation. The technical details essential for success, J. Bone Joint Surg. **38-B**:614, 1956.

Harris, R. I.: The history and development of Syme's amputation, Artif. Limbs **6**:4, 1961.

Hornby, R., and Harris, R. B.: Syme's amputation. Follow-up study of weight-bearing in sixty-eight patients, J. Bone Joint Surg. **57-A**:346, 1975.

Horwitz, T.: The use of the transfibular approach in arthrodesis of the ankle joint, Am. J. Surg. **55**:550, 1942.

Inglis, A. E., Scott, W. N., Sculco, T. P., and Patterson, A. H.: Ruptures of the tendo-achilles. An objective assessment of surgical and non-surgical treatment, J. Bone Joint Surg. **58-A:** 990, 1976.

Ingram, A. J., and Huntley, J. M.: Posterior bone block of the ankle for paralytic equinus, J. Bone Joint Surg. **33-A:**679, 1951.

Irwin, C. E.: The calcaneus foot, American Academy of Orthopaedic Surgeons Instructional Course Lectures, vol. 15, Ann Arbor, Mich., 1958, J. W. Edwards, p. 135.

Jansen, K.: Arthrodesis of the ankle joint, Acta Orthop. Scand. **32:**476, 1962.

Johnson, E. W., Jr., and Boseker, E. H.: Arthrodesis of the ankle, Arch. Surg. **97:**766, 1968.

Johnson, E. W., Jr., and Ortiz, P. R.: Electrodiagnosis of tarsal tunnel syndrome, Arch. Phys. Med. **47:**776, 1966.

Joy, G., Patzakis, M. J., and Harrey, J. P., Jr.: Precise evaluation of the reduction of severe ankle fractures. Technique and correlation with end results, J. Bone Joint Surg. **56-A:**979, 1974.

Keck, C.: The tarsal-tunnel syndrome, J. Bone Joint Surg. **44-A:** 180, 1962.

Klossner, O.: Late results of operative and non-operative treatment of severe ankle fractures, Acta Chir. Scand. (Suppl.) 293, 1962.

Kopell, H. P., and Thompson, W. A.: Peripheral entrapment neuropathies of the lower extremity, N. Engl. J. Med. **262:** 56, 1960.

Lam, S. J. S.: Tarsal-tunnel syndrome, J. Bone Joint Surg. **49-B:** 87, 1967.

Lambotte, A.: The operative treatment of fractures, Br. Med. J. **2:**1530, 1912.

Lane, W. A.: The operative treatment of fractures, London, 1912, Medical Publishing Co.

Laurin, C. A., Ouellet, R., and St. Jacques, R.: Talar and subtalar tilt: an experimental investigation, Can. J. Surg. **11:**270, 1968.

Lawrence, G. H., Cave, E. F., and O'Connor, H.: Injury to the Achilles tendon, Am. J. Surg. **89:**795, 1955.

Lee, H. G.: Surgical repair in recurrent dislocation of the ankle joint, J. Bone Joint Surg. **39-A:**828, 1957.

Leonard, M. H.: Injuries of the lateral ligaments of the ankle. A clinical and experimental study, J. Bone Joint Surg. **31-A:** 373, 1949.

Linscheid, R. L., Burton, R. C., and Fredericks, E. J.: Tarsal-tunnel syndrome, South. Med. J. **63:**1313, 1970.

Lipscomb, P. R., and Sanchez, J. G.: Anterior transplantation of the posterior tibial tendons for persistent palsy of the common peroneal nerve, J. Bone Joint Surg. **43-A:**60, 1961.

Magnusson, R.: On the late results in non-operative cases of malleolar fractures, Acta Chir. Scand. (Suppl.) 84, 1944.

Malka, J. S., and Taillard, W.: Results of nonoperative and operative treatment of fractures of the ankle, Clin. Orthop. **67:**159, 1969.

Marinacci, A. A.: Neurological syndromes of the tarsal tunnels, Bull. Los Angeles Neurol. Soc. **33:**90, 1968.

Mazet, R., Jr.: Syme's amputation. A follow-up study of fifty-one adults and thirty-two children, J. Bone Joint Surg. **50-A:**1549, 1968.

Mazur, J. M., Schwartz, E., and Simon, S. R.: Ankle arthrodesis. Long-term follow-up with gait analysis, J. Bone Joint Surg. **61-A:**964, 1979.

McCauley, J. C.: The early treatment of equinus in congenital club foot, Am. J. Surg. **22:**491, 1933.

McDade, W. C.: Treatment of ankle fractures. I. Diagnosis and treatment of ankle injuries, American Academy of Orthopaedic Surgeons Instructional Course Lectures, vol. 24, St. Louis, 1975, The C. V. Mosby Co., p. 251.

Milgram, J. E.: Office measures for relief of the painful foot, J. Bone Joint Surg. **46-A:**1095, 1964.

Miller, A. J.: Posterior malleolar fractures, J. Bone Joint Surg. **56-B:**508, 1974.

Miller, J. A., Jr.: Joint paracentesis from an anatomic point of view. II. Hip, knee, ankle and foot, Surgery **41:**999, 1957.

Monk, C. J. E.: Injuries of the tibio-fibular ligaments, J. Bone Joint Surg. **51-B:**330, 1969.

Morris, H. D., Hand, W. L., and Dunn, A. W.: The modified Blair fusion for fractures of the talus, J. Bone Joint Surg. **53-A:**1289, 1971.

Murphy, O. B.: Achilles tendon advancement for the spastic equinus foot, Clin. Orthop. **70:**238, 1970.

Ottolenghi, C. E., Animoso, J., and Burgo, P. H.: Percutaneous arthrodesis of the ankle joint, Clin. Orthop. **68:**72, 1970.

Ottosson, L.: Lateral instability of the ankle treated by a modified Evans procedure, Acta Orthop. Scand. **49:**302, 1978.

Pankovich, A. M.: Maisonneuve fracture of the fibula, J. Bone Joint Surg. **58-A:**337, 1976.

Patrick, J.: A direct approach to trimalleolar fractures, J. Bone Joint Surg. **47-B:**236, 1965.

Peabody, C. W.: Tendon transposition in the paralytic foot, American Academy of Orthopaedic Surgeons Instructional Course Lectures, vol. 6, Ann Arbor, Mich., 1949, J. W. Edwards, p. 178.

Pollock, L. J., and Davis, L.: Peripheral nerve injuries, Am. J. Surg. **18:**361, 1932.

Quigley, T. B.: Fractures and ligament injuries of the ankle, Am. J. Surg. **98:**477, 1959.

Ratliff, A. H. C.: Compression arthrodesis of the ankle, J. Bone Joint Surg. **41-B:**524, 1959.

Ratliff, A. H. C.: Syme's amputation: result after forty-four years. Report of a case, J. Bone Joint Surg. **49-B:**142, 1967.

Rosenman, L. D.: Syme's amputation for ischemic disease in the foot, Am. J. Surg. **118:**194, 1969.

Rubin, G., and Witten, M.: The talar tilt angle and the fibular collateral ligaments. A method for determination of talar tilt, J. Bone Joint Surg. **42-A:**311, 1960.

Ruth, C. J.: The surgical treatment of injuries of the fibular collateral ligaments of the ankle, J. Bone Joint Surg. **43-A:**229, 1961.

Sammarco, J. G., Burstein, A. H., and Frankel, V. H.: Biomechanics of the ankle: a kinematic study, Orthop. Clin. North Am. **4:**75, 1973.

Sarmiento, A., Gilmer, R., and Finnieston, A.: A new surgical-prosthetic approach to the Syme's amputation. A preliminary report, Artif. Limbs **10:**52, 1966.

Smith, M. G. H.: Inferior tibio-fibular diastasis treated by cross screwing, J. Bone Joint Surg. **45-B:**737, 1963.

Smith, R. C.: Arthritic patients take first step with ankle prosthesis, J.A.M.A. **228:**11, 1974.

Sneppen, O.: Long-term course in 119 cases of pseudarthrosis of the medial malleolus, Acta Orthop. Scand. **40:**807, 1970.

Speed, J. S.: Ankylosis and deformity. In Crenshaw, A. H., editor: Campbell's operative orthopaedics, vol. 2, ed. 4, St. Louis, 1963, The C. V. Mosby Co.

Staples, O. S.: Injuries to the medial ligaments of the ankle. Result study, J. Bone Joint Surg. **42-A:**1287, 1960.

Staples, O. S.: Ruptures of the fibular collateral ligaments of the ankle. Result study of immediate surgical treatment, J. Bone Joint Surg. **57-A:**101, 1975.

Stauffer, R. N.: Total ankle joint replacement as an alternative to arthrodesis, Geriatrics **31:**79, 1976.

Stauffer, R. N.: Total ankle joint replacement, Arch. Surg. **112:**1105, 1977.

Steindler, A.: Orthopaedic operations, Springfield, Ill., 1940, Charles C Thomas, Publisher.

Stewart, M. J.: Athletic injuries, particularly to the ligaments of the knee. Diagnosis, repair and physical rehabilitation, Am. J. Orthop. **3:**52, 1961.

Syme, J.: Amputation at the ankle-joint, Lond. Edinb. Monthly J. Med. Sci. **3:**93, 1843.

Thomas, F. B.: Arthrodesis of the ankle, J. Bone Joint Surg. **51-B:**53, 1969.

Van Gorder, G. W., and Chen, C. M.: The central graft operation for fusion of tuberculous knees, ankles, and elbows, J. Bone Joint Surg. **41-A:**1029, 1959.

Vasli, S.: Operative treatment of ankle fractures, Acta Chir. Scand. (Suppl.) 226, 1957.

Vichard, Ph., Watelet, F., Leclerc, D., and Lefon, M.: Comparative anatomical result of conservative orthopaedic treatment and surgical treatment in recent severe sprains of the ankle, J. Chir. (Paris) **114:**287, 1977.

Warren, R., et al.: The Syme's amputation in peripheral arterial disease, Surgery **37:**156, 1955.

Watson-Jones, R.: Fractures and joint injuries, ed. 4, vol. 2, Baltimore, 1955, The Williams & Wilkins Co.

White, J. W.: Torsion of the Achilles tendon; its surgical significance, Arch. Surg. **46:**784, 1943.

Wilson, A. B., Jr.: Prosthesis for Syme's amputation, Artif. Limbs **6:**52, 1961.

Wilson, F. C., Jr., and Skilbred, L. A.: Long-term results in the treatment of displaced bimalleolar fractures, J. Bone Joint Surg. **48:**1065, 1966.

Wilson, H. J.: Arthrodesis of the ankle. A technique using bilateral hemimalleolar onlay grafts with screw fixation, J. Bone Joint Surg. **51-A:**775, 1969.

Wood, W. L., Zlotsky, N., and Westin, G. W.: Congenital absence of the fibula. Treatment by Syme amputation—indications and technique, J. Bone Joint Surg. **47-A:**1159, 1965.

Yablon, I. G., Heller, F. G., and Shouse, L.: The key role of the lateral malleolus in displaced fractures of the ankle, J. Bone Joint Surg. **59-A:**169, 1977.

15

FOOT

TRIPLE ARTHRODESIS (Plate 15-1)

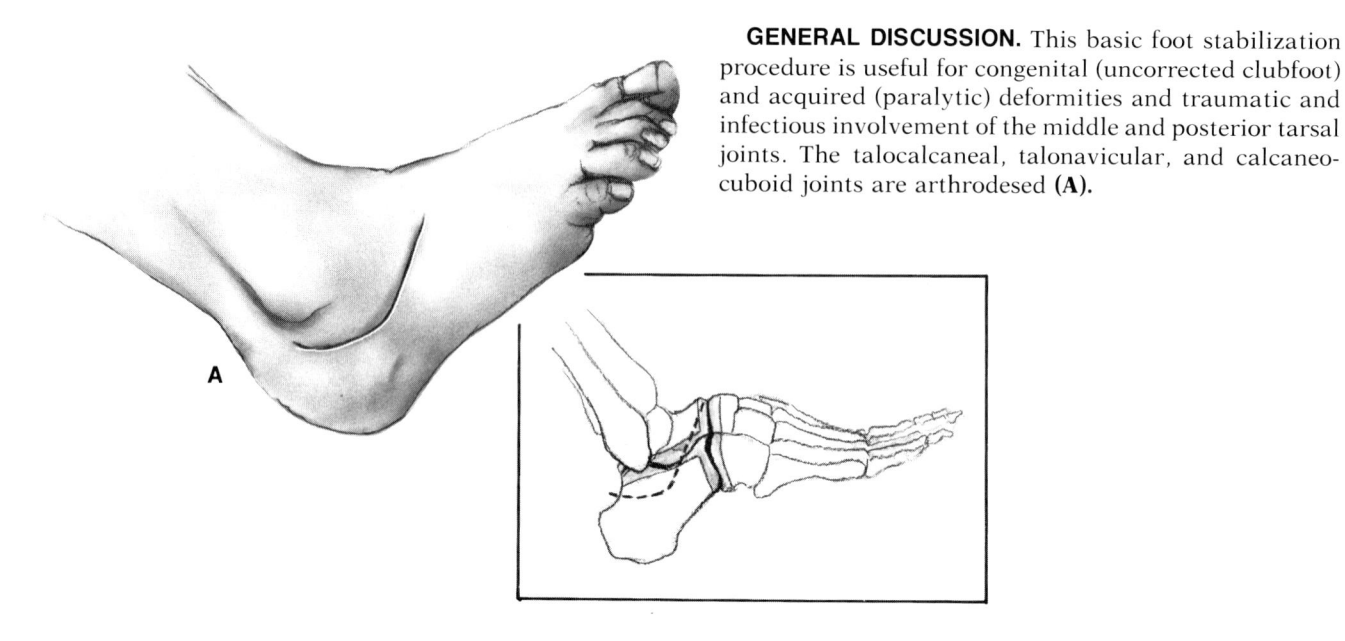

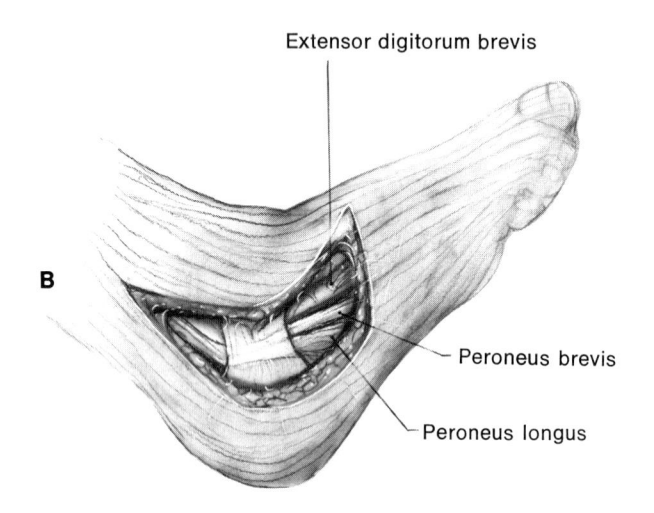

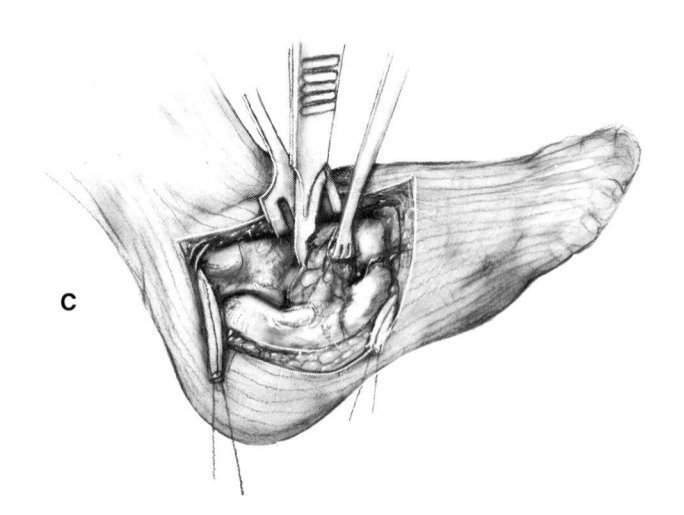

GENERAL DISCUSSION. This basic foot stabilization procedure is useful for congenital (uncorrected clubfoot) and acquired (paralytic) deformities and traumatic and infectious involvement of the middle and posterior tarsal joints. The talocalcaneal, talonavicular, and calcaneocuboid joints are arthrodesed (**A**).

DETAILS OF PROCEDURE. The procedure is carried out under pneumatic tourniquet. The patient is positioned with a large sandbag under the ipsilateral hip. A curvilinear incision is made as illustrated (**A** and **B**). The incision should be of sufficient length to avoid any necessity for heavy retraction. Skin and subcutaneous tissue are reflected jointly to expose the peroneal tendon sheaths. The peroneal sheaths are opened. The peroneus brevis and peroneus longus tendons are divided sharply, tagged with sutures, and held aside to facilitate the exposure. The sinus tarsi is methodically cleaned of its adipose tissue contents. It is helpful to remove the contents of the sinus tarsi in one mass, if possible, making an incision through periosteum superiorly (talar) and inferiorly (calcaneal). Reflecting everything subperiosteally from both bones and sectioning the mass of tissue medially in the depth of the sinus allows removal of the entire contents of the sinus tarsi in continuity (**C**). A portion of the origin of the extensor digitorum brevis is reflected by sharp dissection from the anterosuperior margin of the calcaneus to expose the midtarsal joints.

(Plate 15-1) TRIPLE ARTHRODESIS

The talocalcaneal, talonavicular, and the calcaneocuboid joints are opened, and the foot is turned into varus position until the contiguous surfaces of all joints can be clearly visualized (**D**). The articular cartilage is removed from the adjacent surfaces of the calcaneocuboid, the talonavicular, and the anterior and posterior talocalcaneal joints, exposing subchondral cancellous bone over all these surfaces (**E**). Extra bone is removed as may be necessary for correction of any existing deformity.

The foot is then carefully positioned in very slight valgus position. With the hind foot held in a mild (5°) valgus position with the denuded surfaces apposed in this position, the talocalcaneal and the two midtarsal joints are secured by staples (**F** and **G**). There must be caution to avoid even the slightest degree of varus position of the hind foot, which would inevitably lead to the subsequent development of painful pressure over the plantar aspect of the fifth metatarsal head. The peroneal tendons are reapproximated. The divided portion of the extensor digitorum brevis is resutured, and the remainder of the wound is closed in the usual fashion. The staples maintain the foot in proper position during wound closure. A circular cast is applied from toes to tibial tubercle with the foot in mild valgus position and the ankle in neutral position.

POSTOPERATIVE MANAGEMENT. Immobilization in a short-leg cast is continued until there is roentgenographic evidence that each of the three individual joints fused, usually at about 12 weeks.

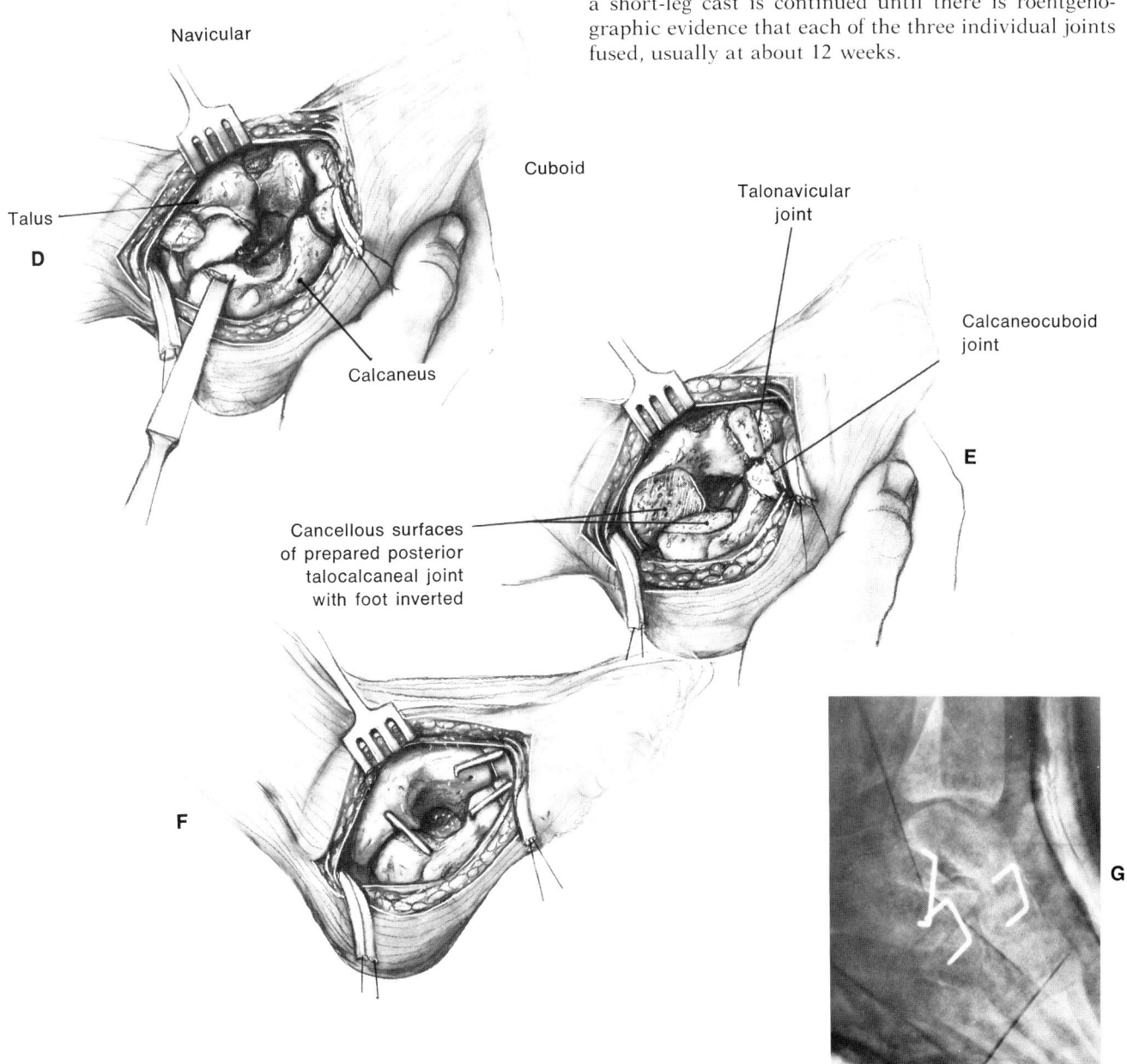

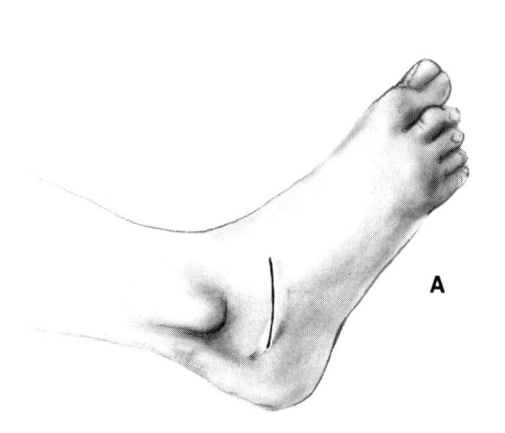

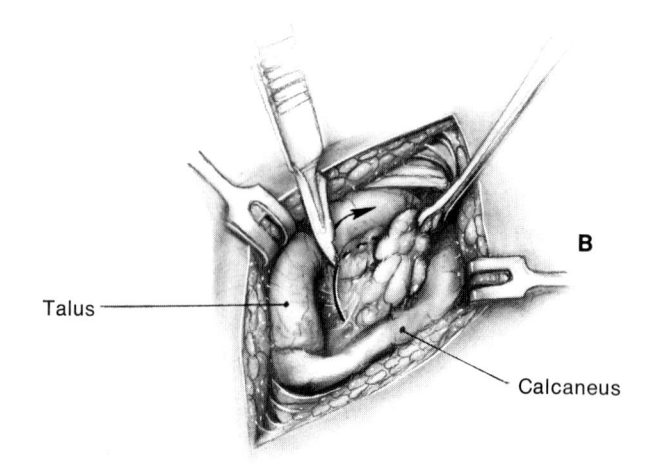

SUBTALAR ARTHRODESIS (GRICE PROCEDURE) (Plate 15-2)

GENERAL DISCUSSION. The extra-articular subtalar arthrodesis is ideally suited to stabilize the subtalar joint in the young patient (4 to 10 years of age) When it is undesirable to perform a triple arthrodesis. Triple arthrodesis generally should be reserved for the patient over 12 years of age when the development of the tarsal bones is more mature. The procedure for extra-articular arthrodesis of the subtalar joint, described by Grice, is useful in the progressive valgus deformity of the foot. It may be combined with forward transfer of a peroneal muscle. Other indications for this type of subtalar arthrodesis are the flail foot that rolls into valgus position and presents a skin pressure problem in the braced shoe and the calcaneus foot in which either posterior tendon transfer or tenodesis is performed to prevent progressive deformity. This type of subtalar arthrodesis is not designed for the varus foot deformity. Any heel cord contracture should be fully corrected preoperatively.

Peroneal tendon transfer may be done at the same time, although it is preferable to do the tendon transfer at a second stage 6 weeks after the subtalar joint stabilization.

Careful placement of the tibial grafts and positioning of the foot after placement of the grafts are important steps in this operative procedure. Varus position of the heel must be avoided because it will result in troublesome symptoms postoperatively and may require revision of the stabilization. Excessive valgus is also undesirable. This procedure will not solve the problem of intrinsic forefoot deformities. It is devised to stabilize the hind foot in good weight-bearing position without disturbing growth of the foot. It is a useful procedure when properly performed in the well-selected patient.

DETAILS OF PROCEDURE. The subtalar joint is exposed through a short, oblique, lateral incision **(A)**. The capsule of the posterior subtalar and the sustentaculum articulation anteriorly are identified. An incision is then made through periosteum on the talus and calcaneus corresponding to the lateral margin of the roof and floor of the sinus tarsi. Then, by subperiosteal reflection, the entire mass of fibro-fatty tissue can be removed from the sinus **(B)**, leaving joint capsule exposed. The cortex is removed with a thin osteotome from the talus (roof of the sinus tarsi) and from the calcaneus (floor of the sinus tarsi) between the anterior and posterior talocalcaneal articulations to provide a mortise for the bone blocks. The most lateral cortical margin of the bony bed is preserved to allow support for the bone blocks and to prevent these from sinking deeply into the soft, cancellous bone. The calcaneus is brought into the position in which the joint is to be stabilized (mild valgus), and the length of the bone blocks required for grafts is estimated with the end of a straight, broad osteotome **(C)**.

A linear incision is then made of the anteromedial aspect of the proximal and midportion of the tibia **(D)**. An H-shaped incision made in the periosteum allows wide exposure of the anteromedial surface of the tibia **(E)**. A bone block 5 cm long and 2 cm wide, enough to provide two grafts, is outlined with drill holes and removed with the bone saw (**F** and **G**).

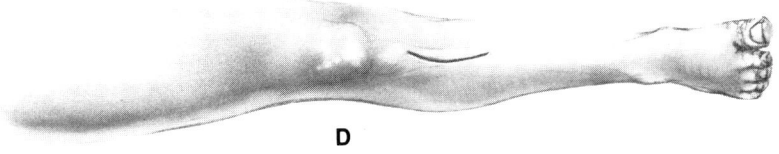

(Plate 15-2) SUBTALAR ARTHRODESIS (GRICE PROCEDURE)

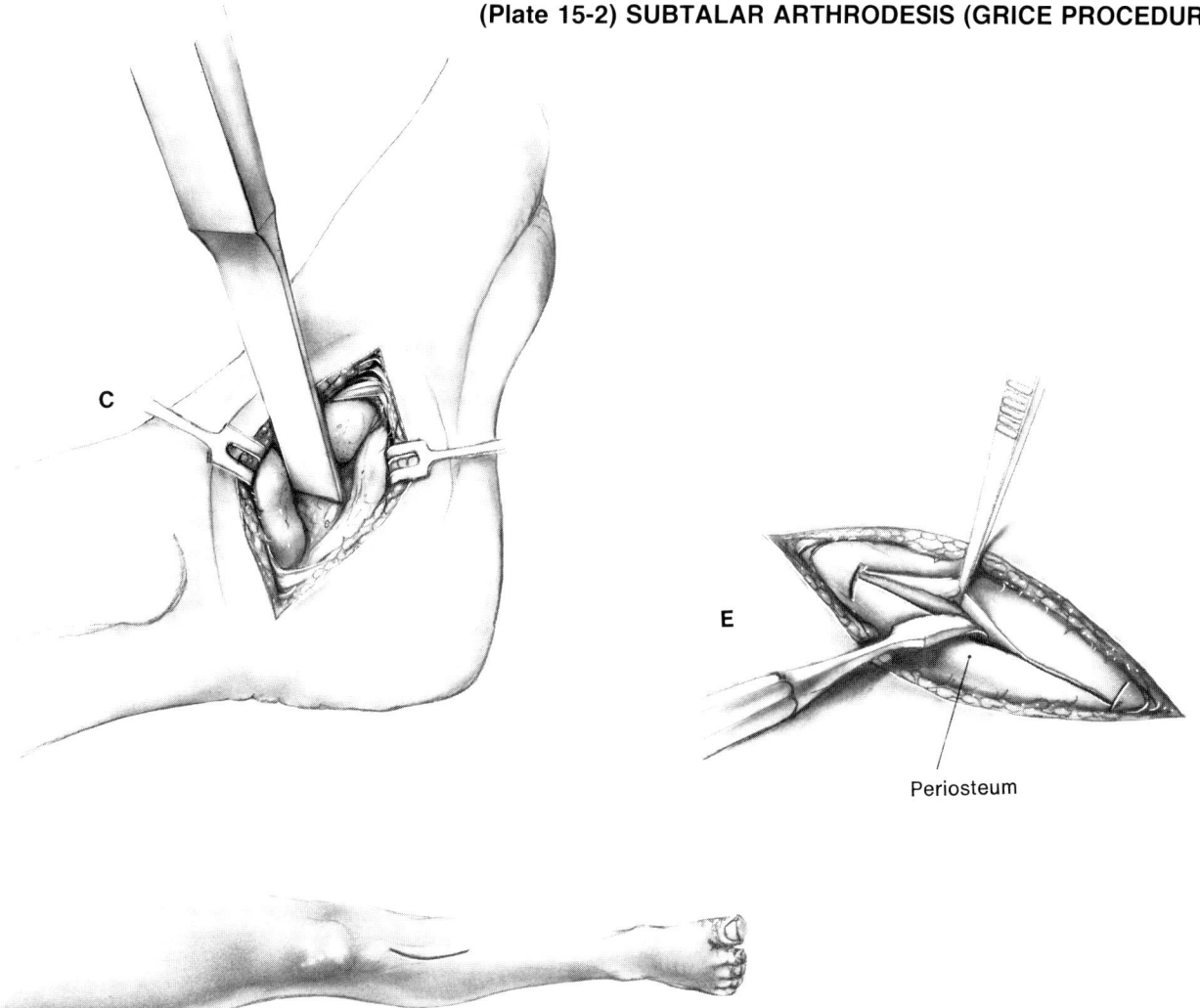

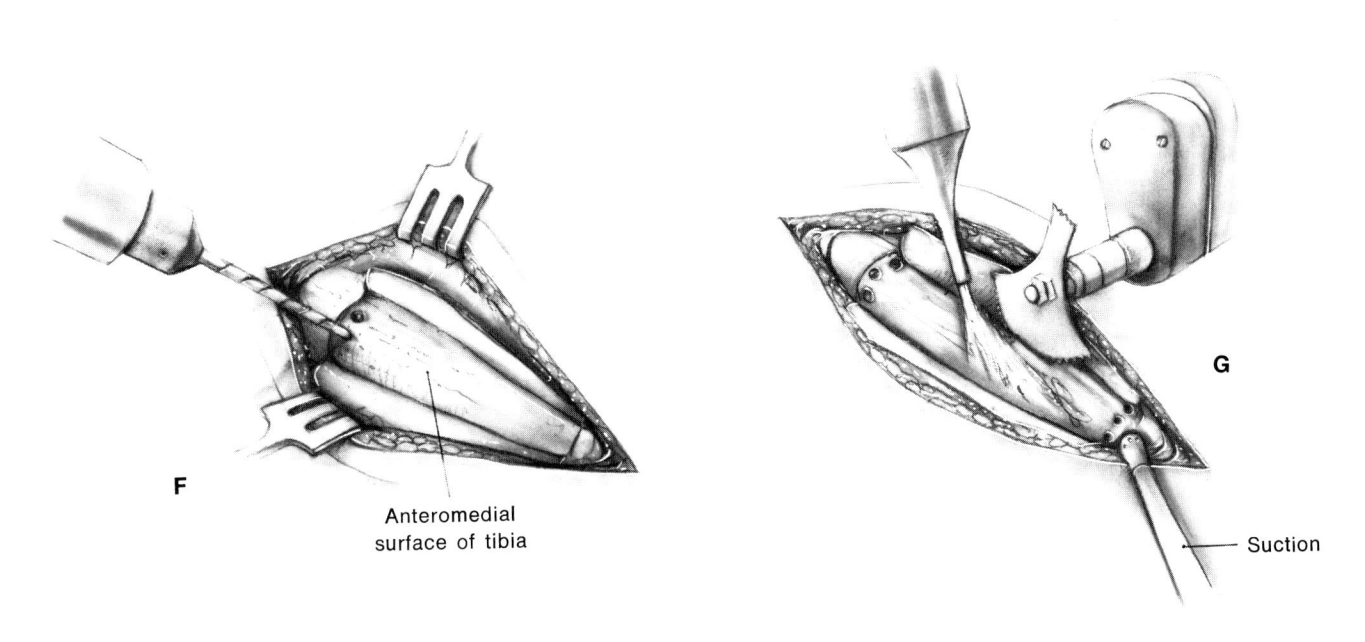

C

E
Periosteum

D

F
Anteromedial surface of tibia

G
Suction

551

SUBTALAR ARTHRODESIS (GRICE PROCEDURE) (Plate 15-2)

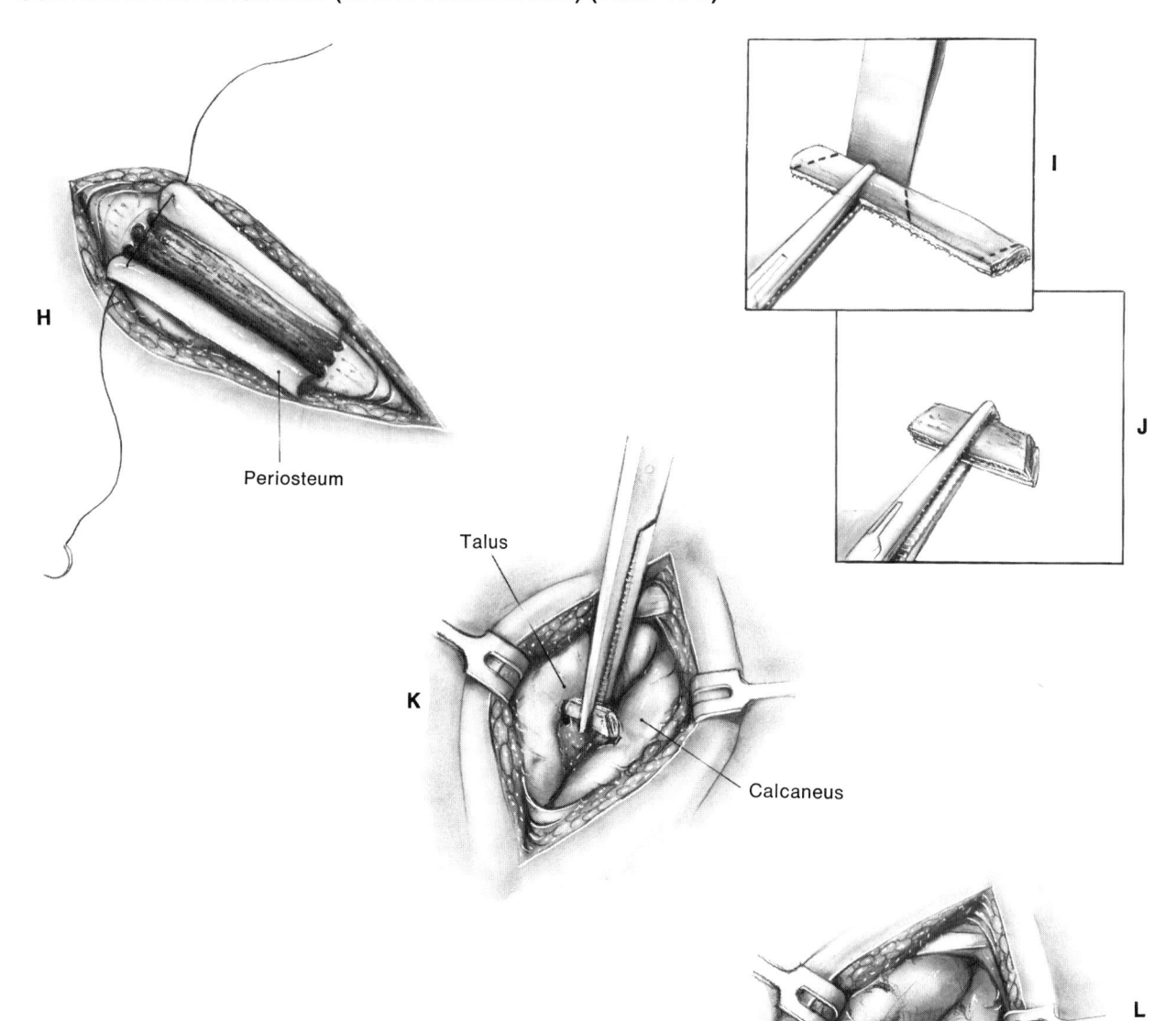

The tibial wound is closed in layers **(H)**. The bone graft is then cut in half. The two remaining fragments (each 2.5 cm long) are then shaped with rongeurs or bone cutters into a trapezoid form and snugly fitted into the prepared bed in the hind foot with the foot held momentarily in slight varus position **(I to K)**. With the cancellous surfaces of the graft in apposition, two corticocancellous grafts are placed so that their long axes are in line with the shaft of the tibia, the proximal ends pointing slightly posterior with the ankle in neutral position **(L and M)**. The foot is then everted gently. If the grafts are correctly placed and of proper length, they will be stable under compression in the subtalar joint with the foot in the desired position of slight valgus. The foot is carefully held in this position until the subcutaneous tissues and skin are closed and the foot and leg have been immobilized in a long-leg cast.

POSTOPERATIVE MANAGEMENT. The foot is immobilized in a long-leg plaster cast for 6 weeks after the subtalar arthrodesis.

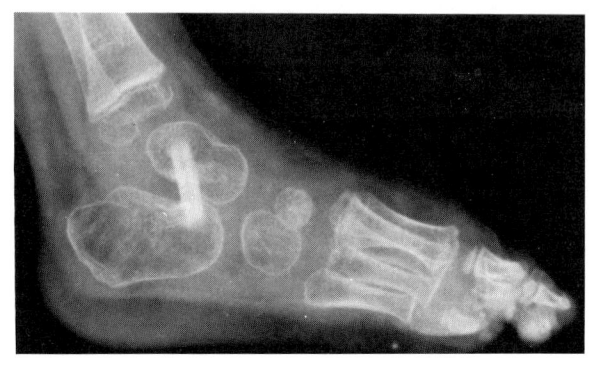

(Plate 15-3) OSTEOTOMY OF CALCANEUS (DWYER PROCEDURE)

GENERAL DISCUSSION. This procedure is useful for the child with persistent varus deformity of the heel or the child with significant pes cavus deformity. Just as the extra-articular subtalar arthrodesis (Grice procedure) is useful for the significant valgus deformity of a child who is too young for triple arthrodesis, osteotomy of the calcaneus as recommended by Dwyer permits an extra-articular correction for varus deformity in the hind foot of a child who may be too old for soft issue correction and yet too young for triple arthrodesis. If there is a significant component of plantar foot contracture, plantar fasciotomy can be carried out simultaneously to improve the overall foot correction.

DETAILS OF PROCEDURE. The patient is placed in a lateral position on the uninvolved side. An oblique incision is made over the lateral aspect of the hind foot **(A)**. The skin incision parallels the course of the peroneus longus tendon but remains 1 cm posterior and inferior to it. A thick layer of adipose tissue is encountered subcutaneously as the dissection is carried down to expose the lateral aspect of the calcaneus. The upper flap is reflected superiorly and anteriorly until the tendon of the peroneus longus is exposed **(B)**. When the lateral surface of the calcaneus has been exposed, a wedge of bone with its base 8 to 12 mm in width on the lateral surface of the calcaneus is mapped out at 45° to the longitudinal axis of the tibia with the ankle in neutral position. The plantar fascia may be divided at this time if necessary. The anterior edge of the wedge osteotomy should be approximately 1 cm posterior and inferior to the peroneus longus tendon. The wedge of calcaneus is osteotomized down to the medial cortex of the calcaneus **(C)**.

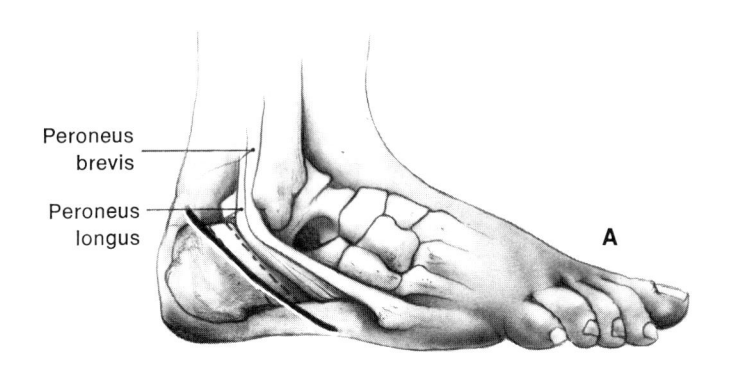

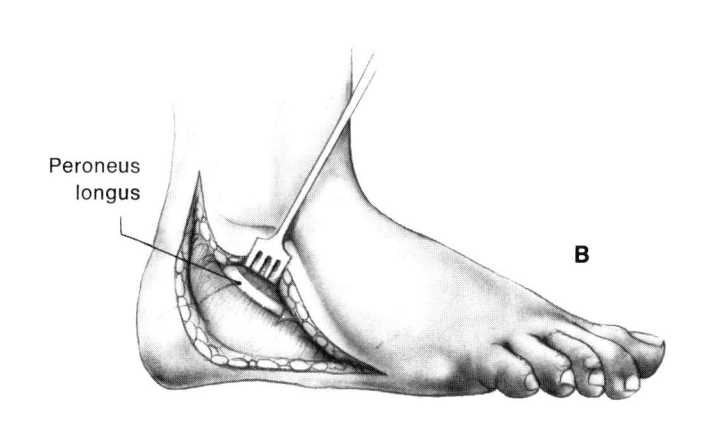

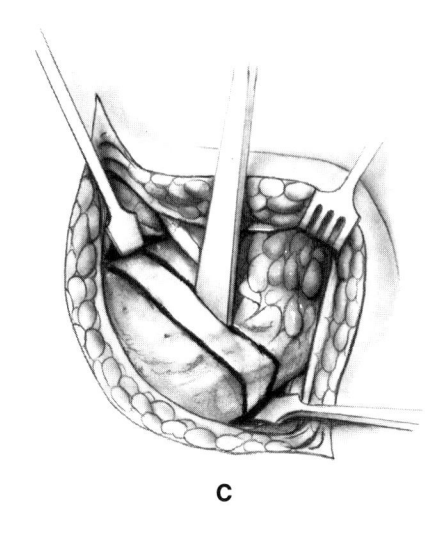

OSTEOTOMY OF CALCANEUS (DWYER PROCEDURE) (Plate 15-3)

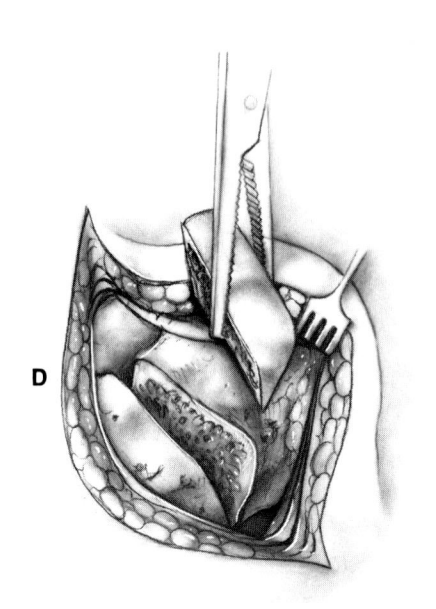

The wedge of bone is removed **(D)** and the medial cortex is broken manually to close the lateral opening and to correct the varus deformity **(E)**. If the superior and inferior cortices of the calcaneus have been completely removed with the wedge osteotomy down to the medial cortex, the osteotomy site can be closed without difficulty **(F)** and held without any internal fixation in the corrected position in a short-leg cast after wound closure **(G)**.

POSTOPERATIVE MANAGEMENT. The patient is maintained in a short-leg cast but is permitted partial weight bearing on the involved heel as soon as wound discomfort subsides and until the osteotomy site is united (approximately 6 weeks).

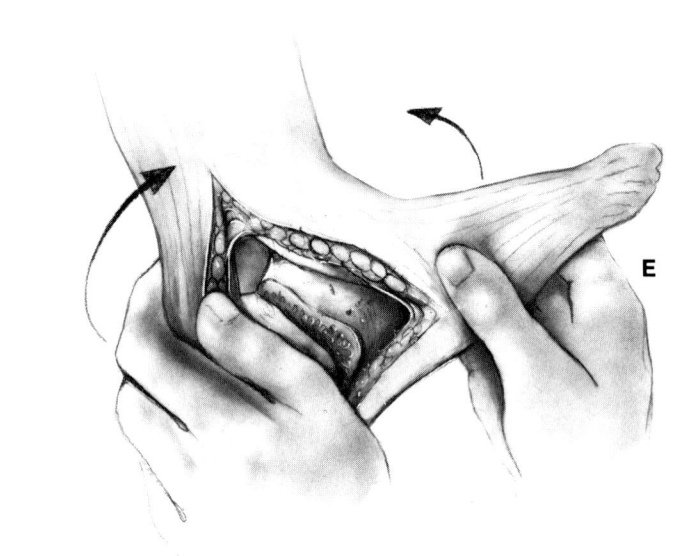

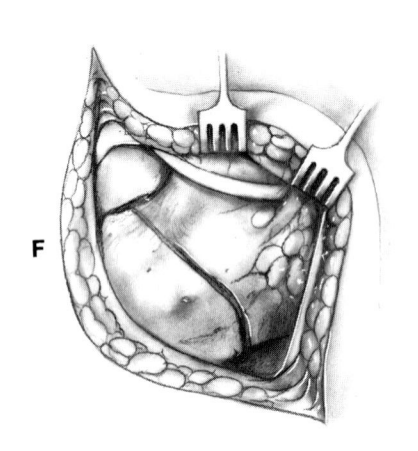

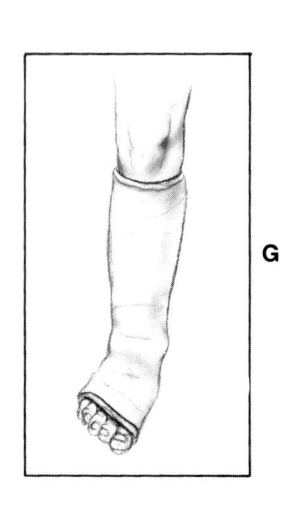

(Plate 15-4) EXCISION OF CALCANEAL SPUR

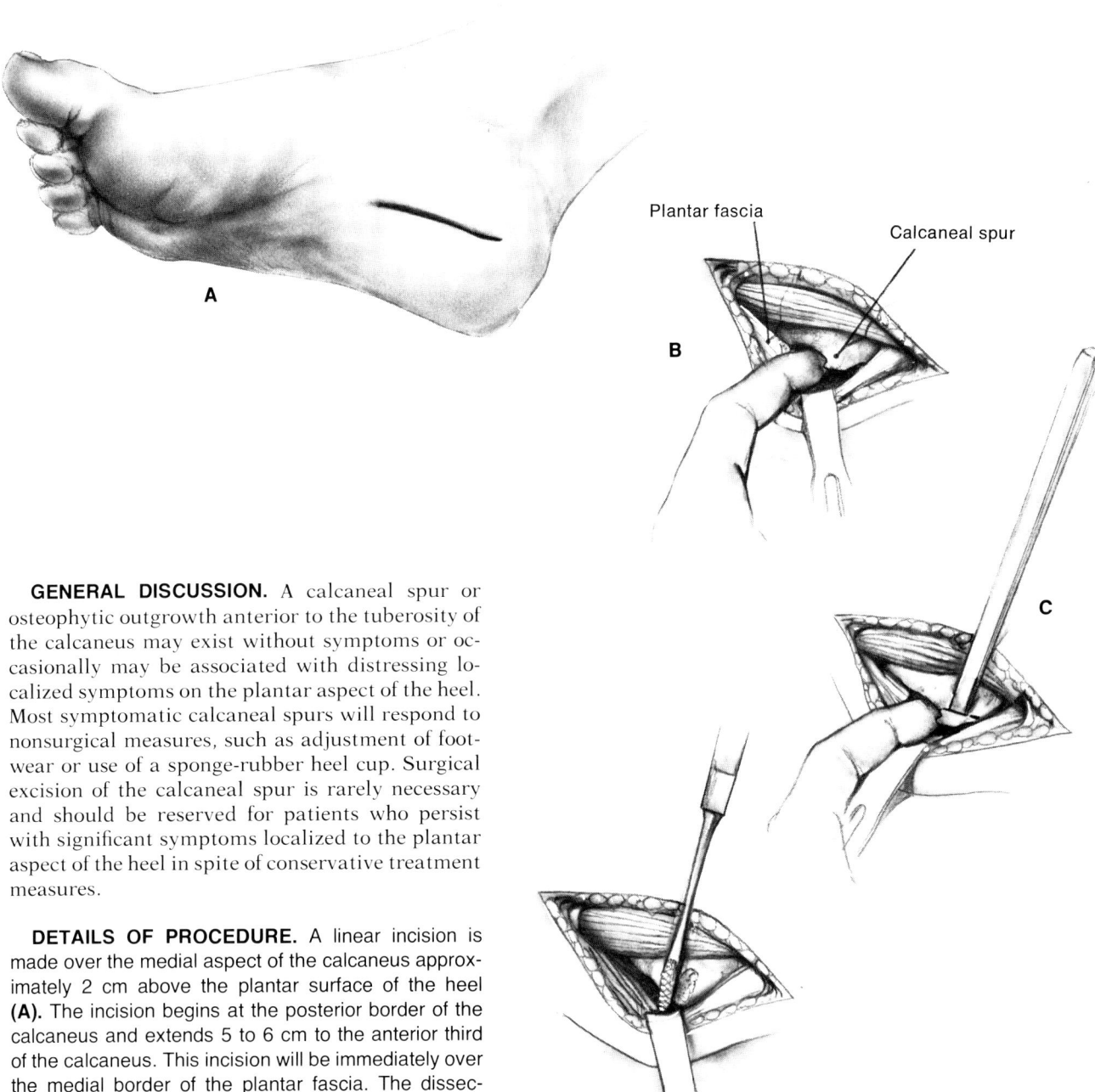

GENERAL DISCUSSION. A calcaneal spur or osteophytic outgrowth anterior to the tuberosity of the calcaneus may exist without symptoms or occasionally may be associated with distressing localized symptoms on the plantar aspect of the heel. Most symptomatic calcaneal spurs will respond to nonsurgical measures, such as adjustment of footwear or use of a sponge-rubber heel cup. Surgical excision of the calcaneal spur is rarely necessary and should be reserved for patients who persist with significant symptoms localized to the plantar aspect of the heel in spite of conservative treatment measures.

DETAILS OF PROCEDURE. A linear incision is made over the medial aspect of the calcaneus approximately 2 cm above the plantar surface of the heel **(A)**. The incision begins at the posterior border of the calcaneus and extends 5 to 6 cm to the anterior third of the calcaneus. This incision will be immediately over the medial border of the plantar fascia. The dissection continues in line with the skin incision to expose the medial border of the plantar fascia. Placing an index finger over the superior surface of the plantar fascia, just anterior to its origin, is helpful **(B)** as the fascia is freed with scissors over and around the calcaneal spur. A small (8 mm) osteotome is placed against the base of the spur, and pressure of the palm of the hand against the osteotome is often sufficient to remove the spur from its base **(C)**. A nasal rasp is used to smooth the surface of the calcaneus where the spur has been removed **(D)**. The wound is closed in layers, and a compression bandage is applied.

POSTOPERATIVE MANAGEMENT. Partial weight bearing with the aid of crutches is resumed 3 to 4 days after surgery. Sutures are removed 10 to 14 days postoperatively. A sponge-rubber heel cup in the patient's shoe is helpful during the early postoperative period. With the aid of a good sponge-rubber heel cup, the patient should be fully weight bearing within 1 month postoperatively.

PLANTAR FASCIOTOMY (Plate 15-5)

GENERAL DISCUSSION. The treatment of claw foot deformity usually depends on the type and severity of the deformity. When mild, it is barely distinguishable form a normal foot with a high arch, since the cavus and slight clawing of the toes disappear with weight bearing. For this type of foot, conservative measures such as a metatarsal bar on the shoe or an insole with a metatarsal pad for use during the day should be all that is necessary. However, these measures will not necessarily prevent the cavus deformity from increasing.

For the more severe deformity that progresses in spite of conservative measures and in a patient too young for tarsal reconstruction, plantar fasciotomy, or the more complete Steindler stripping procedure, may be indicated.

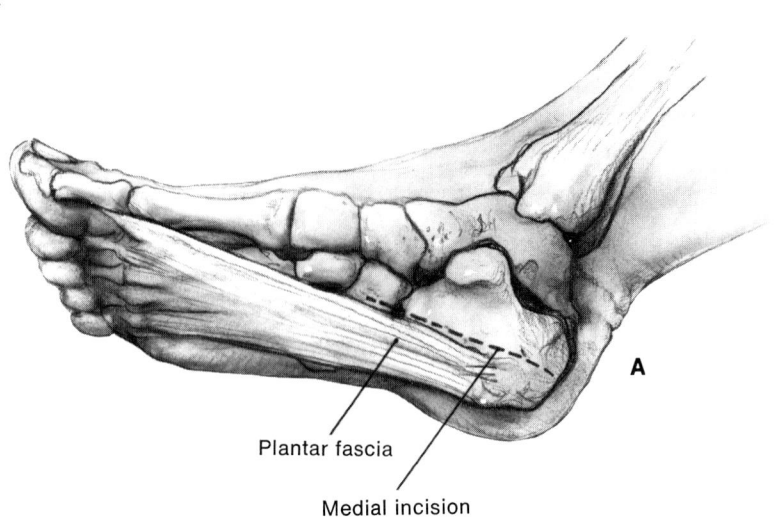

DETAILS OF PROCEDURE. A longitudinal incision is made along the medial aspect of the heel for a distance of approximately 5 cm **(A)**. The layer of fat on the undersurface of the plantar fascia is separated from the plantar fascia from medial to lateral **(B)**. The plantar fascia is then sharply and completely incised transversely near the point where it attaches to the plantar surface of the calcaneus **(C)**. It will be noted that the plantar fascia is much thicker medially than it is laterally. A blunt periosteal elevator is used to strip the muscles from the plantar aspect of the calcaneus extraperiosteally (from medial to lateral—the abductor hallucis, flexor digitorum brevis, and abductor digiti quinti). To avoid the subsequent formation of new bone on the plantar surface of the calcaneus, cortical bone should not be removed as this is done.

Optionally, the soft tissue dissection is continued distally to the calcaneocuboid joint where the long plantar ligament is divided transversely (where it extends from the calcaneus to the cuboid). In the fixed cavus deformity the long plantar ligament is usually contracted. The plantar vessels are protected throughout the procedure by keeping the dissection close to bone. After release of the plantar fascia and the long plantar ligament, the cavus deformity is manually corrected. The wound is closed, and a short-leg cast is applied holding the foot in the corrected position.

POSTOPERATIVE MANAGEMENT. Sutures are removed 10 to 14 days after surgery, and a new short-leg cast is applied with generous padding beneath the metatarsal heads and over the dorsum of the foot to prevent pressure necrosis in these areas. Weight bearing is allowed in this cast, and all plaster immobilization is discontinued 4 weeks postoperatively. Metatarsal bars and/or plantar-stretching exercises may be of additional help to the patient subsequently.

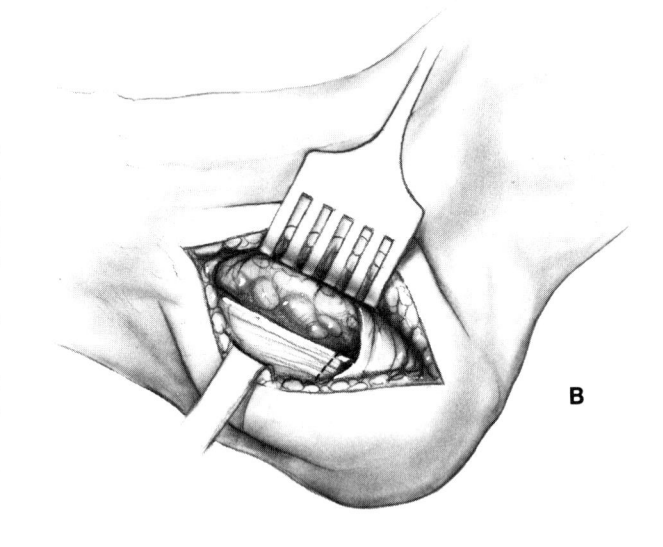

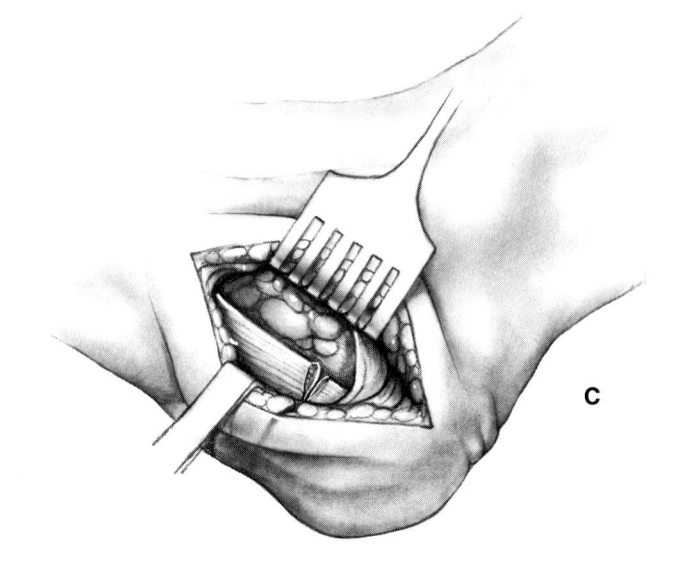

(Plate 15-6) MEDIAL SOFT TISSUE RELEASE (FOR RESISTANT EQUINOVARUS CLUBFOOT)

GENERAL DISCUSSION. There are two principal indications for surgical correction of resistant clubfoot: (1) failure to obtain complete correction after adequate nonoperative treatment and (2) recurrence of deformity or failure to maintain a lasting correction. The one-stage release is most effective in the treatment of resistant clubfoot in children between the ages of 1 and 2 years. The upper age limit should be 6 years. This one-stage method of surgical correction is not recommended in older children because adaptive changes occur in the shape and articular surfaces of the tarsal bones, which prevent reduction of the talus into the ankle mortise and reduction of the talocalcaneonavicular dislocation after that age. It must be emphasized that surgery for clubfoot deformities should be performed only after an adequate trial of nonoperative treatment has failed to accomplish complete correction.

When the soft tissue contractures are released surgically in the clubfoot of a young child, three groups of contractures are generally present: posterior, medial, and subtalar. The posterior contractures involve the posterior capsule of the ankle and subtalar joints, the Achilles tendon, the posterior talofibular, and the calcaneofibular ligaments. The Achilles tendon also inserts more medially on the calcaneus, thereby contributing to the varus deformity of the heel. The medial contracture involved the deltoid and spring ligaments, the talonavicular joint capsule, and the posterior tibial, flexor digitorum longus, and flexor hallucis longus tendons. The subtalar contractures are in the anterior subtalar interosseous ligament and the bifurcate ligament.

In older children the residual clubfoot deformity is often accompanied by a marked cavus deformity caused by contracture of the plantar fascia and the abductor hallucis, intrinsic toe flexors, and abductor digiti quinti muscles.

DETAILS OF PROCEDURE. Adequate surgical exposure is necessary to carry out a careful dissection under direct vision without injuring the articular surfaces, to excise or release all the abnormally contracted soft tissues preventing complete correction of the deformity, and to reduce and stabilize the navicular and calcaneus on the talus by transfixing the talonavicular joint with a Kirschner wire as recommended by Turco. The incision is made as illustrated **(A)**, 8 to 9 cm in length, beginning at the base of the first metatarsal and continuing posteriorly to the tendo Achillis curving slightly under the medial malleolus. A vertical extension of the incision along the tendo Achillis is not necessary and should be avoided.

The dissection in a small deformed foot can be difficult but will be greatly facilitated if the following specific structures are identified and exposed in the following order: posterior tibial tendon, flexor digitorum longus, posterior tibial neurovascular bundle, flexor hallucis longus, and the tendo Achillis **(B)**. As the tendons are exposed, their sheaths should be opened and divided, since the sheaths also are contracted and contribute to the resistance of the deformity. The posterior tibial tendon must be identified and its sheath incised from its insertion to above the ankle. In the child with a clubfoot, this tendon is more anterior and vertically oriented than in a normal foot. Next, the flexor digitorum longus tendon is identified just below the posterior tibial and is freed from its sheath. The posterior tibial vein identifies the neurovascular bundle, which is located below the flexor digitorum longus tendon. The nerve, artery, and vein and their common sheath are carefully mobilized and retracted with a

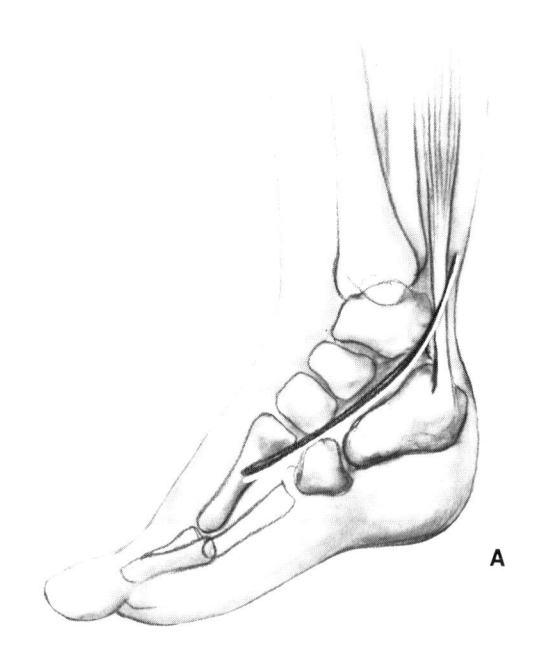

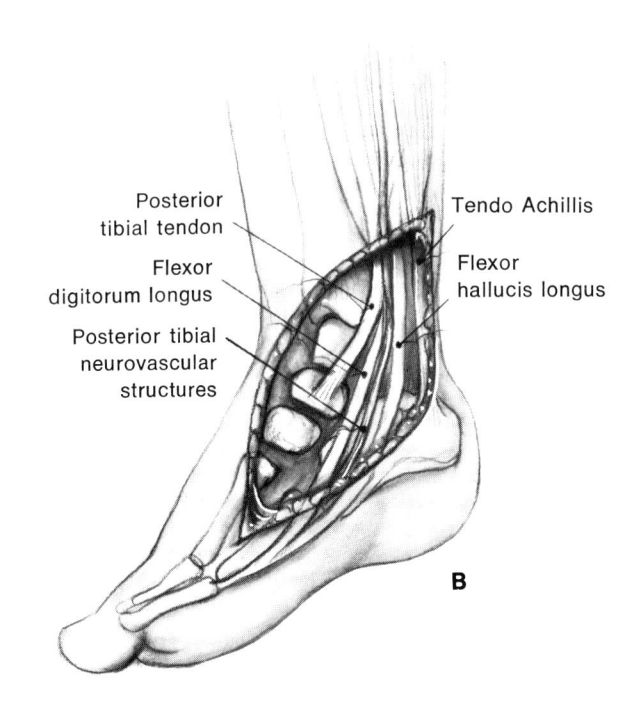

MEDIAL SOFT TISSUE RELEASE (FOR RESISTANT EQUINOVARUS CLUBFOOT) (Plate 15-6)

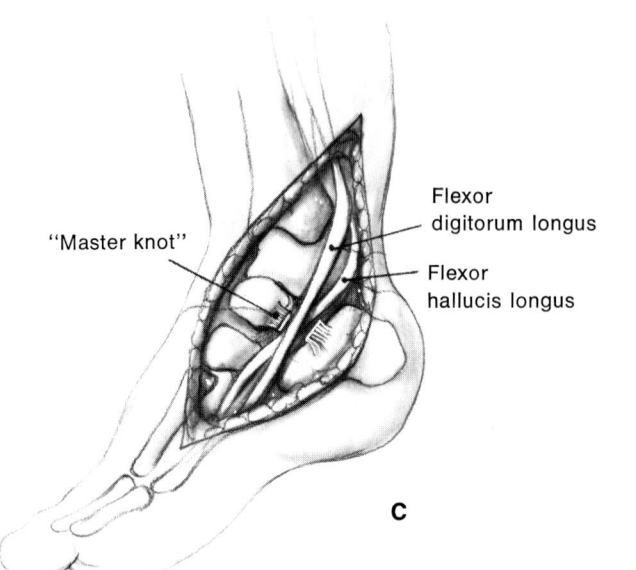

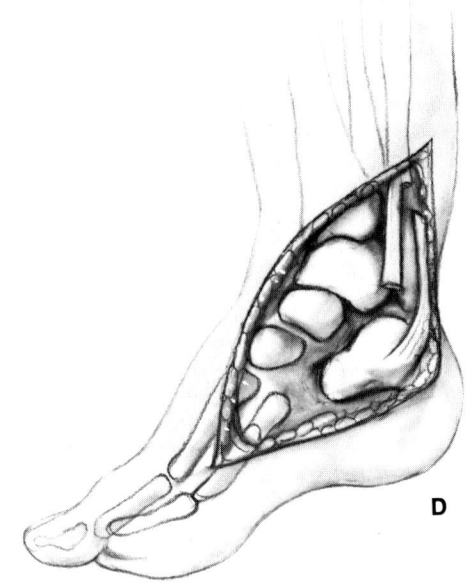

small Penrose drain. The neurovascular bundle must be mobilized proximally and distally so all contracted tissue can be excised by sharp dissection under direct vision. The neurovascular bundle is retracted posteriorly, and the flexor hallucis longus is identified under the sustentaculum tali and freed from its sheath. Next, anterior retraction of the neurovascular bundle brings the tendo Achillis into view. Only the distal 2 or 3 cm of the tendo Achillis needs to be exposed. The last specific step to obtain the necessary exposure is to free the sheaths of the flexor digitorum longus and flexor hallucis longus tendons by dividing the "master knot" of Henry **(C)**. This is a fibrocartilaginous structure that attaches to the undersurface of the navicular and envelops the flexor digitorum longus and flexor hallucis longus tendons where they cross. Excision of the "master knot" is necessary to mobilize the navicular. After these specific structures have been identified and mobilized, excision of the abnormal soft tissue contractures is carried out in the following sequence: the posterior release, the medial release, and then the subtalar release. The posterior release must be done first to facilitate the exposure and incision of the medial and subtalar contractures. The tendo Achillis is lengthened by Z-plasty, detaching the medial one half of its insertion on the calcaneus **(D)**.

Anterior retraction of the neurovascular bundle and flexor hallucis longus, after the tendo Achillis has been divided, then brings the posterior aspect of the ankle into view. The posterior margin of the tibia can now be identified by palpation, and a posterior capsulotomy of the tibiotalar joint is carried out under direct vision **(E)**. If necessary, the posterior talofibular ligament can be transsected by extending the capsulotomy laterally. The posterior capsule of the subtalar joint (which is only a short distance from the ankle joint, separated only by the posterior tubercle of the talus) is identified and divided along with the calcaneofibular ligament, which is accessible in the depth of the wound **(E)**. The calcaneofibular ligament is often contracted and is a significant contributor to the deformity of the heel in older children. Finally, for the posterior release, the neurovascular bundle is retracted posteriorly and the posterior insertion of the deltoid ligament on the calcaneus is divided by extending the incision in the posterior subtalar capsule slightly forward **(E)**. After the posterior subtalar joint has been identified through this capsular incision, attention is directed to correction of the remaining medial and subtalar contractures.

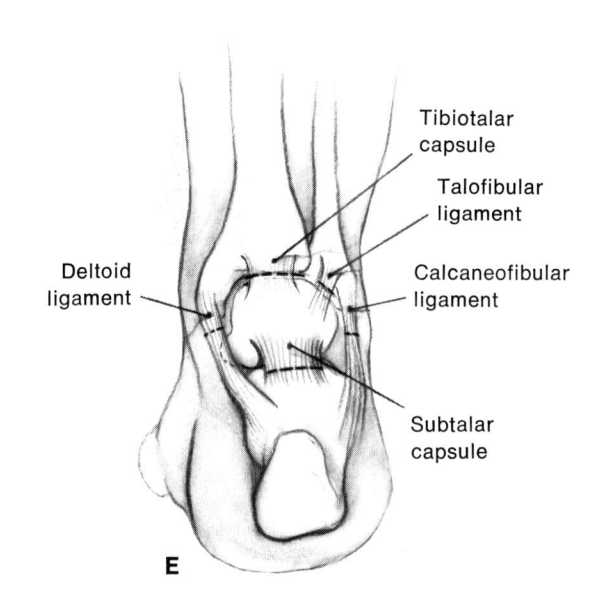

(Plate 15-6) MEDIAL SOFT TISSUE RELEASE (FOR RESISTANT EQUINOVARUS CLUBFOOT)

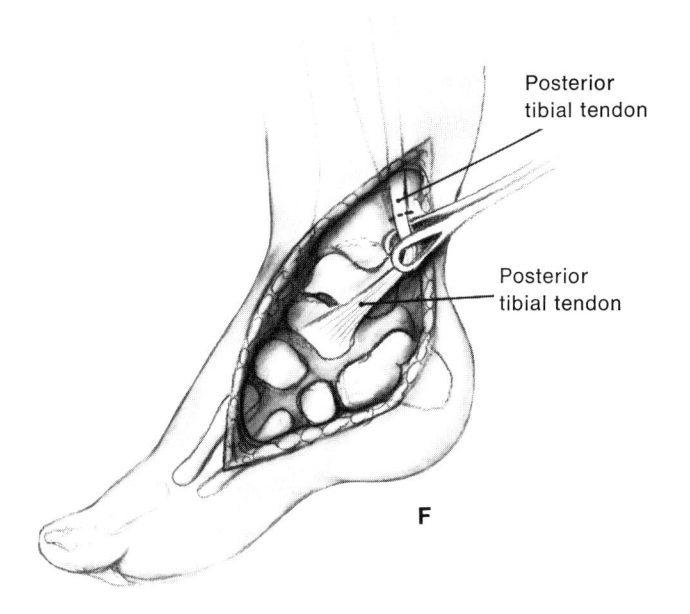

The tendons and the neurovascular bundle are retracted, bringing into view an unidentifiable mass of scar tissue that is composed of the posterior tibial tendon, the superficial deltoid ligament, the capsule of the talonavicular joint, and the spring ligament. This mass usually obscures the joint lines and the neck of the talus. The tarsal navicular is always found to be displaced medially with respect to the head of the talus. Mobilization of the navicular is initiated by dividing the posterior tibial tendon just above the medial malleolus (F). The proximal end of the tendon is allowed to retract while the distal portion attached to the navicular is preserved temporarily to be used as a retractor (G). The mass of scar tissue should be excised with care to avoid damage to the bone and joint surfaces. Traction on the posterior tibial stump opens the talonavicular joint and permits excision of the deltoid ligament insertion on the navicular and the talonavicular capsule. This part of the procedure should be done carefully, avoiding damage to the articular surfaces. The posterior tibial attachments to both the sustentaculum tali and the spring ligament are now incised (G), and the spring ligament is detached from the sustentaculum tali. Mobilization of the medially displaced navicular now brings into view the false articular facet on the proximal and medial aspects of the head of the talus. The talar head usually faces slightly more medially toward the medially displaced navicular than in a normal foot.

The medial release is carried out by returning to the site of the posterior release (which ended at the subtalar joint) and everting the foot. The subtalar joint is thereby exposed. This permits release of the superficial layer of the deltoid ligament from the calcaneus under direct vision. The deep portion of the deltoid ligament that inserts into the body of the talus should be preserved (if this is divided, a flatfoot deformity with tilting of the talus may develop).

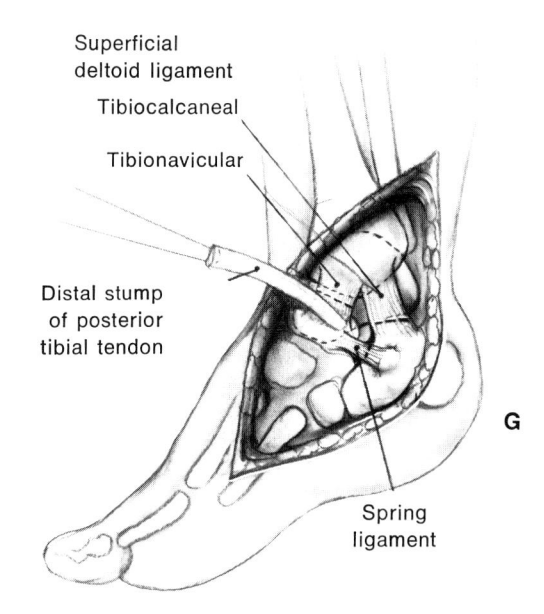

The subtalar release completes the mobilization of the anterior end of the calcaneus and the navicular. The talocalcaneal interosseous ligament located above the sustentaculum tali is exposed by everting the foot and is transected under direct vision. Mobilization of the navicular is completed by dividing the bifurcate ligament, which extends from the calcaneus to the lateral border of the navicular and to the medial border of the cuboid. The distal remnant of the posterior tibial tendon is now excised by dividing its attachment to the navicular.

After completion of the posterior, medial, and subtalar releases, reduction of the deformity should be accomplished without force, When the navicular is reduced onto the head of the talus, the other tarsal bones are carried with it. As the navicular moves forward, the anterior portion of the calcaneus moves laterally while the medially displaced sustentaculum tali assumes a normal position under the talus, and the subtalar joint opens like a book. For this reduction to occur, the anterior end of the calcaneus must evert and move laterally while its posterior tuberosity moves downward and away from both the ankle joint and the posterior ends of the talus. The calcaneus must be released at both ends if complete correction of the deformity is to be accomplished.

MEDIAL SOFT TISSUE RELEASE (FOR RESISTANT EQUINOVARUS CLUBFOOT) (Plate 15-6)

The advantage of a one-stage operation is that all contracted tissues are released simultaneously. Care must be taken not to overcorrect the navicular on the head of the talus. A Kirschner wire, 0.45 mm, is inserted percutaneously on the dorsum of the foot in the region of the first metatarsal shaft, transfixing the talonavicular joint. Before insertion of the Kirschner wire, the relationship of the calcaneus and navicular on the talus must be inspected to be certain that the correction is complete and that the foot is not overcorrected into valgus position **(H)**.

After the talonavicular joint is transfixed, the foot remains in the corrected position without any external force. The sectioned Achilles tendon ends are then approximated to allow dorsiflexion to a right angle and resutured. Excessive lengthening increases atrophy of the calf muscles and should be avoided. The subcutaneous tissues and skin are closed with interrupted fine catgut sutures. The protruding Kirschner wire is bent outside the skin and is not incorporated into the cast. A small piece of sterile felt is placed between the wire and the skin for protection. A well-padded above-knee cast is applied with the knee in slight flexion. Initial dorsiflexion of the foot is limited to a right angle to avoid tension on the skin and subcutaneous tissues and separation of the skin edges.

POSTOPERATIVE MANAGEMENT. Usually there will be a flexion contracture of the big toe, the result of correction of the preoperative medial concavity of the foot. Three weeks following operation the cast is changed under general anesthesia. The sutures are *not* removed at this time. A new above-knee cast is applied, bringing the foot up into further dorsiflexion. At 6 weeks postoperatively, the cast is changed on an outpatient basis. Sutures and Kirschner wire are removed, and a new above-knee plaster cast is applied that maintains full correction of the foot in dorsiflexion and valgus position. Immobilization is continued for a total of 4 months. The cast may be changed as necessary. If the child is old enough to walk, a walking cast is applied after the Kirshner wire is removed. After 4 months of immobilization, the foot is protected in a Denis Browne splint with a 25 cm crossbar that the child wears during his sleeping hours for 1 year. Lateral sole wedges are used during the day for 2 years after cast removal.

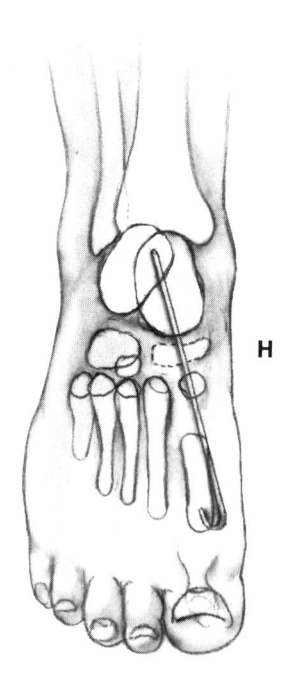

(Plate 15-7) TARSOMETATARSAL MOBILIZATION (FOR RESISTANT FOREFOOT ADDUCTION)

GENERAL DISCUSSION. Tarsometatarsal capsulotomy and release of the intermetatarsal ligaments is an effective procedure in the resistant, or recurrent, adduction deformity of the forepart of the foot in congenital clubfoot and congenital metatarsus adductus in the child 3 to 8 years of age when the hind part of the foot is in neutral alignment and when conservative methods have failed to correct the deformity.

As suggested by Kendrick, Herndon, and others, the following precautions are recommended if good results are to be obtained in tarsometatarsal mobilization: minimum dissection, avoidance of damage to the articular surfaces, division of only the intermetatarsal and tarsometatarsal ligaments, avoidance of division of the lateral capsule of the fifth metatarsal cuboid joint, and the immobilization of the operated foot in a well-molded walking short-leg cast for a minimum of 4 months postoperatively.

DETAILS OF PROCEDURE. A curvilinear incision is made over the dorsal aspect of the foot beginning at the medial side of the first tarsometatarsal joint extending to the base of the fifth metatarsal bone with convexity distally **(A)**. The incision may be extended proximally at the medial side to expose the articulations between the navicular and cuneiform bones in order to divide these capsules if they appear to offer resistance to correction. The skin flaps are retracted to expose the deep fascia covering the tarsometatarsal joints. The anterior tibial tendon is identified and protected. A longitudinal incision is then made through the deep fascia over the first tarsometatarsal joint. The fascia is retracted, exposing the dorsal ligaments. The dorsal and interosseus ligaments and joint capsule are divided with an incision around the base of the first metatarsal with care to avoid injury to the anterior tibial tendon at its insertion. The joint is flexed to allow the scalpel to be inserted to divide the capsule and ligaments of the same joint on its plantar aspect. Another longitudinal incision is made through the deep fascia over the interval between the bases of the second and third metatarsals. These two joints can be exposed by retracting the deep fascia. A deep incision is made around the base of each of these metatarsals, and the joint capsules and the dorsal interosseus and intermetatarsal ligaments of these joints are completely divided **(B)**. In similar fashion an incision is made through the deep fascia over the interval between the bases of the fourth and fifth metatarsals and the corresponding ligaments, and capsules of these joints are divided in similar fashion. With traction and simultaneous flexion on the tarsometatarsal joints, the scalpel is introduced to assure completion of the division of the capsules and ligaments on the plantar aspect of these joints. After complete division of the ligaments and joint capsules of the tarsometatarsal and intermetatarsal articularions, the lateral four metatarsal bones should glide on one another and the forepart of the foot should swing outward or laterally at the tarsometatarsal level without much resistance **(C)**. If the patient is a very young child, the adduction deformity can be overcorrected. Following wound closure, a molded plaster cast is applied with the forepart of the foot held in as much abduction as possible and with the hind foot in neutral position.

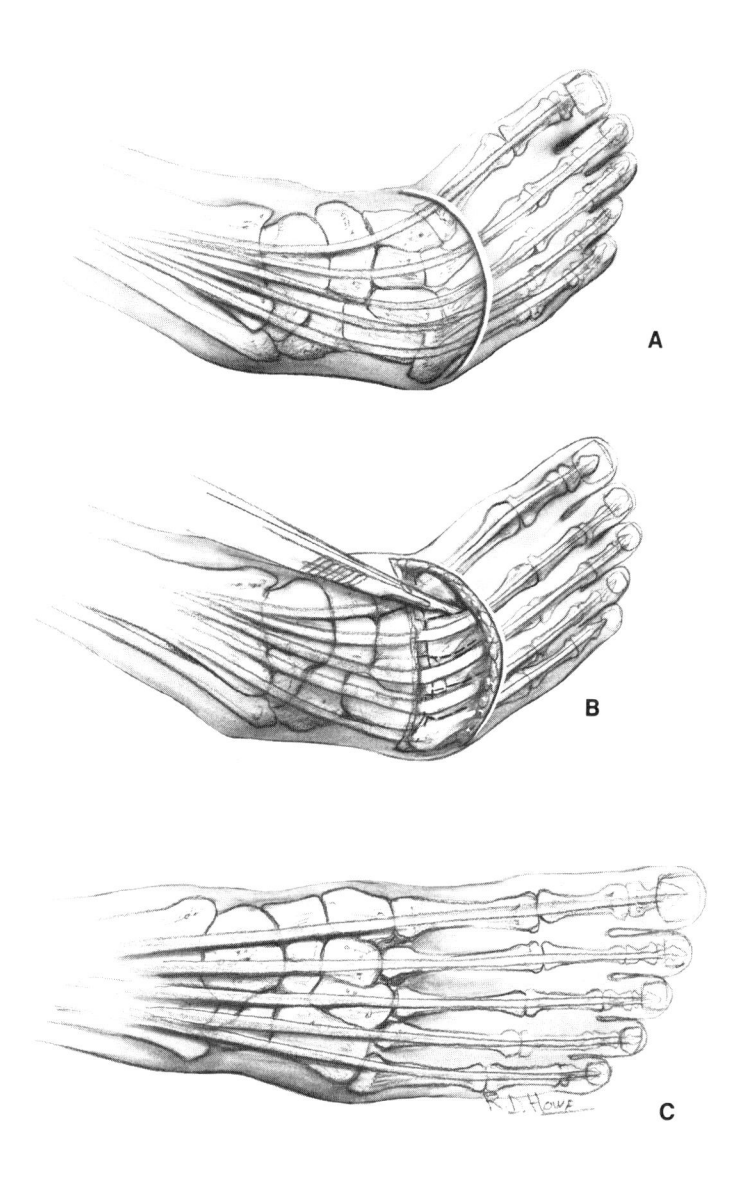

POSTOPERATIVE MANAGEMENT. The cast is changed 2 weeks after surgery and the sutures are removed. If the correction initially was not as complete as desired, a little more stretching of the forefoot can be accomplished at this time. The foot should then be maintained in the corrected position in a plaster cast for an additional 3½ months. Weight bearing in plaster with the foot in the functional position is allowed after the third postoperative week.

MEDIAL TRANSFER OF PERONEUS LONGUS TENDON (Plate 15-8)

GENERAL DISCUSSION. The peroneus longus or brevis muscle, when transferred medially, can substitute adequately for loss of dorsiflexion function at the ankle. The foot may need stabilization with a triple arthrodesis in a child 12 years of age or over. With anterior tibial paralysis, both the peroneus longus and brevis may be transferred to the first cuneiform bone at the same time a triple arthrodesis is performed.

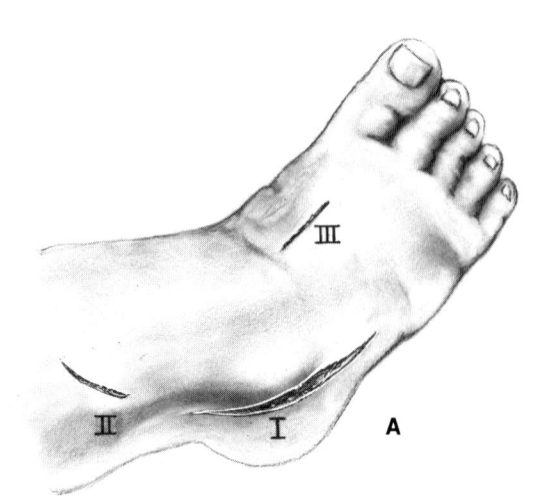

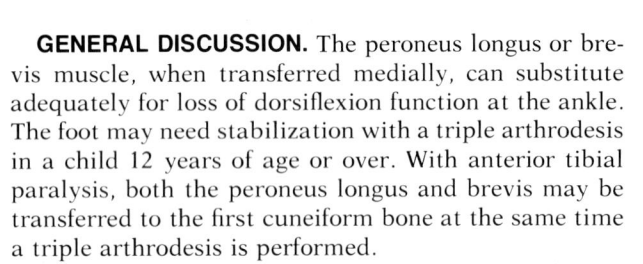

In the child under 12 years of age with an unbalanced foot and progressive deformity, stabilization of the hind foot may be accomplished by subtalar extra-articular arthrodesis (Grice procedure). Then, the peroneus longus is usually transferred through the anterior tibial sheath to the first cuneiform and the peroneus brevis is transferred to the distal stump of the peroneus longus (to provide some plantar flexion effect on the first metatarsal to prevent development of a dorsal bunion).

With a single tendon transfer, the peroneus longus is a better muscle for medial transfer than the peroneus brevis.

DETAILS OF PROCEDURE. The peroneal tendons are exposed through a short incision parallel to their course proximal to the base of the fifth metatarsal (**A**). The tendon sheath is opened, and the peroneus brevis is divided close to its point of insertion into the base of the fifth metatarsal. The peroneus longus is divided as it begins to enter its groove on the plantar aspect of the cuboid. The peroneus brevis tendon is sutured to the distal stump of the peroneus longus tendon (**B** and **C**).

A short, oblique incision is then made on the anterolateral aspect of the leg at the junction of the middle and distal thirds of the lower leg, and the peroneus longus is identified by traction on its distal tendon. A third incision is made over the dorsum of the foot (**A**). The anterior tibial tendon sheath or common extensor tendon sheath is opened depending on where the tendon transfer is to be inserted. A tendon passer is then directed from the dorsum of the foot through the tendon sheath to the proximal wound where the fascia is incised, allowing the tendon passer to emerge in the proximal wound.

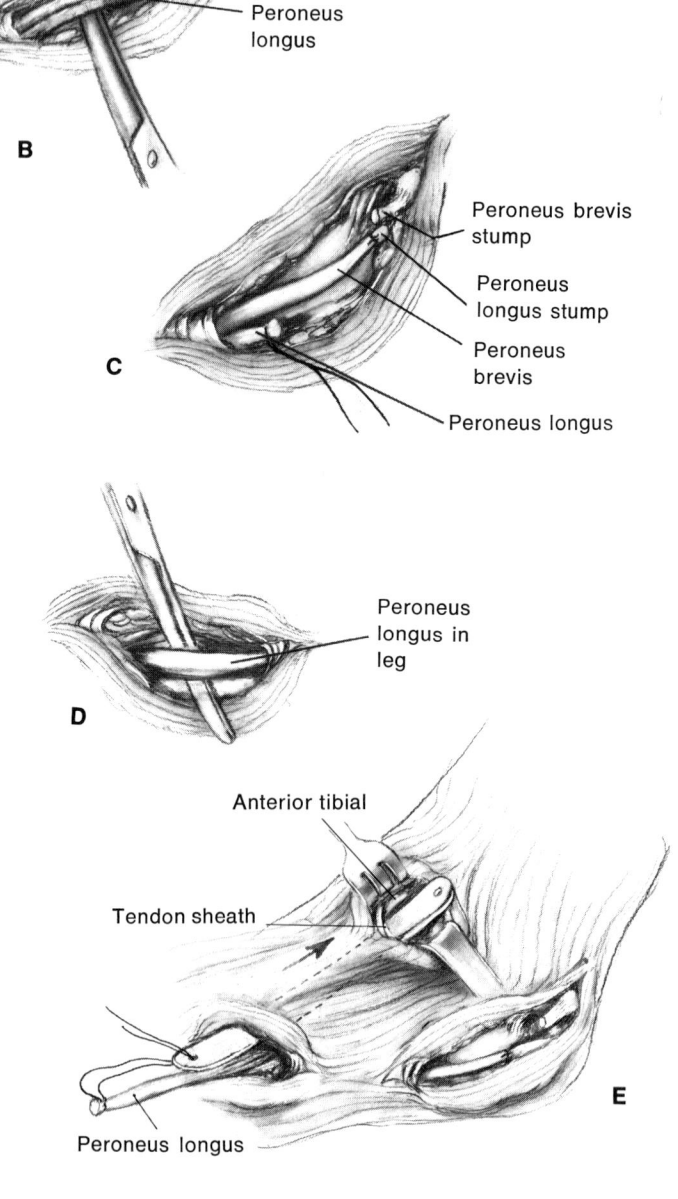

The peroneus longus tendon is mobilized and pulled through to the proximal incision (**D**). A suture is placed in the peroneus tendon, threaded in the hole of the tendon passer, and pulled through to the dorsum of the foot (**E**). The fascia is then incised widely over the dorsum of the foot to allow the transferred tendon and muscle to be directed in a straight line toward their new insertion without angulation over fascial edges.

(Plate 15-8) MEDIAL TRANSFER OF PERONEUS LONGUS TENDON

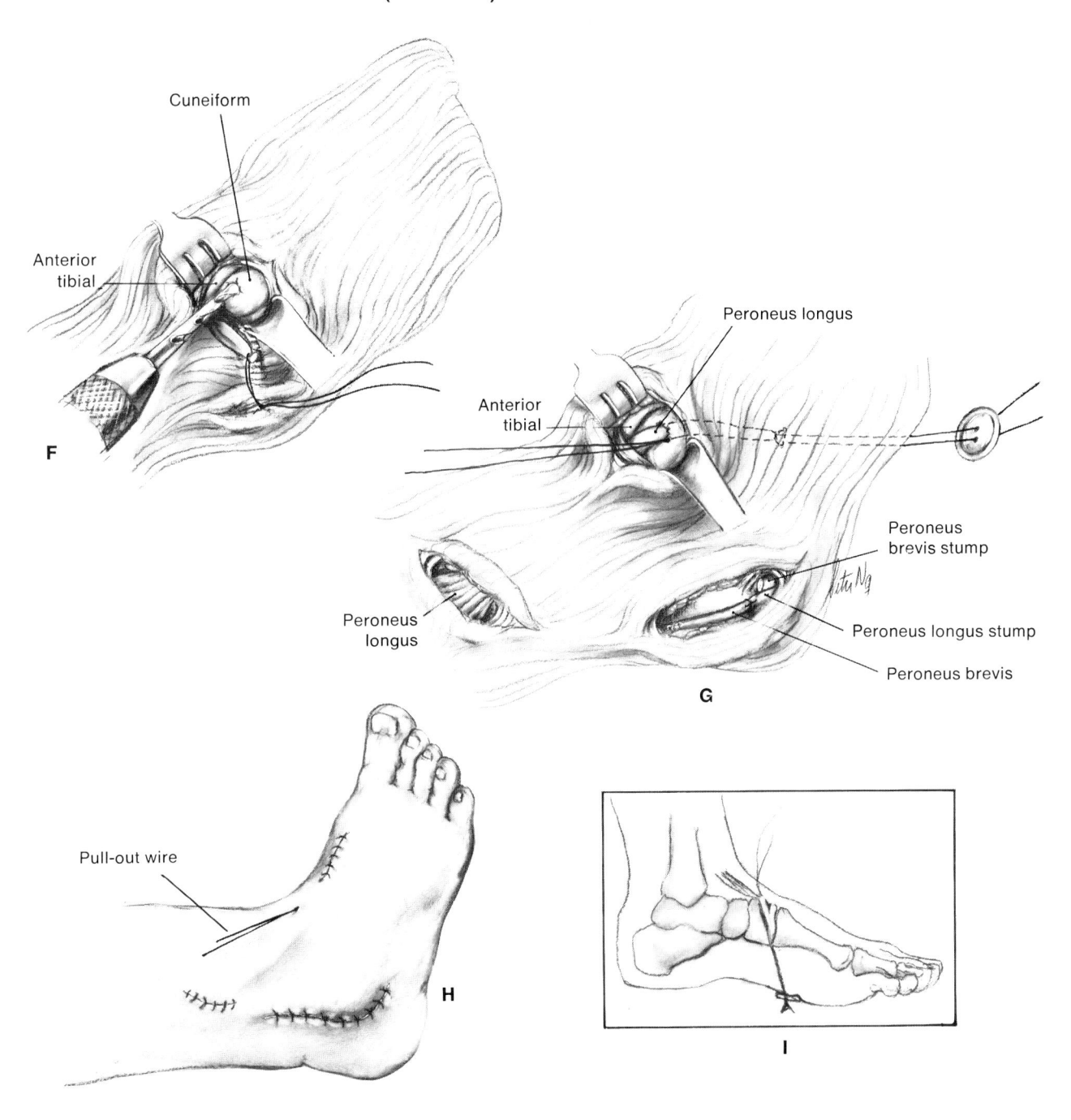

The ankle is held in neutral position. Tension is placed on the peroneus longus tendon, and the exact site of the bony bed is determined (the area of the first or second cuneiform bone is the most common site). This area is then exposed subperiosteally, and a large oblique drill hole is made from the dorsal surface to the plantar surface of the bone **(F)**. The dorsal two thirds of this drill hole is then enlarged with a curet to allow easy accommodation of the end of the transferred tendon. A pull-out, Bunnell-type, stainless-steel wire is placed in the tendon. The two needles on the ends of the Bunnell suture are then passed through the drill hole to the plantar surface of the foot. Again the ankle is held in neutral position, and the tendon is carefully placed into the hole in the selected bone and pulled up snugly as the wire is tied over a padded button on the plantar surface of the foot **(G)**. The pull-out wire is placed through the skin proximally, and the incisions are closed **(H)**. An assistant continues to support the ankle and foot in neutral position **(I)** until a short-leg cast has been applied.

POSTOPERATIVE MANAGEMENT. Plaster immobilization is continued for 6 weeks postoperatively.

563

LATERAL TRANSFER OF ANTERIOR TIBIAL TENDON (Plate 15-9)

GENERAL DISCUSSION. Lateral transfer of the anterior tibial tendon is a useful procedure in recurrent and resistant forefoot adduction deformities. The deformities may be congenital or paralytic. Fixed deformities must be corrected preoperatively. The tendon transfer is carried out when the foot can be passively corrected with ease beyond the neutral position. To avoid the complication of progressive valgus deformity, the new insertion should be made just lateral to the midline of the foot. The tendon should not be transferred to the extreme lateral margin of the foot.

DETAILS OF PROCEDURE. Three skin incisions are made, one over the dorsomedial aspect of the base of the first metatarsal, another 5 cm above the ankle, and the third over the third cuneiform just lateral to the midline of the dorsum of the foot **(A)**. A subcutaneous tunnel is made with a clamp between the second and third incisions to prepare the new course of the tendon. The insertion of the anterior tibial tendon is then detached as far distally as possible, taking a fascial tongue with it. The muscle-tendon structure is identified in the proximal incision by tugging distally on the sectioned tendon stump. The tendon is pulled through into the leg incision **(B)** and subsequently passed through the prepared subcutaneous tunnel to the point of its new insertion **(D)**. The bony bed is prepared after testing the length of the tendon to allow at least 1.5 cm of tendon to be pulled down into the depth of the bed. A drill hole is made through the tarsal bone at the selected point just lateral to the midline of the foot **(C)**. This must be large enough to accommodate the full thickness of the tendon without fraying.

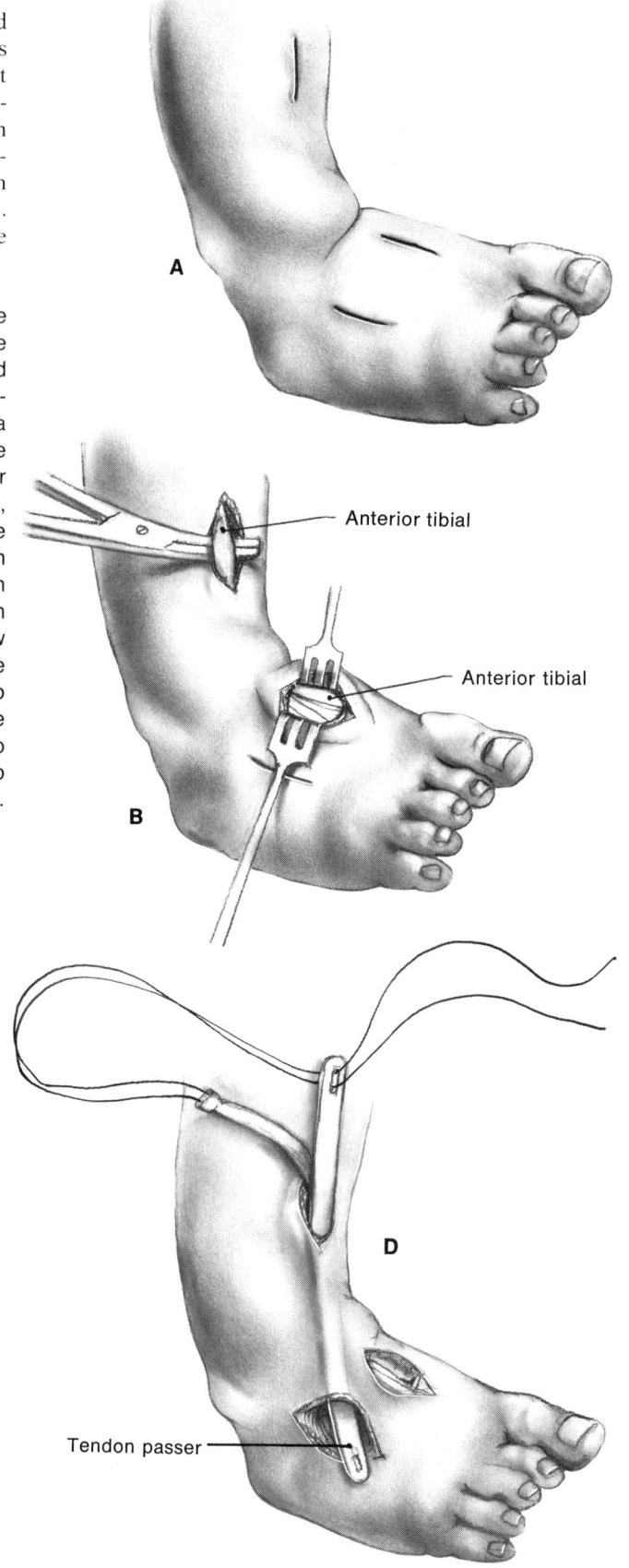

(Plate 15-9) LATERAL TRANSFER OF ANTERIOR TIBIAL TENDON

A pull-out, Bunnell, stainless-steel suture is placed in the transferred tendon (**E** and **F**). The two ends of the Bunnell suture are passed through the drill hole and sole of the foot **(G)**.

The tendon is pulled securely into the bony bed, and the wire suture is tied securely over a small gauze pad and button on the sole of the foot while the foot is held in mild valgus and the ankle in neutral position **(H)**. The pull-out suture is then passed proximally through the skin, and the wounds are closed **(I)**. The foot is held in mild valgus and the ankle in neutral position during wound closure and until after application of the cast, which extends from toes to tibial tubercle.

POSTOPERATIVE MANAGEMENT. Immobilization of the foot in plaster is continued for 6 weeks postoperatively.

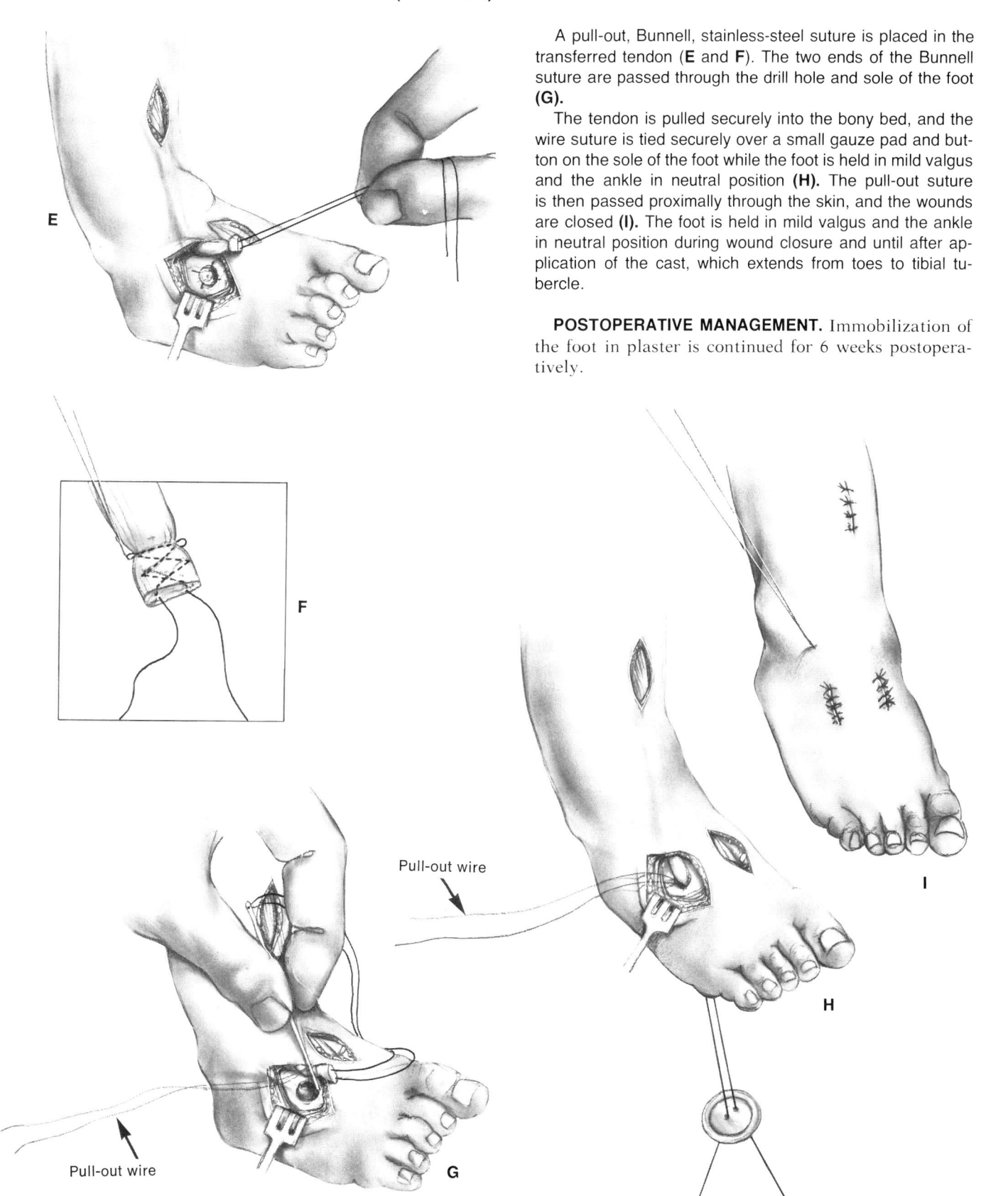

EXCISION OF ACCESSORY TARSAL NAVICULAR (Plate 15-10)

GENERAL DISCUSSION. The accessory tarsal navicular is a congenital anomaly in which the tuberosity develops from a second center of ossification. The occurrence of this anomaly is related to the other inconstant accessory bones of the foot, which, in most instances, are of only academic interest. However, the accessory tarsal navicular may occasionally produce symptoms requiring surgical correction. In this type of foot, the posterior tibial tendon is usually attached to the accessory tarsal navicular and passes across the medial aspect of the tarsal navicular rather than inferior to it. The normal support of the longitudinal arch by the posterior tibial muscle is lacking. There may be local tenderness and discomfort when a bursa, formed over the bone as a result of pressure from the shoe, becomes irritated.

A variant of this type of anomaly is a foot in which the medial end of the tarsal navicular is enlarged and abnormally curved. This can produce the same mechanical abnormality and symptoms. More often than not, the anomaly is bilateral, but symptoms may occur only in one foot.

In patients who do not obtain relief with conservative measures, the Kidner procedure will usually alleviate symptoms. This procedure involves excision of the accessory tarsal navicular and/or the abnormal medial projection of the tarsal navicular and transposition of the posterior tibial tendon into a groove on the inferior surface of the bone.

DETAILS OF PROCEDURE. A curvilinear incision is made from a point just anterior and distal to the medial malleolus to the base of the first metatarsal **(A)**. The fascia is incised along the anterior border of the posterior tibial tendon throughout the length of the incision. By sharp periosteal dissection, the tendinous attachment of the tibialis posterior tendon is reflected inferiorly **(B)** to expose the accessory navicular bone, the body of the navicular, and a portion of the talus. The accessory navicular bone is excised. Manual motion of the accessory bone will help in determining the connecting area of the accessory bone. The accessory bone is excised. The remaining prominent medial portion of the tarsal navicular should also be removed using a curved osteotome (**C** to **E**). The edges of the remaining bone are smoothed with a rasp. The reflected portion of the posterior tibial tendon is resutured to the remainder of the tendon on the plantar surface of the tarsal navicular. Fascia and skin are closed in layers, and a soft dressing is applied.

POSTOPERATIVE MANAGEMENT. Weight bearing is limited for 7 to 10 days and allowed as tolerated thereafter.

(Plate 15-10) EXCISION OF ACCESSORY TARSAL NAVICULAR

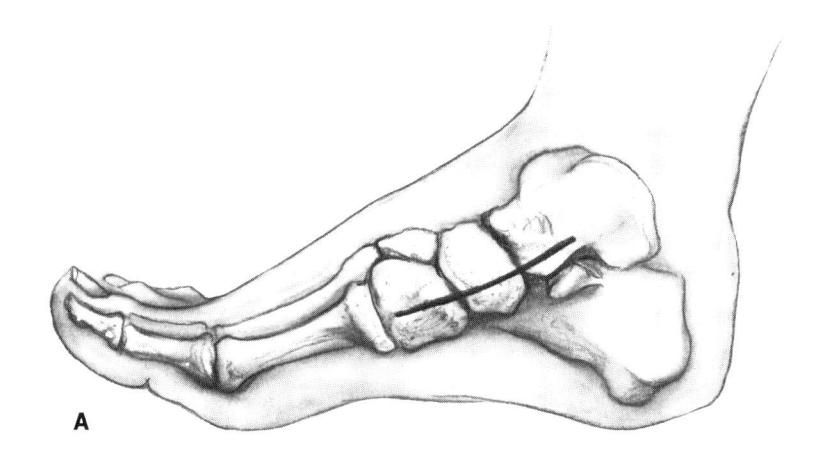

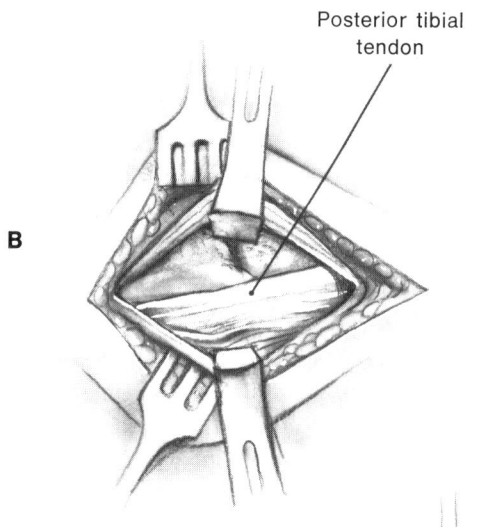

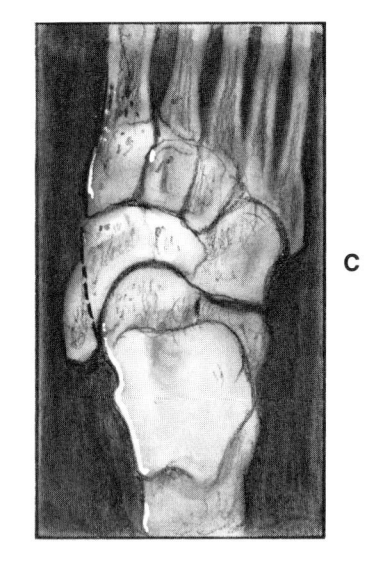

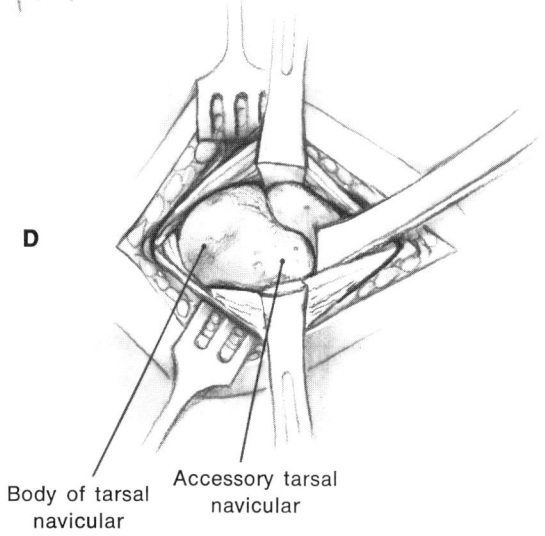

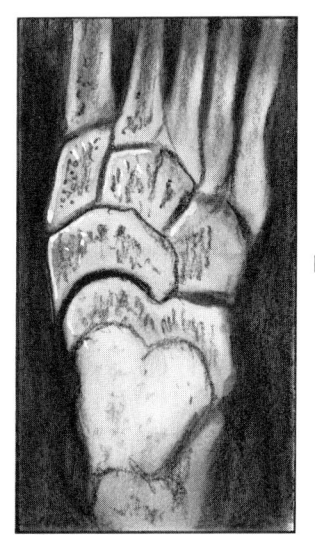

A

B Posterior tibial tendon

C

D Body of tarsal navicular — Accessory tarsal navicular

E

567

EXCISION OF TARSAL COALITION (Plate 15-11)

GENERAL DISCUSSION. Tarsal coalition is the union of two or more tarsal bones. It may be congenital or acquired. Coalition of any tarsal joint can result from trauma or infection, as well as being congenital and hereditary and may, or may not, be associated with symptoms. The union may be cartilaginous, osseous, or fibrous. The commonest coalitions are calcaneonavicular bar, talocalcaneal bridge, and talonavicular and calcaneocuboid bar. Coalition has been demonstrated in the fetus. It is usually fibrous or cartilaginous at birth. Good tarsal motion is feasible in the presence of the fibrous lesions; some limitation of motion occurs with a cartilaginous lesion; with an osseous coalition, there is a complete loss of joint motion.

Symptoms usually appear in the second decade of life. Usually, there is vague discomfort over the talonavicular joint or nearby in the foot. On physical examination, there is limited subtalar motion and often flatfoot with peroneal muscle spasm.

In the adult, a painful rigid flat foot with a tarsal coalition, such as a calcaneonavicular bar, usually requires treatment by triple arthrodesis. In the adolescent, long-standing deformity or adaptive joint changes may also require a triple arthrodesis to alleviate the discomfort. In the younger patient, however, without adaptive joint changes, it is reasonable to consider simple excision of the tarsal coalition.

Tarsal coalition should be suspected in any young patient with a painful flatfoot with limited subtalar joint motion. The presence of degenerative changes at the superior aspect of the talonavicular joint in the lateral roentgenogram is a valuable clue. Although oblique views and axial calcaneal views are often helpful, tomograms can be of further help in making the specific diagnosis. Although the anomaly may begin to develop earlier, limited movement of the subtalar and midtarsal joints usually does not become evident until after 9 years of age. It may be that after this age, ossification of any cartilaginous bar begins.

Calcaneonavicular coalition may be overlooked in regular roentgenographic views of the foot. If a fibrous or cartilaginous coalition is present, the cortical bone surfaces will be indistinct and irregular at their junction. The talar head may be hypoplastic or underdeveloped. Autosomal dominant transmission has been demonstrated. A fibrous or a cartilaginous calcaneonavicular coalition in the young patient should be resected and the origin of the extensor digitorum brevis muscle interposed, as illustrated.

In talocalcaneal coalition, lateral foot roentgenographs are likely to show beaking of the talar head, broadening of the lateral talar process, and narrowing of the posterior talocalcaneal facet. These changes are probably a reflection of abnormal subtalar motion.

It is recognized that patients with symptomatic tarsal coalition can sometimes be relieved indefinitely by conservative treatment, but in view of the simplicity of operation and the short period of treatment after operation, excision of the tarsal coalition in a rigid and painful foot in a young individual merits consideration. To be successful, the operation should be confined to patients under 14 years of age. Long-standing deformity or adaptive changes diminish the likelihood of success with any operative treatment other than triple arthrodesis. The ideal patient for operative excision of tarsal coalition is the young patient with symptoms of recent origin and no adaptive joint changes visible roentgenographically.

DETAILS OF PROCEDURE. A lateral incision is used extending from a point just below the lateral malleolus forward toward the calcaneocuboid joint **(A)**. The dissection is carried down to expose the origin of the extensor digitorum brevis muscle, which is reflected from the anterosuperior margin of the calcaneus, and the long extensor tendons are retracted medially. The calcaneocuboid and talonavicular joints are opened sufficiently to expose the calcaneonavicular bar. An osteotome is used to divide the calcaneal and the navicular ends of the bar **(B)**. The osteotome is almost horizontal in dividing the calcaneal portion of the bar. The osteotome is angled downward as the navicular portion of the bar is divided. The bony synostosis is removed **(C)**. The origin of the extensor digitorum brevis muscle is sutured into the defect formerly occupied by the bony synostosis **(D)**. The wound is closed and the foot is immobilized in a short-leg cast holding the foot in some inversion.

POSTOPERATIVE MANAGEMENT. The cast is removed 3 weeks after surgery. Subsequently, increasing activity is permitted as tolerated.

(Plate 15-11) EXCISION OF TARSAL COALITION

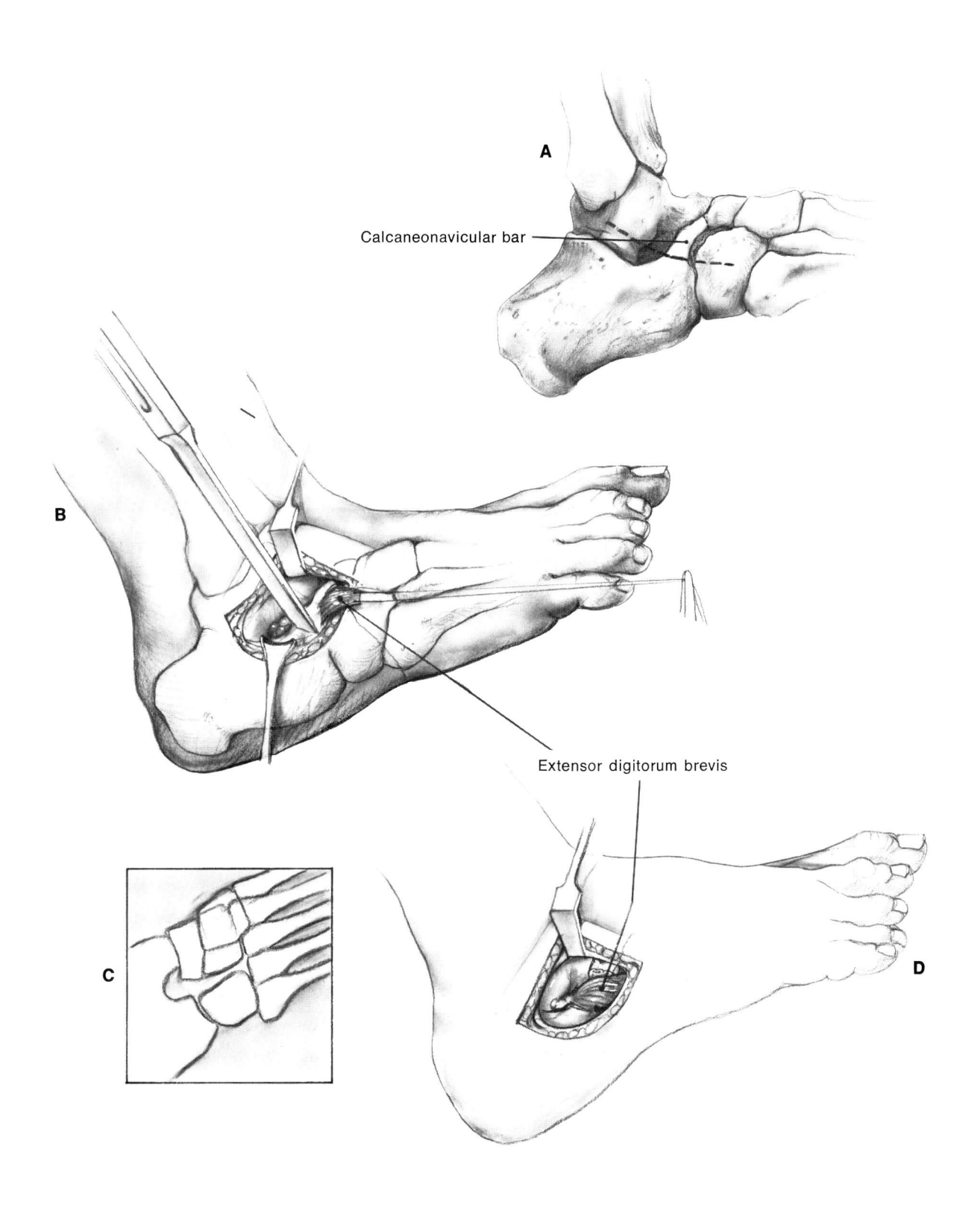

Calcaneonavicular bar

Extensor digitorum brevis

TRANSMETATARSAL AMPUTATION (Plate 15-12)

GENERAL DISCUSSION. For trauma or disease of the foot that is localized to the toes or metatarsal heads and requires amputation, the relatively conservative transmetatarsal amputation may be indicated in preference to an amputation above the ankle joint.

DETAILS OF PROCEDURE. The dorsal incision should begin midway between the dorsal and plantar surfaces near the distal portion of the first metatarsal and is continued in a straight line across the dorsum of the foot to the lateral side of the fifth metatarsal. The plantar incision is then made beginning at either end of the dorsal incision to create a long plantar flap. The plantar incision should be parallel and 1 cm proximal to the flexion crease of the toes **(A)**. The plantar flap, including all soft tissues, is dissected proximally to the level of the transmetatarsal bone amputation. A small saw is used to remove the metatarsal heads one at a time, beginning with the first, to form an even stump. Each individual metatarsal should be rongeured or smoothed with a rasp. Rounding the plantar aspect of the distal end of each transected metatarsal will provide a better weight-bearing surface **(B)**. The first and fifth metatarsals may require beveling. Care should be taken to avoid unnecessary dissection of the dorsal flap, especially in ischemic feet. The plantar tendons are divided at the level of the bone division, and the sesamoids are removed. The plantar flap is sutured to the dorsal soft tissues in one layer with fine steel wire **(C)**. The "dog ears" on the medial and lateral side of the skin flap closure are not removed, since they help to prevent skin sloughing. A bulky dressing is applied, and the foot and ankle are immobilized in a well-padded plaster splint.

POSTOPERATIVE MANAGEMENT. Bed rest is continued for several days, or, in cases of borderline viability, until the sutures are removed 2 to 3 weeks postoperatively. Full weight bearing is allowed only after complete healing has occurred. This may require 4 to 6 weeks. A shoe with a rigid sole and a metatarsal bar is helpful **(D)**.

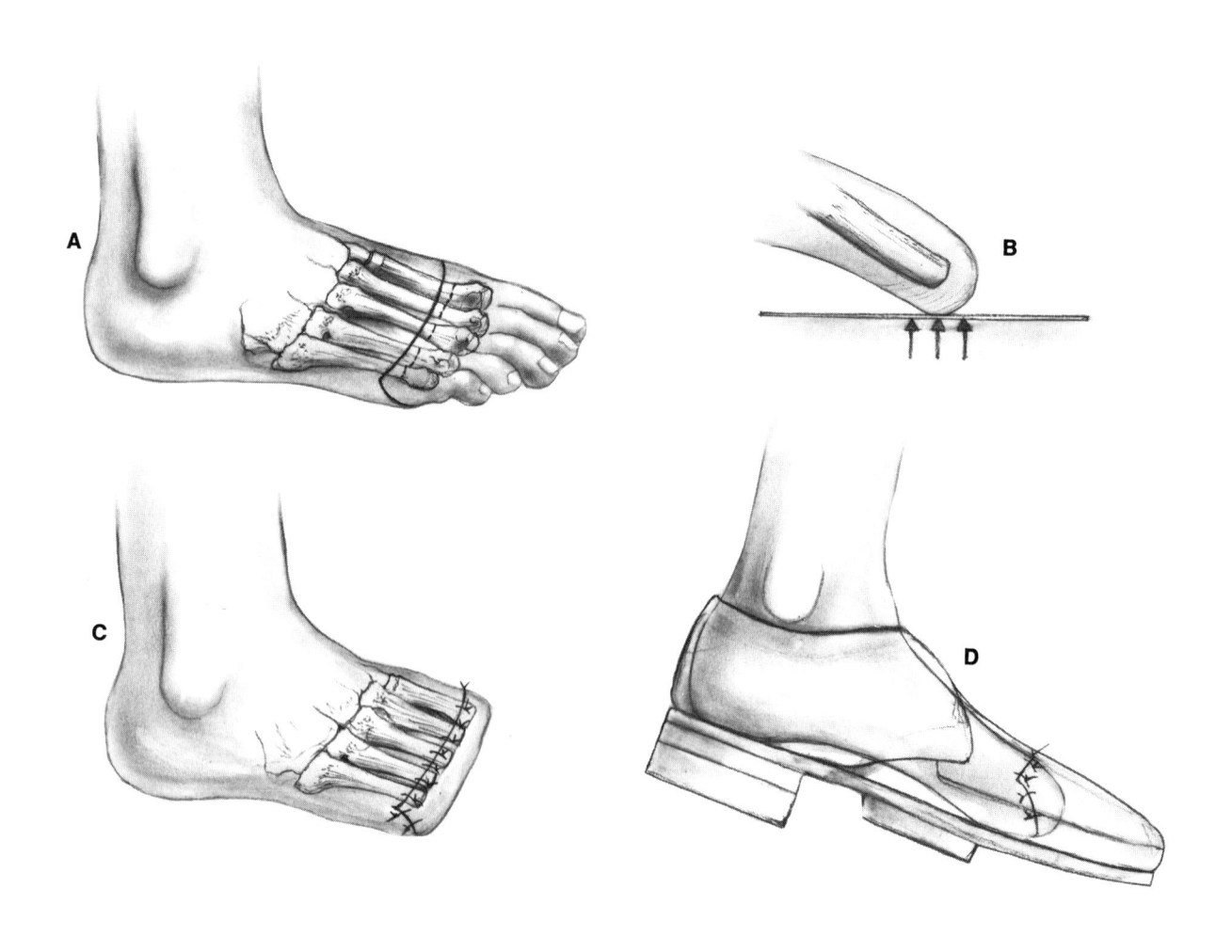

(Plate 15-13) INTRAMEDULLARY FIXATION FOR DISPLACED METATARSAL FRACTURE

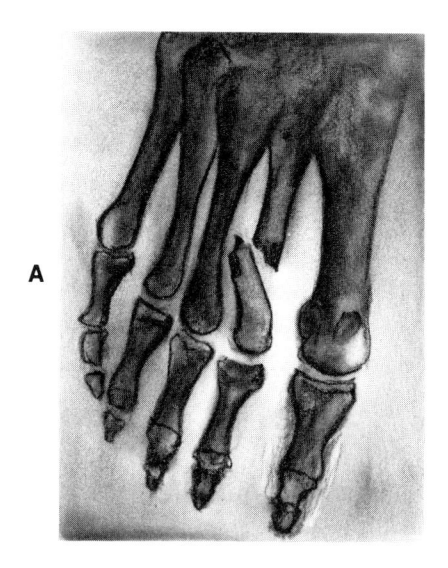

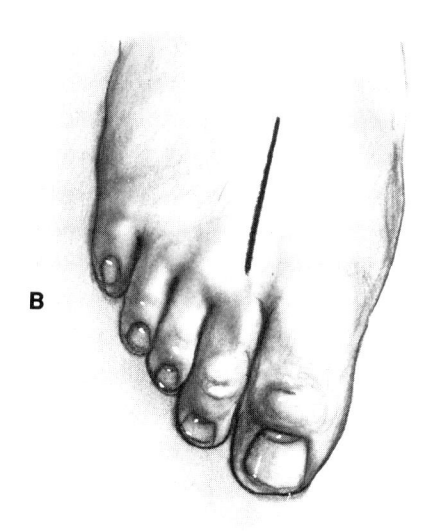

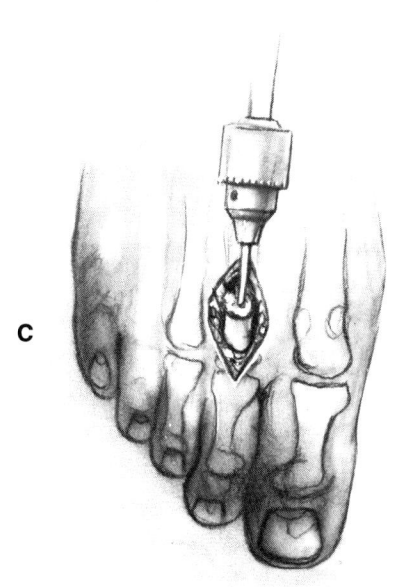

GENERAL DISCUSSION. Generally, metatarsal fractures will not be grossly displaced unless several metatarsals are fractured. Open reduction of a metatarsal fracture may occasionally be indicated when displacement is such that manual reduction or maintenance of reduction is not possible **(A)**.

The small diameter of the metatarsals obviates the use of plates or screws for internal fixation. However, the metatarsals are suitable for intramedullary fixation.

A displaced fracture of the distal shaft of a metatarsal can be difficult to maintain in position without surgery, but, with intramedullary fixation, good position is easily maintained.

DETAILS OF PROCEDURE. A short longitudinal incision is made dorsally to expose the fracture of the metatarsal **(B)**. Dissection of the soft tissues should be held to a minimum. The distal end of the metatarsal is elevated into the dorsal longitudinal wound and, with the toes held in hyperextension, a small Kirschner wire is drilled into the medullary canal of the distal fragment and advanced until it emerges through the skin **(C)**. The drill is then removed and reversed in order to drill it retrograde into the proximal fragment. At this point the Kirschner wire is divided sharply at the fracture level. The ends of the fracture fragments are held reduced while the Kirschner wire is drilled across the fracture until its proximal end is well into the metaphyseal area of the proximal fragment **(D)**. Approximately, 0.5 cm of the wire is left protruding through the skin on the plantar aspect of the foot, and a small dressing is applied after it is sealed with collodion. A short-leg cast is applied over generous padding.

POSTOPERATIVE MANAGEMENT. The patient is kept in bed with the foot elevated for several days. Crutch walking without weight bearing on the involved foot is allowed thereafter. Three to four weeks postoperatively, the Kirschner wire is removed and a new walking short-leg cast is applied with care to mold the plaster well to the transverse and longitudinal arches of the foot. Plaster immobilization is discontinued when there is clinical and roentgenographic evidence that fracture healing is adequate to permit walking in a standard shoe.

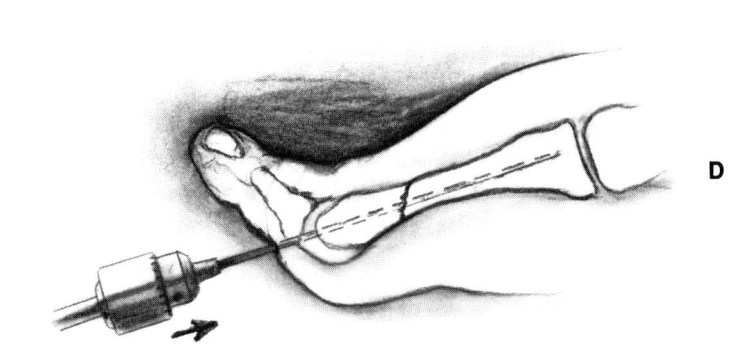

KELLER PROCEDURE (Plate 15-14)

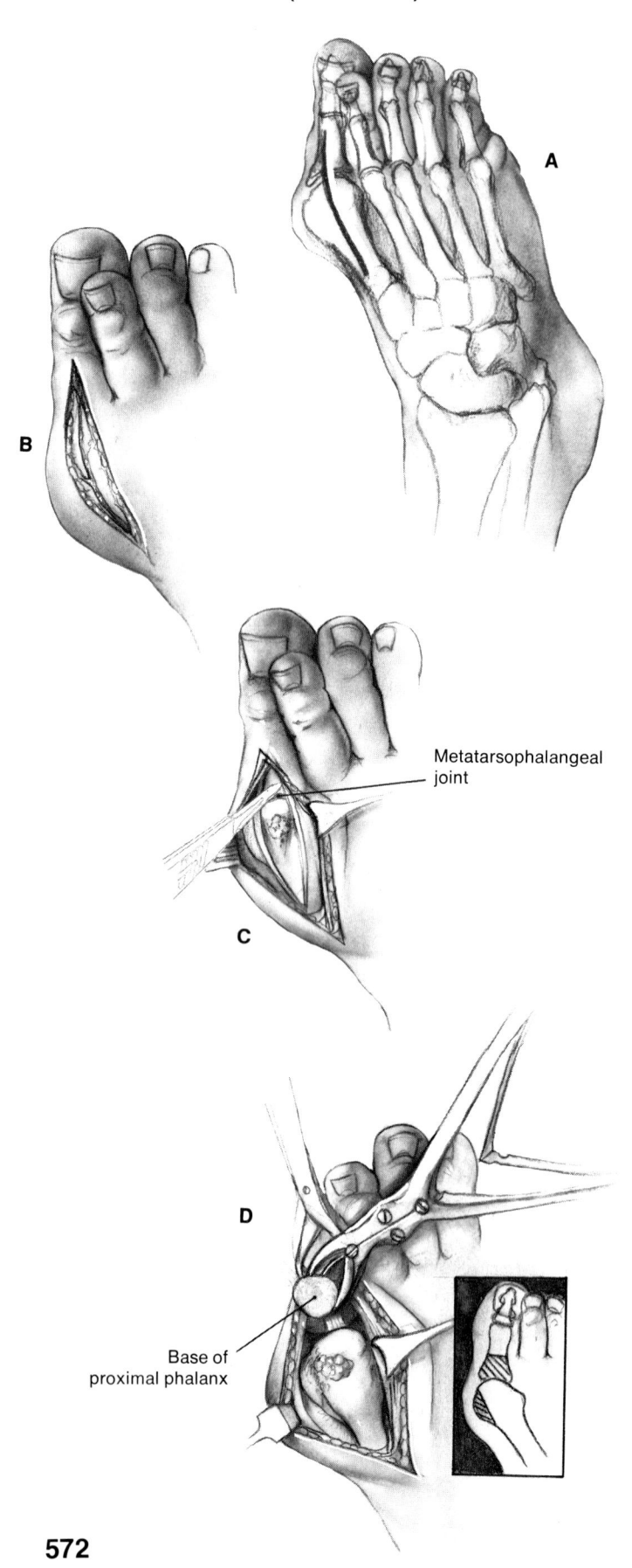

Metatarsophalangeal joint

Base of proximal phalanx

GENERAL DISCUSSION. Hallux valgus is a deformity of the foot that includes lateral deviation of the great toe at the metatarsophalangeal joint (often associated with lateral subluxation of the base of the proximal phalanx), and medial prominence of the first metatarsal head. There may also be varus deviation of the first metatarsal with greater than average widening of the first intermetatarsal space. Less obvious associated changes are lateral displacement of the flexor and extensor tendons to the great toe with bowstringing of these long tendons and plantar displacement of the abductor hallucis tendon. The abductor hallucis muscle is the only force resisting the progressive valgus deformity of the great toe, and its power is greatly decreased by any plantar displacement of its tendon. A considerable proportion of the medial prominence is usually caused by inflammation and a traumatic thickening of the bursa over the medial aspect of the first metatarsal head and any underlying exostosis. Surgical correction for hallux valgus is indicated primarily to relieve pain; seldom for cosmetic reasons alone.

The Keller procedure involves excision of the proximal half of the proximal phalanx of the great toe in addition to the exostosis of the metatarsal head. The toe is thereby shortened, the contracted lateral portion of the joint capsule is relaxed, and the deformity is corrected. The patient should understand, preoperatively, that the great toe may be a little floppy for a few months following surgery, that it will be permanently shortened to a minimal degree, and that active control of it will be slightly impaired.

DETAILS OF PROCEDURE. A curvilinear incision is made over the dorsal and medial aspects of the first metatarsophalangeal joint **(A)**. Dorsal veins may require ligation **(B)**. The capsule and periosteum at the base of the proximal phalanx are incised, and the articular surfaces of the metatarsophalangeal joint are exposed **(C)**. The dissection is continued proximally over the dorsal and medial aspects of the first metatarsal extending proximally over any protuberant exostosis to normal metatarsal shaft. The remainder of the capsule of the metatarsophalangeal joint is incised sufficiently to dislocate the base of the proximal phalanx dorsally. As the plantar aspect of the capsule is divided from its attachment to the proximal phalanx, care must be taken to avoid injury to the flexor hallucis longus tendon. Bone cutters are used to sharply divide the proximal phalanx in its midportion **(D)**.

(Plate 15-14) KELLER PROCEDURE

The protuberant exostosis from the medial, dorsal, and plantar aspects of the first metatarsal head is then exposed and removed with an osteotome back to the normal cortex of the metatarsal shaft (**E** to **G**). The bursa that has developed over the medial aspect of the metatarsal head need not be excised because resection of the protuberant exostosis will lead to spontaneous shrinkage of the bursa postoperatively. Soft tissue of the remaining capsule is sutured into the interval between the raw surface of the remaining portion of proximal phalanx and the first metatarsal head. Optionally, a Kirschner wire may be inserted longitudinally through the great toe and then retrograde into the first metatarsal to stabilize the great toe in the desired position for the early postoperative period (**H**). The wound is closed in layers and should be carefully bandaged to hold the great toe in the desired position (**I** and **J**).

POSTOPERATIVE MANAGEMENT. The patient is kept in bed with the foot elevated for the first 2 days after surgery. Gradual ambulation is then allowed with the patient walking on the heel of the operated foot. Crutches are usually not necessary. Two weeks postoperatively the sutures are removed, and a small bandage is applied. If a Kirschner wire was used for internal stabilization, it should also be removed 2 weeks postoperatively. Beginning 2 weeks after surgery, the patient is encouraged to resume wearing standard shoes or enclosed footwear as soon as possible to minimize subsequent foot swelling. The patient should be wearing normal footwear within 6 weeks postoperatively.

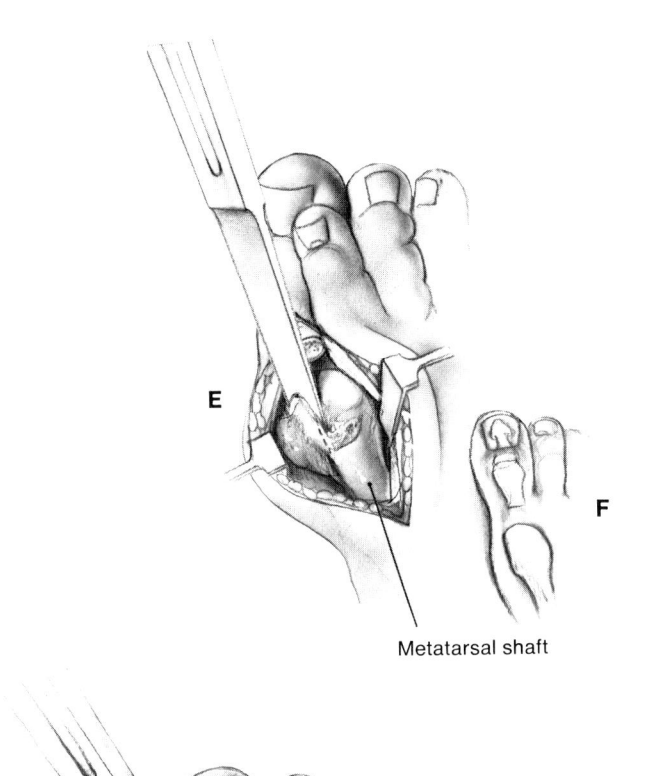

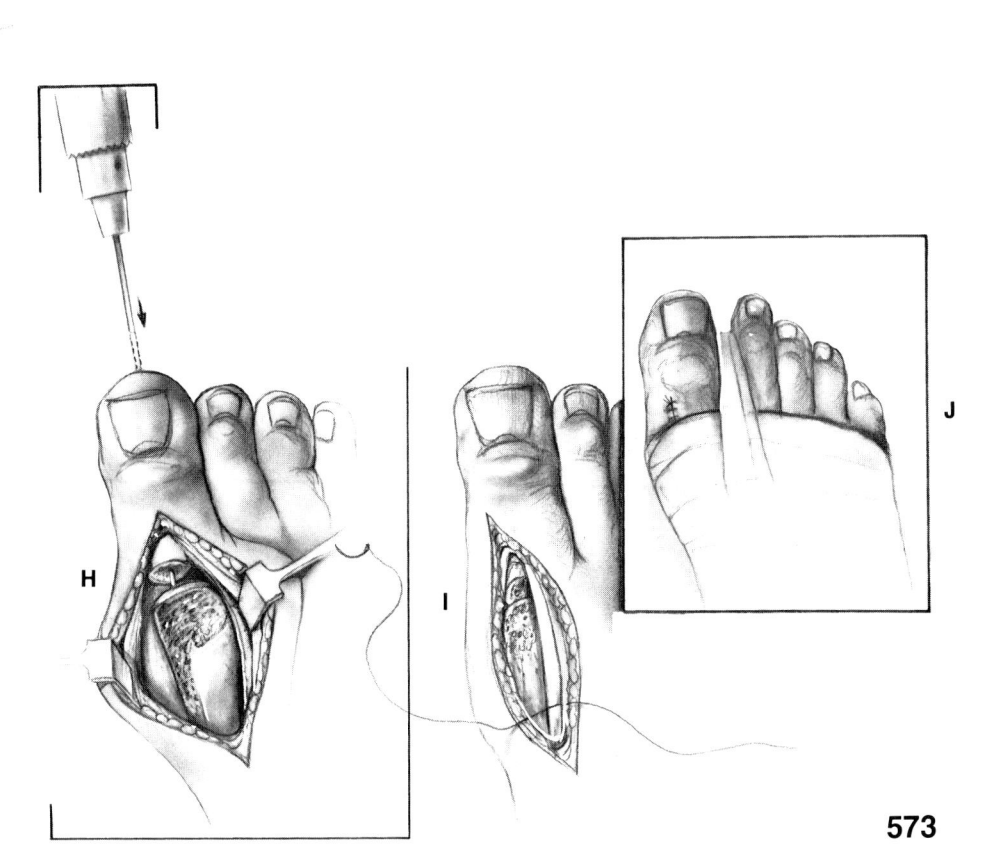

McBRIDE PROCEDURE (Plate 15-15)

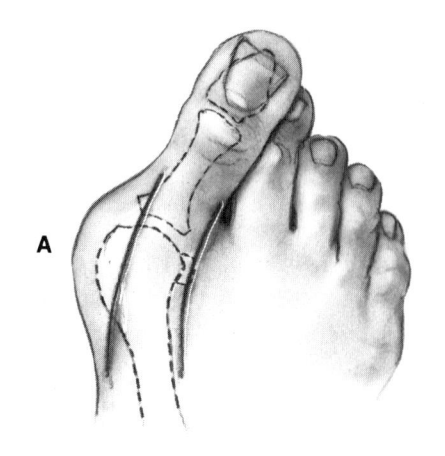

GENERAL DISCUSSION. For the adolescent patient with a hallux valgus deformity requiring surgery, the McBride procedure is recommended. This operation deals principally with the soft tissues.

DETAILS OF PROCEDURE. The operation is carried out under pneumatic tourniquet. The procedure should be done through two incisions (**A**). A 4 cm incision runs proximally from the web in the first intermetatarsal space. The dissection is carried through subcutaneous tissues while the dorsal cutaneous nerve is retracted laterally (**B**). The tendon attachment of the adductor hallucis to the base of the proximal phalanx of the great toe is identified and sectioned (**C** and **D**).

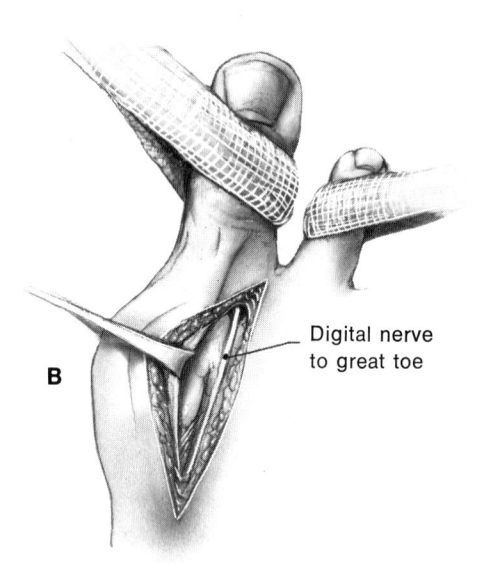

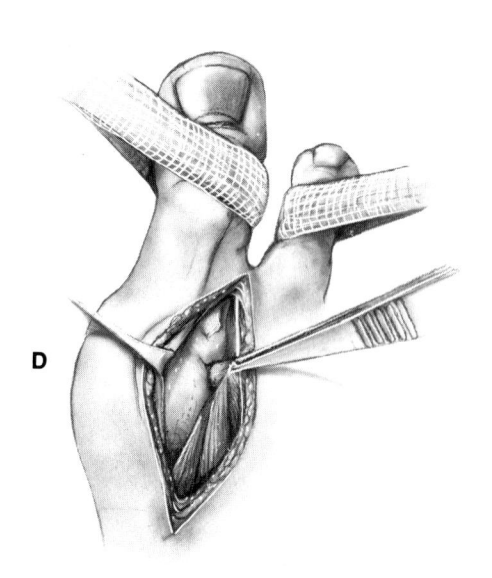

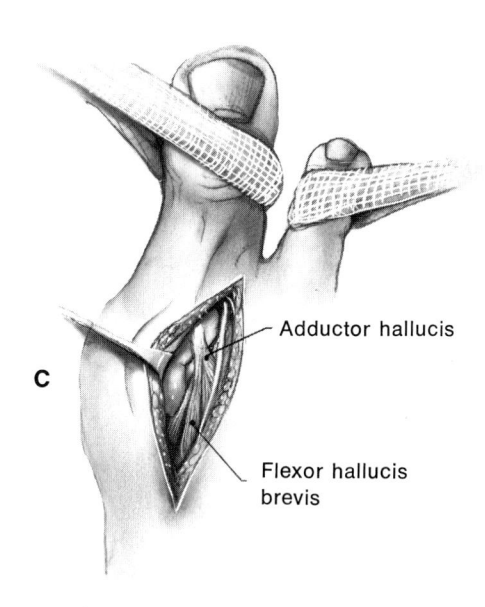

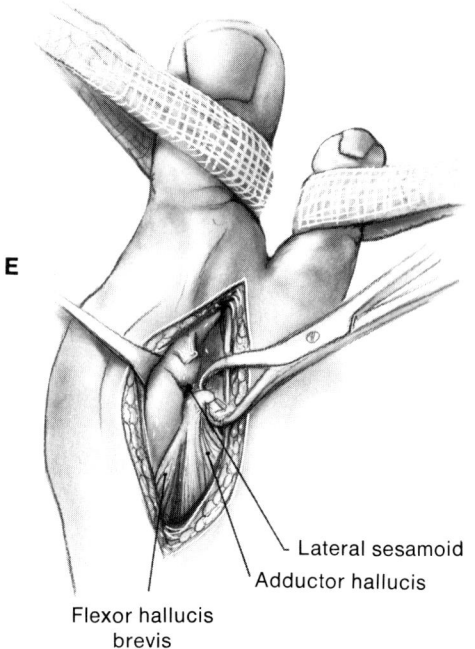

574

(Plate 15-15) McBRIDE PROCEDURE

A clamp is placed on the stump of the adductor tendon, traction is applied, and by sharp dissection, the fibular sesamoid is excised, with sectioning of the remaining adductor and flexor tendon attachment as well as of the capsule (E). A second, slightly curved, dorsomedial incision is then made over the first metatarsophalangeal joint, and at least a 2.5 cm bridge of skin is left between the two incisions. The skin flap is developed plantarward to expose the first metatarsal head. The long extensor tendon to the great toe is exposed and retracted. A periosteal elevator under the metatarsal head allows adequate exposure of the capsule, which is incised proximal to the joint line. This incision is carried through the abductor tendon on the plantar aspect of the capsule. The great toe is then displaced laterally.

With a broad osteotome, the exostosis on the medial surface of the first metatarsal is excised, and the sharp border on the plantar aspect rounded off (F). The joint capsule including the sectioned abductor tendon is then overlapped, compressing the metatarsals and holding the great toe in exactly neutral position in relation to the first metatarsal. The overlapped portion of the capsule is excised, and the edges of the capsule are then sutured (G). At the completion of suturing of the capsule, the deformity is fully corrected, but overcorrection at this stage must be avoided. The adductor hallucis tendon is sutured to the periosteum on the lateral aspect of the first metatarsal head. Three strong chromic catgut sutures are then placed through the adjacent surfaces of the capsules of the first and second metatarsophalangeal joints. The metatarsal area is compressed by an assistant as these sutures, approximating the first and second metatarsal heads, are tied (H and I). The tourniquet is released before the wounds are closed. A pad is placed between the great toe and the second toe, and a compression bandage is applied around the distal metatarsal region, leaving the great toe free.

POSTOPERATIVE MANAGEMENT. Postoperatively the feet are elevated, and ice caps are applied for 48 hours. The patient is ambulated without weight on the involved foot beginning on the third postoperative day. The initial dressing is not changed for 2 weeks unless there is some specific reason to do so. The circular gauze-pressure bandage is retained for 6 weeks. A cut-out shoe is worn for 2 months.

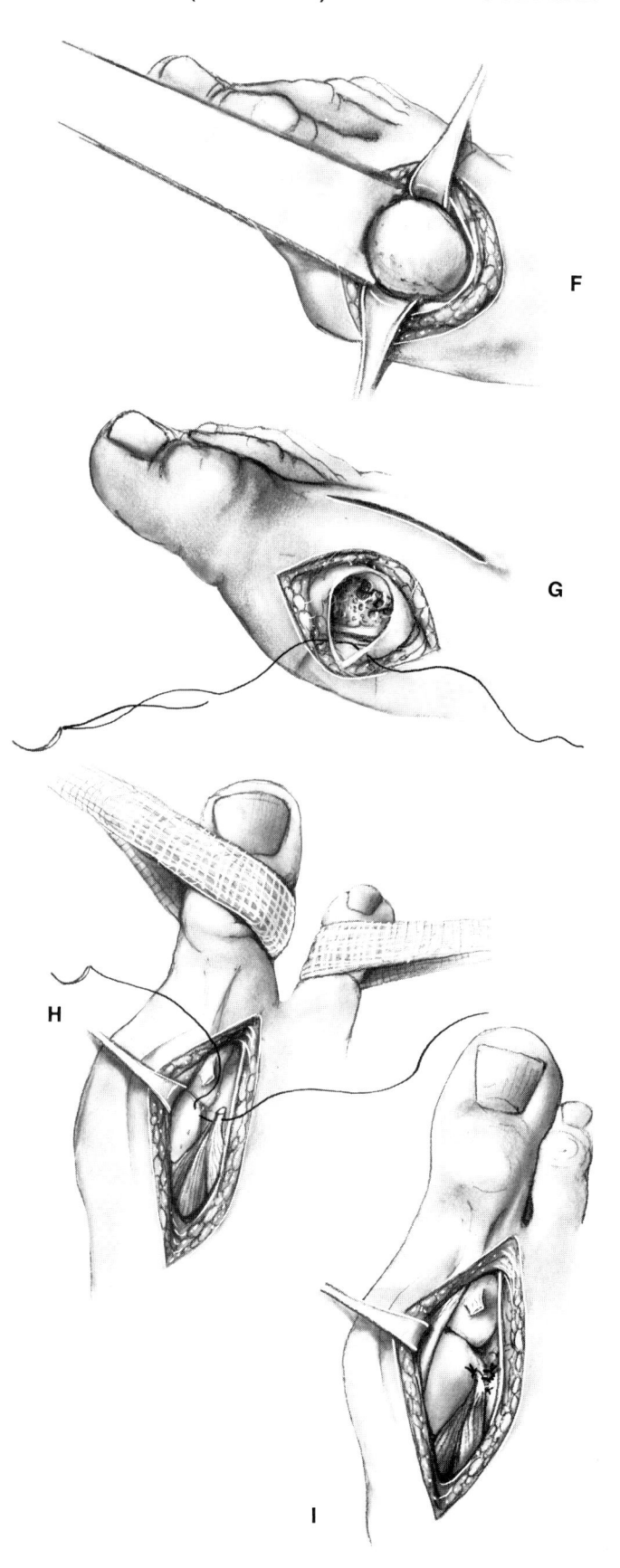

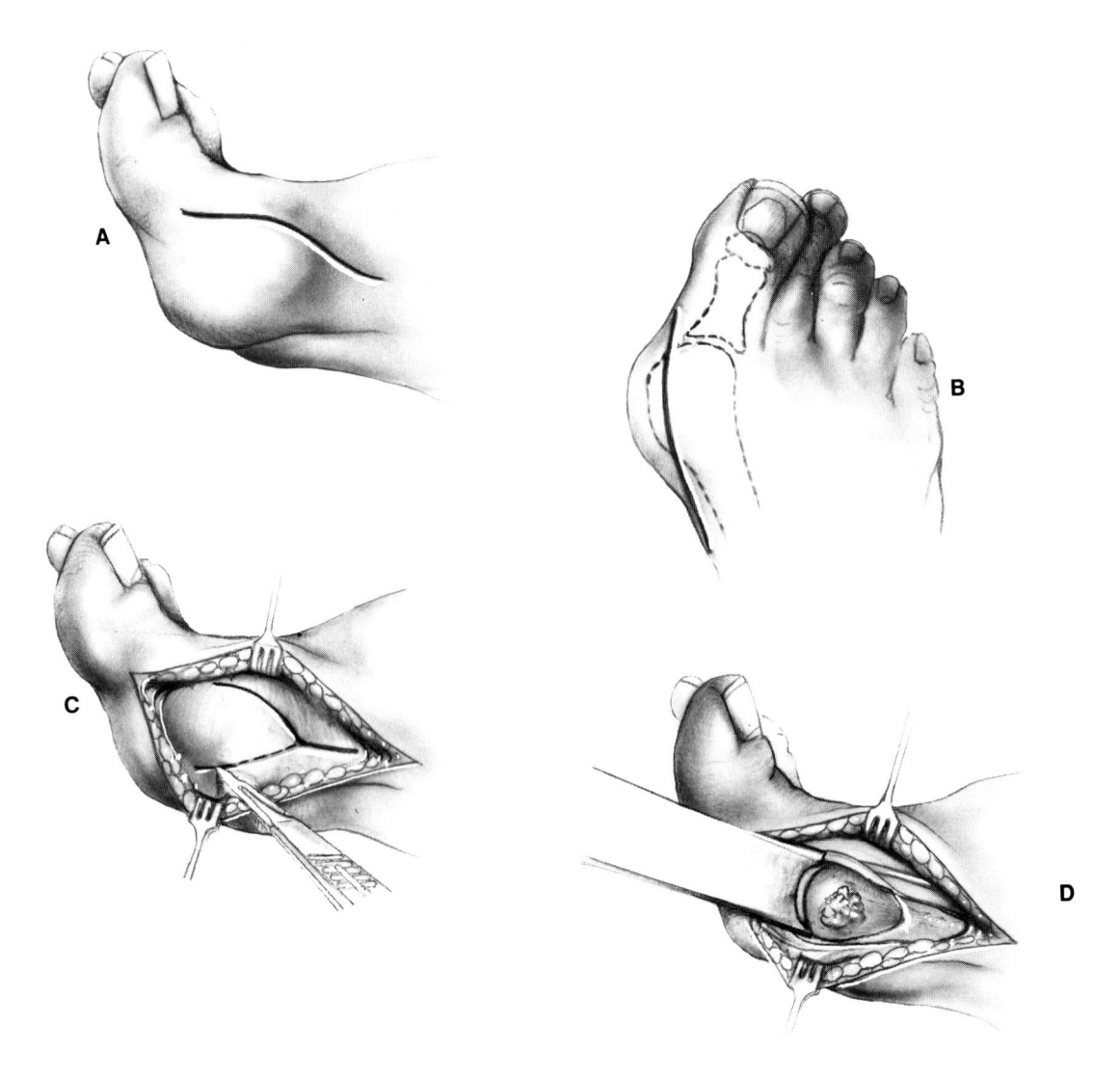

RECONSTRUCTIVE OSTEOTOMY OF FIRST METATARSAL (FOR ADOLESCENT HALLUX VALGUS) (Plate 15-16)

GENERAL DISCUSSION. An alternative operation for the young patient requiring surgery for hallux valgus is reconstructive osteotomy of the first metatarsal as described by Mitchell et al. In this procedure an osteotomy is made through the neck of the first metatarsal and the metatarsal head is displaced laterally. This procedure may be particularly useful when varus deformity of the first metatarsal is a principal cause of the hallux valgus. According to Mitchell et al., osteotomy of the first metatarsal is indicated when the intermetatarsal angle is 10° or more.

The time required for convalescence following reconstructive osteotomy of the first metatarsal is longer than after most other operations for hallux valgus. Significant arthritic change or limitation of motion in the metatarsophalangeal joint makes this operation unsuitable. The most common factors associated with poor results after osteotomy of the first metatarsal are dorsal displacement of the distal fragment or excessive shortening of the first metatarsal.

DETAILS OF PROCEDURE. A curvilinear incision is made over the dorsal and medial aspects of the great toe (**A** and **B**). Skin and subcutaneous tissue are elevated to expose the medial aspect of the joint. A Y-shaped incision is made in the capsule medially with the stem of the Y pointing proximally (**C**). The protuberant portion of the exostosis medially and dorsally is removed with an osteotome (**D**).

The periosteum and soft tissues are reflected over the dorsal surface to permit drilling of two holes completely through the neck of the metatarsal and through its plantar cortex. The metatarsal is osteotomized between these two drill holes, preferably with a power saw. The initial osteotomy cut should stop at a point that leaves one sixth of the width of the shaft laterally, and for a severe deformity, at a level that leaves one third of the shaft laterally. A more proximal osteotomy is then made through the entire metatarsal transverse to the long axis of the metatarsal shaft as illustrated. A short longitudinal osteotomy is made between the two transverse osteotomies leaving a lateral spur

(Plate 15-16) RECONSTRUCTIVE OSTEOTOMY OF FIRST METATARSAL (FOR ADOLESCENT HALLUX VALGUS)

on the distal fragment (**E** and **F**). The distal fragment is now displaced laterally so the spur on the distal fragment overlaps the proximal fragment, and the two fragments of the metatarsal are secured in this position with a heavy chromic catgut suture passed through the holes in the two portions of the metatarsal (**G** and **H**). Optionally the two metatarsal fragments may be stabilized by insertion of a Kirschner wire obliquely (**I**). If there are any remaining prominent portions of bone medially, these should be removed at this time. The wound is closed (**J**), and the toe is splinted in approximately 5° flexion and very slight varus position with splints applied to the dorsal, medial, and plantar aspects of the foot and toe.

POSTOPERATIVE MANAGEMENT. The splints are removed 14 days postoperatively. Skin sutures may be removed at that time or a few days later. A walking short-leg cast is applied at the time the splints are removed, and the walking cast is used for 4 to 8 weeks subsequently or until there is clinical and roentgenographic evidence that the metatarsal osteotomy is solidly united.

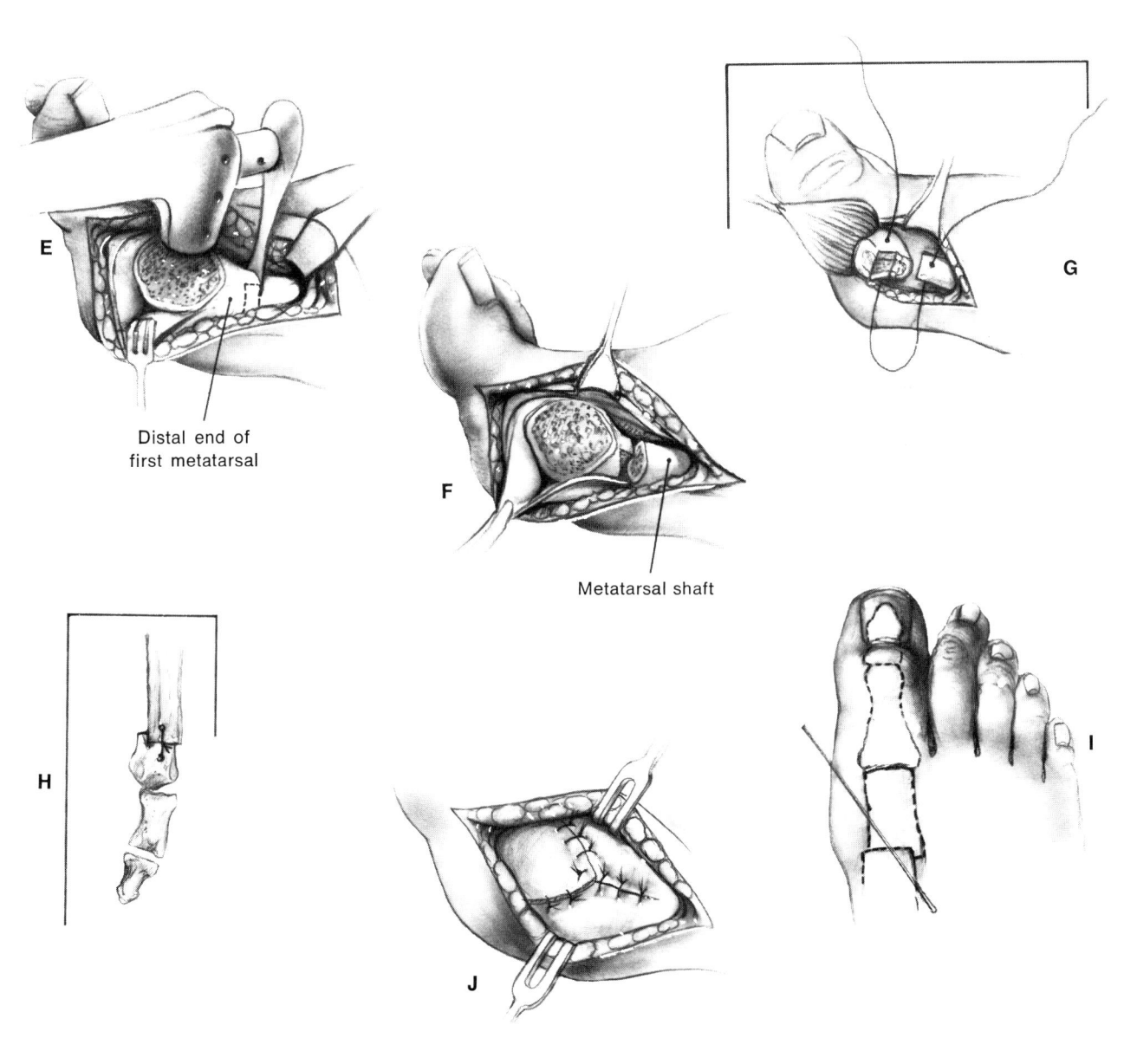

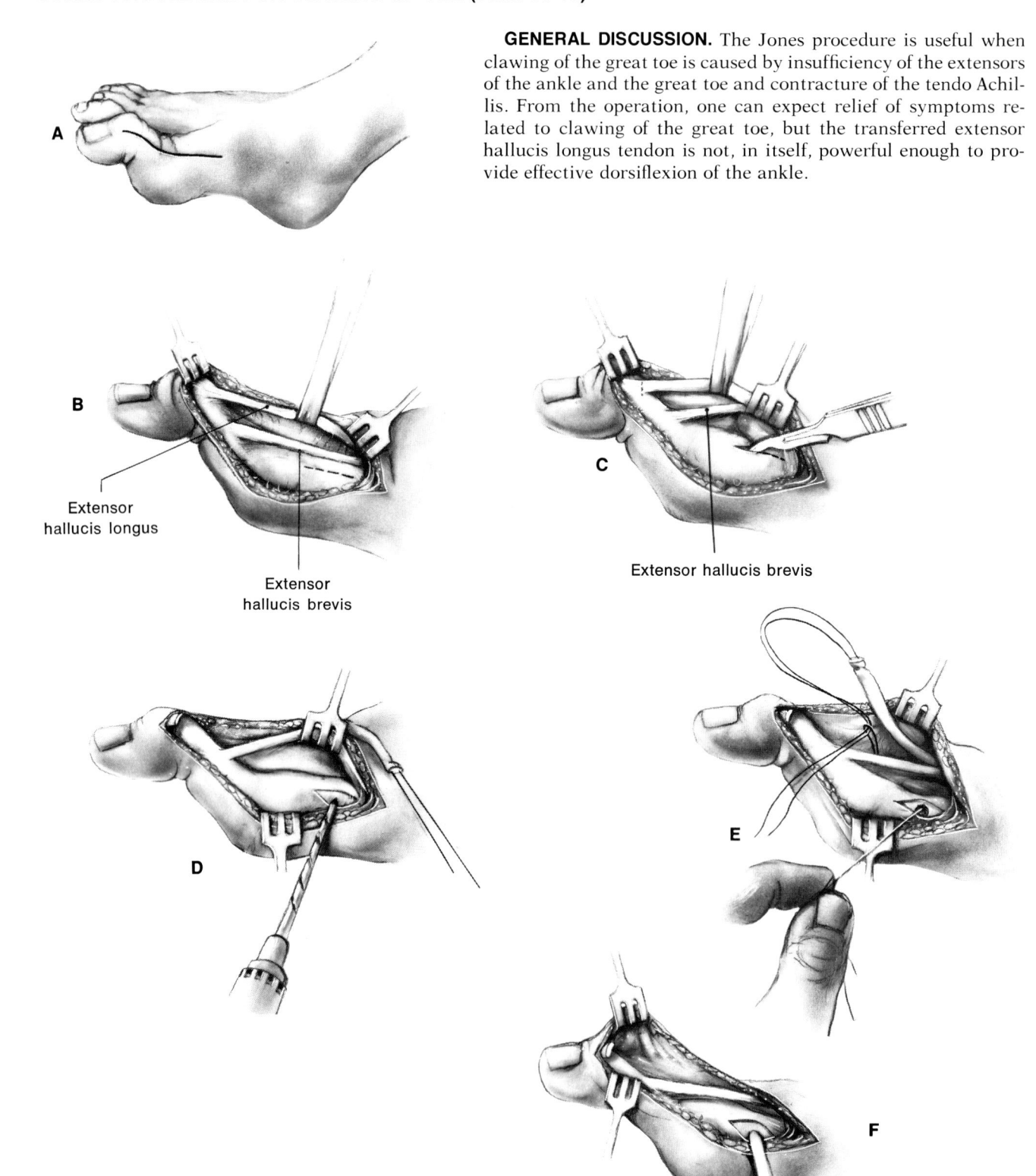

JONES PROCEDURE FOR CLAWING OF TOE (Plate 15-17)

GENERAL DISCUSSION. The Jones procedure is useful when clawing of the great toe is caused by insufficiency of the extensors of the ankle and the great toe and contracture of the tendo Achillis. From the operation, one can expect relief of symptoms related to clawing of the great toe, but the transferred extensor hallucis longus tendon is not, in itself, powerful enough to provide effective dorsiflexion of the ankle.

A

B
Extensor hallucis longus
Extensor hallucis brevis

C
Extensor hallucis brevis

D

E

F

(Plate 15-17) JONES PROCEDURE FOR CLAWING OF TOE

DETAILS OF PROCEDURE. A longitudinal dorsomedial incision is made **(A)**. The extensor hallucis longus is exposed **(B)** and divided near its insertion into the distal phalanx. The head and neck of the first metatarsal are exposed **(C)**. A drill hole is made through the metatarsal neck from medial to lateral and perpendicular to the longitudinal axis of the first metatarsal **(D)**. The divided tendon of the extensor hallucis longus tendon is then passed through this drill hole in the first metatarsal neck (**E** and **F**) and is later turned back and sutured to itself with interrupted nonabsorbable sutures.

The interphalangeal joint of the great toe is then exposed through the distal end of the same incision. The joint capsule is incised **(G)**, and the joint surfaces are resected (**H** and **I**) to allow good apposition of cancellous bone with the joint in neutral position. A Kirschner wire is drilled distally through the distal phalanx and then retrograde into the proximal phalanx as the two phalanges are held in proper apposition, alignment, and rotation **(J)**. The Kirschner wire is divided 3 to 4 mm beyond the toe. After wound closure, a plaster boot is made extending out beyond the end of the Kirschner wire to support and protect the great toe.

POSTOPERATIVE MANAGEMENT. A heel is applied to the cast, and ambulation is permitted as soon as soft tissue discomfort will allow. Plaster immobilization is continued for 4 weeks. The Kirschner wire is removed when there is roentgenographic evidence of bony union at the interphalangeal joint of the great toe.

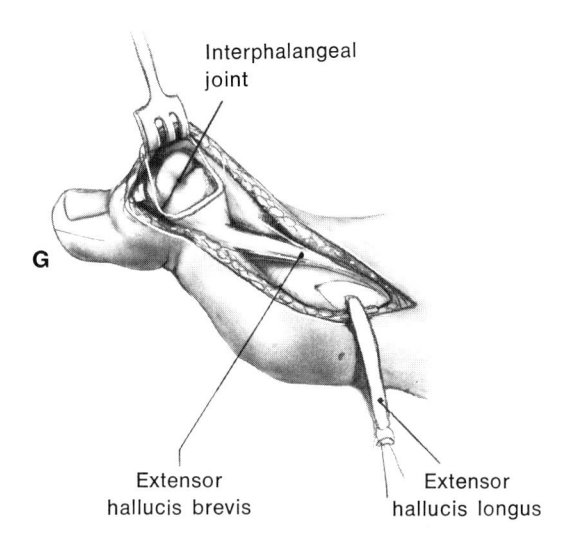

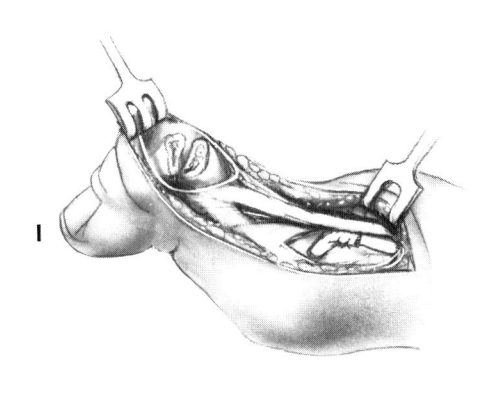

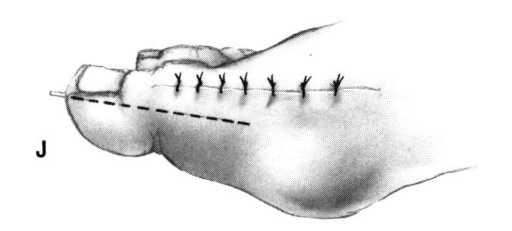

EXCISION OF TIBIAL SESAMOID (Plate 15-18)

GENERAL DISCUSSION. Discomfort associated with a pressure callus under the first metatarsal head is less frequent than pressure symptoms under the middle three metatarsals. When present, it is most likely to occur under the tibial sesamoid of the great toe. The sesamoids are normally embedded in the tendon of the flexor hallucis brevis (**B**, shown in cross section). Any degree of hallux valgus tends to rotate both sesamoids on their long axis and may cause the tibial sesamoid to become a greater weight-bearing pivot. In patients who cannot obtain relief with conservative measures, excision of the tibial sesamoid can provide symptomatic relief.

DETAILS OF PROCEDURE. A curvilinear incision is made along the medial and plantar border of the metatarsophalangeal joint (**A**). Plantar skin and subcutaneous tissue are retracted from the plantar aspect of the same joint. Placing the index finger against the plantar surface of the tibial sesamoid while the great toe is dorsiflexed will aid in outlining this sesamoid. An incision approximately 1 cm long over the medial surface of the involved sesamoid (**C**) will usually permit its plantar aspect to be grasped with an Allis forceps or suitable clamp (**D**). The sesamoid is removed by sharp dissection, with its own outline as a guide. The capsule is closed with interrupted absorbable sutures (**E**), and the skin is closed. A compression bandage is applied.

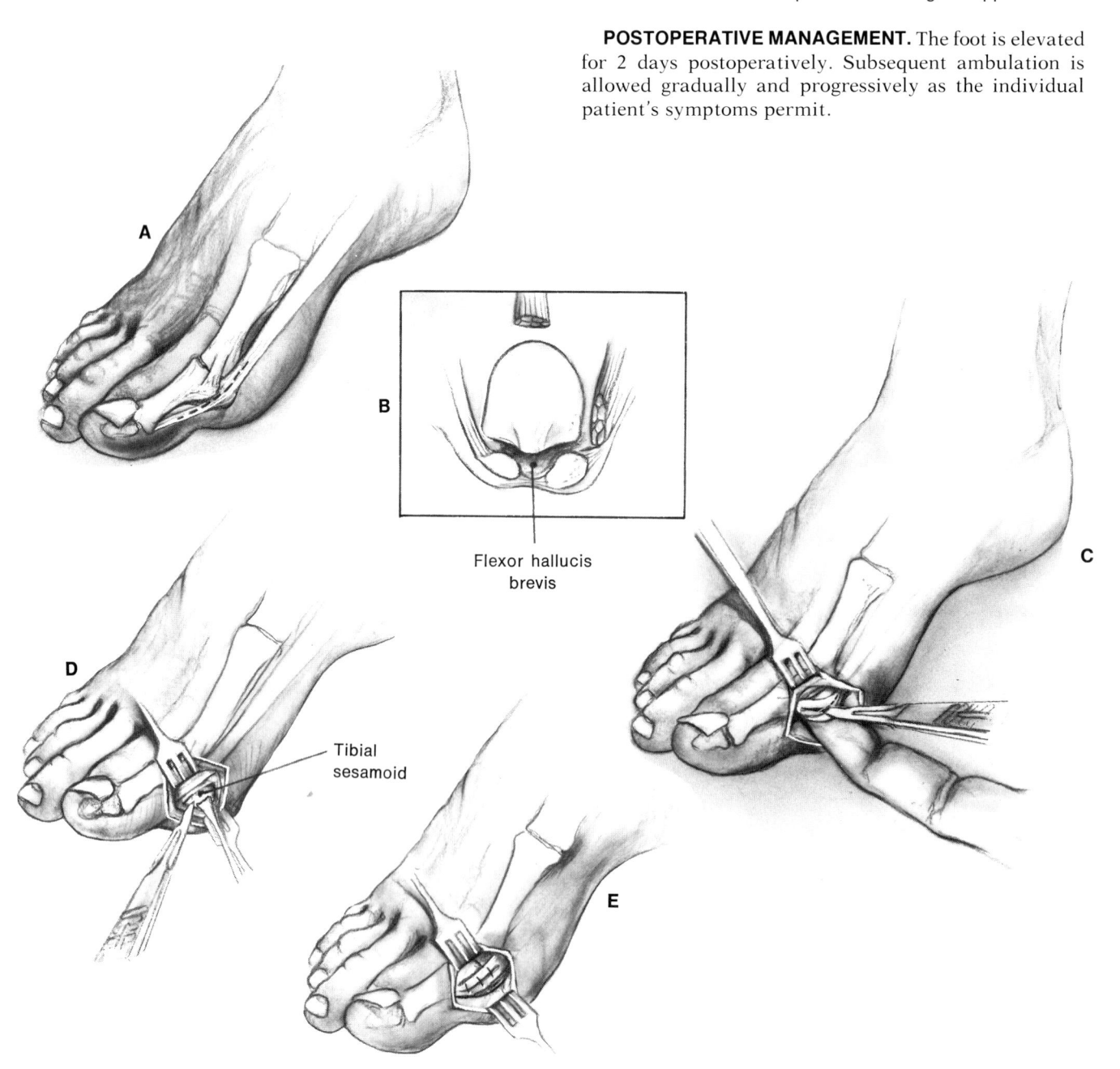

POSTOPERATIVE MANAGEMENT. The foot is elevated for 2 days postoperatively. Subsequent ambulation is allowed gradually and progressively as the individual patient's symptoms permit.

(Plate 15-19) ARTHRODESIS OF PROXIMAL INTERPHALANGEAL JOINT

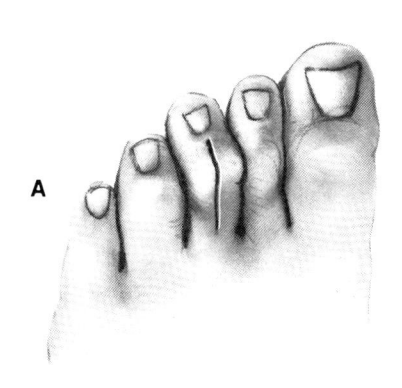

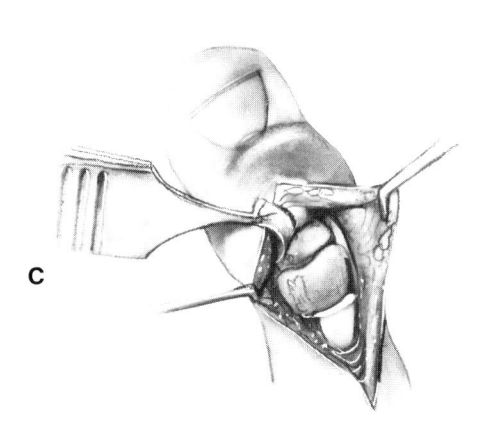

GENERAL DISCUSSION. Arthrodesis of the proximal interphalangeal joint of a toe is effective for the elimination of symptoms and deformity of a hammertoe deformity, that is, flexion of the proximal interphalangeal joint in the lateral four toes or flexion of the interphalangeal joint in the lateral four toes or flexion of the interphalangeal joint of the great toe. Then symptomatic hard corns are present on the dorsal aspect of the proximal interphalangeal joint secondary to this fixed position of the toe, arthrodesis of the interphalangeal joint with realignment of the toe will ensure relief of abnormal pressure areas and of symptoms. However, if flexion of the proximal interphalangeal joint is combined with more than approximately 15° extension of the metatarsophalangeal joint of the great toe. When symptomatic some other procedure or additional tendon surgery with interphalangeal joint fusion may be indicated.

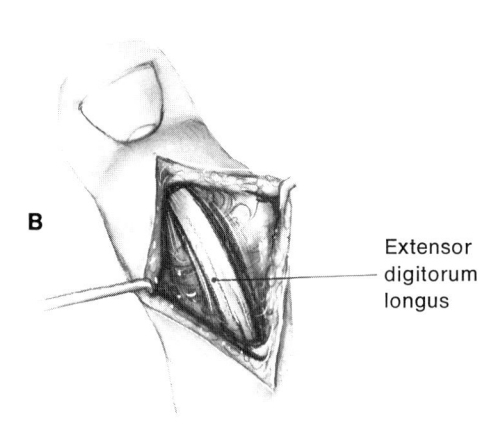

DETAILS OF PROCEDURE. A longitudinal incision is made over the dorsal aspect of the proximal interphalangeal joint adjacent to the tendon of the extensor digitorum longus (**A** and **B**). The dissection is carried down to the proximal interphalangeal joint (**C**). The tendon of extensor digitorum longus can be retracted laterally or divided and subsequently resutured. The neurovascular bundle is protected. In the case of the middle three toes of the foot, the tendon of the extensor digitorum brevis is released at its point of insertion into the middle phalanx. The proximal interphalangeal joint is opened. The articular cartilage is removed from the surfaces of the adjacent phalanges in a manner that permits reapposition with the toe in functional longitudinal alignment (**D**). A high-speed dental burr is technically helpful for this part of the procedure.

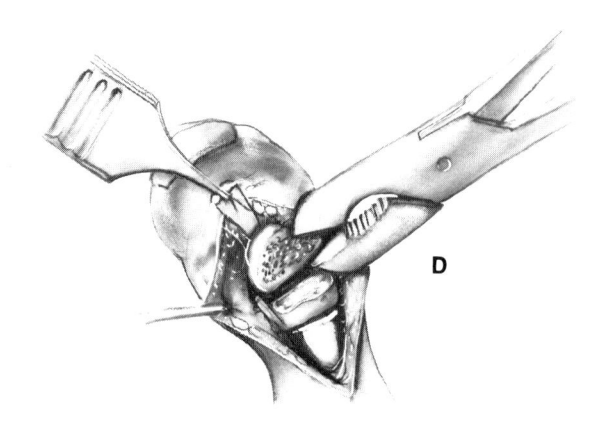

ARTHRODESIS OF PROXIMAL INTERPHALANGEAL JOINT (Plate 15-19)

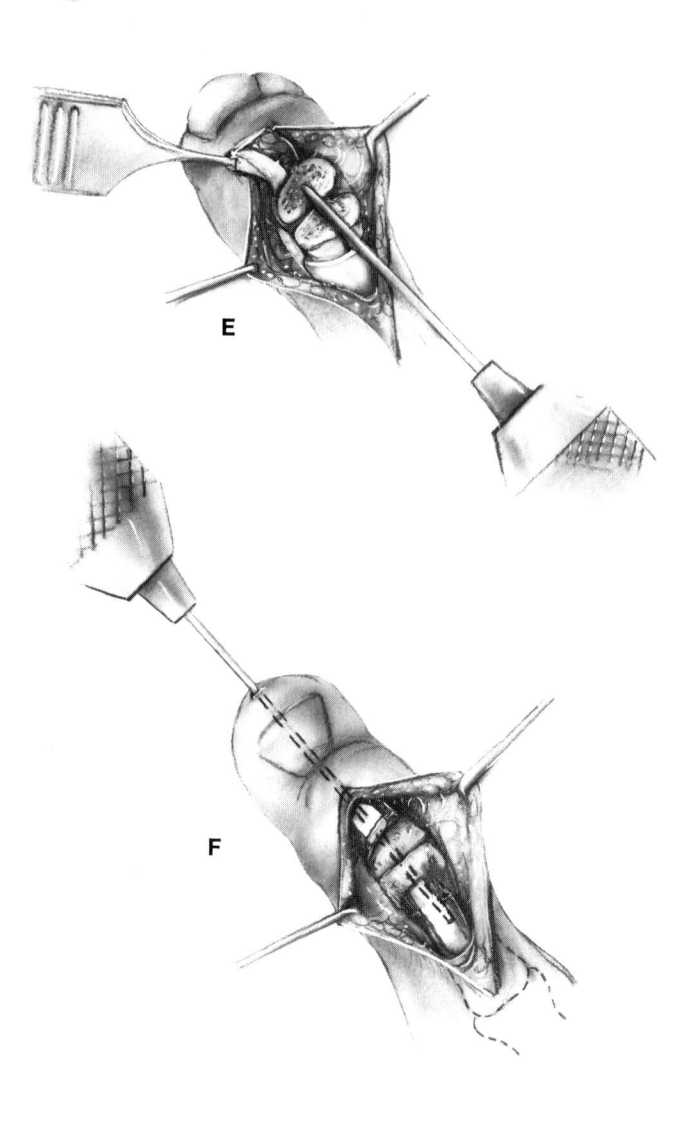

A Kirschner wire is drilled distally through the middle and distal phalanges while the distal interphalangeal joint is held in neutral position (**E**). The denuded surfaces of the proximal interphalangeal joints are then apposed, and the Kirschner wire is drilled into the proximal phalanx for a distance of approximately two thirds the length of the remaining shaft of the proximal phalanx (**F**). After this is done, all phalanges in the toe should have the same alignment, the surfaces of the denuded proximal interphalangeal joint should be in good apposition, and free movement of the metatarsophalangeal joint should be possible, confirming that the Kirschner wire does not cross the metatarsophalangeal joint.

The Kirschner wire is cut off 5 mm from the tip of the toe. If the long extensor tendon had been previously divided, it is now resutured and the wound is closed in routine fashion (**G** and **H**). The toe is immobilized by bandaging to the two adjacent toes, with particular care to see that the two distal phalanges of the operated on toe are left in their proper rotational position.

POSTOPERATIVE MANAGEMENT. The Kirschner wire is removed when there is clinical and roentgenographic evidence of bony union at the site of arthrodesis, usually 3 to 4 weeks postoperatively.

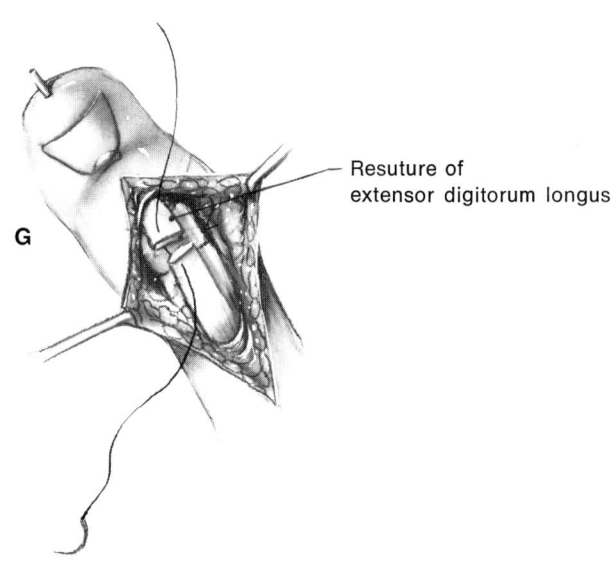

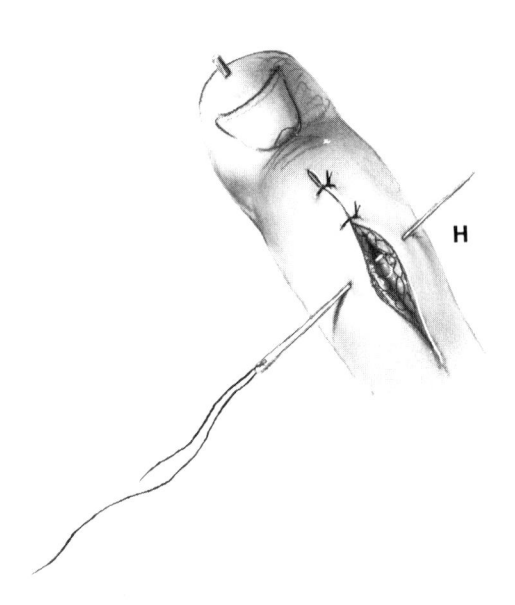

Resuture of extensor digitorum longus

(Plate 15-20) PROXIMAL PHALANGECTOMY

GENERAL DISCUSSION. For the symptomatic claw toe deformity involving any of the lateral four toes, excision of the proximal phalanx is an effective way to relieve symptoms. A distinct advantage of this procedure is the short convalescent period postoperatively.

DETAILS OF PROCEDURE. A dorsal longitudinal incision is made along the medial aspect of the extensor tendon to the involved toe **(A)**. The dissection is continued on the medial aspect of the extensor digitorum longus and extensor digitorum brevis tendons **(B)**. These tendons are reflected laterally at the midshaft of the proximal phalanx. The slip of insertion of the extensor digitorum brevis into the middle phalanx is reflected, and then the capsule of the proximal interphalangeal joint is opened **(C)** with care to protect the flexor tendons.

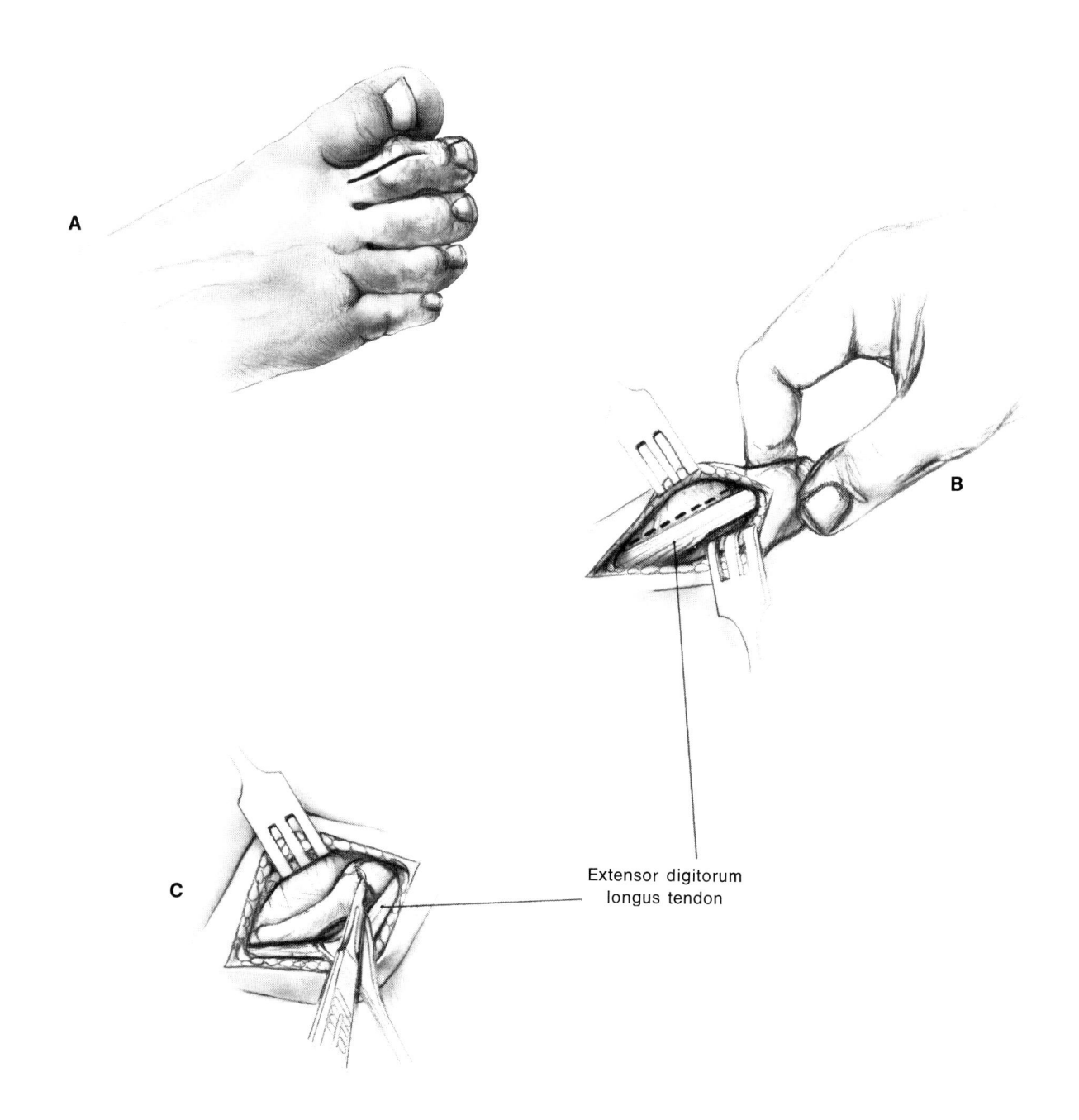

Extensor digitorum longus tendon

PROXIMAL PHALANGECTOMY (Plate 15-20)

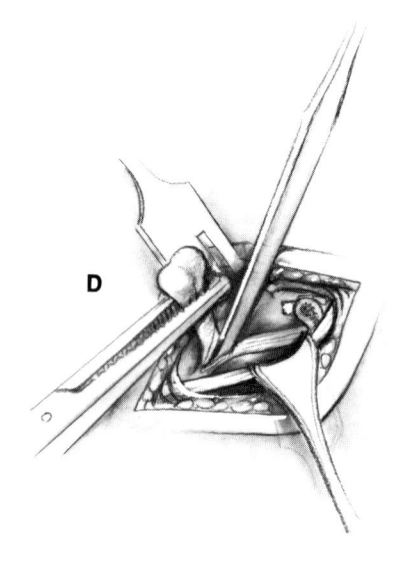

A Kocher clamp is used to hold the distal shaft of the proximal phalanx as the soft tissues are reflected circumferentially from the proximal phalanx with a small periosteal elevator to its base (**D**). A No. 15 scalpel blade is used to divide the capsule of the metatarsophalangeal joint and to completely remove the proximal phalanx. The flexor and extensor tendons are allowed to fall back into place. While longitudinal traction is applied to the distal portion of the toe, the subcutaneous tissues and skin are closed (**E**). The toe is positioned carefully as the foot is bandaged following wound closure (**F**).

POSTOPERATIVE MANAGEMENT. Sutures are removed 10 to 14 days postoperatively, and the patient is encouraged to return to normal footwear as soon as possible thereafter. No other specific protective measures are necessary for the isolated proximal phalangectomy.

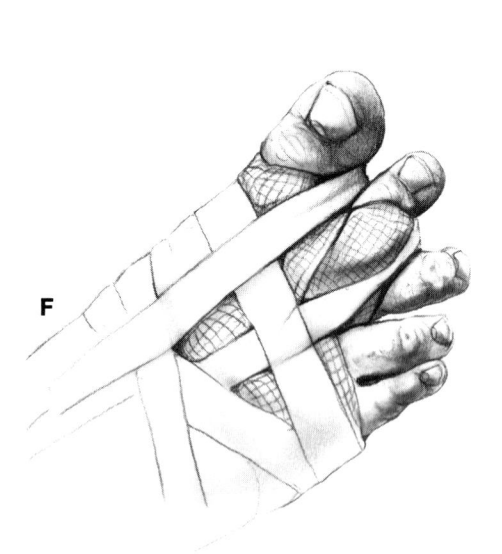

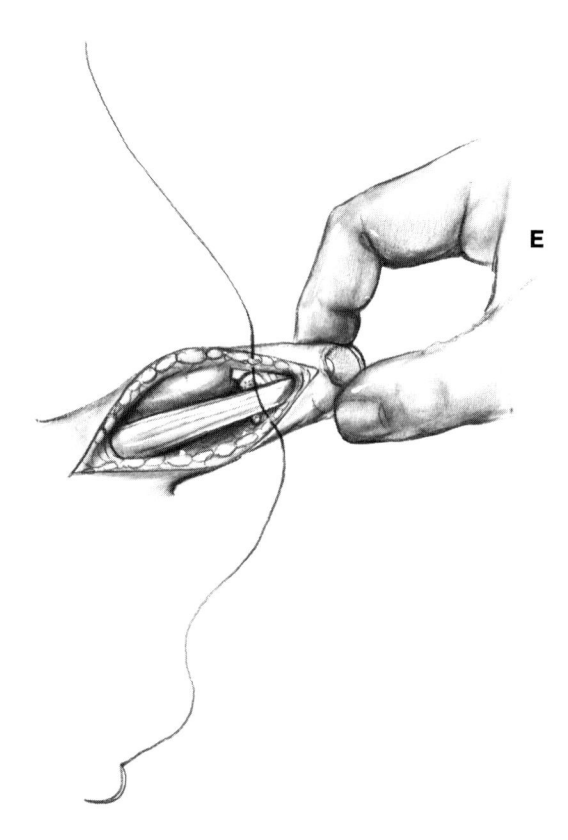

(Plate 15-21) RESECTION OF METATARSAL HEAD

GENERAL DISCUSSION. In chronic rheumatoid arthritis, deformities of the forepart of the foot can be painful and disabling. These deformities are frequently the source of pain on a mechanical as well as an inflammatory basis, whether the arthritis is active or not. The most common foot deformities in rheumatoid arthritis are hallux valgus and bunion, depressed metatarsal heads, and various degrees of cock-up deformities of the toes.

The indication for resection of one or more metatarsal heads is pain on weight bearing that is not relieved by conservative measures (satisfactory arch supports and metatarsal pads in the shoes). Relief of abnormal weight-bearing pressure can be obtained surgically. In advanced cases, the marked contracture of soft tissues accompanying these deformities requires resection of bone for correction of deformity and relief of discomfort. The joints are already damaged, and the feet are weak. The toes will not be functioning normally in these patients. Corrective surgery on the forepart of the foot does not weaken the damaged arthritic foot or impair the patient's gait; rather, the gait is usually improved.

The basic surgical procedure is adequate resection of bone at the metatarsophalangeal joints. The number of joints resected and the extent of resection will depend on the degree of involvement. In severe cases, it is usually necessary to resect all of the metatarsal heads and a portion of the metatarsal necks in addition to all or portions of each of the proximal phalanges. Occasionally, only one or two toes need to be operated on, although generally the deformity is such that all the metatarsal heads should be removed. If three metatarsal heads have to be removed, it will be best to remove all five. Both feet may require treatment at the same time.

DETAILS OF PROCEDURE. A transverse dorsal incision is made at the base of the toes curving proximally over the first interdigital space **(A)**. The extensor tendons are exposed **(B)** and then individually retracted. The second toe should be approached first and then the third, fourth, and fifth. The skin can then be retracted medially to expose what can be the more difficult area on the great toe. The metatarsophalangeal capsule is incised, and the base of each proximal phalanx is delivered into the wound **(C)**.

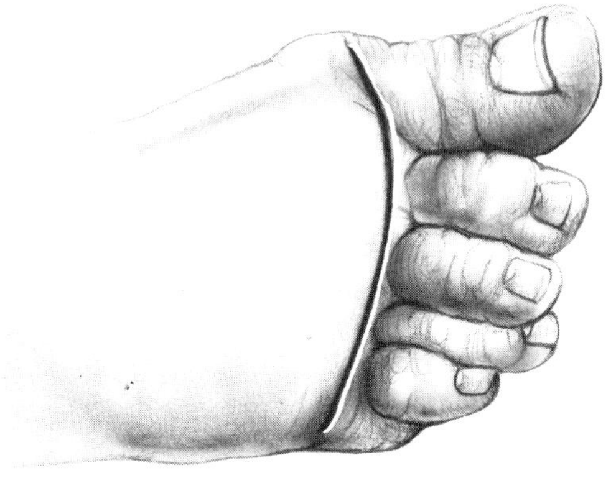

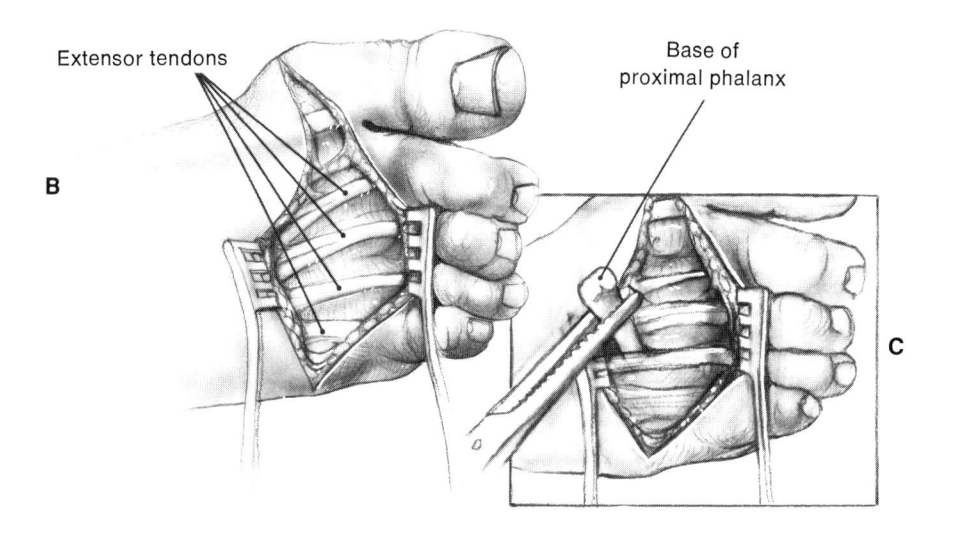

RESECTION OF METATARSAL HEAD (Plate 15-21)

The distal portion of each individual toe is held extended while the proximal phalanx is freed of all remaining soft tissue attachments and then removed **(D)**. The metatarsal head is then easily delivered and resected with bone cutters **(E)**. The plantar aspect of the remaining portion of each metatarsal is beveled to give a smooth weight-bearing surface.

The amount of bone removed depends on the amount of deformity. Through the dorsal incision, it should be relatively easy to estimate the amount of the metatarsal that should be excised. It is preferable to ultimately have the first and second metatarsals approximately the same length, gently tapering from the second to the third, fourth, and fifth metatarsals **(F)**. The capsule of each metatarsophalangeal joint is reapproximated. Subcutaneous tissue and skin of the dorsal transverse wound are sutured. A bulky compression dressing is applied, holding the toes in the desired position.

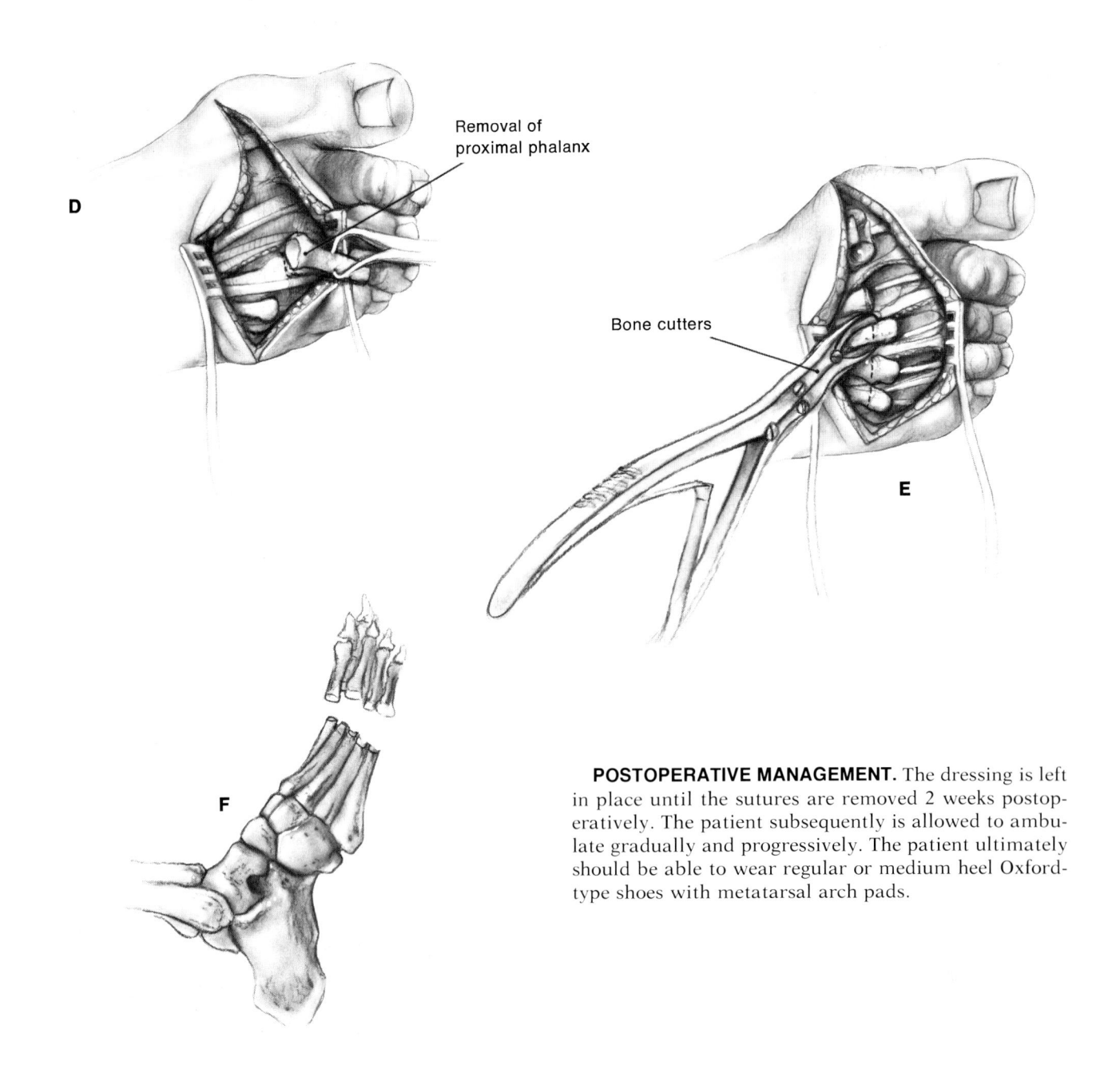

POSTOPERATIVE MANAGEMENT. The dressing is left in place until the sutures are removed 2 weeks postoperatively. The patient subsequently is allowed to ambulate gradually and progressively. The patient ultimately should be able to wear regular or medium heel Oxford-type shoes with metatarsal arch pads.

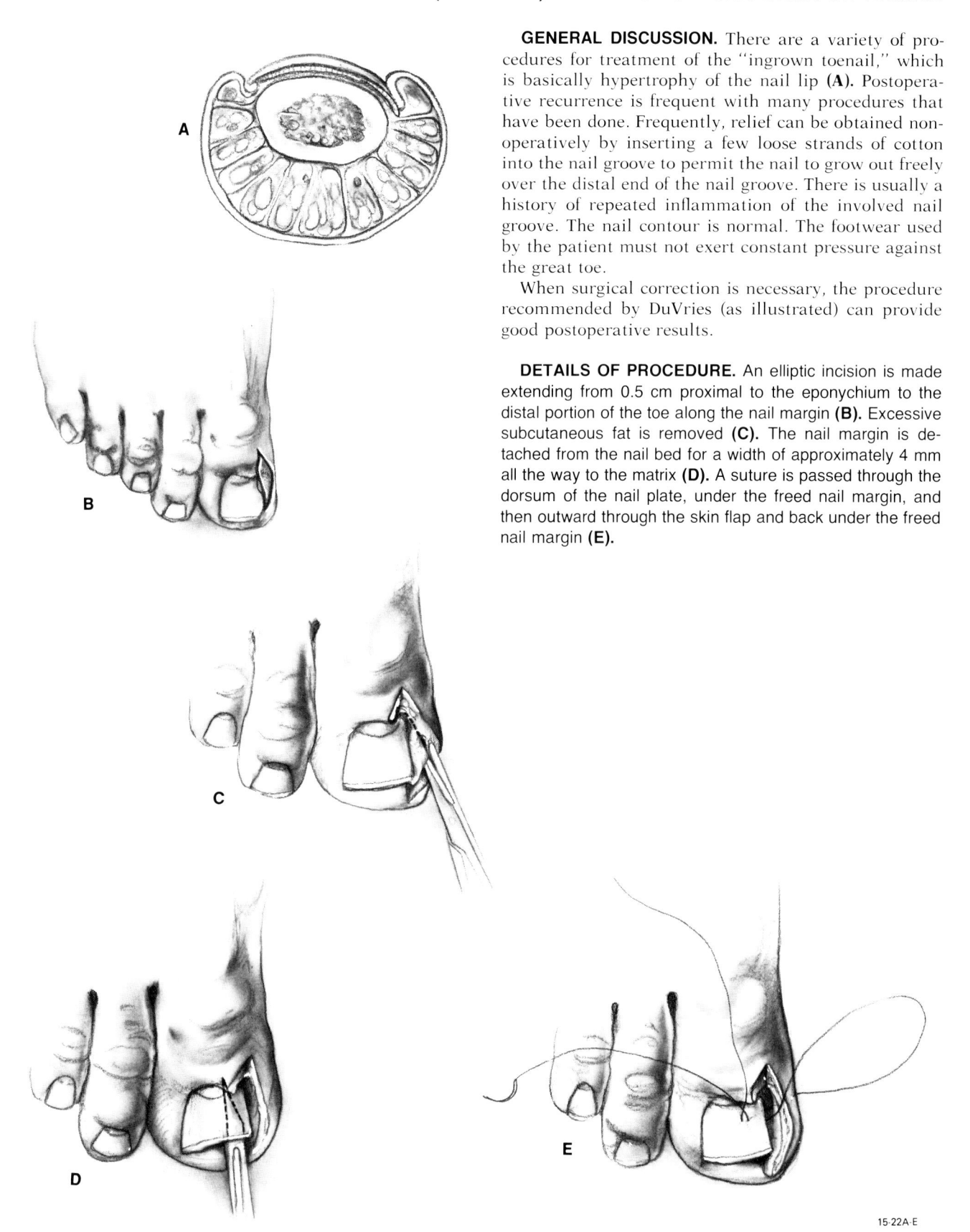

(Plate 15-22) REPAIR FOR CHRONIC INGROWN TOENAIL

GENERAL DISCUSSION. There are a variety of procedures for treatment of the "ingrown toenail," which is basically hypertrophy of the nail lip (**A**). Postoperative recurrence is frequent with many procedures that have been done. Frequently, relief can be obtained nonoperatively by inserting a few loose strands of cotton into the nail groove to permit the nail to grow out freely over the distal end of the nail groove. There is usually a history of repeated inflammation of the involved nail groove. The nail contour is normal. The footwear used by the patient must not exert constant pressure against the great toe.

When surgical correction is necessary, the procedure recommended by DuVries (as illustrated) can provide good postoperative results.

DETAILS OF PROCEDURE. An elliptic incision is made extending from 0.5 cm proximal to the eponychium to the distal portion of the toe along the nail margin (**B**). Excessive subcutaneous fat is removed (**C**). The nail margin is detached from the nail bed for a width of approximately 4 mm all the way to the matrix (**D**). A suture is passed through the dorsum of the nail plate, under the freed nail margin, and then outward through the skin flap and back under the freed nail margin (**E**).

587

REPAIR FOR CHRONIC INGROWN TOENAIL (Plate 15-22)

The ends of the suture are tied to invaginate the skin flap under the nail margin **(F)**. Additional sutures are placed as needed to reapproximate the eponychium and at the distal end of the incision **(G)**. A nonadherent dressing is applied.

POSTOPERATIVE MANAGEMENT. The dressing should be changed on the first or second postoperative day. Subsequently the dressing is changed every 5 to 7 days until healing is complete. If granulation tissue tends to form in the wound during that period, it is cauterized with silver nitrate. It may be necessary to repeat applications of silver nitrate (or painting with a solution of 95% phenol) a number of times until proper healing is assured.

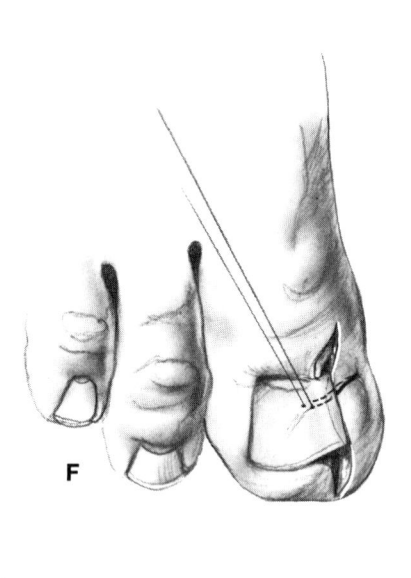

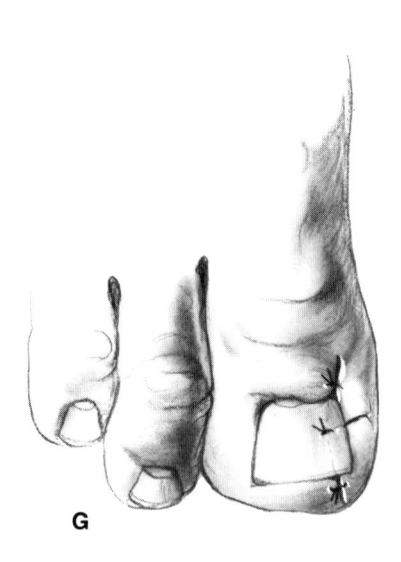

(Plate 15-23) EXCISION OF INTERDIGITAL NEUROMA

GENERAL DISCUSSION. A syndrome, characterized by sudden cramplike discomfort in the region of one or two toes and characteristically between the third and fourth toes as originally described by Morton, may be produced by an interdigital neuroma **(B)**. Typically, the complaint is that while walking, the patient feels a sudden, sharp, burning discomfort or cramping and a numbness in the third and fourth toes. The discomfort may extend into the ball of the foot and may be so severe that the patient removes the shoe in an effort to relieve the discomfort. These symptoms increase gradually in frequency and severity. Conservative treatment includes the use of Oxford shoes of adequate width with moderate heels, a metatarsal arch pad inside the shoe, or a metatarsal bar on the sole of the shoe. Operative treatment consists of excision of the neuroma, which provides complete relief if the diagnosis is correct.

DETAILS OF PROCEDURE. The neuroma can be excised through a longitudinal incision in the cleft between the two involved toes **(A)** or, optionally, through a dorsal incision over the interval between the adjacent metatarsal heads. The dissection extends through a small amount of adipose tissue while the soft tissues are spread horizontally (i.e., in a mediolateral plane) with a hemostat. The neuroma frequently bulges into the wound as an encapsulated lobular mass, especially when pressure is applied to the plantar surface of the foot between the two metatarsal heads **(C)**. The neuroma is excised completely **(D)**. The wound is closed, and a soft dressing is applied **(E)**.

POSTOPERATIVE MANAGEMENT. Weight bearing is resumed immediately or as soon as the minimal wound discomfort subsides.

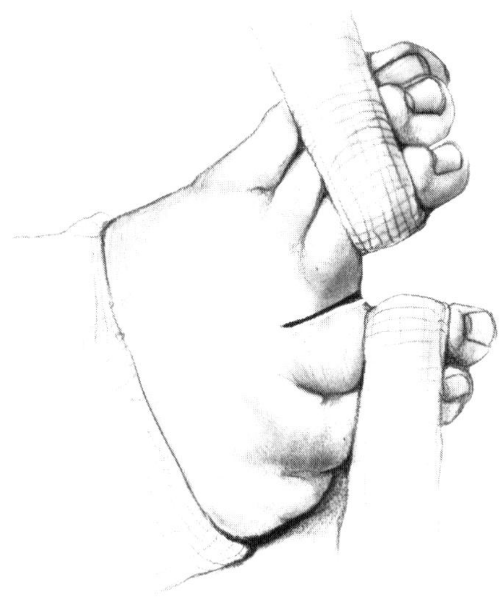

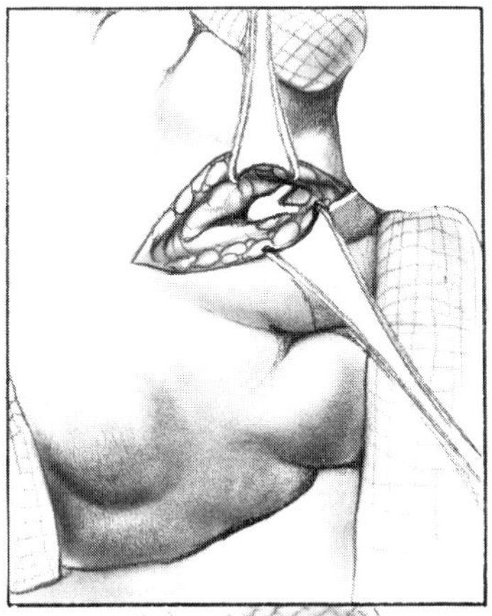

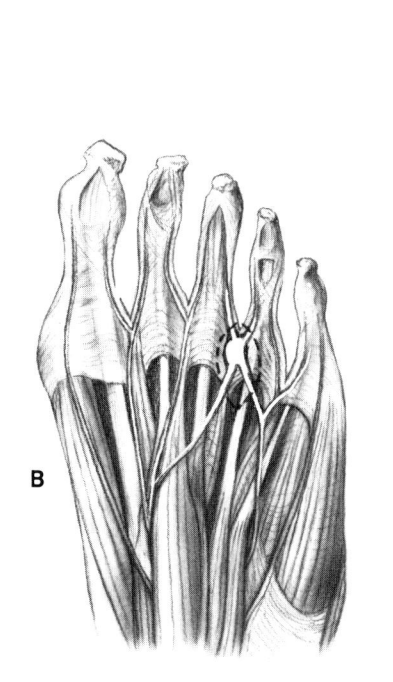

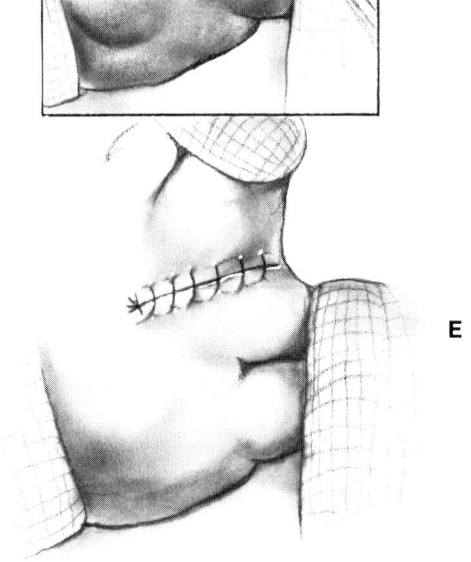

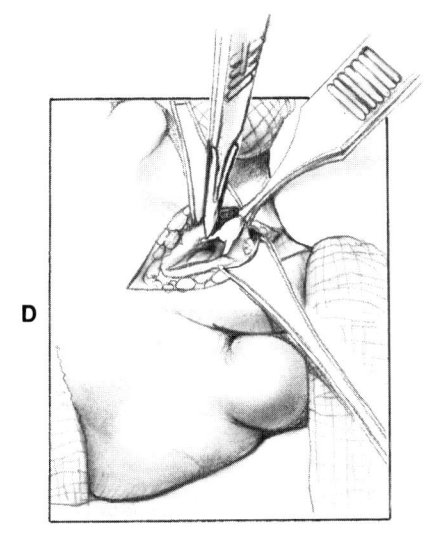

EXOSTECTOMY FOR BUNIONETTE (Plate 15-24)

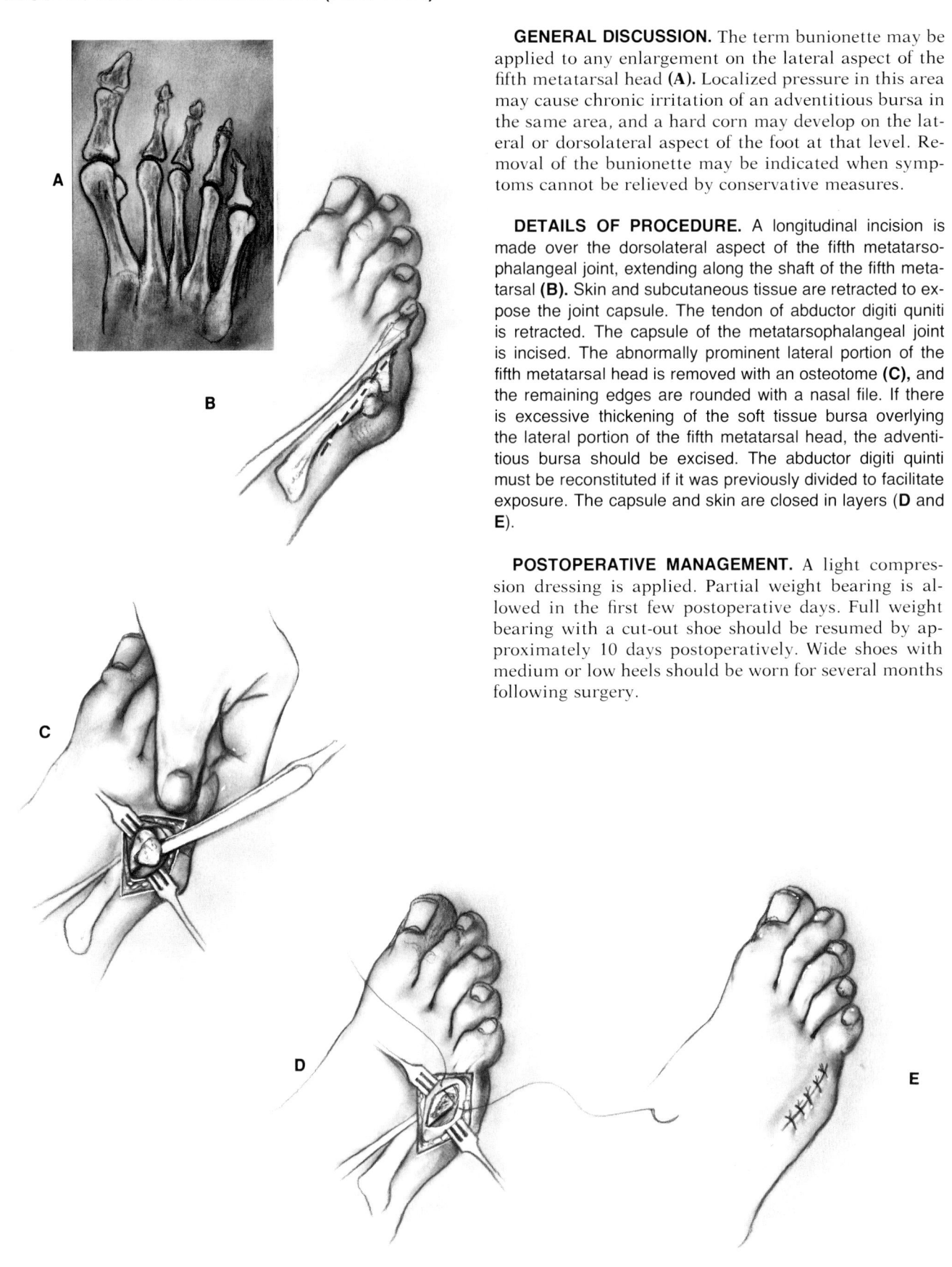

GENERAL DISCUSSION. The term bunionette may be applied to any enlargement on the lateral aspect of the fifth metatarsal head (**A**). Localized pressure in this area may cause chronic irritation of an adventitious bursa in the same area, and a hard corn may develop on the lateral or dorsolateral aspect of the foot at that level. Removal of the bunionette may be indicated when symptoms cannot be relieved by conservative measures.

DETAILS OF PROCEDURE. A longitudinal incision is made over the dorsolateral aspect of the fifth metatarsophalangeal joint, extending along the shaft of the fifth metatarsal (**B**). Skin and subcutaneous tissue are retracted to expose the joint capsule. The tendon of abductor digiti quniti is retracted. The capsule of the metatarsophalangeal joint is incised. The abnormally prominent lateral portion of the fifth metatarsal head is removed with an osteotome (**C**), and the remaining edges are rounded with a nasal file. If there is excessive thickening of the soft tissue bursa overlying the lateral portion of the fifth metatarsal head, the adventitious bursa should be excised. The abductor digiti quinti must be reconstituted if it was previously divided to facilitate exposure. The capsule and skin are closed in layers (**D** and **E**).

POSTOPERATIVE MANAGEMENT. A light compression dressing is applied. Partial weight bearing is allowed in the first few postoperative days. Full weight bearing with a cut-out shoe should be resumed by approximately 10 days postoperatively. Wide shoes with medium or low heels should be worn for several months following surgery.

(Plate 15-25) REPAIR OF OVERLAPPING FIFTH TOE

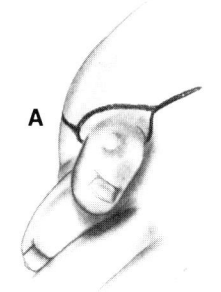

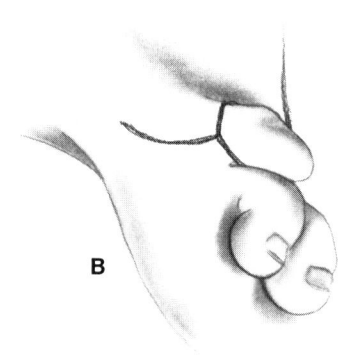

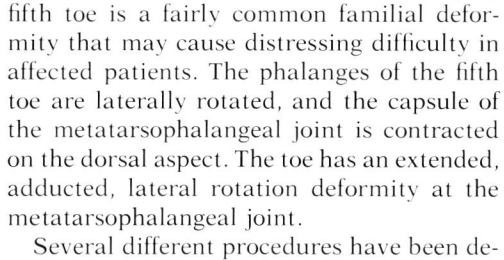

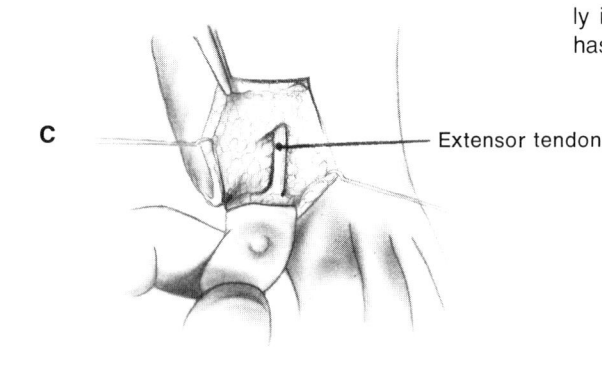

GENERAL DISCUSSION. The overlapping fifth toe is a fairly common familial deformity that may cause distressing difficulty in affected patients. The phalanges of the fifth toe are laterally rotated, and the capsule of the metatarsophalangeal joint is contracted on the dorsal aspect. The toe has an extended, adducted, lateral rotation deformity at the metatarsophalangeal joint.

Several different procedures have been described for the correction of this deformity. The procedure illustrated is similar to that described by Cockin. If the patient is an adult, creation of an artificial syndactyly (Ruiz-Mora) may be preferable.

DETAILS OF PROCEDURE. A racquet-shaped incision is made through the skin only, extending circumferentially about the base of the toe with extensions proximally on the dorsal and plantar aspects of the foot (**A** and **B**). After reflection of the skin flaps, the extensor tendon will be noted to be right (**C**). The neurovascular bundles must be carefully preserved (**D**). The extensor tendon to the toe is divided, and the dorsal capsule of the metatarsophalangeal joint is opened widely (**E**). In many instances, the toe will then go freely downward and laterally into the correct position (**F**). If the deformity has been long-standing, the toe may not move

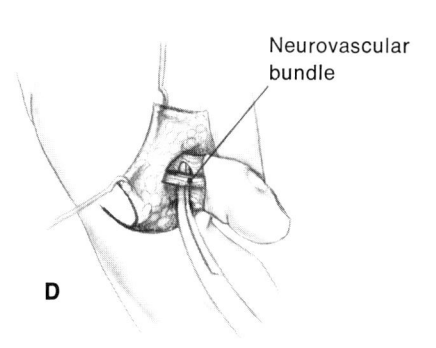

591

REPAIR OF OVERLAPPING FIFTH TOE (Plate 15-25)

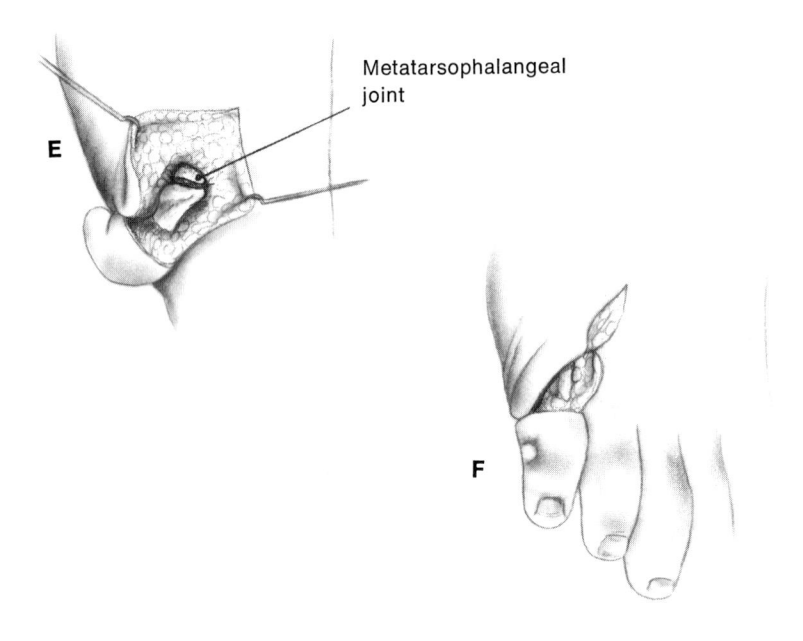

freely around the metatarsal head into the correct position but may hinge, leaving a minimal incongruity at the metatarsophalangeal joint. This will be caused by adherence of the plantar portion of the capsule to the metatarsal head. Any such adherent capsule must be separated from the metatarsal head by blunt dissection, and this should allow the toe to rotate freely. The toe should lie in its fully corrected position without any tension after having been moved downward into the plantar portion of the incision. The skin is sutured to hold the toe securely in its new position (**G** and **H**).

POSTOPERATIVE MANAGEMENT. No splints are needed, since the two should lie correctly at the end of the procedure without tension. Sutures are removed 10 to 14 days postoperatively. No restrictions on activity are necessary.

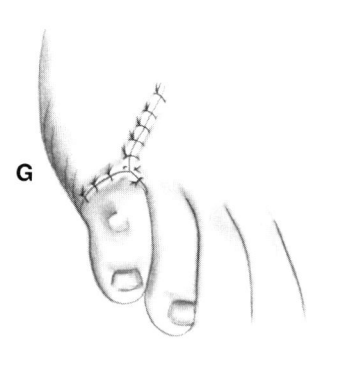

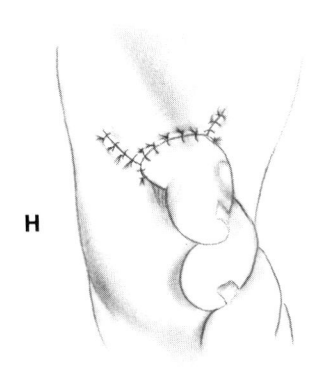

REFERENCES

Auerbach, A. M.: Review of distal metatarsal osteotomies for hallux valgus in the young, Clin. Orthop. **70**:148, 1970.

Axer, A.: Into-talus transposition of tendons for correction of paralytic valgus foot after poliomyelitis in children, J. Bone Joint Surg. **42-A**:1119, 1960.

Baker, L. D.: A rational approach to the surgical needs of the cerebral palsied patient, J. Bone Joint Surg. **38-A**:313, 1956.

Baker, L. D., and Dodelin, C. D.: Extra-atricular arthrodesis of the subtalar joint (Grice procedure), J.A.M.A. **168**:1005, 1958.

Baker, L. D., and Hill, L. M.: Foot alignment in the cerebral palsy patient, J. Bone Joint Surg. **46-A**:1, 1964.

Banks, H. H., and Green, W. T.: The correction of equinus deformity in cerebral palsy, J. Bone Joint Surg. **40-A**:1359, 1958.

Bassett, F. H., and Baker, L. D.: Equinus deformity in cerebral palsy. In Adams, J. P., editor: Current practice in orthopaedic surgery, vol. 3, St. Louis, 1966, The C. V. Mosby Co.

Berman, A., and Gartland, J. J.: Metartarsal osteotomy for the correction of adduction of the fore part of the foot in children, J. Bone Joint Surg. **53-A**:498, 1971.

Bernau, A.: Long-term results following Lambrinudi arthrodesis, J. Bone Joint Surg. **59-A**:473, 1977.

Blockey, N. J., and Smith, M. G. H.: The treatment of congenital club foot, J. Bone Joint Surg. **48-B**:660, 1966.

Bojsen-Møller, F.: Anatomy of the forefoot, normal and pathologic, Corr. **142**:10, 1979.

Bost, F. C., Schottstaedt, E. R., and Larsen, L. J.: Plantar dissection. An operation to release the soft tissues in recurrent or recalcitrant talipes equinovarus, J. Bone Joint Surg. **42-A**:151, 1960.

Bradley, N., Miller, W. A., and Evans, J. P.: Plantar neuroma: analysis of results following surgical excision in 145 patients, South. Med. J. **69**:853, 1976.

Brahms, M. A.: Common foot problems, J. Bone Joint Surg. **49-A**:1653, 1967.

Broms, J. D.: Sub-talar extra-articular arthrodesis—follow-up study, Clin. Orthop. **42**:139, 1965.

Canale, S. T., and Kelly, F. B., Jr.: Fractures of the neck of the talus. Long-term evaluation of seventy-one cases, J. Bone Joint Surg. **60-A**:143, 1978.

Capener, N.: Congenital clubfoot, J. Bone Joint Surg. **44-B**:956, 1962.

Carpenter, E. B., and Huff, S. H.: Selective tendon transfers for recurrent clubfoot, South. Med. J. **46**:220, 1953.

Carr, C. R., and Boyd, B. M.: Correctional osteotomy for metatarsus primus varus and hallux valgus, J. Bone Joint Surg. **50-A**:1353, 1968.

Clayton, M. L.: Surgery of the lower extremity in rheumatoid arthritis, J. Bone Joint Surg. **45-A**:1517, 1963.

Cleveland, M., and Winant, E.: An end result study of the Keller operation, J. Bone Joint Surg. **32-A**:163, 1950.

Cockin, J.: Butler's operation for an over-riding fifth toe, J. Bone Joint Surg. **50-B**:78, 1968.

Conway, J. J., and Cowell, H. R.: Tarsal coalition: clinical significance and roentgenographic demonstration, Radiology **92**:799, 1969.

Cozen, L.: Management of foot drop in adults after permanent peroneal nerve loss, Clin. Orthop. **67**:151, 1969.

Crego, C. H., Jr., and McCarroll, H. R.: Recurrent deformities in stabilized paralytic feet. A report of 1100 consecutive stabilizations in poliomyelitis, J. Bone Joint Surg. **20**:609, 1938.

Curtin, J. W.: Fibromatosis of the planta fascia. Surgical technique and design of skin incision, J. Bone Joint Surg. **47-A**:1605, 1965.

Davies-Colley, N.: Contraction of the metatarsophalangeal joint of the great toe. Br. Med. J. **1**:728, 1887.

Deburge, A., Nordin, J.-Y., and Taussig, G.: Articular fractures of the calcaneus: Therapeutic indications from a series of 105 cases, Rev. Chir. Orthop. **61**:233, 1975.

Duncan, J. W., and Lovell, W. W.: Hoke triple arthrodesis, J. Bone Joint Surg. **60-A**:795, 1978.

Duncan, T. L., and Wright, J. L.: Plantar interdigital neuroma, South. Med. J. **51**:49, 1958.

Dunn, H. K., and Samuelson, K. M.: Flat top talus. A long-term report of twenty clubfeet, J. Bone Joint Surg. **56-A**:57, 1974.

DuVries, H. L.: Heel spur (calcaneal spur), Arch. Surg. **74**:536, 1957.

DuVries, H. L.: Surgery of the foot, ed. 2, St. Louis, 1965, The C. V. Mosby Co.

Dwyer, F. C.: A new approach to the treatment of pes cavus, Société Internationale de Chirurgie Orthopédique, Sixième Congrès International de Chirurgie Orthopédique. Procèsverbaux, rapports, discussions et communications particulières, publiés par M.A. Bailleux, Brussels, 1955, Imp. Lielens, p. 551.

Dwyer, F. C.: Osteotomy of the calcaneum for pes cavus, J. Bone Joint Surg. **41-B**:80, 1959.

Dwyer, F. C.: The treatment of relapsed clubfoot by the insertion of a wedge into the calcaneum. J. Bone Joint Surg. **45-B**:67, 1963.

Essex-Lopresti, P.: The mechanism, reduction technique, and results in fractures of the os calcis, Br. J. Surg. **39**:395, 1952.

Evans, D.: Treatment of cavo varus foot and clubfoot, J. Bone Joint Surg. **39-B**:789, 1957.

Evans, D.: Relapsed clubfoot, J. Bone Joint Surg. **43-B**:722, 1961.

Fisher, R. L., and Shaffer, S. R.: An evaluation of calcaneal osteotomy in congenital clubfoot and other disorders, Clin. Orthop. **70**:141, 1970.

Flinchum, D.: Pathological anatomy in talipes equinovarus, J. Bone Joint Surg. **35-A**:111, 1953.

Freiberg, A. H.: The so-called infraction of the second metatarsal bone, J. Bone Joint Surg. **8**:257, 1926.

Gallie, W. E.: Subastragalar arthrodesis in fractures of the os calcis, J. Bone Joint Surg. **25**:731, 1943.

Garceau, G. J.: Anterior tibial tendon transposition in recurrent congenital clubfoot, J. Bone Joint Surg. **22**:932, 1940.

Garceau, G. J.: Talipes equinovarus, American Academy of Orthopaedic Surgeons Instructional Course Lectures, vol. 12, Ann Arbor, Mich., 1955, J. W. Edwards, p. 90.

Garceau, G. J.: Pes cavus, American Academy of Orthopaedic Surgeons Instructional Course Lectures, vol. 18, St. Louis, 1961, The C. V. Mosby Co., p. 184.

Garceau, G. J., and Manning, K. R.: Transposition of anterior tibial tendon in treatment of recurrent congenital clubfoot, J. Bone Joint Surg. **29**:1044, 1947.

Garceau, G. J., and Palmer, R. M.: Transfer of the anterior tibial tendon for recurrent clubfoot. A long-term follow-up, J. Bone Joint Surg. **49-A**:207, 1967.

Gartland, J. J.: Posterior tibial tendon transplant in the surgical treatment of recurrent clubfoot, J. Bone Joint Surg. **46-A**:1217, 1964.

Goldner, J. L., and Irwin, C. E.: Paralytic deformities of the foot, American Academy of Orthopaedic Surgeons Instructional Course Lectures, vol. 5, Ann Arbor, Mich., 1948, J. W. Edwards.

Goldstein, L. A., and Dickerson, R. C.: Orthopedic surgery. In White, R. R., editor: Atlas of pediatric surgery, New York, 1965, McGraw-Hill Book Co.

Gorman, J. F., and Rosenberg, J. C.: Dry ice refrigeration for above-knee amputations, Am. J. Surg. 113:241, 1967.

Green, W. T., and Grice, D. S.: The surgical correction of the paralytic foot, American Academy of Orthopaedic Surgeons Instructional Course Lectures, vol. 10, Ann Arbor, Mich., 1953, J. W. Edwards.

Grice, D. S.: An extra-articular arthrodesis of the subastragalar joint for correction of paralytic flat feet in children, J. Bone Joint Surg. 34-A:927, 1952.

Grice, D. S.: Further experience with extra-articular arthrodesis of the subtalar joint, J. Bone Joint Surg. 37-A:246, 1955.

Grice, D. S.: The role of subtalar fusion in the treatment of valgus deformities of the feet, American Academy of Orthopaedic Surgeons Instructional Course Lectures, vol. 16, St. Louis, 1959, The C. V. Mosby Co.

Haimovici, H.: Criteria for and results of transmetatarsal amputation for ischemic gangrene, Arch. Surg. 70:45, 1955.

Harris, R. I.: Retrospect—peroneal spastic flat foot (rigid valgus 1956.

Harris, R. I.: Tetrospect—peroneal spastic flat foot (rigid valgus foot), J. Bone Joint Surg. 47-A:1657, 1965.

Harrison, M. H. M., and Harvey, F. J.: Arthrodesis of the first metatarsophalangeal joint for hallux valgus and ridigus, J. Bone Joint Surg. 45-A:471, 1963.

Hawkins, F. B., Mitchell, C. L., and Hedrick, D. W.: Correction of hallux valgus by metatarsal osteotomy, J. Bone Joint Surg. 27:387, 1945.

Hersh, A.: The role of surgery in the treatment of clubfeet, J. Bone Joint Surg. 49-A:1684, 1967.

Heyman, C. H.: The surgical release of fibrous tissue structures resisting correction of congenital clubfoot and metatarsus varus, American Academy of Orthopaedic Surgeons Instructional Course Lectures, vol. 16, St. Louis, 1959, The C. V. Mosby Co.

Heyman, C. H., Herndon, C. H., and Strong, J. M.: Mobilization of the tarsometatarsal and intermetatarsal joints for the correction of resistant adduction of the fore part of the foot in congenital clubfoot or congenital metatarsus varus, J. Bone Joint Surg. 40-A:299, 1958.

Hoover, G. H., and Frost, H. M.: Dynamic correction of spastic rocker-botton foot. Peroneal to anterior tibial tendon transfer and heel-cord lengthening, Clin. Orthop. 65:175, 1969.

Hunt, J. C., and Brooks, A. L.: Subtalar extra-articular arthrodesis for paralytic valgus deformity of the foot, J. Bone Joint Surg. 47-A:1310, 1965.

Ingram, A. J.: Anterior poliomyelitis. In Crenshaw, A. H., editor: Campbell's operative orthopaedics, vol. 2, ed. 4, St. Louis, 1963, The C. V. Mosby Co.

Irani, R. N., and Sherman, M. S.: The pathological anatomy of clubfoot, J. Bone Joint Surg. 45-A:45, 1963.

Irani, R. N., and Sherman, M. S.: The pathological anatomy of clubfoot, J.A.M.A. 189:613, 1964.

James, A. E., Jr.: Tarsal coalitions and peroneal spastic flat foot, Australas. Radiol. 14:80, 1970.

Janecki, C. J., and Wilde, A. H.: Results of phalangectomy of the fifth toe for hamertoe. The Ruiz-Mora procedure, J. Bone Joint Surg. 58-A:1005, 1976.

Jones, R.: The soldiers foot and the treatment of common deformities of the foot, Br. Med. J. 1:749, 1916.

Jones, R., and Lovett, R. W.: Orthopaedic surgery, ed. 2, New York, 1929, William Wood & Co.

Judet, J.: New concepts in the corrective surgery of congenital talipes equinovarus and congenital neurologic flatfeet, Clin. Orthop. 70:56, 1970.

Kates, A., and Kay, A.: Arthoplasty of the forefoot, J. Bone Joint Surg. 49-B:552, 1967.

Keim, H. A., and Ritchie, G. W.: "Nutcracker" treatment of clubfoot, J.A.M.A. 189:613, 1964.

Keller, W. L.: Surgical treatment of bunions and hallux valgus, N. Y. Med J. 80:741, 1904.

Keller, W. L.: Further observations on the surgical treatment of hallux valgus and bunions. N.Y. Med J. 95:696, 1912.

Kelly, P. J., and Sullivan, C. R.: Blood supply of the talus, Clin. Orthop. 30:37, 1963.

Kendrick, R. E., Sharma, N. K., Hassler, W. L., and Herndon, C. H.: Tarsometatarsal mobilization for resistant adduction of the fore part of the foot. A follow-up study, J. Bone Joint Surg. 52-A:61, 1970.

Kidner, F. C.: The prehallux (accessory scaphoid) in its relation to flatfoot, J. Bone Joint Surg. 11:831, 1929.

Kite, J. H.: Non-operative treatment of congenital clubfeet: A review of 100 cases, South. Med. J. 23:337, 1930.

Kite, J. H.: The treatment of congenital club-feet, Surg. Gynecol. Obstet. 61:190, 1935.

Kite, J. H.: Principles involved in the treatment of clubfoot, J. Bone Joint Surg. 21:595, 1939.

Kite, J. H.: Congenital metatarsus varus. Report of 300 cases, J. Bone Joint Surg. 32-A:500, 1950.

Kite, J. H.: The treatment of resistant clubfeet, American Academy of Orthopaedic Surgeons Instructional Course Lectures, vol. 9, Ann Arbor, Mich., 1952, J. W. Edwards, p. 143.

Kite, J. H.: The operative treatment of congenital clubfeet, American Academy of Orthopaedic Surgeons Instructional Course Lectures, vol. 12, Ann Arbor, Mich., 1955, J. W. Edwards, p. 100.

Knight, R. A.: Static or postural affections, In Speed, J. S., and Knight, R. A., editors: Campbell's operative orthopaedics, vol. 2, ed. 3, St. Louis, 1956, The C. V. Mosby Co.

Lam, S. J. S.: Tarsal tunnel syndrome, J. Bone Joint Surg. 49-B: 87, 1967.

Lambrinudi, C.: New operation on drop-foot, Br. J. Surg. 15:193, 1927.

Lapidus, P. W.: Transplantation of the extensor tendon for correction of the overlapping fifth toe, J. Bone Joint Surg. 24:555, 1942.

Lapidus, P. W.: A quarter of a century of experience with the operative correction of the metatarsus varus primus in hallux valgus, Bull. Hosp. Joint Dis. 17:404, 1956.

Larmon, W. A.: Arthrodesis of the joints of the lower extremity, Surg. Clin. North Am. 45:157, 1965.

Last, R. J.: Specimens from the Hunterian collection. The ligaments of the tarsus. The interosseous ligaments of the wrist, J. Bone Joint Surg. 33-B:114, 1951.

Lewin, P.: The foot and ankle, Philadelphia, 1940, Lea & Febiger.

Lipscomb, P. R.: Surgery for rheumatoid arthritis—timing and techniques: summary, J. Bone Joint Surg. 50-A:614, 1968.

Lipscomb, P. R., and Sanchez, J. J.: Anterior transplantation of the posterior tibial tendon for persistent palsy of the common peroneal nerve, J. Bone Joint Surg. 43-A:60, 1961.

Litchman, H. M., Silver, C. M., and Simon, S. D.: Morton's metatarsalgia, J. Int. Coll. Surg. 41:647, 1964.

MacEwen, D. G., Scott, D. J., and Shands, A. R.: Follow-up survey of clubfoot, J.A.M.A. 175:427, 1961.

Mann, R. A., Coughlin, M. J., and DuVries, H. L.: Hallux rigidus. A review of the literature and a method of treatment, Corr. **142:**57, 1979.

Mann, R. A., and Hagy, J. L.: The function of the toes in walking, jogging, and running, Corr. **142:**24, 1979.

Margo, M. K.: Surgical treatment of conditions of the fore part of the foot, J. Bone Joint Surg. **49-A:**1665, 1967.

McBride, E. D.: A conservative operation for bunions, J. Bone Joint Surg. **10:**735, 1928.

McBride, E. D.: Hallux valgus bunion deformity, American Academy of Orthopaedic Surgeons Instructional Course Lectures, vol. 9, Ann Arbor, Mich., 1952, J. W. Edwards. p. 334.

McBride, E. D.: Hallux valgus, J. Int. Coll. Surg. **21:**99, 1954.

McBride, E. D.: The McBride bunion hallux valgus operation. Refinements in the successive surgical steps of the operation, J. Bone Joint Surg. **49-A:**1675, 1967.

McCauley, J. C., Jr.: Surgical treatment of clubfoot, Surg. Clin. North Am. **31:**561, 1951.

McCauley, J. C., Jr.: Triple arthrodesis for congenital talipes equinovarus deformities, Clin. Orthop. **34:**25, 1964.

McCauley, J. C., Jr.: Clubfoot. History of the development and the concepts of pathogenesis and treatment, Clin. Orthop. **44:**51, 1966.

McCormick, D. W., and Blount, W. P.: Metatarsus adductovarus. "Skewfoot," J.A.M.A. **141:**449, 1949.

Mindell, E. R., Cisek, E. E., Kartalian, G., and Dzoib, J. M.: Late results of injuries to the talus. Analysis of forth cases, J. Bone Joint Surg. **45-A:**221, 1963.

Mitchell, C. L., et al.: Osteotomy-bunionectomy for hallux valgus, J. Bone Joint Surg. **40-A:**41, 1958.

Mitchell, G. P., and Gibson, J. M. C.: Excision of calcaneo-navicular bar for painful spasmodic flat foot, J. Bone Joint Surg. **49-B:**281, 1967.

Mooney, V., Perry, J., and Nickel, V.: Surgical and non-surgical orthopaedic care of stroke, J. Bone Joint Surg. **49-A:**989, 1967.

Morris, E., and Morse, T. S.: Aneurysm of the posterior tibial artery after a foot stabilization procedure. A case report, J. Bone Joint Surg. **48-A:**337, 1966.

Morton, T. G.: A peculiar and painful affection of the fourth metatarso-phalangeal articulation, Am. J. Med. Sci., p. 1, 1876.

Nissen, K. I.: Plantar digital neuritis—Morton's metatarsalgia, J. Bone Joint Surg. **30-B:**84, 1948.

Ober, F. R.: An operation for the relief of congenital equinovarus deformity, J. Bone Joint Surg. **2:**558, 1920.

O'Rahilly, R.: A survey of carpal and tarsal anomalies, J. Bone Joint Surg. **35-A:**626, 1953.

Palinacci, J.-Cl., Veran, J., Dexpert, M., and Bourrel, P.: Fractures of the tarsal scaphoid, Rev. Chir. Orthop. **60:**549, 1974.

Pedersen, H. E., and Day, A. J.: The transmetatarsal amputation in peripheral vascular disease, J. Bone Joint Surg. **36-A:**1190, 1954.

Polo, G., and Lechtman, C. P.: Surgical treatment of congenital talipes equinovarus adductus, Clin. Orthop. **70:**87, 1970.

Ponseti, I. V., and Becker, J. R.: Congenital metatarsus adductus: the results of treatment, J. Bone Joint Surg. **48-A:**702, 1966.

Ponseti, I. V., and Smoley, E. M.: Congenital clubfoot: the results of treatment, J. Bone Joint Surg. **45-A:**261, 1963.

Rix, P. R.: Modified Mayo operation for hallux valgus and bunion—a comparison with the Keller procedure. J. Bone Joint Surg. **50-A:**1368, 1968.

Rowe, C. R., et al.: Fractures of the os calcis. A long-term follow-up study of 146 patients, J.A.M.A. **184:**920, 1963.

Ryerson, E. W.: Arthrodesing operations on the feet, J. Bone Joint Surg. **5:**453, 1923.

Salter, R. B.: Present trends in treatment of clubfeet, The American Academy of Orthopaedic Surgeons, Sound-slide program, 1965.

Schottstaedt, E. R.: Symposium: treatment of fractures of the calcaneus. Introduction, J. Bone Joint Surg. **45-A:**863, 1963.

Schurman, D. J.: Ankle-block anesthesia for foot surgery, Anesthesiology **44:**348, 1976.

Schwartz, R. P.: Arthrodesis of subtalus and midtarsal joints of the foot; historical review, preoperative determinations and operative procedure, Surgery **20:**619, 1946.

Semb, H. T.: The treatment of clubfoot and its results. A followup study, Acta Orthop. Scand. **34:**271, 1964.

Settle, G. W.: The anatomy of congenital talipes equinovarus: Sixteen dissected specimens, J. Bone Joint Surg. **45-A:**1341, 1963.

Shands, A. R., Jr., and Wentz, I. J.: Congenital anomalies, accessory bones and osteochondritis in the feet of 850 children, Surg. Clin. North Am. **33:**1643, 1953.

Shapiro, F., and Glimcher, M. J.: Gross and histological abnormalities of the talus in congenital club foot, J. Bone Joint Surg. **61-A:**522, 1979.

Shaw, N. E.: Comparison of three methods for treatment of congenital clubfoot, Br. Med. J. **1:**1084, 1966.

Silver, C. M., et al.: Calcaneal osteotomy for valgus and varus deformities of the foot in cerebral palsy. A preliminary report on twenty-seven operations, J. Bone Joint Surg. **49-A:**232, 1967.

Simmons, E. H.: Tibialis spastic varus foot with tarsal coalition, J. Bone Joint Surg. **47-B:**533, 1965.

Slocum, D. B.: An atlas of amputations, St. Louis, 1949, The C. V. Mosby Co.

Slocum, D. B.: Amputations. In Crenshaw, A. H., editor: Campbell's operative orthopaedics, ed. 4, St. Louis, 1963, The C. V. Mosby Co.

Smith, J. B., and Westin, G. W.: Subtalar extra-articular arthrodesis, J. Bone Joint Surg. **50-A:**1027, 1968.

Steytler, J. C. S., and Van der Walt, I. D.: Correction of resistant adduction of the forefoot in congenital club-foot and congenital metatarsus varus by metatarsal osteotomy, Br. J. Surg. **53:**558, 1966.

Swanson, A. B., Lumsden, R. M., II, and Swanson, G. DeG.: Silicone implant arthroplasty of the great toe. A review of single stem and flexible hinge implants, Corr. **142:**30, 1979.

Szaboky, G. T., and Raghaven, V. C.: Modification of Mitchell's lateral displacement angulation osteotomy, J. Bone Joint Surg. **51-A:**1430, 1969.

Thomas, F. B.: Arthrodesis of the subtalar joint, J. Bone Joint Surg. **49-B:**93, 1967.

Thompson, T. C.: Surgical treatment of disorders of the fore part of the foot, J. Bone Joint Surg. **46-A:**1117, 1964.

Tohen, A., et al.: Extra-articular subtalar arthrodesis. A review of 286 operations, J. Bone Joint Surg. **51-B:**45, 1969.

Turco, V. J.: Surgical correction of the resistant clubfoot. Onestage posteromedial release with internal fixation: A preliminary report, J. Bone Joint Surg. **53-A:**477, 1971.

Turco, V. J.: Resistant congenital clubfoot-one-stage posteromedial release with internal fixation. A follow-up report of a fifteen-year experience, J. Bone Joint Surg. **61-A:**805, 1979.

Vahvanen, V. A., Jr.: Rheumatoid arthritis in the pantalar joints. A follow-up study of triple arthrodesis on 292 adult feet, Acta Orthop. Scand. (Suppl.) 107, 1967.

Vainio, K.: The rheumatoid foot, Ann. Chir. Gynaecol. Fenn. 45 (Suppl.) 1, 1956.

Warren, R., et al.: The transmetatarsal amputation in arterial deficiency of the lower extremity, Surgery **31**:132, 1952.

Waugh, T. R., Wagner, J., and Stinchfield, F. E.: An evaluation of pantalar arthrodesis. A follow-up study of 116 operations, J. Bone Joint Surg. **47-A**:1315, 1965.

Wenger, R. J. J., and Whalley, R. C.: Total replacement of the first metatarsophalangeal joint, J. Bone Joint Surg. **60-B**:88, 1978.

Weseley, M. S., and Barenfeld, P. A.: Mechanism of the Dwyer calcaneal osteotomy, Clin. Orthop. **70**:137, 1970.

Westin, G. W.: Tendon transfers about the foot, ankle, and hip in the paralyzed lower extremity, J. Bone Joint Surg. **47-A**:1430, 1965.

Westin, G. W., and Hall, C. B.: Subtalar extra-articular arthrodesis, J. Bone Joint Surg. **39-A**:501, 1957.

Whellock, F. C., Jr.: Transmetatarsal amputations and arterial surgery in diabetic patients, N. Engl. J. Med. **264**:316, 1961.

Whitman, R.: The classic observations of forty-five cases of flat-foot with particular reference to etiology and treatment, Clin. Orthop. **70**:4, 1970.

Wilson, F. C., Jr., et al.: Triple arthrodesis. A study of the factors affecting fusion after three hundred and one procedures, J. Bone Joint Surg. **47-A**:340, 1965.

Wilson, J. N.: Oblique displacement osteotomy for hallux valgus, J. Bone Joint Surg. **45-B**:552, 1963.

Wolf, M. D.: Metatarsal osteotomy for relief of painful metatarsal callosities, J. Bone Joint Surg. **55-A**:1760, 1973.

Wright, D. J., and Rennels, D. C.: A study of the elastic properties of plantar fascia, J. Bone Joint Surg. **46-A**:482, 1964.

Wyard, G. E., Thompson, W. W., and Eilers, V. E.: Syndactylism, Minn. Med. **61**:177, 1978.

Zadek, I., and Gold, A. M.: The accessory tarsal scaphoid, J. Bone Joint Surg. **30-A**:957, 1948.

16

MISCELLANEOUS OPERATIVE PROCEDURES

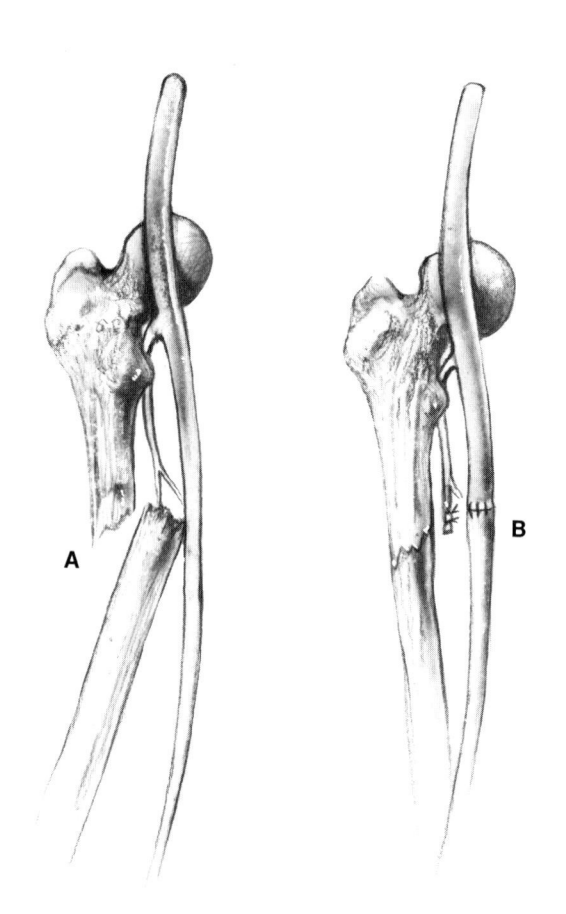

REPAIR OF SEVERED ARTERY (Plate 16-1)

GENERAL DISCUSSION. Arterial injuries can be inflicted in a number of ways by either penetrating or nonpenetrating trauma. The acute result may be laceration, transection, thrombosis, or spasm of the artery. The chronic result may be false aneurysm, true aneurysm, or arteriovenous fistula. The most common arterial injuries are those which result from the penetrating injury, whether it be by a bullet, knife, glass fragment, or other cause. The result is that of laceration or transection of the arterial wall in most instances. Blunt trauma may lead to thrombosis or possible spasm of the arterial wall.

The most common arterial injuries in association with fractures or fracture-dislocations are encountered where the artery is anatomically in close proximity to bone (**A**). The brachial artery, in close association with the humerus, and the superficial femoral artery in Hunter's canal, as well as the popliteal artery, are particularly vulnerable to injury.

The technique of arterial repair is basically the same regardless of the type of injury. Arterial injuries associated with fractures may introduce other factors such as the associated management of bone, nerve, and/or muscle injury. Consideration should be given to restoration of blood volume and hydration of the patient preoperatively whenever arterial surgery is anticipated. The tendency for thrombosis in the dehydrated patient and the necessity for adequate blood pressure to maintain patency of the repaired artery are important factors. Repair of injury to a major artery is an emergency procedure (**B**).

A few specific instruments should be available as minimum requirements for adequate surgical treatment of arterial injuries. These include vascular clamps, Fogarty catheters, suction tips (Frazier type), irrigating cannulae, and arterial suture. Heparinized saline solution (2,000 units of heparin per 150 ml of saline solution) for irrigation should be available.

In preparation of the patient for surgery, if bleeding is a problem, it is best to control hemorrhage with a bulky dressing or direct pressure, which is far better than application of a tourniquet, for a tourniquet will produce total ischemia to the limb by obliterating all collaterals.

DETAILS OF PROCEDURE. Before the site of arterial injury is approached directly, proximal and distal control of the artery must be gained. If there is an associated bone injury, this may need to be stabilized before arterial repair is undertaken. When less than one third of the diameter of the artery is disrupted, particularly when the interruption is clean-cut and there is no adjacent contusion, limited debridement and careful suturing of the defect are effective. If the interruption in the wall of the artery is more extensive and if there is extensive bruising of the wall of the artery, the damaged area must be excised. The debrided ends are united by direct anastomosis or by the use of a graft. Direct anastomosis of the ends is preferable and is usually possible if the gap between the debrided ends of the vessel is less than 2.5 cm.

If the divided ends of the artery cannot be reanastomosed with ease, a graft should be used to restore arterial continuity. A reversed autogenous, saphenous, or cephalic vein graft is the graft of choice. The vein graft is living tissue with an intimal lining, and thrombosis is less likely, particularly if infection is present. If a vein graft is used, it is important to determine the length of the graft so it will equal exactly the length of the arterial defect. If a vein graft is placed under excessive tension, it will increase the likelihood of thrombosis and/or possible rupture of the suture line. However, if a suitable vein is not available, a synthetic arterial prosthesis may be used.

(Plate 16-1) REPAIR OF SEVERED ARTERY

Prior to reconstruction, all clots should be removed from the proximal artery. Residual distal thrombosis may compromise an otherwise successful repair. Distal clot, if present, should be removed from the distal arterial tree with a Fogarty catheter. The Fogarty catheter is also useful in dilating the proximal and distal arterial segments, prior to reconstruction. If it is not possible to be satisfied about distal patency at the time of operation, an arteriogram may be done on the operating table.

When the artery has been transected cleanly, direct anastomosis is the method of choice and is frequently possible if the artery is adequately mobilized. However, the sacrifice of major collateral channels to permit direct approximation of the artery is unwise, and the use of acute joint flexion to permit direct approximation of the artery is not justified. In either circumstance it is better to bridge the gap with a vascular graft. The distal artery may be perfused with a dilute heparin solution along with removal of any distal clots with the Fogarty catheter. When everything is ready for anastomosis of the vessel ends, a stay-suture is placed. A second stay-suture is placed at 180° to the first, and the remainder of the anastomosis is carried out with an ordinary over-and-over continuous arterial suture (**C** to **F**).

The distal occluding clamp is released to reveal whether any bleeding occurs at the anastomosis site. If necessary, additional sutures may be placed with the two segments again isolated between proximal and distal arterial clamps. Following release of both distal and proximal arterial clamps, the pulse through the distal artery should be observed. Papaverine may be used locally if there is any element of vessel spasm. The wound is then closed.

Palpation of pulse at the most distal portion of the extremity may be difficult at first because of arterial spasm. The distal pulse is sometimes not palpated until some hours subsequently. However, the distal portion of the extremity should be warm and pink, even if a distal pulse is not immediately palpable. If not, reexploration to look for residual clot is mandatory.

POSTOPERATIVE MANAGEMENT. Successful arterial repair does not allow the surgeon to relax, for if thrombosis occurs, reexploration is mandatory. Prolonged use of sympathetic blocks or anticoagulation in an effort to avoid a secondary procedure are temporizing measures that delay the steps necessary to preserve tissue function. Anticoagulants generally are not used postoperatively. The need for immobilization of the patient's extremity postoperatively depends mainly on the presence of any associated injury.

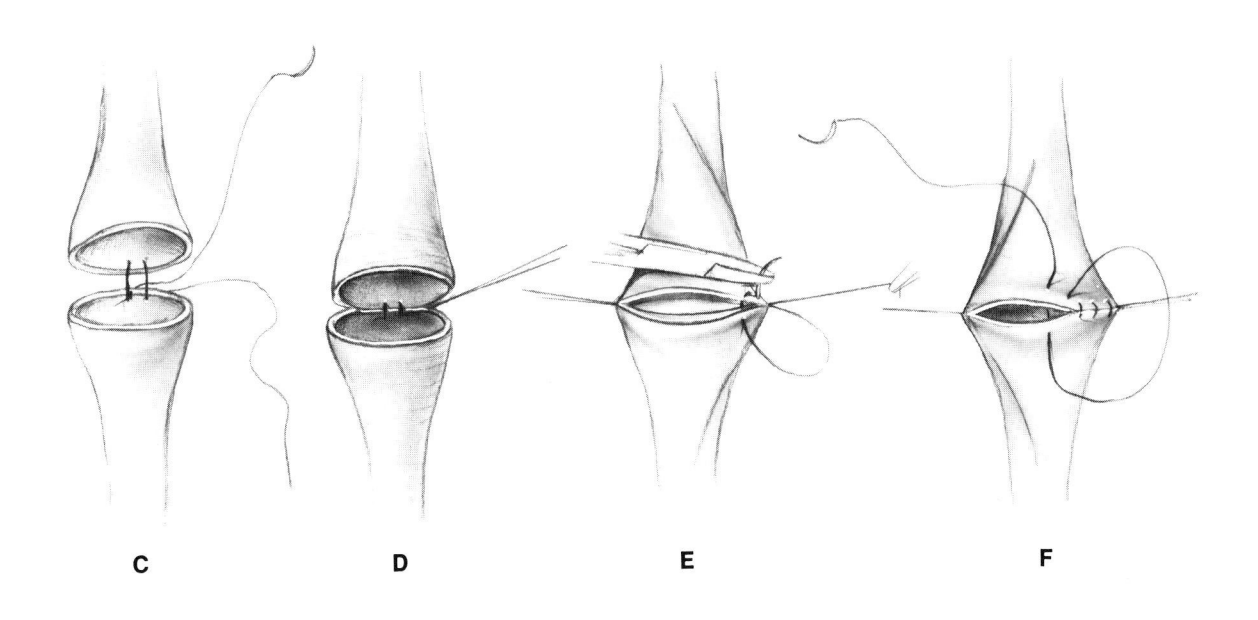

C   D   E   F

RELEASE OF SUPERFICIAL TISSUE CONTRACTURE (Z-PLASTY TECHNIQUE) (Plate 16-2)

GENERAL DISCUSSION. Z-plasty is basically a transposition-plasty carried out to elongate contracted tissue or scar. Its principle is to rotate the scar or contracted tissue that is under tension by roughly 90° by crossing two triangular flaps.

Use of Z-plasty should be restricted to relief of linear contractures. In the hand, as elsewhere, it can increase length in a particular direction and provide exposure of deeper structures. Transposition of Z-plasty flaps results in lengthening in one direction and equal shortening in the other. Increasing the Z-plasty angle will increase the amount of lengthening and shortening. By transposing the two pointed flaps in the Z-plasty, the straight line of tension or contracture is converted to a zigzag line, so the tension expends itself.

Z-plasty may be indicated for web contractures in the axilla, elbow, flexor surfaces of the digits, and elsewhere. In the digits, Z-plasty is best if the scar has formed a true web, for such a contracture means that there is adequate skin fom the sides of the digit so that a circular constriction when the two triangles of the Z-plasty are transposed can be avoided. Multiple Z-plasties may be used when a scar is too long to allow correction with one Z-plasty.

DETAILS OF PROCEDURE. The central limb of the Z-plasty is made along the line of the contracture that is to be released. The other two limbs of the Z-plasty are made equal in length to that of the central limb; the angle between each limb and the central limb must be equal one to the other and is usually about 60° (**A**). If this angle is greater than 60°, it may be difficult to transpose the flap. If the angle is decreased, the Z-plasty will be less effective in releasing tension and the blood supply to each flap may be impaired.

The triangular flaps are transposed as illustrated (**B** to **E**). The point of each flap must be handled with care, since it will be the most likely area to undergo necrosis. The apex of each triangular flap should be sutured with an apical stitch, as illustrated, after transposition.

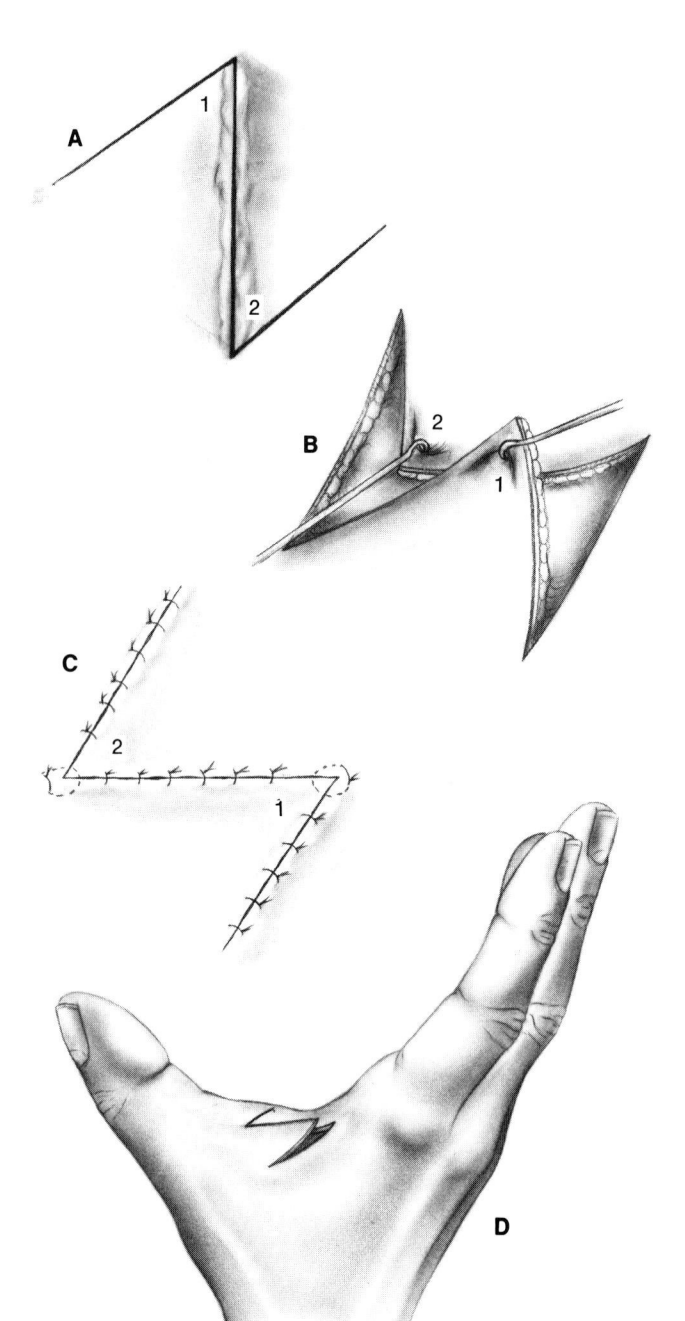

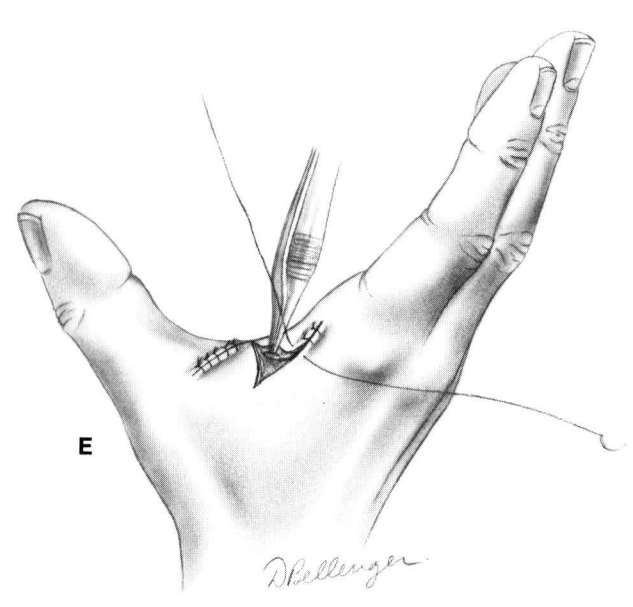

(Plate 16-3) SOFT TISSUE COVERAGE OF INJURED EXTREMITY

GENERAL DISCUSSION. For the injured extremity with an open fracture, early soft tissue coverage will be a critical factor in the management of the fracture and the prognosis for the patient. An open fracture is a true surgical emergency. Adequate antibiotic therapy should be started in the emergency department and continued into the postoperative period. Tetanus antitoxin or a booster of tetanus toxoid should be given. As soon as the patient's general condition will permit, any open fracture should receive definitive treatment, preferably within 4 to 6 hours from the time of injury.

In the operating room, cleansing and extensive irrigation of the open fracture wound is followed by debridement of devitalized soft tissues. It is important to preserve as much overlying skin as possible. If adequate skin remains, the wound should be closed primarily, particularly when the open fracture has been adequately treated in the operating room within the first 8 to 12 hours following injury. In some open fractures that are treated early after injury, internal fixation may be considered. However, metallic internal fixation should be used with great caution in open fractures, that is, only in situations where there is prompt treatment, adequate soft tissue coverage, and when satisfactory reduction of the fracture would be otherwise impossible.

For closure of the soft tissues over an open fracture, tension is one of the greatest hazards to effective wound closure. The length of the laceration or the wound has little relation to healing if tension and infection are avoided. To eliminate tension, some type of skin graft may be necessary.

Occasionally, local flaps may be useful for soft tissue coverage, possibly in conjunction with free grafts. An advancement flap in its simplest form would be direct closure obtained from undermined flaps of wound margins after resection of a wide scar. Rotational flaps are useful for coverage about the knee area or on the plantar surface of the foot.

Free skin grafts alone may provide sufficient permanent coverage or may be used in conjunction with pedicle flaps. The medium thickness skin graft is satisfactory for ordinary wear and tear of lower extremity use except for plantar surfaces. Free grafts should be placed into recipient areas only after all deep scar has been excised and good hemostasis has been obtained.

Loss of skin in the pretibial region of the lower leg is common. Methods of skin coverage in instances of skin loss in this area including a relaxing incision and a bipedicle skin flap, local rotational flaps, and direct split-thickness skin grafts. Muscle also may be helpful for coverage of the tibia.

When a cross leg flap is necessary, it is usually elevated and moved in stages. The most richly vascularized donor areas are the anterior thigh and medial calf. Before initial operation the pattern of the flap and positioning should be accurately determined. The pattern of the donor area should be slightly larger than the area it is to replace. If the flap is to cover an ulcer or bony cavity, freedom from infection must be assured.

Contraindications to cross leg pedicles are the existence of any significant injury within potential donor areas of the opposite leg and stiffness of the hips or knees that prevents the required positioning. Consideration should also be given to the cosmetic defect in the donor thigh or calf of a female patient. Flaps taken from a distance require extensive and often multiple operative stages but can occasionally salvage function of an extremity.

DETAILS OF PROCEDURE. Closure of the skin may be carried out with continuous suture **(A)** or interrupted sutures **(B)**. Nonabsorbable sutures are commonly used, although in children a fine plain catgut suffices and absorbs slowly enough to allow healing. If, from the laceration or from an elective procedure (such as a Z-plasty), there is need to suture a point of skin, damage to the blood supply of the apex can be minimized by using a horizontal suture that should be passed through the subdermal layer of the apical portion of the wound **(C)**. In the palm, or in any area where there is tendency for the skin edges to invert, it is advisable to use a vertical mattress suture **(D)**. If the skin has been widely undermined, leaving a possible space for a hematoma, the deep loop of the vertical mattress suture can be passed through the deeper tissues.

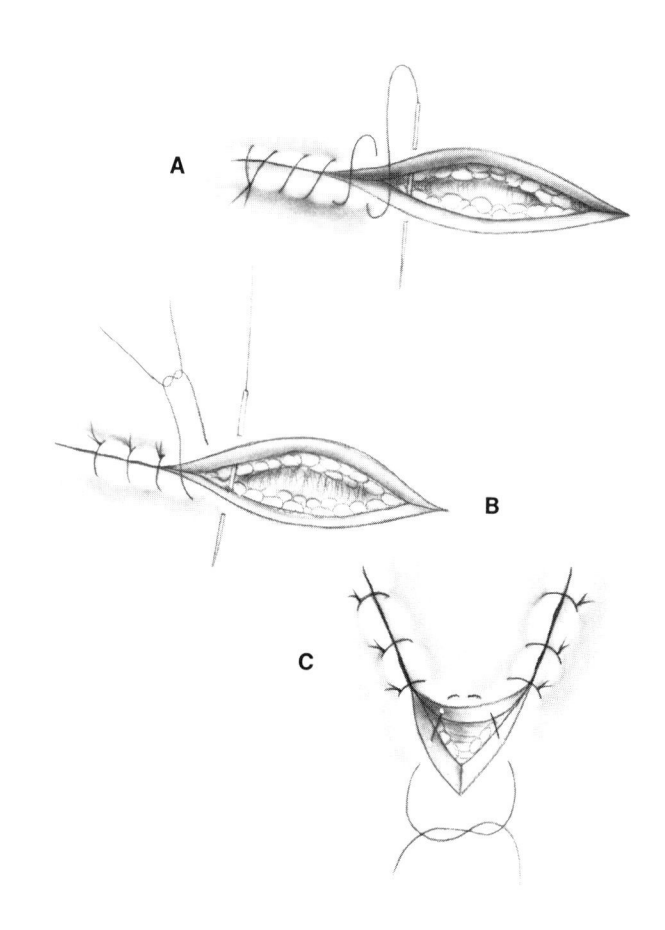

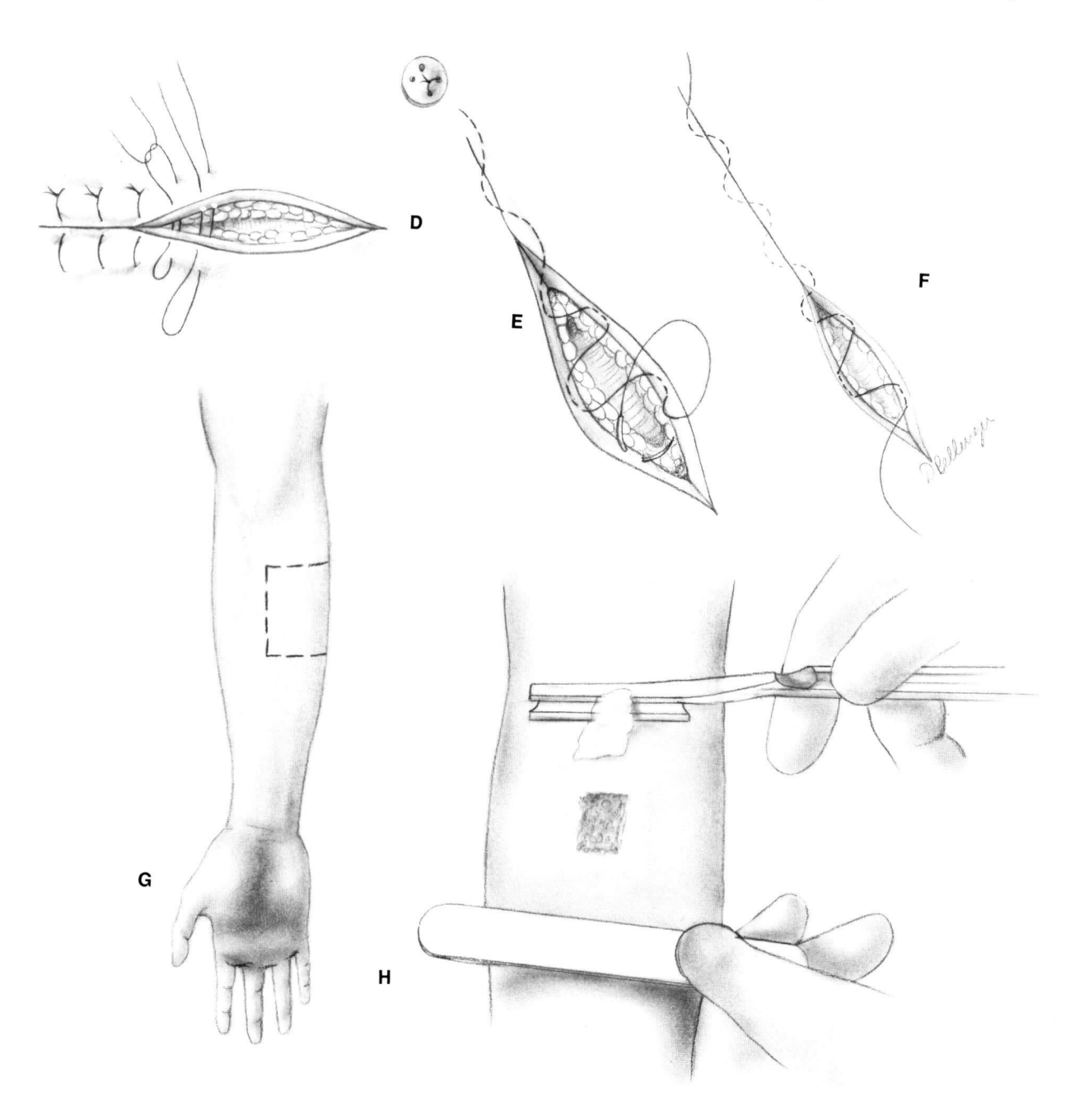

SOFT TISSUE COVERAGE OF INJURED EXTREMITY (Plate 16-3)

A fine cosmetic closure can be obtained by a running subcuticular suture with a stainless-steel wire or other smooth-surfaced suture material. Each end is brought out through the skin and, if necessary, tied to a button (**E** and **F**). To pass this suture, a circular reverse cutting needle is used, taking a shallow bite but engaging the dermis over a long distance, ordinarily 1 to 2 cm. Each bit of the suture enters the opposite side slightly behind the exit point of the alternate suture. Any loop in the suture should be unrolled smoothly to avoid kinking of the suture if stainless-steel wire suture is employed. Intermittently during wound closure and at the completion of wound closure, it will be advisable to test the "running" by moving the wire suture back and forth through the tissues and ultimately to leave a smooth portion of the stainless-steel wire within the wound.

Many wounds of the hand involve loss of skin of only a small area. A splint-skin graft taken from the anterior surface of the forearm with a straight razor (as illustrated) is easily obtained (**G** and **H**). The skin of the forearm, having been cleansed, and shaved if necessary, is lightly greased with a petroleum jelly, as is the razor or scalpel blade. An assistant holds the forearm firmly on the arm board and, with a tongue blade, flattens out the convexity and pulls distalward on the forearm skin. The surgeon also uses a tongue de-

(Plate 16-3) SOFT TISSUE COVERAGE OF INJURED EXTREMITY

pressor just ahead of the scalpel or razor blade to keep the surface flat. The scalpel or razor blade is oscillated back and forth, and a consistent cutting depth is maintained by keeping the back edge of the scalpel or razor blade firmly on the skin and over the freshly cut donor area. Split-thickness grafts vary in thickness, depending on that of the donor skin, and are cut so that only a thin layer of dermis remains. The appearance of the donor area is that of a dull white surface with many punctate oozing points where the papillae of the dermis have been transected. This donor site must be used with caution in the child or female because the residual scar in some patients hypertrophies and is unsightly. The hypothenar area is ideal for small grafts (2 × 2 cm) and the buttock for larger areas.

For large amounts of skin, one may use any of the available powered machines. Split-skin grafts are generally used to cover skin loss where there is some subcutaneous tissue to act as a nutrient bed. Split-skin grafts are not placed over open joints or tendons. After a skin graft is applied, it is covered by a finely meshed nonadherent material and then fluffy gauze (I to L). In the hand, this may be held in place with stockinette and a splint to support the hand in a position of function.

Traumatic fingertip amputations are common injuries, and in some patients may result in many months of disability. Certain guidelines are helpful in selecting the surgical treatment. The simplest solution is usually the best. There are five basic alternatives: (1) simple direct closure if adequate soft tissue is present; (2) skin graft (split or full); (3) local advancement flaps (volar or bilateral); (4) distant flaps from elsewhere on the hand (thenar, cross finger, or neurovascular island); (5) distant flaps from outside the hand (almost never indicated).

Tissue should not be closed under tension. It is important always to accurately approximate the nail matrix. *Absorbable sutures (6-0 or 5-0)* are used in the nail matrix and in children to avoid painful suture removal. If a displaced fracture of the distal phalanx is present, one must be certain that the nail matrix is not interposed; failure to recognize this and reduce the nail matrix will frequently result in osteo-

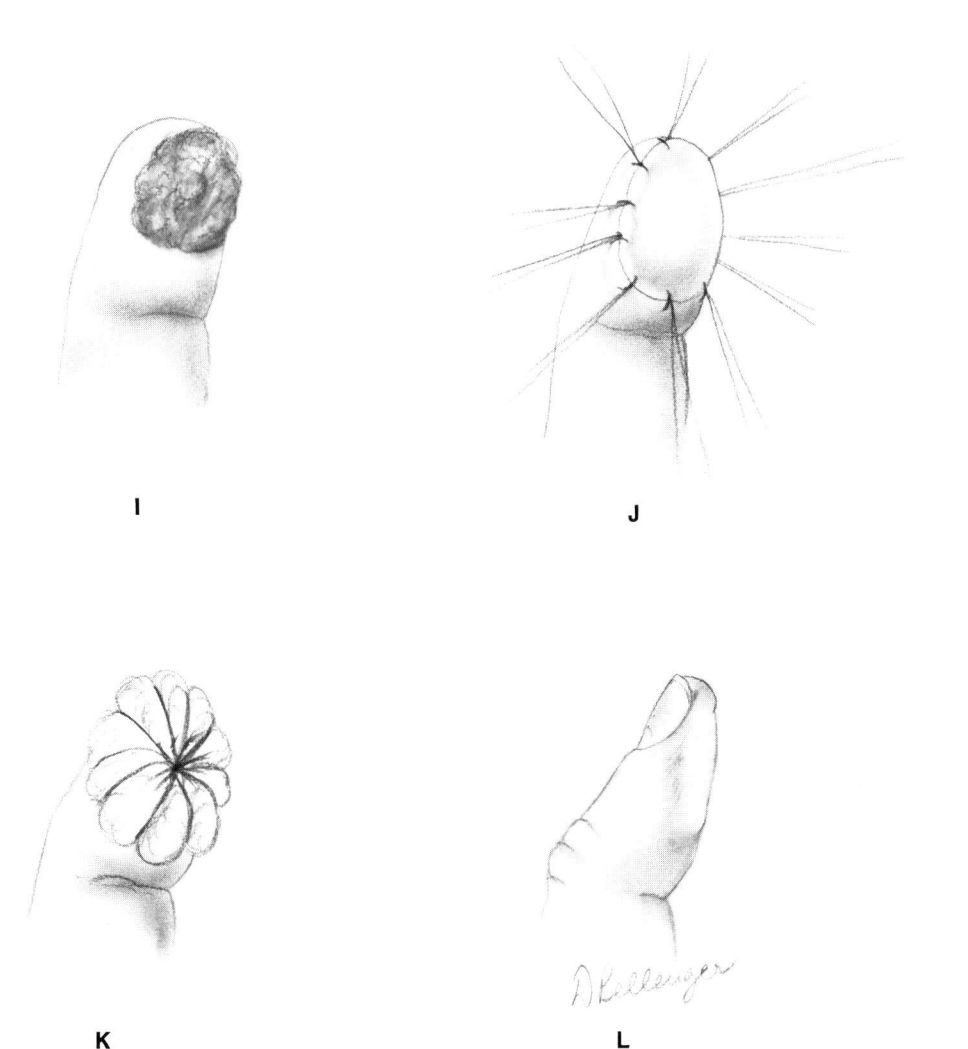

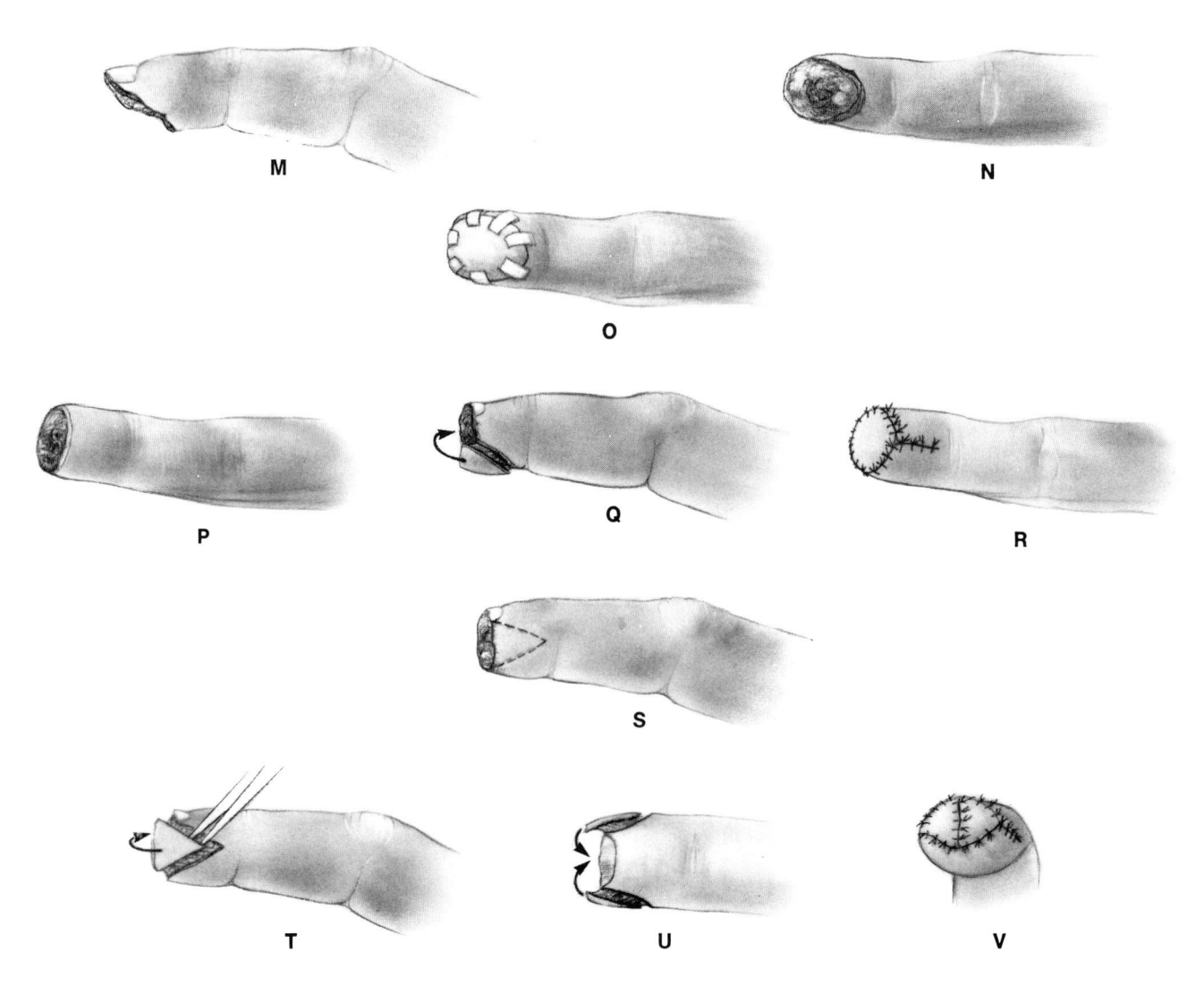

SOFT TISSUE COVERAGE OF INJURED EXTREMITY (Plate 16-3)

myelitis. If the amputation is through bone, the distal bone end should always be smoothed and contoured with a rongeur to avoid subsequent painful bone prominences. If the amputation is more proximal, the nerve ending is resected away from the bone end at the amputation stump.

If the amputation is through the middle or proximal phalanx, the bone is rongeured and smoothed so that a direct primary closure without tension can be done. The one exception for this is amputation of the thumb, when primary reconstruction is sometimes advisable. See also p. 613 for discussion of indications for replantation.

Amputations of the fingertip are usually one of two types: the oblique type as represented in **M,** or the more transverse type shown in **P.** In amputations of the oblique type with loss of the pulp, the best initial primary treatment, and certainly the safest, is that of a split-thickness skin graft applied to achieve primary closure **(N, O).** If the mechanism of amputation has been a sharp injury, frequently the skin from the amputated fingertip can be defatted and applied as a full-thickness skin graft. Cross finger flaps or thenar flaps are best done later as elective procedures, if necessary (they most often are not required).

If this original tissue is not available, or if the mechanism of injury has been a crush, it is more prudent to close this wound with a split-thickness skin graft. This may be obtained from the proximal flexor aspect of the forearm. This donor site should not be used in children or in young women, since this often leaves an unsightly scar. For these people it is more prudent to take the split-thickness skin graft from either the hypothenar or the buttock area. The donor skin should never be taken from a hair-bearing surface. The split graft can be secured with either 5-0 sutures or small Steri-strips; the full-thickness graft is best sutured in place.

Should the amputation be of a transverse type as is seen in **P,** then additional possibilities include the use of local advancement flaps. This can be the anterior YV advancement flap as described by Kleinert et al. (**Q** and **R**), or the bilateral lateral advancement YV-plasty described by Kutler (**S** to **V**).

(Plate 16-3) SOFT TISSUE COVERAGE OF INJURED EXTREMITY

A sterile dressing must be applied that supports the wound, regardless of the type of repair. This should be maintained for 3 to 4 weeks, at which point the patient should be started on an exercise program and gradually increase the use of the hand.

If skin overlying the tibia has been lost or tension on wound closure is excessive, a relaxing incision made medially and/or laterally at an appropriate distance from the wound can permit sliding of full-thickness skin and subcutaneous tissue to cover an open wound over the tibia (**W** to **Y**). Split-thickness skin grafts are used to cover the defect created by the counterincision. The relaxing incision should be made approximately 8 cm (and never less than 4 cm) from the lateral edge of the wound and should generally be approximately 15 cm in length. If the skin defect is large, two relaxing incisions may be necessary. The relaxing incision should be made sufficiently long so the skin and subcutaneous tissue can be easily mobilized to cover the skin defect.

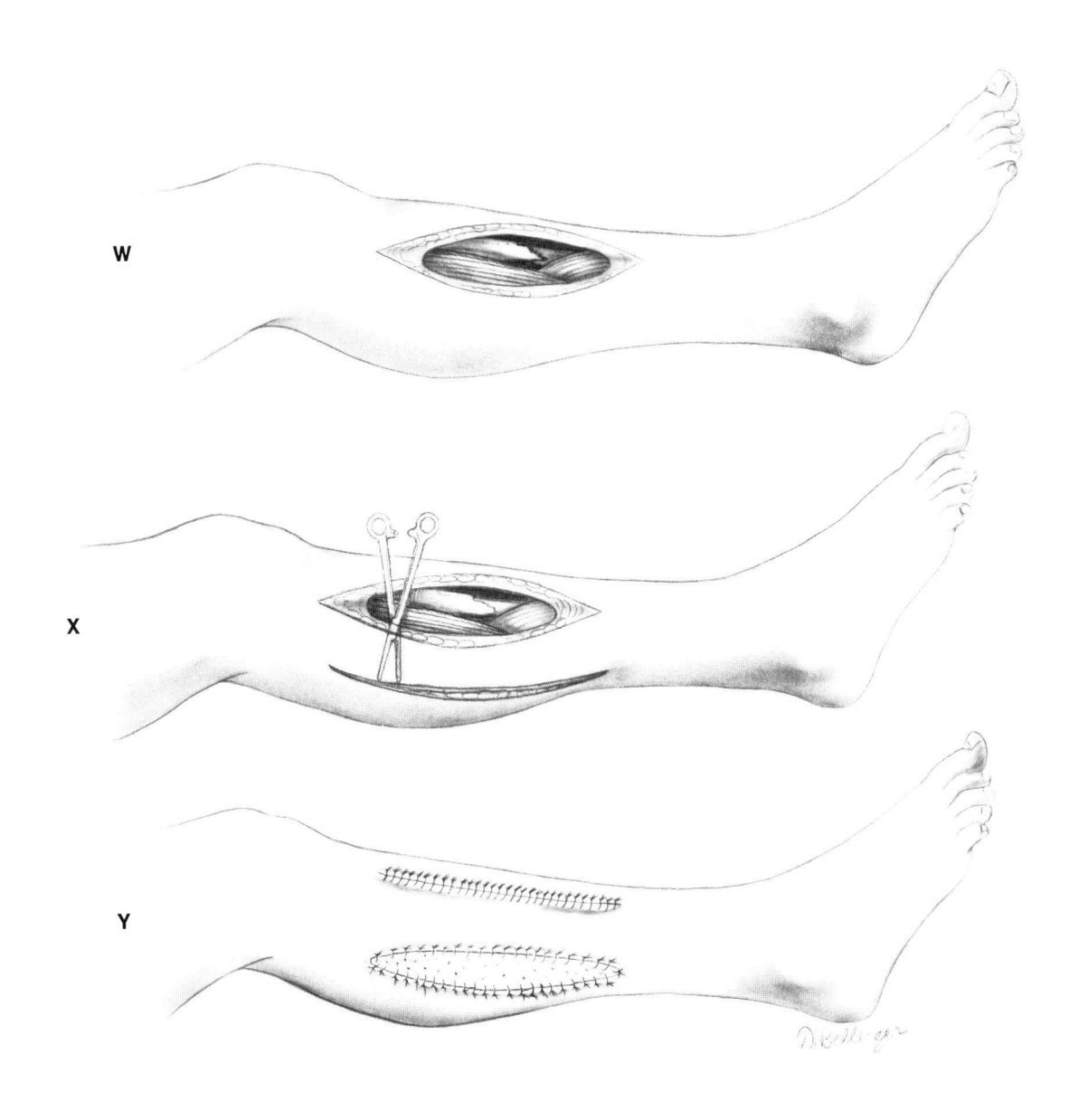

SOFT TISSUE COVERAGE OF INJURED EXTREMITY (Plate 16-3)

It may at times be possible to obtain coverage of the exposed shaft of the tibia by mobilizing and shifting the soleus muscle (**Z** and **AA**). On the rare occasion when soft tissue trauma is so extensive that adequate coverage of the tibia is not possible (even with relaxing incisions), temporary covering of the tibia with a split-thickness graft for 10 to 14 days can be used until a full-thickness cross leg flap or tube graft can be provided. Every means should be used to cover the tibia with viable soft tissue. If skin or soft tissue coverage of the tibia is preserved, it will facilitate the management of any underlying tibial fracture in the future.

Free skin grafting is recognized as a valuable part of primary treatment of traumatized soft tissue defects. However, free skin grafts succeed permanently only when the base of the wound is vascularized. Fascia and muscle are ideal recipient sites.

In some situations a local pedicle flap can be employed to provide coverage, as, for example, for a pressure sore of the posterior surface of the heel (**BB** and **CC**). A split-thickness skin graft is used to cover the secondary defect. In other circumstances, a cross leg pedicle graft may be necessary to obtain adequate soft tissue coverage for the heel **(DD)**.

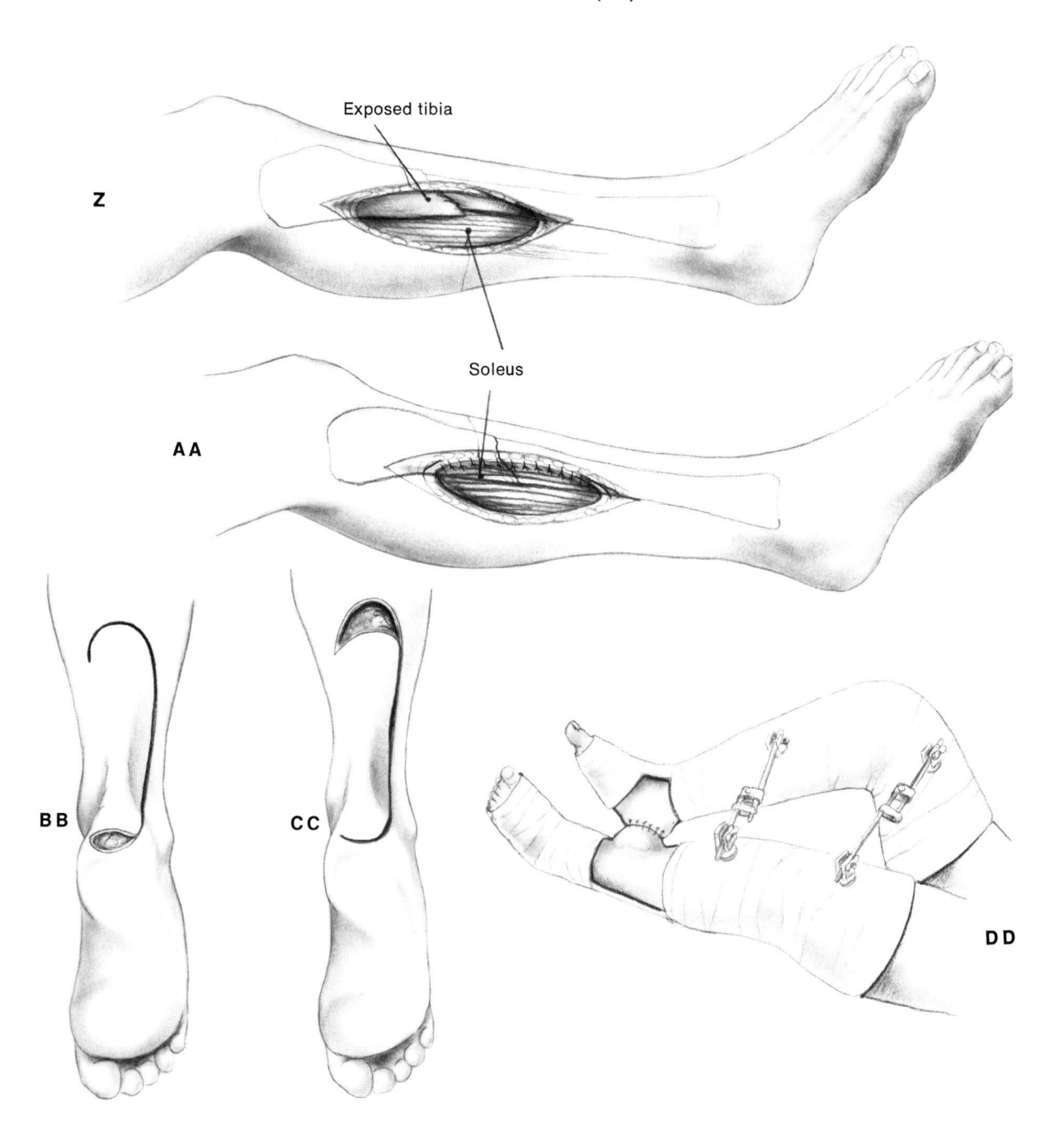

(Plate 16-4) CLOSED TUBE IRRIGATION AND DRAINAGE OF LOCALIZED MUSCULOSKELETAL AREAS

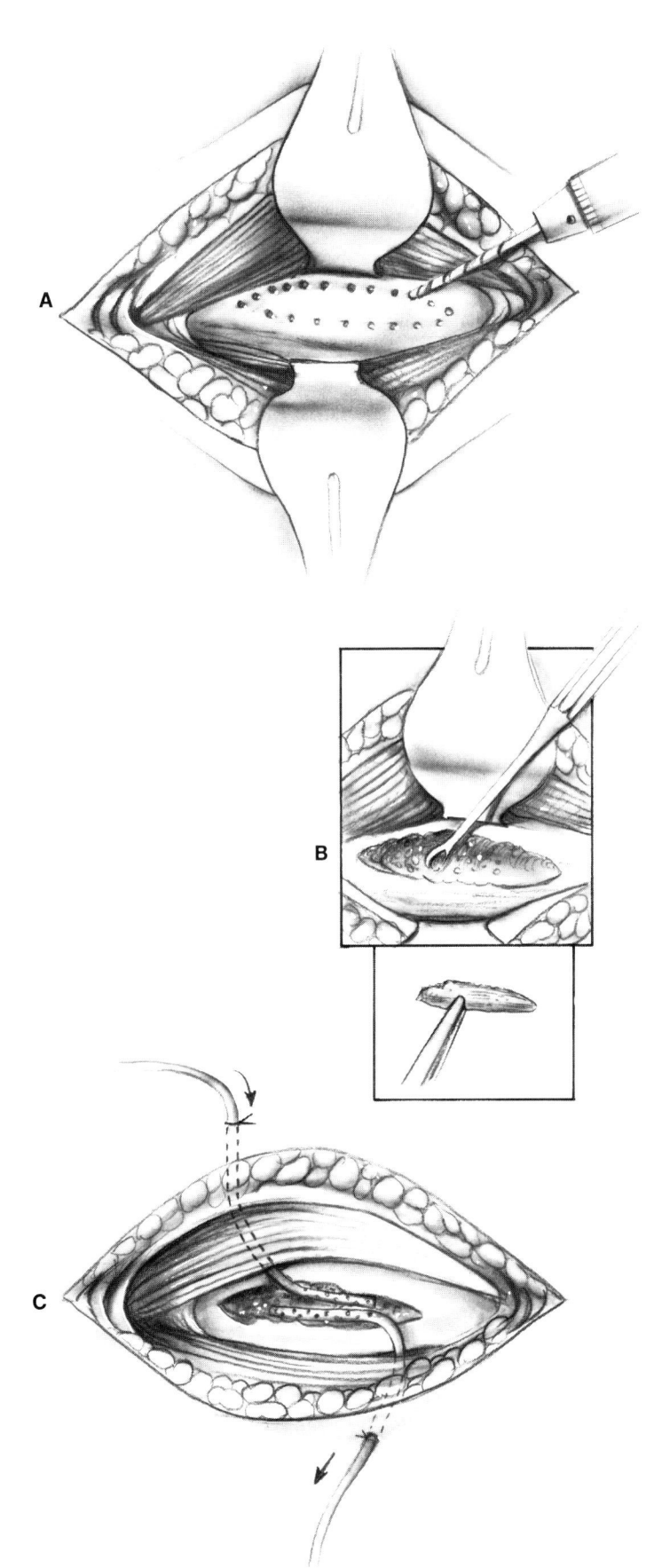

GENERAL DISCUSSION. Closed irrigation with suction can occasionally help in the treatment of chronic osteomyelitis.

DETAILS OF PROCEDURE. After the area of diseased bone has been exposed **(A)** and sequestra removed if necessary **(B)**, suction tubes with multiple perforations are placed so the perforated section of each lies closed to the diseased bone **(C)**. An introducing needle for each tube is passed into the depth of the wound and brought out through the skin 2 to 5 cm from the wound edge for hookup of installation and suction catheters. The wound is closed carefully in layers to avoid leakage. The tubes should be sutured to the skin if it is anticipated that they may have to remain in place for several weeks. The installation tube is connected to a drip bottle or normal saline solution containing the appropriate antibiotic solution and/or detergent solution (for example, Alevaire). The suction tube is connected to a suction source.

POSTOPERATIVE MANAGEMENT. During the first 2 or 3 postoperative days, there will be a certain amount of bleeding into the wound and this, plus bone debris, may tend to cause tube blocking. If the system is working correctly, the wound and dressing should remain dry. Blocking of the tubes can be prevented by reversing the flow in the two tubes at intervals. If a tube still becomes blocked, it may be possible to free it by using a syringe and heparin solution. After the third postoperative day, difficulty with tube blocking should be less frequent and the system should become established and run fairly smoothly thereafter. The rate of circulation of fluid should be regulated between 1,000 and 1,500 ml per day. This treatment may be continued for as long as 6 weeks. When the installation tube is removed, the suction tube is left in place until there is no further drainage. Systemic antibiotics are given concomitantly with the installation-suction treatment of the diseased bone.

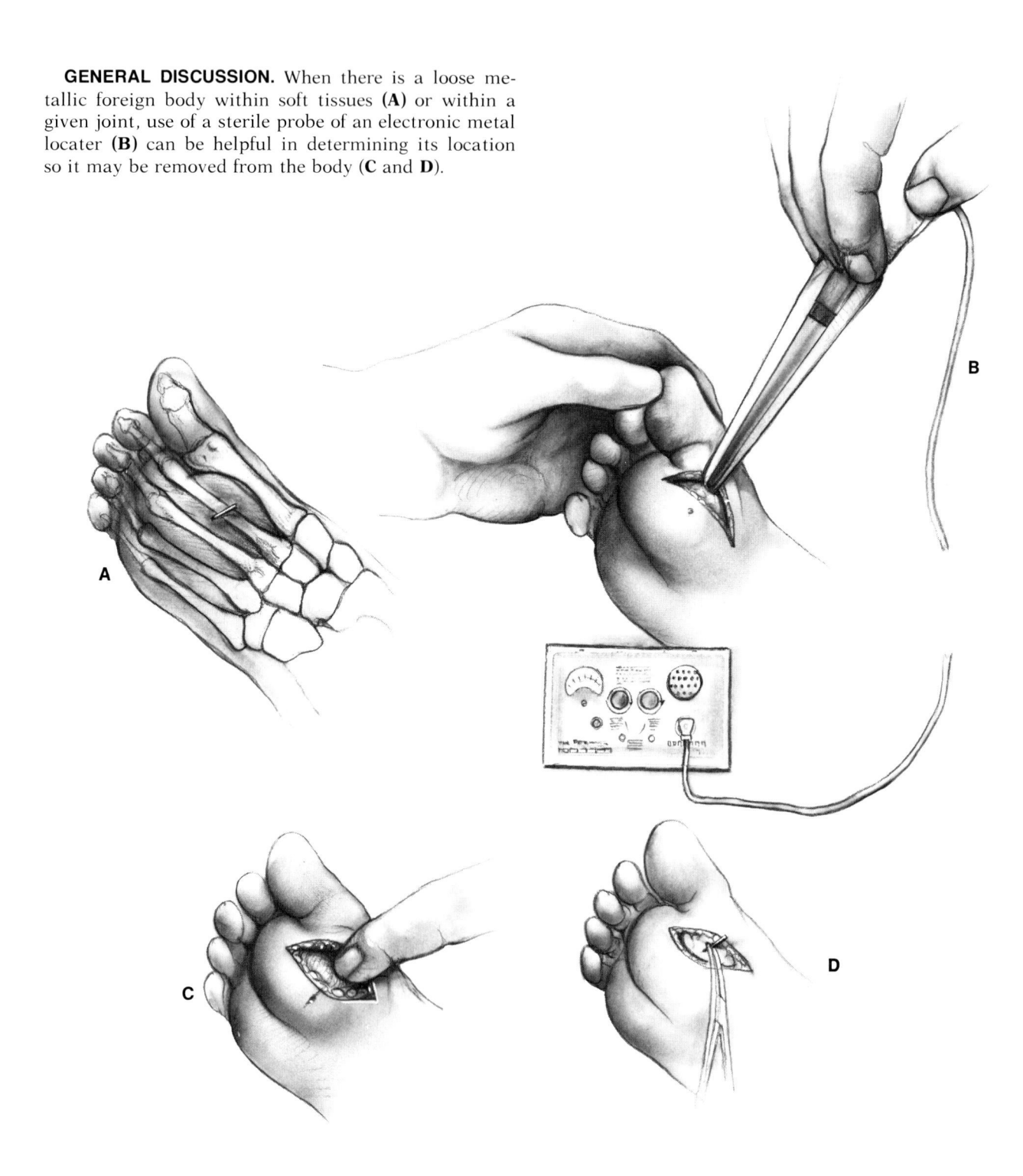

LOCALIZATION OF METALLIC FOREIGN BODY (Plate 16-5)

GENERAL DISCUSSION. When there is a loose metallic foreign body within soft tissues (**A**) or within a given joint, use of a sterile probe of an electronic metal locater (**B**) can be helpful in determining its location so it may be removed from the body (**C** and **D**).

(Plate 16-6) APPLICATION OF SKELETAL COMPRESSION PLATE FIXATION

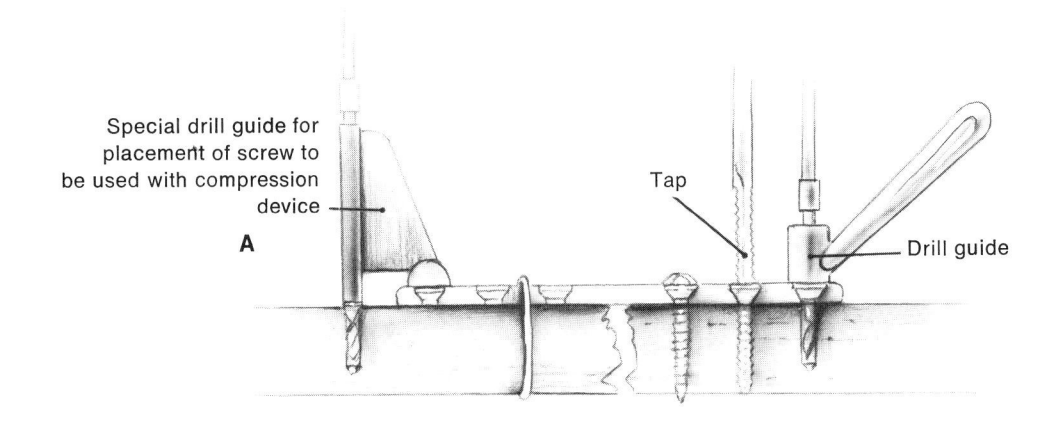

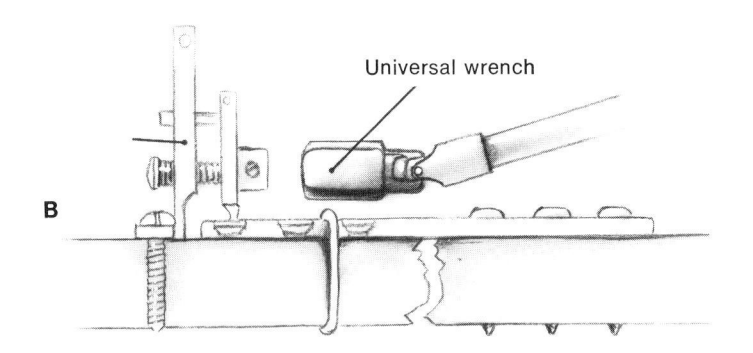

GENERAL DISCUSSION. Skeletal compression plate fixation is a means of obtaining rigid fixation of a fracture or an osteotomy. This can permit early mobilization of adjacent joints and minimize the likelihood of delayed bone union or nonunion.

DETAILS OF PROCEDURE. The straight compression plate has a small horizontal hole on both ends into which the hook of a compression device can be introduced. The plate is fixed to one bone fragment with one or more screws. A special drill guide is inserted into the end hole of the plate over the opposite fragment, and a hole is drilled 20 mm away from the end of the plate **(A)**. The hook of the compression device is inserted into the small horizontal hole in the end of the plate, and the compression device is then fixed firmly to the bone with a screw. After control of the position of the fracture, the tightening screw of the compression device is turned with a universal wrench **(B)**. While compression is maintained, the plate is fixed with screws to the bone fragment adjacent to the compression device **(C)**. A drill guide, a 3.2 mm drill, and a tap are used prior to insertion of each screw. Compression of 60 to 80 kg can be obtained. Finally, the compression device is removed, and the last screw is inserted.

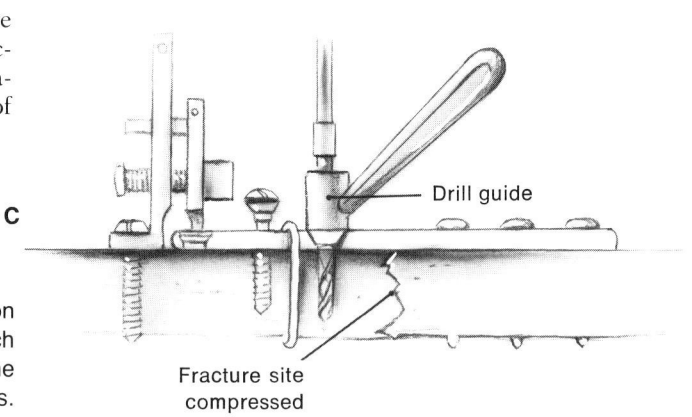

609

BONE BIOPSY (Plate 16-7)

GENERAL DISCUSSION. A bone tumor may appear at any area in the skeletal system. Needle biopsy has limited usefulness in the diagnosis of bone lesions; therefore, if the area in question is surgically accessible, open biopsy is preferable. To afford maximum opportunity to determine the true nature of the lesion, it is desirable that the biopsy be carried out before any local radiation has been given lest there be additional changes in the structure and appearance of the cells.

DETAILS OF PROCEDURE. A tourniquet is used whenever possible to permit clear excision of a representative section, as well as to control profuse bleeding that may be encountered. Electrocautery is avoided, if possible, to render a specimen free of thermal tissue necrosis that may affect microscopic study. Subperiosteal stripping is avoided. An adequate section is removed that includes periosteum with overlying soft tissue, bone cortex, and subjacent medullary tissue—all in continuity (**A** to **C**). If there is any question about the precise location of the lesion, roentgenograms should be obtained in the operating room for accurate localization of the lesion. Permanent tissue sections should be prepared. The biopsy is closed without drains or packing to permit healing of the wound (**D**).

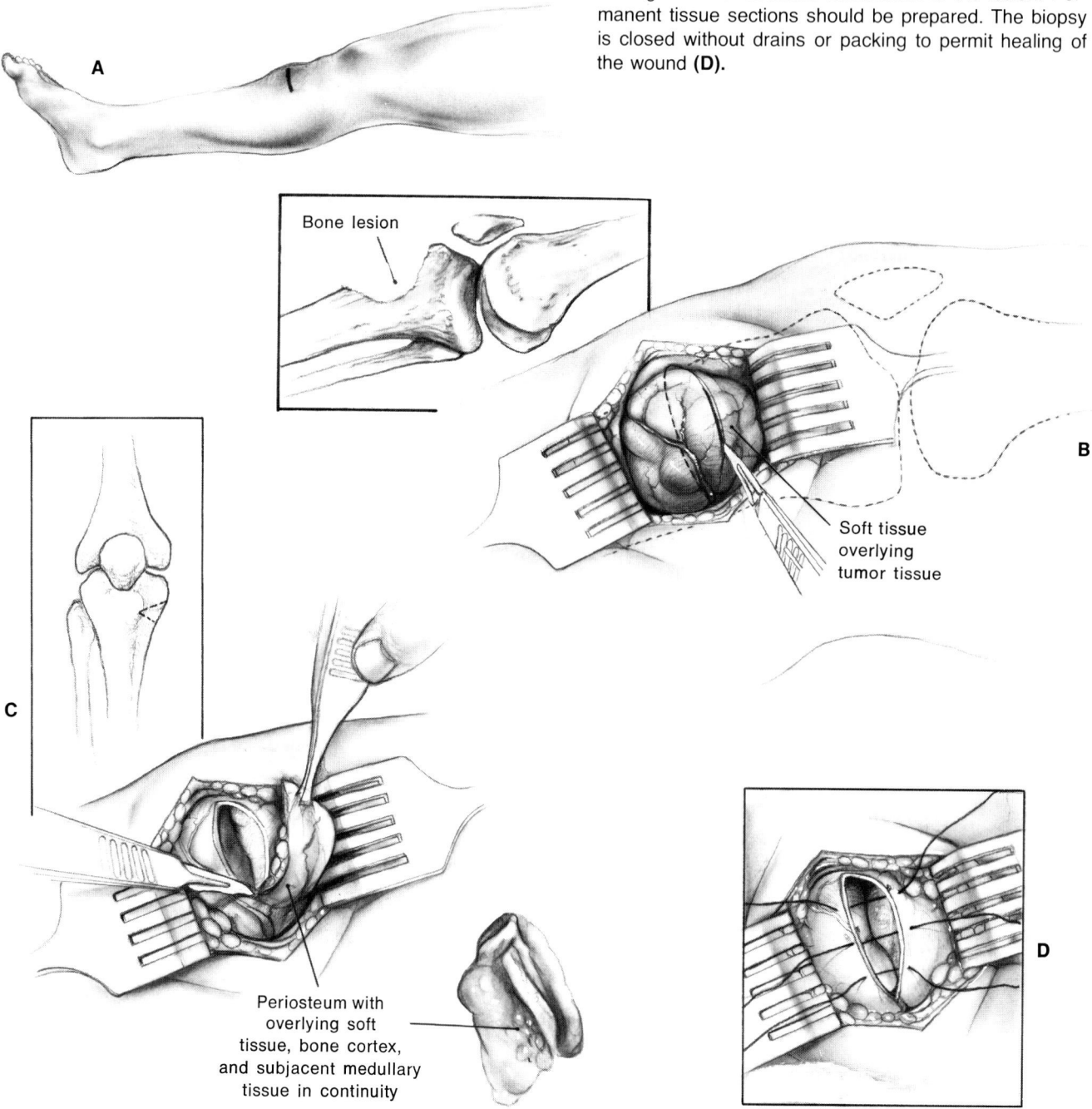

(Plate 16-7) BONE BIOPSY

If the procedure is performed for diagnostic biopsy of an intramedullary lesion, only enough tissue for histologic diagnosis should be obtained (**E** and **F**). Unless the cortex is very thin, it is best to outline the biopsy section with cortical drill holes to facilitate removal of the cortex with minimal tissue disturbance. If the lesional tissue is soft tissue, a frozen section may be helpful to at least provide assurance that the specimen contains the pathologic tissue. Permanent sections of the same specimen can then be expected to provide a definitive diagnosis.

611

MUSCLE BIOPSY (Plate 16-8)

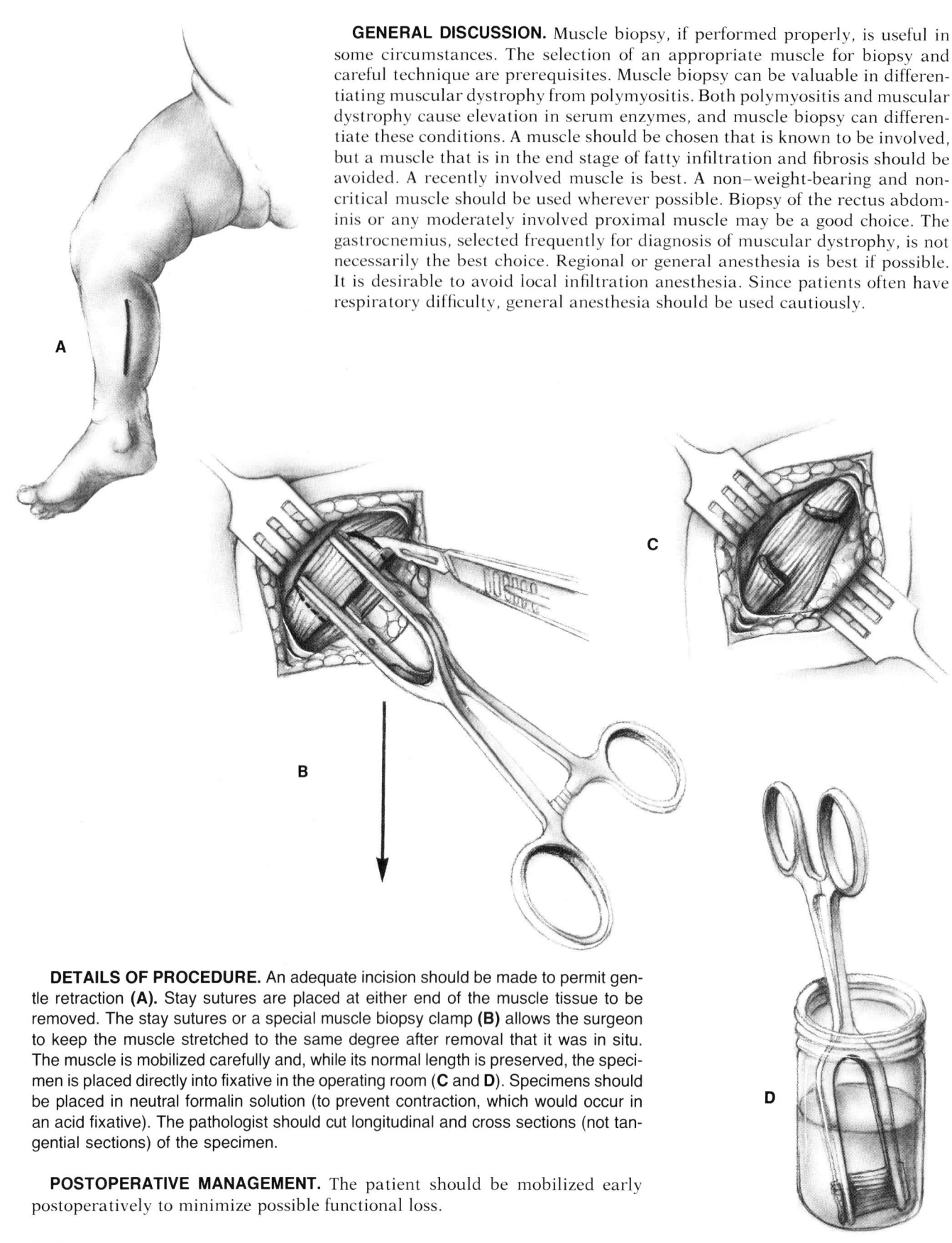

GENERAL DISCUSSION. Muscle biopsy, if performed properly, is useful in some circumstances. The selection of an appropriate muscle for biopsy and careful technique are prerequisites. Muscle biopsy can be valuable in differentiating muscular dystrophy from polymyositis. Both polymyositis and muscular dystrophy cause elevation in serum enzymes, and muscle biopsy can differentiate these conditions. A muscle should be chosen that is known to be involved, but a muscle that is in the end stage of fatty infiltration and fibrosis should be avoided. A recently involved muscle is best. A non–weight-bearing and non-critical muscle should be used wherever possible. Biopsy of the rectus abdominis or any moderately involved proximal muscle may be a good choice. The gastrocnemius, selected frequently for diagnosis of muscular dystrophy, is not necessarily the best choice. Regional or general anesthesia is best if possible. It is desirable to avoid local infiltration anesthesia. Since patients often have respiratory difficulty, general anesthesia should be used cautiously.

DETAILS OF PROCEDURE. An adequate incision should be made to permit gentle retraction **(A)**. Stay sutures are placed at either end of the muscle tissue to be removed. The stay sutures or a special muscle biopsy clamp **(B)** allows the surgeon to keep the muscle stretched to the same degree after removal that it was in situ. The muscle is mobilized carefully and, while its normal length is preserved, the specimen is placed directly into fixative in the operating room **(C** and **D)**. Specimens should be placed in neutral formalin solution (to prevent contraction, which would occur in an acid fixative). The pathologist should cut longitudinal and cross sections (not tangential sections) of the specimen.

POSTOPERATIVE MANAGEMENT. The patient should be mobilized early postoperatively to minimize possible functional loss.

MICROSURGERY AND REPLANTATION

Since 1970 the rapidly developing techniques using the operating microscope have found widespread application in orthopaedic surgery. The feasibility of replantation of the amputated parts as pioneered by Kleinert, Buncke, Acland, Urbaniak, and others has now been firmly established. Moreover, the exacting operative techniques possible with the microscope have allowed improvement in peripheral nerve surgery. Finally, the use of free tissue transfer, with vascular anastomoses at recipient sites, is rapidly being developed and shows great promise for the future.

NERVE REPAIRS. It has been widely accepted that more accurate orientation of fascicular patterns in their axial alignment gives better results in repair of peripheral nerves. Using the operating microscope, the surgeon can separate nerves into bundles of fascicles. With these patterns visible, and with the aid of the alignment of external blood vessels, extremely accurate placement of 8-0 or 9-0 nylon sutures through the epineurium is possible. With more accurate alignment and accurate placement of a minimum number of fine structures, the results of nerve repairs have improved. The bundle approximation technique appears to be the most satisfactory; approximation of individual fascicles does not appear to improve the results further. It is essential that nerve repairs be done under minimal tension. If, with some nerve mobilization proximally and distally, the nerve ends cannot be approximated with 8-0 suture, an intercalated fascicular nerve graft may be advisable.

REPLANTATION. Replantation series now report a 90% success rate in salvage of completely amputated parts of the hand. Success requires careful patient selection, exacting microsurgical technique, and meticulous postoperative care. Most replantations are best done with a team approach in which several skilled surgeons are available, since replanting multiple digits may require up to 18 hours of surgery. Special instruments required include an operating microscope (with dual optical heads for surgeon and assistants), adequate microsurgical instruments, and special suture material. Vessels of 1 mm outside diameter can be joined reliably with practice, using sutures 20 μm in diameter and needles 70 μm in diameter. Vein grafts to bridge arterial gaps and/or vein gaps are often required in traumatic amputations. In digits, two veins are generally anastomosed for each artery anastomosed. Standard techniques of bone fixation and tendon repair are used.

Patient selection is extremely important. Young patients with sharp amputations are the best candidates. Age, smoking history, associated diseases, and occupation weigh heavily in the decision of whether to replant. Single digits (except the thumb) and double digits amputated through "no man's land" are generally not replanted. These guidelines are occasionally waived in children.

Patients thought to be candidates for replantation should be transported as quickly as possible to the center where the operation will be performed. Blood loss may be considerable, and volume replacement must be adequate. Antibiotics are used routinely. The amputated part should be placed in a plastic bag, which in turn is placed on ice for transport, while the amputation site is dressed. No perfusion of the parts should be attempted. One should not clamp or attempt to identify vessels or nerves in the amputated part or in the amputation stump. To do so may damage vessels and/or nerves, and thus jeopardize the possibility of a good functional result from the replantation. In many centers, aspirin (10 grains every 12 hours) and/or low molecular weight dextran 40 are used preoperatively, intraoperatively, and postoperatively to decrease platelet adhesion at the anastomosis site. Heparin may cause further hemorrhage and is generally not given.

Careful attention to preoperative management and methods of transportation have a significant effect on the replantation attempt. Where possible, protocols should be available in advance to facilitate triage and patient care process.

FREE VASCULARIZED TISSUE GRAFTS. The details of free vascularized tissue grafts are beyond the scope of this work. Recent clinical research has made it possible to transfer living vascularized grafts of skin, bone, nerve, and combinations of these (composite grafts) without delay techniques. (An example of the latter is the transfer of the iliac crest with its overlying soft tissue and skin as a composite free vascularized bone graft for segmental defect of a long bone.) These are extremely difficult procedures and require isolating the tissue on a vascular pedicle, separating out vessels in the recipient area, and transferring the tissue, anastomosing its vessels into the recipient vessels. End-to-end or end-to-side techniques may be used. Muscles can be similarly transferred, with repair of vessels and nerves to replace paralyzed forearm muscles and provide recovery of some active finger flexion. As in replantation, extreme attention to detail is necessary, and a team approach is helpful. The scope of these techniques is continually expanding, and they promise help for problems previously considered unsolvable.

SUMMARY. The possibilities of microsurgery in orthopaedics are still being explored. The success of replantation has been most helpful in the development of the operative techniques, which are now being expanded to include transfer of free vascularized tissue. This is an exciting advance and promises much for the future.

REFERENCES

Ackerman, L. V., and Spjut, H. J.: Tumors of bone and cartilage. In Armed Forces Institute of Pathology, sect. II, fasc. 4, Washington, D.C., 1962, National Research Council, Committee on Pathology.

Aegerter, E. E., and Kirkpatrick, J. A.: Orthopedic diseases: physiology, pathology, radiology, ed. 3, Philadelphia, 1968, W. B. Saunders Co.

Aitken, G. T.: Amputation as a treatment for certain lower-extremity congenital abnormalities, J. Bone Joint Surg. **41-A:** 1267, 1959.

Aitken, G. T., and Frantz, C. H.: The juvenile amputee, J. Bone Joint Surg. **35-A:**659, 1953.

Alldredge, R. H.: Artificial limbs. A consideration of aids employed in the practice of orthopaedic surgery. In American Academy of Orthopaedic Surgeons, Inc.: Orthopaedic appliances atlas, vol. 2, Artificial limbs, Ann Arbor, Mich., 1960, J. W. Edwards.

Almquist, E. E.: The changing epidemiology of septic arthritis in children, Clin. Orthop. **68:**96, 1970.

Ambrose, G. B., Alpert, M., and Neer, C. S.: Vertebral osteomyelitis. A diagnostic problem, J.A.M.A. **197:**619, 1966.

Anderson, L. D.: Compression plate fixation and the effect of different types of internal fixation on fracture healing, J. Bone Joint Surg. **47-A:**191, 1965.

Anderson, L. D., and Horn, L. G.: Irrigation-suction technic in the treatment of acute hematogenous osteomyelitis chronic osteomyelitis and acute and chronic joint infections, South. Med. J. **63:**745, 1970.

Artz, C. P., and Howard, J. M.: Initial care of the severely wounded, J.A.M.A. **156:**488, 1954.

d'Aubigne, R. M.: Surgical treatment of non-union of long bones, J. Bone Joint Surg. **31-A:**256, 1949.

d'Aubigne, R. M.: Infection in the treatment of ununited fractures, Clin. Orthop. **43:**77, 1965.

Badgley, C. E., and Harris, H. W.: The treatment of old ununited infected fractures, J. Int. Coll. Surg. **3:**413, 1940.

Banks, S. W., and Laufman, H.: An atlas of surgical exposures of the extremities, Philadelphia, 1953, W. B. Saunders Co.

Bardenheier, J. A., III, Morgan, H. C., and Stamp, W. G.: Treatment and sequelae of experimentally produced septic arthritis, Surg. Gynecol. Obstet. **122:**249, 1966.

Barford, B., and Pers, M.: Gastrocnemius plasty for primary closure of compound injuries of the knee, J. Bone Joint Surg. **52-B:**124, 1970.

Baitch, A.: Recent observations of acute suppurative arthritis, Clin. Orthop. **22:**157, 1962.

Bechtol, C. O.: Engineering principles applied to orthopaedic surgery, American Academy of Orthopaedic Surgeons Instructional Course Lectures, vol. 9, Ann Arbor, Mich., 1952, J. W. Edwards.

Bechtol, C. O., Ferguson, A. B., and Laing, P. G.: Metals and engineering in bone and joint surgery, Baltimore, 1959, The Williams & Wilkins Co.

Benner, E. J.: The use and abuse of antibiotics—1967, J. Bone Joint Surg. **49-A:**977, 1967.

Bickel, W. H., Bateman, J. G., and Johnson, W. E.: Treatment of chronic hematogenous osteomyelitis by means of saucerization and bone grafting. Surg. Gynecol. Obstet. **96:**265, 1953.

Björkesten, G.: Suture of war injuries to peripheral nerves. Clinical studies of results, Acta Chir. Scand. (Suppl.) 119, 1947.

Blount, W. P.: Fractures in children, Baltimore, 1954, The Williams & Wilkins Co.

Böhler, L.: The treatment of fractures, ed. 4 (translated by Groves, E. W. H.), Baltimore, 1936, William Wood & Co.

Böhler, L.: The treatment of fractures, ed. 5 (translated by Tretter, H., et al.), 3 vols., New York, 1956-1958, Grune & Stratton, Inc.

Borella, L., Goobar, J. E., Summits, R. L., and Clark, G. M.: Septic arthritis in childhood, J. Pediatr. **62:**742, 1963.

Boswick, J. A., Jr., and Stromber, W. B., Jr.: Isolated injury to the median nerve above the elbow, J. Bone Joint Surg. **49-A:** 653, 1967.

Bowden, R. E. M., and Napier, J. R.: The assessment of hand function after peripheral nerve injuries, J. Bone Joint Surg. **43-B:**3, 1961.

Boyd, H. B.: The treatment of difficult and unusual nonunions: With special reference to the budging of defects, J. Bone Joint Surg. **25:**535, 1943.

Boyd, H. B., Anderson, L. D., and Johnston, D. S.: Changing concepts in the treatment of nonunion, Clin. Orthop. **43:**37, 1965.

Boyd, H. B., and Lipinski, S. W.: Causes and treatment of nonunion of the shafts of the long bones, with a review of 741 patients, American Academy of Orthopaedic Surgeons Instructional Course Lectures, vol. 17, St. Louis, 1960, The C. V. Mosby Co.

Boyd, H. B., Lipinski, S. W., and Wiley, J. H.: Observations on nonunion of the shafts of the long bones, with a statistical analysis of 842 patients, J. Bone Joint Surg. **43-A:**159, 1961.

Boyes, J. H.: Bunnell's surgery of the Hand, ed. 5, Philadelphia, 1964, J. B. Lippincott Co.

Boyes, J. H.: Suture technics for wounds of the hand, 1970, Ethicon, Inc., Somerville, N.J.

Boyes, J. H., and Stark, H. H.: Flexor-tendon grafts in the fingers and thumb. A study of factors influencing results in 1000 cases, J. Bone Joint Surg. **53-A:**1332, 1971.

Brashear, H. R.: Diagnosis and prevention of nonunion, J. Bone Joint Surg. **47-A:**174, 1965.

Brav, E. A.: The management of open fractures of the extremities, American Academy of Orthopaedic Surgeons Instructional Course Lectures, vol. 13, Ann Arbor, Mich., 1956, J. W. Edwards, p. 227.

Brav, E. A., et al.: Cineplasty. An end result study, J. Bone Joint Surg. **39-A:**59, 1957.

Bristow, W. R.: Injuries of peripheral nerves in two world wars, Br. J. Surg. **34:**333, 1947.

Brooks, D.: The place of nerve-grafting in orthopaedic surgery, J. Bone Joint Surg. **37-A:**299, 1955.

Brown, P. W.: The time factor in surgery of upper extremity peripheral nerve injury, Clin. Orthop. **68:**14, 1970.

Brown, P. W., and Urban, J. G.: Early weight-bearing treatment of open fractures of the tibia. An end-result study of sixty-three cases, J. Bone Joint Surg. **51-A:**59, 1969.

Bunnell, S.: Hand surgery: the surgery of nerves of the upper extremity, American Academy of Orthopaedic Surgeons Instructional Course Lectures, vol. 13, Ann Arbor, Mich., 1956, J. W. Edwards, p. 101.

Burchman, J., and Blair, J. E.: The surgical management of chronic osteomyelitis, J. Bone Joint Surg. **33-A:**118, 1951.

Burstein, A. H., and Frankel, V. H.: The viscoelastic properties of some biological materials, Ann. N.Y. Acad. Sci. **146:**158, 1968.

Campbell, C. J.: The healing of cartilage defects, Clin. Orthop. **64:**45, 1969.

Carrel, A.: The operative technique of vascular anastomoses and the transplantation of viscera, Clin. Orthop. **29:**3, 1963.

Carter, J., Dickerson, R., and Needy, C.: Angiosarcoma of bone, Ann. Surg. **144**:107, 1956.

Casscells, S. W.: Arthroscopy of the knee joint. A review of 150 cases, J. Bone Joint Surg. **53-A**:287, 1971.

Cave, E. F.: Fractures and other injuries, Chicago, 1958, The Year Book Medical Publishers, Inc.

Cave, E. F.: Technique of bone grafting. In Cave, E. F., editor: Fractures and other injuries, Chicago, 1958, The Year Book Medical Publishers, Inc.

Chandler, G. N., and Wright, V.: Deleterious effect of intra-articular hydrocortisone, Lancet **2**:661, 1958.

Clawson, D. K., and Dunn, A. W.: Management of common bacterial infections of bones and joints, J. Bone Joint Surg. **49-A**:164, 1967.

Clawson, D. K., and Stevenson, J. K.: Treatment of chronic osteomyelitis, Surg. Gynecol. Obstet. **120**:59, 1965.

Clayton, M. L., Miles, J. S., and Abdulla, M.: Experimental investigations of ligamentous healing, Clin. Orthop. **61**:146, 1968.

Cleveland, M., Manning, J. G., and Stewart, W. J.: Care of battle casualties and injuries including bones and joints, J. Bone Joint Surg. **33-A**:517, 1951.

Clippinger, F. W.: Immediate postsurgical fitting of prosthesis in children, Inter-Clin. Inform. Bull. **5**:7, 1966.

Clippinger, F. W., Goldner, J. L., and Roberts, J. M.: Use of the electromyogram in evaluating upper extremity peripheral nerve lesions, J. Bone Joint Surg. **44-A**:1047, 1962.

Cohen, J.: Performance and failure in performance of surgical implants on orthopedic surgery, J. Mater. **1**:354, 1966.

Cohen, J., and Lindenbaum, B.: Fretting corrosion in orthopedic implants, Clin. Orthop. **61**:167, 1968.

Cohen, S. M., and Schulenburg, C. A. R.: Treatment of war wounds of the limbs. Experience in 266 cases, Lancet **2**:351, 1940.

Coleman, C. C.: Surgical treatment of peripheral nerve injuries, Surg. Gynecol. Obstet. **78**:113, 1944.

Coley, B. L., and Higinbotham, N. L.: Diagnosis and treatment of metastatic lesions in bone, American Academy of Orthopaedic Surgeons Instructional Course Lectures, vol. 7, Ann Arbor, Mich., 1950, J. W. Edwards.

Collins, H. A., and Jacobs, J. K.: Acute arterial injuries due to blunt trauma, J. Bone Joint Surg. **43-A**:193, 1961.

Compere, E. L.: Treatment of osteomyelitis and infected wounds by closing irrigation with a detergent-antibiotic solution, Acta Orthop. Scand. **32**:325, 1962.

Compere, E. L., Metzger, W. I., and Mitra, R. N.: The treatment of pyogenic bone and joint infections by closed irrigation (circulation) with a non-toxic detergent and one or more antibiotics, J. Bone Joint Surg. **49-A**:614, 1967.

Conwell, H. E., and Ryenolds, F. C.: Key and Conwell's management of fractures, dislocations, and sprains, ed. 7, St. Louis, 1961, The C. V. Mosby Co.

Copeland, C. X., Jr., and Enneking, W. F.: Incidence of osteomyelitis in compound fractures, Am. J. Surg. **31**:156, 1965.

Copeland, M. M.: Benign tumors of bone, Surg. Gynecol. Obstet. **90**:697, 1950.

Copeland, M. M.: Primary malignant tumors of bone. Evaluation of current diagnosis and treatment, Cancer **20**:738, 1967.

Cottingham, G., et al.: Osteomyelitis since the advent of antibiotics: a study of infants and children, Clin. Orthop. **14**:97, 1959.

Cozen, L.: Positioning in surgery of the extremities, Surg **11**:605, 1942.

Crikelair, G. F.: The corss-leg pedicle in chronic osteomyelitis of the lower limb, Plast. Reconstr. Surg. **38**:404, 1966.

Curtis, B.: Orthopaedic management of muscular dystrophy and related disorders, American Academy of Orthopaedic Surgeons Instructional Course Lectures, vol. 19, St. Louis, 1970, The C. V. Mosby Co., p. 78.

Curtiss, P. H., Jr., and Klein, L.: Destruction of articular cartilage in septic arthritis. II. In vivo studies, J. Bone Joint Surg. **47-A**:1595, 1965.

Dahlin, D. C.: Bone tumors, Springfield, Ill., 1967, Charles C Thomas, Publisher.

Daland, E. M.: The management of 236 compound fractures treated at Massachusetts General Hospital, N. Engl. J. Med. **10**:983, 1934.

Dale, W. A.: Salvage of arteriosclerotic legs by vascular repair, Ann. Surg. **165**:844, 1967.

Davis, A. G.: Primary closure of compound fracture wounds with immediate internal fixation, skin graft and compression dressing, J. Bone Joint Surg. **30-A**:405, 1948.

Davis, G. L.: Management of open wounds of joints during the Vietnam War. A preliminary study, Clin. Orthop. **68**:3, 1970.

Davis, L.: Peripheral nerve surgery, Surg. Gynecol. Obstet. **80**:444, 1945.

Dehne, E., and Kirz, F. K., Jr.: Slow arterial leak consequent to unrecognized arterial laceration: Report of five cases, J. Bone Joint Surg. **49-A**:372, 1967.

Dickerson, R. C.: The diversion of arterial blood flow to growing bone, Surg. Gynecol. Obstet. **123**:103, 1966.

Dickerson, R. C.: An improved method for diversion of arterial blood flow to bone, J. Bone Joint Surg. **50-A**:1036, 1968.

Dickerson, R. C.: Recent developments in the study and treatment of fractures. A collective review, Surg. Gynecol. Obstet. **131**:537, 1970.

Dickerson, R. C., and Duthie, R. B.: The diversion of arterial blood flow to bone. A preliminary report, J. Bone Joint Surg. **45-A**:356, 1963.

Dickson, F. D., Dively, R. L., and Kiene, R. H.: Subacute and chronic osteomyelitis. Treatment with use of chemotherapeutic agents, antibiotics and primary closure; follow-up report, Arch. Surg. **66**:60, 1963.

Dilmaghani, A., Close, J. R., and Rhinelander, F. W.: A method for closed irrigation and suction therapy in deep wound infections. A preliminary report, J. Bone Joint Surg. **51-A**:323, 1969.

Dombrowski, E. T., and Dunn, A. W.: Treatment of osteomyelitis by debridement and closed wound irrigation-suction, Clin. Orthop. **43**:215, 1965.

Drutz, D. J., Schaffner, W., Hillman, J. W., and Koenig, M. J.: The penetration of penicillin and other antimicrobials into joint fluid. Three case reports with a reappraisal of the literature, J. Bone Joint Surg. **49-A**:1415, 1967.

Dunn, A. W., and Dombrowski, E. T.: Treatment of osteomyelitis by debridement and closed wound irrigation-suction, Clin. Orthop. **43**:215, 1965.

Edshage, S.: Peripheral nerve injuries: diagnosis and treatment, N. Engl. J. Med. **278**:1431, 1968.

Eggers, G. W. N., Ainsworth, W. H., Shindler, T. O., and Pomerat, C. M.: Clinical significance of contactcompression factor in bone surgery, Arch. Surg. **62**:467, 1951.

Eggers, G. W. N., Shindler, T. O., and Pomerat, C. M.: The influence of the contact-compression factor on osteogenesis in surgical fractures, J. Bone Joint Surg. **31-A**:693, 1949.

Emery, M. A., and Murakami, H.: The fracture healing in cats after immediate and delayed open reduction, J. Bone Joint Surg. **49-B:**571, 1967.

Evans, E. M., and Davies, D. M.: The treatment of chronic osteomyelitis by saucerisation and secondary skin grafting, J. Bone Joint Surg. **51-B:**454, 1969.

Evarts, C. M.: Emerging concepts of fat embolism, Clin. Orthop. **33:**183, 1964.

Evarts, C. M., and Feil, E. J.: Prevention of thromboembolic disease after elective surgery of the hip, J. Bone Joint Surg. **53-A:**1271, 1971.

Eyring, E. J., and Murray, W. R.: The effect of joint position on the pressure on intra-articular effusion, J. Bone Joint Surg. **46-A:**1235, 1964.

Fahey, J. J.: Surgical approaches to bone and joints, Surg. Clin. North Am. **29:**65, 1949.

Fisher, R. H.: The Kutler method of repair of finger-tip amputations, J. Bone Joint Surg. **49-A:**317, 1967.

Frackelton, W. H.: Surface covering of traumatic lower extremity defects, Surg. Clin. North Am. **38:**1093, 1958.

Frankel, V. H., and Burstein, A. H.: The biomechanics of refracture of bone, Clin. Orthop. **60:**221, 1968.

Frantz, C. H., and Aitken, G. T.: Management of the juvenile amputee, Clin. Orthop. **14:**30, 1959.

Ger, R.: The management of pretibial skin loss, Surgery **63:**757, 1968.

Geschickter, C. F., and Copeland, M. M.: Tumors of bone, ed. 3, Philadelphia, 1919, J. B. Lippincott Co.

Glattly, H. W.: A statistical study of 12,000 new amputees, South. Med. J. **57:**1373, 1964.

Glenn, F.: Tetanus, a preventable disease; including an experience with civilian casualties in the Battle for Manila (1945), Ann. Surg. **124:**1030, 1946.

Godfrey, J. D.: Major and extensive soft-tissue injuries complicating skeletal fractures, J. Bone Joint Surg. **44-A:**753, 1962.

Goldner, J. L.: Amputation pain, Inter-Clin. Inform. Bull. **5:**1, 1966.

Grabb, W. C.: Median and ulnar nerve suture. An experimental study comparing primary and secondary repair in monkeys, J. Bone Joint Surg. **50-A:**964, 1968.

Griffin, P.: Fractures in children. Part I, American Academy of Orthopaedic Surgeons Instructional Course Lectures, vol. 19, St. Louis, 1970, The C. V. Mosby Co., p. 170.

Gustilo, R. B., et al.: Analysis of 511 open fractures, Clin. Orthop. **66:**148, 1969.

Hampton, O. P., Jr.: The management of penetrating wounds and suppurating arthritis of the knee joint in the Mediterranean theater of operations, J. Bone Joint Surg. **28:**659, 1946.

Hampton, O. P., Jr.: Wounds of the extremities in military surgery, St. Louis, 1951, The C. V. Mosby Co.

Hampton, O. P., Jr.: Management of open fractures and open wounds of joint, J. Trauma **8:**475, 1968.

Hardy, J. D.: Surgery of the aorta and its branches. Part VII: Traumatic injuries, Am. Practit. **11:**621, 1960.

Harris, W. H., Salzman, E. W., and Desanctis, R. W.: The prevention of thromboembolic disease by prophylatic anticoagulation. A controlled study in elective hip surgery, J. Bone Joint Surg. **49-A:**81, 1967.

Harrison, W. E., Jr., Chakales, H. H., Eppright, R. H., and DeBakey, M. E.: Recent progress in the management of gunshot fractures of the femur, J. Trauma **3:**52, 1963.

Heberling, J.: A review of 201 cases of suppurative arthritis, J. Bone Joint Surg. **23:**917, 1941.

Heiple, K. G., Chase, S. W., and Herndon, C. H.: A comparative study of the healing process following different types of bone transplantation, J. Bone Joint Surg. **45-A:**1593, 1963.

Henderson, M. S.: The massive bone graft in ununited fractures, J.A.M.A. **107:**1104, 1936.

Herndon, C. H., and Chase, S. W.: Experimental studies in the transplantation of whole joints, J. Bone Joint Surg. **34-A:**564, 1952.

Higinbotham, N. L., and Marcove, R. C.: The management of pathological fractures, J. Trauma, **5:**792, 1965.

Hinman, F., Jr.: The rational use of tourniquets, special contribution, Int. Abstr. Surg. **81:**357, 1945.

Hitchcock, C. R., Haglin, J. J., and Arnar, O.: The treatment of cloistridial infections with hyperbaric oxygen, Surgery **62:**759, 1967.

Hohl, M.: Symposium: treatment of ununited fractures of the long bones: surgical treatments and technique, J. Bone Joint Surg. **47-A:**179, 1965.

Hughes, C. W.: Arterial repair during the Korean War, Ann. Surg. **147:**555, 1958.

Inoue, T., et al.: Replantation of severed limbs, J. Cardiovasc. Surg. **8:**31, 1967.

Jaffe, H. L.: Tumors and tumorous conditions of the bones and joints, Philadelphia, 1958, Lea & Febiger.

Johnson, L. C.: A general theory of bone tumors, Bull. N.Y. Acad. Med. **29:**164, 1953.

Keiser, H., Ruben, F. L., Wolinsky, E., and Kushner, I.: Clinical forms of gonococcal arthritis, N. Engl. J. Med. **279:**234, 1968.

Kelly, P. J., and James, J. M.: Criteria for determining the proper level of amputation in occlusive vascular disease. A review of 323 amputations, J. Bone Joint Surg. **39-A:**883, 1957.

Kelly, P. J., Martin, W. J., and Coventry, M. B.: Chronic osteomyelitis: II. Treatment with closed irrigation and suction, J.A.M.A. **213:**1843, 1970.

Kelly, P. J., Weed, L. A., and Lipscomb, P. R.: Infection of the tendon sheaths, bursae, joints and soft tissues by acid-fast bacilli other than tubercle bacilli, J. Bone Joint Surg. **45-A:**327, 1963.

Kelly, R. P.: Skin grafting in the treatment of osteomyelitic war wounds, J. Bone Joint Surg. **28:**681, 1946.

Key, J. A.: Electrolytic absorption of bone due to the use of stainless steels of different composition for internal fixation, Surg. Gynecol. Obstet. **82:**319, 1946.

Key, J. A.: Fixation of tendons, ligaments and bone by Bunnell's pull-out wire suture, Ann. Surg. **123:**656, 1946.

King, T.: Compression of the bone ends as an aid to union in fractures: A report on 49 ununited and 4 recent fractures, J. Bone Joint Surg. **39-A:**1238, 1957.

Knight, M. P., and Wood, G. O.: Surgical obliteration of bone cavities following traumatic osteomyelitis, J. Bone Joint Surg. **27:**547, 1945.

Koskinen, E. V. S.: Restoration of blood flow in severely injured limbs by direct surgical techniques, Vasc. Dis. **5:**13, 1968.

Laing, P. G.: The significance of metallic transfer in the corrosion of orthopedic screws, J. Bone Joint Surg. **40-A:**853, 1958.

Laing, P. G.: The timing of definitive nerve repair, Surg. Clin. North Am. **40:**363, 1960.

Lam, S. J. S.: The place of delayed internal fixation in the treatment of fractures of the long bones, J. Bone Joint Surg. **46-B:**393, 1964.

Lance, E. M., Inglis, A. E., Figarola, F., and Veith, F. J.: Transplantation of the canine hind limb. Surgical technique and methods of immunosuppression for allotransplantation. A preliminary report, J. Bone Joint Surg. **53-A:**1137, 1971.

Lewin, M. L.: Repair of digital nerves in lacerations of the hand and the fingers, Clin. Orthop. **16**:227, 1960.

Lichtenstein, L.: Bone tumors, ed. 3, St. Louis, 1965, The C. V. Mosby Co.

Linton, R. R.: Arterial injuries associated with fractures of the extremity, J. Bone Joint Surg. **46-A**:575, 1964.

Lipscomb, P. R.: Tumors of the tendons and tendon sheaths including ganglia and xanthomas, American Academy of Orthopaedic Surgeons Instructional Course Lectures, vol. 11, Ann Arbor, Mich., 1954, J. W. Edwards.

Lipscomb, P. R., and Wakim, K. G.: Further observations in the healing of severed tendons: an experimental study, Proc. Staff Meet. Mayo Clin. **36**:277, 1961.

Lipscomb, P. R., and Wakim, K. G.: Regeneration of severed tendons: an experimental study, Proc. Staff Meet. Mayo Clin. **36**:271, 1961.

Lister, J.: On a new method of treating compound fractures, abscess, etc., Lancet **1**:357, 1867.

Lloyd, R. G. C.: Suppurative arthritis of infancy. Some observations upon prognosis and management, J. Bone Joint Surg. **42-B**:706, 1960.

Lumpkin, M. B., Logan, W. D., Couves, C. M., and Howard, J. M.: Arteriography as an aid in the diagnosis and localization of acute arterial injuries. Ann. Surg. **147**:353, 1958.

Lusskin, R., Grynbaum, B. B., and Dhir, R. S.: Rehabilitation surgery in adult spastic hemiplegia, Clin. Orthop. **63**:132, 1969.

Marmor, L.: Surgery of rheumatoid arthritis, London, 1967, Henry Kimpton.

Mason, M. L., and Shearon, C. G.: The process of tendon suture and tendon graft, Arch. Surg. **25**:615, 1932.

Mayer, L.: Repair of severed tendons, Am. J. Surg. **42**:714, 1938.

Mazet, R., Jr.: Cineplasty. Historical review, present status, and critical evaluation of sixty-four patients, J. Bone Joint Surg. **40-A**:1389, 1958.

Mazet, R., Jr., and Chupurdia, R.: Pylons and peg legs, Clin. Orthop. **57**:117, 1968.

McCarroll, H. R.: Practical considerations in the management of malignant bone tumors, J.A.M.A. **152**:297, 1953.

McCarroll, H. R.: Orthopedic management of the severely injured patient, J.A.M.A. **165**:1913, 1957.

McElvenny, R. T.: The tourniquet, its clinical application, Am. J. Surg. **69**:94, 1945.

McElvenny, R. T.: The use of closed circulation and suction in the treatment of chronically infected, acutely infected and potentially infected wounds, Am. J. Orthop. **3**:86, 1961.

McNeur, J. C.: The management of open skeletal trauma with particular reference to internal fixation, J. Bone Joint Surg. **52-B**:54, 1970.

Mercer, W., and Duthie, R. B.: Orthopaedic surgery, ed. 6, Baltimore, 1964, The Williams & Wilkins Co.

Milford, L.: The hand. In Crenshaw, A. H., editor: Campbell's operative orthopaedics, vol. 1, ed. 5, St. Louis, 1971, The C. V. Mosby Co.

Miller, J. A., Jr.: Joint paracentesis from an anatomic point of view. I. Shoulder, elbow, wrist and hand, Surgery **40**:993, 1956.

Miller, J. A., Jr.: Joint paracentesis from an anatomic point of view. II. Hip, knee, ankle and foot, Surgery **41**:999, 1957.

Moberg, E.: Evaluation and management of nerve injuries in the hand, Surg. Clin. North Am. **44**:1019, 1964.

Moellering, R. C., Jr., Tratt, G., and Weinberg, A. N.: The In Vitro antibacterial effectiveness of antibiotic-detergent combinations. Preliminary studies using Alevaire, penicillin G, methicillin and oxacillin, J. Bone Joint Surg. **53-A**:30, 1971.

Mooney, V., Nickel, V. L., and Snelson, R.: Fitting of temporary prosthetic limbs immediately after amputation, Calif. Med. **107**:330, 1967.

Mooney, V., Perry, J., and Nickel, V. L.: Surgical and nonsurgical orthopaedic care of stroke, J. Bone Joint Surg. **49-A**:989, 1967.

Moore, F. D.: Metabolic care of the surgical patient, Philadelphia, 1959, W. B. Saunders Co.

Morton, D. L., and Malmgren, R. A.: Human osteosarcomas: immunologic evidence suggesting an associated infectious agent, Science **162**:1279, 1968.

Morton, J. H., Southgate, W. A., and DeWeise, J.: Arterial injuries of the extremities, Surg. Gynecol. Obstet. **123**:611, 1966.

Muller, M. E.: Internal fixation for fresh fractures and for nonunion, Proc. R. Soc. Med. **56**:455, 1963.

Muller, M. E.: Treatment of nonunions by compression, Clin. Orthop. **43**:83, 1965.

Muller, M. E., Allgöwer, M., and Willenegger, H.: Technique of internal fixation of fractures, New York, 1965, Springer-Verlag, Inc.

Naffziger, H. C.: Methods to secure end-to-end suture of peripheral nerves, Surg. Gynecol. Obstet. **32**:193, 1921.

Naiman, P. T., Schein, A. J., and Siffert, R. S.: Use of ASIF compression plates in selected shaft fractures of the upper extremity. A preliminary report, Clin. Orthop. **71**:208, 1970.

Nelson, J. D., and Koontz, W. C.: Septic arthritis in infants and children: a review of 117 cases, Pediatrics **38**:966, 1966.

Nicholson, O. R., and Seddon, H. J.: Nerve repair in civil practice—results of treatment of median and ulnar nerve lesions, Br. Med. J. **2**:1065, 1957.

Obletz, B. E.: Vertical traction in the early management of certain compound fractures of the femur, J. Bone Joint Surg. **28**:113, 1946.

O'Donoghue, D. H.: Treatment of injuries to athletes, Philadelphia, 1962, W. B. Saunders.

Omer, G. E., Jr.: Evaluation and reconstruction of the forearm and hand after acute traumatic peripheral nerve injuries, J. Bone Joint Surg. **50-A**:1451, 1968.

Onne, L.: Recovery of sensibility and sudomotor activity in the hand after nerve suture, Acta Chir. Scand. (Suppl.) **300**:1, 1962.

Orr, H. W.: The treatment of acute osteomyelitis by drainage and rest, J. Bone Joint Surg. **9**:733, 1927.

Orr, H. W.: Compound fractures with special reference to the lower extremity, Am. J. Surg. **46**:733, 1939.

Osgood, R. B.: Classification and etiology of chronic rheumatism or arthritis, Acta Chir. Scand. **67**:634, 1930.

Ottolenghi, C. E.: Diagnosis of orthopaedic lesions by aspiration biopsy. Results of 1061 punctures, J. Bone Joint Surg. **37-A**:443, 1955.

Owens, J. C.: The management of arterial trauma, Surg. Clin. North Am. **43**:371, 1963.

Padgett, E. C.: Full-thickness skin graft in correction of soft tissue deformities, J.A.M.A. **98**:18, 1932.

Paget, J.: Healing of cartilage, Clin. Orthop. **64**:7, 1969.

Patrick, J.: Aneurysm of the popliteal vessels after meniscectomy, J. Bone Joint Surg. **45-B**:570, 1963.

Peterson, L. T.: Principles of internal fixation with plates and screws, Arch Surg. **64**:345, 1952.

Phemister, D. B.: Treatment of ununited fractures by onlay bone grafts without screw or tie fixations and without breaking down of the fibrous union, J. Bone Joint Surg. **29**:946, 1947.

Phemister, D. B.: Biologic principles in healing of fractures and their bearing on treatment, Ann. Surg. **133**:433, 1951.

Platt, H.: On the peripheral nerve complications of certain fractures, J. Bone Joint Surg. **10**:403, 1928.

Platt, H., and Bristow, W. R.: The remote results of operations for injuries of the peripheral nerves, Br. J. Surg. **11**:535, 1924.

Pulvertaft, R. G.: Suture material and tendon junctures, Am. J. Surg. **109**:346, 1965.

Pyka, R. A., and Lipscomb, P. R.: Fractures in amputees, J. Bone Joint Surg. **42-A**:499, 1960.

Ramirez, Z. M. A., et al.: Reimplantation of limbs, Plast. Reconstr. Surg. **40**:315, 1967.

Rapp, G. F., Griffith, R. S., and Hebble, W. M.: The permeability of traumatically inflamed synovial membrane to commonly used antibiotics, J. Bone Joint Surg. **48-A**:1534, 1966.

Ray, R. D.: Needle biopsy of the lumbar vertebral bodies. A modification of Valls' technique, J. Bone Joint Surg. **35-A**:760, 1953.

Ray, R., Sankaran, B., and Fetrow, K. O.: Delayed union and nonunion of fractures, J. Bone Joint Surg. **46-A**:627, 1964.

Record, E. E.: Surgical amputation in the geriatric patients, J. Bone Joint Surg. **45-A**:1742, 1963.

Rich, N. M., Baugh, J. H., and Hughes, C. W.: Popliteal artery injuries in Vietnam, Am. J. Surg. **118**:531, 1969.

Riordan, D. C.: Emergency treatment of compound injury of the hand, Orthopaedics **1**:30, 1958.

Ropes, M. E., et al.: Revision of diagnostic criteria for rheumatoid arthritis, Bull. Rheum. Dis. **9**:221, 1958.

Rush, L. V.: Atlas of Rush pin technics. A system of fracture treatment, Meridian, Miss., 1955, The Berivon Co.

Saad, M. N.: The problems of traumatic skin loss of the lower limbs, especially when associated with skeletal injury, Br. J. Surg. **57**:601, 1970.

Sakellarides, H.: A follow-up study of 172 peripheral nerve injuries in the upper extremity in civilians, J. Bone Joint Surg. **44-A**:140, 1962.

Saletta, J. D., and Freeark, R. J.: The partially severed artery, Arch. Surg. **97**:198, 1968.

Salter, R. B., and Fiela, P.: The effect of continuous compression on living aticular cartilage, J. Bone Joint Surg. **42-A**:31, 1960.

Salter, R. B., and Harris, W. R.: Injuries involving the epiphyseal plate, J. Bone Joint Surg. **45-A**:587, 1963.

Samilson, R. L., Bersani, F. A., and Watkins, M. B.: Acute suppurative arthritis in infants and children, Pediatrics **21**:798, 1958.

Scales, J. T., and Winter, G. D.: Corrosion of orthopedic implants, J. Bone Joint Surg. **41-B**:810, 1959.

Schajowicz, F.: Aspiration biopsy in bone lesions. Cytological and histological techniques, J. Bone Joint Surg. **37-A**:465, 1955.

Scuderi, C.: Atlas of orthopedic traction procedures, St. Louis, 1954, The C. V. Mosby Co.

Seddon, H. J.: The practical value of peripheral nerve repair, Proc. R. Soc. Med. **42**:427, 1949.

Seddon, H. J.: War injuries of peripheral nerves, Br. J. Surg. (Suppl.) **36**:325, 1949.

Seddon, H. J.: Peripheral nerve injuries: Medical Research Council. Special report series. No. 282, London: Her Majesty's Stationery Office, 1954,

Seddon, H. J.: Nerve grafting, J. Bone Joint Surg. **45-B**:447, 1963.

Sherman, M. S.: Benign lesions simulating malignancy, American Academy of Orthopaedic Surgeons Instructional Course Lectures, vol. 9, Ann Arbor, Mich., 1952, J. W. Edwards.

Sherman, W. O. N.: Vandium steel bone plates and screws, Surg. Gynecol. Obstet. **14**:629, 1912.

Siffert, R. S., and Arkin, A. M.: Trephine biopsy of bone with special reference to the lumbar vertebral bodies, J. Bone Joint Surg. **31-A**:146, 1949.

Slocum, D. B.: Atlas of amputations, St. Louis, 1949, The C. V. Mosby Co.

Speed, K.: Growth problems following osteomyelitis of adolescent long bones, Surg. Gynecol. Obstet. **34**:469, 1922.

Stevens, D. B.: Postoperative orthopaedic infections. A study of etiological mechanisms, J. Bone Joint Surg. **46-A**:96, 1964.

Stout, A. P.: Tumors of the soft tissues. In Armed Forces Institute of Pathology: Atlas of Tumor Pathology, sect. II, fasc. 5, Washington, D.C., 1953, National Research Council.

Stromberg, W. B., et al.: Injury of the median and ulnar nerves, J. Bone Joint Surg. **43-A**:717, 1961.

Sturman, M. J.: Late results of finger-tip injuries, J. Bone Joint Surg. **45-A**:289, 1963.

Swanson, A. B.: Bone overgrowth in the juvenile amputee and its control by the use of silicone rubber, Inter-Clin. Inform. Bull. **8**:9, 1969.

Tachdijan, M. O., and Compere, E. L.: Postoperative wound infections in orthopaedic surgery: evaluation of prophylactic antibiotics, Int. Surg. **28**:797, 1957.

Taylor, A. R., and Maudsley, R. H.: Installation-suction technique in chronic osteomyelitis, J. Bone Joint Surg. **52-B**:88, 1970.

Tedeschi, C. G., Walter, C. E., and Tedeschi, L. G.: Shock and fat embolism: an appraisal, Surg. Clin. North Am. **48**:431, 1968.

Thomson, J. E. M.: The treatment of nonunion and malunion by intramedullary nailing, American Academy of Orthopaedic Surgeons Instructional Course Lectures, vol. 11, Ann Arbor, Mich., 1954, J. W. Edwards, p. 87.

Tinel, J.: Nerve wounds. In Joll, C. A., editor: Symptomatology of peripheral nerve lesions caused by war wounds. (translated by Rothwell, F.), London, 1917, Bailliere, Tindall, and Cox, Ltd.

Trueta, J.: Principles and practice of war surgery, St. Louis, 1943, The C. V. Mosby Co.

Trueta, J., and Morgan, J. D.: Late results in the treatment of one hundred cases of acute haematogenous osteomyelitis, Br. J. Surg. **41**:449, 1954.

Urist, M. R., Mazet, R., Jr., and McLean, F. C.: The pathogenesis and treatment of delayed union and nonunion, J. Bone Joint Surg. **36-A**:931, 1954.

Venable, C. S., and Stuck, W. G.: Electrolysis controlling factor in the use of metals in treating fractures, J.A.M.A. **111**:1349, 1938.

Venable, C. S., and Stuck, W. G.: Result of recent studies and experiments concerning metals used in the internal fixation of fractures, J. Bone Joint Surg. **30-A**:247, 1948.

Venable, C. S., Stuck, W. G., and Beach, A.: The effects on bone of the presence of metals; based upon electrolysis; an experimental study, Ann. Surg. **105**:917, 1937.

Watanabe, M., Takeda, S., and Ikeuchi, H.: Atlas of arthroscopy, ed. 2, Tokyo, 1969, Igaku Shoin, Ltd.

Watkins, M. B.: Acute suppurative arthritis: Follow-up notes, J. Bone Joint Surg. **47-A**:428, 1966.

Watkins, M. B., Samilson, R. L., and Winters, D. M.: Acute suppurative arthritis, J. Bone Joint Surg. **38-A:**1313, 1956.

Watson-Jones, R.: Fractures and joint injuries, Baltimore, 1962, The Williams & Wilkins Co.

Waugh, T. R., and Stinchfield, F. E.: Suction drainage of orthopaedic wounds, J. Bone Joint Surg. **43-A:**939, 1961.

Wessler, S., and Auioli, L. V.: Tetanus, J.A.M.A. **207:**123, 1969.

White, W. L.: Tendon grafts: a consideration of their source, procurement and suitability, Surg. Clin. North Am. **40:**403, 1960.

Wilgis, E. F. S.: Observations on the effects of tourniquet ischemia, J. Bone Joint Surg. **53-A:**1343, 1971.

Williams, G. R., Carter, D. R., Frank, G. R., and Price, W. E.: Replantation of amputated extremities, Ann. Surg. **163:**788, 1966.

Wilson, A. B., Jr.: Limb prosthetics—1967, Artif. Limbs **2:**1, 1967.

Wilson, P. D., and Lance, E. M.: Surgical reconstruction of the skeleton following segmental resection for bone tumors, J. Bone Joint Surg. **47-A:**1629, 1965.

Woodhall, B.: Peripheral nerve injuries. II. Basic data from the peripheral nerve registry concerning 7,050 nerve sutures and 67 nerve grafts, J. Neurosurg. **4:**146, 1947.

Woodhall, B.: The surgical repair of acute peripheral nerve injury, Surg. Clin. North Am. **31:**1669, 1951.

Woodhall, B.: Common injuries of peripheral nerves, American Academy of Orthopaedic Surgeons Instructional Course Lectures, vol. 11, Ann Arbor, Mich., 1954, J. W. Edwards, p. 269.

Woodhall, B., and Beebe, G. W., editors: Peripheral nerve regeneration. A follow-up study of 3,656 World War II injuries, Veterans Administration Medical Monograph, Washington, D.C., 1956, United States Government Printing Office.

Woodhall, B., and Lyons, W. R.: Peripheral nerve injuries. I. The results of "early" nerve suture: A preliminary report, Surgery **19:**757, 1946.

Young, J. M., and Funk, F. J.: Incidence of tumor metastasis to the lumbar spine, J. Bone Joint Surg. **35-A:**55, 1953.

AUTHOR INDEX

A
Aadalen, R. J., 369
Abbott, J. C., 369
Abbott, L. C., 45, 46, 64, 90, 135, 298, 369, 486
Abdulla, M., 615
Abernathy, P. J., 134
Abrami, G., 370
Ackerman, L. V., 614
Ackerson, T., 509
Ackerson, T. T., 213
Ackroyd, C. E., 486
Acland, 613
Adamkiewicz, A., 278
Adams, J. C., 369, 543
Adams, J. P., 112, 184, 593
Adler, J. B., 45, 133
Adler, S., 90
Adson, A. W., 45, 277
Aegerter, E. E., 614
Agerholm, J. C., 64, 133, 136
Aglietti, P., 488
Ahlbäck, S. O., 369
Ahlberg, A., 486
Ahstrom, J. P., 486
Ainsworth, W. H., 615
Aitken, G. T., 508, 543, 614, 616
Akeson, W. H., 277
Albee, F. H., 277, 298, 369, 543
Albert, S. M., 133
Albright, J. A., 134, 184, 213, 491
Alexakis, P. G., 401
Alexander, H., 112
Alexander, H. H., 188
Alexander, J. P., 369
Alkhudairy, H., 90
Alldred, A. J., 45, 184
Alldredge, R. H., 64, 543, 614
Allen, H. S., 185, 186
Allen, W. C., 401
Allgower, M., 508, 617
Allman, F. L., 9
Allman, F. L., Jr., 45
Almquist, E. E., 614
Alms, M., 508
Alpert, M., 614

Althoff, B., 213
Alvarez, A., 136
Ambrose, G. B., 614
Amstutz, H. C., 326, 369, 401
Anas, P. P., 213
Anderson, C. E., 486
Anderson, K. J., 543
Anderson, L. D., 90, 112, 213, 369, 370, 614
Anderson, M., 433, 486, 488
Anderson, T. P., 277
Andersson, G. B. J., 277
Andersson, K., 189
Andren, L., 189
Andrews, J. R., 462, 464, 486, 488, 490
Andrews, P. S., 491
Animoso, J., 544
Ansell, B. M., 369
Antonelli, E. E., 403
Apley, A. G., 369
Appel, H., 486
Apuzzo, M. L. J., 213
Arden, G. P., 369
Arden, H. P., 486
Arkin, A. M., 618
Armbrust, E. N., 279
Armstrong, J. R., 45
Arnar, O., 616
Arner, O., 543
Arnot, J. P., 373
Aronson, H. A., 277
Artz, C. P., 614
Arzimanoglow, A., 508
Asher, M. A., 490
Asherman, E. G., 47
Ashworth, C. R., 189
Athanasoulis, C. A., 186
Atlas, S., 134
d'Aubigne, R. M., 369, 401, 508, 614
Auerbach, A. M., 593
Aufranc, O. E., 64, 135, 369, 370, 372, 374, 377, 401, 486
Auioli, L. V., 619
Aune, S. L., 189
Axer, A., 593

B
Babbitt, D. P., 45
Babcock, J. L., 45
Baber, L. D., 486
Bachmann, F., 490
Backdahl, M., 134
Backhouse, K. M., 190
Badger, F. G., 90
Badgley, C. E., 45, 369, 614
Bado, J. L., 90
Bagg, R. J., 280
Bailey, R. W., 45, 280
Bailey, S. I., 213
Bailey, W. H., 489
Baitch, A., 369, 614
Bakalim, G., 45
Baker, G. C. W., 543
Baker, L. D., 543, 593
Baker, S. L., 487
Baker, W. M., 486
Ball, J., 190
Bankart, A. S., 45
Banks, H. H., 112, 369, 488, 543, 593
Banks, S. W., 614
Barber, J. R., 374
Bardenheier, J. A., III, 486, 614
Bardenstein, M. B., 369
Barenfeld, P. A., 91, 596
Barford, B., 614
Bargary, R. A., 509
Bargen, J. H., 486
Barlow, T. G., 369
Barnard, L., 133
Barne, H. C., 509
Barnes, R., 369
Barnes, S. N., 298
Barr, J. S., 90, 133, 213, 277, 369, 486, 543
Barrett, A. M., 401
Barrington, T. W., 45
Barron, D. W., 369
Bartolozzi, P., 280
Barton, J. R., 133
Bassett, F. H., 491, 593
Batchelor, J. S., 362, 369
Bateman, J. E., 45
Bateman, J. G., 614

621

Batson, O. V., 277
Bauer, G. C. H., 486
Baugh, J. H., 618
Baum, J., 134
Beach, A., 378, 491, 618
Beal, J. M., 374
Beals, R. K., 401
Beaupre, A., 487
Bechtol, C. O., 64, 112, 369, 614
Beckenbaugh, R. D., 134, 188, 369, 371
Becker, G. E., 491
Becker, J. R., 595
Becton, J. L., 486
Beebe, G. W., 619
Beighton, P., 213
Bell, D. M., 373
Bell, G. D., 213
Bell, H. G., 46
Bell, J. L., 184, 185
Bell, J. P., 402
Bell Tawse, A. J. S., 90
Beltran, J. E., 136
Ben-Hur, N., 489
Benjamin, H., 298
Benner, E. J., 614
Bennett, E. H., 168, 184
Bennett, G. A., 64
Bennett, J. E., 45
Bentley, G., 486
Benton, B. F., 277
Bergfield, J. A., 491
Bergofsky, E. H., 278
Berman, A., 593
Bernau, A., 593
Bersani, F. A., 377, 618
Bianco, A. J., 280, 369
Bianco, A. J., Jr., 277
Bickel, W. H., 64, 369, 376, 486, 614
Bingold, A. C., 543
Birkeland, I. W., 277
Bishop, R. E. D., 487
Björkesten, G., 614
Black, J. R., 188
Blair, H., 491
Blair, J. E., 614
Bland, J., 135
Bland, W. G., 491
Blandy, J. P., 508
Blazina, M. E., 486, 487
Bleck, E. E., 369, 508
Blockey, N. J., 136, 593
Blount, W. P., 90, 278, 279, 369, 433, 436, 491, 508, 595, 614
Bluhm, M. M., 374
Blum, B., 486
Blumberg, L., 509
Blumenfeld, I., 401
Boals, J. C., 90
Böhler, J., 213, 401
Böhler, L., 401, 614
Bohler, N., 374
Bojsen-Møller, F., 593
Bollinger, J. A., 190

Bolton, P. E., 189
Bonaquist, M., 279
Bonfiglio, M., 369
Bonnett, C. A., 280
Bonney, G., 401
Bora, F. W., 184
Bora, F. W., Jr., 127, 136
Borden, J., 370
Borella, L., 614
Bose, K. S., 508
Boseker, E. H., 64, 544
Bost, F. C., 45, 90, 370, 486, 593
Boswick, J. A., 47
Boswick, J. A., Jr., 614
Bosworth, D. M., 45, 277, 279, 370, 487
Boucher, P., 543
Bourland, W. L., 370
Bourrel, P., 595
Bowden, R. E. M., 614
Bowker, J. H., 486
Boxall, D., 279
Boyd, B. M., 593
Boyd, H. B., 45, 90, 91, 112, 136, 370, 401, 486, 508, 614
Boyd, R. J., 370
Boyes, J. H., 184, 185, 187, 189, 614
Bradford, D. S., 279, 280
Bradley, N., 593
Brady, L. P., 277
Brady, W. M., 64, 112
Brahms, M. A., 593
Brain, W. R., 135
Brand, P. W., 185, 186
Brandfass, W. T., 375
Brånemark, P.-I., 134
Brannon, E. W., 188
Brantigan, O., 508
Brantigan, O. C., 486
Brashear, H. R., 614
Brattstrom, H., 90
Braun, R. M., 112
Braund, R. R., 298
Brav, E. A., 45, 401, 614
Bremmer, R. A., 491
Brett, M. S., 90
Brewerton, D. A., 133, 188
Brewster, R. C., 370
Bridgman, C. F., 371
Briggs, B. T., 45
Bright, D. S., 186
Bristow, 9
Bristow, W. R., 486, 614, 618
Brittain, H. A., 298, 370
Briyan, S., 135
Broders, A. C., 188
Broderson, M. P., 486
Broms, J. D., 593
Brooks, A. L., 213, 594
Brooks, D., 614
Brooks, D. B., 487
Brown, F. W., 45
Brown, G. C., 372
Brown, J. C., 280

Brown, J. E., 90
Brown, J. T., 370
Brown, P. W., 186, 508, 614
Brown, R. H., 64
Brown, R. L., 188
Brown, T., 277
Brown, T. D., 487
Browne, W. E., 187
Bruce, H. E., 112
Bruce, J., 486
Bruner, J. M., 167, 184
Bruton, W., 186
Bryan, R. S., 90, 188, 369, 486, 487, 489
Buck, C. A., 213
Buck, R. M., 91
Bulmer, J. H., 370
Buncke, 613
Bunin, J. J., 190
Bunnell, S., 90, 133, 139, 184, 185, 186, 188, 614
Bunnell, W. P., 374
Burchman, J., 614
Burgess, E. M., 401, 508
Burgo, P. H., 544
Burke, J. R., 370
Burkhalter, W. E., 64, 112, 508
Burleson, R. J., 486
Burstein, A. A., 213, 616
Burstein, A. H., 401, 487, 544, 614
Burton, R. C., 544
Burton, R. I., 133, 135, 184, 185, 187, 188, 189, 190
Burwell, H. N., 112, 508, 543
Bush, L. F., 90
Bushell, G. R., 277
Butt, W. P., 486
Byers, P. D., 486

C

Cabaud, H. E., 370
Calandriello, B., 377
Calandruccio, R. A., 277
Caldwell, A. B., 277
Callahan, J. J., 371, 543
Callander, C. L., 401
Callery, G., 64
Callery, G. E., 64
Callison, J. R., 185
Cameron, H., 46
Cameron, H. V., 372
Camitz, H., 135, 186
Campbell, C. J., 134, 543
Campbell, C. S., 184
Campbell, J. C., 614
Campbell, R. D., Jr., 133, 134, 370, 510
Campbell, R. E., 508
Campbell, W. C., 90, 277, 370, 486
Canale, S. T., 370, 593
Cannon, B. W., 135
Canty, T. J., 508
Capello, W. N., 326, 370
Capener, N., 184, 593
Carbonara, P. N., 64

Cargill, A. O., 136
Cargill, A. O'R., 486
Carlson, C. E., 375
Carlsson, A. S., 370
Carmona, L. S., 64, 112
Carnesale, P. G., 298
Carpenter, E. B., 45, 486, 508, 593
Carpenter, W. F., 486
Carr, C. C., 401
Carr, C. R., 593
Carrel, A., 614
Carrell, B. C., 134
Carroll, N., 46
Carroll, N. C., 112, 370
Carroll, R. E., 84, 90, 134, 188, 189, 377
Carroll, R. W., 177, 188
Carstam, N., 189
Carter, A. B., 508
Carter, D. R., 619
Carter, J., 615
Carter, S. J., 185
Carvalho, B. C., 134
Casey, M. J., 401
Casscells, S. W., 615
Cassidy, R. H., 45
Cattell, H. S., 213
Catterall, R. C. F., 543
Cavadias, A. X., 403
Cavallaro, W. V., 47, 377
Cave, E. F., 133, 370, 377, 401, 403, 486, 508, 544, 615
Chacha, P. B., 90, 370
Chakales, H. H., 616
Chalmers, J., 91, 136, 543
Chamberlin, A. C., 377
Chan, D. P. K., 278
Chan, K. P., 370
Chan, R. N. W., 490
Chandler, F. A., 370, 486
Chandler, G. N., 615
Chao, E. Y., 91
Chapchal, G., 370
Chapman, W. C., 112
Chapman, M. W., 401
Charif, P., 486
Charnley, A. D., 112, 543
Charnley, J., 45, 319-325, 370, 372, 484, 486, 487, 540, 543
Chase, C., 277
Chase, R. A., 134, 184
Chase, S. W., 616
Cheema, H. M., 127, 136, 184
Chen, C. M., 491, 545
Chen, H.-T., 370
Childress, H. M., 487, 543
Choi, B. Y., 185
Chou, P. K., 280
Chou, S. N., 280
Chrisman, O. D., 508, 543
Christensen, I., 370
Christie, J., 369
Chuinard, E. G., 370, 543
Chung, S. M. K., 214

Chupurdia, R., 617
Cirincione, R. J., 280
Cisek, E. E., 595
Clancy, G. L., 490
Clancy, W. J., 452, 487
Clark, B. L., 543
Clark, G. L., Jr., 213
Clark, G. M., 614
Clark, G. R., 486
Clark, J. G., 48
Clark, J. M. P., 64
Clark, W., 489
Clark, W. K., 213
Clarke, I. C., 369
Clawson, D. K., 370, 401, 615
Clayton, M. D., 188
Clayton, M. L., 133, 134, 188, 189, 487, 488, 543, 593, 615
Cleveland, M., 370, 487, 593, 615
Clippinger, F. W., 184, 189, 615
Close, J. R., 615
Clouse, M. E., 370
Cloutier, G. E., 135
Cobb, J. R., 217, 278
Cockin, J., 591, 593
Codman, E. A., 45
Coffey, J. R., 45
Cofield, R. H., 45
Cohen, J., 64, 370, 615
Cohen, S. H., 487
Cohen, S. M., 615
Coker, T. P., 487
Coker, T. P., Jr., 377
Cole, J. M., 133
Cole, T. M., 277
Coleman, C. C., 615
Coleman, C. R., 377
Coleman, S. S., 370
Coley, B. L., 615
Collins, H. A., 615
Collins, H. R., 371, 372, 487, 491
Collis, 217
Collis, D. K., 370
Collon, D. J., 374
Colonna, P. C., 370, 371
Colton, C. L., 543
Colton, T., 370
Colville, J., 185
Compere, C., 508
Compere, C. L., 487
Compere, E. L., 277, 615, 618
Connelly, S., 370
Conner, A. N., 90
Converse, J. M., 184
Conway, F. M., 401
Conway, H., 184, 187
Conway, J. J., 593
Conwell, H. E., 45, 615
Cooke, A. J., 45
Cooley, S. G. E., 186, 187
Coonrad, R. W., 184, 185
Cooper, P., 190
Cooper, P. R., 213

Cooper, W., 112, 186
Cooperman, B., 377
Cope, C., 487
Copeland, C. X., Jr., 615
Copeland, M. M., 615, 616
Copeland, S. A., 90
Corban, M. S., 403
Corcoran, P. J., 509
Corss, M. J., 488
Cotrel, Y., 234, 236, 278
Cottingham, G., 615
Cotton, F. J., 543
Cotton, R. E., 45
Cottrell, G. W., 45
Coughlin, M. J., 45, 595
Coutte, A., 491
Couves, C. M., 617
Coventry, M. B., 64, 277, 278, 370, 371, 374, 472, 486, 487, 616
Coventry, M. D., 487
Cowan, D. J., 487
Cowan, R. J., 185
Cowell, H. R., 593
Cozen, L., 593, 615
Cracchiolo, A., III, 487
Craig, J., 213
Craig, W. A., 279, 280
Cram, R. H., 371
Cramer, L. M., 135
Crampton, R. S., 47
Cranley, J. J., 45
Crauener, E. K., 487
Crawford, H. B., 371
Crawford, H. R., 45
Crawford, W. J., 370
Cregan, J. C. F., 133
Crego, C. H., Jr., 371, 375, 401, 402, 593
Crenshaw, A. H., 64, 184, 371, 486, 594, 617
Crenshaw, A. W., 595
Crikelair, G. F., 615
Croft, C., 376
Cross, H., 134
Cross, M. J., 488
Crothers, O. D., 372
Crowe, J. F., 371
Cruess, R. L., 135, 278, 371
Cseuz, K. A., 135
Cubbins, W. R., 371, 543
Cunha, B. A., 371
Curtin, J. W., 593
Curtis, B., 615
Curtis, B. H., 401
Curtis, R. M., 135, 184
Curtiss, P. H., 371
Curtiss, P. H., Jr., 615

D

Dahlin, D. C., 64, 376, 486, 615
Daland, E. M., 615
Dale, G. M., 543
Dale, W. A., 615
Dall, D., 277

D'Alonzo, R. T., 213
Dalton, J. B., Jr., 486
Dameron, F. D., 213
Danckwardt-Lillieström, G., 402
Dandy, D. J., 487, 489
Danzig, L. A., 543
D'Arcy, J., 487
Dargan, E. L., 185
Darrach, W., 134
Datta, S. R., 508
Davidson, A. J., 90
Davies, D. M., 616
Davies-Colley, N., 593
Davis, A. G., 615
Davis, G. L., 615
Davis, I. S., 280
Davis, J. B., 45
Davis, J. R., 371
Davis, L., 544, 615
Davis, P. H., 371
Davis, W. M., 90
Dawson, E. G., 213
Day, A. J., 45, 595
Day, P. L., 373
Day, W. H., 486
De Jour, J., 491
DeBakey, M. E., 616
DeBelder, K. R. J., 401
Debeyre, J., 47
Deburge, A., 593
Decoulx, J., 134
Decoulx, P., 134
Deffer, P. A., 508
DeFiore, J. D., 136
Dehne, E., 401, 508, 615
DeHaven, K., 487
DeHaven, K. B., 487
DeHaven, K. E., 371, 487, 491
Déjerine-Klumpke, A., 45
Delorme, T. L., 127, 133, 136, 401
Demarest, L., 279
Demottaz, J. D., 543
Demuth, R. J., 186
Denham, R. A., 487, 543
Dennyson, W. G., 134
DePalma, A. F., 45, 64, 277, 371
Derby, A. C., 543
Derennes, R., 189
Desanctis, R. W., 373, 616
Devanny, J. R., 278, 280
Devas, M. B., 45, 487
Dewald, R. L., 210, 278
Dewar, F. P., 45
DeWeese, J. W., 185
DeWeise, J., 617
Dexpert, M., 595
Deyerle, W. M., 371
Dhir, R. S., 617
DiChiro, G., 278
Dickerson, R., 615
Dickerson, R. C., 46, 371, 594, 615
Dickson, F. D., 371, 508, 615
Dickson, J. A., 280, 371

Dickson, J. H., 280, 486
Dickson, J. W., 45
Dietrichson, G. J. F., 508
Dilmaghani, A., 615
Dimon, J. H., III, 45, 371
Dingman, P. V. C., 134
Dion, M. A., 135
Dively, R. L., 615
Dobbie, R. P., 90
Dobechko, W. P., 280
Dobyns, J. H., 90, 188
Dodelin, C. D., 593
Dolan, J., 188
Dolphin, J. A., 187
Dombrowski, E. T., 615
Dommisse, G. F., 278
Donovan, J. F., 369
Doobie, J. J., 508
Dooley, B. J., 134
Doolittle, R. C., 508
Doppman, J. O., 278
Doren, W. W., 189
Dow, N. J., 213
Dow, S., 373
Dowsett, D. J., 375
Doyle, J. R., 188
Drennan, D. B., 487
Drutz, D. J., 371, 615
Du Toit, G. T., 46
Duchenne, G. B., 46
Duckworth, T., 490
Duncan, J. W., 593
Duncan, T. L., 593
Dunlop, J., 90
Dunlop, K., 510
Dunn, A. W., 90, 544, 615
Dunn, D. M., 371
Dunn, E. J., 213, 543
Dunn, H. K., 48, 593
Dunoyer, J., 373
Dunsmore, R. H., 277
Dupont, C., 135
Dupont, M., 134
Dupuytren, G., 187, 543
Duquennoy, A., 134
Duthie, H. L., 487
Duthie, R. B., 294, 298, 371, 615, 617
DuVries, H. L., 587, 593, 595
Dwyer, A. F., 251, 253, 268-271, 278
Dwyer, F. C., 553-554, 593
Dzoib, J. M., 595

E

Eaton, R. G., 90, 112, 135, 156, 158, 167, 184, 185, 187, 189, 190, 402
Eberhart, H. D., 403
Ecker, M. L., 371
Eden, R., 46
Edshage, S., 615
Edwards, P., 508
Edwards, W. G., 543
Eggers, G. W. N., 371, 392-393, 401, 508, 615

Ehrlich, G. E., 190, 487
Ehrlich, H. E., 376
Ehrlich, M. G., 490
Eicher, 326
Eicher, P., 370
Eilers, A. F., 488
Eilers, V. E., 279, 596
Eisenstein, A. L., 91
Ekholm, R., 134
Ellis, B. W., 91
Ellis, H., 508
Ellis, J., 134
Ellis, V. H., 46
Ellison, A. E., 487
Ellison, M. R., 188, 190
Elliston, W. A., 133
Elmelik, E., 47
Elmslie, 422-423, 427
Elmslie, R. C., 46, 543
Emery, M. A., 615
English, T. A., 402
Enneking, W. F., 371, 376, 615
Entin, M. A., 133, 185
Eppright, R. H., 616
Epstein, H. C., 371
Erikson, 452
Eriksson, E., 487
Eshrage, A., 46
Essex-Lopresti, P., 593
Evans, D., 593
Evans, D. L., 543
Evans, E. B., 371, 401
Evans, E. D., 403
Evans, E. M., 90, 371, 616
Evans, J. A., 134
Evans, J. P., 593
Evarts, C. M., 213, 278, 371, 487, 490, 491, 616
Eversmann, W. W., 135
Ewald, F. C., 213
Eyler, D. L., 133
Eyre-Brook, A. L., 298, 372, 491
Eyring, E. J., 616

F

Fahey, J. J., 90, 91, 190, 372, 487, 616
Fairbank, H. A. T., 46, 487
Fairbank, T. J., 401, 487
Fairchild, R. D., 372
Fairen, M. F., 136
Falvo, K. A., 488
Fang, H. S. Y., 278
Fay, G. F., 90
Feil, E. J., 371, 616
Femi-Pearse, D., 278
Fenton, R., 190
Ferciot, C. F., 372
Ferguson, A. B., 279, 369, 614
Ferguson, A. B., Jr., 133, 372, 487
Fetrow, K. O., 185, 618
Fidler, W. J., 298
Fiela, P., 618
Fielding, J. W., 213, 277, 279, 372

Figarola, F., 616
Fiken, O., 189
Fink, C. W., 134
Finkestein, H., 136
Finnieston, A., 544
Fischer, F. J., 369, 401
Fisher, R. H., 372, 616
Fisher, R. L., 401, 593
Fishman, A. P., 278
Fisk, J., 280
Fitzgerald, R. H., 372, 486
Flatt, A. E., 112, 133, 184, 185, 188, 190
Flesch, J. R., 277
Flinchum, D., 593
Florence, D. W., 369
Flynn, J. C., 90
Flynn, J. E., 184, 185, 190
Foix, C., 135
Follacci, F. M., 372
Forrester-Brown, M., 372
Forsythe, M., 213
Forward, A. D., 185
Foster, Y. C., 372
Fourniee, A., 187
Fowler, P. J., 489
Fowler, S. B., 133, 188
Fox, J. M., 185
Frackelton, W. H., 616
Francis, J. D., 491
Francis, K. C., 64, 372, 401, 402, 489
Francis, W. R., 213
Frangakis, E. K., 372
Frank, G. R., 619
Frankel, B. A., 213
Frankel, V. H., 401, 487, 544, 614, 616
Frantz, C. H., 487, 488, 614, 616
Fredericks, E. J., 544
Fredin, H., 46
Freeark, R. J., 618
Freehafer, A. A., 112, 187
Freeland, A. E., 508
Freeman, A. W., 508
Freeman, M. A. R., 326, 372, 486, 543
Freeman, P. A., 509
Freiberg, A. H., 487, 593
Freiberg, J. A., 372
Frejka, B., 372
French, G., 508
French, P. R., 64
Frey, C., 298
Fried, A., 402
Friedenberg, Z. B., 372, 508
Friedman, B., 134
Frigerio, E., 376
Froimson, A. I., 90, 189, 372
Frontino, G., 280
Frost, H. M., 594
Fryer, C. M., 403
Frymoyer, J. W., 135, 371
Fu, F. H., 487
Fuller, R., 508
Fullerton, P. M., 135, 521, 543
Funk, F. J., 401, 619

Furlong, R., 184
Furya, 326

G

Gabrielsen, T. O., 213
Gaenslen, F. J., 298, 372
Galante, J. O., 490
Galante, R., 372
Gallie, W. E., 46, 543, 593
Gallo, G. A., 487
Galway, R. D., 459, 487
Ganguli, S., 508
Ganosa, A. C., 508
Garceau, G. J., 64, 593
Garcia, A., 487
Garcia, A., Jr., 64
Gardner, W. J., 136
Gariépy, R., 487
Garner, R. W., 133
Garnes, A. L., 508
Garrett, A., 207, 279
Garrett, A. L., 187, 278
Garrett, J. C., 372
Garrett, R. G., 45
Gartland, J. J., 593
Gaspar, M. B., 402
Gatellier, J., 543
Gazioglu, K., 278
Gear, M. W. L., 487
Gedda, K.-O., 169, 185
Geens, S., 487, 488
George, I. L., 370
Ger, R., 508, 616
Gerard, 326
Gertzbein, S. D., 277
Gervis, W. H., 189
Geschickter, C. F., 616
Geuss, L. F., 489
Ghormley, R. K., 277, 372, 374, 487
Ghosh, P., 277
Gibson, A., 372
Gibson, D. A., 46
Gibson, J. M. C., 595
Gill, A. B., 46, 372
Gill, B., 298
Gill, G. G., 486
Gill, L. H., 186
Gillespie, H. S., 543
Gillespie, R., 280
Gillies, H., 487, 543
Gilmer, R., 544
Ginsburg, H., 278
Girdlestone, G. R., 362-363, 372
Girzadas, D. V., 188, 488
Gjerdrum, T. C., 402
Glattly, H. W., 616
Gleave, J. A. E., 401
Glenn, F., 616
Glimcher, M. J., 595
Godfrey, J. D., 616
Godsil, R. D., 46
Goergen, T. G., 543
Golbranson, F. L., 401, 508

Gold, A. M., 596
Goldie, I., 134, 373, 488
Goldie, I. F., 213, 375
Goldner, J. L., 112, 133, 184-189, 593, 615, 616
Goldstein, L. A., 46, 136, 278, 280, 594
Goldstein, M. N., 135
Goldstone, J., 509
Goldthwait, J. E., 277, 488
Gonzalez, E. G., 509
Goobar, J. E., 614
Goodfellow, J. W., 64, 136
Goodgold, J., 135, 543
Goodman, A. H., 372
Goodrich, E. R., 277
Gordon, M. L., 90
Gordon, S. L., 543
Gorman, J. F., 594
Gothman, L., 509
Gould, J. S., 188
Grabb, W. C., 616
Graff-Radford, A., 369
Graham, C. E., 543
Graham, J. H., 185
Graham, W. P., 188
Grana, L., 377
Graner, O., 134
Granowitz, S., 188
Grant, B. D., 509
Grant, J. C. B., 184
Grantham, S. A., 135, 402
Green, D. P., 134, 488
Green, J. P., 488, 489
Green, W. T., 46, 112, 369, 372, 433, 486, 488, 543, 593, 594
Greenbaum, E. I., 509
Greene, W., 91
Gregg, T., 489
Gregory, C. F., 64
Greunlich, W. W., 488
Grice, D. S., 524, 543, 550-552, 553, 562, 594
Griffin, P., 616
Griffith, R. S., 376, 618
Griffiths, J. C., 185, 509
Griffiths, S. C., 213
Grimes, O. F., 46
Griswold, D. M., 213
Grogono, B. J. S., 489
Gross, H. P., 373
Groves, E. W. H., 372, 488
Gruen, T. A., 369
Grunwald, A., 509
Grynbaum, B. B., 617
Guhl, J. F., 377
Guidotti, F. P., 46
Guinto, F. C., Jr., 213
Gullickson, G., 277
Gunn, A. L., 488
Gunn, D. R., 401, 488
Gurd, F. B., 46
Gustilo, R. B., 279, 374, 616

625

H

Haake, P. W., 278, 280
Haddad, R. J., 187
Haddad, R. J., Jr., 134
Hageman, W. F., 488
Hagey, H., 45
Haggart, G. E., 372
Haglin, J. J., 616
Hahn, D., 372
Hahns, S. Y., 213
Haimovici, H., 594
Hakstian, R. W., 188
Haldeman, K. O., 134
Hall, C. B., 64, 112, 596
Hall, J. E., 213, 279, 372
Hall, R. M., 508
Hallberg, D., 185
Hamlin, C., 189
Hammond, G., 46, 509
Hamon, G., 134
Hampole, M. K., 186
Hampton, A. O., 277
Hampton, O. P., Jr., 488, 616
Hamsa, W. R., Jr., 369
Hancock, D. D., 213
Hand, W. L., 544
Hanelin, J., 133
Hanger, H. B., 403
Hansen, S. T., 401
Hansen-Street, 380
Haraldsson, S., 46
Hardacre, J. A., 90
Hardin, C. A., 46
Hardy, J. D., 616
Harmon, P. H., 46, 509
Harrey, J. P., Jr., 544
Harrington, K. D., 372
Harrington, P. R., 229, 237-248, 249, 251, 278, 279, 280
Harris, C., 187
Harris, C., Jr., 187
Harris, C. M., 135, 371
Harris, H. W., 614
Harris, N. H., 372
Harris, R. B., 543
Harris, R. I., 277, 280, 543, 594
Harris, W. H., 330, 369, 372, 373, 375, 401, 618
Harris, W. R., 488, 618
Harrison, M. H. M., 373, 378, 594
Harrison, S. H., 185
Harrison, W. E., Jr., 616
Hart, D. L., 213
Hartman, J. T., 213
Harty, M., 46, 90, 488
Hartz, M., 373
Harvey, F. J., 594
Harvey, J. P., 213, 509
Harvey, J. P., Jr., 112
Haskell, D. S., 279
Haslam, T., 48
Hassler, W. L., 594
Hastings, D., 46

Hastings, D. E., 134
Hauser, E. D. W., 420-421, 488
Haverson, S. B., 488
Hawkins, B. L., 486
Hawkins, F. B., 594
Hawkins, J. R., 213
Hayden, J. W., 135
Hayes, J. R., 135
Hayes, J. T., 373
Hayes, T. D., 280
Hays, M. B., 490
Hazelman, B. L., 133
Hebble, W. M., 376, 618
Heberling, J., 616
Heberling, J. A., 373
Hedrick, D. W., 594
Heiple, K. G., 184, 616
Heitn, J. S., 213
Helfet, A. J., 9, 46, 488
Heller, F. G., 545
Helton, D. O., 490
Henderson, E. D., 133
Henderson, E. W., 188
Henderson, M. S., 298, 373, 488, 489, 616
Hennessy, C. A., 489
Henning, C. E., 445, 488
Henrikson, B., 373
Henry, A. K., 112
Hensinger, R. N., 213, 280
Henson, G. F., 46
Heppenstall, M., 207, 279
Herndon, C. H., 369, 370, 373, 401, 561, 594, 616
Herndon, J. H., 135, 189
Herron, L. D., 213
Herschel, H., 90, 133, 490
Hersh, A., 594
Hesketh, K. T., 402
Heuston, J. T., 187, 188
Hewitson, W. A., 134
Heyman, C. H., 298, 373, 594
Heywood, A. W. B., 187
Hibbs, R. A., 279, 373
Hicks, J. H., 509
Hiertonn, T., 373
Higinbotham, N. L., 615, 616
Higmans, W., 490
Hijmans, W., 90, 133
Hilal, S. K., 279
Hilgenreiner, H., 373
Hill, A. G. S., 213
Hill, B. J., 213
Hill, H. A., 46
Hill, J. A., 487
Hill, L. J., 509
Hill, L. M., 593
Hill, N. A., 84, 90, 177, 188, 189
Hillman, J. W., 615
Hinchey, J. J., 373
Hindenach, 12
Hinman, F., Jr., 616
Hirsch, C., 277, 373

Hislop, H., 403
Hitchcock, C. R., 616
Hitchcock, H. H., 64
Hoaglund, F. T., 373, 509
Hodgen, J. T., 488
Hodgson, A., 213
Hodgson, A. R., 213, 278, 279, 280
Hoerner, E. F., 277
Hogshead, H. P., 373
Hohl, M., 134, 488, 616
Hoi, F. C., 91
Holden, C. E. A., 112
Holden, N., 375
Holden, W. D., 402
Holdsworth, D. E., 133
Holdsworth, F. W., 277
Holmes, J. C., 213
Holscher, E. C., 277
Holstein, P., 373
Holster, A., 64
Holt, E. P., 309, 373
Honner, R., 112, 187
Hoover, G. H., 594
Hoover, N. W., 491
Horelius, L., 46
Horn, C. E., 509
Horn, L. G., 614
Hornby, R., 543
Horwich, J. P., 91
Horwitz, M. T., 90
Horwitz, T., 543
Høstrup, H., 488
Hotchkiss, B., 403, 510
House, K., 403
Houston, J. K., 45
Howard, F. M., 46, 135
Howard, J. M., 614, 617
Howard, L. D., Jr., 187, 189
Howard, N. J., 186
Howe, W., Jr., 371
Howe, W. M., 488
Howorth, B., 277, 488
Howorth, M. B., 46, 277, 288, 373
Hoyt, W., 369
Huber, E., 140, 186
Hudgens, M. S. W., 277
Huebert, H. T., 279
Huff, S. H., 593
Hughes, C. W., 616, 618
Hughes, J. R., 509
Hughston, J. C., 112, 371, 373, 462, 464, 486, 488
Hundley, J. M., 64
Hungerford, D. S., 490
Hunt, D. D., 373
Hunt, H. L., 45
Hunt, J. C., 594
Hunter, G. A., 298, 373
Hunter, J. M., 186
Huntley, J. M., 544
Hutchinson, J. R., 487
Hutchinson, R. H., 280
Hutchison, R. H., 48

Hyatt, J. W., 64
Hybbinette, C.-H., 135
Hybbinette, S., 46
Hyman, I., 375

I

Ikeuchi, H., 618
Ilstrup, D. M., 369, 371
Immerman, E. W., 401
Inge, G., 488
Inge, G. A. L., 373
Ingersoll, R. E., 90
Inglis, A. E., 90, 112, 186, 189, 544, 612
Ingram, A. J., 544, 594
Inman, V. T., 23, 45, 46, 375, 402
Inoue, T., 616
Insall, J., 486, 488
Insall, J. N., 488, 490
Ionescu, L., 378
Irani, R. N., 594
Ireland, P. H., 370
Irstram, L. K. H., 375
Irwin, C. E., 488, 544, 593
Ivins, J. C., 373

J

Jack, E. A., 488
Jackson, D. W., 280
Jackson, J. P., 486, 489
Jackson, R. W., 489
Jacobs, B., 46, 378
Jacobs, J. K., 615
Jacobs, R. J., 64, 112
Jacobsen, T., 112
Jaffe, H. F., 64
Jaffe, H. L., 616
Jaffe, S., 112, 186
Jahr, J., 509
James, A. E., Jr., 594
James, C. C. M., 279
James, J. I. P., 187, 279
James, J. M., 616
James, S. L., 491
James, U., 373
Jamieson, W. G., 188
Janecki, C. J., 594
Janes, J. M., 47, 91
Jansen, K., 544
Janzen, J., 375, 377
Jeffress, V. H., 401
Jenkins, A. W., 213
Jenkins, J. A., 280
Jensen, J. S., 373
Jessing, P., 90
Jewett, E. L., 373
Jinkins, W. J., Jr., 46
Johansson, O., 64
Johnson, E. V., 508
Johnson, E. W., 369, 370, 373, 489, 544
Johnson, J. T. H., 489
Johnson, L. C., 64, 616
Johnson, L. H., 377

Johnson, L. L., 373, 406, 489
Johnson, M., 112
Johnson, R., 213
Johnson, R. A., 377
Johnson, R. J., 489
Johnson, R. M., 213, 214
Johnson, T. R., 489
Johnson, W. E., 614
Johnston, D. S., 614
Johnston, J. O., 372
Johnston, R. C., 373
Joll, C. A., 618
Jones, E. W., Jr., 45
Jones, F. E., 187
Jones, H. T., 488
Jones, J. B., 489
Jones, J. M., 373
Jones, J. R., 376
Jones, K. G., 452, 489, 509
Jones, R., 112, 578-579, 594
Jones, R. E., 489
Jones, W. N., 369, 401
Jordan, H. H., 489
Jordan, L. R., 376
Jouvinvoux, P., 279
Joy, G., 544
Joyce, J. J., 373
Joyce, J. J., III, 46, 90, 91, 371
Judet, J., 298, 373, 594
Judet, R., 298, 373
Justis, E. J., Jr., 134

K

Kalamchi, A., 213
Kalenak, A., 543
Kamanger, A., 370
Kambin, P., 277
Kampner, S. L., 133
Kanavel, A. B., 187, 190
Kaplan, E. B., 184, 185, 187, 189
Kaplan, S. S., 90
Kartalian, G., 595
Karuse, R. J., 45
Kates, A., 594
Katz, M. P., 489
Kaufer, H., 373, 489, 491
Kauffman, M. S., 487
Kaushal, S. P., 490
Kay, A., 594
Kaye, J., 280
Keats, S., 186, 373
Keats, T. E., 48
Keck, C., 544
Keggi, K. J., 374
Keim, H. A., 279, 594
Keiser, E., 616
Kelikian, H., 184, 489
Keller, W. L., 572-573, 594
Kelly, A. P., Jr., 186
Kelly, F. B., Jr., 593
Kelly, K. J., 188, 190
Kelly, P. J., 134, 374, 594, 616
Kelly, R. P., 616

Kelsey, J. L., 374
Kempkin, T. G., 491
Kendrick, J. I., 136
Kendrick, R. E., 561, 594
Kendrick, R. R., 509
Kennedy, J. C., 46, 489
Kennelly, B. M., 509
Kent, M., 487
Keokarn, T., 134
Kessler, I., 134, 185, 186
Kettelkamp, D. B., 90, 112, 184, 188, 489, 491
Kettlewell, J., 370
Key, J. A., 46, 90, 277, 278, 298, 402, 489, 509, 616
Keyes, D. C., 277
Kick, H. M., 134
Kidner, 566
Kidner, F. C., 374, 566, 594
Kienböck, R., 134
Kiene, R. H., 615
Kihn, R. B., 510
Kilburn, P., 374
Kilgor, E. S., 188
Kilgore, E. S., 188
Kilgore, W. E., 64
Killgren, J. H., 190
Kindling, P. H., 186
Kindred, R. G., 64
King, D., 64, 374, 490
King, P., 298
King, T., 509, 616
Kini, M. G., 90
Kinnunen, P., 374
Kirkpatrick, J. A., 614
Kirkup, J. R., 402
Kirwan, E., 372
Kirz, F. K., Jr., 615
Kite, J. H., 594
Klassen, R. A., 374
Klein, L., 371, 615
Kleinert, 604, 613
Kleinert, H. F., 135
Klemek, J. S., 371
Klossner, O., 544
Knight, R. A., 46, 90, 112, 134, 298, 374, 594, 616
Knodt, H., 374
Knowles, F. L., 374
Knutsson, B., 277, 402, 509
Koch, S. L., 185, 186, 187
Kohl, E. J., 371
Koenig, M. J., 615
Koontz, W. C., 617
Kopell, H. P., 135, 543, 544
Kopits, S. E., 213
Korn, M. W., 374
Koshino, T., 486
Koskinen, E. V. S., 616
Kostuik, J. P., 488
Kraus, D., 214
Krida, A., 489
Kruper, J. S., 45

Krupp, S., 508
Kuczynski, K., 188
Kuderna, H., 374
Kuhns, J. G., 190
Küntscher, G., 380, 402
Kurtz, J. F., 90
Kurze, T., 213
Kushner, I., 616
Kutler, 604
Kyle, R. F., 374

L

Lacey, T., III, 136
Lagrange, J., 373
Laine, V., 90
Laine, V. A., 188
Laine, V. A. I., 188, 190
Laing, P. G., 369, 614, 616
LaLonde, A. A., 136
Lam, S. J., 112, 186
Lam, S. J. S., 489, 544, 594, 616
Lamb, D. W., 48, 91, 136, 187
Lamb, R. H., 509
Lambert, C. N., 64
Lambert, E. H., 135
Lambotte, A., 544
Lambrinudi, C., 594
LaMont, R. L., 509
Lance, E. M., 133, 616, 619
Landmark, J. J., 374
Landry, R. M., 189
Landsmeer, J. M. F., 133, 187
Lane, W. A., 544
Lang, A. G., 374
Lang, J. R., 280
Langenskiöld, A., 374, 489
Lansche, W. E., 491
Lapidus, P. W., 46, 190, 594
Larmon, W. A., 90, 594
Larsen, J., 486
Larsen, L. J., 90, 370, 593
Larsen, R. D., 187
Larson, C. B., 90, 135, 373, 374, 377
Larson, R. L., 408, 445, 448, 472, 491
Larsson, K., 510
Lasda, N. A., 374
Lasserre, C., 189
Lassman, L. T., 279
Last, R. J., 133, 489, 594
Lauder, C. H., 279, 280
Laufman, H., 614
Laurent, L. E., 280
Laurin, C. A., 489, 490, 544
Laurnen, E. L., 64
Lovell, W. W., 593
Law, W. A., 374, 377
Lawrence, G. H., 544
Lazansky, M. G., 374
Leach, R. E., 91, 189, 489, 509
Leadbetter, G. W., 374
Leaf, E., 374
Leaverton, P., 489
Lechtman, C. P., 595

Leclerc, D., 545
LeCocq, J. F., 543
Lee, H. G., 544
Lee, M. L. H., 133, 185
Lee, T.-S., 370
L'Episcopo, J. B., 34-35, 46
Leffert, R. D., 46, 186
Lefon, M., 545
Leider, L., 279
Leidholt, J. D., 488
LeMesurier, A. B., 46
Leonard, M. H., 544
Leslie, J. T., Jr., 46
Letournel, E., 298
Leukens, C. A., 280
Levin, M., 136
Lewinnek, G. E., 487
Levisohn, E. M., 374
Levy, M., 402
Levy, S. J., 46
Lewin, M. L., 617
Lewin, P., 594
Lewis, G. B., 64
Lewis, M. H., 135
Lewis, N. R., 491
Lewis, R., 376
Lewis, R. C., Jr., 374
Li, C. S., 135, 186
Liao, S. J., 402
Lichtenstein, L., 617
Lichter, R. L., 112
Lichtman, D. M., 136
Lidge, R. T., 489
Liebolt, F. L., 373, 374
Lievano, A., 185
Liljedahl, S., 489
Lim, R. C., Jr., 509
Lindahl, O., 369
Lindenbaum, B., 615
Lindblom, K., 277
Lindholm, A., 185, 543
Lindholm, R. V., 374
Lindsay, W. K., 186
Lindström, J., 134
Lindvall, N., 489
Linscheid, R. L., 46, 90, 133, 134, 188, 544
Linton, P., 374
Linton, R. R., 617
Lipinski, S. W., 370, 401, 508, 614
Lipke, J., 491
Lippmann, R. K., 374
Lipscomb, P. R., 133, 134, 135, 136, 184, 188, 374, 489, 544, 594, 616, 617, 618
Lipscomb, P. R., Jr., 489
Lipscomb, P. R., Sr., 489
Lipson, S. J., 213
Lister, J., 617
Litchman, H., 489
Litchman, H. M., 46, 594
Littler, 110
Littler, J. W., 135, 156, 158, 184-187, 189, 190

Lévesque, H. P., 490
Livingstone, S. M., 90
Lloyd, R. G. C., 617
Lloyd-Roberts, G. C., 279, 374
Lockie, L. M., 375
Logan, N. D., 370
Logan, W. D., 617
Lombardo, S. J., 46
Longfield, M. D., 370
Longstein, J. E., 279, 280
Lopes, E. I., 134
Lorenz, A., 374
Losee, R. E., 489
Lottes, J. O., 373, 402, 500, 509
Love, J. G., 135, 278
Lovett, R. W., 594
Lowe, H. G., 487
Lowe, R. W., 280
Lowell, H. A., 279
Lowell, J. D., 298, 374
Lowman, C. L., 46
Lowry, J. H., 491
Lozano, J. C., 508
Lucas, D. B., 45, 369, 375, 402
Luck, J. V., 188, 374, 488
Ludloff, K., 340, 345, 374
Lugnegård, H., 134
Lumpkin, M. B., 617
Lumsden, R. M., II, 595
Lunceford, E. M., 375
Lunceford, E. M., Jr., 374
Lurie, M., 402
Lusskin, R., 46, 617
Lynch, A. C., 135
Lyons, W. R., 619

M

MacAusland, R., 90
MacAusland, W. R., 90, 91, 134
MacAusland, W. R., Jr., 402
MacCallum, P., 188
MacDonell, J. A., 45
MacEwen, 216
MacEwen, D. G., 594
MacEwen, G. D., 280, 374
Macey, H. B., 91
MacIntosh, D. L., 451, 459-461, 487, 489
MacKay, I. M., 238, 279
MacKenzie, I. G., 374
MacKinnon, W. B., 279
MacLellan, D. I., 47
Macnab, I., 46, 48, 277, 489
MacNab, I., 280, 378
Macnicol, M. F., 91
Madden, J., 188
Madelung, O. W., 136
Madsen, E., 186
Maeck, B. H., 64
Magliato, H. J., 372
Magnuson, P. B., 46, 489
Magnusson, R., 544
Mahoney, J. R., 489
Maisels, D. O., 184

Makin, M., 489
Malin, T. H., 543
Malka, J. S., 544
Mallock, J. D., 489
Malmgren, R. A., 617
Mani, V. S., 371
Mann, R. A., 595
Mann, T. S., 91
Mannerfelt, L., 135, 189, 190
Manning, C. W. S. F., 213
Manning, J. G., 615
Manning, K. R., 593
Mantz, F. A., 490
Maor, P., 402
Maravilla, K. R., 213
Marcove, R. C., 64, 376, 616
Margo, M. K., 595
Marie, P., 135
Marin, J. C., 136
Marinacci, A. A., 544
Markee, J. E., 133
Marmor, L., 91, 188, 402, 487, 489, 509, 617
Marrin, R. A., 489
Marsden, F. W., 508
Marshall, 449
Marshall, J. L., 491
Martell, W., 213
Martin, W. J., 374, 616
Martinek, H., 402
Mason, M. L., 184, 185, 186, 187, 617
Massie, W. K., 305, 374
Mast, W. A., 112
Matchett, F., 374
Maten, I., 187
Mather, C., 489
Matthews, L. S., 298, 373, 491
Matthewson, M. H., 91
Mauck, H. P., 489
Maudsley, R. H., 618
Mavor, G. E., 509
Maxwell, J. A., 213
May, B. J., 402, 509
May, V. R., Jr., 46
Mayer, L., 46, 91, 184, 375, 489, 617
Mayer, V., 488
Mayfield, G., 64, 112
Maylahn, D. J., 91, 487
Mayne, J. A., 46
Mazet, R., Jr., 134, 489, 544, 617, 618
Mazur, J. M., 543, 544
McBride, E., 509
McBride, E. D., 574-575, 595
McCarroll, H. R., 298, 375, 384-385, 402, 509, 596, 617
McCash, C. R., 188
McCaslin, F. E., Jr., 374
McCauley, J. C., 544
McCauley, J. C., Jr., 595
McClain, E. J., 136
McClain, E. J., Jr., 90
McCloy, N. P., 402
McCollough, N. C., III, 402

McCollum, D. E., 188
McCormack, R. M., 136, 184, 186
McCormick, D. W., 595
McCreath, S. W., 91
McCue, F. C., 112
McDade, W. C., 544
McDaniels, J. M., 403
McDonough, J. M., 375
McDougall, E. P., 186
McElvenny, R. T., 375, 617
McEwen, C., 133, 135
McFarland, B., 375, 489
McFarland, R. M., 188
McFarlane, R. M., 186, 189
McGinty, J. B., 489
McIntyre, J. L., 486
McIvor, R. R., 401
McJeraw, R. W., 213
McKee, G. K., 375
McKeever, D. C., 489
McKeever, F. M., 48, 91
McKenna, R., 490
McKenzie, D. S., 112
McLaughlin, H. L., 12, 23, 46, 47, 134, 402
McLean, F. C., 618
McLearie, M., 91
McLeod, W. D., 488
McMaster, M., 189
McMurray, T. P., 375
McNeill, T. W., 279
McNeur, J. C., 617
McPhee, I. B., 280
McPhee, I. D., 213
McReynolds, I. S., 402
Meadows, V., 403, 510
Medbö, I., 490
Medgyesi, S., 375
Medici, V., 509
Meisterling, R. C., 490
Menelaus, M. B., 375, 490
Mensor, M. C., 375
Mercer, W., 617
Merkow, W., 403
Merrill, E. F., 371
Mersheimer, W. L., 185
Merson, R. D., 91
Messner, M. B., 486
Metz, C. W., 508
Metz, C. W., Jr., 375
Metzger, W. I., 615
Meyer, A. W., 47
Meyer, T. L., 375
Meyerding, H. W., 91, 136, 188, 254, 277, 490
Meyers, M. H., 375
Michele, A. A., 375
Mikic, Z., 112
Milbourn, E., 47
Milch, H., 47, 112, 134, 362, 363, 375
Miles, J. S., 376, 615
Milford, L., 184, 617
Milford, L. W., 298, 377

Milgram, J. E., 402, 490, 544
Millar, E. A., 402, 510
Millard, D. R., Jr., 91
Millender, L. H., 133, 135, 187, 189, 190
Miller, A. J., 544
Miller, D. S., 47
Miller, E., 48
Miller, J. A., Jr., 375, 490, 544, 617
Miller, T. R., 298, 376
Miller, W. A., 593
Miller, W. E., 91
Millner, W. F., 369
Mindell, E. R., 595
Mister, W. J., 277
Mital, M. A., 91, 112
Mitchell, C. L., 576, 594, 595
Mitchell, N. S., 135
Mitra, R. N., 615
Mixter, W. J., 277
Moberg, E., 133, 169, 185, 617
Mobley, J. E., 91
Mochizuki, R. M., 490
Moe, J. H., 217, 278, 279, 280
Moellering, R. C., Jr., 617
Monk, C. J. E., 544
Montalbo, F. J., 280
Monteggia, G. B., 78-79, 91
Moody, S. F., 213
Mooney, V., 112, 509, 595, 617
Moore, A. T., 375
Moore, F. D., 617
Moore, F. H., 490
Moore, J. F., 189
Moore, R. D., 375
Moore, T. M., 375
Moore, W. S., 509
Morchio, F. J., 136
Morel, G., 278
Moretz, W. H., 509, 510
Morgan, H. C., 486, 614
Morgan, J. D., 618
Morgese, A. N., 373
Morley, T. R., 375
Morrey, B. F., 47, 91
Morris, E., 595
Morris, H. D., 544
Morris, J. de L. S., 135
Morris, J. M., 45, 112, 187
Morris, J. R., 486
Morse, T. S., 595
Mortens, J., 187
Morton, D. L., 617
Morton, J. H., 617
Morton, K. S., 509
Morton, T. G., 589, 595
Moschi, A., 488
Moseley, H. F., 47
Moseley, R. V., 510
Mouradian, W. H., 378
Mowat, A. G., 133, 486
Mozan, L., 375
Mozes, M., 509
Mubarak, S. J., 112

629

Mueller, K. H., 375
Mulder, J. D., 134, 187
Muldoon, S. M., 374
Muller, G. E., 402
Muller, G. M., 189
Muller, M. E., 319-325, 375, 617
Muller, W., 370
Mulroy, R. D., 375
Mumenthaler, A., 509
Mumford, E. B., 47
Murakami, H., 615
Murley, A. H. G., 189
Murphy, A. F., 185
Murphy, M. J., 213
Murphy, O. B., 544
Murphy, R. W., 277
Murray, G., 134
Murray, W. R., 375, 402, 616
Musnick, H., 133
Mussleman, J. P., 213
Mustard, W. T., 348-351, 352, 375
Mutz, S. B., 508
Myerding, H. W., 280

N

Nachemson, A., 217, 277, 279, 280
Nadel, C. I., 279
Naffziger, H. C., 617
Nagel, D. A., 184
Nahigian, S. H., 90
Naiman, P. T., 112, 375, 617
Nalebuff, E. A., 133, 135, 187, 189, 190
Napier, J. R., 189, 614
Narquist, D. H., 279
Navigato, W. J., 45
Needy, C., 615
Neer, C. S., II, 20, 22, 26, 47, 64, 402, 487, 614
Neibauer, J. J., 490
Nelson, C. L., Jr., 371, 487, 490, 491
Nelson, J. D., 617
Neufeld, A. J., 375, 377
Neugebauer, F. L., 280
Neviaser, J. S., 15, 23, 47, 490
Neviaser, R. J., 144, 185
Newman, J., 402
Newman, P. H., 213, 280, 375
Newton, N. C., 278
Nicholas, J. A., 490
Nichols, P. J. R., 491
Nicholson, J. D., 214
Nicholson, J. T., 127, 136, 184
Nicholson, O. R., 617
Nickel, V. L., 47, 112, 187, 207, 278, 279, 377, 595, 617
Nicola, T., 47
Nicoll, E. A., 375, 402, 509
Niebauer, J. J., 188, 189
Nimberg, G. A., 402
Nirschal, R. P., 91
Nishio, 326
Nissen, K. I., 375, 595
Nolan, D. R., 371

Nolan, N. G., 374
Nordin, J.-Y., 593
Norman, O., 135, 190
Norquist, D. H., 280
Norquist, D. M., 280
Norton, P. L., 277
Norwood, L. A., Jr., 490
Noyes, F. R., 490

O

Ober, F. R., 375, 595
Obletz, B. E., 133, 375, 617
O'Brien, E. T., 90, 372
O'Brien, J. P., 213, 280
O'Brien, J. T., 214
O'Connor, H., 544
Odell, R. I., 278
O'Donoghue, D. H., 47, 443, 445, 490, 617
Oh, I., 375
O'Hara, L. J., 136
Oka, M., 189
Olerud, S., 402
Oliver, C. H., 377
Olix, M. L., 377
O'Loughlin, B. J., 509
Olsson, S. S., 375
Omer, G. E., 136
Omer, G. E., Jr., 112, 186, 617
Omerod, J. A., 136
Omnaya, A. K., 278
Ong, G. B., 278
Onne, L., 617
O'Rahilly, R., 595
Orr, H. W., 490, 617
Ortengren, R., 277
Ortiz, A. C., 91
Ortiz, P. R., 544
Ortolani, M., 376
Osborne, G., 375
Osgood, R. B., 378, 617
Osmond-Clarke, H., 47
Osterman, K., 280
Ottolenghi, C. E., 376, 544, 617
Ottosson, L., 544
Ouellet, R., 490, 544
Övergaard, B., 47
Owen, C. A., 543
Owen, R., 47, 509
Owens, J. C., 617
Oyston, J. K., 47

P

Pack, G. T., 47, 298, 376
Padgett, E. C., 617
Page, P. W., 213
Paget, J., 136, 617
Pahle, J. A., 135
Palinacci, J.-Cl., 595
Palmer, R. M., 593
Palumbo, F., 213
Panjabi, M. M., 214, 280
Pankovich, A. M., 91, 544

Pankratz, D. G., 91
Paradies, L. H., 134, 490
Pardee, M. L., 490
Park, W. I., III, 112
Parker, L. B., 277
Parkes, J. C., II, 488
Parr, P. L., 376
Parrish, T. F., 376
Pasila, M., 45
Paterson, D. C., 376
Patrick, J., 490, 544, 617
Patterson, A. H., 544
Patterson, R. J., 376
Patterson, W. R., 47
Patte, D., 47, 48
Patzakis, M. J., 544
Paul, W. D., 90, 133, 490
Pauwels, F., 376
Pauzat, D., 189
Peabody, C. W., 544
Peacock, E. E., Jr., 184, 186
Pedersen, H. E., 45, 509, 595
Pegington, J., 91
Pellicci, P. M., 376
Pemberton, P. A., 298, 376
Penrose, J. H., 91
Perry, J., 187, 207, 278, 279, 403, 595, 617
Pers, M., 614
Peterson, C. D., 376
Peterson, H. A., 135
Peterson, L. F. A., 90, 486, 490
Peterson, L. T., 190, 376, 617
Peterson, R. E., 543
Pettee, D. S., 135
Pettrone, F. A., 91
Phalen, G. S., 136, 280
Phelps, W. M., 376
Phemister, D. B., 298, 433, 436, 490, 617, 618
Pierce, D. S., 48, 213
Pigott, J. D., 298
Pilcher, M. F., 279, 490
Pilgaard, S., 488
Pilliar, R. M., 378
Pillin, B., 279
Piotrowski, G., 401
Pistevos, G., 490
Platou, E., 376
Platt, H., 618
Pohlman, M. H., 184
Poigenfurst, J., 376
Poirier, H., 490
Pollock, G. A., 402
Pollock, L. J., 544
Polo, G., 595
Polyzoides, A. J., 486
Pomeranz, M. M., 376
Pomerat, C. M., 508, 615
Ponseti, 217
Ponseti, I. V., 373, 376, 595
Porter, B. B., 490
Porter, D. S., 369

Posch, J. L., 187
Postel, M., 369
Potenza, A. D., 186
Potter, R. A., 190
Potter, T. A., 190, 490
Potterson, R. K., Jr., 45
Power, G. R. I., 543
Predecki, P. K., 376
Prevost, Y., 135
Price, W. E., 619
Probhakar, M., 45
Protzman, R., 508
Pugh, W. L., 376
Pulkki, T., 133, 189
Pulvertaft, R. G., 150, 186, 618
Puranen, J., 374
Purvis, G. D., 112
Putti, V., 376
Pyka, R. A., 618
Pyle, S. I., 488

Q

Quigley, T. B., 47, 48, 490, 544

R

Radin, E. L., 91
Raghaven, V. C., 595
Ralston, E. L., 378
Ramirez, Z. M. A., 618
Ramon, Y., 509
Ramsay, R. H., 402, 509
Ramsby, G. R., 213
Ramselaar, J. M., 187
Rana, N. A., 213
Ranawat, C. S., 90, 135, 136, 371, 376, 488
Rank, B. K., 184, 186
Ransford, A. O., 213
Rapp, G. F., 376, 618
Ratliff, A. H. C., 544
Raunio, P., 48, 135
Ray, R., 618
Ray, R. D., 210, 277, 278, 618
Ray, R. L., 490
Razzano, C. D., 371
Rechtman, A. M., 133
Reckling, F. W., 90, 490
Record, E. E., 509, 543, 618
Redhead, R. G., 510
Reed, J. R., 184
Regan, J. M., 491
Regan, T., 488
Reich, R. S., 376
Reichelderfer, T. E., 486
Reid, S. F., 136
Reiman, I., 189
Rein, B. I., 488
Reisch, J. S., 489
Relton, J. E. S., 279
Rennels, D. C., 596
Resnick, D., 543
Retzan, S. A., 213

Reyes, R. L., 509
Reynolds, F. C., 45, 374, 402, 490, 615
Rhinelander, F. W., 509, 615
Rich, N. M., 618
Richards, J. F., 90
Richards, R. L., 508
Richards, V., 298
Riddell, D. M., 186
Rideout, D. F., 45
Riley, L. H., Jr., 490
Rinehard, W. T., 543
Ring, P. A., 376
Riordan, D. C., 112, 133, 134, 136, 187, 188, 618
Riseborough, E. J., 91, 280
Riska, E. B., 489
Risser, J. C., 234, 279, 280
Ritchie, G. W., 594
Ritter, M. A., 376
Rix, P. R., 595
Rob, C., 90, 279
Robbins, H., 136
Roberts, A. H., 277
Roberts, J. B., 91
Roberts, J. M., 490, 615
Robins, R. H. C., 184
Robinson, H. J., 376
Robinson, R. A., 508
Robinson, S., 278
Robinson, W. C., 378
Roca, J., 136
Roche, M. B., 280
Rodrigo, J. J., 188
Rogers, S. P., 508
Rogers, W. A., 213
Rokkanen, P., 402, 509
Romano, R. L., 401, 508
Roon, A. J., 509
Roos, 195
Roosth, H. P., 376
Ropes, M. E., 618
Rosen, S. von, 376
Rosenberg, J. C., 594
Rosenberg, N. J., 280, 490
Rosenfeld, H., 402
Rosenman, L. D., 544
Rosenthal, J. J., 402
Rosianu, I., 378
Rothman, R. H., 213, 214, 278, 371
Roux, D., 490
Rowe, C. R., 12, 23, 47, 48, 298, 486, 595
Rower, C. R., 48
Rowland, S. A., 185
Royle, N. D., 187
Ruben, F. L., 616
Rubin, G., 544
Rubin, R., 376
Ruiz-Mora, 591
Rusch, R. M., 213
Rush, H. L., 112, 402
Rush, L. V., 402, 509, 618
Rusk, L. V., 112

Russe, O., 134
Russe, O. A., 376
Russell, E., 490
Russin, L. D., 213
Ruth, C. J., 544
Rutherford, R. E., 402
Rutkowski, R., 487
Ryan, T. J., 46
Rybka, V., 48
Ryder, C. T., 376, 377
Ryerson, E. W., 595

S

Saad, M. N., 618
Sachs, M. D., 46
Sage, F. P., 112, 402
St. Jacques, R., 544
Sairanin, E., 188
Sakellarides, H., 64, 618
Sakellarides, H. T., 48, 185, 187, 509
Salama, R., 378
Salenius, P. A., 376
Saletta, J. D., 618
Salisbury, R. E., 186
Salter, R. B., 288, 298, 344, 376, 377, 595, 618
Salvati, E. A., 376, 377
Salvatori, J. E., 370
Salzman, E. W., 373, 616
Samilson, R. L., 48, 112, 187, 377, 618, 619
Sammarco, J. G., 544
Samuelson, K. M., 593
Sanchez, J. G., 544
Sanchez, J. J., 594
Sankaran, B., 618
Sargent, J. P., 112
Sarmiento, A., 377, 402, 544
Sarpio, O., 374
Saunders, J. B. de C. M., 45, 46, 64, 135, 486
Sayre, R. H., 184
Schein, A. J., 112, 375, 617
Scaglietti, O., 254, 280, 377
Scal, P. V., 490
Scales, J. T., 618
Schaffner, W., 615
Schajowicz, F., 373, 618
Scham, S., 486
Schantz, A., 377
Scheck, M., 375, 377
Schecter, L., 378
Scheller, S., 373
Schenck, R., 187
Scheuermann, H. W., 248, 280
Schiffman, E., 213
Schlesinger, P. T., 278
Schlossman, D., 488
Schmid, L., 402
Schmidt, G. H., 112
Schneider, H. W., 402
Schneider, L. H., 187
Schnell, A., 402

Schottstaedt, E. R., 90, 370, 486, 593, 595
Schrey, E. L., 402
Schrock, R. D., 48, 508
Schrock, R. D., Jr., 509
Schulenburg, C. A. R., 615
Schultz, R. T., 185
Schurman, D. J., 490, 595
Schwartz, D. I., 48
Schwartz, E., 544
Schwartz, R. P., 595
Schwartzmann, J. R., 371, 377, 402
Schweigel, J. F., 213
Scott, D. J., 594
Scott, D. J., Jr., 12, 48
Scott, J. C., 377
Scott, P. J., 377
Scott, W. N., 488, 544
Scuderi, C., 390, 402, 618
Scuderi, C. S., 112, 371, 543
Sculco, T. P., 544
Secor, C., 64
Seddon, 110
Seddon, H., 46
Seddon, H. J., 136, 370, 374, 617, 618
Seelenfreund, M., 402
Seinscheimer, F., III, 377
Seligson, D., 487
Sell, K. W., 64
Semb, H. T., 595
Semple, J. C., 136
Sengelmann, R. P., 189
Settle, G. W., 595
Sever, J. W., 48
Shafer, S. J., 46
Shaffer, S. R., 593
Shands, A. R., 594
Shands, A. R., Jr., 374, 595
Shapiro, F., 595
Shapiro, J. S., 135, 189
Sharma, N. K., 594
Sharp, N., 377
Sharrard, W. J. W., 348, 352-355, 370, 377
Shaw, J. L., 64, 89
Shaw, N. E., 595
Shaw, P. C., 186
Shea, C. E., Jr., 377
Shea, J. D., 136
Shearon, C. G., 617
Shelton, M. L., 402
Sherik, S. K., 112
Sherk, H. H., 214
Sherman, C. D., Jr., 294, 298
Sherman, M. S., 372, 594, 618
Sherman, W. O. N., 618
Sherwood, A. A., 278
Shin, J. S., 370
Shindler, T. O., 508, 615
Shine, J., 488
Shinno, N., 491
Shoji, H., 488, 490
Short, M. D., 375

Shouse, L., 545
Shriber, W. J., 401
Siber, F. J., 489
Siberman, Z., 509
Sideman, S., 490
Siegel, I., 490
Siewers, C. F., 508
Siffert, R. S., 112, 375, 617, 618
Silver, C., 489
Silver, C. M., 46, 594, 595
Simeone, F. A., 278
Simmons, E. F., 213
Simmons, E. H., 595
Simon, S., 489
Simon, S. D., 46, 594
Simon, S. R., 543, 544
Simon, W. H., 377
Simpson, D. C., 48
Sinclair, W. F., 402
Sisk, T. D., 45, 112, 403
Skiadaressis, G., 508
Skilbred, L. A., 545
Sklar, F. H., 213
Skoog, T., 185, 188
Skownund, H. H. V., 213
Slager, R. F., 375, 377
Slätis, P., 402, 509
Sledge, C. B., 543
Slocum, D. B., 64, 112, 133, 408, 445, 448, 472, 491, 509, 595, 618
Smillie, I. S., 490, 491
Smith, B., 491
Smith, D. M., 377
Smith, E. C., 489
Smith, F. G., 377
Smith, F. M., 91
Smith, H., 112, 134, 298, 402
Smith, J. B., 595
Smith, J. E. M., 402
Smith, J. M., 277
Smith, J. W., 135, 185
Smith, L., 64, 134, 213
Smith, M. G. H., 90, 544, 593
Smith, R., 90, 279
Smith, R. C., 544
Smith, R. F., 401
Smith, R. J., 185, 189
Smith, R. W., 134
Smith, T. K., 213
Smith, W. S., 377
Smith-Petersen, M. N., 135, 292, 298, 377
Smoley, E. M., 595
Smyth, M. J., 278
Snelson, R., 509, 617
Sneppen, O., 544
Snook, G. A., 508, 543
Snyder, B., 214
Sofield, H. A., 402, 509, 510
Sokoloff, L., 190
Sollars, R., 402, 509
Solomons, C., 376
Somerville, E. W., 298, 377

Sones, D. A., 133
Sonstegard, D., 373
Sonstegard, D. A., 490, 491
Soper, K. P., 489
Sorenson, R. I., 377
Soto-Hall, R., 64, 134, 377, 402, 491
Sotos, L. N., 378
Southgate, W. A., 617
Southmayd, W. W., 48
Southwick, W. O., 184, 213, 214, 374, 489, 491
Souter, W. A., 187
Soutter, R., 377
Spademan, R., 510
Speed, J. S., 91, 134, 491, 544, 594
Speed, K., 48, 377, 618
Speer, D. S., 374
Spence, K. F., 64
Spence, K. F., Jr., 298
Spencer, G. E., Jr., 370, 510
Spielholz, N. I., 543
Spinner, M., 136, 185
Spjut, H. J., 614
Sprague, B., 134
Sprecher, E. E., 190
Stableforth, P. G., 543
Stack, H. G., 135, 188
Stack, J. K., 46, 136
Stagnara, P., 229, 279, 280
Stahl, F., 402, 509
Stamp, W. G., 486, 491, 614
Staples, O. S., 91, 544
Stark, H. H., 185, 189, 614
Stark, R. B., 184
Stark, W. A., 510
Starr, D. E., 491, 509
States, J. D., 374, 509
Stauffer, R. N., 278, 545
Steel, H. H., 298
Stein, I., 135
Steindler, 556
Steindler, A., 48, 82, 84, 91, 135, 279, 545
Steingass, N. H., 213
Stellbrink, G., 190
Stelling, F. H., 133, 184
Stener, B., 48, 165, 185
Stephen, J., 280
Stephens, J. S., 376
Sternach, R. A., 278
Stevens, D. B., 618
Stevens, J., 491
Stevenson, J. K., 615
Stewart, M., 134, 491
Stewart, M. J., 64, 134, 298, 377, 402, 403, 545
Stewart, R., 489
Stewart, W. J., 615
Steytler, J. C. S., 595
Still, J. M., Jr., 510
Stinchfield, F. E., 278, 375, 377, 488, 596, 619
Stock, F. E., 279

Stöffel, A., 510
Stone, K. H., 280
Stone, M. M., 136
Stören, G., 508
Stougård, J., 491
Stout, A. P., 618
Strachan, J. C. H., 91
Straub, L. R., 90, 133, 134, 135, 136, 188, 189, 190, 491
Strayer, L. M., Jr., 504-505, 510
Street, D. M., 401, 402, 403
Streitz, W., 280
Stroot, J. H., 64
Stromber, W. B., Jr., 614
Stromberg, W. B., 618
Stromberg, W. B., Jr., 185
Strong, J. M., 187, 373, 594
Stryker, W. S., 489, 509
Stuart, D., 190
Stubbins, S. G., 133
Stuck, W. G., 378, 491, 510, 618
Sturman, M. J., 618
Sudeck, P., 184
Suk, S., 278
Sullivan, C. R., 594
Summits, R. L., 614
Sunzel, H., 510
Sutro, C. J., 185
Sutton, F. S., Jr., 491
Swan, M., 374
Swanson, A. B., 112, 133, 135, 157, 161, 184, 185, 187, 189, 403, 510, 595, 618
Swanson, G. DeG., 595
Swanson, S. A. V., 486
Sweet, E. D., 369
Sweetnan, R., 213
Syme, J., 535-536, 545
Szaboky, G. T., 595

T

Taber, T. H., 188
Tachdjian, M. O., 377, 618
Taddonio, R. F., 279
Taillard, W., 544
Taillard, W. F., 280
Takeda, S., 618
Taleisnik, J., 134
Tambornino, J. M., 279
Tanner, E., 135
Tanzer, R. C., 136
Tapper, E. M., 491
Taussig, G., 593
Taylor, A. R., 213, 369, 618
Taylor, G. M., 375, 377
Taylor, J. G., 90
Taylor, L. W., 403
Taylor, R. G., 377
Taylor, T. C., 280
Taylor, T. K. F., 277
Taylor, W. F., 486
Tedeschi, C. G., 618
Tedeschi, L. G., 618
Teipner, W. A., 112

Telfer, N., 375
Terwilliger, C. K., 374
Terz, J., 64
Thibodeau, A., 298
Thibodeau, A. A., 133
Thomas, C. L., 280
Thomas, F. B., 545, 595
Thomas, J. E., 135
Thomas, W. H., 490, 543
Thompkins, F., 490
Thompson, 516
Thompson, C. H., 491
Thompson, E. B., 486
Thompson, F. R., 370, 377
Thompson, M. S., 403
Thompson, R. G., 375, 403, 487, 510
Thompson, T. C., 133, 187, 189, 403, 491, 595
Thompson, W. A., 544
Thompson, W. A. L., 48, 278
Thompson, W. W., 596
Thomson, J. E. M., 618
Thorling, J., 46
Thorndike, A., 48, 403
Thorndike, A., Jr., 48
Tinel, J., 618
Tobin, C. E., 136
Tobin, W. J., 378
Todd, T. W., 91, 491
Tohen, A., 595
Tøjner, H., 280
Tomford, W. W., 375
Tompkins, D. G., 91
Torgerson, W. R., 91, 491
Tooms, R. E., 112
Tosberg, W. A., 510
Trammel, T. R., 370
Tratt, G., 617
Traub, J. E., 401, 508
Tredwell, S. J., 214
Tregunning, R. J., 489
Trentani, 326
Tressler, H. A., 369
Trevor, D., 374
Trillat, A., 422-423, 427, 462, 491
Trott, A. W., 543
Trout, P. C., 491
Truchly, G., 48, 278
Trueta, J., 373, 378, 403, 491, 618
Trumble, H. C., 378
Tsimboukis, B., 509
Tubiana, R., 186, 187, 188
Tullos, H. S., 279, 280, 488
Turco, V. J., 557, 595
Turner, R. H., 280
Turnio, G. M., 278
Turnipseed, D., 401

U

Ulin, R., 543
Unander-Scharin, L., 486
Urban, J. G., 614
Urbaniak, 613

Urbaniak, J. R., 186, 188
Uriburu, I. J. F., 136
Uricchio, J. V., Jr., 509
Urist, M. L., 378
Urist, M. R., 48, 618
Uthus, D., 488

V

Vahvanen, V. A., Jr., 595
Vainio, K., 48, 90, 134, 188, 189, 190, 596
Valentin, P., 187
Van Der Linden, W., 510
Van der Walt, I. D., 595
Van Gorder, G. W., 91, 377, 378, 491, 545
Van Nes, C. P., 510
Van Wagoner, F. H., 508
VanDemark, R. E., 490
Vanderpool, D. W., 91, 136
VanGrouw, A., Jr., 279
Vankka, E., 402
Vanzelle, C., 279
Vasli, S., 545
Vaughan, B. A., 376
Vaughan-Jackson, O. J., 133, 135, 190
Vaughen, J., 277
Veith, F. J., 616
Veleanu, C., 378
Venable, C. S., 378, 491, 618
Veran, J., 595
Verdan, C. E., 184, 186
Vesely, D. G., 133, 135, 378, 403
Vichard, Ph., 545
ViGario, G. D., 48
Vise, G. T., Jr., 403
Vitale, M., 510
Voshell, A. F., 377, 486, 508
Voss, C., 378

W

Waddell, J. P., 510
Waddell, J., 509
Wade, P. A., 46, 510
Wagner, C. S., 185
Wagner, F. W., Jr., 509
Wagner, H., 326, 378
Wagner, J., 596
Wakefield, A. R., 184, 186
Wakim, K. G., 617
Walker, D. M., 489
Wallace, S. L., Jr., 403
Waller, A., 298
Walmsley, R., 486
Walter, C. E., 618
Wang, J. F., 279
Waring, T. L., 369
Waring, W., 47
Warren, L. F., 491
Warren, R., 510, 545, 596
Warren, W. D., 509
Washington, E. R., 214
Watanabe, M., 491, 618

633

Watelet, F., 545
Waters, R. L., 403
Watkins, 254, 258
Watkins, M. B., 377, 618, 619
Watson, H. K., 135, 184
Watson-Farrar, J., 375
Watson-Jones, R., 48, 91, 319, 378, 403, 510, 532, 545, 619
Waugh, T. R., 278, 596, 619
Waugh, W., 488, 489
Weaver, J. K., 48
Weber, A. L., 370
Weber, B. G., 378
Weckesser, E., 186
Weckesser, E. C., 184, 185
Weed, L. A., 616
Weeks, P. M., 189
Weierman, R. J., 279
Weiland, A. J., 190
Weinberg, A. N., 617
Weinberg, H., 489
Weinberg, H. W., 489
Weiner, D. S., 48, 369
Weinfeld, M. S., 490
Weiss, C., 186
Weiss, C. A., 46
Weiss, N. H., 213
Weissman, S. L., 378
Wells, R. E., 401
Welsh, R. P., 378
Wenger, D. R., 280
Wenger, R. J. J., 596
Wentworth, E. T., 491
Wentz, I. J., 595
Weseley, M. S., 91, 596
Wessler, S., 619
West, F. E., 401, 491
West, W. F., 45
Westerborn, A., 298
Westin, G. W., 213, 370, 403, 510, 545, 595, 596
Wetterfors, J., 489
Wetzler, S. H., 403
Whalley, R. C., 596
Whellock, F. C., Jr., 596
Whipple, T. L., 491
Whiston, T. B., 91, 136
White, 433
White, A. A., III, 214, 280
White, J. W., 545
White, R. R., 46, 594
White, W. L., 152, 185, 619
Whitefield, G. A., 491

Whitman, A., 48
Whitman, R., 378, 596
Whittaker, R. P., 378
Wiberg, G., 378, 491
Wickstrom, J., 48, 403
Widell, E. H., 280
Wiesal, S., 214
Wiesman, H. J., Jr., 378
Wilber, M. C., 403
Wilbur, M. C., 64
Wilde, A. H., 371, 491, 594
Wilde, A. M., 371
Wiles, P., 378, 491
Wiley, J. H., 401, 508, 614
Wiley, J. J., 91
Wilgis, E. F. S., 619
Wilkinson, J., 491
Wilkinson, M., 135
Wilkinson, M. C., 491
Willenegger, H., 617
Williams, E. M., 377, 402
Williams, G. R., 619
Williams, P. F., 403
Williams, R., 187
Willien, L. J., 371
Willis, T. A., 278
Willner, P., 491
Wilson, A. B., 403, 508
Wilson, A. B., Jr., 401, 545, 619
Wilson, A. B. K., 48
Wilson, A. S., 489
Wilson, E. H., 190
Wilson, F. C., Jr., 545, 596
Wilson, H. J., 545
Wilson, J. C., 48
Wilson, J. C., Jr., 112
Wilson, J. N., 91, 185, 491, 596
Wilson, P. D., 91, 376, 378, 491, 619
Wilson, P. D., Jr., 376, 377, 401
Wiltse, L. L., 254, 258, 278, 280
Winant, E., 593
Winer, J., 46
Wingate, K., 112
Wingo, C. H., 401
Winter, G. D., 618
Winter, R. B., 279, 280
Winters, D. M., 619
Wise, D. W., 488
Wissinger, A., 190
Witten, D. M., 213
Witten, M., 544
Wohl, M. A., 133
Wolf, M. D., 596

Wolinsky, E., 616
Woltman, H. W., 136
Wong, S. K., 280
Wong, W. L., 373
Woo, S. L-Y., 277
Wood, G. O., 616
Wood, W. L., 510, 545
Woodhall, B., 619
Woods, G. W., 488
Woodward, J. W., 48
Wray, C. H., 510
Wray, J. B., 45, 510
Wright, A. D., 135
Wright, D. J., 596
Wright, H. A., 277
Wright, J. L., 593
Wright, T. A., 185
Wright, V., 615
Wright, V. J., 278
Wu, J. T., 213
Wyard, G. E., 596
Wyatt, G. M., 488
Wyman, E. T., Jr., 377
Wynn, P. C. B., 491

Y

Yablon, I. G., 545
Yamada, K., 491
Yassini, Z., 90
Yau, A. C., 213, 373
Yee, L. B. K., 12, 48, 486
Yeoh, C. B., 133
Young, H. H., 278, 486, 491
Young, J. M., 619
Yount, C. C., 339, 378, 403
Yu, P. N., 278
Yuan, H. A., 374

Z

Zachary, R. B., 34-35, 48, 112, 508
Zadek, I., 596
Zancolli, E. A., 112, 184, 187
Zeier, F., 486
Zettl, J. H., 401, 508
Zickel, R. E., 378
Zielke, K., 271, 279
Zlotsky, N., 510, 545
Zohn, D. A., 489
Zorab, P. A., 279
Zuck, F. N., 112
Zuege, R. C., 279, 491

SUBJECT INDEX

A

Abductor pollicis longus tendon, tenosynovitis of, tenolysis for, 114-115
Abductors, hip, paralysis of; see Paralysis of hip abductors
Above-elbow amputation, 59-61
Above-knee amputation, 398-400
Accessory tarsal navicular, excision of, 566-567
Acetabular fracture, displaced, open reduction and internal fixation for, 292-293
Acetabuloplasty, 284-287
Achilles tendon; see Tendo Achillis
Acromioclavicular separation, repair of, 15-16
Acromioplasty, anterior, Neer, 20-22
Acrosyndactyly, 180
Adduction, forefoot, resistant, tarsometatarsal mobilization for, 561
Adduction contracture
  and internal rotation of shoulder, release of, Sever procedure for, 32-33
  thumb, release of, 164
Adductor longus and brevis, origin of, transfer of, to ischial tuberosity, 358
Adductor tenotomy, 336
Adolescent hallux valgus, reconstructive osteotomy of first metatarsal for, 576-577
Adolescent idiopathic scoliosis, 216
Advancement
  patellar, 428
  volar plate, for dorsal fracture-dislocation of proximal interphalangeal joint, 167
Amputation
  above-elbow, 59-61
  above-knee, 398-400
  below-elbow, 102-103
  below-knee, 506-507
  fingertip, traumatic, 603-605

Amputation—cont'd
  Syme, modified, 535-536
  transmetatarsal, 570
Animetric total knee replacement (nonconstrained), 477-480
Ankle, 511-542
  arthrodesis of
    compression, anterior approach to, 540-542
    lateral approach to, 537-539
  drainage of, 534
  lateral ligaments of, reconstruction of, 532-533
Anterior acromioplasty, Neer, 20-22
Anterior approach
  to compression arthrodesis of ankle, 540-542
  to open reduction and bone graft for fracture of scaphoid, 121-122
Anterior cervical spine fusion, 205-206
Anterior cruciate ligament of knee
  reconstruction of, 452-454
  repair of, 449-451
Anterior dislocation of shoulder, recurrent, repair of, 2-8
  Bristow procedure for, 9-11
Anterior drainage of hip joint, 359-360
Anterior impingement syndrome, 20
Anterior interbody fusion with Dwyer instrumentation, 268-271
Anterior spine fusion
  by retroperitoneal approach to lumbar spine, 261-263
  by thoracoabdominal approach, 264-267
Anterior tibial compartment, fasciotomy of, 502-503
Anterior tibial compartment syndrome, acute, 502
Anterior tibial tendon
  lateral transfer of, 564-565
  rupture of, repair of, 519-520
Anterior transplantation of ulnar nerve, 88-89

Anterolateral approach
  to insertion of femoral head prosthesis, 316
  to open reduction for tibial shaft fracture, 494-496
Anterolateral rotatory instability of knee, chronic, modified MacIntosh reconstruction for, 459-461
Antibiotics, prophylactic, for posterior spine fusion and Harrington instrumentation, 248
Appliance, telescoping, for pinning of subcapital fracture of femur, 304-305
Arm, upper, 49-63
Arrest, epiphyseal, of distal femur
  by epiphysiodesis, 433-435
  by stapling, 436-438
Artery, severed, rupture of, 598-599
Arthritis
  degenerative, at carpometacarpal joint of thumb, 175
  rheumatoid, of wrist, 128, 129
Arthrodesis
  of ankle
    compression, anterior approach to, 540-542
    lateral approach to, 537-539
  of carpometacarpal joint of thumb, 175-176
  of foot
    subtalar (Grice procedure), 550-552
    triple, 548-549
  of hip, 366-368
  of knee, compression, 484-485
  of proximal interphalangeal joint, 581-584
    for claw toe, 583-584
    for hammertoe, 581-582
  shoulder, 43-44
  of small joints of hand, 177-179
  of wrist, 129-131
Arthroplasty
  of carpometacarpal joint of thumb, 175
  cup, 330-335

635

Arthroplasty—cont'd
  replacement, of metacarpophalangeal joint, 161-163
Arthroscopy of knee, 406-407
Arthrotomy of knee, 410, 415
Asymptomatic spondylolisthesis, 232
Atlantoaxial spine fusion, 201-202
Axillary approach to resection of first rib, 195-197

B

Baker's cyst, excision of, 470-471
Base of thumb metacarpal, fracture of, open reduction and internal fixation for, 168-169
Below-elbow amputation, 102-103
Below-knee amputation, 506-507
Benign bone cyst of humerus, curettage and bone graft for, 54-56
Bennett's fracture, 168-169
Biceps, long head of, tendon of, tenodesis of, 57-58
Biceps brachii muscle, distal tendon of, rupture of, repair of, 80-81
Bicipital tenosynovitis, 57
Bilateral lateral approach, posterolateral spine fusion by, 258-260
Biopsy
  bone, 610-611
  muscle, 612
Blood replacement and monitoring during posterior spine fusion and Harrington instrumentation, 247
Bone
  donor, removal of, from iliac wing for bone graft, 282-283
  sesamoid, tibial, excision of, 580
  tarsal navicular, accessory, excision of, 566-567
Bone biopsy, 610-611
Bone cyst, benign, of humerus, curettage and bone graft for, 54-56
Bone graft
  curettage and, for benign bone cyst of humerus, 54-56
  open reduction and, for fracture of scaphoid, anterior approach to, 121-122
  removal of donor bone from iliac wing for, 282-283
Boutonniere deformity of finger, repair of, 158
Bristow procedure for repair of recurrent anterior dislocation of shoulder, 9-11
Bunionette, exostectomy for, 590
Bursitis, calcific, of shoulder, 18

C

Calcaneal spur, excision of, 555
Calcaneocuboid joint, arthrodesis of, 548-549
Calcaneonavicular coalition, 568
Calcaneus
  osteotomy of, Dwyer procedure for, 553-554
  transfer of posterior tibial and peroneus brevis tendons to, 524-526
Calcific bursitis of shoulder, 18
Calcific deposit of shoulder, excision of, 18-19
Capsulotomy of knee, posterior, 418-419
Caput ulnae syndrome, 159
Carpal ligament, transverse, release of, for carpal tunnel syndrome, 116-117
Carpal tunnel syndrome, release of, transverse carpal ligament for, 116-117
Carpometacarpal joint of thumb
  arthrodesis of, 175-176
  arthroplasty of, 175
Cast, localizer, for correction of scoliosis, 234-237
Cerebral palsy, release of flexor-pronator origin of forearm for, 94-95
Cervical spine, neck and, 191-212
Cervical spine fusion
  anterior, 205-206
  posterior, 198
    C3 and below, 203-204
Charnley-Müller method of total hip reconstruction, 319-325
Classification
  of lumbosacral spondylolisthesis, 254
  of spine deformity, 216
Clavicle
  lateral end of, resection of, 17
  open reduction and internal fixation of, 28-29
Clawing
  of fingers secondary to ulnar nerve palsy, tendon transfers for, 142-143
  of toe, Jones procedure for, 578-579
Closed tube irrigation and drainage of localized musculoskeletal areas, 607
Clubfoot, equinovarus, resistant, medial soft tissue release for, 557-560
Clubhand, radial, surgical correction of, 126-127
Coalition, tarsal, excision of, 568-569
Coccygectomy, 297
Collateral ligament
  medial, of knee
    reconstruction of, 445-448
    torn, repair of, 443-444
  of metacarpophalangeal joint of thumb, repair of, 165-166
Colles' fracture, malunited, 118, 120
Compartment, tibial, anterior, fasciotomy of, 502-503

Compression
  costoclavicular, 195
  neurovascular, 193, 195
Compression arthrodesis
  of ankle, anterior approach to, 540-542
  of knee, 484-485
Compression plate, skeletal, fixation of, application of, 609
Compression plate fixation of intertrochanteric displacement osteotomy of femur, 317-318
Compression screw fixation for hip pinning for peritrochanteric fracture of femur, 306-308
Condylar fractures, T, of humerus, open reduction for, 76-77
Condyles
  femoral, transplantation of hamstring tendons to, Eggers procedure for, 392-393
  lateral, of humerus, displaced fracture of, open reduction for, 72-73
Congenital dislocation of hip, open reduction for, 343-344
Congenital elevation of scapula, repair of, 36-37
Congenital spine deformity
  classification of, 216
  correction of, 251-253
  surgical management of, guidelines for, 253
Constrictive tenosynovitis, 147
Contracture
  adduction
    and internal rotation of shoulder, release of, Sever procedure for, 32-33
    of thumb, release of, 164
  Dupuytren's, fasciectomy for, 154-155
  flexion, of hip, release of, 337
  superficial tissue, release of, Z-plasty technique for, 600
  Volkmann's, 110
    ischemic, impending, forearm decompression for, 110-111
Costoclavicular compression syndrome, 195
Coverage, soft tissue, of injured extremity, 601-606
Cranial halo, application of, 207-209
Cruciate ligament
  anterior, of knee
    reconstruction of, 452-454
    repair of, 449-451
  posterior, of knee, torn, repair of, 455-456
Cubitus valgus deformity, 62
Cuff, rotator, of shoulder, tear of, repair of, 23-25
Cup arthroplasty, 330-335
Curettage and bone graft for benign bone cyst of humerus, 54-56

Curve(s)
  lumbar, major thoracic curve with compensatory structural upper thoracic and compensatory nonstructural or mild structural, 220-224
  structural, thoracic and lumbar, associated with fractional lumbosacral structural curve and spondylolisthesis, 232-233
  thoracic
    convex transverse processes of, osteotomy of, 244
    major, with compensatory structural upper thoracic and compensatory nonstructural or mild structural lumbar curve, 220-224
  thoracolumbar and lumbar, 227-229
Curve pattern
  major, double, 228, 229
  thoracic, 217, 218
    double major, 224-225
    single major, 217-220
  of thoracolumbar spine, 217-226
Cyst, bone, benign, of humerus, curettage and bone graft for, 54-56

D
Darrach procedure, 118-119
Decompression, forearm, for impending Volkmann's ischemic contracture, 110-111
Decortication of posterior elements of spine, 241-244
Deformity
  boutonniere, of finger, repair of, 158
  rotational, osteotomy of phalanx for, 174
  spine; see Spine deformity
  swan neck, repair of, 156-157
  thumb-in-palm, 164
Degenerative arthritis at carpometacarpal joint of thumb, 175
Degenerative lumbosacral spondylolisthesis, 254
Deltoid muscle, paralysis of, transfer of trapezius for, 30-31
Deposit, calcific, of shoulder, excision of, 18-19
Derotation osteotomy
  subtrochanteric, 346-347
  supracondylar, McCarroll procedure for, 384-385
Diastasis, tibiofibular, internal fixation for, 531
Digital incisions in hand, 138
Disarticulation
  of hip, 364-365
  of shoulder, 38-39
Disc, intervertebral, lumbar, lesion of, laminectomy for, 274-276

Disease, Scheuermann's, treatment of, 248-251
Dislocation
  of hip, congenital, open reduction for, 343-344
  of patella, recurrent, repair of
    Hauser technique for, 420-421
    Insall technique for, 426-427
    semitendinosus tenodesis for, 424-425
  of shoulder, recurrent
    anterior, repair of, 2-8
    Bristow procedure for, 9-11
    posterior, repair of, 12-14
Displaced acetabular fracture, open reduction and internal fixation for, 292-293
Displaced fracture
  of lateral condyle of humerus, open reduction for, 72-73
  of medial epicondyle, open reduction for, 74-75
Displaced metatarsal fracture, intramedullary fixation for, 571
Displaced proximal humeral fractures, open reduction for, 26-27
Distal femur, epiphyseal arrest of
  by epiphysiodesis, 433-435
  by stapling, 436-438
Distal radius, osteotomy of, for correction of malunion, 120
Distal tendon of biceps brachii muscle, rupture of, repair of, 80-81
Distal ulna, excision of, Darrach procedure for, 118-119
Donor bone, removal of, from iliac wing for bone graft, 282-283
Donor tendon, removal of, for tendon grafting of hand, 152-153
Dorsal fracture-dislocations of proximal interphalangeal joint, volar plate advancement for, 167
Dorsal incisions in hand, 138
Dorsal interosseous tendon, first, weak or absent, tendon transfers for, 144
Double major curve pattern, 228, 229
Double major thoracic curve pattern, 224-225
Drainage
  of ankle joint, 534
  of felon, 183
  of hip joint
    anterior, 359-360
    posterior, 361
  of knee joint, 467
  of localized musculoskeletal areas, closed tube irrigation and, 607
  of paronychia, 182
Dressings, hand, basic principles of, 139
Dupuytren's contracture, fasciectomy for, 154-155

Dwyer instrumentation, anterior interbody fusion with, 268-271
Dwyer procedure for osteotomy of calcaneus, 553-554
Dysplastic lumbosacral spondylolisthesis, 254

E
Eggers procedure for transplantation of hamstring tendons to femoral condyles, 392-393
Elbow, 65-89
  amputation below, 102-103
  synovectomy of, 86-87
Elevation of scapula, congenital, repair of, 36-37
Elmslie-Trillat patellar realignment, 422-423
Epicondyle, medial, displaced fracture of, open reduction for, 74-75
Epiphyseal arrest of distal femur
  by epiphysiodesis, 433-435
  by stapling, 436-438
Epiphysiodesis
  epiphyseal arrest of distal femur by, 433-435
  of proximal tibia and fibula, 439-442
Equinovarus clubfoot, resistant, medial soft tissue release for, 557-560
Erb's palsy, transfer of latissimus dorsi and teres major for, L'Episcopo-Zachary procedure for, 34-35
Excision
  of accessory tarsal navicular, 566-567
  of calcaneal spur, 555
  of calcific deposit of shoulder, 18-19
  of distal ulna, Darrach procedure for, 118-119
  of interdigital neuroma of foot, 589
  of lateral meniscus, 415-416
  of medial meniscus, 410-413
  of patella, 431
  of popliteal cyst, 470-471
  of proximal ulna following olecranon fracture with reattachment of triceps, 70-71
  of radial head, 66-67
  of tarsal coalition, 568-569
  of tibial sesamoid, 580
Exostectomy for bunionette, 590
Exposure, knee, 408-409
Extension, knee, forward transfer of hamstrings to reinforce, 394-397
Extensor carpi radialis brevis, transfer of flexor carpi ulnaris to, 108-109
Extensor digiti quinti tendon, rupture of, 159, 160
Extensor digitorum communis tendon, rupture of, 159, 160
Extensor or flexor tenodesis, 145-146

637

Extensor indicis proprius tendon, transfer of, 142, 144
Extensor pollicis brevis tendon, tenosynovitis of, tenolysis for, 114-115
Extensor pollicis longus tendon, rupture of, 159
Extensor tendons of hand
  lacerations of, repair of, 149
  ruptured, repair of, by tendon transfer, 159-160
Extensor tightness of hand tendons
  extrinsic, 151
  intrinsic, 150
External oblique muscle, transfer of, for paralysis of hip abductors, 356-357
Extrapelvic obturator neurectomy, 337-338
Extremity
  injured, soft tissue coverage of, 601-606
  upper, surgery on, tourniquet use in, 139
Extrinsic extensor tightness of hand tendons, repair of, 151

F

Fasciectomy for Dupuytren's contracture, 154-155
Fasciotomy
  of anterior tibial compartment, 502-503
  plantar, 556
Felon, drainage of, 183
Femoral condyles, transplantation of hamstring tendons to, Eggers procedure for, 392-393
Femoral head prosthesis, insertion of, 312-315
  anterolateral approach to, 316
Femoral shaft fracture, open reduction and internal fixation for, 380-383
Femur
  distal, epiphyseal arrest of
    by epiphysiodesis, 433-435
    by stapling, 436-438
  fracture of; *see* Fracture of femur
  intertrochanteric displacement osteotomy of, compression plate fixation for, 317-318
Fibula and tibia, proximal, epiphysiodesis of, 439-442
Fifth toe, overlapping, repair of, 591-592
Finger
  boutonniere deformity of, repair of, 158
  clawing of, secondary to ulnar nerve palsy, tendon transfers for, 142-143
  snapping, tenolysis for, 147-148
Fingertip, traumatic amputation of, 603-605

First dorsal interosseous tendon, weak or absent, tendon transfers for, 144
First metatarsal, reconstructive osteotomy of, for adolescent hallux valgus, 576-577
First rib, resection of, axillary approach to, 195-197
Fixation
  compression plate, for intertrochanteric displacement osteotomy of femur, 317-318
  compression screw, for hip pinning for peritrochanteric fracture of femur, 306-308
  internal, for tibiofibular diastasis, 531; *see also* Open reduction and internal fixation
  intramedullary
    for displaced metatarsal fracture, 571
    for fracture of shaft of humerus, 52-53
  medullary, for fracture of shaft of ulna, including Monteggia fracture dislocation, 78-79
  nail and bolt, extrastrong, for hip pinning for peritrochanteric fracture of femur, 309-311
  pin, multiple, for subcapital fracture of femur, 300-303
  plate, open reduction and, for fracture of shaft of humerus, 50-51
  skeletal compression plate, application of, 609
Flexion contracture of hip, release of, 337
Flexor carpi ulnaris, transfer of, to extensor carpi radialis brevis, 108-109
Flexor digitorum superficialis, transfer of, 142
Flexor or extensor tenodesis, 145-146
Flexor tendons of hand, lacerations of, repair of, 149
Flexorplasty, Steindler, 82-83
Flexor-pronator origin of forearm, release of, for cerebral palsy, 94-95
Foot, 547-592
  arthrodesis of
    subtalar, Grice procedure for, 550-552
    triple, 548-549
  interdigital neuroma of, excision of, 589
  Keller procedure of, 572-573
  McBride procedure on, 574-575
Forearm, 93-111
  decompression of, for impending Volkmann's ischemic contracture, 110-111
  flexor-pronator origin of, release of, for cerebral palsy, 94-95

Forefoot adduction, resistant, tarsometatarsal mobilization for, 561
Foreign body, metallic, localization of, 608
Forward transfer of hamstring tendons to reinforce knee extension, 394-397
Fracture
  acetabular, displaced, open reduction and internal fixation for, 292-293
  of base of thumb metacarpal, open reduction and internal fixation for, 168-169
  Bennett's, 168-169
  Colles' malunited, 118-120
  femoral shaft, open reduction and internal fixation for, 380-383
  of femur
    peritrochanteric, hip pinning for compression screw fixation for, 306-308
    extrastrong nail and bolt fixation for, 309-311
    subcapital, hip pinning for
      using multiple pin fixation, 300-303
      using telescoping appliance, 304-305
  humeral
    displaced proximal, open reduction of, 26-27
    supracondylar or T condylar, open reduction for, 76-77
  of lateral condyle of humerus, displaced, open reduction for, 72-73
  of medial epicondyle, displaced, open reduction for, 74-75
  of medial malleolus, open reduction and internal fixation for, 527-528
  of metacarpal shaft, open reduction and internal fixation for, 170-171
  metatarsal, displaced, intramedullary fixation for, 571
  olecranon
    excision of proximal ulna following, with reattachment of triceps, 70-71
    open reduction and internal fixation for, 68-69
  open, treatment of, 601
  of patella, repair of, 429-430
  phalangeal shaft, open reduction and internal fixation for, 172-173
  of posterior lip of tibia, open reduction and internal fixation for, 529-530
  of proximal radius, open reduction for, 96-98
  of radius and ulna, midshaft, open reduction for, 99-101
  of scaphoid, open reduction for, 123
    and bone graft for, anterior approach to, 121-122

Fracture—cont'd
  of shaft of humerus
    intramedullary fixation for, 52-53
    open reduction and plate fixation for fracture of, 50-51
  of shaft of ulna, medullary fixation for, 78-79
  tibial plateau, open reduction and internal fixation for, 465-466
  tibial shaft
    intramedullary nailing for, 500-501
    open reduction for
      anterolateral approach to, 494-496
      posterolateral approach to, 497-499
Fracture-dislocation
  Monteggia, medullary fixation for, 78-79
  of proximal interphalangeal joint, dorsal, volar plate advancement for, 167
Free vascularized tissue grafts, 613
"Frozen shoulder" syndrome, 18
Fusion
  cervical spine
    anterior, 205-206
    posterior, 198
    C3 and below, 203-204
  interbody, anterior, with Dwyer instrumentation, 268-271
  occipitocervical, 199-200
  spine; see Spine fusion
Fusion area of thoracolumbar spine, selection of, 217-233

G

Gastrocnemius muscle, recession of, Strayer method for, 504-505
Genu recurvatum, proximal tibial osteotomy for, 474-476
Girdlestone procedure for resection of hip, 362-363
Graft
  bone
    curettage and, for benign bone cyst of humerus, 54-56
    open reduction and, for fracture of scaphoid, anterior approach to, 121-122
    removal of donor bone from iliac wing for, 282-283
  skin, 601, 602-603
  tissue, vascularized, free, 613
Grafting, tendon, of hand, removal of donor tendon for, 152-153
Grice procedure for subtalar arthrodesis of foot, 550-552

H

Hallux valgus
  adolescent, reconstructive osteotomy of first metatarsal for, 576-577

Hallux valgus—cont'd
  Keller procedure for, 572-573
  McBride procedure for, 574-575
Halo, cranial, application of, 207-209
Halo-pelvic hoop apparatus, 210
Hamstring tendons
  forward transfer of, to reinforce knee extension, 394-397
  transplantation of, to femoral condyles, Eggers procedure for, 392-393
Hand, 137-183
  dressings for, basic principles of, 139
  extensor tendons of, ruptured, repair of, by tendon transfer, 159-160
  hinged, 145-146
  incisions in, 138
  median palsy of, opponens transfer for, 140-141
  small joints of, arthrodeses of, 177-179
  tendon grafting of, removal of donor tendon for, 152-153
  tendon repair of, 149-151
  tendons of
    lacerations of, repair of, 149
    tightness of
      extrinsic extensor, 151
      intrinsic extensor, 150
Harrington instrumentation, posterior spine fusion and, for correction of scoliosis, 237-248
Hauser technique for repair for recurrent dislocation of patella, 420-421
Head
  of biceps, long, tendon of, tenodesis of, 57-58
  metatarsal, resection of, 585-586
  radial, excision of, 66-67
Hemipelvectomy, 294-296
Hemivertebra, excision of, 253
High tibial osteotomy for osteoarthritis of knee, 472-473
Hinged hand, 145-146
Hip, 299-368
  adductor tenotomy of, 336
  arthrodesis of, 366-368
  congenital dislocation of, open reduction for, 343-344
  cup arthroplasty of, 330-335
  disarticulation of, 364-365
  drainage of
    anterior, 359-360
    posterior, 361
  medial appraoch to, 345
  osteotomy of, 317-318
  resection of, Girdlestone procedure for, 362-363
  resurfacing of, 326-329
Hip abductors, paralysis of; see Paralysis of hip abductors
Hip flexion contracture, release of, 337

Hip pinning
  for peritrochanteric fracture of femur
    compression screw fixation for, 306-308
    extrastrong nail and bolt fixation for, 309-311
  for subcapital fracture of femur
    using multiple pin fixation, 300-303
    using telescoping appliance, 304-305
Hip reconstruction, total
  Charnley-Müller method for, 319-325
  resurfacing and, 326-329
Hoop, pelvic, application of, 210-212
Humerus
  benign bone cyst of, curettage and bone graft for, 54-56
  fractures of, displaced proximal, open reduction for, 26-27
  lateral condyle of, displaced fracture of, open reduction for, 72-73
  shaft of, fracture of
    intramedullary fixation for, 52-53
    open reduction and plate fixation for, 50-51
  supracondylar or T condylar fractures of, open reduction for, 76-77
  supracondylar osteotomy of, 62-63
Hydrocortisone for coccygodynia, 297

I

Idiopathic scoliosis
  classification of, 216
  indications for operation on, 216-217
Iliac wing, removal of donor bone from, for bone graft, 282-283
Iliopsoas, release of, 340-342
Iliopsoas tendon, transfer of, for paralysis of hip abductors
  Mustard procedure for, 348-351
  posterior, Sharrard procedure for, 352-355
Incisions
  hand, 138
  knee, 408-409
Infantile idiopathic scoliosis, 216
Ingrown toenail, chronic, repair of, 587-588
Injured extremity, soft tissue coverage of, 601-606
Innominate osteotomy, 288-291
Insall technique for repair of recurrent dislocation of patella, 426-427
Insertion of femoral head prosthesis, 312-315
  anterolateral approach to, 316
Instability, rotatory, of knee
  anterolateral, chronic, modified MacIntosh reconstruction for, 459-461
  lateral and posterolateral, lateral ligament reconstruction for, 462-464

639

Instrumentation
  Dwyer, anterior interbody fusion with, 268-271
  Harrington, posterior spine fusion and, for correction of scoliosis, 237-248
Interbody fusion, anterior, with Dwyer instrumentation, 268-271
Interdigital neuroma of foot, excision of, 589
Internal fixation
  open reduction and; *see* Open reduction and internal fixation
  for tibiofibular diastasis, 531
Internal rotation and adduction contracture of shoulder, release of, Sever procedure for, 32-33
Interosseous tendon, dorsal, first, weak or absent, tendon transfers for, 144
Interphalangeal joints, proximal
  arthrodesis of
    for claw toe, 583-584
    for hammertoe, 581-582
  dorsal fracture dislocations of, volar plate advancement for, 167
Interscapulothoracic resection, 40-42
Intertrochanteric displacement osteotomy of femur by compression plate fixation, 317-318
Intervertebral disc lesion, lumbar, laminectomy for, 274-276
Intramedullary fixation
  for displaced metatarsal fracture, 571
  for fracture of shaft of humerus, 52-53
Intramedullary nailing for tibial shaft fracture, 500-501
Intrapelvic obturator neurectomy, 337-338
Intrinsic extensor tightness of hand tendons, repair of, 150
Irrigation, closed tube, and drainage of localized musculoskeletal areas, 607
Ischial tuberosity, transfer of origin of adductor longus and brevis to, 358
Isthmic lumbosacral spondylolisthesis, 254

J

Joint; *see also* specific joint
  carpometacarpal, of thumb
    arthrodesis of, 175-176
    arthroplasty of, 175
  of hand, small, arthrodesis of, 177-179
  interphalangeal, proximal
    arthrodesis of
      for claw toe, 583-584
      for hammertoe, 581-582
    dorsal fracture dislocation of, volar plate advancement for, 167

Joint—cont'd
  metacarpophalangeal
    replacement arthroplasty of, 161-163
    of thumb, collateral ligament of, repair of, 165-166
Jones procedure for clawing of toe, 578-579
Juvenile idiopathic scoliosis, 216
Juvenile kyphosis, treatment of, 248-251

K

Keller procedure on foot, 572-573
Knee, 405-485
  amputation above, 398-400
  amputation below, 506-507
  anterior cruciate ligament of
    reconstruction of, 452-454
    repair of, 449-451
  arthroscopy of, 406-407
  arthrotomy of, 410, 415
  chronic anterolateral rotatory instability of, modified MacIntosh reconstruction for, 459-461
  compression arthrodesis of, 484-485
  drainage of, 467
  exposures of, 408-409
  incisions in, 408-409
  lateral ligaments of
    reconstruction of, for lateral and posterolateral rotatory instability, 462-464
    torn, repair of, 457-458
  lateral and posterolateral, rotatory instability of, lateral ligament reconstruction for, 462-464
  medial collateral ligament of
    reconstruction of, 445-448
    torn, repair of, 443-444
  osteoarthritis of, high tibial osteotomy for, 472-473
  posterior capsulotomy of, 418-419
  posterior cruciate ligament of, torn, repair of, 455-456
  synovectomy of, 468-469
Knee extension, forward, transfer of hamstrings to reinforce, 394-397
Knee replacement, total
  animetric (nonconstrained), 477-480
  spherocentric (semiconstrained), 481-483
Kyphosis, juvenile, treatment of, 248-251

L

Lacerations of tendons of hand, repair of, 149
Laminectomy for lumbar intervertebral disc lesions, 274-276
Lateral approach to arthrodesis of ankle, 537-539
Lateral condyle of humerus, displaced fracture of, open reduction for, 72-73

Lateral exposures of knee, 409
Lateral ligament reconstruction for lateral and posterolateral rotatory instability of knee, 462-464
Lateral ligaments
  of ankle, reconstruction of, 532-533
  of knee, torn, repair of, 457-458
Lateral meniscectomy, 415-416
Lateral meniscus
  excision of, 415-416
  peripheral reattachment of, 417
Lateral and posterolateral rotatory instability of knee, lateral ligament reconstruction for, 462-464
Lateral transfer of anterior tibial tendon, 564-565
Latissimus dorsi and teres major, transfer of, for Erb's palsy, L'Episcopo-Zachary procedure for, 34-35
Leg, lower, 493-507
Lengthening
  quadriceps, 388-389
  tendo Achillis, 512-513
Lesion, lumbar intervertebral disc, laminectomy for, 274-276
Ligament
  of ankle, lateral, reconstruction of, 532-533
  carpal, transverse, release of, for carpal tunnel syndrome, 116-117
  collateral
    of metacarpophalangeal joint of thumb, repair of, 165-166
    medial, of knee
      reconstruction of, 445-448
      torn, repair of, 443-444
  cruciate, of knee
    anterior
      reconstruction of, 452-454
      repair of, 449-451
    posterior, torn, repair of, 455-456
  lateral, of knee
    reconstruction of, for lateral and posterolateral rotatory instability of knee, 462-464
    torn, repair of, 457-458
Lip of tibia, posterior, fracture of, open reduction and internal fixation for, 529-530
Localization of metallic foreign body, 608
Localized musculoskeletal areas, closed tube irrigation and drainage of, 607
Localizer cast technique of correcting scoliosis, 234-237
Long head of biceps, tendon of, tenodesis of, 57-58
Lower leg, 493-507

Lumbar curve, major thoracic curve with compensatory structural upper thoracic and compensatory nonstructural or mild structural, 220-224
Lumbar disc syndrome, 274
Lumbar intervertebral disc lesion, laminectomy for, 274-276
Lumbar scoliosis, thoracolumbar or, structural, associated with spondylolisthesis, 232, 233
Lumbar spine, retroperitoneal approach to, anterior spine fusion by, 261-263
Lumbar and thoracic structural curves associated with fractional lumbosacral structural curve and spondylolisthesis, 232-233
Lumbar and thoracolumbar curves, 227-229
Lumbosacral spine fusion, posterior, 254-257
Lumbosacral spondylolisthesis
　classification of, 254
　scoliosis with, 229-233
Lumbosacral structural curve and spondylolisthesis, thoracic and lumbar structural curve associated with, 232-233

M

MacIntosh reconstruction for chronic anterolateral rotatory instability of knee, modified, 459-461
Major curve pattern, double, 228-229
Major thoracic curve with compensatory structural upper thoracic and compensatory nonstructural or mild structural lumbar curve, 220-224
Major thoracic curve pattern
　double, 224-225
　single, 217-220
Malleolus, medial, fracture of, open reduction and internal fixation for, 527-528
Malunion of wrist, osteotomy of distal radius to correct, 120
Malunited Colles' fracture, 118, 120
McBride procedure on foot, 574-575
McCarroll procedure for supracondylar derotation osteotomy, 384-385
Medial approach to hip joint, 345
Medial collateral ligament of knee
　reconstruction of, 445-448
　torn, repair of, 443-444
Medial epicondyle, displaced fracture of, open reduction for, 74-75
Medial exposures of knee, 408
Medial malleolus, fracture of, open reduction and internal fixation for, 527-528

Medial meniscectomy, 410-413
Medial meniscus
　excision of, 410-413
　peripheral reattachment of, 414
Medial soft tissue release for resistant equinovarus clubfoot, 557-560
Medial transfer of peroneus longus tendon, 562-563
Median palsy, opponens transfer for, 140-141
Medullary fixation for fracture of shaft of ulna, including Monteggia fracture-dislocation, 78-79
Meniscectomy
　lateral, 415-416
　medial, 410-413
　partial, 410
Meniscus
　lateral
　　excision of, 415-416
　　peripheral reattachment of, 417
　medial; see Medial meniscus
Mesenchymal disorders of thoracolumbar spine, classification of, 216
Metacarpal, thumb, base of, fracture of, open reduction and internal fixation for, 168-169
Metacarpal shaft, fracture of, open reduction and internal fixation for, 170-171
Metacarpophalangeal joint
　replacement arthroplasty of, 161-163
　of thumb, collateral ligament of, repair of, 165-166
Metallic foreign body, localization of, 608
Metatarsal, first, reconstructive osteotomy of, for adolescent hallux valgus, 576-577
Metatarsal fracture, displaced, intramedullary fixation for, 571
Metatarsal head, resection of, 585-586
Methicillin, prophylactic, for scoliosis fusion patients, 248
Microsurgery and replantation, 613
Midshaft fracture of radius and ulna, open reduction for, 99-101
Mobilization, tarsometatarsal, for resistant forefoot adduction, 561
Modified Syme amputation, 535-536
Monitoring, blood replacement and, during posterior spine fusion and Harrington instrumentation, 247
Monteggia fracture-dislocation, medullary fixation for, 78-79
Multiple pin fixation for subcapital fracture of femur, 300-303
Muscle(s)
　adductor longus and brevis, origin of, transfer of, to ischial tuberosity, 358

Muscle(s)—cont'd
　biceps brachii, distal tendon of, rupture of, repair of, 80-81
　deltoid, paralysis of, transfer of trapezius for, 30-31
　extensor carpi radialis brevis, transfer of flexor carpi ulnaris to, 108-109
　flexor carpi ulnaris, transfer of, to extensor carpi radialis brevis, 108-109
　gastrocnemius, recession of, Strayer method for, 504-505
　latissimus dorsi and teres major, transfer of, for Erb's palsy, L'Episcopo-Zachary procedure for, 34-35
　oblique, external, transfer of, for paralysis of hip abductors, 356-357
　quadriceps, lengthening of, 388-389
　scalenus anterior, release of, 193-194
　sternocleidomastoid, release of, for torticollis, 192
Muscle biopsy, 612
Musculoskeletal areas, localized, closed tube irrigation and drainage of, 607
Mustard procedure for transfer of iliopsoas tendon for paralysis of hip abductors, 348-351

N

Nail and bolt fixation, extrastrong, for hip pinning for peritrochanteric fracture of femur, 309-311
Nailing, intramedullary, for tibial shaft fracture, 500-501
Navicular bone, tarsal, accessory, excision of, 566-567
Neck and cervical spine, 191-212
Neer anterior acromioplasty, 20-22
Nerve
　radial, palsy of, tendon transfers for, 104-107
　ulnar
　　anterior transplantation of, 88-89
　　palsy of, clawing of fingers secondary to, tendon transfers for, 142-143
Nerve repairs, microsurgical, 613
Neurectomy, obturator, 338-339
Neuroma, interdigital, of foot, excision of, 589
Neuromuscular scoliosis, treatment of, 251, 252
Neuromuscular spine deformity, classification of, 216
Neurovascular compression syndromes, 193, 195
Nonconstrained total knee replacement, 477-480

641

O

Oblique muscle, external, transfer of, for paralysis of hip abductors, 356-357
Obliquity, pelvic, correction of, 251
Obturator neurectomy, 338-339
Occipitocervical fusion, 199-200
Olecranon, fracture of
  excision of proximal ulna following, with reattachment of triceps, 70-71
  open reduction and internal fixation for, 68-69
Open fracture, treatment of, 601
Open reduction
  and bone graft for fracture of scaphoid, anterior approach to, 121-122
  for congenital dislocation of hip, 343-344
  for displaced fracture
    of lateral condyle of humerus, 72-73
    of medial epicondyle, 74-75
  for displaced proximal humeral fractures, 26-27
  for fracture
    of proximal radius, anterior exposure, 96-98
    of scaphoid, 123
  and internal fixation
    of clavicle, 28-29
    for displaced acetabular fracture, 292-293
    for femoral shaft fracture, 380-383
    for fracture
      of base of thumb metacarpal, 168-169
      of medial malleolus, 527-528
      of metacarpal shaft, 170-171
      of olecranon, 68-69
      of posterior lip of tibia, 529-530
    for phalangeal shaft fracture, 172-173
    for tibial plateau fracture, 465-466
    for midshaft fracture of radius and ulna, 99-101
  and plate fixation for fracture of shaft of humerus, 50-51
  for supracondylar or T condylar fractures of humerus, 76-77
  for tibial shaft fracture
    anterolateral approach to, 494-496
    posterolateral approach to, 497-499
Operative procedures, miscellaneous, 597-613
Opponens transfer for median palsy, 140-141
Origin of adductor longus and brevis, transfer of, to ischial tuberosity, 358
Osteoarthritis of knee, high tibial osteotomy for, 472-473

Osteotomy
  of calcaneus, Dwyer procedure for, 553-554
  of convex transverse processes of thoracic curve, 244
  derotation
    subtrochanteric, 346-347
    supracondylar, McCarroll procedure for, 384-385
  of distal radius for correction of malunion, 120
  innominate, 288-291
  intertrochanteric displacement, of femur, compression plate fixation for, 317-318
  of phalanx for rotational deformity, 174
  reconstructive, of first metatarsal for adolescent hallux valgus, 576-577
  supracondylar, of humerus, 62-63
  tibial
    high, for osteoarthritis of knee, 472-473
    proximal, for genu recurvatum, 474-476
Overlapping fifth toe, repair of, 591-592

P

Palmar incisions in hand, 138
Palsy
  Erb's, transfer of latissimus dorsi and teres major for, L'Episcopo-Zachary procedure for, 34-35
  median, opponens transfer for, 140-141
  radial nerve, tendon transfers for, 104-107
  ulnar nerve, clawing of fingers secondary to, tendon transfers for, 142-143
Paralysis
  of deltoid muscle, transfer of trapezius for, 30-31
  of hip abductors
    transfer of external oblique muscle for, 356-357
    transfer of iliopsoas tendon for Mustard procedure for, 348-351
    posterior, Sharrard procedure for, 352-355
Paronychia, drainage of, 182
Partial meniscectomy, 410
Patella
  advancement of, 428
  dislocation of, recurrent, repair of
    Hauser technique for, 420-421
    Insall technique for, 426-427
    semitendinosus tenodesis for, 424-425
  excision of, 431
  fracture of, repair of, 429-430
Patellar realignment, Elmslie-Trillat, 422-423

Patellectomy, 431-432
Pathologic lumbosacral spondylolisthesis, 254
Pelvic hoop, application of, 210-212
Pelvic obliquity, correction of, 251
Pelvis, 281-297
Peripheral reattachment
  of lateral meniscus, 417
  of medial meniscus, 414
Peritrochanteric fracture of femur, hip pinning for
  compression screw fixation for, 306-308
  extrastrong nail and bolt fixation for, 309-311
Peroneus brevis tendon, transfer of, to calcaneus, 524-526
Peroneus longus tendon, medial transfer of, 562-563
Phalangeal shaft fracture, open reduction and internal fixation for, 172-173
Phalanx, osteotomy of, for rotational deformity, 174
Pin fixation, multiple, for subcapital fracture of femur, 300-303
Pinning, hip; see Hip pinning
Plantar fasciotomy, 556
Plate
  compression, skeletal, fixation of, application of, 609
  volar, advancement of, for dorsal fracture dislocation of proximal interphalangeal joint, 167
Plate fixation
  compression, for intertrochanteric displacement osteotomy of femur, 317-318
  open reduction and, for fracture of shaft of humerus, 50-51
Plateau, tibial, fracture of, open reduction and internal fixation for, 465-466
Popliteal cyst, excision of, 470-471
Posterior capsulotomy of knee, 418-419
Posterior cervical spine fusion, 198
  C3 and below, 203-204
Posterior cruciate ligament of knee, torn, repair of, 455-456
Posterior dislocation of shoulder, recurrent, repair of, 12-14
Posterior drainage of hip joint, 361
Posterior elements of spine, decortication of, 241-244
Posterior lip of tibia, fracture of, open reduction and internal fixation for, 529-530
Posterior lumbosacral spine fusion, 254-257
Posterior spine fusion and Harrington instrumentation for correction of scoliosis, 237-248

Posterior tibial and peroneus brevis tendons, transfer of, to calcaneus, 524-526
Posterior transfer of iliopsoas tendon for paralysis of hip abductors, Sharrard procedure for, 352-355
Posterolateral approach to open reduction for tibial shaft fracture, 497-499
Posterolateral and lateral rotatory instability of knee, lateral ligament reconstruction for, 462-464
Posterolateral spine fusion by bilateral, lateral approach, 258-260
Prosthesis, femoral head, insertion of, 312-315
  anterolateral approach to, 316
Proximal humeral fractures, displaced, open reduction for, 26-27
Proximal interphalangeal joint
  arthrodesis of
    for claw toe, 583-584
    for hammertoe, 581-582
  dorsal fracture dislocations of, volar plate advancement for, 167
Proximal radius, fracture of, open reduction of, 96-98
Proximal tibia and fibula, epiphysiodesis of, 439-442
Proximal tibial osteotomy for genu recurvatum, 474-476
Proximal ulna, excision of, following olecranon fracture with reattachment of triceps, 70-71
Putti-Platt type of repair of anterior dislocation of shoulder, 2

Q

Quadriceps lengthening, 388-389
Quadriceps tendon, rupture of, repair of, 390-391
Quadricepsplasty, 386-387
de Quervain's tenosynovitis, tenolysis for, 114-115

R

Radial clubhand, surgical correction of, 126-127
Radial nerve palsy, tendon transfers for, 104-107
Radial styloidectomy, 124-125
Radius
  distal, osteotomy of, for correction of malunion, 120
  head of, excision of, 66-67
  midshaft fracture of, open reduction for, 99-101
  proximal, fracture of, open reduction of, 96-98
Realignment, patellar, Elmslie-Trillat, 422-423

Reattachment, peripheral
  of lateral meniscus, 417
  of medial meniscus, 414
Recession of gastrocnemius muscle, Strayer method of, 504-505
Reconstruction
  of anterior cruciate ligament of knee, 452-454
  for chronic anterolateral rotatory instability of knee, MacIntosh, modified, 459-461
  hip, total
    Charnley-Müller method for, 319-325
    resurfacing and, 326-329
  of lateral ligaments
    of ankle, 532-533
    for lateral and posterolateral rotatory instability of knee, 462-464
  of medial collateral ligament of knee, 445-448
Reconstructive osteotomy of first metatarsal for adolescent hallux valgus, 576-577
Recurrent anterior dislocation of shoulder, repair of, 2-8
  Bristow procedure for, 9-11
Recurrent dislocation of patella, repair of
  Hauser technique for, 420-421
  Insall technique for, 426-427
  semitendinosus tenodesis for, 424-425
Recurrent posterior dislocation of shoulder, repair of, 12-14
Reduction
  open; see Open reduction
  of severe spondylolisthesis associated with scoliosis, 229-233
Release
  of hip flexion contracture, 337
  of iliopsoas, 340-342
  soft tissue, medial, for resistant equinovarus clubfoot, 557-560
  of superficial tissue contracture, Z-plasty technique for, 600
  tarsal tunnel, 521-523
  of thumb adduction contracture, 164
  of transverse carpal ligament for carpal tunnel syndrome, 116-117
Replacement, knee, total
  animetric (nonconstrained), 477-480
  spherocentric (semiconstrained), 481-483
Replacement arthroplasty of metacarpophalangeal joint, 161-163
Replantation, microsurgery and, 613
Resection
  of first rib, axillary approach to, 195-197
  of hip, Girdlestone procedure for, 362-363
  interscapulothoracic, 40-42
  of lateral end of clavicle, 17
  of metatarsal head, 585-586

Resistant equinovarus clubfoot, medial soft tissue release for, 557-560
Resistant forefoot adduction, tarsometatarsal mobilization for, 561
Resurfacing of hip joint, 326-329
Retroperitoneal approach to lumbar spine, anterior spine fusion by, 261-263
Rheumatoid arthritis of wrist, 128, 129
Rib, first, resection of, axillary approach to, 195-197
Rotation, internal, and adduction contracture of shoulder, release of, Sever procedure for, 32-33
Rotational deformity, osteotomy of phalanx for, 174
Rotator cuff tear of shoulder, repair of, 23-25
Rotatory instability of knee
  anterolateral, chronic, modified MacIntosh reconstruction for, 459-461
  lateral and posterolateral, lateral ligament reconstruction for, 462-464
Rupture
  of anterior tibial tendon, repair of, 519-520
  of distal tendon of biceps brachii muscle, repair of, 80-81
  of quadriceps tendon, repair of, 390-391
  of rotator cuff of shoulder, repair of, 23-25
  of ulnar collateral ligament of metacarpophalangeal joint of thumb, 165
Ruptured extensor tendons of hand, repair of, by tendon transfer, 159-160
Ruptured tendo Achillis, repair of, 516-518

S

Scalenus anterior muscle, release of, 193-194
Scaphoid, fractures of, open reduction for, 123
  and bone graft for, anterior approach to, 121-122
Scapula, congenital elevation of, repair of, 36-37
Scheuermann's disease, treatment of, 248-251
Scoliosis
  correction of, methods of, 234-248
  general considerations of, 216
  idiopathic
    classification of, 216
    indications for operation on, 216-217
  with lumbosacral spondylolisthesis, 229-233
  neuromuscular, treatment of, 251, 252

643

Scoliosis—cont'd
  severe spondylolisthesis associated with, reduction of, 229-233
  structural thoracolumbar or lumbar, associated with spondylolisthesis, 232, 233
  thoracolumbar nonstructural, associated with spondylolisthesis, 232
Screw fixation, compression, for hip pinning for peritrochanteric fracture of femur, 306-308
Semitendinosus tenodesis for repair of recurrent dislocation of patella, 424-425
Separation, acromioclavicular, repair of, 15-16
Sesamoid bone, tibial, excision of, 580
Sever procedure for release of internal rotation and adduction contracture of shoulder, 32-33
Severed artery, repair of, 598-599
Shaft
  femoral, fracture of, open reduction and internal fixation for, 380-383
  of humerus, fracture of
    intramedullary fixation for, 52-53
    open reduction and plate fixation for, 50-51
  metacarpal, fracture of, open reduction and internal fixation for, 170-171
  phalangeal, fracture of, open reduction and internal fixation for, 172-173
  tibial, fracture of
    intramedullary nailing for, 500-501
    open reduction for
      anterolateral approach to, 494-496
      posterolateral approach to, 497-499
  of ulna, fracture of, medullary fixation for, 78-79
Sharrard procedure for posterior transfer of iliopsoas tendon for paralysis of hip abductors, 352-355
Shoulder, 1-44
  anterior dislocation of, recurrent, repair of, 2-8
    Bristow procedure for, 9-11
  arthrodesis of, 43-44
  calcific bursitis of, 18
  calcific deposit of, excision of, 18-19
  disarticulation of, 38-39
  "frozen," 18
  internal rotation and adduction contracture of, release of, Sever procedure for, 32-33
  posterior dislocation of, recurrent, repair of, 12-14
  rotator cuff of, tear of, repair of, 23-25
Single major thoracic curve pattern, 217-220

Skeletal compression plate fixation, application of, 609
Skin grafts, 601, 602-603
Small joints of hand, arthrodesis of, 177-179
Soft tissue coverage of injured extremity, 601-606
Soft tissue release, medial, for resistant equinovarus clubfoot, 557-560
Snapping finger or thumb, tenolysis for, 147-148
Spherocentric total knee replacement (semiconstrained), 481-483
Spine
  cervical; see Cervical spine
  lumbar, retroperitoneal approach to, anterior spine fusion by, 261-263
  lumbosacral, posterior, fusion of, 254-257
  posterior elements of, decortication of, 241-244
  thoracic, transthoracic approach to, 272-273
  thoracolumbar, 215-276
    curve patterns in, 217-226
    fusion area of, selection of, 217-233
Spine deformity
  classification of, 216
  congenital, correction of, 251-253
Spine fusion
  anterior
    by retroperitoneal approach to lumbar spine, 261-263
    by thoracoabdominal approach, 264-267
  atlantoaxial, 201-202
  posterior, and Harrington instrumentation for correction of scoliosis, 237-248
  posterolateral, by bilateral, lateral approach, 258-260
Spondylolisthesis
  asymptomatic, 232
  lumbosacral
    classification of, 254
    scoliosis with, 229-233
  mild, 232
  severe, associated with scoliosis, reduction of, 229-233
  structural thoracolumbar or lumbar scoliosis associated with, 232, 233
  thoracic and lumbar structural curve associated with fractional lumbosacral structural curve and, 232-233
  thoracolumbar nonstructural scoliosis associated with, 232
Sprain of metacarpophalangeal joint of thumb, 165
Spur, calcaneal, excision of, 555

Stapling, epiphyseal arrest of distal femur by, 436-438
Steindler flexorplasty, 82-83
Steindler stripping procedure, 556
Stenosing tenosynovitis, 147
Sternocleidomastoid muscle, release of, for torticollis, 192
Strayer method for recession of gastrocnemius muscle, 504-505
Stripping procedure, Steindler, 556
Styloidectomy, radial, 124-125
Subacute Volkmann's contracture, 110
Subcapital fracture of femur, hip pinning for
  using multiple pin fixation, 300-303
  using telescoping appliance, 304-305
Subtalar arthrodesis of foot, Grice procedure for, 550-552
Subtotal fasciectomy for Dupuytren's contracture, 154-155
Subtrochanteric derotation osteotomy, 346-347
Superficial tissue contracture, release of, Z-plasty technique for, 600
Supracondylar derotation osteotomy, McCarroll procedure for, 384-385
Supracondylar fractures of humerus, open reductions for, 76-77
Supracondylar osteotomy of humerus, 62-63
Surgery, upper extremity, tourniquet use in, 139
Surgical correction of radial clubhand, 126-127
Swan neck deformity, repair of, 156-157
Syme amputation, modified, 535-536
Syndactyly, repair of, 180-181
Syndrome
  anterior impingement, 20
  anterior tibial compartment, acute, 502
  caput ulnae, 159
  carpal tunnel, release of transverse carpal ligament for, 116-117
  costoclavicular compression, 195
  "frozen shoulder," 18
  lumbar disc, 274
  neurovascular compression, 193, 195
  tarsal tunnel, 521-523
  "thoracic outlet," 193, 195
Synovectomy
  of elbow, 86-87
  of knee, 468-469
  of tendons at wrist, 128

T

T condylar fractures of humerus, open reduction for, 76-77
Talocalcaneal coalition, 568
Talocalcaneal joint, arthrodesis of, 548-549
Talonavicular joint, arthrodesis of, 548-549

Tarsal coalition, excision of, 568-569
Tarsal navicular, accessory, excision of, 566-567
Tarsal tunnel release, 521-523
Tarsal tunnel syndrome, 521-523
Tarsometatarsal mobilization for resistant forefoot adduction, 561
Tear, rotator cuff, of shoulder, repair of, 23-25
Telescoping appliance for pinning of subcapital fracture of femur, 304-305
Tendo Achillis
　lengthening of, 512-513
　ruptured, repair of, 516-518
　tenodesis of, 514-515
Tendon
　distal, of biceps brachii muscle, rupture of, repair of, 80-81
　donor, removal of, for tendon grafting of hand, 152-153
　extensor indicis proprius, transfer of, 142, 144
　flexor digitorum superficialis, transfer of, 142
　hamstring
　　forward transfer of, to reinforce knee extension, 394-397
　　transplantation of, to femoral condyles, Eggers procedure for, 392-393
　of hand
　　extensor, ruptured, repair of, by tendon transfer, 159-160
　　lacerations of, repair of, 149
　　tightness of
　　　extrinsic extensor, 151
　　　intrinsic extensor, 150
　iliopsoas
　　release of, 340-342
　　transfer of, for paralysis of hip abductors
　　　Mustard procedure for, 348-351
　　　posterior, Sharrard procedure for, 352-355
　interosseous, first dorsal, weak or absent, tendon transfers for, 144
　of long head of biceps, tenodesis of, 57-58
　peroneus longus, medial transfer of, 562-563
　posterior tibial and peroneus brevis, transfer of, to calcaneus, 524-526
　quadriceps, rupture of, repair of, 390-391
　tibial, anterior
　　lateral transfer of, 564-565
　　rupture of, repair of, 519-520
　triceps, transfer of, 84-85
　at wrist, synovectomy of, 128
Tendon grafting of hand, removal of donor tendon for, 152-153

Tendon repair of hand, 149-151
Tendon transfers
　for clawing of fingers secondary to ulnar nerve palsy, 142-143
　of extensor indicis proprius, 142, 144
　using flexor digitorum superficialis tendon, 142
　for radial nerve palsy, 104-107
　repair of ruptured extensor tendons of hand by, 159-160
　for weak or absent first dorsal interosseous, 144
Tenodesis
　flexor or extensor, 145-146
　semitendinosus, for repair of recurrent dislocation of patella, 424-425
　of tendo Achillis, 514-515
　of tendon of long head of biceps, 57-58
Tenolysis
　for de Quervain's tenosynovitis, 114-115
　for snapping finger or thumb, 147-148
Tenosynovitis
　bicipital, 57
　constrictive, 147
　de Quervain's, tenolysis for, 114-115
　stenosing, 147
Tenotomy, adductor, 336
Teres major and latissimus dorsi, transfer of, for Erb's palsy, L'Episcopo-Zachary procedure for, 34-35
Thigh, 379-400
Thoracic curve
　convex transverse processes of, osteotomy of, 244
　major, with compensatory structural upper thoracic and compensatory nonstructural or mild structural lumbar curve, 220-224
Thoracic curve patterns, 217, 218
　double major, 224-225
　single major, 217-220
Thoracic and lumbar structural curve associated with fractional lumbosacral structural curve and spondylolisthesis, 232-233
"Thoracic outlet syndrome," 193, 195
Thoracic spine, transthoracic approach to, 272-273
Thoracoabdominal approach, anterior spine fusion by, 264-267
Thoracolumbar and lumbar curves, 227-229
Thoracolumbar or lumbar scoliosis associated with spondylolisthesis, structural, 232, 233
Thoracolumbar nonstructural scoliosis associated with spondylolisthesis, 232
Thoracolumbar spine, 215-276
　curve patterns in, 217-226
　fusion area of, selection of, 217-233

Thumb
　adduction contracture of, release of, 164
　carpometacarpal joint of
　　arthrodesis of, 175-176
　　arthroplasty of, 175
　metacarpophalangeal joint of, collateral ligament of, repair of, 165-166
　snapping, tenolysis for, 147-148
　"trigger," 148
Thumb-in-palm deformity, 164
Thumb metacarpal, base of, fracture of, open reduction and internal fixation for, 168-169
Tibia
　and fibula, proximal, epiphysiodesis of, 439-442
　posterior lip of, fracture of, open reduction and internal fixation for, 529-530
　soft tissue coverage of, 605-606
Tibial compartment, anterior, fasciotomy of, 502-503
Tibial osteotomy
　for genu recurvatum, proximal, 474-476
　for osteoarthritis of knee, high, 472-473
Tibial plateau fracture, open reduction and internal fixation for, 465-466
Tibial sesamoid, excision of, 580
Tibial shaft fracture
　intramedullary nailing for, 500-501
　open reduction for
　　anterolateral approach to, 494-496
　　posterolateral approach to, 497-499
Tibial tendon
　anterior
　　lateral transfer of, 564-565
　　rupture of, repair of, 519-520
　posterior, transfer of, to calcaneus, 524-526
Tibiofibular diastasis, internal fixation for, 531
Tightness of hand tendons
　extrinsic extensor, 151
　intrinsic extensor, 150
Tinel's sign in carpal tunnel syndrome, 116
Tissue
　soft; see Soft tissue
　superficial, contracture of, release of, Z-plasty technique for, 600
Tissue grafts, vascularized, free, 613
Toe
　clawing of, Jones procedure for, 578-579
　fifth, overlapping, repair of, 591-592
Toenail, ingrown, chronic, repair of, 587-588
Torn lateral ligaments of knee, repair of, 457-458

645

Torn medial collateral ligament of knee, repair of, 443-444
Torn posterior cruciate ligament of knee, repair of, 455-456
Torticollis, release of sternocleidomastoid muscle for, 192
Total hip reconstruction
  Charnley-Müller method of, 319-325
  resurfacing and, 326-329
Total knee replacement
  animetric (nonconstrained), 477-480
  spherocentric (semiconstrained), 481-483
Tourniquet use in upper extremity surgery, 139
Traction, cranial halo, 207-209
Transfer
  of external oblique muscle for paralysis of hip abductors, 356-357
  of hamstring tendons, forward, to reinforce knee extension, 394-397
  of iliopsoas tendon for paralysis of hip abductors
    Mustard procedure for, 348-351
    posterior, Sharrard procedure for, 352-355
  lateral, of anterior tibial tendon, 564-565
  medial, of peroneus longus tendon, 562-563
  opponens, for median palsy, 140-141
  of origin of adductor longus and brevis to ischial tuberosity, 358
  of posterior tibial and peroneus brevis tendons to calcaneus, 524-526
  tendon; see Tendon transfers
Transmetatarsal amputation, 570

Transplantation
  of hamstring tendons to femoral condyles, Eggers procedure for, 392-393
  of ulnar nerve, anterior, 88-89
Transthoracic approach to thoracic spine, 272-273
Transverse carpal ligament, release of, for carpal tunnel syndrome, 116-117
Transverse processes of thoracic curve, convex, osteotomy of, 244
Trapezius, transfer of, for paralysis of deltoid muscle, 30-31
Traumatic fingertip amputations, 603-605
Traumatic lumbosacral spondylolisthesis, 254
Triceps
  reattachment of, excision of proximal ulna following olecranon fracture with, 70-71
  transfer of, 84-85
"Trigger thumb," 148
Triple arthrodesis of foot, 548-549
Tube, closed, irrigation via, and drainage of localized musculoskeletal areas, 607
Tuberosity, ischial, transfer of origin of adductor longus and brevis to, 358
Tunnel, tarsal, release of, 521-523

U

Ulna
  distal, excision of, Darrach procedure for, 118-119

Ulna—cont'd
  midshaft fracture of, open reduction for, 99-101
  proximal, excision of, following olecranon fracture with reattachment of triceps, 70-71
  shaft of, fracture of, medullary fixation for, 78-79
Ulnar collateral ligament of metacarpophalangeal joint of thumb, rupture of, 165
Ulnar nerve, anterior transplantation of, 88-89
Ulnar nerve palsy, clawing of fingers secondary to, tendon transfers for, 142-143
Upper arm, 49-63
Upper extremity surgery, tourniquet use in, 139

V

Vascularized tissue grafts, free, 613
Volar plate advancement for dorsal fracture-dislocations of proximal interphalangeal joint, 167
Volkmann's contracture, 110
  ischemic, impending, forearm decompression for, 110-111

W

Wrist, 113-132
  arthrodesis of, 129-132
  rheumatoid arthritis of, 128, 129
  tendons at, synovectomy of, 128

Z

Z-plasty technique for release of superficial tissue contracture, 600